ESSENTIALS OF PAIN MEDICINE

ESSENTIALS OF
PAIN MEDICINE
FOURTH EDITION

EDITORS

Honorio T. Benzon, MD
Professor of Anesthesiology
Department of Anesthesiology
Northwestern University Feinberg School of Medicine
Chicago, Illinois

Srinivasa N. Raja, MD
Professor of Anesthesiology and Critical Care Medicine, and Neurology
Director of Pain Research
Division of Pain Medicine
Johns Hopkins University School of Medicine
Baltimore, Maryland

Spencer S. Liu, MD
Clinical Professor of Anesthesiology
Attending Anesthesiologist
Hospital for Special Surgery
Weill Cornell Medical College
New York, New York

Scott M. Fishman, MD
Professor of Anesthesiology and Pain Medicine
Chief
Division of Pain Medicine
Vice Chair
Department of Anesthesiology and Pain Medicine
Director
Center for Advancing Pain Relief
University of California, Davis School of Medicine
Sacramento, California

Steven P. Cohen, MD
Chief of Pain Medicine
Professor of Anesthesiology, Neurology and Physical Medicine & Rehabilitation
Johns Hopkins School of Medicine
Professor of Anesthesiology and Physical Medicine & Rehabilitation
Director of Pain Research
Walter Reed National Military Medical Center
Uniformed Services University of the Health Sciences
Bethesda, Maryland

ASSOCIATE EDITORS

Robert W. Hurley, MD, PhD
Professor
Department of Anesthesiology
Wake Forest School of Medicine
Executive Director
Pain Shared Service Line
Wake Forest Baptist Medical Center
Winston-Salem, North Carolina

Khalid Malik, MD, FRCS
Professor of Anesthesiology
University of Illinois Chicago
Chicago, Illinois

Philip Peng, MBBS, FRCPC, Founder (Pain Med)
Professor
Department of Anesthesia and Pain Management
University Health Network & Mount Sinai Hospital
University of Toronto
Toronto, Ontario

ELSEVIER

ELSEVIER

1600 John F. Kennedy Blvd.
Ste 1800
Philadelphia, PA 19103-2899

ESSENTIALS OF PAIN MEDICINE, FOURTH EDITION ISBN: 978-0-323-40196-8

Library of Congress Cataloging-in-Publication Data

Names: Benzon, Honorio T., editor. | Raja, Srinivasa, editor. | Liu, Spencer S., editor. | Fishman, Scott, 1959- editor. | Cohen, Steven P. (Steven Paul), 1963- editor.
Title: Essentials of pain medicine / editors, Honorio T. Benzon, Srinivasa N. Raja, Spencer S. Liu, Scott M. Fishman, Steven P. Cohen, ; associate editors, Robert W. Hurley, Khalid Malik, Philip Peng.
Description: Fourth edition. | Philadelphia, PA : Elseiver, [2018] | Includes bibliographical references and index.
Identifiers: LCCN 2017039957 | ISBN 9780323401968 (hardcover : alk. paper)
Subjects: | MESH: Pain--drug therapy | Anesthesia, Conduction
Classification: LCC RD84 | NLM WL 704.6 | DDC 617.9/64--dc23
LC record available at https://lccn.loc.gov/2017039957

Executive Content Strategist: Michael Houston
Content Development Specialist: Angie Breckon
Publishing Services Manager: Catherine Jackson
Senior Project Manager: Daniel Fitzgerald
Designer: Ashley Miner

Printed in India

Last digit is the print number: 9 8 7 6 5

To my wife, Juliet, for your love, understanding, and counsel.
To our children and their spouses: Hazel and Paul, Hubert and Natalie.
To our grandchildren: Annalisa, Jonathan, and Hunter.
To my co-editors, associate editors, and contributors, for their hard work.
To my previous and present colleagues at Northwestern, it has been an enjoyable ride.

Honorio T. Benzon

To my wife and best friend, Geetha: Thanks for your constant support, immense sacrifice, and enthusiastic encouragement of my educational activities.

To my daughters, Pushpa and Meera: Thanks for bringing JOY to my life with your infinite love and ardent affection.

To my Johns Hopkins colleagues and friends: Thanks for the intellectual stimulation and being my extended family.

Srinivasa N. Raja

To my wonderful wife, Roja, darling daughter, Anais, and my parents, Paul and Grace Liu.

Spencer S. Liu

To my patients, who continually inspire my work. To my colleagues at the UC Davis Center for Pain Medicine, who make my work a joy. To my wife and children, who give so much to support me and my work.

Scott M. Fishman

In loving memory of my father, my greatest advocate, who guided me onto a path of wisdom and responsibility.
To my wife, Karen, for her unwavering patience and support.
To my mother, Harriet, for teaching me what is important in life.
To my children, Berklee, Zared and Seffrah, for providing me with happiness and inspiration.
To my fellow service members—all gave some, and some gave all, in defense of our freedom and lifestyle.

Steven P. Cohen

To my wife and best friend, Meredith, for her unending support.
To my daughter, Alexandra, and sons, Sebastian and Gibson, my greatest joys.
To my parents, Morrison and Brenda, and my sister, Erin, who have always kept me grounded.
To my mentors, Donna Hammond and Chris Wu, for fostering my interests and, at times, reining me in.
To my collaborators, for questioning every sentence I put down on paper.

Robert W. Hurley

To my wife, Bonnie, for her love and patience; my son, Jahan, for the delight; and my daughter, Zara, for the vigor she brings to my life.
In fond remembrance of my parents.
To Dr. Benzon, for his kind and steadfast mentorship.

Khalid Malik

To my wife, Carol, for her continued support, encouragement, and understanding;
To my children, Julia and Michael, who fill me with joy and love;
To my sister, Rita, who keeps reminding me to be strong and assertive.

Philip Peng

CONTENTS

SECTION VII
THERAPEUTIC INTERVENTIONS

SECTION VIII
INTERVENTIONAL TECHNIQUES FOR PAIN MANAGEMENT

SECTION IX
OTHER NERVE BLOCKS IN PAIN MEDICINE

PREFACE

The fourth edition of this book reflects the continuing advances in our subspecialty. All the chapters have been revamped and new chapters have been added including cannabinoids, TNF-alpha inhibitors, tai chi, dorsal root ganglion stimulation, ultrasound-guided pain procedures, and risk of infection in interventional procedures. Dr. Samer Narouze exited as an Associate Editor, and we thank him for his past and ongoing contributions. Dr. Philip Peng, our new Associate Editor, assisted with the chapters on ultrasound and nontraditional treatments of pain. We hope that this edition continues the outstanding quality of the previous editions, which is a reflection of the hard work of our contributors and editor, Ms. Angie Breckon.

The completion of any medical text has become more challenging, and this book is no exception. Given the growing number of textbooks devoted to pain medicine, writing book chapters does not have the allure it once had and at many institutions, chapters do not count towards academic promotion. However, the feedback of this textbook sets it apart from other books in this field, which has enabled us to continue to recruit an exceptional cadre of authors. Collectively, we believe that books will continue to play a role in the education of trainees and the continuing education of clinicians globally. We therefore thank the contributors who, in spite of their busy schedules, submitted authoritative and up-to-date reviews of their topics.

This is the last edition in which Drs. Benzon and Raja will serve as Editors. In 1998, Dr. Benzon recruited Drs. Srinivasa Raja, David Borsook, Robert Molloy, and Gary Strichartz as co-editors and persuaded Mr. Michael Houston, now an Executive Content Strategist of Elsevier, to have Churchill-Livingstone publish the book. When this book originally came out in 1999, it was the first one of its kind in pain medicine. It then went through subsequent revisions in 2005 and 2011. The third edition was translated into a Chinese version, which enabled us to expand its outreach to a much larger audience. The next edition will be under the tutelage of Dr. Steven P. Cohen. The remarkable quality of this book, and its continued availability as an authoritative reference to future residents, fellows, and clinicians, is therefore assured.

The Editors and Associate Editors

LIST OF CONTRIBUTORS

Samer Abdel-Aziz, MD
Division of Pain Medicine
Department of Anesthesiology
Medical College of Wisconsin
Milwaukee, Wisconsin
United States

Meredith C. B. Adams, MD, MS
Division of Pain Medicine
Department of Anesthesiology
Medical College of Wisconsin
Milwaukee, Wisconsin
United States

Moustafa Ahmed, MD
Assistant Professor of Anesthesia and Critical Care
Department of Anesthesiology
UT Health–McGovern Medical School
Houston, Texas
United States

Abbas Al-Qamari, MD
Department of Anesthesiology
Northwestern University Feinberg School of Medicine
Chicago, Illinois
United States

Magdalena Anitescu, MD, PhD
Associate Professor
Anesthesia and Critical Care
University of Chicago Medical Center
Chicago, Illinois
United States

Juan Francisco Asenjo, MD, FRCPC
Professor of Anesthesia and Pain Management
McGill University Health Center
Montreal, Quebec
Canada

Michael Lynn Ault, MD, FCCP, FCCM
Associate Professor of Anesthesiology, Neurological Surgery, Surgery and Medical Education
Department of Anesthesiology
Chief and Fellowship Program Director
Section of Critical Care Medicine
Department of Anesthesiology
Northwestern University Feinberg School of Medicine
Medical Director
Cardiac Transplant Intensive Care Unit
Medical Director
Blood Gas Services and Emergency Response Teams
Northwestern Memorial Hospital
Chicago, Illinois
United States

Jeanette Bauchat, MD, MS
Associate Professor
Department of Anesthesiology
Northwestern University Feinberg School of Medicine
Chicago, Illinois
United States

Rena Beckerly, MD, MBA
Visiting Associate Professor
University of Illinois
Chicago, Illinois
United States

Dawn Belvis, MD
Pediatric Anesthesiologist
Advocate Lutheran General Hospital
Park Ridge, Illinois
United States

Honorio T. Benzon, MD
Professor of Anesthesiology
Department of Anesthesiology
Northwestern University Feinberg School of Medicine
Chicago, Illinois
United States

Hubert A. Benzon, MD, MPH, FAAP
Assistant Professor of Anesthesiology
Department of Pediatric Anesthesiology
Ann & Robert H. Lurie Children's Hospital of Chicago
Chicago, Illinois
United States

Charles B. Berde, MD, PhD
Chief
Division of Pain Medicine
Professor of Pediatrics
Children's Hospital Boston
Boston, Massachusetts
United States

Anuj Bhatia, MBBS, MD, FRCA, FFPMRCA, FIPP, FRCPC, EDRA, CIPS
Associate Professor
University of Toronto
Staff
Department of Anesthesia and Pain Management
University Health Network
Mount Sinai Hospital
Women's College Hospital
Toronto, Ontario
Canada

Sadiq Bhayani, MBBS, FRCA
Consultant Pain Medicine and Anesthesia
University Hospitals
Leicester NHS Trust
Leicester
United Kingdom

Mark C. Bicket, MD
Assistant Professor
Department of Anesthesiology and Critical Care Medicine
Baltimore, Maryland
United States

Patrick K. Birmingham, MD, FAAP
Professor
Northwestern University Feinberg School of Medicine
Executive Vice-Chair
Department of Pediatric Anesthesiology
Chief
Division of Pain Medicine
Ann & Robert H. Lurie Children's Hospital of Chicago
Chicago, Illinois
United States

Jessica Boyette-Davis, PhD
Department of Pain Medicine
The University of Texas MD Anderson Cancer Center
Houston, Texas
United States

Thomas H. Brannagan III, MD
Professor of Neurology
Director
Peripheral Neuropathy Center
Columbia University, College of Physicians and Surgeons
Co-Director
Electromyography Lab
New York, New York
United States

Chad Brummett, MD
Associate Professor of Anesthesiology
The University of Michigan
Ann Arbor, Michigan
United States

Alejandra Camacho-Soto, MD
Instructor of Neurology
Department of Neurology
Division of NeuroRehabilitation
Washington University in St. Louis School of Medicine
St. Louis, Missouri
United States

Kiran Chekka, MD
Partner
Multidisciplinary Pain Medicine
Premier Pain and Spine, LLC
Chicago, Illinois
United States

Sandy Christiansen, MD
Assistant Professor of Anesthesiology and Perioperative Medicine
Comprehensive Pain Center
Oregon Health & Science University
Portland, Oregon
United States

Brian A. Chung, MD
Assistant Professor
Anesthesiology
Northwestern University Feinberg School of Medicine
Chicago, Illinois
United States

Michael R. Clark, MD, MPH, MBA
Vice Chair
Clinical Affairs
Psychiatry and Behavioral Sciences
Johns Hopkins University School of Medicine
Director
Chronic Pain Treatment Program
Psychiatry and Behavioral Sciences
Johns Hopkins Hospital
Baltimore, Maryland
United States

Daniel J. Clauw, MD
Professor of Anesthesiology, Medicine (Rheumatology)
and Psychiatry
The University of Michigan
Ann Arbor, Michigan
United States

Marc Samuel Cohen, MS, MD
Anesthesiology
Montefiore Hospital
Bronx, New York
United States

Steven P. Cohen, MD
Chief of Pain Medicine
Professor of Anesthesiology, Neurology and Physical Medicine & Rehabilitation
Johns Hopkins School of Medicine
Professor of Anesthesiology and Physical Medicine & Rehabilitation
Director of Pain Research
Walter Reed National Military Medical Center
Uniformed Services University of the Health Sciences
Bethesda, Maryland
United States

Nikki Conlin, MD
Senior Instructor of Anesthesiology
The Johns Hopkins School of Medicine
Baltimore, Maryland
United States

Matthew Crooks, MD
Pain Management Specialist
Anesthesiology and Critical Care
Pinnacle Pain & Spine Consultants
Scottsdale, Arizona
United States

Miles Day, MD
Professor
Anesthesiology and Pain Medicine
Texas Tech University HSC
Lubbock, Texas
United States

Sheetal K. DeCaria, MD
Clinical Associate
Anesthesia and Pain Medicine
University of Chicago
Chicago, Illinois
United States

Timothy R. Deer, MD
The Center for Pain Relief, Inc.
Charleston, West Virginia
United States

Patrick M. Dougherty, PhD
Professor
Department of Pain Medicine
Division of Anesthesiology and Critical Care
The University of Texas MD Anderson Cancer Center
Houston, Texas
United States

Shravani Durbhakula, MD
Clinical Instructor, Anesthesiology & Pain Management
Johns Hopkins University
Baltimore, Maryland
United States

Robert H. Dworkin, PhD
Professor of Anesthesiology, Neurology, and Psychiatry
University of Rochester School of Medicine and Dentistry
Rochester, New York
United States

Robert R. Edwards, PhD
Clinical Psychologist
Associate Professor Department of Anesthesiology, Perioperative, and Pain Medicine
Brigham and Women's Hospital
Harvard Medical School
Boston, Massachusetts
United States

Nick Elbaridi, MD
Anesthesiology and Pain Medicine
Pain Management Center
Brigham and Women's Hospital
Boston, Massachusetts
United States

Sarah A. Endrizzi, MD
Clinical Assistant Professor
Department of Anesthesiology
Medical College of Wisconsin
Milwaukee, Wisconsin
United States

Michael Erdek, MD
Associate Professor of Anesthesiology and Critical Care Medicine
Associate Professor of Oncology
School of Medicine
Johns Hopkins University
Baltimore, Maryland
United States

F. Michael Ferrante, MD
Director
UCLA Comprehensive Pain Center
Professor of Clinical
Anesthesiology and Medicine
David Geffen School of Medicine at UCLA
Los Angeles, California
United States

Nanna Brix Finnerup, MD, PhD
Danish Pain Research Center
Department of Clinical Medicine
Aarhus University
Aarhus
Denmark

David Flamer, MD, FRCPC
Department of Anesthesiology and Pain Management
Mount Sinai Hospital and University Health Network
University of Toronto
Toronto, Ontario
Canada

Timothy J. Furnish, MD
Associate Clinical Professor
Pain Fellowship Director
Division of Pain Medicine
Department of Anesthesiology
UC San Diego School of Medicine
La Jolla, California
United States

Aaron M. Gilson, MS, MSSW, PhD
Senior Scientist
Research Program Manager
Pain & Policy Studies Group
Carbone Cancer Center
School of Medicine and Public Health
University of Wisconsin-Madison
Madison, Wisconsin
United States

Michael Gofeld, MD
Associate Professor
University of Toronto & McMaster University
Toronto, Ontario
Canada

Michael C. Grant, MD
Assistant Professor
Anesthesiology and Critical Care Medicine
The Johns Hopkins Hospital
Baltimore, Maryland
United States

Karina Gritsenko, MD
Department of Anesthesiology
Montefiore Medical Center
Bronx, New York
United States

Anthony Guarino, MD
Associate Professor
Anesthesiology
Washington University
St. Louis, Missouri
United States

Omar I. Halawa, MD
Pain Fellow
Division of Pain Medicine
Department of Anesthesiology
UC San Diego School of Medicine
La Jolla, California
United States

Charity Hale, PharmD
Pharmacy
University of California Davis Medical Center
Sacramento, California
Assistant Clinical Professor
Clinical Pharmacy
University of California, San Francisco
San Francisco, California
United States

Haroon Hameed, MD
Director of Neuromodulation
KURE Pain Management
Annapolis, Maryland
United States

Mariam Hameed, MD
Assistant Professor
Division of Pain Medicine
George Washington University
Washington, DC
United States

Michael C. Hanes, MD
Jacksonville Spine Center
Jacksonville, Florida
United States

Simon Haroutounian, MScPharm, PhD
Assistant Professor
Anesthesiology
Washington University
St. Louis, Missouri
United States

Jennifer Haythornthwaite, PhD
Professor
Psychiatry and Behavioral Sciences
Johns Hopkins University School of Medicine
Baltimore, Maryland
United States

Kimberly J. Henderson, MD, JD
Attending Physician
Department of Emergency Medicine
Beth Israel Mount Sinai Medical Center
New York, New York
United States

Gabriel A. Hernandez, MD
Senior Instructor
Anesthesiology and Critical Care Medicine
The Johns Hopkins Hospital
Baltimore, Maryland
United States

J. Gregory Hobelmann, MD, MPH
Attending Psychiatrist
Ashley Addiction Treatment
Adjunct Faculty
Psychiatry and Behavioral Sciences
Johns Hopkins University School of Medicine
Baltimore, Maryland
United States

Mark Holtsman, PharmD
Co-Director
Inpatient Pain Service
Pharmacy
University of California, Davis Medical Center
Clinical Professor
Anesthesiology and Pain Medicine
University of California, Davis
Sacramento, California, Clinical Professor
Clinical Pharmacy
University of California, San Francisco
San Francisco, California
United States

Megan Hosey, PhD
Assistant Professor
Department of Physical Medicine and Rehabilitation
Johns Hopkins School of Medicine
Baltimore, Maryland
United States

Eric S. Hsu, MD
Clinical Professor
Anesthesiology
David Geffen School of Medicine at UCLA
Los Angeles, California
United States

Julie H. Huang-Lionnet, MD, MBA
Interventional and Cancer Pain Management
Department of Anesthesiology and Pain Medicine
Greenwich Hospital—Yale New Haven Health
Greenwich, Connecticut
United States

Marc Alan Huntoon, MD
Professor of Anesthesiology
Virginia Commonwealth University
Director of Pain Management
VCU Neuroscience, Orthopaedic and Wellness Center
Richmond, Virginia
United States

Robert W. Hurley, MD, PhD
Professor
Department of Anesthesiology
Wake Forest School of Medicine
Executive Director
Pain Shared Service Line
Wake Forest Baptist Medical Center
Winston-Salem, North Carolina
United States

Brian M. Ilfeld, MD, MS (Clinical Investigation)
Professor of Anesthesiology, In Residence
Director of Clinical Research
Division of Regional Anesthesia
University of California San Diego
San Diego, California
United States

Mohammed A. Issa, MD
Medical Director for Pain Medicine
Department of Anesthesiology, Perioperative, and Pain Medicine
Department of Psychiatry
Brigham and Women's Hospital/Brigham and Women's Faulkner Hospital
Clinical Instructor, Harvard Medical School
Boston, Massachusetts
United States

Michael B. Jacobs, MD, MPH
Walter Reed National Military Medical Center
Uniformed Services University of the Health Sciences
Bethesda, Maryland
United States

David E. Jamison, MD
Department of Anesthesiology
Walter Reed National Military Medical Center
Department of Anesthesiology
Uniformed Services University of Health Sciences
Bethesda, Maryland
United States

Rafael Justiz, MD
Clinical Associate Professor in Anesthesiology
University of Oklahoma
Oklahoma Pain Physicians
Oklahoma City, Oklahoma
United States

Dost Khan, MD
Clinical Instructor
Department of Anesthesiology
Northwestern University Feinberg School of Medicine
Chicago, Illinois
United States

David J. Krodel, MD, MS
Assistant Professor
Northwestern University Feinberg School of Medicine
Attending Physician
Department of Pediatric Anesthesiology
Division of Pain Medicine
Ann & Robert H. Lurie Children's Hospital of Chicago
Chicago, Illinois
United States

Brian Lai, MD
Physician
Advanced Pain Medical Group, Inc.
West Hills, California
United States

Asimina Lazaridou, PhD
Department of Anesthesiology
Perioperative and Pain Medicine
Brigham and Women's Hospital
Harvard Medical School
Boston, Massachusetts
United States

Sheera F. Lerman, PhD
Postdoctoral Fellow
Department of Psychiatry and Behavioral Sciences
Johns Hopkins University School of Medicine
Baltimore, Maryland
United States

Benjamin P. Liu, MD
Assistant Professor of Radiology
Section of Neuroradiology
Department of Radiology
Northwestern Memorial Hospital
Northwestern University Feinberg School of Medicine
Chicago, Illinois
United States

Spencer S. Liu, MD
Clinical Professor of Anesthesiology
Attending Anesthesiologist
Hospital for Special Surgery
Weill Cornell Medical College
New York, New York
United States

Britni L. Lookabaugh, MD
OhioHealth Hospice and Palliative Medicine
Columbus, Ohio
United States

Gagan Mahajan, MD
Professor
Anesthesiology and Pain Medicine
University of California, Davis
Sacramento, California
United States

Khalid Malik, MD, FRCS
Professor of Anesthesiology
University of Illinois Chicago
Chicago, Illinois
United States

Edward R. Mariano, MD, MAS (Clinical Research)
Chief
Anesthesiology and Perioperative Care Service
Associate Chief of Staff for Inpatient Surgical Services
VA Palo Alto Health Care System
Professor of Anesthesiology, Perioperative and Pain Medicine
Stanford University School of Medicine
Palo Alto, California
United States

Zwade Marshall, MD, MBA
Director of Medical Outcomes
Alliance Spine and Pain
Atlanta, Georgia
United States

James Mathews, MD
Professor Emeritus of Emergency Medicine
Northwestern University Feinberg School of Medicine
Department of Emergency Medicine
Chicago, Illinois
United States

Colin J.L. McCartney, MBChB, PhD, FRCA, FCARCSI, FRCPC
Chair of Anesthesiology
Department of Anesthesiology and Pain Medicine
University of Ottawa
Ottawa, Ontario
Canada

Jessica Wolfman McWhorter, PhD, ABPP/RP
Rehabilitation Neuropsychologist
The Sandra and Malcolm Berman Brain & Spine Institute at Lifebridge Health
Sinai Hospital of Baltimore
Baltimore, Maryland
United States

Michael M. Minieka, MD
Assistant Professor of Clinical Neurology
Department of Neurology
Northwestern University Feinberg School of Medicine
Chicago, Illinois
United States

Arthur Moore, MD
Resident in Emergency Medicine
Northwestern University Feinberg School of Medicine
Department of Emergency Medicine
Chicago, Illinois
United States

Antoun Nader, MD
Professor of Anesthesiology and Orthopedic Surgery
Anesthesiology
Northwestern University
Chicago, Illinois
United States

Samer Narouze, MD, PhD
Clinical Professor of Anesthesiology and Pain Management
Ohio University
Clinical Professor of Neurological Surgery
Ohio State University
Chairman
Center for Pain Medicine
Western Reserve Hospital
Cuyahoga Falls, Ohio
United States

Ariana Nelson, MD
Assistant Professor
Anesthesiology and Perioperative Care
University of California-Irvine
Orange, California
United States

Andrea L. Nicol, MD, MSc
Assistant Professor
Anesthesiology
University of Kansas School of Medicine
Kansas City, Kansas
United States

Takashi Nishida, MD
Assistant Professor of Clinical Neurology
Department of Neurology
Northwestern University Feinberg School of Medicine
Chicago, Illinois
United States

Kent H. Nouri, MD
Department of Pain Medicine
The University of Texas MD Anderson Cancer Center
Houston, Texas
United States

Uzondu Osuagwu, MD
The University of Texas Health Medical School at Houston
Houston, Texas
United States

Judith A. Paice, PhD, RN
Director
Cancer Pain Program
Division Hematology/Oncology
Northwestern University Feinberg School of Medicine
Chicago, Illinois
United States

Philip Peng, MBBS, FRCPC, Founder (Pain Med)
Professor
Department of Anesthesia and Pain Management
University Health Network & Mount Sinai Hospital
University of Toronto
Toronto, Ontario
Canada

Stacy Peterson, MD
Division of Pain Medicine
Department of Anesthesiology
Medical College of Wisconsin
Milwaukee, Wisconsin
United States

Jason E. Pope, MD
Napa Pain Institute
Napa, California, Assistant Professor
Vanderbilt University Medical Center
Nashville, Tennessee
United States

Heidi Prather, DO
Professor of Physical Medicine and Rehabilitation
Chief
Section of Physical Medicine and Rehabilitation
Department of Orthopaedic Surgery
Washington University School of Medicine
St. Louis, Missouri
United States

Joel Press, MD
Professor of Clinical Rehabilitation Medicine
Weill Cornell Medical College
Physiatrist-in-Chief
Hospital for Special Surgery
New York, New York
United States

David A. Provenzano, MD
Pain Diagnostics and Interventional Care
Sewickley, Pennsylvania
United States

Rohit Rahangdale, MD
Assistant Professor of Anesthesiology
Northwestern University Feinberg School of Medicine
Chicago, Illinois
United States

Srinivasa N. Raja, MD
Professor of Anesthesiology and Critical Care Medicine, and Neurology
Director of Pain Research
Division of Pain Medicine
Johns Hopkins University School of Medicine
Baltimore, Maryland
United States

James P. Rathmell, MD
Chief
Division of Pain Medicine
Massachusetts General Hospital
Associate Professor of Anesthesiology
Harvard Medical School
Boston, Massachusetts
United States

Ben A. Rich, JD, PhD
Emeritus Professor of Internal Medicine (Bioethics)
UC Davis School of Medicine
Sacramento, California
United States

Matthias Ringkamp, MD
Associate Professor
Department of Neurosurgery
Johns Hopkins University
Baltimore, Maryland
United States

W. Evan Rivers, DO
Assistant Professor
Department of Neurosurgery
Chief
Division of Physical Medicine and Rehabilitation
University of New Mexico
Albuquerque, New Mexico
United States

Meghan Rodes, MD
Assistant Professor
Anesthesiology
Northwestern University Feinberg School of Medicine
Chicago, Illinois
United States

Joshua Rosenow, MD, FAANS, FACS
Director of Functional Neurosurgery
Northwestern Memorial Hospital
Professor of Neurosurgery, Neurology, and Physical Medicine and Rehabilitation
Northwestern University Feinberg School of Medicine
Chicago, Illinois
United States

Jack M. Rozental, MD, PhD, MBA
Medical Director and Vice Chair
Department of Neurology
Feinberg School of Medicine
Chief
Neurology Service
Jesse Brown Veterans Affairs Medical Center
Chicago, Illinois
United States

Eric J. Russell, MD, FACR, FSIR
Professor and Chairman
Department of Radiology
Northwestern Memorial Hospital
Northwestern University Feinberg School of Medicine
Chicago, Illinois
United States

Leslie Rydberg, MD
Assistant Professor
Physical Medicine and Rehabilitation
Rehabilitation Institute of Chicago
Northwestern University Feinberg School of Medicine
Chicago, Illinois
United States

Kashif Saeed, MD
Division of Pain Medicine
Department of Anesthesiology
Medical College of Wisconsin
Milwaukee, Wisconsin
United States

Kenneth Schmader, MD
Director
Geriatric Research Education and Clinical Center
Durham VA Medical Center
Professor of Medicine-Geriatrics
Duke University Medical Center
Durham, North Carolina
United States

Paul Scholten, MD
Assistant Professor
Department of Physical Medicine and Rehabilitation
Northwestern University Feinberg School of Medicine
Pain Management Center
Shirley Ryan AbilityLab
Chicago, Illinois
United States

Ravi D. Shah, MD
Assistant Professor of Anesthesiology
Department of Pediatric Anesthesiology
Ann & Robert H. Lurie Children's Hospital of Chicago
Chicago, Illinois
United States

Hariharan Shankar, MD
Professor
Anesthesiology
Medical College of Wisconsin
Staff Physician
Anesthesiology
Clement Zablocki VA Medical Center
Milwaukee, Wisconsin
United States

Samir Sheth, MD
Associate Professor
Anesthesiology and Pain Medicine
Director of Neuromodulation
Director of Student and Resident Training
University of California, Davis
Sacramento, California
United States

Ellen M. Soffin, MD, PhD
Assistant Professor of Anesthesiology
Department of Anesthesiology
Hospital for Special Surgery
Associate Director
Clinical Research
Department of Anesthesiology
Hospital for Special Surgery
Assistant Professor of Anesthesiology
Department of Anesthesiology
New York Presbyterian Hospital
New York, New York
United States

Gwendolyn A. Sowa, MD, PhD
Associate Professor Physical Medicine and Rehabilitation
University of Pittsburgh School of Medicine
Pittsburgh, Pennsylvania
United States

Eric M. Spitzer, MD
Clinical Instructor, Fellow in Neuroradiology
Department of Radiology
Northwestern Memorial Hospital
Northwestern University Feinberg School of Medicine
Chicago, Illinois
United States

Christina M. Spofford, MD, PhD
Associate Professor of Anesthesiology
Regional Anesthesia and Acute Pain Medicine
Fellowship Director
Medical College of Wisconsin
Milwaukee, Wisconsin
United States

Brett Stacey, MD
Professor
Anesthesiology & Pain Medicine
Medical Director
UW Center for Pain Relief
University of Washington
Seattle, Washington
United States

Steven P. Stanos, DO
Medical Director
Swedish Pain Services
Swedish Health System
Seattle, Washington
United States

Santhanam Suresh, MD, FAAP
Professor and Chair
Pediatric Anesthesia
Ann & Robert H. Lurie Children's Hospital of Chicago
Professor of Anesthesiology and Pediatrics
Northwestern University Feinberg School of Medicine
Chicago, Illinois
United States

Steven Tremblay, BScPT, MD, FRCPC
Department of Anesthesiology and Pain Medicine
University of Ottawa
Ottawa, Ontario
Canada

Luminita Tureanu, MD
Assistant Professor of Anesthesiology
Northwestern University Feinberg School of Medicine
Chicago, Illinois
United States

Jean Pierre Van Buyten, MD, PhD
Multidisciplinary Pain Center
AZ Nikolaas
Sint-Niklaas
Belgium

Murugusundaram Veeramani, MBBS
Clinical Instructor, Fellow in Neuroradiology
Department of Radiology
Northwestern Memorial Hospital
Northwestern University Feinberg School of Medicine
Chicago, Illinois
United States

Charles F. Von Gunten, MD, PhD
Vice President
Medical Affairs
Hospice and Palliative Care
OhioHealth
Editor-in-Chief
Journal of Palliative Medicine
Columbus, Ohio
United States

David Richard Walega, MD, MSCI
Chief
Division of Pain Medicine
Northwestern Medicine
Associate Professor
Anesthesiology
Northwestern University Feinberg School of Medicine
Chicago, Illinois
United States

Matthew T. Walker, MD
Professor and Vice Chairman
Department of Radiology
NorthShore University HealthSystem
University of Chicago
Evanston, Illinois
United States

Mark S. Wallace, MD
Professor of Clinical Anesthesiology
Chair of Division of Pain Medicine
Division of Pain Medicine
Department of Anesthesiology
UC San Diego School of Medicine
La Jolla, California
United States

Ajay D. Wasan, MD, MSc
Vice Chair for Pain Medicine
Department of Anesthesiology
University of Pittsburgh School of Medicine
Professor of Anesthesiology and Psychiatry
University of Pittsburgh
Pittsburgh, Pennsylvania
United States

Lynn R. Webster, MD
Vice President of Global Scientific Affairs
PRA Health Sciences
Salt Lake City, Utah
United States

Stephen T. Wegener, PhD
Professor
Physical Medicine and Rehabilitation
Johns Hopkins School of Medicine
Baltimore, Maryland
United States

Debra K. Weiner, MD
Staff Physician
Geriatric Research, Education and Clinical Center
VA Pittsburgh Healthcare System
Professor
Medicine, Psychiatry, Anesthesiology
University of Pittsburgh School of Medicine
Pittsburgh, Pennsylvania
United States

Indy Wilkinson, MD
Pain Medicine Fellow
Johns Hopkins School of Medicine
Department of Anesthesiology and Critical Care Medicine
Baltimore, Maryland
United States

Bryan S. Williams, MD, MPH
Metro Spine Pain Centers
Oxon Hill, Maryland
United States

Kayode Williams, MD, MBA, FFARCSI
Associate Professor and Vice Chair for System Integration
Anesthesiology and Critical Care Medicine
Johns Hopkins School of Medicine
Associate Professor
Johns Hopkins Carey Business School
Baltimore, Maryland
United States

Cynthia A. Wong, MD
Professor
Chair and DEO
Department of Anesthesia
University of Iowa Carver College of Medicine
Iowa City, Iowa
United States

Christopher L. Wu, MD
Professor of Anesthesiology
Department of Anesthesiology and Critical Care Medicine
The Johns Hopkins University
Baltimore, Maryland
United States

Irene Wu, MD
Assistant Director
UCLA Comprehensive Pain Center
Assistant Clinical Professor
Department of Anesthesiology
UCLA David Geffen School of Medicine
Los Angeles, California
United States

Jiang Wu, MD
Assistant Professor of Anesthesiology & Pain Medicine
Center for Pain Relief
UWMC Acute Pain Service
University of Washington
Seattle, Washington
United States

Sophy C. Zheng, MD
Assistant Professor
Department of Anesthesiology
Northwestern University Feinberg School of Medicine
Chicago, Illinois
United States

SECTION I

BASIC CONSIDERATIONS

SECTION OUTLINE HEAD

CHAPTER 1

Anatomy and Physiology of the Pain Signaling Process

Matthias Ringkamp, MD ◎ Patrick M. Dougherty, PhD ◎ Srinivasa N. Raja, MD

Pain is a physiologic consequence of tissue injury and serves a vital protective function. For example, clinical observations of patients with congenital insensitivity to pain and patients with leprosy have clearly demonstrated that the absence of pain results in repeated injuries and disabilities. However, pain can become a disease when it occurs or persists in the absence of tissue damage or following appropriate healing of injured tissues. This chronic pain is disabling, has considerable negative impact on quality of life of the individual, and has profound economic impact on the family and society.

The International Association for the Study of Pain defines pain as "an unpleasant sensory and emotional experience associated with actual or potential tissue damage, or described in terms of such damage."[1] This definition acknowledges that pain is not only a sensory experience but may be associated with affective and cognitive responses. The definition also recognizes that the intensity of pain and the severity of tissue damage are not necessarily correlated. Thus, an understanding of the anatomic substrates and physiologic mechanisms by which noxious and nonnoxious stimuli are perceived provides the essential background to apprehend the mechanisms of acute and chronic pain and the sites of action of pharmacologic therapies for pain.

SOMATOSENSATION, NOCICEPTION, AND PAIN

Somatosensation is the physiologic process by which neural substrates are activated by physical stimuli resulting in the perception of what we describe as touch, pressure, and pain. Nociception is the physiologic process of activation of neural pathways by stimuli that are potentially or currently damaging to tissue. A stimulus is considered nociceptive when it induces behavioral avoidance or escape response in animals and humans or when the stimulus evokes activity in specialized groups of afferent fibers (i.e., nociceptors). Clinically, the degree of nociception is inferred by overt evidence of tissue damage. In contrast to nociception, pain is a conscious experience. Although the stimulus-induced activation of afferent neural pathways plays an important role, other factors such as alterations in somatosensory processing after injury to tissues and/or nerves and psychosocial factors may influence the overall perception of pain. The experience of pain, particularly chronic pain, often results in suffering. Suffering results from a multitude of factors that includes loss of physical function, social isolation, family distress, and a sense of inadequacy or spiritual loss. This chapter briefly reviews the basic anatomy and physiology of the neural pathways that respond to somatosensory stimuli, especially nociceptive stimuli, and emphasizes the plasticity in this system following an injury. This knowledge is fundamental in the evaluation and subsequent management of patients with painful disorders.

The sequence of events by which a stimulus is perceived involves four processes: (1) transduction, (2) transmission, (3) modulation, and (4) perception (Fig. 1.1). *Transduction* occurs in the peripheral terminals of primary afferent neurons, where different modes of stimuli (e.g., mechanical, heat, chemical, or cold) induce a generator potential through activation of transduction channels expressed on the axonal membrane. If the generator potential is sufficient, it will generate action potentials that are then transmitted through the nervous system. There are three major components of the transmission system. The peripheral sensory neurons with their cell bodies residing in the dorsal root ganglia transmit impulses from the site of transduction at their peripheral terminal to the spinal cord where the central terminals synapse with second-order neurons. The spinal neurons are the *second* component in the transmission network. These cells send projections to the thalamus and various brainstem and diencephalic structures. Finally, neurons of the brainstem and diencephalon form the *third* component of the transmission network as they project to various cortical sites. Modulation is the process whereby neural activity may be altered along the pain transmission pathway. A major site of modulation occurs within the dorsal horn of the spinal cord. *Modulation* at this level of processing involves a multitude of neurotransmitter systems that will be discussed in Chapter 2. Activation of pain modulation systems usually results in less activity in the pain transmission pathway after a noxious stimulus. Examples of activation of this process include stress-induced analgesia. However, in some circumstances, modulation can also result in an enhancement of pain signaling. *Perception* is the final stage of the nociceptive process by which neural activity in the somatosensory transmission pathway results in a subjective sensation of pain. It is presumed that this process results from the concerted activation of primary and secondary somatosensory and limbic cortices.

PERIPHERAL MECHANISMS

In general, somatosensation begins with activation of primary afferent neurons. These neurons are part of the peripheral nervous system, with cell bodies located in the dorsal root ganglia, from which the neurons project with a peripheral axon into the target tissue (skin, muscles, joints) and a central axon into the spinal cord. Primary afferent fibers are classified based on their conduction velocity and the stimuli by which they are activated. Much of our knowledge about the physiology of primary afferents including nociceptors originates from studies on cutaneous afferents (i.e., those that innervate the skin). Many of the principal

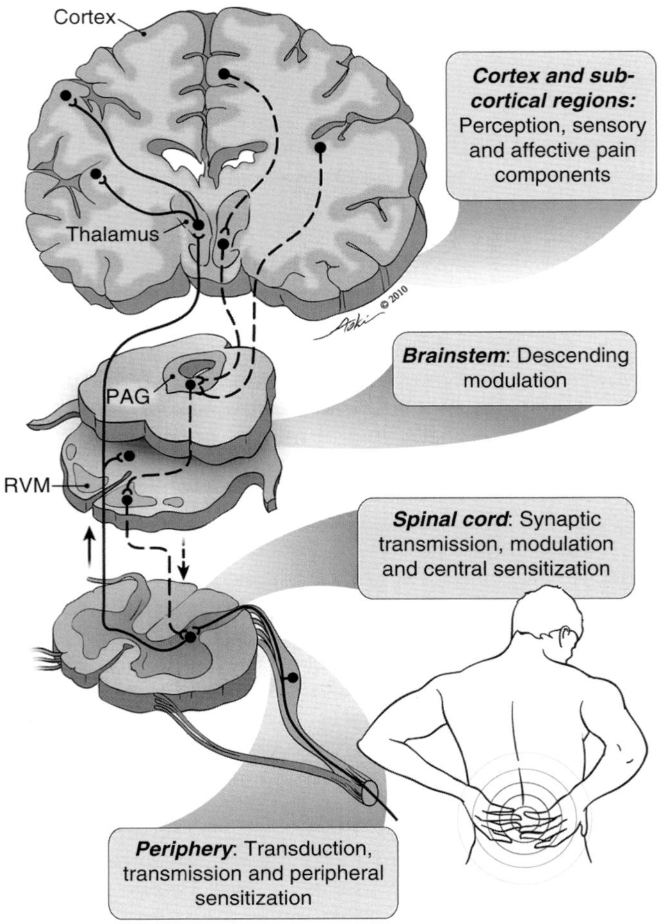

FIG. 1.1 Schematic of pain-signaling mechanisms involved in transduction, transmission, modulation, and perception of pain. Ascending afferent and descending modulatory pathways are shown. *PAG*, Periaqueductal gray; *RVM*, rostral ventromedial medulla.

findings made on cutaneous afferents extend to primary afferents innervating other peripheral tissues. Among cutaneous afferents, three classes of primary afferent fibers can be differentiated.[2,3] The fastest-conducting fibers (>20 m/s) are the large-diameter myelinated A beta (Aβ) fibers. These afferents are activated by nonnociceptive stimuli that evoke the sensation of light touch, pressure, or hair movement. The axons of nociceptive neurons are generally thinly myelinated A delta (Aδ) fibers or unmyelinated C fibers, which conduct between 2 and 20 m/s and less than 2 m/s, respectively. Many nociceptors have the capacity to respond to intense heat, cold, mechanical, and chemical stimuli (i.e., they respond to different stimulus modalities and are therefore "polymodal"). The functional role of the Aδ- and C-fiber nociceptors may be different. The C fibers are the predominant (75%) type of afferent fiber in peripheral nerves. Recordings from C fibers in humans suggest that C-fiber activity is associated with a prolonged burning sensation. In contrast, activation of faster-conducting Aδ fibers evokes a sharp, intense, tingling sensation. The combined activation of these two groups of afferents, such as by an intense brief heat stimulus, results in a dual-pain sensation as Aδ fibers convey the rapid-onset *first pain* sensation, a pricking pain, whereas C fibers mediate the slower-onset, burning *second pain* sensation that follows brief intense heat stimulation to the skin.[4] Combined, Aδ- and C-fiber nociceptors encode and transmit information to the central nervous system (CNS) concerning the intensity, location, and duration of noxious stimuli. Although polymodal nociceptors are the most common type, a functionally distinct and important subgroup of nociceptors is insensitive to mechanical stimuli. These mechanically insensitive nociceptors ("MIAs") likely act as chemonociceptors, and input from these afferents is thought to be crucial for the induction and maintenance of central sensitization.

Nociceptive afferents are further subclassified based on the molecules expressed on their cell surface (e.g., receptors, glycoconjugates), based on the molecules they store and release (e.g., peptides), and based on the enzymes they contain. Although none of these cell markers is completely specific for the peripheral target tissue innervated, the percentage of dorsal root ganglion cells positive for a given marker differs significantly among target tissues. For example, almost all visceral afferents are peptidergic, but only approximately half of the afferents projecting to the skin are,[5] and only a small percentage of the nonpeptidergic afferents, characterized by binding the plant isolectin B4 (IB4) from *Griffonia simplicifolia*,[6] project to muscle.[7,8] Similarly, the central projection areas of peptidergic and nonpeptidergic afferents differ, with peptidergic fibers mainly projecting to lamina I and lamina II outer, and IB4 binding (nonpeptidergic) afferents projecting preferably to lamina II inner (e.g., Silverman and Kruger,[6] but see also Woodbury et al.[9]). Most peptidergic neurons express the tyrosine kinase receptor A (trk A), suggesting that they depend on nerve growth factor (NGF) for survival.[10–12] In contrast, most IB4-positive dorsal root ganglion cells do not express trk A but express one of the glial cell-derived neurotrophic factor (GDNF) family receptors (GDNFRa1–4) together with receptor tyrosine kinase Ret.[13,14] Peptidergic and nonpeptidergic neurons also express different patterns of receptors involved in signal transduction, and they may therefore display different sensitivities to a given stimulus. Thus the P2X3 receptor, which mediates nociceptor excitation by ATP, is primarily expressed in IB4-positive neurons.[15] In contrast, the vanilloid receptor 1 (VR1/TRPV1), which mediates responses to heat, capsaicin, and protons, is expressed in only a minority of IB4-positive cells in mice,[16] and IB4-positive neurons are less responsive to these stimuli than their IB4-negative counterparts.[16–18] The role of these various peptides and receptors, in addition to others, in pain transmission is discussed in greater detail in Chapter 2. Another class of receptors primarily expressed in small primary afferent neurons are mas-related G protein–coupled receptors (Mrgprs). In mice, different Mrgprs are expressed in nonoverlapping neuronal populations, some of which have been linked to mediating specific behavior. For example, MrgprD neurons are thought to mediate nociceptive behavior to mechanical stimuli, whereas neural activity in neurons expressing MrgprA3 induces scratching behavior in response to itch-producing stimuli. In primary afferent nerve fibers, including nociceptors, information on the intensity of a given stimulus is coded by the number of action potentials in a population of primary afferents, with a generally monotonic relationship between the stimulus intensity and the number of impulses generated by afferent fibers. The sensitivity of nociceptors to different stimuli is not fixed but can change considerably under pathologic conditions. For example, mediators released during inflammation can dramatically decrease the threshold for activation and increase responses to suprathreshold stimuli. This peripheral sensitization of nociceptive afferents is a major contributor to increased pain that can be elicited from a site of injury. In addition to this *primary hyperalgesia* from the injury site, increased pain responses may also be elicited from the surrounding area. This so-called *secondary hyperalgesia* involves mechanisms residing in the CNS and leads to the sensitization of central neurons (i.e., central sensitization).

Voltage-gated sodium channels are crucial for the generation and conduction of action potentials in central and peripheral neurons. The different channel isoforms (Na_V1.1-1.9) are broadly classified as tetrodotoxin (TTX) sensitive and TTX insensitive. Among these channels, the TTX-sensitive Na_V1.7 isoform and the TTX-insensitive isoforms (Na_V1.8, Na_V1.9) are of major interest in nociception and pain. Thus loss-of-function mutations in the gene *(SCN9A)* that encodes Na_V1.7 lead to congenital insensitivity to pain (CIP)[19] and anosmia.[20] Conversely, gain-of-function mutations in the same gene can lead to severe spontaneous pain episodes in patients, for example, with inherited erythromelalgia (IEM) or extreme paroxysmal pain disorder (for review see Dib-Hajj et al. [21]). Gain-of-function mutations of Na_V1.7 have also been observed in patients with small fiber neuropathy.[22] In contrast to Na_V1.7, which, in addition to primary afferent fibers, is also expressed in sympathetic nerve fibers and olfactory epithelium, the TTX-insensitive isoforms Na_V1.8 and Na_V1.9 appear to be selectively expressed in nociceptive afferents. Similar to Na_V1.7, gain-of-function mutations in Na_V1.8 have been found to contribute to painful peripheral neuropathy,[23] and a gain-of-function mutation for Na_V1.9 leads, paradoxically, to CIP.[24] It should be noted that Na_V1.7, Na_V1.8, and Na_V1.9 differ significantly in channel properties, and they contribute differently to cell excitability and action potential generation (for review see Dib-Hajj et al.[25]).

SPINAL MECHANISMS

The first synapse in somatosensory processing of information from the body surface occurs at either the spinal dorsal horn or in the dorsal column nuclei at the spinal cord–brainstem junction.[26] Somatosensory processing for information from the face is similarly processed either in the spinal trigeminal nucleus (pain and temperature) or in the chief sensory nucleus of the trigeminal nerve located in the mid-pons region of the brainstem. Both nociceptive and nonnociceptive fibers provide inputs to both of these initial targets. However, under normal circumstances the dorsal column nuclei and the chief sensory nucleus can be considered to selectively process inputs from large myelinated Aβ fibers related to light touch, whereas the spinal dorsal horn and spinal trigeminal nucleus process inputs of nociceptive Aδ and C fibers. This separation of modalities in the somatosensory system is the basis for the localization of neural lesions through neurologic examination in patients.

Nociceptive primary afferent fibers terminate in a highly ordered way in the spinal dorsal horn on the same side of the body of their origin.[27,28] The dorsal horn is anatomically organized in the form of layers or laminae, as first recognized by Rexed in the cat (Fig. 1.2).[29] The unmyelinated C fibers terminate primarily in the most superficial lamina (I and II outer), whereas the thinly myelinated Aδ fibers end in lamina I, and in laminae III to V. Collaterals of the large myelinated fibers (Aβ) terminate in laminae III to V of the dorsal horn. Lamina I is also known as the *marginal nucleus* and lamina II as the *substantia gelatinosa* of Rolando.

Two predominant types of second-order nociceptive spinal and spinal trigeminal projection neurons have been identified: wide dynamic range (WDR) neurons and nociceptive-specific (NS) neurons. WDR cells are especially concentrated in the deeper laminae of the dorsal horn (III to V), where they receive input from both low-threshold Aβ and nociceptive Aδ and C fibers, and hence are activated by both innocuous and noxious stimuli. However, the responses of WDR cells to these stimuli are graded such that the noxious stimuli evoke a greater response than nonnoxious stimuli. WDR spinal projection neurons (i.e., neurons whose axons terminate in supraspinal targets) have a spontaneous discharge (average rate of approximately 11 Hz in monkeys), and their activity is increased by innocuous cutaneous (average rate of approximately 25 Hz after brushing skin with a hair brush), and noxious mechanical stimulation (approximately 50 Hz after a small arterial clip is applied to the skin) (Fig. 1.3).

In contrast to WDR cells, NS projection cells respond only to noxious stimuli under physiologic conditions. The majority of NS cells are found in the superficial laminae of the dorsal horn (I and outer II). These cells have a lower rate of spontaneous activity than do WDR cells, averaging approximately 3 to 5 Hz. The discharge rates to the noxious stimuli of NS cells are comparable to those of WDR cells, averaging approximately 50 Hz (Fig. 1.4).

The axons of both the WDR and NS second-order neurons cross the midline near the level of the cell body, gather into bundles of ascending fibers in the contralateral, anterolateral spinal region, and then ascend toward targets in the brainstem and diencephalon (Fig. 1.5). The conduction velocity of the WDR cells is usually faster than that of the NS cells (approximately 30 m/s vs. 12 m/s). In addition, the axons of the NS cells that largely arise from laminae I of the dorsal horn and those of the WDR cells arising primarily from laminae III to V tend to run in slightly different positions in the anterolateral spinal funiculus. In the anterolateral spinal column, the NS cell axons are found in the dorsal medial region, whereas axons of WDR cells are more concentrated in the ventral lateral region.

SPINAL MODULATION

The concept of modulation of noxious inputs at spinal levels was highlighted by the gate control theory of Melzack and Wall.[30] This theory suggested that input along low-threshold (Aβ) fibers inhibits the responses of WDR cells to nociceptive input. The theory was offered as an explanation for the efficacy of transcutaneous electrical stimulation for pain relief. Subsequent studies have identified intrinsic spinal neurons that release a plethora of neurotransmitters in the spinal cord that play a role in the modulation of nociceptive impulses. Furthermore, a number of inputs

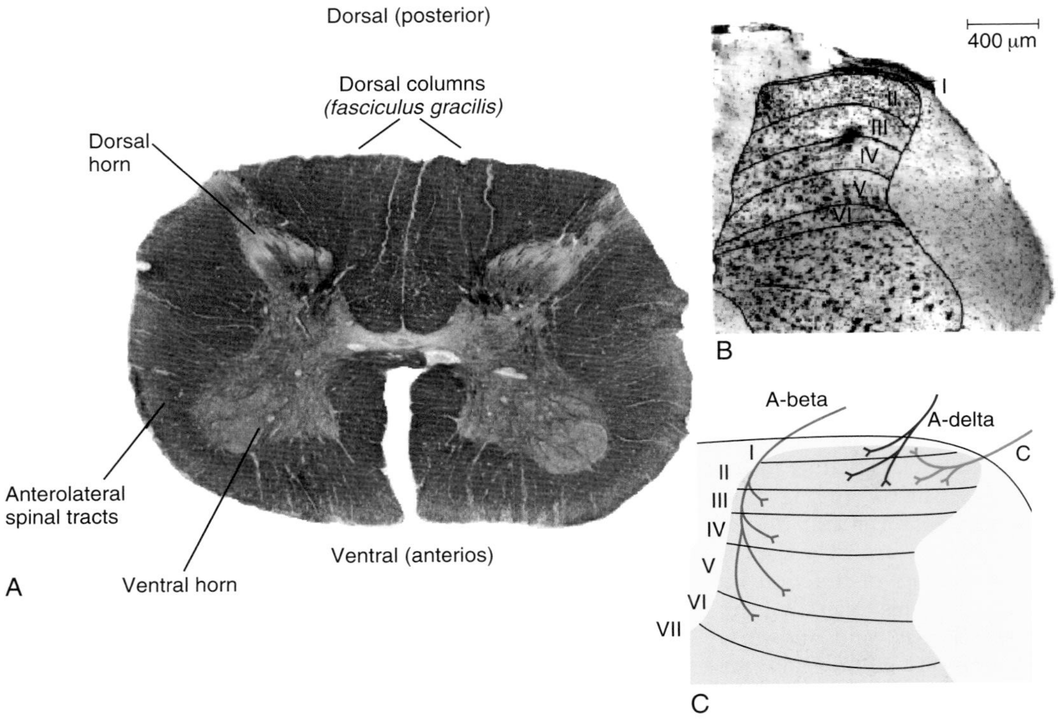

FIG. 1.2 Histologic sections and schematic diagrams of the spinal dorsal horn. (A) Human lumbar spinal cord is labeled to show the relationship between the major spinal somatosensory structures. (B) From rat spinal cord. The outer heavy lines show the boundary of the spinal gray matter, and the inner heavy lines show the boundaries of Rexed laminae. These boundaries are established by the histologic characteristics of each zone, and the layers are identified by the numerals at the right of the dorsal horn boundary. (C) Pattern of primary afferent innervation to the nonhuman primate spinal dorsal horn. The large myelinated (Aβ) fibers segregate to the dorsal aspect of an entering rootlet and then course medially in the dorsal horn and terminate in layers III to V. The small myelinated (Aδ) fibers and C fibers, which carry nociceptive information, segregate ventrally in the entering roots, course laterally in the dorsal horn, and then largely terminate in the more superficial layers (I and II) of the dorsal horn.

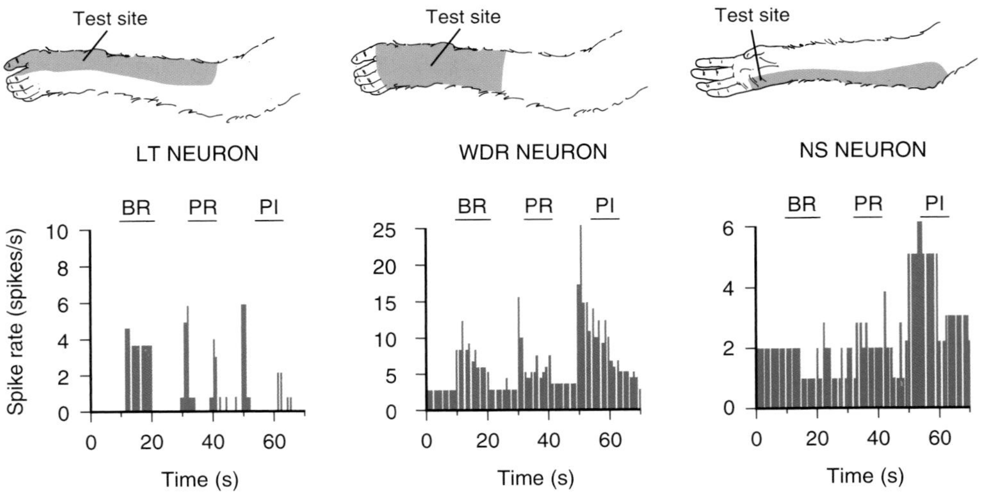

FIG. 1.3 Rate histograms show responses of primate spinothalamic tract neurons representative of low threshold (LT), wide dynamic range (WDR), and nociceptive-specific (NS) classes. The responses of these cells were evoked by application of a series of mechanical stimuli of graded intensity to multiple sites across the receptive field for each cell. The times and sites of each stimulus application are indicated by the lines and labels at the top of each histogram. The brush stimulus (BR) was provided by a soft, camel-hair brush, whereas a large arterial clip was used to produce innocuous pressure (PR), and a small arterial clip was used to produce a noxious pinch (PI) sensation. The WDR cell in the center shows responses that are graded with the intensity of the stimuli. The NS neuron at the right shows no significant responses to any stimuli but the most intense, whereas the LT neuron on the left responds to innocuous brushing of the skin alone (the transient responses with the application and removal of the arterial clips are due to the touch stimuli provided at contact). The diagrams of the hind limbs show the receptive field locations of each neuron *(shaded region)* and the site on the skin where each of the mechanical stimuli was applied (test site).

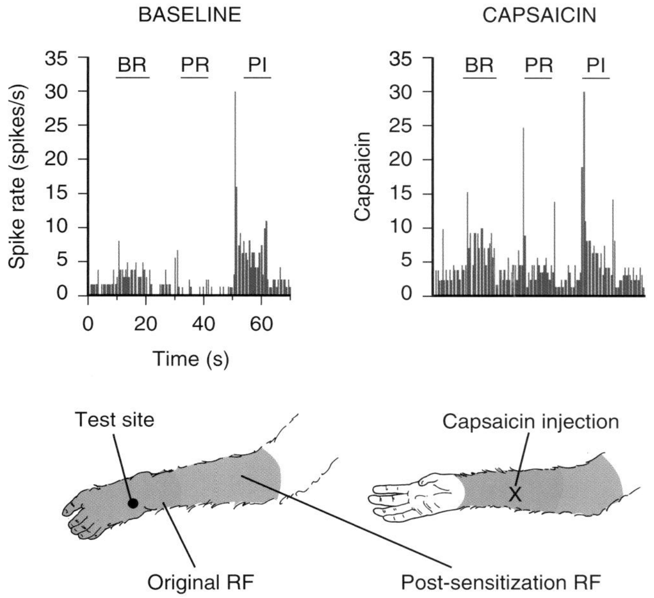

FIG. 1.4 Rate histograms show the background activity and responses of a representative wide dynamic range, spinothalamic tract neuron to mechanical stimulation of the hind limb before and after sensitization by an intradermal injection of capsaicin. The baseline responses to the mechanical stimuli are shown on the left, and the matching records after capsaicin are shown on the right. The mechanical stimuli were applied to the spot shown on the drawing of the leg at the bottom. The *X* shows the site at which capsaicin was delivered. The *blue area* shows the receptive field during the baseline recordings, whereas the *purple area* shows the expansion in the receptive field induced by capsaicin. *BR*, Brush stimulus; *PI*, pinch; *PR*, pressure; *RF*, receptive field.

to the dorsal horn from various brainstem sites have been shown to also modulate peripheral inputs, as well as outputs, of intrinsic cells.[31,32] Both types of modulation, that arising in the local network of cells at the spinal levels as well as that from the descending inputs, can result in either augmented or inhibited output from spinal cord nociceptive neurons. It is the combined effects of spinal excitatory and inhibitory systems that determine what messages are delivered to the higher levels of the CNS.

A special type of spinal modulation that is observed under certain circumstances is known as *central sensitization*.[33] In this phenomenon, the capacity for transmission in the nociceptive system is changed or shows neuronal plasticity. The result of this plasticity is that after a noxious stimulus of sufficient intensity and duration, such as a surgical incision, the coding of pain-signaling neurons for a given stimulus may be increased. One example of central plasticity is the phenomenon of *wind-up*, whereby repeated stimulation of C fibers at intervals of 0.5 to 1 Hz results in a progressive increase in the number of discharges evoked by each volley.[34] In addition to an increase in discharges evoked by a given stimulus, sensitized spinal neurons also show an expansion of receptive field size and an increase in spontaneous discharge rate. WDR cells tend to become sensitized more readily than NS cells. However, in circumstances in which NS cells do show sensitization, they often acquire novel responsiveness to innocuous stimuli and hence could be recategorized as WDR neurons. The neurochemistry of central sensitization is discussed in Chapter 2. Better understanding of the pharmacology of this and other types of plasticity will have profound consequences in the development of new analgesic pharmacotherapies.

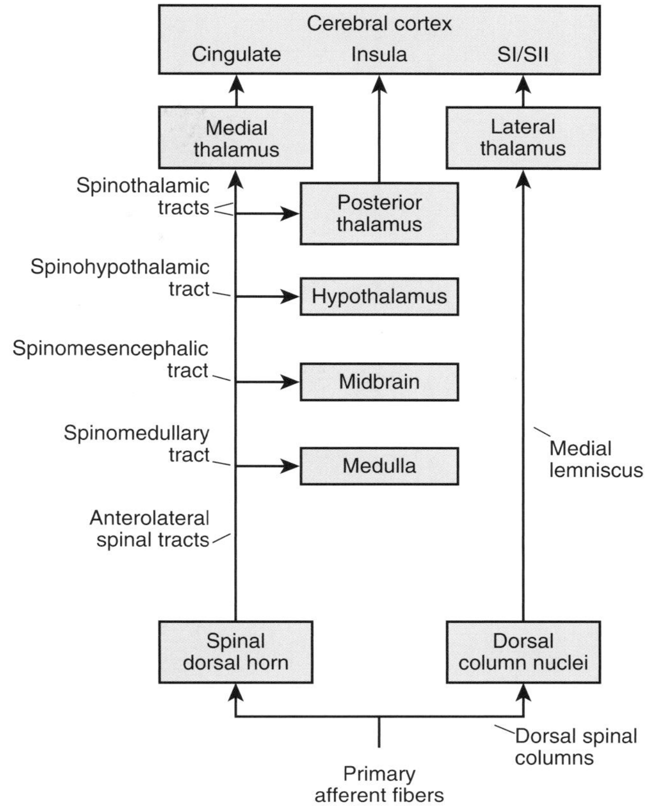

FIG. 1.5 Schematic diagram summarizing the central nociceptive pathways. Each box represents the discrete anatomic locations at which noxious stimuli are processed and/or registered. The lines indicate the neural pathways that interconnect each of the anatomic locations.

A different form of spinal modulation is exerted by glial cells (microglia, astrocytes, and oligodendrocytes). Microglia, the macrophages of the CNS, and astrocytes become activated after different insults including nerve injury, inflammation, or chronic opioid therapy. Upon activation, these cells can release a number of substances, including cytokines, inflammatory mediators, and growth factors, which then can affect neuronal function in multiple ways (for review see Ji et al.[35] and Tiwari et al.[36]). After nerve injury, for example, activated microglia release brain-derived neurotrophic factor (BDNF), which leads to the downregulation of potassium-chloride cotransporter KCC2 in lamina I neurons. As a consequence, a shift in transmembrane anion gradient can occur such that normally inhibitory input becomes excitatory.[37] Although animal studies have provided substantial evidence for a role of glia in chronic pain, it should be noted that the contribution and role of glia in chronic pain states in humans are less clear.

SUPRASPINAL MECHANISMS

Supraspinal structures involved in somatosensory processing include brainstem, diencephalic, and cortical sites.[38] There are two sets of somatosensory inputs to the brainstem and diencephalon. First, many axons and axon collaterals of the spinal projection neurons that ascend in the anterolateral spinal quadrant depart this ascending tract to terminate in a number of nuclei of the brainstem and midbrain (see Figs. 1.5 and 1.6). These target sites include

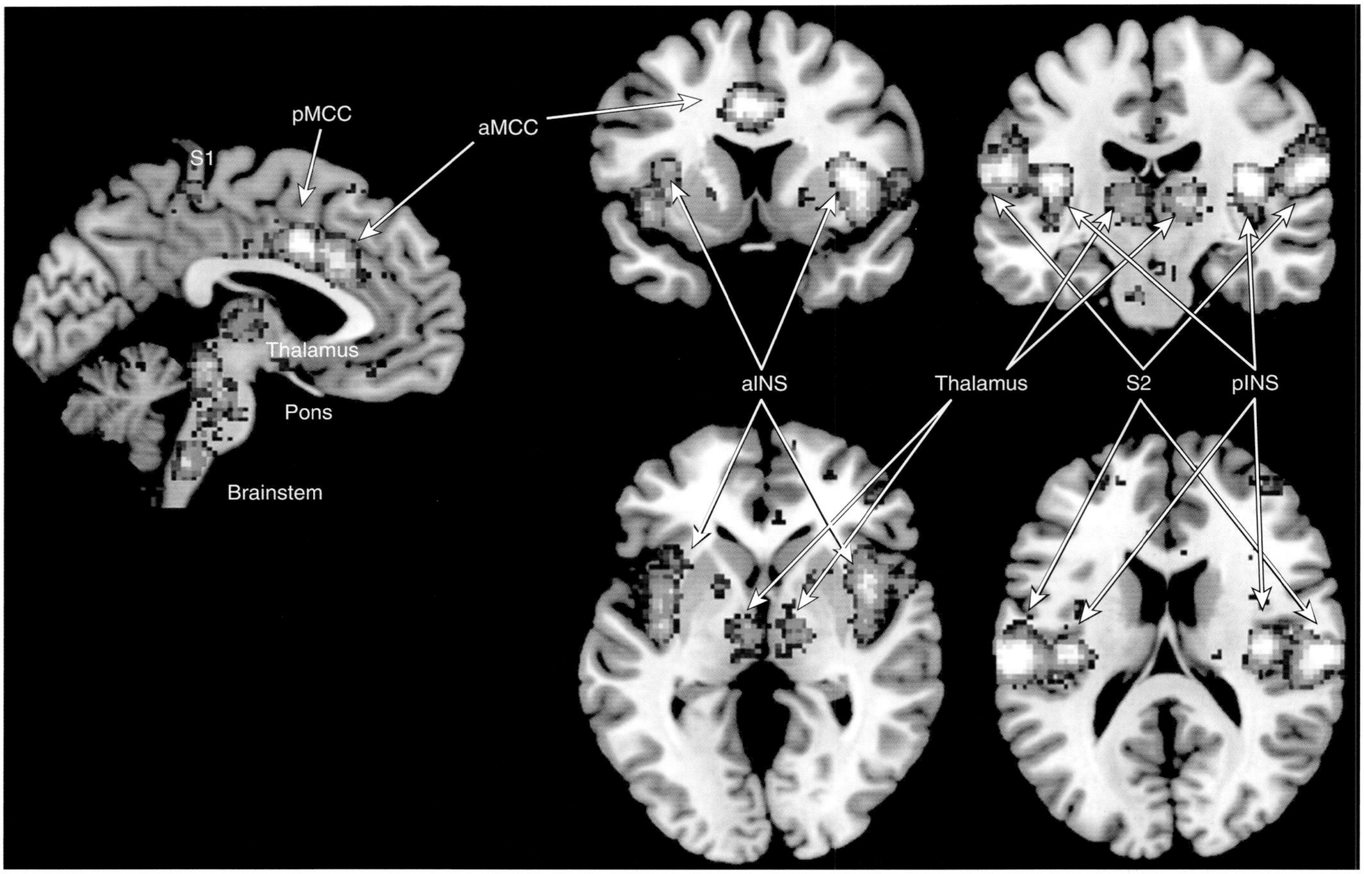

FIG. 1.6 Brain regions involved in pain signaling, based on imaging studies. Meta-analytic reverse inference statistical map of 420 fMRI studies with the term "pain" created on Neurosynth.org. *a/pINS*, Anterior/posterior insula; *a/pMCC*, anterior/posterior midcingulate cortex; *PAG*, periaqueductal gray; *S1/2*, primary/secondary somatosensory cortex. *(Courtesy of Dr. David A. Seminowicz.)*

brainstem autonomic regulatory sites that influence cardiovascular and respiratory functions, whereas in the midbrain there are multiple inputs to centers from which both descending and ascending (e.g., to thalamus) modulation of somatosensory processing is evoked. The remainder of the so-called anterolateral system fibers continue through the brainstem and midbrain to terminate in diencephalic structures, including the hypothalamus and posterior, lateral, and medial regions of the thalamus (see Figs. 1.5 and 1.6).

The second set of somatosensory inputs to the brainstem includes those primary afferent fibers that ascend in the dorsal (posterior) columns of the spinal cord to form their first synapse at the dorsal column nuclei. These inputs are organized so that the fibers from the lower extremities synapse most medially in the nucleus gracilis and inputs from the upper extremities synapse laterally in the nucleus cuneatus. The trunk is represented in regions of both nuclei. Comparative inputs from the face are processed in the chief sensory nucleus of the trigeminal nerve located at the origin site of cranial nerve five in the midpons of the brainstem. The axons of the second-order cells in the dorsal column nuclei cross the midline and form the medial lemniscus on the contralateral side of the brainstem. These fibers then ascend through the brainstem and midbrain, acquiring the functionally related fibers from the trigeminal nerve as they pass and continue on to provide the second somatosensory input to the diencephalon as they terminate in the ventral posterior lateral (VPL) nucleus (inputs from the body) and ventral posterior medial (VPM) nucleus (inputs from the face) of the thalamus.

The somatosensory inputs to the cortex include the third-order projections from thalamic somatosensory relay neurons of VPL and VPM as well as third- (and higher-) order neurons projecting from brainstem and midbrain relay neurons.[39,40] Some of these projections are highly organized and quite specific. For example, the cells in the core of VPL that receive inputs from the dorsal column–medial lemniscus fibers project to cortical areas SI and SII. The neurons in the posterior region of the lateral thalamus that receive inputs from the anterolateral system project to SII and the retroinsular areas of cortex, whereas medial thalamic nuclei ultimately project to the anterior cingulate cortex. Similarly, somatosensory relay neurons of the midbrain parabrachial nucleus project specifically to the amygdaloid nucleus of the neocortex. On the other hand, other third-order projections into cortex are quite diffuse. Outputs from cells of the brainstem reticular activating system that receive somatosensory inputs from the spinoreticular tract, for example, project throughout the neocortex.

In addition to peripheral and spinal mechanisms of nociceptive processing and modulation, there are several cortical regions that consistently have been shown to be involved in acute and chronic pain states. Although the exact brain areas included in what has been coined the "pain matrix" have been the focus of debate, the primary and secondary somatosensory cortices, insula, anterior cingulate cortex, prefrontal cortex, and several nuclei of the thalamus have consistently been shown to be active in imaging studies of acute and chronic pain states (see Fig. 1.6). In addition, pharmacologically induced analgesia has been shown to have effects in these brain regions. The "pain matrix" has further been categorized as comprising the lateral pathway, which encodes for the sensory-discriminative aspect of pain perception, and the medial pathway, which encodes for the affective component of pain perception. Brain structures involved in the affective component of pain processing are required for encoding the unpleasant and aversive aspects of pain, which is critical for self-preservation. A case study of several patients with unilateral ischemic damage to the insular cortex exhibited pain *asymbolia*, as evidenced by a lack of or inappropriate emotional response to multiple painful stimuli applied over the entire body. Moreover, these patients failed to learn appropriate escape or protective responses in response to the painful stimuli.[41] Another example of the role of cortical structures in the experience of pain is the placebo analgesic effect. Previous studies have shown that the placebo effect is at least partially mediated by activation of the endogenous opioid system, and μ-opioid receptors are highly localized within structures of the pain matrix.[42,43] Studies using positron emission tomography and the selective μ-opioid radiotracer[11] [^{11}C] carfentanil have shown that the placebo-mediated activation of the endogenous opioid system is predominantly located in the pain matrix structures, such as the anterior cingulate, prefrontal cortex, insula, medial thalamus, amygdala, and periaqueductal gray (PAG).[44,45]

SUPRASPINAL MODULATION OF NOCICEPTION

Several lines of research have clearly indicated that plasticity and modulation of somatosensory signaling occur at brainstem, midbrain, and diencephalic levels. Examples of plasticity of responses of dorsal column neurons after intradermal injection of the irritant capsaicin have been documented in the rat and monkey. Similarly, with the development of acute inflammation and after deafferentation, neurons of the thalamus alter their patterns of spontaneous discharge so that a large increase in bursting of these cells is observed. Ascending modulation from the brainstem dorsal raphe nucleus also influences signaling of thalamic neurons.

Descending modulation of nociception at the supraspinal level is a well-established phenomenon that can have both inhibitory and facilitatory effects on neurons in the dorsal horn. This modulation is important for the attenuation of acute pain, and the facilitatory aspect has been implicated in the establishment and maintenance of chronic pain states. There are many different sites and pathways involved in descending modulation. Highlighting the complexity of this phenomenon, the vast majority of these anatomic sites have been shown to have inhibitory and facilitatory effects. The best characterized pathway is the PAG and rostral ventromedial medulla (RVM) pathway. The PAG and RVM receive descending projections from a variety of cortical and limbic sites known to be involved in the affective component of pain processing, such as the anterior cingulate cortex, amygdala, and prefrontal cortex. Activation of these structures results in pronociceptive or antinociceptive effects and requires the PAG and RVM.[46,47] The PAG has few direct projections to the spinal cord and instead projects to the RVM, which sends either inhibitory or excitatory impulses to nociceptive projection and WDR neurons in the superficial and deep layers of the dorsal horn of the spinal cord.

It is hypothesized that the RVM is able to facilitate both inhibitory and facilitatory effects on the dorsal horn via different types of neurons termed "ON" and "OFF" cells.[48] These contrasting cell types have distinctly different functional characteristics. OFF cells are tonically active except during nociceptive input and activated by known analgesics, such as morphine. In contrast, ON cells become more active during nociceptive input and are inhibited by morphine.[48–50] It is generally accepted that OFF cells are required for descending inhibition.

Although the evidence supporting the role of ON cells in descending facilitation is mixed, several studies have shown that activation of ON cells within the RVM induces hyperalgesia. For example, the peptide cholecystokinin (CCK) induces mechanical and thermal hyperalgesia when directly injected into the RVM, and this direct CCK administration has been shown to preferentially activate ON cells.[51,52] In addition, ON cells are activated and OFF cells suppressed in models of chronic pain.[53,54] Descending facilitation via ON cell activation is thought to induce hyperalgesia by upregulating spinal dynorphin, which is linked to the increased release of excitatory neurotransmitters from primary afferent neurons, which can lead to central sensitization and chronic pain.[55] ON cells activation and the subsequent cascade of facilitatory effects in the spinal cord are also implicated in opioid-induced hyperalgesia resulting from chronic opioid exposure.[56,57]

Studies indicate that in addition to functional changes in neurons, microglia and astrocytes may also play an important role in the central sensitization process. Other central neuroplastic changes that may contribute to neuropathic pain states include deafferentation hyperactivity that may occur following spinal cord or avulsion injuries, loss of large-fiber afferent inhibition, reorganization of central connections of primary afferent fibers, and excitatory descending modulatory mechanisms. Central and, to a lesser extent, peripheral sensitization are considered to be the prime culprits responsible for pain induced by innocuous stimuli *(allodynia)* and increased pain to normally noxious stimuli *(hyperalgesia)*, which are commonly observed in neuropathic pain states.

KEY POINTS

- The processes resulting in a noxious stimulus-inducing pain are transduction, transmission, modulation, and perception.
- Nociceptors in the periphery respond to intense heat, cold, mechanical, or chemical stimuli and encode the intensity, location, and duration of noxious stimuli.
- The dorsal horn is anatomically organized in laminae. Unmyelinated C fibers terminate in Rexed laminae I and II, and large myelinated fibers terminate in laminae III to V.

- Two types of second-order nociceptive spinal and spinal trigeminal projection neurons are wide dynamic range (WDR) and nociceptive specific (NS). WDR cells receive input from both Aβ and nociceptive (C and Aδ) fibers.
- The somatosensory system is composed of two main signaling channels. The anterolateral system is the primary pain-signaling channel. In contrast, the dorsal column–medial lemniscal system is primarily a high-speed, very discrete signaling channel for innocuous stimuli.
- Several cortical regions, referred to as the "pain matrix," have been shown to be involved in acute and chronic pain states. These regions include the primary and secondary somatosensory cortices, insula, anterior cingulate cortex prefrontal cortex, amygdala, and several nuclei of the thalamus.
- Descending modulation of nociception from supraspinal level sites can have both inhibitory and facilitatory effects on spinal dorsal horn neuronal activity. Descending modulation may be important for the attenuation of acute pain. However, descending facilitatory activity has been implicated in the establishment and maintenance of chronic pain states.
- Derangements can occur in both the ascending and descending signaling systems at any and all levels that result in the generation of chronic pain.

REFERENCES

Access the reference list online at ExpertConsult.com.

CHAPTER 2

Neurochemistry of Somatosensory and Pain Processing

Kent H. Nouri, MD ◎ Uzondu Osuagwu, MD ◎ Jessica Boyette-Davis, PhD ◎ Matthias Ringkamp, MD ◎ Srinivasa N. Raja, MD ◎ Patrick M. Dougherty, PhD

Expertise in the neurochemistry of somatosensory processing provides clinicians the knowledge needed to control pain at the site of transduction of injury-related signals by nociceptors in the periphery and, secondly, by modification of signal transmission through the central nervous system.

NEUROCHEMISTRY OF PAIN TRANSDUCTION

Numerous chemicals are released in skin following tissue injury that either directly activate nociceptors or that increase their excitability. The graphical summary shown in Fig. 2.1 reveals that there are numerous mediators, frequently referred to simply as the "inflammatory soup."

Inflammatory Soup: Several of the key "ingredients" of this soup include the following components.

Bradykinin, a potent vasodilating peptide, plays a critical role in inflammatory pain and hyperalgesia via actions on two G protein–coupled receptors (GPCRs): the constitutively expressed B2 receptor and the B1 receptor, expression of which is increased following tissue injury (see Petho and Reeh[1] for reviews). Following injury, bradykinin is released by kininogens and produces acute pain in humans by activation of unmyelinated and myelinated nociceptors. Bradykinin also produces transient heat hyperalgesia in humans by sensitization of nociceptors through activation of phospholipase C (PLC), protein kinase C (PKC), the production of eicosanoids and nitric oxide (NO), and modulation of the transient receptor potential vanilloid 1 (TRPV1).[2]

Low pH (excess free H^+) of inflamed tissue also contributes to the pain and hyperalgesia associated with inflammation. Low pH selectively causes activation and sensitization of nociceptors to mechanical stimuli by opening dorsal root ganglion neuron–specific acid-sensing ion channels (DRASIC/ASIC-3; see Dussor[3] and Sluka and Gregory[4] for reviews). Excitation of nociceptors by protons does not undergo tachyphylaxis or adaptation, and a synergistic excitatory effect of protons and a combination of inflammatory mediators has been reported.[3,4]

Serotonin, which is released from platelets in response to platelet-activating factor derived from mast cell degranulation, leads to pain by directly activating nociceptors.[5] In humans, direct application of serotonin to a blister base produced pain, and serotonin also potentiates bradykinin-induced pain and nociceptor activation.[5]

Histamine is released from mast cells by *substance P* and *calcitonin gene–related peptide (CGRP)*. These neuropeptides are derived from activated nociceptors and produce a variety of responses, including vasodilation and edema.[6–8] Exogenous histamine applied to the skin produces itch but not pain when binding at the histamine 1 (H1) receptor. Nevertheless, histamine excites polymodal visceral nociceptors and potentiates the responses of nociceptors to bradykinin and heat. Histamine H3 and H4 receptors have been implicated in pain signaling. Both are Gi/o protein–coupled receptors found in various tissues. In the spinal cord, activation of these receptors attenuates the transmission of nociceptive information. Specifically, H3 receptor agonists have been proposed as potentially beneficial in treatment of neuropathic pain.[6] H4 receptor activation was shown to decrease pain in a nerve injury model in mice. Further research to elucidate the site of action and drug targets is ongoing.[9]

Eicosanoids are a large family of arachidonic acid metabolites that includes the *prostaglandins*, *thromboxanes*, and *leukotrienes*. Eicosanoids directly activate joint afferents and sensitize these, as well as those in skin and viscera, to natural stimuli and other endogenous chemicals (for reviews see Noguchi and Okubo[10] and Chen et al.[11]). Prostaglandins, synthesized by the constitutive enzyme cyclo-oxygenase-1 (COX-1) and by the inducible enzyme cyclo-oxygenase-2 (COX-2), reduce the activation threshold of tetrodotoxin-resistant Na^+ currents in nociceptors, increase intracellular cyclic AMP (cAMP) levels, and increase the excitability of sensory neurons. Leukotrienes, metabolites of the lipoxygenase pathway, are released by macrophages and mast cells, contribute to hyperalgesia and sensitization to mechanical stimuli by acting on GPCR and by serving as chemoattractants for cytokine-producing cells, and result in further sensitization of primary afferents.

Oxidized linoleic acid metabolites are relatives of the eicosanoids, given that they derive from arachidonic acid and have also emerged as new peripheral mediators of pain sensitization.[12] These contribute to inflammatory and thermal injury pain and interact with the sensitizing effects of nerve growth factor (NGF) at the TRPV1 receptor.

NO released by damaged afferents and acting on soluble guanylyl cylase (sGC) can further sensitize nearby neurons, augmenting pain and inflammation in both GPCR- and non-GPCR-mediated pathways.[1] Direct injection of NO into the skin produces acute pain in humans, and mechanical sensitivity in animal models of neuropathic pain are decreased following administration of the NO synthase inhibitor N(G)-Nitro-L-arginine methyl ester (L-NAME).[1] Further research on NO has uncovered a dual role: one as a mediator of nociceptive information and the other as a mediator of analgesia. NO has been shown to have analgesic properties both centrally and peripherally and may mediate the analgesic effects of drugs, such as opioids and nonsteroidal antiinflammatory drugs (NSAIDs).[13,14]

Adenosine and its monophosphate and polyphosphate derivatives (AMP, ADP, adenosine triphosphate [ATP]) are increased in the extracellular space with tissue injury and inflammation (for review see Sawynok[15]). Like serotonin, adenosine induces pain in humans by direct activation of

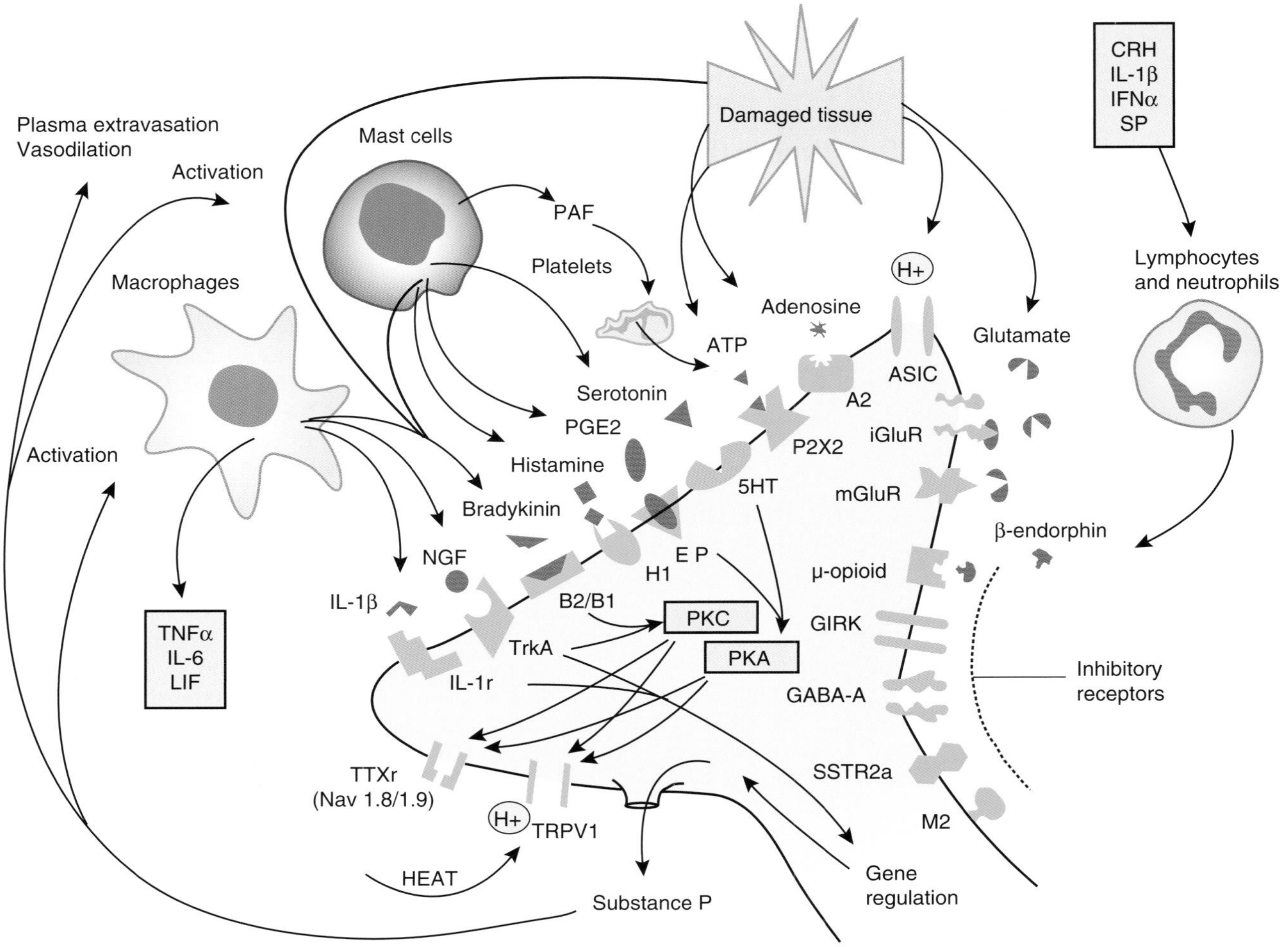

FIG. 2.1 Schematic diagram of the neurochemistry of somatosensory processing at peripheral sensory nerve endings. *5HT*, Serotonin receptor; *A2*, adenosine 2 receptor; *ASIC*, acid-sensing ion channels; *ATP*, adenosine triphosphate; *B2/B1*, bradykinin 2/1 receptors; *CRH*, corticotropin-releasing hormone; *EP*, eiconsanoid receptor; *GABA*, gamma amino butyric acid; *GIRK*, G-protein coupled inward rectifying potassium channel; *H1*, histamine 1 receptor; *IFN*, interferon; *iGluR*, iontotropic glutamate receptors; *IL*, interleukin; *LIF*, leukemia inhibitory factor; *M2*, muscarinic 2 receptor; *mGluR*, metabotropic glutamate receptor; *NGF*, nerve growth factor; *P2X2*, ATP activated ion channels; *PAF*, platelet activating factor; *PGE2*, prostaglandin E2; *PKA*, protein kinase A; *PKC*, protein kinase C; *SSTR*, somatostatin receptor; *TNF*, tumor necrosis factor; *TrkA*, tropomyosin receptor kinase A; *TRPV1*, transient receptor potential vanilloid 1; *TTXr*, tetrodotoxin resistant (channel).

nociceptors. ATP also induces pain in humans and activates C-nociceptors in healthy human skin but does not sensitize C fibers to mechanical or heat stimuli. It is thought that ATP activates nociceptive neurons in normal skin via the *purinergic receptors* $P2X_3$ and the heteromeric $P2X_2/P2X_3$ receptor (discussed later).[15]

Cytokines (e.g., interleukin-1β [IL-1β], tumor necrosis factor α [TNFα], IL-6) are released by a variety of cells, such as macrophages, microglia, astrocytes, and Schwann cells, to regulate inflammatory cell responses (see Ji et al.,[16] Tiwari et al.,[17] and Clark et al.[18] for reviews) but also modulate pain signaling. Cytokines can largely be classified as either proinflammatory or antiinflammatory, with those in the proinflammatory category more associated with different pain syndromes. Both IL-1β and TNFα directly excite and sensitize nociceptive afferent fibers to thermal and mechanical stimuli, and IL-6 in combination with its soluble IL-6 receptor also sensitizes nociceptors to heat. Clinical studies show that TNFα levels are increased in synovial fluid of painful joints and that treatment with antibodies against TNFα improves symptoms accompanying rheumatoid arthritis, including pain. Schwann cells express receptors for certain cytokines, such as TNF, interferon (IFN), IL-1, and IL-6. Activation of these receptors triggers a cascade of downstream reactions, including downregulation of myelin synthesis, increased expression of NGF receptors, dedifferentiation, and proliferation. The activated Schwann cells then begin to synthesize and release proinflammatory cytokines, affecting neighboring Schwann cells and thus closing a positive feedback loop that can exacerbate and sustain pain. IL-18, a member of the IL-1 family, plays a significant role in neuropathic pain; inhibition of IL-18 in the spinal cord also reduced bone cancer pain in rats.[19] In contrast, the antiinflammatory cytokine IL-10 has shown antinociceptive properties in both neuropathic and inflammatory pain.[20]

Furthermore, a subset of chemotactic cytokines, the *chemokines*, plays a role in the development of ongoing pain.[18] Dorsal root ganglion (DRG) neurons coexpress chemokine and opioid receptors, and chemokine activation can enhance or prevent opioid-induced analgesia and even promote tolerance.[21] Monocyte chemoattractant protein 1 (MCP1) and its receptor CCR2 are upregulated in primary afferent fibers and DRG cells following nerve injury, and injection of MCP1 in control animals creates a state of mechanical allodynia.[22] In addition, mice lacking the CCR2 receptor are less susceptible to neuropathic pain.[23]

Excitatory amino acid (EAA) receptors play a role in the modulation of nociception. EAA receptors are present on dorsal root ganglion cells and on the presynaptic terminals of primary afferents (see Miller et al.[24] for review). Peripheral injection of glutamate activates nociceptors by binding to both ligand-gated ion channels (ionotropic glutamate receptors, iGluRs) and G protein–coupled metabotropic (mGlu) type 1 and 5 receptors (mGluR1 and mGluR5, respectively) on unmyelinated axons. Neurons in the DRG labeled for mGluR5 also express TRPV1 that are characteristic of nociceptive neurons.

NGF may contribute to inflammatory pain via direct and indirect mechanisms. Inflammatory mediators, such as cytokines, increase NGF production in inflamed tissues (see Mizumura and Murase[25] and Lewin et al.[26] for reviews). In turn, NGF stimulates mast cells to release histamine and serotonin, which can sensitize primary afferent fibers. Furthermore, NGF itself may directly sensitize nociceptors and can alter the distribution of Aδ fibers such that a greater proportion of fibers have nociceptor properties. Heat hyperalgesia can be induced by NGF acting directly on the peripheral terminals of primary afferent fibers. NGF is implicated in the inflammation-induced changes in nociceptor response properties, such as an increase in the incidence of ongoing activity, increase in maximum fiber frequency, and changes in the configuration of the action potential of DRG neurons. NGF-induced hyperalgesia may be mediated via its actions on the TTX resistant sodium channel Nav1.8 and by potentiating the responses of the VR1 receptor.

Proteinases, such as thrombin, trypsin, and tryptase, which are traditionally not considered part of the inflammatory soup, are gaining increasing attention as mediators of pain and inflammation for their actions on *proteinase-activated receptors (PARs)*.[27,28] There are four classes of PARs, with PAR1 and PAR2 being implicated strongly in pain and inflammation. Both receptor types are located in the periphery on nerve fiber endings. Activation of PAR1 via thrombin leads to the release of histamine, substance P, CGRP, and cytokines. Activation of PAR2 by trypsin and tryptase creates a cascade of inflammatory reactions, including prostaglandin and bradykinin release, which would further sensitize unmyelinated primary afferents. The net effect of activation of these receptors is increased sensitivity to both mechanical and thermal stimuli. Neutrophil elastase activates PAR2 and TRPV4, resulting in nociceptor hyperexcitability and inflammation.[29]

Matrix metalloproteinases (MMPs) are a large family of endopeptidases that have only recently been found to contribute to pain. MMP-2, and possibly MMP-9, has been suggested to be related to diabetic neuropathy. MMPs serve as a macrophage chemoattractant and convert the cytokine TNFα into its active form. Following injury, microglia release MMPs, and at least one MMP, MMP-3, is upregulated in DRG cells.[30] Use of the MMP-3 inhibitor minocycline protects against chemotherapy-induced hypersensitivity. Furthermore, research using other MMP antagonists has found decreased MMP-mediated degradation of myelin basic protein, decreased macrophage infiltration, and subsequent decreased mechanical sensitivity.[31] At this time, the mechanisms and receptors involved in MMP-related pain induction have not been fully explored. Research regarding this family of proteins has made some progress and distinct roles for both MMP-9 and MMP-2 have been shown including: (1) transient MMP-9 upregulation after nerve injury in the early phase of development of neuropathic pain, (2) steady MMP-2 upregulation leading to maintenance of neuropathic pain, and (3) MMP-9/MMP-1-induced cleavage of IL-1β in the early and late phases of nerve injury, respectively.[32] There is also some thought that upregulation of MMP-9 in the spinal cord is implicated in chronic opioid-induced withdrawal syndrome.[33]

Peripheral AntiHyperalgesic Mechanisms: In contrast to the mediators discussed previously, there are also numerous mediators released into inflamed or injured tissue that act to limit pain transmission.

Opioids are also a component in inflammatory soup (see Stein[34,35] for review). The peripheral terminals of afferent fibers contain receptors for opioids, but the number of receptors present is upregulated during inflammation. Furthermore, inflammatory cells such as macrophages, monocytes, and lymphocytes may be induced to increase the amount of endogenous opioids released by IL-1β and corticotropin-releasing hormone (CRH) originating from the inflamed tissue. Peripheral endogenous opioids may also be activated by endothelin-1 (ET-1), which is a potent vasoactive peptide, synthesized and released by epithelia after tissue injury.[36] Paradoxically, ET-1 can trigger pain by activating ET_A receptors on nociceptors or analgesia through its actions on ET_B receptors. Activation of ET_B receptors on keratinocytes by ET-1 results in release of β-endorphins and analgesia that is mediated via peripheral μ- and κ-opioid receptors that are linked to G protein–coupled inward rectifying potassium channels (GIRKs).

Acetylcholine (Ach) is released into injured tissue from nonneuronal sources and modulates pain via its effects on nicotinic or muscarinic receptors. Nonspecific nicotinic agonists have weak excitatory effects on C-nociceptors and induce a mild sensitization to heat but no alterations in mechanical responsiveness, but more recently selective agonist for the alpha 5 and 9 subunits have been reported to produce analgesia.[37,38] In contrast, muscarinic agonists desensitizes C-nociceptors to mechanical and heat stimuli. Mice with targeted deletions of the M2 receptor show enhanced responsiveness of nociceptive fibers to noxious stimuli (see Fiorino and Garcia-Guzman[39] for review), indicating a tonic inhibitory role for this mediator.

Gamma-aminobutyric acid (GABA) may have a peripheral role in pain transmission similar to the bimodal actions of Ach. GABA type A ($GABA_A$) receptors are located on unmyelinated primary afferents, and activation of these receptors by low doses of the agonist muscimol decreases pain, whereas high doses potentiate pain. $GABA_A$ receptors have also been found in DRG cells and on their central terminals in the dorsal horn, and direct application of GABA antagonists to DRG cells decreases hypersensitivity in an animal model of neuropathic pain.[40]

Somatostatin (SST) is a peptide commonly associated with the gastrointestinal (GI) system that may also serve as an antinociceptive agent. Type 2a receptors (SSTR2a) are present in approximately 10% of unmyelinated primary afferent fibers innervating the glabrous skin of the rat, and intraplantar administration of an SST receptor agonist, octreotide, reduces the phase II response after formalin injection (see Malcangio[41] for review). In addition, octreotide reduces the response of CMHs to heat stimuli and attenuates the thermal responses of nociceptors sensitized by bradykinin. SST also inhibits the release of cholecystokinin (CCK), which has been shown to have nociceptive properties. The peripheral effects of SST agonists may be mediated by a direct effect on primary afferents or by its antiinflammatory effects. The SSTR4 has also been implicated as a possible therapeutic target. Studies indicate that an SSTR4–δ-opioid receptor complex exists with varying functions. In neuronal cells, activation of this complex led to greater inhibition of cAMP/protein kinase A (PKA)-induced nociception.[42]

Angiotensin II type 2 receptor (AT_2R) is a relatively newly reported potential analgesic target (see Rice and Smith[43] and Smith and Muralidharan[44] for reviews). Angiotensin II is the primary effector in the renin-angiotensin system and is produced from angiotensin I in the lungs by angiotensin-converting enzyme, whereas angiotensin I is produced from angiotensinogen by the renal enzyme renin. Angiotensin II has well-known effects in the regulation of blood pressure acting at the type 1 receptor, whereas a physiologic role for the AT_2R has remained elusive. The discovery of both angiotensin II and the AT_2R in DRG neurons suggested a potential role in the modulation of sensory information and additional studies indicated an excitatory role on both peptidergic and larger DRG neurons. AT_2R antagonists subsequently were shown to have antinociceptive properties in experimental animals, and this has subsequently been validated in a phase IIa proof-of-concept double-blind, placebo-controlled study in postherpetic neuralgia patients.

Peripheral Second Messenger Pathways: Inflammation is associated with the release of a host of chemical mediators. These agents may mediate pain by directly activating nociceptors, such as is primarily discussed previously. However, they may also produce more enduring changes in the sensory neuron, such as early posttranslational changes or even longer-lasting transcription-dependent changes in effector genes in DRG cells. The early posttranslational changes include phosphorylation of transducer molecules (e.g., TRPV1 receptor) and voltage-gated ion channels (e.g., sodium channels) in the peripheral terminals of nociceptors (peripheral sensitization). A classic example of these changes is seen in a *VR*, TRPV1 (also known as VR1).[45,46] This receptor is present on a subpopulation of primary afferent fibers that are activated by capsaicin, heat, and protons. Inflammatory mediators, such as bradykinin and NGF, lower the threshold of TRPV1-mediated heat-induced currents in DRG neurons and increase the proportion of DRG cells that respond to capsaicin. These changes occur by PLC-dependent phosphorylation by PKC, by phosphorylation by PKA, and by hydrolysis of the membrane phospholipid, phosphatidylinositol-4-5-biphosphate (PIP_2).[45,46] PKA and PKC also induce a short-term sensitization of nociceptors to heat by modulating the activity of tetrodotoxin-resistant sodium currents.[47] In addition, increases in the activity of various transcription factors, including cAMP response element–binding protein (CREB) and the mitogen-activated protein kinase (MAPK), most especially the extracellular signal–regulated kinases (ERKs), the c-Jun amino-terminal kinases (JNKs), and the p38 enzymes produce even longer-term changes in TRPV1 following inflammation in primary afferent fibers.[48,49] All of these signal cascades may be engaged by activation of Toll-like receptors on dorsal root ganglion neurons in mediating chemotherapy– and peripheral inflammation–related hyperalgesia.[50–53]

NEUROCHEMISTRY OF PAIN TRANSMISSION

As reviewed in the previous chapter, the anterolateral and dorsal column-medial lemniscal pathways transmit nociceptive signals from spinal cord to supraspinal sites, with differences between these paths being determined by anatomy and physiology of constituent neurons. However, unlike the differences in anatomy and physiology between the anterolateral and dorsal column-medial lemniscal systems, the neurochemistry of somatosensory processing in both is very similar. Both systems involve three classes of transmitter compounds, excitatory neurotransmitters, inhibitory neurotransmitters, and neuropeptides, that are found in three anatomic compartments: sensory afferent terminals, local circuit terminals, and descending (or ascending) modulatory circuit terminals. A graphical summary is found in Fig. 2.2.

Excitatory Neurotransmitters: The amino acids *glutamate* and *aspartate* constitute the main excitatory neurotransmitters found at synapses throughout the somatosensory system. Thus transmission between primary afferent fibers and spinal neurons, between spinal neurons and thalamic neurons, and so on are dependent on the four receptor types for glutamate and aspartate in the somatosensory system.[54,55] These receptors are named for the synthetic agonists that best activate them and include the N-methyl-D-aspartate (NMDA), the kainate, the AMPA ([R,S]-α-amino-3-hydroxy-5-methlyisoxazole-4-propionic acid) receptor and the metabotropic receptors. The latter three are often collectively referred to as the non-NMDA receptors. The AMPA and kainate receptors gate sodium channels and mediate the majority of the fast synaptic afferent signaling for all modalities and intensities of stimuli. The NMDA receptor is recruited only by intense and/or prolonged somatosensory stimuli that are sufficient to remove the magnesium ion that normally blocks the channel pore. Persistent activation of NMDA receptors leads to sensitization of dorsal horn neurons that includes an increase in receptive field size, decreased activation threshold, and prolonged depolarization. Multiple factors influence NMDA receptor-related sensitization. For instance, the release of bradykinin leads to increases in spinal glutamate released by astrocytes and neurons. This glutamate activates NMDA receptors, augmenting central sensitization.

In addition to the release of glutamate from neurons, activated glial cells can release glutamate. In certain pain conditions, such as chemotherapy-induced neuropathy, glial glutamate transporters GLAST and GLT-1 are downregulated, leading to decreased reuptake of spinal glutamate and subsequent spillover of glutamate to extrasynaptic receptor sites.[56]

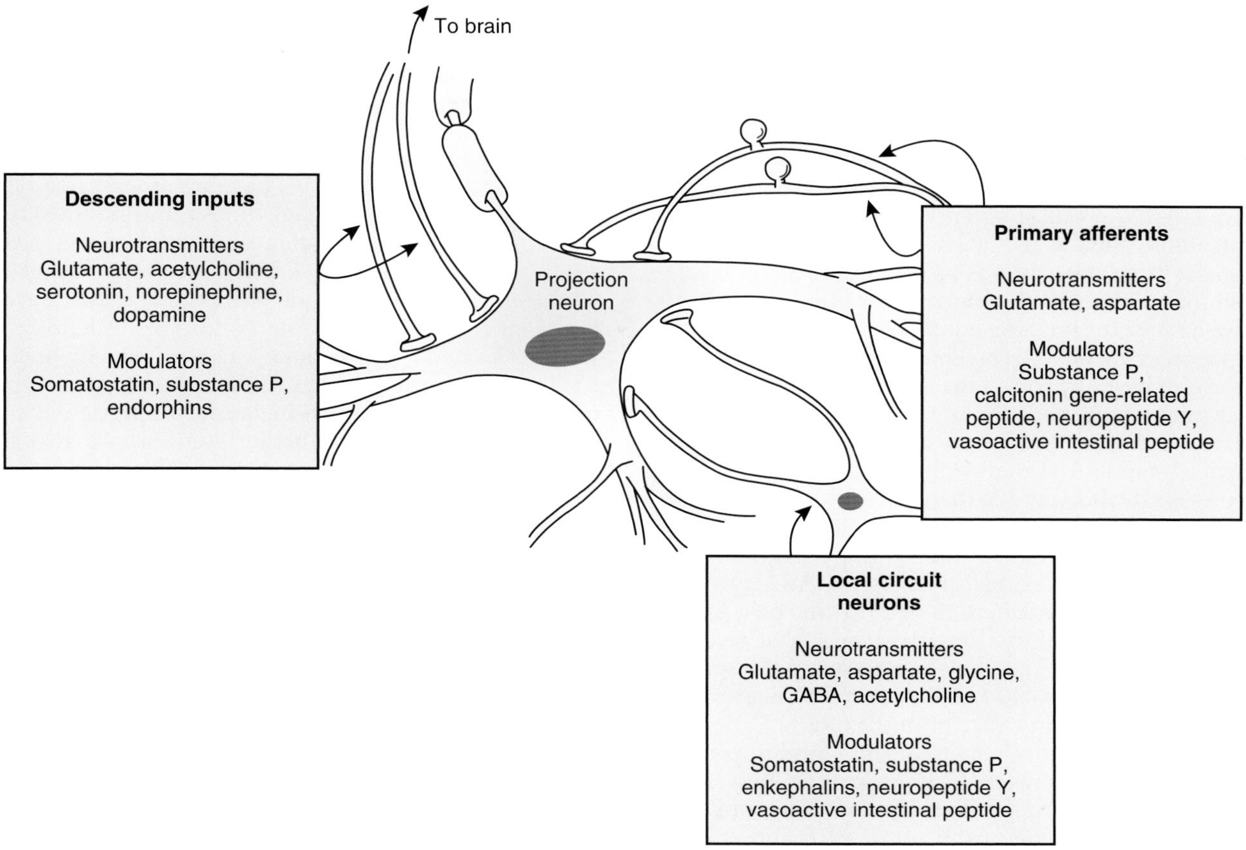

FIG. 2.2 Schematic diagram of the neurochemistry of somatosensory processing in the spinal dorsal horn. *GABA*, Gamma amino butyric acid.

The metabotropic glutamate receptors (mGluRs) are a family of G protein–linked sites involved in more long-term cellular changes.[57] The group I mGluRs when activated are coupled to $G_{q/11}$ that activate PLC-liberating inositol phosphate, which in turn results in the release of cytosolic calcium and activation of PKC. The group II and III metabotropic receptors are negatively coupled by G_i/G_o to adenylyl cyclase and so reduce intracellular cyclic AMP and PKA activity. Given the complexity of these receptor transduction mechanisms, it should come as no surprise that activation of mGluRs can result in the modulation of multiple cellular kinases, receptors, ion channels, and transcription factors and so have complex and sometimes variable effects on somatosensory and pain processing. However, as a general rule the group I mGluRs have cooperative effects with NMDA receptors in promoting cellular excitability and signaling, whereas the group II and III mGluRs most often have inhibitory effects on transmission.

ATP also modulates somatosensory transmission. The primary receptor for ATP is the P2X family of receptors, which is composed of seven subunits expressed in six homomeric and at least four heteromeric subtypes.[58] These receptors are present on the central terminals of primary afferent fibers innervating neurons in lamina V and II of the dorsal horn, where they function to increase the release of glutamate. The P2 class of receptors, both the ionotropic P2X and the GPCR P2Y classes, further play a unique role in glial-mediated pain sensitivity. The binding of ATP to P2 receptors on microglia changes the phenotype of these cells to include increased expression of P2 and cytokine receptors. These now-activated microglia begin to secrete inflammatory mediators, such as cytokines, NGF, and NO. These factors serve to sustain pain and inflammation.[59] In support of these findings, researchers have found that mice lacking either $P2X_4$ or $P2X_7$ showed decreased sensitivity to mechanical and thermal stimulation in an animal model of pain. ATP may play a central role in pain perception in head and neck cancers as a result of expression of $P2X_2/P2X_3$ on nerve fibers supplying these cancers.[60]

Inhibitory Neurotransmitters: The amino acids *glycine* and *GABA* are the chief inhibitory neurotransmitters in the somatosensory system (for review see Prescott[61]). Glycine is the chief inhibitory amino acid at spinal levels, whereas GABA predominates at higher levels. There are two receptor sites for glycine, a chloride-linked strychnine-sensitive receptor and a strychnine-insensitive regulatory site on the NMDA glutamate receptors. GABA is found in local circuit neurons of spinal laminae I, II, and III. Three types of GABA receptors have been identified. The $GABA_A$ receptor is linked to a chloride channel and modulated by barbiturates, benzodiazepines, and alcohol. Selective $GABA_A$ agonists include muscimol, and selective antagonists include gabazine. A $GABA_A$-mediated link between large myelinated fibers and C-fiber nociceptors has been proposed as a mechanism for the development of allodynia following intradermal injection of the irritant capsaicin.[62] In addition, a selective loss of inhibitory interneurons at both spinal and thalamic levels has been suggested as contributing to some neuropathic pain conditions; and alternatively a shift in the chloride potential such that $GABA_A$ channels assume an excitatory function has also been proposed.[63] The $GABA_B$ receptor has been associated with both a potassium ionophore and with a G protein–linked complex. Baclofen is a selective $GABA_B$ receptor agonist and phaclofen is a selective antagonist. Finally, the newly described $GABA_C$ receptor has also been described as associated with a potassium channel ionophore. Cis-4-aminocrotonic acid (CACA) is a selective agonist for this site, but there is currently no selective antagonist for $GABA_C$ receptors. $GABA_C$ receptors do not appear to have any role in the modulation of somatosensory information. Application of CACA has been shown to induce an antinociceptive effect that is blocked by 1,2,5,6–tetrahydropyridine-4-yl methylphosphinic acid (TPMPA). It was previously thought that these receptors did not appear to have any role in the modulation of somatosensory information, but this recent study indicates a potential role at this receptor site.[64] Decreased spinal cord GABAergic inhibition is thought to contribute to neuropathic pain following peripheral nerve injury. Reports suggest that restoring spinal cord GABAergic signaling by intraspinal transplantation of cortical precursors of GABAergic interneurons can reverse neuropathic pain behavior in the mouse.[65]

Norepinephrine is another abundant inhibitory neurotransmitter and is especially important in descending brainstem projections to the dorsal horn.[66] The inhibitory effects of norepinephrine in the spinal cord appear to be twofold by directly activating inhibitory GABAergic interneurons and by also inhibiting excitatory interneurons.[67] The adrenergic receptors include two broad classes termed the alpha and beta receptors, each of which in turn have several subtypes. The alpha2-adrenergic receptor is the primary form found in the spinal dorsal horn that has an inhibitory role on the processing of sensory information. However, it should be noted that the function of norepinephrine following injury to the nervous systems might reverse from an inhibitory, analgesic role into one of promoting and/or sustaining an ongoing chronic pain state.

Serotonin is also expressed in descending pathways to the spinal dorsal horn, predominately in those originating from the midbrain raphe nuclei.[66] There are multiple serotonin (5-HT) receptor subtypes, including 5-HT-1, 2, and 3 receptors, and each of these major types also has several subtypes. Due to controversy concerning which of these subtypes mediates the analgesic properties of serotonin, interest in serotonin as a clinically useful target for the treatment of pain has weaned. In part, this controversy may be because some serotonin receptor subtypes in fact promote nociception, whereas others are inhibitory. If more selective tools are developed with which to dissect this pharmacology, serotonin may regain its former status as a potentially useful clinical target. Serotonin-norepinephrine reuptake inhibitors, such as duloxetine and amitryptiline, have been used to treat assorted pain conditions, with variable rates of success. The inhibitory and antinociceptive nature of norepinephrine and serotonin is further evidenced by the abundance of literature showing that many antidepressants that modulate both of these neurotransmitters, including duloxetine and amitriptyline, have analgesic properties in humans and in animal models of pain. Currently, it is thought that the antinociceptive effects are mediated by activation of α-1adenoreceptors and 5-HT2 receptors,[68] leading to facilitation of descending inhibition.

Adenosine is another important inhibitory neurotransmitter at the spinal level.[15] There are at least two types of adenosine receptors, termed the A1 and A2 sites. Occupation of these sites by adenosine results in G protein–mediated alterations of cAMP levels in target cells. However, both elevations and decreases in cAMP formation have been reported in various conditions. Adenosine may mediate a portion of the analgesia produced by brainstem norepinephrine projections to the spinal cord and appears to have especially robust analgesic properties in neuropathic pain conditions. Further studies have also shown that the adenosine A1 receptor (A1R) plays a role in transmission of pain signals. Activation of this receptor is believed to produce postsynaptic inhibition by activation of potassium (K^+) channels, thus causing hyperpolarization of the neuronal membrane. It has been demonstrated that mice that lack this A1 receptor have increased nociceptive responses to different pain stimuli.[69]

Ach is yet another neurotransmitter that mediates antinociception at the level of the spinal dorsal horn.[70] Stimulation of the vagus nerve results in inhibition of pain transmission, and it is likely that this effect is mediated by Ach. Ach may also contribute to the analgesia produced by the alpha2-adrenergic receptor agonist clonidine. It was previously thought that the antinociceptive effects of Ach were mediated by the muscarinic and not by the nicotinic Ach receptor subtypes. However, findings have shown that several nicotinic receptor subtypes play a role in a variety of pain states, their efficacy often limited by adverse effects. It was shown that coadministration of ABT-594 (an antiallodynic nicotinic Ach receptor agonist) with NS-9283 (a positive allosteric modulator of the $\alpha4\beta2$ nicotinic Ach receptor subtype) resulted in potentiation of the analgesic effect without concomitant potentiation of adverse effects. Many other nicotinic receptor subtypes are being identified as potential therapeutic targets.[71]

Neuropeptides: In addition to the excitatory and inhibitory neurotransmitters discussed previously, there are multiple neuropeptides that contribute to signaling of somatosensory information. Although some of these could be classified as excitatory compounds and others as inhibitory, we have separated these into a section of their own because of the distinct profile of action of these compounds as opposed to the neurotransmitters. Unlike the very rapid onset and termination of action of the transmitters, neuropeptides tend to have a more gradual onset and a more prolonged duration of action once released.

Substance P and *neurokinin A* serve as excitatory neuropeptides in the somatosensory system.[72] The receptors for these peptides include the neurokinin 1 and 2 sites, each of which have been associated with elevation of intracellular calcium levels, perhaps through liberation of inositol phosphate. These two peptides may be present in intrinsic neurons of the spinal dorsal horn and thalamus but are especially concentrated in primary afferent fibers. At the spinal level, these peptides are only released following application of noxious stimuli that are sufficient to produce sustained discharges in C-nociceptors, although some small myelinated (Aδ) fibers may also contain substance P. Instead of signaling as synaptic transmitters, these peptides tend to spread throughout the dorsal horn, potentially acting on multiple synapses some distance from their point of release. It has been suggested that stimuli of particular modalities (e.g., mechanical vs. thermal) are associated with selective release of one peptide versus another; however, this suggestion has not been corroborated. Activation of neurokinin 1 and/or 2 receptors by substance P and/or neurokinin A is regarded as a key step needed for the induction of sensitization and hence the expression of hyperalgesia following cutaneous injury. It has been further proposed that the mechanism of neurokinin receptor involvement in the expression of sensitization is through facilitation of the synaptic actions of the EAA neurotransmitters.

CGRP, like substance P, is expressed predominately by small, unmyelinated primary afferent fibers, and it is also found in DRG cells and in the superficial layers of the spinal cord.[72] Both CGRP and substance P synthesis and release are increased by another excitatory peptide, neuropeptide Y. Spinal release of CGRP has an excitatory effect on wide dynamic range neurons, and administration of the CGRP antagonist CGRP8-37 reverses this activity. Intrathecal administration of CGRP has been shown by some researchers to produce mechanical hypersensitivity, although it should be noted that others have failed to replicate this finding. Interestingly, the function of CGRP released within the brain seems to be antithetic to the peripheral and spinal effects, with release of this peptide within the PAG producing antinociceptive results.

CCK is a hormone peptide normally involved in digestion; however, it is also involved in the maintenance of pain. Some researchers contend that this effect is achieved via descending facilitation of nociceptive output from the rostral ventromedial medulla,[73] whereas others propose that CCK blocks the descending antinociceptive effects of endogenous opioids within the periaqueductal grey.[74] Coadministration of a CCK antagonist along with traditional exogenous opioids results in augmented analgesia and even opioid tolerance reversal. CCK also caused release of both prostaglandin E2 (PGE2) and 5-HT in the lumbar spinal cord that was attenuated by naproxen and ondansetron, respectively.[75] Continued work is needed to better understand the mechanisms and therapeutic uses of CCK antagonists.

SST, the *enkephalins*, and possibly *dynorphin* are included as inhibitory neuropeptides at the spinal level. These peptides are contained in both intrinsic neurons of the dorsal horn and in the fibers descending to the dorsal horn from various brainstem nuclei. The *endorphins* are another class of inhibitory neuropeptides. The receptor types for the opioid peptides include the μ, δ, and κ receptor subtypes, and these receptors are found at all levels of the somatosensory system. These receptors are associated with modulation of both intracellular cAMP and potassium levels. There is also an important cooperative functional link between μ-opioid and alpha2-adrenergic receptors that have yet to be fully exploited for clinical applications.

Cannabinoids are present in the peripheral and central nervous systems and play a role in inhibiting pain. At this point, the CB1 receptor within the central nervous system seems to be a likely target for pharmacologic interventions. The CB1 receptor agonist Sativex is very effective at decreasing neuropathic pain but has sedative side effects. CB1 receptors are highly expressed in the DRG, and their activation at this level decreases the release of neurotransmitters involved in pain transmission and attenuates mechanical and heat hypersensitivity.[76] Agarwal et al. showed that specific loss of CB1 receptors in *peripheral* nociceptive neurons leads to a major reduction in the antihyperalgesic effects of endocannabinoids and systemically administered cannabinoids.[77] CT3 has decreased central nervous system bioavailability, and therefore fewer side effects, and yet is still efficient at producing analgesia. Lately, research has focused on a potential role of the CB2 receptor because activation of this receptor is associated with fewer adverse effects. Research has demonstrated that AM1710, an agonist at the CB2 receptor, decreased allodynia induced by paclitaxel in a mouse model. Furthermore, this same effect was not seen in mice in which the CB2 receptor was knocked out.[78] A separate study showed that the CB2 agonist, JWH133, was able to attenuate pain responses in a model of osteoarthritis-associated pain.[79]

Peroxisome proliferator-activated receptors (PPARs): The receptors discussed up to this point have been limited to those contained on the cell surface; however, the PPARs represent a class of nuclear receptors that serve as transcription factors.[80,81] Within this family, three different isoforms exist (PPARα, PPARβ/δ, and PPARγ), which are localized to different tissues and serve different functions. Of these, PPARγ has been studied most extensively regarding the role it plays in attenuating inflammation. Rosiglitazone has been shown to possibly modulate neuropathic pain by acting on the PPARγ receptor to reduce expression of MCP-1 and its receptor, CCR2, in the DRG.[82] Based on this line of research, it follows that PPARs may offer a novel means to decrease pain. As previously mentioned, future research attempting to use these receptor agonists as analgesics will have to overcome the serious side effects of increased adiposity and fluid retention.[83] PPARs, such as PPARγ, are located in the brain and spinal cord. Although it is currently unclear how these receptors become activated following injury, once activated they mediate inflammatory substances, such as substance P, CGRP, and cytokines. In turn, mediation of these and other factors allows for inhibition of inflammation and pain.

Central Signal Propagation and Second Messenger Systems: The movement of various ions and the activity of cellular enzymes and metabolites are essential in the propagation of bioelectric signals in the central nervous system. Alterations to these factors can drastically reduce or augment signal propagation and ultimately somatosensory perception. Ion movement relies on proteins that form ion channels and function as second messenger enzymes. The actions of these proteins can be blocked by a number of agents, and many of these have been studied as putative analgesics. However, because ion channels and second messengers are found in all neural elements, the effects of compounds acting at these sites are not specific to pain circuitry. Side effects are therefore often encountered with these drugs, which limit their usefulness. There are four ion channels involved in pain signal propagation in the central nervous system, those for sodium, calcium, potassium, and chloride.

Sodium channels serve as the key to propagation of neural impulses throughout the nervous system because the opening of these channels is the primary event underlying the depolarization of nerve membranes, and sodium currents in dorsal horn neurons are mediated by at least three types of tetrodotoxin-sensitive channels.[84,85] The local anesthetics lidocaine and bupivacaine physically block sodium channels, preventing the movement of sodium across the membrane. Prolonged infusions of local anesthetics for postoperative pain in humans became widespread in the 1990s, and cancer and chronic nonmalignant pain are treated with continuous infusions of intraspinal local anesthetics outside of the hospital. However, side effects are common and include delayed urinary retention, paresthesia, paresis/gait impairment, periods of orthostatic hypotension, bradypnea, and dyspnea.[84] Advances in the understanding of sodium channel subtypes present novel means of achieving pain relief. Both the Nav1.7 and Nav1.8 subtypes are expressed throughout the central and peripheral nervous system and are critical in action potential generation in peripheral nociceptors. Clinically, patients with absent or nonfunctioning Nav1.7 channels experience congenital insensitivity to pain, and overactivity of this subtype is associated with certain chronic pain conditions. The anticonvulsant carbamazepine produces analgesia, presumably by inhibiting Nav1.7. Furthermore, mice lacking Nav1.8 display decreased pain responding, and the Nav1.8 selective blocker A-803467 alleviates neuropathic and inflammatory pain in animals. The Nav1.9 subtype is also involved in pain transmission.[86] Evidence indicates a possibility that Nav1.9 plays a role in the development of pain secondary to trigeminal neuralgia. Each of these subtypes has been found to have genes that produce gain-of-function mutations leading to transmission of pain signals.[87] As such, current research is focusing on genomics as a basis for possible therapeutic interventions (for reviews see Waxman[88] and Moldovan et al.[89]).

Potassium channels are the second main cation channels of the neuronal action potential. There are four families of potassium channels, with the voltage-gated channels and the inwardly rectifying channels being strongly implicated to play a role in pain.[90–92] Opening of voltage-gated potassium channels allows outward positive current flow from neurons, such as during repolarization following an action potential. Blockade of these channels initially prolongs generation of action potentials. However, continued application prevents repolarization and so ultimately produces a failure to generate action potentials. The inwardly rectifying channels establish and regulate the resting membrane potential. Evidence has implicated a potential for potassium channels to serve as targets for the treatment of pain. NO has been found to activate ATP-sensitive potassium channels (K[ATP]) and contribute to the maintenance of neuropathic pain, although the exact mechanisms of this effect are yet to be uncovered. Administration of the potassium channel blocker retigabine reversed surgically induced neuropathic pain in an animal model. Two-pore potassium (K2P) channels have emerged as potential therapeutic targets. This group of potassium channels has many different members. For instance, the TRESK and TREK subtypes have been shown to have a role in nociception. Studies have shown that mice in which the K2P was knocked out had silencing of heat nociceptors.[91] Li and Toyoda also described several K2P channels, their role in pain signaling, and the potential for the development of new therapeutics.[92]

Calcium ions are not directly involved in action potential propagation but instead are essential for the release of neurotransmitters following synaptic depolarization.[90,93] At least four different types of calcium channels, the L-, N-, T-, and P-types, have been identified in dorsal horn neurons. There are numerous chemical antagonists of L-type calcium channels, whereas N-type calcium channels are blocked using toxins of *Conus magus*. P-type channels are especially prevalent in Purkinje cells and are sensitive to venom toxins of the funnel web spider *(Agelenopsis aperta)*. T-type channels are involved in the regulation of neuronal excitability and pacemaker activity and are blocked by some omega conotoxins. Antinociceptive effects have been shown for N-, L-, T- and P-type calcium channels in animals and for L- and N-type channels in humans.[94]

Chloride ions are also a major contributor to signal propagation, and three major classes of chloride channels have been identified. The first class identified was the ligand-gated chloride channels, including those of the GABAA and glycine receptors, and these are common in dorsal horn neurons.[95] The second class, also likely common at spinal levels, is the voltage-gated chloride channel.[96] The final chloride channel class is activated by cyclic adenosine monophosphate and may include only the cystic fibrosis transmembrane regulator.[97] Activation of chloride currents usually results in hyperpolarization of neurons, and facilitation of these hyperpolarizing currents underlies the mechanisms of many depressant drugs. However, the GABAA receptors on primary afferent terminals gate a chloride channel that allows efflux, instead of the normal influx, of chloride with a net effect therefore of depolarizing primary afferent terminals. Chloride channel antagonists such as bicuculline and strychnine have not been given to relieve pain but instead to produce an experimental pain state characterized by a pronounced opiate-refractory allodynia.[63,95] These compounds were also used to exacerbate the anatomic consequences of nerve constriction injury. A group of chloride channels known as calcium-activated chloride channels (CACCs) have been studied more recently. As their name implies, these channels are activated by increases in intracellular calcium, which then leads to an increase in chloride conductance. Pineda-Farias showed that anoctamin-1 and bestrophin-1, CACCs subtypes, may play a role in neuropathic pain. They specifically showed that anoctamin-1 mRNA was increased in rats that underwent L5/L6 spinal nerve ligation.[98] Cho et al. also studied anoctamin-1 activity and demonstrated that it may function as a heat sensor, detecting thermal information and mediating nociceptive information; knockout of Ano-1 resulted in decreased nociception.[99]

Finally, the role of *second messenger systems* on pain sensitivity has been examined in a number of studies. Increases in the levels of membrane-bound PKC have been found following both nerve injury and intraplantar injection of formalin.[100] Spinal infusion of phorbol esters to activate PKC increases the behavioral response to intraplantar formalin and increases the spontaneous and evoked activity of primate spinothalamic tract neurons. In contrast, antagonists for PKC decrease pain behavior following nerve injury, intraplantar formalin, intraspinal NMDA, and intradermal capsaicin. Similarly, inhibition of PLC or phospholipase A (needed for release of cofactors to PKC) reduced hyperalgesia following intraplantar formalin and zymosan, respectively. Further evidence comes from the finding that animals engineered with defects in PKC had less pain following nerve injury, whereas those engineered with defects in PKA had decreased responses to formalin, capsaicin, and hind paw inflammation.[101]

Based on this abundance of research, many second messenger systems could become targets for clinical pain treatment. However, the current role of these systems in pain management is indirect through the action of various drugs that interact with surface receptors linked to G proteins.[102] Receptors linked to GS (receptors associated with βγα S subunits) include the beta1-adrenergic, dopaminergic type 1, and adenosine type 2 receptors. Those that activate Gq,12 (βγα q,12) include the serotonin 2c, alpha1-adrenergic, histamine, thromboxane A2, metabotropic glutamate, and the muscarinic type 1, 3, and 5 receptors. Finally, GI-(βγα i)-linked receptors include the adenosine 1, serotonin 1B, GABAB, muscarinic 2, μ-, δ- and κ-opioid receptors. Neurotransmitter receptors linked to GS and Gq,12 generally increase pain transmission, whereas GI-linked receptors inhibit pain signaling.

SUMMARY

Throughout the nervous system, many interrelated factors contribute to pain. In the periphery, mediators such as bradykinin, cytokines, and second messenger pathways facilitate the mechanisms of each other and lead to increased nociceptive transmission to the spinal cord. Within the spinal cord, many of these same elements work to convert acute pain into chronic conditions. This transition may occur via changes in gene regulation, receptor expression, and glial activation and through central sensitization. Attempts to alleviate pain have been made by interfering with many of the chemical mediators involved in pain, with various levels of success. Future research will continue to expand our understanding of the neurochemistry of pain and will add to the means by which pain can be alleviated.

KEY POINTS

- The EAAs glutamate and aspartate are the key excitatory neurotransmitters in the somatosensory system.
- The four types of EAA receptors are the NMDA, AMPA, kainite, and metabotropic receptors.
- GABA and glycine are the key inhibitory neurotransmitters.
- Substance P is the key excitatory neuropeptide in the somatosensory system.
- The enkephalins and SST are the key inhibitory neuropeptides in the somatosensory system.
- Potential novel targets in the periphery and central nervous system include sodium channel subtypes, adenosine, Ach, and cannabinoid receptors and second messenger systems.

REFERENCES

Access the reference list online at ExpertConsult.com.

CHAPTER 3

Taxonomy: Definition of Pain Terms and Chronic Pain Syndromes

Kiran Chekka, MD ◎ Honorio T. Benzon, MD

Acute pain—Pain resulting from nociceptor activation due to damage or potential damage to tissues. Acute pain typically resolves after the tissue damage is repaired.

Allodynia—Pain due to a stimulus that does not normally provoke pain.

Analgesia—Absence of pain in response to stimulation that would normally be painful.

Anesthesia—Absence of all sensory modalities.

Anesthesia dolorosa—Pain in an area or region that is anesthetic.

Budapest criteria—An empirically driven and statistically derived criteria developed to objectively diagnose complex regional pain syndrome (CRPS) using the patient's history and physical examination findings.

Carpal tunnel syndrome—Pain in the hand, usually occurring at night, due to entrapment of the median nerve in the carpal tunnel area. The quality of the pain is a "pins-and-needles" sensation, stinging, burning, or aching. There may be decreased sensation on the tips of the first to third fingers, positive Tinel sign, and, rarely, atrophy of the thenar muscles. A nerve conduction study shows delayed conduction across the carpal tunnel. The syndrome is caused by compression of the median nerve in the wrist between the carpal bones and the flexor retinaculum (transverse carpal ligament).

Central pain—Pain caused by a lesion or disease of the central somatosensory nervous system. Central pain is usually associated with abnormal sensibility to temperature and to noxious stimulation.

Chronic pain—Pain that persists beyond the course of an acute disease or a reasonable time for an injury to heal or that is associated with a chronic pathologic process that causes continuous pain or the pain recurs at intervals of months or years. Some investigators use duration of ≥6 months to designate pain as chronic.

Claudication pain—Crampy, achy lower extremity pain precipitated by ambulation and activity, caused by vascular insufficiency. This is to be differentiated from neurogenic claudication, which presents with similar symptoms but due to significant central spinal canal stenosis.

Complex regional pain syndrome (CRPS; Budapest criteria definition)—An array of painful conditions that are characterized by a continuing (spontaneous and/or evoked) regional pain that is seemingly disproportionate in time or degree to the usual course of any known trauma or other lesion. The pain is regional (not in a specific nerve territory or dermatome) and usually has a distal predominance of abnormal sensory, motor, sudomotor, vasomotor, and/or trophic findings. The syndrome shows variable progression over time.[1] There is an International Association for the Study of Pain (IASP)[2,3] and Budapest[1] criteria for CRPS (Tables 3.1 and 3.2).

Comprehensive pain center—Center dedicated to managing a full spectrum of chronic pain syndromes using multiple disciplines and modalities.

Cubital tunnel syndrome—Entrapment of the ulnar nerve in a fibro-osseous tunnel formed by the trochlear groove between the olecranon process and the medial epicondyle of the humerus. A myofascial covering converts the groove to a tunnel, which causes the nerve entrapment. There is pain, numbness, and paresthesia in the distribution of the ulnar nerve and, sometimes, weakness and atrophy in the same distribution. Tinel sign is positive at the elbow. Nerve conduction velocity shows slowing of conduction in the ulnar nerve across the elbow. The intrinsic muscles of the hand may show signs of denervation. Surgery may be required to decompress the entrapment or to transpose the ulnar nerve.

Deafferentation pain—Pain due to loss of sensory input into the central nervous system. This may occur with lesions of peripheral nerves, such as avulsion of the brachial plexus, or due to pathology of the central nervous system.

Disability—Loss of ability to perform a specific task in a standard or normal fashion.

Discogenic pain—Vague, achy low back pain emanating from the disc itself and not attributed to compression of adjacent nerves likely attributable to nociceptor ingrowth into the disc itself. The pain is usually axial in character and worse on standing. Magnetic resonance imaging (MRI) may help in the diagnosis (presence of a "high-intensity zone") and discography may help to localize the affected vertebral level.

Dysesthesia—An unpleasant abnormal evoked sensation, whether spontaneous or evoked.

TABLE 3.1 IASP Diagnostic Criteria for Complex Regional Pain Syndrome[2,3]

Presence of an initiating noxious event or a cause of immobilization
Continuing pain, allodynia, or hyperalgesia in which the pain is disproportionate to any known inciting event
Evidence at some time of edema, changes in skin blood flow, or abnormal sudomotor activity in the region of pain (can be sign or symptom)
Diagnosis is excluded by the existence of other conditions that would otherwise account for the degree of pain and dysfunction
CRPS type I: seen without "major nerve damage" diagnose CRPS I CRPS type II: seen in the presence of "major nerve damage"

CRPS, *Complex regional pain syndrome;* IASP, *International Association for the Study of Pain.*

TABLE 3.2 Budapest Criteria for Complex Regional Pain Syndrome[1]

*To make the **clinical diagnosis**, the following criteria must be met:*

1. Continuing pain that is disproportionate to any inciting event
2. Must report at least one symptom in ***three of the four*** following categories:

Sensory: Reports of hyperesthesia and/or allodynia

Vasomotor: Reports of temperature asymmetry and/or skin color changes and/or skin color asymmetry

Sudomotor/edema: Reports of edema and/or sweating changes and/or sweating asymmetry

Motor/trophic: Reports of decreased range of motion and/or motor dysfunction (weakness, tremor, dystonia) and/or trophic changes (hair, nail, skin)

3. Must display at least one sign *at time of evaluation* in *two or more* of the following categories:

Sensory: Evidence of hyperalgesia (to pinprick) and/or allodynia (to light touch and/or temperature sensation and/or deep somatic pressure and/or joint movement)

Vasomotor: Evidence of temperature asymmetry (>1°C) and/or skin color changes and/or asymmetry

Sudomotor/edema: Evidence of edema and/or sweating changes and/or sweating asymmetry

Motor/trophic: Evidence of decreased range of motion and/or motor dysfunction (weakness, tremor, dystonia) and/or trophic changes (hair, nail, skin)

4. There is no other diagnosis that better explains the signs and symptoms.

For ***research purposes,*** diagnostic decision rule should be at least one symptom in ***all four*** symptom categories and at least one sign (observed at evaluation) in two or more sign categories.

Eagle syndrome (stylohyoid syndrome)—Elongated or deviated styloid process and/or calcification of the stylohyoid ligament, which interferes with adjacent anatomical structures giving rise to pain. Pain may be precipitated by trauma to the region.

FIBROMYALGIA

The original American College of Rheumatology (ACR) criteria were proposed in 1990. The criteria required tenderness on pressure (tender points) in at least 11 of 18 specified sites and the presence of widespread pain.[4] (*Widespread pain* is axial pain, left- and right-sided pain, and upper and lower segment pain). Most physicians did not look for trigger points, and when they did, they performed incorrectly. Realizing this deficiency, and with better understanding of the disease, the ACR proposed a new criteria in 2010 (Table 3.3).[5] The presence of tender points are not required. Rather, a score of 7 or greater in the widespread pain index (WPI) and symptom severity (SS) score of 5 or greater (or WPI 3-6 and SS score ≥9) are required for diagnosis (see Table 3.3).

Hyperalgesia—Increased pain from a stimulus that normally provokes pain.

Hyperesthesia—Increased sensitivity to stimulation; this excludes the special senses.

Hyperpathia—A painful syndrome, characterized by increased reaction to a stimulus, especially a repetitive stimulus, as well as increased threshold.

Hypoalgesia—Diminished pain in response to a normally painful stimulus.

Hypoesthesia—Diminished sensitivity to stimulation; this excludes the special senses.

Lateral epicondylitis (tennis elbow)—Pain in the region of the lateral epicondyle of the elbow due to strain or partial tear of the extensor tendon of the wrist. The pain may radiate to the lateral forearm or to the upper arm. There is pain in the elbow during grasping and supination of the wrist and on repeated wrist dorsiflexion. Physical examination shows tenderness of the wrist extensor tendon approximately 5 cm distal to the epicondyle.

Modality-oriented pain center—Facility that offers one specific therapeutic modality for an array of chronic pain disorders. For example, an interventional center may provide nerve blocks and other procedures for back pain, neck pain, CRPS, and other syndromes.

Multidisciplinary pain management—Treatment of chronic pain by professionals from multiple disciplines (physical therapy, psychology, rehabilitation medicine, anesthesiology, and others) in a group setting. Pain centers are usually quite large due to the amount of space needed to perform multidisciplinary evaluations and therapies in groups.

Neuralgia—Pain in the distribution of a nerve or nerves.

Neuritis—Inflammation of a nerve or nerves. (Not to be used unless inflammation is thought to be present.)

Neuropathic pain—Pain initiated or caused by a primary lesion or disease in the peripheral or central somatosensory nervous systems.

Central neuropathic pain—A lesion or disease in the central nervous system causing pain. These include thalamic pain syndrome, poststroke pain, and post-spinal cord injury pain.

Peripheral neuropathic pain—Pain caused by a lesion or disease of the peripheral somatosensory nervous system. Examples are postherpetic neuralgia (PHN), painful diabetic neuropathy (PDN), and CRPS.

Neuropathy—A disturbance of function or pathologic change in a nerve. This may involve one nerve (mononeuropathy), several nerves (mononeuropathy multiplex), or it may be bilateral or symmetrical (polyneuropathy).

Nociceptive pain—Pain caused by activation of nociceptive afferent fibers. This type of pain satisfies the criteria for pain transmission (i.e., transmission to the spinal cord, thalamus, and then to the cerebral cortex).

Somatic pain—Pain carried along the sensory fibers; this pain is usually discrete and intense.

Visceral pain—Pain carried by the sympathetic fibers; this pain is diffuse and poorly localized.

Nociceptor—A receptor preferentially sensitive to a noxious stimulus or to a stimulus that would become noxious if prolonged.

Noxious stimulus—A stimulus that is actually or potentially damaging to body tissue.

Pain—An unpleasant sensory and emotional experience associated with actual or potential tissue damage, or described in terms of damage.

TABLE 3.3 American College of Rheumatology Diagnostic Criteria for Fibromyalgia[5]

Criteria			
A patient satisfies diagnostic criteria for fibromyalgia if the following three conditions are met:			
1. WPI ≥7 and SS scale score ≥5 or WPI 3–6 and SS scale score ≥9.			
2. Symptoms have been present at a similar level for at least 3 months.			
3. The patient does not have a disorder that would otherwise explain the pain.			
Ascertainment			
1. WPI: note the number areas in which the patient has had pain over the last week. In how many areas has the patient had pain? Score will be between 0 and 19.			
Shoulder girdle, left	Hip (buttock, trochanter), left	Jaw, left	Upper back
Shoulder girdle, right	Hip (buttock, trochanter), right	Jaw, right	Lower back
Upper arm, left	Upper leg, left	Chest	Neck
Upper arm, right	Upper leg, right	Abdomen	
Lower arm, left	Lower leg, left		
Lower arm, right	Lower leg, right		
2. SS scale score:			
Fatigue			
Waking unrefreshed			
Cognitive symptoms			
For each of the three symptoms above, indicate the level of severity over the past week using the following scale:			
0 = no problem			
1 = slight or mild problems, generally mild or intermittent			
2 = moderate, considerable problems, often present and/or at a moderate level			
3 = severe: pervasive, continuous, life-disturbing problems			
Considering somatic symptoms in general, indicate whether the patient has[a]:			
0 = no symptoms			
1 = few symptoms			
2 = a moderate number of symptoms			
3 = a great deal of symptoms			
The SS scale score is the sum of the severity of the three symptoms (fatigue, waking unrefreshed, cognitive symptoms) plus the extent (severity) of somatic symptoms in general. The final score is between 0 and 12.			

[a]*Somatic symptoms that might be considered: muscle pain, irritable bowel syndrome, fatigue/tiredness, thinking or remembering problem, muscle weakness, headache, pain/cramps in the abdomen, numbness/tingling, dizziness, insomnia, depression, constipation, pain in the upper abdomen, nausea, nervousness, chest pain, blurred vision, fever, diarrhea, dry mouth, itching, wheezing, Raynaud phenomenon, hives/welts, ringing in ears, vomiting, heartburn, oral ulcers, loss of/change in taste, seizures, dry eyes, shortness of breath, loss of appetite, rash, sun sensitivity, hearing difficulties, easy bruising, hair loss, frequent urination, painful urination, and bladder spasms.*

SS, *Symptom severity;* WPI, *widespread pain index.*

From Wolfe F, Clauw DJ, Fitzcharles MA, et al. The American College of Rheumatology preliminary diagnostic criteria for fibromyalgia and measurement of symptom severity. Arthritis Care Res (Hoboken) *2010;62:600-610.*

PAIN OF PSYCHOLOGICAL ORIGIN

- Delusional or hallucinatory: pain of psychological origin and attributed by the patient to a specific delusional cause.
- Hysterical, conversion, or hypochondriac: pain specifically attributable to the thought process, emotional state, or personality of the patient in the absence of an organic or delusional cause or tension mechanism.
- Pain associated with depression: pain occurring in the course of a depressive illness, not preceding the depression and not attributable to any other cause.

Pain threshold—The least intensity of pain that a subject can recognize.

Pain tolerance level—The greatest level of pain that a subject is willing to tolerate.

Paresthesia—An abnormal sensation, whether spontaneous or evoked. (Note: Paresthesia is an abnormal sensation that is not unpleasant, whereas dysesthesia is an abnormal sensation that is considered unpleasant. Dysesthesia does not include all abnormal sensations, only those that are unpleasant.)

Peripheral neuropathy—Constant or intermittent burning, aching, or lancinating limb pain due to generalized or focal diseases of peripheral nerves.

Phantom pain—Pain referred to a surgically removed limb or portion thereof.

Piriformis syndrome—Pain in the buttock and posterior thigh due to myofascial injury of the piriformis muscle itself or pain in the posterior leg and foot, due to entrapment of the sciatic or other nerves by the piriformis muscle within the greater sciatic foramen, or a combination of these causes.

Platelet-rich plasma—A concentrated injectate of autologous platelets used frequently in a variety of pain syndromes, although data for its use are limited.

Postthoracotomy pain syndrome—Pain along a thoracotomy scar persisting at least 2 months after a thoracotomy. There is an aching sensation in the distribution of the surgical incision. Sensory loss and tenderness may be present along the thoracotomy scar. A trigger point may be present, secondary to a neuroma, which responds to a trigger-point injection.

Radicular pain—Pain perceived as arising in a limb or the trunk wall caused by ectopic activation of nociceptive afferent fibers in a spinal nerve or its roots or other neuropathic mechanisms. The pain is usually lancinating and travels in a narrow band. Etiologic causes include anatomic lesions affecting the spinal nerve and dorsal root ganglion including herniated intervertebral disc and spinal stenosis.

Radiculopathy—Objective loss of sensory and/or motor function as a result of conduction block in axons of a spinal nerve or its roots. Symptoms include numbness and weakness in the distribution of the affected nerve. Neurologic examination and diagnostic tests confirm the neurologic abnormality. (Note: Radicular pain and radiculopathy are not synonymous. The former is a symptom caused by ectopic impulse generation. The latter relates to objective neurologic signs due to conduction block. The two conditions may coexist and may be caused by the same lesion.)

Raynaud disease—Episodic attacks of aching, burning pain associated with vasoconstriction of the arteries of the extremities in response to cold or emotional stimuli.

Raynaud phenomenon—Attacks like those of Raynaud disease but related to one or more other disease processes. Systemic and vascular diseases such as collagen disease, arteriosclerosis obliterans, nerve injuries, and occupational trauma may all contribute to the development of Raynaud phenomenon.

Referred pain—Pain perceived as occurring in a region of the body topographically distinct from the region in which the actual source of pain is located.

Sensitization—Increased responsiveness of nociceptive neurons to their normal input and/or recruitment of a response to normally subthreshold inputs. Sensitization can be associated with a drop in threshold to stimulation of the receptive field, an increase in response to suprathreshold stimuli, spontaneous discharges, and/or increase in receptive field size. Sensitization can occur in the peripheral nervous system (peripheral sensitization) or in the central nervous system (central sensitization).

Somatic—Derived from the Greek word for "body." Although somatosensory input refers to sensory signals from all tissues of the body including skin, viscera, muscles, and joints, it usually signifies input from body tissue other than the viscera.

Stump pain—Pain in the residual limb, at the site of an extremity amputation.

Suffering—A state of severe distress associated with events that threaten the intactness of the person; it may or may not be associated with pain.

Syndrome-oriented pain center—A center that is specialized to provide thorough and wide-reaching care for patients suffering from a specific chronic pain syndrome. Examples include fibromyalgia clinics and back pain centers.

Tarsal tunnel syndrome—Irritation of the posterior tibial nerve as it passes through the fibrous tarsal tunnel in the foot, resulting in foot pain with neuropathic features.

Thoracic outlet syndrome—Pain in the root of the neck, head, and shoulder, radiating down the arm into the hand, due to compression of the brachial plexus by a hypertrophied scalene or pectoralis muscle, congenital bands, posttraumatic fibrosis, cervical rib or band, or a malformed first thoracic rib.

REFERENCES

Access the reference list online at ExpertConsult.com.

SECTION II

CLINICAL EVALUATION AND DIAGNOSTIC EXAMINATIONS

SECTION OUTLINE HEAD

CHAPTER 4

Physical Examination of the Patient With Pain

Paul Scholten, MD ◎ Kiran Chekka, MD ◎ Honorio T. Benzon, MD

The physical examination of a patient with pain is the most significant diagnostic tool, surpassed in importance only by the pain history. The goals of the physical examination include developing the patient's trust, gaining insight into the impact of pain on the patient's level of functioning, and ultimately identifying potential pain generators and other neuromusculoskeletal derangements. To simplify and focus what can be a complex physical examination, a logical and systematic approach should be followed (Table 4.1). The pain physical examination is a comprehensive neuromusculoskeletal evaluation that begins with general observations and a mental status examination. This is followed by inspection; palpation; range-of-motion (ROM) evaluation; and testing of strength, sensation, and reflexes. Finally, provocative maneuvers of the affected body region(s) are performed. This chapter outlines each of these components in detail, but every joint or extremity need not be evaluated exhaustively. Instead, the nature of the patient's complaint should be sufficiently established through history taking so that the physical examination can be efficiently directed toward the affected region.

An in-depth knowledge and understanding of the examined region is vital to integrate the results of sensory, motor, and reflex examinations and come to a meaningful conclusion about the localization and nature of the lesion. The differential diagnosis established at the conclusion of the physical examination can be further narrowed through an appropriate diagnostic work-up.

GENERAL OBSERVATIONS

The physical examination should begin as soon as the patient walks into the office. Observations of the patient's mannerisms, coordination, interpersonal interactions, and gait can provide insight into their mental, emotional, and physical status. Early observations in a less obvious setting (such as the waiting room) provide a basis against which to compare information collected during more formal portions of the examination. In particular, patients with chronic pain often display behaviors that communicate to others that they are experiencing pain and suffering, such as guarding, restlessness, audible sighs, altered gait, lack of eye contact, and use of unnecessary assistive devices. Any inconsistencies in gait or behavior should be noted.

Depending on practitioner preference and the magnitude of perceived impairment, evaluation of gait may be conducted informally as part of the general observation process or more formally during the motor portion of the neurologic examination. In general terms, gait is divided into two main phases: stance and swing. By definition, stance phase is the portion of the gait cycle during which the limb is in contact with the ground, and swing phase is the portion during which the limb has no points of contact with the ground. Although there are numerous detailed descriptions of normal and pathologic gaits, for a directed pain physical examination, the initial goal is to simply categorize the gait pattern as normal or abnormal. One specific type of abnormal gait that should be identified by the pain practitioner is antalgic gait, which is characterized by the avoidance of bearing weight on an affected limb or joint secondary to pain. This results in decreased time in stance phase for the affected limb. Other abnormal nonantalgic gait patterns may be caused by poor balance, neurologic deficits, or musculoskeletal disorders (Box 4.1). Gait analysis should include observation of the width of the basis of support, stride length, cadence, and pelvic motion and tilt. Because most gait abnormalities are not specific for a particular pathology, further investigation is almost always indicated to detect the cause.[1]

The general assessment should also include measurement of vital signs because they provide an objective indication of the patient's general health status and, if abnormal (fever, uncontrolled hypertension), may be a relative contraindication to interventions.

MENTAL STATUS EXAMINATION

During history taking, it is key to develop trust and basic insight into cognition to determine how detailed of a mental status examination is warranted. A basic mental examination is described in Table 4.2. Descriptors of the general mental status include the patient's level of consciousness; alertness; orientation to person, place, and time; and demeanor toward the examiner.[2] Signs of mental deterioration should correlate with the patient's history or prompt a search for an underlying pathology. The examiner should be especially vigilant for signs of undiagnosed depression, which is frequently associated with chronic pain.

INSPECTION

After completing general observations and the mental status examination, attention should turn to the neuromusculoskeletal examination. This begins with inspection of the affected region. Signs of trauma including erythema, swelling, bruising, peripheral joint effusion, or lacerations, as well as evidence of more remote trauma such as scarring should be noted in the affected body region. In addition, examiners should be mindful of evidence of rashes, infection, herpetic lesions, edema, sudomotor alterations, cutaneous discoloration, and abnormal hair growth. The identification of any surgical scars is also important, particularly in the cervical, thoracic, or lumbar spine, where their presence may indicate a history of spine surgery that

TABLE 4.1 Components of the Neuromusculoskeletal Examination

Examination	Observation
Inspection	Cutaneous landmarks, symmetry, temperature, trauma, muscle bulk
Palpation/percussion	Tenderness, masses, trigger points, pulses Tinel sign, fractures
Range of motion	Described in degrees, reason for motion limitation
Strength	Graded 0–5
Sensation	Gain or loss of sensory function is tested and findings described in terms of dermatomal versus peripheral nerve distribution
Reflexes	Graded 0–4
Provocative maneuvers	Performed for appropriate symptomatic region to further narrow differential diagnosis

BOX 4.1 Types of Gait Abnormalities

Antalgic gait—Avoidance of weight bearing on the affected limb due to pain (i.e., short stance phase). Seen in patients with radicular pain or painful lower extremity conditions, such as hip or knee osteoarthritis or other trauma to the affected limb.
Ataxic gait—Unsteady, uncoordinated ambulation, with a wide base and the feet thrown out, coming down first on the heel and then on the toes with a double tap.
Propulsive gait—Stooped, rigid posture with head/neck bent forward. Seen with Parkinson disease, CO poisoning, antipsychotics, such as haloperidol and chlorpromazine.
Scissoring gait—Crossing of the legs while advancing with slow, small steps. Seen with CVA, SCI, syringomyelia, MS, liver failure, cervical myelopathy, cerebral palsy.
Spastic gait—Indicates central lesion or head trauma.
Steppage gait—Caused by foot drop, so toes scrape the ground. Seen with lumbar HNP, peroneal atrophy, peroneal neuropathy or polyneuropathy, Guillain-Barré, MS, SCI, poliomyelitis.
Vaulting—Compensatory strategy to clear an advancing lower extremity that cannot be shortened, such as in the case of weak hip flexion, knee flexion, or ankle dorsiflexion that involves rising up on the toes of the stance limb so that the swing limb may clear the floor.
Circumduction—Swing limb is advanced in a semicircular arc to create extra clearance when the functional length of the advancing limb cannot be shortened in the usual fashion with hip flexion, knee flexion, or ankle dorsiflexion.
Waddling gait—Like a duck. Muscular dystrophy, gluteus medius weakness, spinal muscle atrophy, hip problems.

CVA, Cerebral vascular accident; *HNP,* herniated nucleus pulposus; *MS,* multiple sclerosis; *SCI,* spinal cord injury.

is a relative contraindication for certain interventions. Inspection of muscular structures should focus on evaluation of bulk and symmetry and should identify any atrophy, hypertrophy, fasciculations, or masses that are present. Hypertrophy suggests overuse, whereas atrophy and fasciculations may indicate a lower motor neuron disorder. In addition to visual inspection, the cutaneous temperature should be measured peripherally in suspected cases of sympathetically maintained pain.

Inspection of the head and face should be performed similarly to other regions of the body and should always include the oral cavity because intraoral lesions that frequently refer pain to distant facial regions may be missed if only external structures are examined. Furthermore, any facial asymmetry should be noted and investigated in subsequent portions of the examination to better elucidate the underlying etiology.

TABLE 4.2 Brief Mental Status Examination

Orientation to person, place, and date
Ability to name objects (e.g., pen, watch)
Memory immediate at 1 min, and at 5 min; repeat the names of three objects
Ability to calculate serial 7s, or if patient refuses have them spell "world" backward
Signs of cognitive deficits, aphasia

When the cervical spine, shoulders, or upper back are the regions of suspected pathology, inspection should focus on identifying any postural abnormalities, such as a forward protruding head or protracted shoulders, that may be contributing to the patient's symptoms, because these may be amenable to postural re-education in physical therapy. Similarly, when pathology is suspected in the low back, hips, or sacrum, any abnormal pelvic obliquity, tilt, or rotation should be identified. More distally, alignment at the hips, knees, and ankles should be evaluated for any varus or valgus deformities that place bony and soft tissue structures under abnormal stresses that may predispose to chronic conditions, such as osteoarthritis or tendinopathy. With regard to the spine, inspection should focus on establishing the presence of abnormal curvatures in the coronal and sagittal planes, such as increased kyphosis in the cervicothoracic region, accentuated or reduced lordosis in the lumbar region, and scoliosis in any region of the spine. For example, reduced lordosis or functional scoliosis may signify severe paraspinal muscle spasm, whereas exaggerated lumbar lordosis may indicate weakened abdominal musculature or a tethered cord. Usually, these curvatures can be identified and assessed by thorough inspection and palpation, except in the very obese.

In each region, the mechanical alterations that result from the observed abnormal curvature should be considered and interpreted in conjunction with information from the history to establish a differential diagnosis for the patient's symptoms. In the thorax, the spine and rib cage essentially function as one unit to transmit loads and torque into the lumbosacral spine. Because loads are shared and there is not a great deal of mobility in this region, in the absence of trauma, surgery, and congenital defects, clinically significant thoracic degenerative changes are not very common. When observed, thoracic kyphosis or scoliosis is an important indicator of thoracic alignment and possible neural and intrathoracic compression. The lumbar spine is less restricted than the thoracic spine, and greater curvatures can be observed in this region.

PALPATION

Palpation of superficial structures follows inspection and can help to further narrow the cause of the patient's pain. Lymph nodes, discrete trigger points, and lipomas can look very similar, but with palpation each lesion can be distinguished. Tenderness to palpation over specific structures suggests that these entities are pain generators. For example, tenderness to palpation over the greater trochanter may be suggestive of trochanteric bursitis. Patients with allodynia, dysesthesia, hyperesthesia, or other sensory derangements often are unable to tolerate this portion of the examination. When tolerated, palpation should be performed in a systematic, comprehensive manner from the least to most painful area with standard pressure. This permits an appreciation of the normal tissues against which to compare the painful region. The objectives of palpation are to identify and delineate subcutaneous masses, edema, and muscle contractures; assess pulses; and to localize tender myofascial trigger points. Remember that unless the pain is bilateral, there is a contralateral structure that can be palpated and used as a control in most patients.

Percussion of specific structures also reveals useful information but, like palpation, is dependent on the patient being able to tolerate it. Pain on percussion of bony structures can indicate a fracture, abscess, or infection. Percussion of spinous processes is often performed to determine whether a vertebral body fracture is a true pain generator or an incidental magnetic resonance imaging (MRI) finding. Pain on percussion over a sensory nerve, or Tinel sign, can indicate nerve entrapment or the presence of a neuroma. Specific nerves commonly tested with this technique are discussed in the section on provocative maneuvers.

Facial palpation is important to identify masses or tenderness over the sinuses. The only major articulation in the face is the temporomandibular joint (TMJ), which can dislocate or freeze and should be palpated to detect any bony asymmetry when patients complain of pain or dysfunction in this region. A detailed facial examination should be performed in patients being evaluated for headache to identify referred pain patterns (supraorbital neuralgia, sinus headache, or headache secondary to TMJ syndrome).[3,4]

Palpation in the cervical and trunk region can identify muscle spasms, myofascial trigger points, enlarged lymph nodes, occipital nerve entrapment, and pain over the bony posterior spine elements that suggests facet arthropathy. Upper extremity palpation should identify gross sensory changes and pulse symmetry.

Thoracic palpation should mainly focus on ruling out rib and spine fractures. Palpation of the abdominal wall may differentiate between superficial and deep pain generators. Deep palpation can detect pulsatile masses consistent with an abdominal aortic aneurysm that can present as low thoracic back pain.

Palpation in the lumbar spine begins with identification of the bony landmarks, specifically the iliac crests. The horizontal line connecting the iliac crests approximately estimates the L4–L5 level. Severe tenderness to midline palpation may be present with supraspinous or interspinous ligamentous rupture. Moreover, the location of tenderness may provide important clues as to the etiology of lumbar spine pain. For example, discogenic low back pain is nearly always associated with midline tenderness and in most cases paraspinal tenderness, whereby facetogenic pain is associated with paraspinal tenderness in a large majority of cases but is infrequently associated with prominent midline tenderness. In contrast, sacroiliac joint pain is predominantly associated with unilateral pain situated predominantly below L5.[5] Common bony pain generators in the lumbar region include the facet joints, sacroiliac joints, and the coccyx. For piriformis syndrome or coccydynia, a digital rectal examination is a valuable tool for diagnosis. Soft tissue palpation is important to evaluate paraspinous muscle tone, the localization of trigger points, and the presence of masses or lipomas.

RANGE OF MOTION

ROM testing is important to help to identify soft tissue restrictions, functionally limiting deficits in ROM and hypermobility and laxity that may be a risk factor for specific injuries. Active ROM is that brought about by the patient's own effort, whereas passive ROM is generated by the examiner moving a body part through its arc of motion. The possibilities of ROM depend on the body location or joint. For example, in the shoulder the movements include flexion, extension, abduction, adduction, and external and internal rotation. The ROM for each possible movement is described in terms of maximum degrees of movement through which the body part was moved either actively or passively and the reported reason for any limitations. Alternatively, when arcs are not formally measured it may be helpful to classify ROM as increased, full, or mildly, moderately, or severely restricted. It is important to be aware that ROM may also be greater than expected. Joint, connective tissue, or ligamentous laxity can result in supranormal ROM, whereas pain and structural abnormalities (strictures, arthritis) can limit ROM.

Tone, the sensation of resistance felt as one manipulates a joint through its expected ROM with the patient relaxed, is described in terms of hypotonia and hypertonia. Hypotonia, a decrease in the normal expected muscular resistance to passive manipulation, is due to a depression of alpha or gamma motor unit activity either centrally or peripherally. Hypotonia can be seen in polyneuropathy, myopathy, and certain spinal cord lesions. Hypertonia, a greater-than-expected normal resistance to passive joint manipulation, is divided into spasticity and rigidity. Spasticity is defined as a velocity-dependent increase in tone with joint movement. Spasticity is seen with excitation of spinal reflex arcs or with loss of descending inhibitory control in the reticulospinal or rubrospinal tracts. Spasticity is commonly seen after brain and spinal cord injury and stroke and in multiple sclerosis. It is commonly assessed using the Modified Ashworth Scale (Table 4.3). Rigidity, a generalized increase in muscle tone, is characteristic of extrapyramidal diseases, and is due to lesions in the nigrostriatal system.

In the head, when testing the TMJ, it is important to note any crepitus during active or ROM testing. In the neck, normal cervical active ROMs are flexion of 0–60 degrees; extension of 0–25 degrees; bilateral lateral flexion of 0–25 degrees; and bilateral lateral rotation of 0–80 degrees.[4] Any reduction in active ROM should be documented with the reported reason for limitation.

The normal lumbar spine ROMs are flexion of 0–90 degrees; extension of 0–30 degrees; bilateral lateral flexion of 0–25 degrees; and bilateral lateral rotation of 0–60

TABLE 4.3 Modified Ashworth Scale Scoring

Score	Clinical Finding
0	No increase in muscle tone
1	Slight increase in muscle tone, manifested by a catch and release or minimal resistance at the end of range of motion when the affected part is moved in flexion or extension
1+	Slight increase in muscle tone, manifested by a catch, followed by minimal resistance throughout the remainder (less than half) of the range of movement.
2	More marked increase in muscle tone through most of the range of movement, but affected part(s) easily moved.
3	Considerable increase in muscle tone, passive movement difficult
4	Affected part(s) rigid in flexion or extension

degrees.[4,6] Chapter 24 provides a review of the possible causes of limitation of ROM and pain. In general, pain on flexion hints at a possible disc lesion, whereas pain on extension can indicate spinal stenosis, spondylosis, or a myofascial pain generator.

The remainder of the examination of the face, cervical, and lumbar regions is based on motor, sensory, and reflex examinations, which are best reviewed in an integrated manner. A directed examination of the face is largely based on cranial nerve testing, for which a detailed strategy is presented in Table 4.4. Table 4.5 lists appropriate tests for the C4–T1 nerve roots and Table 4.6 provides an outline for the L2–S1 roots.[4,6]

STRENGTH

Identifying a deficit in motor function and then comparing this with known motor innervation charts can help isolate a neurologic lesion. Usually, isolated voluntary muscle strength is tested and graded from 0 to 5 (normal strength). Table 4.7 describes the standard muscle strength grading system. This test is effort dependent, and a patient in pain may not be able to give full effort. If a "giveaway" component to muscle weakness is suspected, this should be documented because the classic scoring system may then overestimate the degree of weakness. Comparing bilateral muscle groups can identify even more subtle deficits. Even when muscle strength is 5/5 on both sides, relative weakness of the dominant limb can suggest pathology. For example, a weak right-hand grip (vs. the left hand) in a right-hand dominant patient may suggest a right-sided radiculopathy or carpal tunnel syndrome. Greater proximal muscle weakness, in contrast to distal muscle weakness, is suggestive of myopathy, whereas greater distal muscle weakness may indicate polyneuropathy. Single innervation muscle weakness indicates a peripheral nerve lesion or a radiculopathy (if one nerve root provides all motor innervation for the given muscle).[4,7,8] In addition, two complementary tests for evaluation of lumbosacral myotomes are heel walk (dorsiflexion), which tests L4–L5 function, and toe walk (plantar flexion), which tests S1–S2 integrity. It is important to distinguish between pain-induced weakness and true neurologic weakness (which is usually accompanied by decreased deep tendon reflexes or muscle atrophy).

SENSATION

Understanding the basic mechanisms of sensation changes, whether they cause loss or gain of function, is essential to interpreting the findings on examination. One major goal of sensory testing is determining which fibers, neuronal types, or neural tracts are involved in the transmission of each patient's specific pain. Logically, when damage occurs to the nervous system one expects loss of function; however, clinically what is sometimes observed is a gain of function in which there is increased neural transmission resulting in neuropathic pain.

To better interpret physical examination findings, it is important to understand the transmission of pain signals. Classically, pain starts with activation of peripheral nociceptors. There are three broad classes of nociceptors differentiated based on the type of noxious stimuli they detect: mechanical nociceptors respond to pinch and pinprick, heat nociceptors respond to a temperature greater than 45°C, and polymodal nociceptors respond equally to mechanical, heat, and chemical noxious stimuli. After the nociceptor is activated, the generated impulse is then transmitted to the central nervous system (CNS) via Aδ and C fibers. Aδ fibers are responsible for "fast" or quickly sensed pain, whereas C fibers are responsible for "slow" pain. Fast pain is transmitted by small myelinated Aδ fibers at a rate of 2–30 m/s and is typically characterized as a sharp, shooting pain. Slow pain is transmitted by even smaller unmyelinated C fibers at a rate of less than 2 m/s and is characterized as a dull, poorly localized burning pain. The patient's description of symptoms can help to elucidate the type of pain fibers being activated. For example, a dull and diffuse nonfocal pain complaint would be more suggestive of C-fiber activation.

Sensory alterations should be described in standardized terms to create a more universal record of symptoms. *Hyperesthesia* is a sensation out of proportion to the stimulus applied. Hyperesthesia can be further divided into hyperalgesia and allodynia. *Hyperalgesia* is severe pain in response to a mild noxious stimuli, such as a pinprick. *Allodynia* is the sensation of pain in response to a nonnoxious stimuli (e.g., light touch, fabric on skin). Allodynia is a physical examination finding in many neuropathic pain states, and its distribution, which is frequently nondermatomal, should be documented.

If a deficit is identified during an initial gross sensory examination, a more in-depth investigation of the affected region should be performed using the contralateral side as a control, whenever possible. C fibers can be tested using both a painful stimulus (pinprick) and warm temperature. Aδ fibers are tested using pinprick and cold.

One state to be mindful of during examination is sensory dissociation in which patients present with loss of fine touch and proprioception in the same region in which pain and temperature sensation are intact. Patients may report a sharp sensation to pinprick in an area without being able to perceive fine touch or proprioception. This constellation of symptoms (or the converse—intact proprioception and fine touch with loss of temperature and pain perception)

TABLE 4.4 Cranial Nerve Examination: Summary of Cranial Nerve Functions and Tests

Cranial Nerve	Function	Test
I. Olfactory	Smell	Use coffee, mint, etc. held to each nostril separately; consider basal frontal tumor in unilateral dysfunction
II. Optic	Vision	Assess optic disc, visual acuity; name number of fingers in central and peripheral quadrants; direct and consensual pupil reflex; note Marcus-Gunn pupil (paradoxically dilating pupil)
III, IV, and VI. Oculomotor, trochlear, and abducens	Extraocular muscles	Pupil size; visually track objects in eight cardinal directions (abduction, abduction/elevation, elevation, adduction/elevation, adduction, adduction/depression, depression, abduction/depression); note diplopia (greatest on side of lesion); accommodation; note Horner pupil (miosis, ptosis, anhidrosis)
V. Trigeminal: motor and sensory	Facial sensation, muscles of mastication	Cotton-tipped swab/pinprick to all three branches; recall bilateral forehead innervation (peripheral lesion spares forehead, central lesion affects forehead); note atrophy, jaw deviation to side of lesion
VII. Facial	Muscles of facial expression	Wrinkle forehead, close eyes tightly, smile, purse lips, puff cheeks; corneal reflex
VIII. Vestibulocochlear (acoustic)	Hearing, equilibrium	Use tuning fork, compare side to side; Rinne test for AC versus BC (BC > AC); Weber test for sensorineural hearing
IX. Glossopharyngeal	Palate elevation; taste to posterior third of tongue; sensation to posterior tongue, pharynx, middle ear, and dura	Palate elevates away from the lesion; check gag reflex
X. Vagus	Muscles of pharynx, larynx	Check for vocal cord paralysis, hoarse or nasal voice
XI. Spinal accessory	Muscles of larynx, sternocleidomastoid, trapezius	Shoulder shrug, sternocleidomastoid strength
XII. Hypoglossal	Intrinsic tongue muscles	Protrusion of tongue; deviates toward lesion

AC, *Air conduction;* BC, *bone conduction.*

TABLE 4.5 Cervical Region Nerve Root Testing

Root Level	Nerve	Muscle(s) Tested	Position	Movement	Sensory	Reflex
C4	Dorsal scapular	Levator scapulae	Sitting	Shrug shoulder	Shoulders	None
C5	Musculocutaneous (C5–6)	Biceps	Forearm fully supinated, elbow flexed 90°	Patient attempts further flexion against resistance	Lateral forearm, first and second finger	Biceps
C6	Radial (C5–6)	Extensor carpi, radialis, longus, and brevis	Elbow flexed at 45°, wrist extended	Maintain extension against resistance	Middle finger	Brachioradialis
C7	Radial (C6–8)	Triceps	Shoulder slightly abducted, elbow slightly flexed	Extend forearm against resistance	Middle finger	Triceps
C8	Anterior interosseous (median) (C7–8)	Flexor digitorum profundus	Finger extended at MCP and PIP, flexed at DIP	Maintain flexion at DIP against resistance	Fourth, fifth finger; medial forearm	None
T1	Ulnar, deep branch (C8–T1)	Dorsal interossei	Patient extends and spreads all fingers	Examiner pushes patient's fingers together, patient resists	Medial arm	None

DIP, *Distal interphalangeal joint;* MCP, *metacarpophalangeal joint;* PIP, *proximal interphalangeal joint.*

can occur with lesions that interrupt fibers at the spinal cord level. The symptoms can be explained by the geography of the respective neural tracts in the spinal cord. For example, the posterior columns house the tracts that transmit proprioception and light touch, whereas the anterolateral cord carries the spinothalamic tract (pain, temperature) and motor tract. A syrinx can cause a progressive myelopathy that presents as a central high cervical cord syndrome with a sensory deficit in a cape or shawl distribution, and neck, shoulder, and arm muscle wasting.

Aβ fibers are examined through light touch, vibration, and joint position. Vibration is tested with a 128-Hz tuning fork and has increased value when combined with joint position testing. Isolated decreased vibratory sense is an

TABLE 4.6 Lumbar Region Nerve Root Testing

Root Level	Nerve	Muscle(s) Tested	Position	Movement	Sensory	Reflex
L2	Femoral (L2–L4)	Psoas, iliacus	Hip and knee flexed at 90°	Flex hip against resistance applied at distal femur	Anterior upper thigh	Patellar
L3	Femoral (L2–L4)	Quadriceps femoris	Supine, hip flexed, knee flexed at 90°	Extend knee against resistance	Anterior lower thigh	Patellar
L4	Deep peroneal (L4–L5)	Tibialis anterior	Ankle dorsiflexed	Maintain dorsiflexion against resistance	Medial shin and medial malleolus	Patellar[a]
L5	Deep peroneal (L4–L5)	Extensor hallucis longus	Great toe extended	Maintain extension against resistance	Web between big and second toe dorsum of foot	Medial hamstring
S1	Tibial (S1–S2)	Gastrocnemius, soleus	Ankle plantarflexed (to test gastrocnemius extend the knee, to test soleus flex to the knee)	Maintain plantar flexion against resistance applied over plantar surface of foot	Lateral malleolus	Achilles

[a]*Patellar reflex is mainly secondary to L4.*

TABLE 4.7 Standard Muscle Grading System

Grade	Description
0	No movement
1	Trace movement, no joint movement
2	Full range of motion with gravity eliminated
3	Full range of motion against gravity
4	Full range of motion against gravity and partial resistance
5 (normal)	Full range of motion against gravity and full resistance

early sign of large-fiber (Aβ) neuropathy and, if combined with position sensation deficits, indicates posterior column disease or peripheral nerve involvement. Posterior column disease can also be suggested by the loss of graphesthesia or the ability to interpret a number outlined on the patient's palm or calf. The inability to perceive isolated joint position is indicative of parietal lobe dysfunction or a peripheral nerve lesion.[9,10]

Lesions can be divided anatomically into central (brain and spinal cord), spinal nerve root (dermatomal), and peripheral nerve lesions. Careful comparison of an individual patient's sensory deficits relative to classic dermatome charts and known peripheral cutaneous nerve maps (Figs. 4.1 and 4.2) allows practitioners to identify potential causative lesions. Dermatomes are most accurate and exhibit the least variability distally (in the digits). Through comparison with established maps, it is possible to first differentiate between central and peripheral lesions, and then perhaps pinpoint the anatomic location of a lesion (Table 4.8) without expensive and invasive testing and imaging.

Although not yet fully validated and accepted, quantitative sensory testing (QST) can be helpful with complex patients; currently QST is predominantly used in research. QST involves using computer-guided precise measured sensory stimuli and then recording the responses objectively (i.e., the patient pushes a button when he/she feels pain, and the computer records at what level of stimulation the patient's pain threshold was reached). QST should increase interrater reliability and create easily reproducible and comparable exams, although the equipment is costly and the techniques are time consuming.

REFLEXES AND COORDINATION

Deep tendon reflexes (muscle stretch reflexes) can also help the clinician to localize a neurologic lesion. Similar to motor and sensory tests, specific reflexes are activated at specific spinal levels. The most commonly tested reflexes are listed in Table 4.9. A standardized grading system for deep tendon reflexes from 0 to 4+ is presented in Table 4.10. In cases of hypoactive reflexes, distraction techniques such as *Jendrassik maneuver* (hooking the digits of both hands together and attempting to forcibly separate both hands) can be used to better elucidate between true loss of reflex and examination artifact. The voluntary contraction of muscles not being tested results in facilitation of underactive reflexes and can provide a more accurate assessment of the reflex. *Clonus*, a grade-four reflex, is characterized by rhythmic, uniphasic muscle contractions in response to sudden sustained muscle stretch. Clonus is not always an abnormal finding but may be indicative of an upper motor neuron disease. *Plantar reflex testing* (elicited with a sharp stimulus on the lateral aspect of the sole of the foot) should be documented in terms of an upgoing *(Babinski sign)* or downgoing great toe. Babinski first noted the great toe moving upward and the toes fanning outward in response to a key scratch along the lateral plantar surface of the foot in patients with pyramidal lesions. It is now well established that Babinski sign can be seen with many upper motor neuron diseases and is also a normal variant in children up until 12 to 18 months of age. In the hand, one can elicit a *Hoffmann sign*, which is thumb and index finger flexion that is observed with flicking of the terminal phalanx of the third or fourth digit. This is indicative of an upper motor neuron disease. Ultimately, the confidence level in

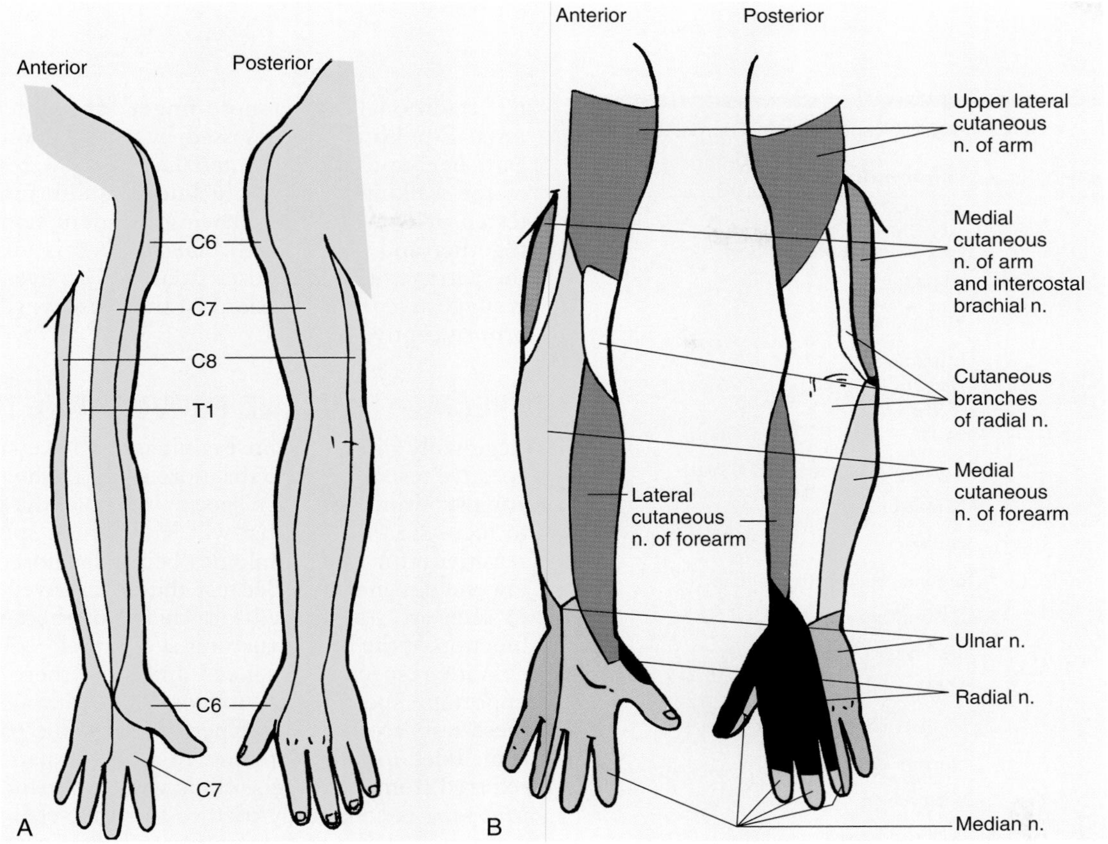

FIG. 4.1 (A) Cutaneous distribution of the cervical roots. (B) Cutaneous distribution of the peripheral nerves of the upper extremity. *(Redrawn from Wedel DJ. Nerve blocks. In: Miller RD, ed.* Anesthesia. *4th ed. New York: Churchill Livingstone; 1994:1537.)*

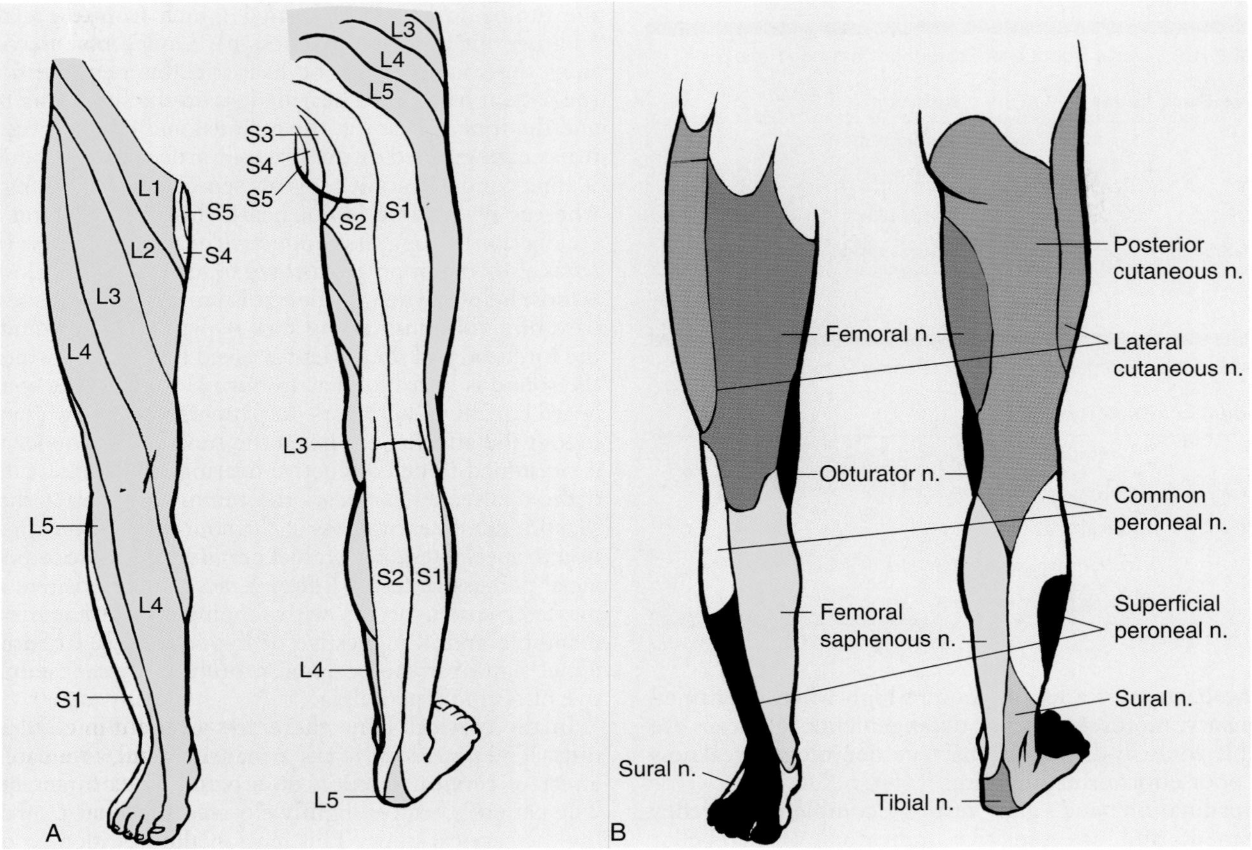

FIG. 4.2 (A) Cutaneous distribution of the lumbosacral nerves. (B) Cutaneous distribution of the peripheral nerves of the lower extremity. *(Redrawn from Wedel DJ. Nerve blocks. In: Miller RD, ed.* Anesthesia. *8th ed. Philadelphia: Saunders, 2015.)*

TABLE 4.8 Sensory Innervation Landmarks by Dermatome

Dermatome	Landmark
C4	Shoulder
C5	Lateral aspect of the elbow
C6	Thumb
C7	Middle finger
C8	Little finger
T1	Medial aspect of the elbow
T2	Axilla
T3–T11	Corresponding intercostal space
T4	Nipple line
T10	Umbilicus
T12	Inguinal ligament at midline
L1	Halfway between T12 and L2
L2	Mid-anterior thigh
L3	Medial femoral condyle
L4	Medial malleolus
L5	Dorsum of foot
S1	Lateral heel
S2	Popliteal fossa at midline
S3	Ischial tuberosity
S4–S5	Perianal area

TABLE 4.9 Nerve Root Level Tested for Common Reflexes

Nerve Root Level	Reflex
S1–S2	Achilles reflex
L3–L4	Patellar reflex
C5–C6	Biceps reflex
C7–C8	Triceps reflex

TABLE 4.10 Deep Tendon Reflex Grading System

Grade	Description
0	No response
1+	Reduced, less than expected
2+	Normal
3+	Greater than expected, moderately hyperactive
4+	Hyperactive with clonus

the localization of a lesion is quite high when confirmed by sensory, motor, and reflex derangements.[4] Reflexes are valuable tools in distinguishing true neurologic weakness from poor effort or malingering.

Coordination and gait testing complement reflex assessment and are sensitive indicators of cerebellar function and equilibrium. Cerebellar function is tested by traditional finger-nose-finger and heel-knee-shin tests. Equilibrium is assessed by observation of normal gait, heel-and-toe walk, and tandem gait testing (heel-to-toe walking in a straight line). Equilibrium is further tested by Romberg test (having a patient stand with feet together and eyes closed). *Romberg test* is positive when the patient sways and loses balance with eyes closed and is suggestive of mild lesions of the sensory, vestibular, or proprioceptive systems.

SPECIAL TESTS AND PROVOCATIVE TESTING

Regionally directed pain examinations have specific provocative tests to help to diagnose many of the pain-generating syndromes. Region specificity allows the practitioner to focus on the tests that will have a high specificity and sensitivity for the pathologies being diagnosed and avoid low-yield maneuvers. Because these maneuvers are unique to each area, a detailed knowledge of the anatomy and function of the local structures is essential.[11]

With respect to the head and face, there are several important special tests to consider. Although most of these tests are not usually performed in the pain clinic, it is included for completeness. In addition, patients may be referred from a headache clinic with results of these tests. *Rinne test* is commonly used to test the vestibulocochlear nerve (CN VIII) and differentiate between sensorineural and conductive hearing loss. To perform the test, the base of a vibrating tuning fork is placed on the mastoid process (bone conduction). When the sound is no longer appreciated through bone conduction, the vibrating portion of the tuning fork is repositioned 1 inch from the external auditory meatus (air conduction). Under normal conditions the sound should be heard in this new position. If the patient has known hearing loss on the side being tested and the tone is heard at the external auditory meatus after it has extinguished at the mastoid process (air conduction > bone conduction), it suggests sensorineural hearing loss, whereas if the tone is not heard (bone conduction > air conduction) it suggests conductive hearing loss. The *Weber test* is also commonly performed to test for hearing loss and is most helpful when the deficit is unilateral. In this test the base of a vibrating tuning fork is placed in the middle of the forehead and the patient is asked to report in which ear the sound is heard louder. In normal patients the sound is heard equally in both ears. In patients with known hearing loss, if the affected ear hears the tuning fork louder there is presumed to be conductive hearing loss in that ear, and if the unaffected ear hears the tuning fork better there is sensorineural hearing loss in the contralateral ear. In addition to special tests for cranial nerve testing, one important facial percussive test is *Chvostek test*. This is positive when masseter spasm occurs with tapping of the angle of the mandible and is suggestive of hypocalcemia. In addition, Tinel sign over the occipital protuberance can be indicative of occipital neuralgia.

In the cervical spine there are several clinically useful tests. The *distraction test* is a maneuver that evaluates the effect of cervical traction on a patient's pain perception. The patient's head is slightly elevated superiorly, off-loading the cervical spine. This motion allows widening of the neural foramina, relieving compression caused by neural foraminal stenosis. In contrast, the cervical compression test involves downward pressure on the head, causing compression of the cervical spine and narrowing of the foramina. A *Spurling test*, which is performed by gently axially loading the cervical spine while extending the neck and rotating the head toward the affected side, is considered positive if it elicits ipsilateral radicular symptoms and indicates foraminal stenosis. A Valsalva maneuver may also be helpful in delineating pathology in the cervical spine. An increase in intrathecal pressure develops with this maneuver, and increased pain may be worsened by compression secondary to the presence of protruding disc material or tumor.

There are numerous painful musculoskeletal conditions in the shoulder region that can be differentiated, to a certain extent, based on several helpful provocative maneuvers. The *drop arm test* can help identify the presence of a tear in the rotator cuff. In this test, the patient with rotator cuff dysfunction will not be able to retain the arm in an abducted position. A full-thickness rotator cuff tear is likely with a combination of three positive findings: painful arc with ROM testing, the drop arm sign, and external rotation weakness. Additional helpful tests for rotator cuff impingement are the Neer, Hawkins, and "empty can" tests. The *Neer test* is performed with the patient in a comfortable standing position, with the arm being tested by the side with the elbow fully extended. The examiner passively internally rotates the arm to keep the thumb pointing downward while flexing the shoulder past 90 degrees to an overhead position. It is considered positive if pain is reported in the anterior or lateral aspect of the shoulder. *Hawkins test* is performed with the patient in a comfortable sitting position, with the arm being tested positioned with 90 degrees of both shoulder and elbow flexion. Stabilizing the shoulder with one hand, the examiner uses their other hand to passively internally rotate the shoulder through the joint's ROM or until the patient reports pain. Pain in the superior and lateral aspects of the shoulder indicates a positive test. The *empty can test* is more specific for supraspinatus pathology and is performed by placing the shoulder being examined in a position of 90 degrees of flexion, approximately 30 degrees of abduction and with full internal rotation with the thumb pointing downward as if emptying a beverage can. The examiner stabilizes the scapula with one hand and applies a downward force to the arm, which is resisted by the patient. Significant pain at the shoulder or weakness is considered a positive test. The *Yergason test* examines the integrity of the biceps tendon in its bony groove in the humerus. In this maneuver the patient flexes the elbow. The examiner grasps the elbow and wrist of the patient and attempts to rotate the arm externally while the patient resists the maneuver. Instability of the tendon is manifested by the presence of pain in the area of the tendon.

More distally in the upper extremities, elbow and wrist tests can also provide helpful information. Patients with lateral epicondylitis (tennis elbow) can have their symptoms reproduced by the *Cozen test*. For this test, the patient's forearm is stabilized laterally with the elbow in 90 degrees of flexion, the forearm in pronation, and the hand radially deviated. The patient then actively extends the wrist while the examiner attempts to resist this motion. Reproduction of the patient's pain on the lateral epicondyle is considered a positive test. A positive ulnar Tinel sign is elicited at the elbow by tapping over the groove between the olecranon and the medial epicondyle and causing pain or numbness in the ulnar nerve distribution. A positive median nerve Tinel sign is elicited by tapping on the carpal tunnel and is suggestive of carpal tunnel syndrome. Similarly, Phalen sign, paresthesias, or pain in the fingers when flexing the patient's wrists and placing the dorsal hand surfaces together for a minute may also indicate median nerve dysfunction at the level of the carpal tunnel.

Multiple provocative tests described for the lumbar region are presented in Chapter 24. The majority of tests are directed toward pathology in the disc and nerve roots, facet joints, sacroiliac joint, hip, and piriformis muscle. The most frequently performed test for nerve root irritation is the straight leg raise, which is specific for a radicular pathology when pain radiates distal to the knee with passive hip flexion between 30 and 70 degrees with the knee in full extension and the patient supine. This test provokes lumbar radicular symptoms by stretching these nerves and is accentuated by ankle dorsiflexion. The *slumped seat test* is similar except it is performed in the seated position. For facet-mediated pain, pain on facet loading is not a reliable criteria.[12] Patrick's test (FABER—flexion, abduction, and external rotation), Gaenslen test, Yeoman test, and posterior shear test are helpful in identifying sacroiliac joint dysfunction. If a patient exhibits at least three of these findings, sacroiliac joint dysfunction should be considered. Patrick's test may also indicate intraarticular hip pathology when it elicits groin pain. Tests for piriformis syndrome include the Pace and Freiberg signs, described in detail in Chapter 67 on piriformis syndrome. General tests for intrathecal lesions include the Kernig test for meningeal irritation and the Milgram test for intrathecal pathology. In the *Kernig test* the examiner flexes a supine patient's hip to 90 degrees and then extends the knee. If this causes pain it is considered to be positive. The *Milgram test* involves a supine patient raising both legs a few inches off the examination table, with the knees fully extended. If this can be sustained for 30 seconds, intrathecal lesions are unlikely to be present.[13]

Provocative tests, by their nature, rely on honest patient cooperation and effort, and their validity can be greatly diminished by lack of patient participation, abnormal pain behaviors, and secondary gain. The Hoover test and Waddell signs can be helpful in cases of suspected poor effort. The *Hoover test* may be used to differentiate true leg paresis from psychogenic weakness caused by conversion disorder, malingering, or factitious disorder. In this test, the patient is supine and the examiner's palms are placed beneath each of the patient's heels to assess for downward force. To perform the test the patient attempts to lift the weak or affected limb off the table by actively flexing the hip with the knee in extension. When the patient is making an honest effort, the contralateral limb is expected to extend at the hip and the examiner will be able to detect a downward force. If no downward force is felt, the possibility of psychogenic causes for the pain should be suspected.[14] Although controversial, Waddell signs are a measurement of patient pain behaviors and provide indications of a nonorganic source for the patient's back pain. There are five potential *Waddell signs;*

the presence of three or more positive signs is a strong indication of a nonorganic source for the patient's pain. The five signs or tests involve evaluation of (1) tenderness, (2) simulation testing, (3) distraction testing, (4) regional disturbances, and (5) overreaction. Tenderness is a deep or diffuse nondermatomal report of pain to a superficial stimulus, often a light skin roll or pinch. Simulation testing is based on simulating movements that a patient may believe should worsen their pain but that are known not to exacerbate the suspected pain generator. Two examples would be pain experienced in the lumbar spine while pressing downward on the shoulders or head, or body rotation with the head and shoulders in line to simulate lumbar rotation for the patient, without actually rotating the lumbar spine. Distraction testing is repetition and comparison of the results of a provocative movement in an obvious and less obvious nonstandard fashion. One example is sitting versus supine straight-leg raise tests. Another would be formal lumbar flexion testing and lumbar ROM observed during a task such as picking up a dropped object off the floor. If the results are contradictory, this is considered a positive finding. Regional disturbances include motor weakness and sensory deficits that cannot be localized to a single or reasonable combination of neuroanatomic structures. Examples include nondermatomal sensory changes or complete limb weakness. Finally, overreaction includes disproportionate verbal and facial expressions, unconventional anatomic movements and postures, and inappropriate responses to the examination.[4,14]

CONCLUSION

The physical examination is secondary in importance only to the pain history. In addition to developing the patient's trust, a complementary physical examination should explore the complaints raised in the history and provide information that confirms or rejects the proposed explanations for the symptoms. (The physical examination signs are summarized in Table 4.11.) Often, costly imaging studies and painful invasive testing can be avoided by performing a simple yet thorough physical examination. To gain a meaningful understanding of the patient's symptoms, the physical examination should be based on anatomic and physiologic principles. Following a brief global assessment of the patient's health, the pain examination should be focused toward the affected region and consistently performed in a structured pattern. Supported by confirmatory physical examination findings and appropriate provocative testing, one can have a high degree of confidence in the working diagnosis. Ultimately, a physical examination that fulfills these criteria is an invaluable component in establishing the correct diagnosis in a pain patient.

KEY POINTS

- The pain physical examination is a comprehensive neuromusculoskeletal evaluation that begins with general observations and a mental status examination. This is followed by inspection; palpation; ROM evaluation; and testing of strength, sensation, and reflexes. Finally, provocative maneuvers of the affected body region(s) are performed.
- The physical examination should begin as soon as the patient walks into the office. Observations of the patient's mannerisms, coordination, interpersonal interactions, and gait can provide insight into their mental, emotional, and physical status.
- Gait is divided into two main phases: stance and swing. Stance phase is the portion of the gait cycle during which the limb is in contact with the ground, and swing phase is the portion during which the limb has no points of contact with the ground. Antalgic

TABLE 4.11 Physical Examination Signs

Sign	Definition/Performance of Test	Possible Causes/Significance
Hypotonia	Decrease in the normal expected muscular resistance to passive manipulation	Polyneuropathy, myopathy, and certain spinal cord lesions
Hypertonia	Greater-than-expected normal resistance to passive joint manipulation, divided into spasticity and rigidity	
Spasticity	Velocity-dependent increase in tone with joint movement	Brain and spinal cord injury, stroke, multiple sclerosis
Rigidity	Generalized increase in muscle tone	Extrapyramidal diseases
Tinel sign	Pain on percussion over a sensory nerve	Nerve entrapment or neuroma
Jendrassik maneuver	Hooking the digits of both hands together and attempting to forcibly separate both hands during elicitation of a deep tendon reflex	Polyneuropathy, myopathy, and certain spinal cord lesions
Babinski sign	Upgoing of great toe in response to plantar reflex testing (elicited with sharp stimulus on the lateral aspect of the sole of the foot)	Seen with many upper motor neuron diseases, also a normal variant in children up until 12–18 months of age
Hoffmann sign	Thumb and index finger flexion with flicking of the terminal phalanx of the third or fourth digit	Upper motor neuron disease
Romberg test	A patient stands with feet together and eyes closed. Positive result: patient sways and loses balance with eyes closed	Test of equilibrium, suggestive of mild lesions of the sensory, vestibular, or proprioceptive systems

TABLE 4.11 Physical Examination Signs—cont'd

Sign	Definition/Performance of Test	Possible Causes/Significance
Rinne test	Base of a vibrating tuning fork is placed on the mastoid process (bone conduction). When the sound is no longer appreciated through bone conduction the vibrating portion of the tuning fork is repositioned 1 inch from the external auditory meatus (air conduction). The sound should be heard in this new position.	Test the vestibulocochlear nerve (CN VIII) and differentiate between sensorineural and conductive hearing loss. If the patient has known hearing loss on the side being tested and the tone is heard at the external auditory meatus after it is extinguished at the mastoid process (air conduction > bone conduction) it suggests sensorineural hearing loss, whereas if the tone is not heard (bone conduction > air conduction) it suggests conductive hearing loss.
Weber test	Base of a vibrating tuning fork is placed in the middle of the forehead and the patient is asked to report in which ear the sound is heard louder. In normal patients the sound is heard equally in both ears.	In patients with known hearing loss, if the affected ear hears the tuning fork louder there is presumed to be conductive hearing loss in that ear, and if the unaffected ear hears the tuning fork better there is sensorineural hearing loss in the contralateral ear.
Chvostek test	Positive when masseter spasm occurs with tapping of the angle of the mandible	Hypocalcemia
Spurling test	Gently axially load the cervical spine while extending the neck and rotating the head toward the affected side.	It is considered positive if it elicits ipsilateral radicular symptoms and indicates foraminal stenosis.
Drop arm test	Patient attempts to retain the arm in an abducted position.	Patient with rotator cuff dysfunction will not be able to retain the arm in an abducted position.
Neer test	Patient in a comfortable standing position with the arm being tested at their side with the elbow fully extended. Examiner passively internally rotates the arm to keep the thumb pointing downward while flexing the shoulder past 90° to an overhead position.	Considered positive for rotator cuff impingement if pain is reported in the anterior or lateral aspect of the shoulder
Hawkins test	Patient in a comfortable sitting position with the arm being tested positioned with 90° of both shoulder and elbow flexion. Stabilizing the shoulder with one hand, the examiner uses the other hand to passively internally rotate the shoulder to the end of their available range of motion or until the patient reports pain.	Pain in the superior and lateral aspects of the shoulder indicate a positive test for rotator cuff impingement.
Empty can test	Place the shoulder being examined in a position of 90° of flexion, approximately 30° of abduction and full internal rotation with the thumb pointing downward as if emptying a beverage can. The examiner stabilizes the scapula with one hand and applies a downward force to the arm, which is resisted by the patient.	Pain or weakness at the shoulder is considered a positive test for supraspinatus pathology.
Yerguson test	Patient flexes the elbow. The examiner grasps the elbow and wrist of the patient and attempts to rotate the arm externally while the patient resists the maneuver.	Instability of the biceps tendon is manifested by the presence of pain in the area of the tendon in its bony groove in the humerus.
Cozen test	Patient's forearm is stabilized laterally with the elbow in 90° of flexion, the forearm in pronation, and the hand radially deviated. The patient then actively extends the wrist while the examiner attempts to resist this motion.	Reproduction of the patient's pain on the lateral epicondyle is considered a positive test for lateral epicondylitis (tennis elbow)
Slumped seat test	Similar to straight leg raise except the patient is in seating position. Pain radiates distal to the knee with passive hip flexion between 30° and 70° with the knee in full extension. Pain is accentuated by ankle dorsiflexion.	Test for nerve root irritation
Kernig test	Examiner flexes a supine patient's hip to 90° and then extends the knee.	Presence of pain is considered positive for meningeal irritation.
Milgram test	Supine patient raises both legs a few inches off the examination table with the knees fully extended. If this can be sustained for 30 s intrathecal lesions are unlikely to be present.	If sustained for 30 s, presence of intrathecal lesion is unlikely
Hoover test	Patient is supine and the examiner's palms are placed beneath each of the patient's heels to assess for downward force. Patient attempts to lift the weak (affected) limb off the table. When the patient is making an honest effort, the contralateral limb is expected to extend at the hip and the examiner will be able to detect a downward force. If no downward force is felt, the possibility of psychogenic causes for the pain is suspected.	Differentiates true leg paresis from psychogenic weakness, for example, conversion disorder, malingering, or factitious disorder.

The tests are not arranged alphabetically but are grouped according to topic or location.
Patrick FABER test, Gaenslen, Yeoman, and posterior shear tests are discussed in the chapter on sacroiliac joint syndrome. Pace and Freiberg signs are explained in the chapter on piriformis syndrome.
See text for Waddell signs, which may indicate nonorganic source of back pain.

gait, which is characterized by the avoidance of bearing weight on an affected limb or joint secondary to pain.

- Descriptors of the general mental status include the patient's level of consciousness; alertness; orientation to person, place, and time; and demeanor toward the examiner.
- Tone, the sensation of resistance felt as one manipulates a joint through its expected ROM with the patient relaxed, is described in terms of hypotonia and hypertonia. Hypertonia, a greater-than-expected normal resistance to passive joint manipulation, is divided into spasticity and rigidity.
- Proximal muscle weakness, in contrast to distal muscle weakness, is suggestive of myopathy, whereas greater distal muscle weakness may indicate polyneuropathy.
- Aδ fibers are responsible for "fast" or quickly sensed pain, whereas C fibers are responsible for "slow" pain.
- Regionally directed pain examinations have specific provocative tests to help to diagnose many of the pain-generating syndromes. Several special and provocative tests in the head and face, cervical spine, lumbar spine, and extremities have been described.
- For Waddell signs the presence of three or more positive signs is a strong indication of a nonorganic source for the patient's pain. The five signs or tests involve evaluation of (1) tenderness, (2) simulation testing, (3) distraction testing, (4) regional disturbances, and (5) overreaction.

REFERENCES

Access the reference list online at ExpertConsult.com.

CHAPTER 5

Pain Assessment

Asimina Lazaridou, PhD ◦ **Nick Elbaridi, MD** ◦ **Robert R. Edwards, PhD** ◦ **Charles B. Berde, MD, PhD**

INTRODUCTION

By its very definition, pain is an internal, subjective experience that cannot be directly observed by others or measured by the use of physiologic markers or bioassays. The assessment of pain therefore relies largely (often exclusively) on the use of self-report. Though self-report of pain or any other construct is subject to a number of biases, a good deal of effort has been invested in testing and refining self-report methodology within the field of human pain research.[1] The purpose of this chapter is to provide an overview of this research, to critically evaluate pain assessment tools, and to assist clinicians and researchers in selecting the pain assessment methods best suited to serve their purposes.

CHALLENGES OF PAIN MEASUREMENT

Assessing pain requires measurement tools that are valid and reliable, as well as an ability to communicate (using language, movements, etc.). However, even when these basic requirements are met, additional challenges abound. For example, over what time frame is pain to be measured? By nature, most pain conditions are fairly variable, and it is sometimes unclear how representative (of a patient's global pain experience) ratings of current or recent pain might be.[2] Many ratings scales do query current pain, or pain over the past week, but longer time frames are often used, and these may introduce additional memory biases. In addition, pain is a multidimensional experience incorporating sensory and affective components that are correlated, but which may be assessed separately. Generally, most self-report pain assessment tools described here focus on pain intensity ratings over a relatively brief and recent period of time (e.g., the past week).

One major challenge in pain assessment is the inability of an evaluator to corroborate, using objective signs or indicators, a patient's subjective report of pain.[3] Clinicians have been trained to ask patients about their pain level at each encounter, and use that number as a vital sign. These methods, used within a health care environment that encourages patient-centered care, have potentially led practitioners to overprescribe pain medications, as argued in recent reviews of the field.[4] Measurement of pain should be multifaceted, and may benefit from the inclusion of functional capacity evaluations (FCE).[5] FCE protocols generally include anthropometric measurements, range of motion testing, static strength testing, cardiovascular endurance, muscle recruitment, stance, and end range of motion movements. FCE can be used for global function measurement or more specifically for selected body regions. Results can be analyzed using both normative and criterion-referenced testing. Moreover, FCE allows assessment of the level of physical effort provided by the subject during an evaluation, which affects both the reliability and the validity of the result.[6] Effort testing at its peak gives the reader of the functional evaluation report confidence that the results represent a true picture of the individual's ability on the day of the evaluation. Reports compromised by less than full effort are read as representing the injured person's minimum ability.

TYPES OF SELF-REPORT PAIN SCALES

A variety of pain assessment scales are available for evaluating the intensity of acute and chronic pain. Multiple types of scales are widely used and well validated in both research and clinical settings. The three most commonly used methods to quantify the pain experience (pain intensity, usually) are verbal rating scales (VRSs), numerical rating scales (NRSs), and visual analog scales (VASs).[7]

VERBAL RATING SCALES

A VRS generally consists of a series of adjectives (or phrases), ordered from least intense (or unpleasant) to most intense (or unpleasant). An adequate VRS should span a maximum possible range of the pain experience (e.g., from "no pain" to "extremely intense pain"). Patients are asked to select the adjective or phrase that best characterizes their level of pain. Dozens of VRS have been described and validated; one of the more common examples appears in Table 5.1.

In general, a VRS is scored by assigning each adjective or phrase a number according to its rank (e.g., 0–4 in the example in Table 5.1). The strengths of the VRS include simplicity, ease of administration and scoring, as well as face validity (i.e., they appear to directly measure exactly what they purport to measure, such as the intensity of pain). In addition, because they are so easy to comprehend, compliance rates for the VRS can be superior to the rates obtained with other scales, especially within certain

TABLE 5.1 Verbal Rating Scale for Pain Intensity

None	0
Mild	1
Moderate	2
Severe	3
Very severe	4

populations such as the elderly. The VRS has demonstrated good reliability (e.g., consistency over short periods of time) in a number of studies. The validity of the VRS has also been repeatedly established; these scales correlate positively with other self-report measures of pain intensity and with pain behaviors.[8]

Despite its substantial strengths, the VRS also exhibits a number of weaknesses, based on which other pain researchers have hesitated to recommend these scales. First, the scoring method for VRS assumes equal intervals between adjectives. That is, the change in pain from "none" to "mild" is quantified identically with the change in pain from "moderate" to "severe." This assumption is rarely tested, and is likely often violated. This property of the VRS poses difficulties in both the interpretation and analysis of VRS-derived data. Second, to properly use a VRS, a patient must both be familiar with all of the words used on the scale, and must be able to find one that accurately describes his or her pain. Some past reviews of the pain assessment literature have indicated that the VRS is being used less often in pain outcome research than has been the case in the past.

NUMERICAL RATING SCALES

An NRS typically consists of a series of numbers with verbal anchors representing the entire possible range of pain intensity. Generally, patients rate their pain from 0 to 10, from 0 to 20, or from 0 to 100.[9] Zero represents "no pain," whereas 10, 20, or 100 represents the opposite end of the pain continuum (e.g., "the most intense pain imaginable," "pain as intense as it could be," "maximum pain"). See Fig. 5.1 for an example. Like VRSs, the NRS have well-documented validity; they correlate positively with other measures of pain and show sensitivity to treatments that are expected to affect pain. The NRS can be administered verbally or in a written format, is simple and easily understood, and is easily administered and scored. The principal weakness of the NRS is that, statistically, it does not have ratio qualities. That is, numerically equal intervals on the scale (e.g., the difference between 1 and 3 and the difference between 7 and 9) may not represent equivalent intervals in terms of scaling the intensity of pain. One other limitation of most NRS measures of pain is that individuals' ratings of a given pain experience can be altered in idiosyncratic ways by the choice of anchors on the upper end of the scale. For example, women and men use systematically different events to contextualize the anchor of "most intense pain imaginable," and this can significantly affect studies of gender differences in the experience of pain.

VISUAL ANALOG SCALES

A VAS consists of a line, often 10 cm long, with verbal anchors at either end, similar to an NRS (e.g., "no pain" on the far left and "the most intense pain imaginable" on the far right). The patient places a mark at a point on the line corresponding to the patient's rating of pain intensity.[8] The line may be depicted with a horizontal or vertical orientation, though a horizontal line is generally preferred (Fig. 5.2). Recent versions include the mechanical VAS, which uses a sliding marker superimposed on a horizontal VAS drawn on a ruler, and is easily scored from the back, which includes numbers for each marker placement. The VAS has often been recommended as the measure of choice for assessment of pain intensity. Substantial evidence supports its validity, and the VAS is sensitive to treatment effects. Though most studies suggest minimal differences in sensitivity among rating scales, significant differences that do emerge generally favor a VAS over a VRS or an NRS.[10] In addition, VAS scores correlate with pain behaviors, and VAS scores do show ratio-level scoring properties. The VAS does possess some limitations, however. It can be difficult to administer to patients with perceptual-motor problems, which are rather common in the context of chronically painful conditions. In addition, a VAS is generally scored using a ruler (the score is the number of centimeters or millimeters from the end of the line), making scoring more time consuming and adding additional possible sources of bias or error. Finally, relative to other rating scales, use of a VAS produces higher noncompletion rates among certain populations, primarily among those with cognitive limitations and among *elderly samples* (discussed later).

MCGILL PAIN QUESTIONNAIRE

The McGill Pain Questionnaire (MPQ) and its brief analog, the short-form MPQ, are among the most widely used measures of pain. In general, the MPQ is considered to be a multidimensional measure of pain quality; however, it also yields numerical indices of several dimensions of the pain experience.[11] Researchers have proposed three dimensions of the experience of pain: sensory-discriminative, affective-motivational, and cognitive-evaluative. The MPQ was created to assess these multiple aspects of pain. It consists of 20 sets of verbal descriptors, ordered in intensity from lowest to highest. These sets of descriptors are divided into those assessing the sensory (10 sets), affective (5 sets), evaluative (1 set), and miscellaneous (4 sets) dimensions of pain. Patients select the words that describe their pain, and their word selections are converted into a pain-rating index, based on the sum of all of the words after they are assigned a rank value, as well as the total number of words chosen.[11,12] In addition, the MPQ contains a present pain intensity VRS (i.e., the Present Pain Intensity [PPI]), ordered from "mild" to "excruciating."

The more frequently used short form of the MPQ consists of 15 representative words that form the sensory (11 items) and affective (4 items) categories of the original MPQ. Each descriptor is ranked on a 0 ("none") to 3 ("severe") intensity scale. The PPI, along with a VAS, are also included (Fig. 5.3). The short form correlates highly with the original scale, can discriminate among different pain conditions, and may be easier than the original scale for geriatric patients to use.

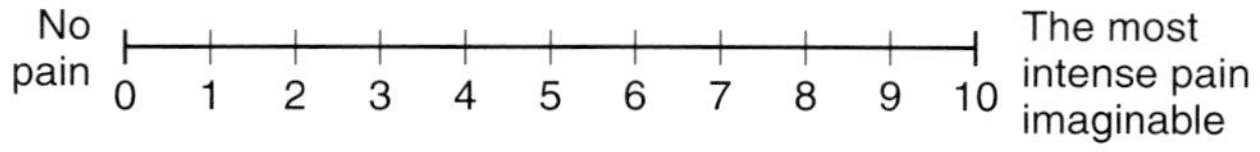

FIG. 5.1 Sample numerical rating scale for pain intensity.

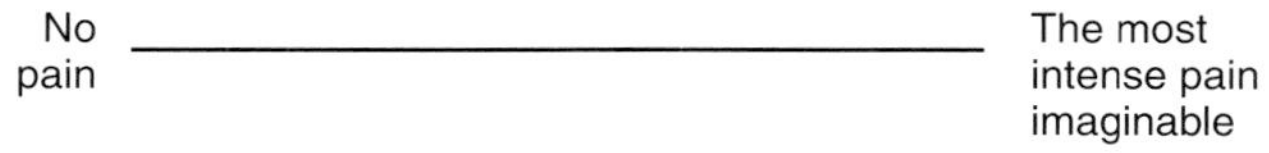

FIG. 5.2 Sample visual analog scale for pain intensity.

PAIN RELIEF

Studies of interventions designed to reduce pain often include a posttreatment assessment of pain relief in addition to measures of pain intensity obtained at both baseline and posttreatment. Pain relief is often measured using a VAS, a VRS with gradations of relief (e.g., "none," "slight," "moderate," "complete"), or an NRS assessing the percentage of relief. Studies showed VAS and VRS responses to be highly correlated and the scales demonstrated similar effect sizes after treatment, though administration and interpretation of VRS was reported to be easier than with other types of scales.[13] Although conceptually attractive, measures of pain relief have demonstrated problems with validity. For example, a significant minority of patients reports at least moderate relief on these scales when an analysis of sequential pain ratings (i.e., pretreatment compared with posttreatment) reveals *increases* in reported pain intensity. In one trial, whereas average pain ratings increased by 28%

	None	Mild	Moderate	Severe
Throbbing	0)_____	1)_____	2)_____	3)_____
Shooting	0)_____	1)_____	2)_____	3)_____
Stabbing	0)_____	1)_____	2)_____	3)_____
Sharp	0)_____	1)_____	2)_____	3)_____
Cramping	0)_____	1)_____	2)_____	3)_____
Gnawing	0)_____	1)_____	2)_____	3)_____
Hot-burning	0)_____	1)_____	2)_____	3)_____
Aching	0)_____	1)_____	2)_____	3)_____
Heavy	0)_____	1)_____	2)_____	3)_____
Tender	0)_____	1)_____	2)_____	3)_____
Splitting	0)_____	1)_____	2)_____	3)_____
Tiring-exhausting	0)_____	1)_____	2)_____	3)_____
Sickening	0)_____	1)_____	2)_____	3)_____
Fearful	0)_____	1)_____	2)_____	3)_____
Punishing-cruel	0)_____	1)_____	2)_____	3)_____

Rate the intensity of your pain on the two scales below. Make a mark on the line to indicate where your pain falls between *No pain* and *Worst possible pain* and then circle the appropriate number on the second scale.

No pain |————————————————| Worst possible pain

Circle one of the following words that best describes your current pain:

0 No pain
1 Mild
2 Discomforting
3 Distressing
4 Excruciating

FIG. 5.3 The short-form McGill Pain Questionnaire. *(Reprinted from Melzack R. The short form McGill Pain Questionnaire.* Pain *1987;30:191-197.)*

early in the study, approximately 90% of patients reported some degree of relief on a VAS. This phenomenon (i.e., the apparent overreporting of relief) seems to be due in part to a memory for past pain as being substantially greater than previous ratings would indicate.

MULTIDIMENSIONAL ASSESSMENT IN CLINICAL TRIALS

Although a full exploration of recommendations for outcome assessment in analgesic trials is beyond the scope of this chapter, the Initiative on Methods, Measurement, and Pain Assessment in Clinical Trials (IMMPACT) has produced a series of publications on this issue. Interested readers should consult one of the IMMPACT position papers (e.g., Dworkin et al.). In brief, this group of experts has reviewed measures of pain intensity, physical functioning, emotional functioning, and other pain-relevant outcome domains, making recommendations for the selection of outcome measures for clinical trials of pain treatments.

ADDITIONAL CONSIDERATIONS

Differentiating Types of Pain: There has been a good deal of interest in the development of self-report measures of neuropathic pain; indeed, the MPQ has been studied in this context, and over recent years several screening tools for distinguishing neuropathic from nociceptive pain have been validated. The Pain DETECT assessment system, which relies on a set of self-report questions about symptoms, was designed to detect neuropathic pain in patients with low back pain; it has been validated in large studies with thousands of patients, and has been reported to achieve reasonable sensitivity and specificity in identifying patients with neuropathic back pain. Other questionnaires such as the Leeds Assessment of Neuropathic Symptoms and Signs (LANSS) scale and the Neuropathic Pain Questionnaire (NPQ) have also been studied as indicators of the presence of neuropathic pain. However, whereas some validity studies suggest good results, several persistent issues have plagued the research in this area. The first is that while the definition of neuropathic pain indicates that a lesion or dysfunction must be present in the nervous system, this can often be difficult to establish in patients with chronic pain, creating a questionable "gold standard" against which the diagnostic accuracy of a questionnaire can be measured. Second, multiple studies strongly suggest that the endorsement of classically "neuropathic" symptoms (e.g., shooting pain, numbness and tingling, etc.) is strongly influenced by other patient characteristics, such as emotional distress, indicating that a wide variety of factors are likely to contribute to self-report of the presence of neuropathic pain.

Daily Diaries: In trials of pain treatments, daily diaries are gradually becoming the standard for assessing pain-related symptoms to minimize memory biases that threaten the validity of global retrospective ratings of pain.[14] Participants are generally asked to complete measures of pain and related symptoms one or more times per day, often for 1 to 2 weeks. Because pain reports can have substantial day-to-day variability, aggregated (averaged) ratings have been demonstrated to be more reliable and sensitive to treatment effects than retrospective measures of pain. In general, recent research has favored electronic diaries; in comparison with paper-and-pencil diaries, electronic diaries (e.g., usually implemented using a PDA, cell phone, or similar tool) have been repeatedly shown to demonstrate superior compliance rates and patient satisfaction. Electronic diaries incorporate several features that enhance reliability, including: date/time stamping of all diary entries, and automatic rejection of erroneous data. Pain drawing has also been applied to the field of pain evaluation, offering patients the ability to provide information on the location and type of pain they are experiencing on a human body map. Such topographical representation of pain was suggested to be very useful in summarizing patients' nature of their pain in an interpretable way for clinicians, and it can be further used to keep track of changes in patients' pain experiences. More recently, a novel three-dimensional (3D) approach is used for the purpose of reporting pain characteristics as an alternative to the conventional 2D pain drawing.

BEHAVIORAL OBSERVATION

Though pain is by definition a private and subjective experience, its manifestations are often apparent to others. People in pain may communicate their discomfort by vocalizations, facial expressions, body postures, and actions. These verbal and nonverbal behaviors have been termed pain behaviors, and they have emerged as an important component of behavioral models of pain. Numerous pain behavior coding systems have been developed, though many of them are specific to particular pain conditions. For example, the osteoarthritis (OA) pain behavior coding system[15] assesses the position, movement, and specific pain behaviors (e.g., guarding, rubbing, flexing) observed in OA patients during standardized tasks. Assessment of pain behaviors can be valuable in establishing a patient's level of physical functioning (e.g., the amount of activity engaged in), in analyzing the factors that may reinforce displays of pain (e.g., solicitous responses from others), or in assessing pain in nonverbal individuals. A review of the literature[16] in this area concluded that although pain behaviors and self-report of pain are moderately related, these measures are not interchangeable. Interestingly, correspondence between pain report and pain behavior was lower in the context of chronic pain than acute pain and, not surprisingly, was highest when observation and verbal report of pain were recorded at the same time.

Many recent behavioral observation studies have focused on facial expressions in response to pain. To date, a number of observational systems have been developed for evaluating pain-related facial expressions in a relatively "objective" manner. Early studies used the Facial Action Coding System (FACS) to characterize the facial expressions of adults responding to a variety of pain induction tasks.[17] Numerous elements of facial expressions (e.g., upper lip raising, mouth opening, and eye closure) were found to be related to pain ratings, and the relative consistency with which the same actions were associated with pain across numerous samples supported the concept of a potentially universal set of "pain expressions." Indeed, striking similarities have been observed between the facial actions associated with pain in middle-aged adults, the elderly, children, and neonates. This commonality of pain-related facial expression suggests that it may be a crucial assessment tool in situations in which verbal report is unavailable, as is the case with very young children, or individuals with verbal communication deficits.

However, behavioral pain indicators often might be troublesome to identify in people with intellectual disabilities; in particular, it has been challenging to demonstrate the pain specificity of many of these behaviors. In a recent review, 14 behavior categories were identified for pain detection. However, the authors pointed out the difficulty in differentiating behaviors caused by fear and stress versus pain. Future research validating these assessment tools can be vital for pain management.

EXPERIMENTAL PAIN ASSESSMENT

Administration of standardized noxious stimulation under controlled conditions constitutes an important subdiscipline within the field of pain. Several modalities of noxious stimulation are commonly used to induce pain (e.g., thermal, mechanical, electrical, chemical, ischemic); typical parameters that are measured include pain threshold, pain tolerance, and ratings of suprathreshold noxious stimuli using an NRS, VAS, or VRS. The clinical relevance of experimental pain assessment is gradually being established; quantitative sensory testing can be used to subtype patients with chronically painful conditions, to identify mechanisms of chronic pain, and to prospectively predict postoperative pain.[18]

FUNCTIONAL NEUROIMAGING

Imaging of pain processing in the human brain has attracted considerable research attention over the past 10 to 15 years. Functional neuroimaging methods such as functional magnetic resonance imaging (fMRI) and positron emission tomography (PET) allow noninvasive assessment of the neurophysiology of pain processing in the brain (and, recently, the spinal cord as well). Most of these studies have been based on measurement of brain responses to acute pain stimuli (often in healthy subjects); brain activity is measured during periods of pain and pain-free periods, and the difference between these two measurements is considered an index of pain-related neurophysiologic processes in the brain. Although the cost and the necessity of sophisticated, expensive equipment make it unlikely that functional neuroimaging will become a routine part of clinical assessment in the near future, these brain imaging studies have rapidly advanced our understanding of the central nervous system's processing of pain-related information, and functional neuroimaging methods show great promise in several key areas of pain assessment.[19] These include refining the mechanism-based classification of pain syndromes, evaluating abnormalities of pain processing in individuals with communication or cognitive deficits, studying the pharmacokinetic and pharmacodynamic properties of analgesic drugs, identifying dysfunctional areas of processing in the nervous system that can serve as analgesic drug targets, and finally, revolutionizing preclinical drug development. This last application is the subject of much current interest, and many experts have proposed using functional neuroimaging as a primary preclinical tool to study, in healthy volunteers, the effects of various putative analgesic agents on pain-related brain activation.

More recent efforts have sought to integrate fMRI and support vector machine (SVM) learning to create a cerebral signature of the experience of pain.[20] Such methods appear to hold great promise for deepening our understanding of the complex interplay among brain regions that mediate the experience of pain. Additional applications of functional neuroimaging include the potential to develop neurofeedback techniques; several studies of real-time fMRI (rt-fMRI) neurofeedback for chronic pain have been conducted, but further research and additional clinical trials are still needed. The efficacy and benefits of real-time neurofeedback for an individual may be strengthened in the future by combining real-time neurofeedback fMRI and machine-learning classifiers (MVPA) to identify spatiotemporal patient-tailored brain maps.[21,22] However, MRI-based methods are restricted by the need for nonuser-friendly, expensive equipment involving artifacts influencing data specificity and sensitivity. Therefore they have limited use in daily clinical assessment of pain.

SPECIAL POPULATIONS

CHILDREN

The assessment of pain in children obviously presents a number of challenges to health care professionals. Many providers may (inaccurately) assume that children cannot reliably provide information about their pain.[23,24] In fact, many pain assessment tools for use specifically in children have been developed and validated, and factors similar to those that influence pain in adults (e.g., the presence and magnitude of tissue damage, affective state, social responses) have been shown to relate in similar ways to children's pain.

Over a dozen behavioral pain rating scales for infants have been developed. Although demonstration of the validity of these scales is often difficult, many have been shown to be consistently reliable. As an example, one of the more commonly used measures is the Neonatal Infant Pain Scale (NIPS),[25] which codes the presence and intensity of six pain-related behaviors: facial expressions, crying, breathing, arm movement, leg movement, and arousal state. Among older children who can more readily self-report sensory and affective experiences, researchers have suggested that direct questioning (e.g., "How is your pain today?"), although clinically useful, is particularly susceptible to bias and demand characteristics. Standardized pain assessment scales have been developed for children of various ages, some of them specific to particular ethnic groups.[26,27] For example, among these are the FACES scale and the Oucher scale, which do not require language and are used for younger children. Pain thermometers, consisting of a vertical NRS superimposed on a VAS shaped to resemble a thermometer, have also been widely used, while for children over 6 years, a standard VAS is a valid and reliable measure of pain.[24,26]

COGNITIVELY IMPAIRED

Several studies have now shown that older adults report less pain on the MPQ (i.e., choose fewer words), even when NRS- or VRS-rated pain does not differ. These findings may suggest that the MPQ assesses the construct of pain differently across age groups, and caution may be warranted before using this instrument with older samples.

Recent findings suggest that a VRS produces the fewest "failure" responses among samples of cognitively intact and cognitively impaired elderly subjects while a VAS produces the largest number. It is therefore recommended that studies of pain in the elderly use, at minimum, a VRS to assess pain intensity. Moreover, some research suggest that the use of behavioral pain indicators may be preferable as among individuals with cognitive impairments, as these patients tend to underreport pain intensity on standard self-report measures, but show preserved indices of pain behaviors. Other pain assessment tools for cognitively compromised patients are the FACS,[28] the Mobilization-Observation-Behavior-Intensity-Dementia Pain Scale, the Certified Nursing Assistant tool, the Elderly Pain Caring Assessment, and the Pain Assessment in Advanced Dementia Scale.[29] Mostly these tools focus on noncoded facial expression, vocalization, motor behavior, social behavior, and mood. In early stages of dementia, when cognitive impairment is limited and communication ability is mostly intact, self-report of pain is usually possible.

USING TECHNOLOGY FOR PAIN ASSESSMENT

Real-time data capture using electronically based pain assessments represents a promising method for the field. Mobile devices such as tablets or smartphones can (1) easily collect pain reports in natural settings, (2) be patient-tailored, (3) create date and time stamped pain reports, and (4) easily export data to secure electronic databases for review or data analysis. When applied to self-report pain assessment, electronic platforms have the benefit of reducing human error and recall bias and improving adherence and cooperation.[30] Pain apps allow patients to enter details of pain episodes and record them in a manner similar to pain diaries. Pain scale apps allow users to input daily the severity of pain usually on a VAS and its nature (e.g., radiating, itching, burning, and pain). Another unique characteristic of electronic pain assessment is the 3D pain mapping programs that can enable patients to represent the location and intensity of their pain with greater accuracy. For instance, "painometer" is a recent smartphone app for assessing pain that contains four pain intensity scales: the Faces Pain Scale–Revised (FPS-R), the Numerical Rating Scale (NRS-11), the Colored Analogue Scale (CAS), and VAS.[31] Collectively, further developing such multifaceted, valid, and reliable pain assessment apps will be an important step for establishing ways to merge user needs with evidence-based content.

ASSESSING PAIN CROSS-CULTURALLY

It is well documented that some other factors that affect an individual's experience and report of pain are culture, and an individual's social and personal history. When the patient's first language is not the same as the health care provider's, it can be challenging to assess pain and provide good quality care. This likely contributes to the finding that minority populations are at risk of poor pain outcomes compared to the general population. For example, a patient that is coming from an Asian background may often express stoicism in the face of pain, which relates directly to strong cultural values about the self. Acting in a dignified manner is considered vital, and a person who is assertive or complains openly is considered to have poor social skills.

In the United States, most of the studies on pain assessment and cultural effects have examined differences between African Americans and non-Hispanic whites. It is well documented that differences in a variety of sociocultural patient-related factors such as family values and religious beliefs influence disparities in pain. Ethnicity is also an important factor in pain response and appraisal, and African Americans report increased levels of depression and disability, as well as pain severity, from various chronic pain conditions. One contributor to these ethnic differences in pain outcomes appears to be ethnic differences in the choice of pain-coping strategies, with African American patients reporting a greater likelihood of using strategies that are classically considered "passive," such as prayer.[32,33]

SUMMARY AND RECOMMENDATIONS

Pain assessment is a critical step in the process of pain management. Any study of pain should include at least one self-report measure, and it is often beneficial to use either multiple measures or a multidimensional measure of pain (e.g., the short form of the MPQ, which includes both verbal descriptors and a VAS). A review of the extensive cancer pain literature indicated that single-item VAS, VRS, and NRS all showed good validity and reliability, and it was concluded that no one of these measures was consistently superior. However, we can advise that in studies of elderly or cognitively compromised subjects, use of a VRS or NRS is strongly preferable to use of a VAS. Pain relief should be measured using sequential ratings (i.e., changes from pretreatment to posttreatment), rather than a retrospective impression. Electronic assessment and daily diaries may be extremely useful in reducing the memory biases associated with recall of pain, and in obtaining a more precise sense of the variability in day-to-day pain symptoms. Behavioral observation and experimental pain assessment are all useful and potentially informative adjunctive measures of pain responses, but none can substitute for self-report of the pain experience. The one exception to this standard is infants, in whom coding of behavioral or facial responses is the current gold standard for pain assessment. For slightly older children, a pictorial scale such as the FACES Scale or Oucher Scale may be used, whereas in children who are 6 years or older, a standard VAS may be the optimal choice. Finally, substantial research suggests that health care professionals, no matter how expert, are not reliable judges of patients' report of pain. Their estimates are both inaccurate and systematically biased in the direction of underestimation. In this chapter, we have attempted to provide those with an interest in treating or studying pain with some of the requisite information on which to base choices regarding pain assessment. Measures should be selected with as complete knowledge as possible of their properties, strengths, and limitations.

KEY POINTS

- Pain is a subjective, private, internal experience; there is no single best tool for pain assessment, and the choice of measure should be guided by the needs of the study or the clinical setting.
- While there is no "objective" measure of pain, a number of self-report pain assessment tools have proven to be valid and reliable.
- For pain assessment, categorical scales with NRSs appear to be preferable compared with traditional visual analogue scales.
- Specialized pain assessment scales are available for special populations (e.g., children, cognitive impaired).
- Psychophysiologic, behavioral, and functional neuroimaging-based assessment methods cannot substitute for an individual's self-reported pain experience.
- Pain is not synonymous with function or quality of life, and other tools assessing these important outcome dimensions are recommended.

REFERENCES

Access the reference list online at ExpertConsult.com.

CHAPTER 6

Psychological Evaluation and Testing

Sheera F. Lerman, PhD ◎ Jennifer Haythornthwaite, PhD

Chronic pain is a multifaceted, subjective experience that is best understood as a complex interaction of physiological, psychological, and environmental variables. Extensive research has documented the role cognitive, emotional, and social factors play in the etiology and maintenance of chronic pain.[1] Thus comprehensive assessment of chronic pain typically includes a psychological evaluation that can significantly improve the overall understanding of the patient and contribute to improved treatment outcomes. This chapter provides an overview of the key components of a psychological evaluation for chronic pain—the clinical interview, including behavioral observation, and the use of standardized assessment instruments.

CLINICAL INTERVIEW

While structured clinical interviews are available, most practitioners elect to conduct semistructured interviews that address multiple aspects of the individual's cognitive, medical, educational, social, employment, and psychiatric history. The interview will include an assessment of mental status to determine if the individual is sufficiently cognitively intact to participate in the assessment and future treatments. Should concerns regarding cognitive impairments emerge, closer examination of cognitive functioning or a referral for a full neuropsychological evaluation is appropriate. If available, the practitioner may draw on collateral sources of information, such as significant others or family members. As part of the clinical interview, the psychologist will gather extensive information regarding the individual's pain history and experience.

The clinical interview is the cornerstone of the psychological evaluation due to the subjective nature of the pain experience and the relatively limited set of standardized psychological measures that have normative data for chronic pain patients. Some individuals with chronic pain may be reluctant to participate in a psychological evaluation, due to the stigma associated with psychiatric illness or the concern that the provider may be suggesting that the pain is psychologically based. Referring physicians and other providers can reduce these concerns by informing patients that psychological evaluation is a routine component of comprehensive pain management. The practitioner conducting the psychological evaluation can establish credibility by beginning the interview with a focus on the patient's pain experience and its impact on daily life and function. Once rapport is established, it is easier to progress to cognitive, social, and psychological aspects of the pain experience, including cognitive-affective variables involved in chronic pain.[2] Symptoms of depression and anxiety are common among patients with chronic pain, and closely correlated are cognitions that render the person more vulnerable to increased pain and suffering.[3] An important objective of the interview is to identify any psychiatric conditions that might exacerbate pain or complicate treatment, such as psychosis, substance dependence, or a personality disorder. Additionally, it is valuable to assess the patient's sleeping patterns, specifically inquiring about any difficulties initiating or maintaining sleep as well as the presence of substantial fatigue or sleepiness impairing daily functioning. Finally, observation of pain behaviors can provide important information about the person's overall pain experience, coping, and the extent of pain-related disability. Pain behaviors—such as ability to sit through the interview, verbal complaints, and other sounds (e.g., grunting and moaning), facial expressions (e.g., grimacing, wincing), and bodily gestures (e.g., bracing when changing positions, moving in a distorted fashion)—are noted during the interview.

STANDARDIZED TESTING

One of the important elements a psychologist contributes in the overall assessment of a pain patient is expertise in the use of standardized testing instruments, which can provide data on the individual's functioning relative to normative samples. Key assessment domains are presented here, along with instruments commonly used (the assessment of pain is included in other chapters of this volume). Important assessment domains include pain-related disability and behavior, psychological function and sleep, and pain-related beliefs, cognitions, and behaviors.

MULTIDIMENSIONAL INSTRUMENTS

When clinicians do not have the need, or opportunity, to administer a battery of assessment instruments, multidimensional measures might be used in the evaluation of pain and its emotional and behavioral correlates. One of the most widely used and studied of these instruments is the Multidimensional Pain Inventory (MPI; 56 items; Box 6.1).[4] This multidimensional scale assesses psychosocial, cognitive, and behavioral aspects of pain, including pain severity and interference; activity levels, including household chores and work; impact of pain on family relationships and social activities; pain-specific support from spouse or partner; perceived life control; and negative affect. This measure is valuable in its ability to assess multiple dimensions of pain, its relative brevity, and its demonstrated responsivity to treatment effects. In addition, the MPI provides overall classification of the individual's function as being "dysfunctional," "interpersonally distressed," or "adaptive coper." However, research on the validity, utility, and distinctiveness of these classifications has yielded mixed results.[5,6]

BOX 6.1 Selected Measurement Tools

BEHAVIORAL ASPECT OF PAIN	MEASUREMENT TOOL
Multidimensional	Multidimensional Pain Inventory
Disability and behavior	Brief Pain Inventory Pain Disability Index Roland-Morris Disability Questionnaire Chronic Disability Index Oswestry Low Back Disability Questionnaire
Sleep	Pittsburgh Sleep Quality Index Insomnia Severity Index
Depression	Center for Epidemiological Studies Depression Scale Patient Health Questionnaire Depression Module
Anxiety	Generalized Anxiety Disorder Scale Hospital Anxiety and Depression Scale Pain Anxiety Symptoms Scale
Psychopathology	Symptom Checklist-90-Revised Minnesota Multiphasic Personality Inventory
Coping	Coping Strategies Questionnaire Chronic Pain Coping Inventory
Beliefs, attitudes, and expectations	Survey of Pain Attitudes-Revised Pain Beliefs and Perceptions Inventory
Catastrophizing	Pain Catastrophizing Scale Coping Strategies Questionnaire (catastrophizing subscale)
Kinesiophobia	Tampa Scale of Kinesiophobia Fear-Avoidance Beliefs Questionnaire
Self-efficacy	Pain Self-Efficacy Questionnaire Chronic Pain Self-Efficacy Scale Arthritis Self-Efficacy Scale
Locus of control	Pain Locus of Control
Acceptance	Chronic Pain Acceptance Questionnaire

PAIN-RELATED DISABILITY AND BEHAVIOR

A number of validated questionnaires are available to assess a person's perceived disability. The Brief Pain Inventory (BPI; 11 items) was developed to measure pain severity and pain-related interference in patients diagnosed with cancer.[7] Later research extended its use to noncancer pain assessment, including heterogeneous pain conditions,[8] osteoarthritis,[9] and neuropathic pain.[10] The most widely used version of this scale uses an 11-point numeric rating scale (where 0 = no interference and 10 = interferes completely) to assess pain-related interference in seven areas: general activity, mood, walking ability, normal work including outside the home and housework, relations with other people, enjoyment of life, and sleep. The BPI has been used to demonstrate the efficacy of pain medication in a variety of chronic painful conditions[9] and appears to be responsive to treatment-related change. Formatted in a similar way, the Pain Disability Index (PDI; seven items)[11] provides an alternative to the BPI. It consists of seven questions assessing disability due to pain in the following domains: family/home, recreation, social activities, occupation, sexual behavior, self-care, and life support activities. Each item is rated on an 11-point scale (0 = no disability to 10 = total disability) and the responses are summed. The PDI is also responsive to change following pain treatment.[12]

The Roland-Morris Disability Questionnaire (24 items) was developed from the Sickness Impact Profile (SIP)[13] and tailored for more focused use with chronic low back pain patients. This measure has become one of a select group of standard outcome measures in the back pain literature.[14,15] Although primarily used for the assessment of function in low back pain, some investigators have used this shorter scale to assess function in heterogeneous groups of patients seen through multidisciplinary programs. Other instruments in common usage include the Chronic Disability Index (9 items), a yes/no checklist covering nine general activities that are typically difficult for people with back pain, such as walking, sleeping, putting on footware[16]; and the Oswestry Low Back Pain Disability Questionnaire (10 items), a brief scale that provides a percentage score reflecting the amount of restriction that pain imposes on the individual. Scores have been shown to be responsive to treatment.[17]

SLEEP

Sleep disturbances are common in chronic pain patients and are known to be risk factors for both the development and exacerbation of pain. There are a number of validated assessment tools available to measure the severity of sleep disorders such as insomnia. The Pittsburgh Sleep Quality Index (19 items)[18] is a widely used and well-validated measure of sleep quality. It assesses disturbances in seven domains of sleep during the past month, including subjective sleep quality, sleep latency, sleep duration, sleep efficiency, sleep disturbance, use of sleep medication, and degree of daytime dysfunction. The Insomnia Severity Index (7 items)[19] identifies severity of sleep continuity disturbance, defined as difficulty: initiating sleep, staying asleep and early morning awakenings, as well as related distress, which are rated on a five-point Likert scale.

Since these measures of sleep patterns evaluate sleep retrospectively, they are prone to bias and error. Daily sleep diaries completed every night before bedtime and in the morning upon awakening can provide more accurate information. Ideally diaries should be collected for at least a week and include the documentation of bedtime, how long it takes to fall asleep, number of nightly awakenings, time spent awake in the middle of the night after initially falling asleep, time of final awakening, and time out of bed. These questions can help determine whether the primary problem is initiating sleep, maintaining sleep, early morning awakening, or poor/irregular sleep habits. It is also informative to have patients rate the quality of their sleep on a scale of 0 (poor quality) to 10 (excellent quality).

PSYCHOLOGICAL FUNCTION AND EMOTIONAL DISTRESS

The extent of disability in pain patients does not correlate strongly with the extent of physical impairment.[20] The biopsychosocial pain model suggests this discrepancy is related to the psychological, social, and contextual variables that interact with physical factors to determine the individual's experience with pain and disability. Thus the assessment of psychological function, specifically negative affect, such as depression and anxiety, as well as negative cognitions is an essential component of pain assessment.

There are several commonly used standardized measures for depressive symptoms. The Center for Epidemiological Studies Depression Scale (CES-D; 20 items)[21] was originally developed for use in general-population epidemiologic studies. Respondents are asked to report the frequency with which they have experienced each symptom during the past week on a four-point scale. The CES-D is brief and has excellent psychometric properties, but has also been criticized for possibly overestimating the prevalence and severity of depression among pain populations.[22] The Patient Health Questionnaire Depression Module (PHQ-9; 9 items)[23] is a newer scale that uses criteria from the Diagnostic and Statistical Manual of Mental Disorders (DSM) for diagnosing depression, using a 2-week time frame, and can be used as a measure of likely depression diagnosis as well as to track severity of symptoms. The PHQ-9 shows adequate sensitivity, specificity, and accuracy in diagnosing depression in chronic pain populations.[24]

Anxiety is a negative affective experience that can exacerbate the pain experience and complicate recovery. Despite the importance of anxiety in chronic pain, there are few studies validating standardized anxiety measures in chronic pain populations. The Generalized Anxiety Disorder scale (GAD-7; 7 items) is a valid and short scale for screening and assessing severity of anxiety in the general population. Common symptoms of anxiety are rated on a scale from 0 ("not at all") to 3 ("nearly every day").[25] The Hospital Anxiety and Depression Scale (HADS; 14 items)[26] is a screening tool for depression and anxiety in medical settings. It is commonly used in chronic pain patients and provides a depression and anxiety subscale with good psychometric properties.[27] An instrument designed to measure anxiety specific to pain patients is the Pain Anxiety Symptoms Scale (PASS; 40- and 20-item versions).[28] The PASS uses a six-point scale and asks respondents to rate the frequency with which they experience several dimensions of anxiety, including somatic, cognitive, fear, and escape/avoidance concerns.

The Symptom Checklist-90-Revised (SCL-90-R; 90 items)[29] is used for assessing psychopathology among chronic pain patients. The SCL-90-R assesses nine different types of psychological disturbance and yields three global measures of distress. This questionnaire is often favored since there is a reduced likelihood of patient resistance due to focus on symptoms; however, it has not demonstrated predictive validity with regard to treatment outcome.

Other instruments are useful when the clinician needs a broader assessment of psychiatric illnesses and personality variables that might impact the functioning of pain patients. The Minnesota Multiphasic Personality Inventory (MMPI)[30] and its successor, the MMPI-2, is the most widely used, and extensively researched, instrument for measuring psychopathology and personality variables. The three core validity scales assess the patient's response set and motivation. The 10 clinical scales tap dimensions such as concern with bodily symptoms, depression, defensive strategies, rebelliousness and antisocial tendencies, suspiciousness, worry and anxiety, and odd thinking. Additional subscales measure more specific symptoms, traits, and behaviors, including anger, family problems, social alienation, addiction potential, and negative treatment indicators.

PAIN-RELATED BELIEFS, COGNITIONS, AND BEHAVIORS

The beliefs and thoughts patients hold regarding their pain can significantly impact their daily functioning and quality of life. In general, the positive or negative content of these cognitions incurs risk or builds resiliency for effectively adjusting to daily life with chronic pain, influencing the impact of pain on mood, social relationships, and other aspects of life.

Coping is a term that typically refers to diverse range of strategies, techniques, and behaviors that people use to manage stressors, including pain, regardless of whether they are successful or not.[31] Some pain-specific coping strategies, like pain catastrophizing (discussed later), are consistently related to a wide range of poor outcomes,[2] and psychological interventions can improve these strategies. Several measures of pain-specific coping are available. The Coping Strategies Questionnaire (50 items)[32] assesses the extent to which patients engage in a variety of cognitive and behavioral coping strategies when they experience pain, including diverting attention, reinterpreting pain sensations, coping self-statements, ignoring the pain, praying or hoping, increasing activity, and perceiving a measure of control over the pain. The Chronic Pain Coping Inventory (65 items)[33] focuses on behavioral strategies of coping that might be encouraged, or discouraged, in a multidisciplinary pain treatment program, including guarding, resting, asking for assistance, relaxation, task persistence, exercise/stretch, seeking social support, coping self-statements, and medication use.

Negative Beliefs and Cognitions

Negative cognitions are the person's habitually maladaptive ways of perceiving and thinking about situations, and can contribute to a cascade of negative emotions and behaviors. Among pain patients, examples might include a tendency to overfocus on the pain, fearful anticipation of extreme pain, or the belief that any amount of pain signals tissue damage or reinjury, and should be avoided at all costs. Indeed, data suggest that a strong anticipation of pain and reinjury or negative thoughts about pain, referred to as catastrophizing,[34] can lead to fear-related avoidance of activity and increased pain-related disability.[35] These fears can produce a negative reinforcement loop supporting the persistence of avoidance behaviors (e.g., lying down) and functional limitations (e.g., work-related disability).[36–38]

Several instruments are available to measure various beliefs, attitudes, and expectancies about pain, including some that are multidimensional. The Survey of Pain Attitudes—Revised (57 items)[33] assesses seven pain-specific attitudes, including perceptions of pain control, disability, and harm, as well as beliefs surrounding pain medication, the role of emotions in their pain experience, and the expectation that other people should be more supportive of their pain concerns. The Pain Beliefs and Perceptions Inventory (16 items)[39] taps three dimensions of pain-related beliefs: future expectancies about pain and its persistence, the nature of pain and its symptomatology, and self-blame surrounding pain.

Catastrophizing is a negative cognitive and emotional response to pain and one of the most widely studied psychological constructs in the pain literature. Pain-related catastrophizing is associated with pain, disability, and emotional distress in both cross-sectional and longitudinal studies, as well as with prolonged hospital stay, use of pain medication and treatment outcome.[40,41] Catastrophizing is most commonly measured using the Pain Catastrophizing Scale (13 items),[42] designed to measure individuals' tendencies to focus on pain-related thoughts and exaggerate the significance of painful stimuli. It contains three subscales: magnification, rumination, and helplessness. The catastrophizing subscale of the Coping Strategies Questionnaire (6 items)[32] is also commonly used and measures primarily pain-related helplessness. Both questionnaires have been extensively used and validated in various pain populations.

When pain is experienced repeatedly, as occurs in chronic pain, individuals can develop a conditioned fear response to activities or events that may evoke pain. Kinesiophobia is the term for excessive fear of pain and reinjury with physical movement, which can lead to avoidance behaviors and may serve to exacerbate and maintain pain-related disability and decrease engagement in meaningful daily activities.[43] The Tampa Scale of Kinesiophobia (17 items)[44] assesses excessive fear of physical activity related to the perceived threat of pain. Similarly, the Fear-Avoidance Beliefs Questionnaire (16 items)[45] measures beliefs concerning the risk of harm from general physical activities and also from work-specific activities.

Positive Beliefs and Cognitions

Self-efficacy is one's confidence that they will persist in activities despite obstacles or negative experiences. In the context of pain, it is the belief that one can successfully carry on with daily life despite pain and its consequences.[46] Self-efficacy is consistently associated with pain-related outcomes such as depression, disability, and treatment benefit.[47] A number of questionnaires have been developed to measure self-efficacy in chronic pain patients. The Pain Self-Efficacy Questionnaire (10 items)[46] is widely used and well-validated scales in which patients are asked to rate their level of confidence (0, "not at all," to 6, "completely") that they can perform different activities despite their pain. The Chronic Pain Self-Efficacy Scale (22 items)[48] is also a commonly used and valid scale that includes three subscales: self-efficacy regarding pain, physical function, and coping. Patients are asked to rate how certain they are in their ability to cope with their pain and other symptoms, as well as their ability to engage in different activities on a 10-point Likert scale (10-very uncertain to 100-very certain). The Arthritis Self-Efficacy Scale (there are 20-, 11-, and 8-item versions)[49] is one of the most widely used scales for measuring self-efficacy in patients with arthritis. Patients rate their ability to cope with pain and disability as a result of arthritis using 10-point Likert scales (1, "very uncertain," to 10, "very certain").

Locus of control refers to an individual's belief about his or her ability to influence outcomes in life. As applied to chronic pain, locus of control refers to the extent to which patients believe they can influence or ameliorate the intensity and impact of their pain experience. The Pain Locus of Control Scale (18 items)[50] was adapted from the Health Locus of Control Scale (54 items) for this purpose, and may be useful in predicting pain treatment outcomes.[51]

When efforts to control pain are unsuccessful or problematic, an alternative approach is acceptance. Acceptance of pain (and pain-related suffering) is the ability to accept the changing nature of present moment thoughts and emotions without judgment. This approach has been combined with a focus on the pursuit of valued goals and activities in a third generation of interventions called Acceptance and Commitment Therapies.[52] The Chronic Pain Acceptance Questionnaire (there are 20-item and 8-item versions) is a validated scale that measures two dimensions of acceptance: activity engagement despite pain and willingness to experience pain.[53,54]

SPECIAL TOPICS
PREINTERVENTIONAL PAIN PROCEDURE EVALUATIONS

There has been an increase in the use of interventional pain procedures including surgically implanted spinal cord stimulators (SCS) for treating chronic or intractable pain. Pain intervention specialists have found, however, that despite meeting appropriate medical criteria for this class of interventions, a significant number of patients fail to find benefit from these therapies, leading to the consideration of how psychosocial factors may impact outcomes.[55]

In 1998, the European Federation of the International Association for the Study of Pain (IASP) Chapters developed a consensus document on neuromodulation treatment of pain[56] that established psychosocial exclusion criteria for SCS implantation (Box 6.2): (1) major psychiatric disorders (active psychosis, severe depression, hypochondriasis, or

BOX 6.2 Psychological Evaluation for Implantation of Spinal Cord Stimulation

EXCLUSION CRITERIA

Major psychiatric disorder
Poor compliance and/or insufficient understanding of the therapy
Lack of appropriate social support
Drug and alcohol abuse
Drug-seeking behavior

ADDITIONAL CONSIDERATIONS

Cognitive deficits impairing the ability to understand or manage an implantable device
Unrealistic expectations for pain relief
Severe sleep disturbance
Presence of suicidal ideation
Pain-related litigation

somatization disorder); (2) poor compliance and/or insufficient understanding of the therapy; (3) lack of appropriate social support; (4) drug and alcohol abuse; or (5) drug-seeking behavior. As these are relatively old criteria, it is recommended that they be considered guidelines rather than exclusion criteria. Other recommendations include the assessment of cognitive deficits that can impair ability to understand or manage an implantable device, as well as unrealistic expectations for pain reduction, the presence of active suicidal or homicidal intentions, severe sleep disturbance, the presence of personality disorders, and pain-related litigation.[57] While none of the above criteria necessarily serves as permanent exclusion from SCS surgery, these guidelines suggest areas that require additional evaluation and intervention to minimize the risk for complications and maximize likelihood of good outcomes. Thus increasingly preinterventional psychological assessment is being included as part of the treatment planning for SCS and related procedures and many third-party payers in the United States require psychological evaluation prior to SCS. These evaluations have several goals, including (1) screening for major psychopathology and cognitive impairments, (2) assessing treatment expectations and ability to follow through on postintervention care and rehabilitation, (3) recommending interventions to address psychosocial factors that may impede optimal outcome, (4) educating the patient as to the procedure and their role in maximizing treatment outcome, and (5) identifying the individual's psychosocial strengths that aid in recovery. It is important to note that both physical and psychological criteria for patient selection for surgery are somewhat imprecise and the predictive ability of psychological measures is relatively mixed. Excellent detailed discussions of these procedures are available elsewhere.[58–60]

SUICIDE

Individuals with chronic pain are at increased risk for suicidal thoughts and behaviors.[61–63] Comorbid psychiatric disorders like depression, prevalent in chronic pain, also increase the risk for suicidality. While thoughts about end of life and death are common, especially in individuals suffering from chronic medical conditions, it is important to make the distinction between these and thoughts of suicide that include wishing one were dead, thoughts about taking one's life, creating a specific plan, or having the means to complete the plan. There are a number of factors that increase the risk for an individual to attempt suicide in the general population such as past suicide attempts, family history of suicide, lack of social support, and access to means of suicide such as weapons or medication. For chronic pain patients, additional risk factors include the presence of comorbid depression, high pain intensity and duration, the presence of sleep-onset insomnia, high catastrophizing, and feelings of hopelessness.[64] When assessing suicide risk, it is important to consider these factors and decide on a proper course of action based on the level of suicide risk (see McDowell et al.[65] for a comprehensive framework for suicide risk assessment).

Depression assessment tools such as the PHQ-9 include an item that addresses suicidality. There are a number of questionnaires that can be used to supplement this assessment and focus specifically on suicidal thoughts and behaviors. The P4 Screener (four items)[66] screens patients who endorse having thoughts about hurting themselves. It uses an algorithm based on responses to questions about past attempts, current plans, probability of an attempt, and preventive factors to determine the level of suicide risk. It has been validated in medical populations treated in primary care and oncology. An additional screening tool is the Suicide Behaviors Questionnaire—Revised (four items)[67] that assesses lifetime suicidal ideation or attempts, frequency of suicidal ideation, threat, and likelihood of suicidal attempts and behaviors in the future. This scale has good sensitivity and specificity and has validated cutoff scores for the general population.

SUBSTANCE USE AND OPIOID MEDICATION MISUSE

The prevalence of alcohol/substance use and prescription opioid misuse in persons with chronic pain is significant; thus a comprehensive evaluation should include screening for alcohol, substance, and prescription opioid use. For alcohol screening, two widely used measures are the CAGE and AUDIT. The CAGE (four items)[68] is the most widely used, typically administered verbally, and includes the following screening questions: (1) Have you ever tried to cut down on your alcohol or drug use? (2) Do you get annoyed when people comment on your drinking or drug use? (3) Do you feel guilty about things you have done while drinking or using drugs? (4) Do you need an eye opener to get started in the morning? A positive response to two or more of these questions is indicative of substance abuse. The Alcohol Use Disorders Identification Test (AUDIT; 10 items)[69] is a screening tool developed by the World Health Organization to assess alcohol consumption and related problematic behaviors. It can be administered either by a clinician or as a self-report questionnaire, and a score of 8 or more indicates harmful alcohol use.

Assessment of alcohol and substance abuse is important in the context of treatment for chronic pain since individuals with substance use disorders are at an increased risk for opioid misuse.[70] Opioid medications are a common tool in the management of both acute and chronic pain; however, the use of these drugs, particularly for long periods of time, may give rise to concerns, in both patients and providers, regarding the potential of misuse. Precise rates of opioid medication misuse have been difficult to establish, but estimates of the prevalence of opioid dependence in primary care settings are as high as 26%[71] and in pain clinic settings to be as high as 14%.[72] When physicians become reluctant to prescribe opiate pain medication out of fear of fostering addiction, this can result in the undertreatment of pain. Poorly controlled pain, in turn, might prompt drug-seeking behavior by patients. Such behavior has been termed pseudoaddiction, because it is not a true signal of opiate misuse, as much as it reflects inadequate pain relief.[73] Nevertheless, the risk for addiction exists with opiate pain medications, and physicians are challenged to minimize this risk while finding the optimum dosing for adequate pain control. If questionable behaviors arise, such as overusing pain medications or requesting early refills, the physician must assess if these behaviors represent misuse. Recently published CDC guidelines address the growing issue of opioid misuse and recommend risk assessment and ongoing discussion with patients regarding the risks and realistic benefits of opioid therapy.[74]

Ideally, before the initiation of opioid therapy, the patient should be assessed as to their level of risk for developing aberrant medication-related behaviors (behaviors that differ from the prescribed medical plan) and abuse or misuse of their medication. These can be evaluated through patient interviews, questionnaires, and lab tests; however, the assessment process is not precise, and clinical judgment is required. The Screener and Opiate Assessment of Patients With Pain—Revised (SOAPP-R; 24 items) is a self-report questionnaire designed to assess the risk for drug abuse and aberrant medication-related behavior. It has been validated in a number of studies on chronic pain patients and is one of the most widely used screening tools for opioid misuse in chronic pain patients.[75] An additional screening tool is the Opioid Risk Tool (five items), which is a screener that uses risk factors such as family and personal history of substance abuse, age, and psychiatric conditions to calculate a risk score. It has shown good sensitivity and specificity in determining which chronic pain patients are at risk for opioid abuse.[76] The Current Opioid Misuse Measure (17 items)[77] is a tool developed to monitor patient's aberrant medication-related behaviors during opioid treatment. Patients rate how often they engage in different behaviors that fall into six potentially problematic domains such as signs and symptoms of intoxication, emotional volatility, addiction, and problematic medication behavior. While validation studies have demonstrated some promise for these instruments in identifying problematic usage of opioid medications, they have not yet progressed in their development to stand as reliable predictors of opiate misuse.

A list of the measurement tools discussed previously is given in Box 6.1.

SYMPTOM EXAGGERATION AND MALINGERING

It is not unusual for clinicians to suspect that some pain complaints and behaviors exceed what might reasonably be expected for the person's medical status. When symptom exaggeration is suspected, it is important to consider that this might occur for a range of reasons related to internal psychological processes or environmental factors that shape the person's presentation or response to pain. While there is no one assessment tool that can definitely establish symptom exaggeration or malingering, multiple strategies, including both behavioral observations and standardized testing, can be used. These include (1) inconsistencies between physical findings and the patient's self-presentation, (2) overly impaired performance, (3) lack of specific diagnostic signs of impairment, (4) nonorganic physical findings, and (5) evidence derived from psychological testing. Some investigators have cautioned that behavioral inconsistencies can be a misleading indicator of symptom exaggeration, as individuals in pain can normally present with some behavioral inconsistencies.[78] Psychological test data including the validity and clinical scales on the MMPI-2[79] and patterns of responding to cognitive testing[80–82] can be useful in identifying patients who are engaged in symptom exaggeration or malingering.

CONCLUSION

A comprehensive, multidisciplinary assessment is needed to develop a helpful treatment plan for most persons with chronic pain, and this evaluation should include an evaluation of psychological, behavioral, and social factors. The psychological evaluation includes both the clinical interview and the use of instruments that are reliable and valid. Effective psychological evaluation should provide a case formulation and specific recommendations that are useful to both the patient and their health care providers.

KEY POINTS

- Conceptualizing psychological evaluation as a routine component of comprehensive pain management can help reduce patients' possible feelings of stigma surrounding psychological assessment.
- Psychological evaluations typically include a clinical interview, as well as the use of standardized self-report scales and questionnaires.
- Key domains for assessment include pain-related disability and behavior, emotional distress such as depression and anxiety, psychopathology, pain-related cognitions and beliefs, coping strategies, sleep disturbance, suicide risk, and substance use.
- When interventional pain therapy is being considered, it is advisable to obtain a specialized psychological consultation that includes evaluation, education, and if necessary, intervention.
- Individuals with chronic pain have an increased risk for suicidal thoughts and behaviors that should be specifically assessed as part of pain management.
- Psychological evaluation of the risk for opioid misuse and abuse as part of chronic opioid therapy can provide valuable information to both the patient and provider by addressing concerns about addiction and promoting realistic expectation from treatment.

REFERENCES

Access the reference list online at ExpertConsult.com.

CHAPTER 7

Diagnostic and Statistical Manual of Mental Disorders and Pain Management

Meghan Rodes, MD

INTRODUCTION

Since the third edition of *Essentials of Pain Medicine*, a fifth edition of the Diagnostic and Statistical Manual of Mental Disorders was published in 2013 (henceforth referred to as DSM-5). The nomenclature has changed significantly with regard to this chapter involving the relationship between psychiatric diagnoses and pain-related complaints. Entities previously classified as somatoform disorders (e.g., somatization disorder, pain disorder, hypochondriasis, and others) have been reorganized and reclassified, and are currently characterized under the heading of somatic symptom and related disorders. This category now includes diagnoses of somatic symptom disorder, illness anxiety disorder, conversion disorder (functional neurological symptom disorder), psychological factors affecting other medical conditions, factitious disorder, other specified somatic symptom and related disorder, and unspecified somatic symptom and related disorder, while pain disorder only made an appearance in DSM-IV and does not appear again in DSM-5. These diagnoses are grouped together by the presence of physical symptoms associated with significant distress and functional impairment. These patients often present to primary care providers, as well as pain specialists, as opposed to psychiatrists/psychologists, and the reorganization of diagnoses was done for the benefit of nonpsychiatry trained clinicians. The term *somatoform disorders* was often confusing to providers because there was too much overlap within this group of diagnoses. Therefore the authors of the DSM-5 reduced both the number of diagnoses in this category, as well as eliminated many sub-diagnoses. In the DSM-IV, there was a focus on unexplained medical symptoms, whereas the DSM-5 recognizes that somatic symptoms and disorders may actually accompany diagnosed medical conditions, and that psychiatric disorders can be present alongside medical diagnoses. There has been difficulty relying on a diagnosis of exclusion as the basis for a psychiatric disorder, in addition to the inappropriateness of making a psychiatric diagnosis merely because a medical diagnosis cannot be made. A negative connotation often accompanies the lack of a medical diagnosis, and patients may feel they are not being understood or believed. Again, the DSM-5 seeks to change this by focusing on the presence of positive symptoms: "however, medically unexplained symptoms remain a key feature in Conversion Disorder and Pseudocyesis (a false belief of being pregnant that is associated with objective signs and reported symptoms of pregnancy, classified as an Other Specified Somatic Symptom and Related Disorder) because it is possible to demonstrate definitively in such disorders that the symptoms are not consistent with medical pathophysiology."[1] It is important to consider entities that influence these types of disorders, including biological predisposition to pain (e.g., fibromyalgia), prior life experiences (particularly those of the emotionally traumatic variety), secondary gain, and/or cultural differences regarding somatic complaints and pain. In this chapter, we will cover somatic symptom and related disorders that are pertinent to pain management, including somatic symptom disorder, conversion disorder, and factitious disorder, as well as malingering.

SOMATIC SYMPTOM DISORDER

In the DSM-IV, patients with somatoform symptom disorder may have been classified as having somatization disorder (an often confusing diagnosis), hypochondriasis, or pain disorder. Undesired and unpleasant bodily experiences may unfortunately be common features of everyday life, with up to 60% to 80% of the general population experiencing one or more somatic symptoms in any given week.[2] Typically these symptoms include pain, fatigue, nausea, imbalance, dystonia, dyspnea, and/or paresthesias. For the vast majority of people, these episodes are transient. A minority of individuals decides to seek medical help, typically when the experience persists, becomes severe or disabling, or is accompanied by the fearful belief that the sensation is a symptom of a more significant medical diagnosis.

The approach to patients with many symptoms must include a thorough history and examination, consisting at a minimum of medical history, individual and family psychiatric history, social history, current medications, and laboratory or diagnostic imaging results. The somatic symptoms can be numerous and overwhelming for the time-constrained clinician. Objective physical examination findings are often lacking, and laboratory results are typically unrevealing. Nonetheless, it remains imperative to rule out general medical conditions that may manifest with vague somatic symptoms. It has become increasingly common in pain management for patients to present with more than the typical complaints of back and neck pain, and the pain practitioner must either be comfortable diagnosing and managing these other types of pain, or have a plan for referral to another physician with expertise in the area of the complaint.

The DSM-5 diagnosis of somatic symptom disorder places greater emphasis on the presence of positive symptoms (often unpleasant or distressing symptoms and resultant abnormal behaviors), as opposed to the lack of a medical explanation for the patient's complaints. The dysfunctional way of thinking and behaving in response to these positive symptoms, and not merely the presence of the complaints themselves, is what distinguishes this diagnosis. According to the DSM-5 diagnostic criteria, patients with somatic symptom disorder typically have multiple symptoms that are distressing or result in significant disruption of daily life (Criterion A), although pain alone is enough to satisfy this criterion. Individuals with this diagnosis often have excessive thoughts, feelings, or behaviors related to the somatic symptoms, as manifested by either disproportionate and persistent thoughts about the seriousness of one's symptoms, persistently high level of anxiety about health or symptoms, or excessive time and energy devoted to the these symptoms (Criterion B). Patients who persist in searching for a medical cause for their functional symptoms risk invasive diagnostic procedures and unnecessary surgery, in addition to the fact that these tests rarely alleviate any concerns, and the unwarranted costs of these examinations may further strain limited medical resources. Patients do not need to have the same complaint continuously, but they must have a symptom present chronically (Criterion C). If the primary complaint is pain, then the somatic symptom disorder should be specified with predominant pain, which was previously classified as pain disorder in the DSM-IV. Table 7.1 lists the diagnostic criteria for somatic symptom disorder.

According to the DSM-5, the differential diagnosis for somatic symptom disorder should also include:

- Depressive disorders—where poor mood is prominent
- Panic disorder—more acute
- Generalized anxiety disorder—patients worry about many things, but not often illness
- Illness anxiety disorder—worries about health with minimal somatic complaints
- Conversion disorder—predominant complaint is a loss of function rather than the associated distress
- Unrecognized organic disease
- Substance abuse
- Cognitive dysfunction

Somatic symptom disorder is more common in women than men (as was somatization disorder), with a possible prevalence of 5% to 7% in adults.[3]

TABLE 7.1 Somatic Symptom Disorder

Diagnostic Criteria

A. One or more somatic symptoms that are distressing or result in significant disruption of daily life.
B. Excessive thoughts, feelings, or behaviors related to the somatic symptoms or associated health concerns as manifested by at least one of the following:
  1. Disproportionate and persistent thoughts about the seriousness of one's symptoms
  2. Persistently high level of anxiety about health or symptoms
  3. Excessive time and energy devoted to these symptoms or health concerns
C. Although any one somatic symptom may not be continuously present, the state of being symptomatic is persistent (typically more than 6 months).

Specify if:

With predominant pain (previously pain disorder): This specifier is for individuals whose somatic symptoms predominantly involve pain.

Specify if:

Persistent: A persistent course is characterized by severe symptoms, marked impairment, and long duration (more than 6 months).

Specify current severity:

Mild: Only one of the symptoms specified in Criterion B is fulfilled.
Moderate: Two or more of the symptoms specified in Criterion B are fulfilled.
Severe: Two or more of the symptoms specified in Criterion B are fulfilled; plus there are multiple somatic complaints (or one very severe somatic symptom).

Modified from American Psychiatric Association. Diagnostic and Statistical Manual of Mental Disorders. *5th ed. Arlington, VA: American Psychiatric Association; 2013.*

CONVERSION DISORDER (FUNCTIONAL NEUROLOGICAL SYMPTOM DISORDER)

The hallmark of conversion disorder is the presence of neurological symptoms that are incompatible with neurological pathophysiology. There may be one or several symptoms, usually involving sensory or motor function. Motor symptoms or deficits include impaired coordination or balance, paralysis, aphonia, dysphagia, and/or urinary retention. Sensory symptoms include loss of touch or pain sensation, diplopia, blindness, deafness, and/or hallucinations. Symptoms may also include seizures or convulsions, or episodes of unresponsiveness. Presenting symptoms may seem implausible and may strongly depend on the patient's level of education. Conversion symptoms typically do not conform to anatomic pathways and physiologic mechanisms but instead follow the individual's conceptualization of a condition. For example, "paralysis" may involve an inability to perform a specific movement or move an entire body part, rather than a deficit corresponding to patterns of motor innervation. There may be unacknowledged strength in antagonistic muscles, normal muscle tone, and intact reflexes. Electromyography (EMG), evoked responses of vision and hearing, fundoscopic examinations, pulmonary function tests, and barium swallows are examples of tests that should be normal. A diagnosis of conversion disorder should only be made after a thorough medical investigation has been performed to rule out an etiologic, neurologic, or general medical condition. Performing repeated exams, changing the examiner, or use of distracting techniques may be helpful in elucidating somewhat feigned symptoms. A few examples include Hoover sign, in which weakness of hip extension returns to normal strength with contralateral hip flexion against resistance, weakness of ankle plantar flexion in a patient that can walk on his toes, or alteration in a functional tremor when a patient is asked to copy an examiner's movements with the nontremulous hand, such that the functional tremor changes or entrains to the unaffected extremity.[4,5] With regard to psychogenic seizures, the presence of closed eyes with resistance to opening may be present.[6] True disability may result from disuse of extremities. A general medical etiology for an apparent diagnosis of conversion disorder may take years to manifest; therefore it is important to reevaluate this diagnosis periodically. The presence of a neurologic condition does not preclude a diagnosis of conversion disorder, and as many as one-third of individuals with conversion symptoms have a current or prior neurological diagnosis. Conversion disorder may be diagnosed in the presence of a neurological disorder if the symptoms are not fully explained given the severity of the organic diagnosis. Table 7.2 lists the diagnostic criteria for conversion disorder. A history of trauma or stress may be present, but is not necessary for the diagnosis of conversion disorder. Dissociative symptoms may manifest, particularly during acute episodes. Patients with conversion disorder may or may not be feigning symptoms, but this is not part of the diagnostic criteria for the disorder (as it was in the DSM-IV).

According to the DSM-5, the differential diagnosis for conversion disorder includes:

- Organic neurological disease
- Somatic symptom disorder—where symptoms are not clearly incompatible with a pathophysiological condition, and thoughts and behaviors are abnormal and excessive
- Factitious disorder and malingering—requires definite evidence of feigning to assume a sick role (factitious disorder) or for external gain (malingering)

The incidence of individual persistent conversion symptoms is estimated to be 2 to 5/100,000 per year.[7,8] Conversion disorder is two to three times more common in females. There is an association between conversion disorder and antisocial personality disorder in males. Conversion disorder has been reported to be more common in rural populations, individuals of lower socioeconomic status, and individuals less knowledgeable about medical and psychological concepts. Factors associated with a good prognosis include acute onset, presence of stress at time of onset, a short interval between onset and treatment, and higher intelligence level. Symptoms of paralysis, aphonia, and blindness portend a good prognosis, whereas tremor and seizures do not.

FACTITIOUS DISORDER

The overarching theme of factitious disorder (sometimes also referred to as Munchausen syndrome) is the intentional production of physical or psychological symptoms. Diagnosis requires proof that the patient is purposefully falsifying symptoms in the absence of obvious rewards (e.g., financial, sick role, secondary gain). Table 7.3 lists the diagnostic criteria for factitious disorder. Examples of actions an individual may take include reporting false symptoms, altering medical records, taking steps to produce false laboratory results, ingesting substances to create a medical abnormality, or physically injuring oneself or another individual to produce illness and the need for medical attention. Patients may complain about nonexistent symptoms, create objective signs (e.g., warming skin to create erythema, using psychoactive drugs to suggest a mental disorder), or exaggerate symptoms of a previous diagnosis. Components of the history suggesting this diagnosis include the following: multiple hospital admissions or office visits, knowledge of medical terminology, vague and unverifiable history, chronic illness at a young age, difficulty with interpersonal relationships and few visitors in the inpatient setting, comorbid personality disorders, or substance abuse disorder.

The differential diagnosis of factitious disorder includes other disorders in the somatic symptom and related disorders spectrum; however, the main differentiating factor is the presence of intentional deception or falsification of symptoms. The prevalence of factitious disorder is unknown.

MALINGERING

Malingering is not classified as a mental illness. Malingering was included under the heading of somatoform disorders in the DSM-IV, but has received a V code in the DSM-5 as one of the other conditions that may be of clinical interest (and is not classified under somatic symptom and related disorders). The DSM-IV defines malingering as "the intentional production of false or grossly exaggerated physical or psychological symptoms, motivated by external incentives such as avoiding military duty, avoiding work, obtaining financial compensation, evading criminal prosecution, or obtaining drugs."[9]

TABLE 7.2 Conversion Disorder (Functional Neurological Symptom Disorder)

Diagnostic Criteria
A. One or more symptoms of altered voluntary motor or sensory function.
B. Clinical findings provide evidence of incompatibility between the symptom and recognized neurological or medical conditions.
C. The symptom or deficit is not better explained by another medical or mental disorder.
D. The symptom of deficit causes clinically significant distress or impairment in social, occupational, or other important areas of functioning or warrants medical evaluation.

Modified from American Psychiatric Association. Diagnostic and Statistical Manual of Mental Disorders. *5th ed. Arlington, VA: American Psychiatric Association; 2013.*

TABLE 7.3 Factitious Disorder

Diagnostic Criteria
Factitious disorder imposed on self
A. Falsification of physical or psychological signs or symptoms, or induction of injury or disease, associated with identified deception
B. The individual presents himself or herself to others as ill, impaired, or injured.
C. The deceptive behavior is evident, even in the absence of obvious external rewards.
D. The behavior is not better explained by another mental disorder, such as delusional disorder or another psychotic disorder.
Factitious disorder imposed on another (previously factitious disorder by proxy)
A. Falsification of physical or psychological signs or symptoms, or induction of injury or disease, in another, associated with identified deception
B. The individual presents another individual (victim) to others as ill, impaired, or injured.
C. The deceptive behavior is evident, even in the absence of obvious external rewards.
D. The behavior is not better explained by another mental disorder, such as delusional disorder or another psychotic disorder.
Note: The perpetrator, not the victim, receives this diagnosis.

Modified from American Psychiatric Association. Diagnostic and Statistical Manual of Mental Disorders. *5th ed. Arlington, VA: American Psychiatric Association; 2013.*

TABLE 7.4 Waddell Signs

Scoring: Any individual sign counts as a positive sign for that type; a finding of three or more of the five types is clinically significant. Isolated positive signs are ignored. Multiple signs suggest that the patient requires a more detailed evaluation, including psychological evaluation.

Category	Signs
Tenderness If related to physical disease, tenderness is usually localized to a particular skeletal or neuromuscular structure.	**Superficial:** Skin is tender to light pinch over a wide area of lumbar skin. **Nonanatomic:** Deep tenderness is felt over a wide area, is not localized to one structure, and often extends to the thoracic spine, sacrum, or pelvis.
Simulation These tests give the patient the impression that a particular examination is being carried out when in fact it is not. A painful movement is simulated without actually being performed.	**Axial loading:** Low-back pain is reported on vertical loading over the standing patient's skull by the examiner's hands. **Rotation:** Back pain is reported when shoulders and pelvis are passively rotated in the same plane as the patient stands relaxed with the feet together.
Distraction A positive physical finding is demonstrated in the routine manner; this finding is then checked while the patient's attention is distracted.	**Straight Leg Raising:** The patient whose back pain has a nonorganic component shows marked improvement in straight leg raising on distraction, as compared with formal testing.
Regional Disturbances Involves a widespread region of neighboring parts such as the leg below the knee, the entire leg, or a quarter or half the body.	**Weakness:** Demonstrated on formal testing by a partial cogwheel "giving way" of many muscle groups that cannot be explained on a localized neurologic basis **Sensory:** Diminished sensation to light touch, pinprick, and sometimes other modalities fitting a "stocking" rather than a dermatomal pattern
Overreaction	Takes the form of disproportionate verbalization, facial expression, muscle tension and tremor, collapsing, or sweating during examination

Modified from Waddell G, McCulloch JA, Kummel E, Venner RM. Nonorganic physical signs in low back pain. Spine (Phila Pa 1976) *1980;5(2):117-125.*

Resnick further classified malingering into three types. In pure malingering, patients fabricate symptoms that do not exist at all, whereas in partial malingering, symptoms that do exist are exaggerated.[10] Lastly, in false imputation, patients attempt to blame real symptoms on an unrelated event. For example, a patient may injure his hand during a home repair project but attempts to blame the injury on a motor vehicle accident that he is involved in a week later. In addition, some cases of malingering may involve a parent fabricating an illness in his or her child, again for the purpose of external gain (such as social benefits). The phrase "malingering by proxy" has been suggested to describe this scenario. Clues that suggest a diagnosis of malingering include the following: medico-legal context of the presentation, marked discrepancy between claimed stress or disability and objective findings, lack of cooperation during the diagnostic evaluation, and the presence of antisocial personality disorder. The prevalence of malingering in the population of chronic pain patients who are seeking compensation has been estimated to be 25% to 50%. Malingering can be extremely difficult to diagnose and, according to an estimate from the Texas Department of Insurance, adds up to $150 billion in costs to the health insurance industry.[11] Feigning illness may often be done to receive disability compensation. In 2011 the estimated cost of malingering in medical court cases was $20.02 billion.[12]

Successful identification of the malingering patient remains difficult. Some advocate looking for inconsistencies in the physical exam and making use of Waddell signs (see Table 7.4).[13,14] While Waddell signs may be predictors of poor response to medical interventions, they are not thought to be able to discriminate between organic and nonorganic pain. The term "pain behavior" can be used to describe a number of aspects of the patient's response to pain, but "behavioral signs" should be used only to describe specifically how the patient responds to examination.[15] Other suggestions for detecting malingering include checking shoes for uneven wear in patients with a limp, examining hands for calluses or cuts in patients claiming an inability to work, or observing an absence of associated injury in patients claiming to have fainted or fallen. Table 7.5 provides a summary of examination maneuvers for the detection of malingering and the relative strength of recommendation of these tests.[16] In the absence of objective evidence of malingering, psychological testing such as the Minnesota Multiphasic Personality Inventory or the Symptom Checklist-90—Revised can be helpful in detecting exaggerations and inconsistencies in a history.[17]

ACKNOWLEDGMENTS

The author would like to acknowledge Jason L. Hennes, MD, for his contribution to the previous edition chapter.

KEY POINTS

- Nomenclature has changed significantly for somatic complaint focused disorders between the DSM-IV and DSM-5.
- Somatic symptom and related disorders share in common somatic symptoms associated with significant distress and functional impairment.
- The DSM-5 diagnosis of somatic symptom disorder places greater emphasis on the presence of positive symptoms (often unpleasant or distressing symptoms and resultant abnormal behaviors) as opposed to the lack of a medical explanation for the patient's complaints.

TABLE 7.5 Summary of Tests for the Detection of Malingering

Test	Symptoms	Description	Evidence/Outcomes	Strength of Recommendation
McBride	Back pain with radicular symptoms	Stand on one leg. Flex symptomatic leg and raise to chest. Refusal or pain = nonorganic	No published studies	C (expert opinion)
Mankopf	Back pain	1700 g pressure applied to the middle phalanx of the 2nd finger of the nondominant hand. True pain should increase heart rate.	Did not correlate with organic pain	C (small inconclusive diagnostic case-control study)
Waddell	Back pain	Positive signs from three or more categories. Associated with poorer treatment outcomes. Not associated with secondary gain.	Cannot discriminate organic from nonorganic	C (from systematic review)
Hoover	Leg paresis	Cup heels and have patient press down with paretic limb. Then have the patient raise the opposite limb. True paresis if no difference in downward pressure at heels.	Indicates nonorganic paresis	C (extrapolated from small diagnostic case-control study using strain gauge)
Abductor	Leg paresis	Ask patient to abduct paretic leg to resistance. In true paresis, opposite leg should abduct.	Indicates nonorganic paresis	C (small, lower-quality case-control study)
Arm Drop	Arm paresis	Hold paretic hand above face and drop it. If hand misses face, paresis is nonorganic.	No published studies	C (expert opinion)
Midline split	Sensory loss	Test facial sensation to pinprick. Nonorganic loss of sensation is delineated by the midline.	Very weakly indicated nonorganic cause	C (small diagnostic case-control study)

Modified from Greer S, Chambliss L, Mackler L. What physical exam techniques are useful to detect malingering? J Fam Pract *2005;54:719-722.*

- A significant number of patients in the chronic pain setting are likely to meet criteria for a diagnosis of somatic symptom disorder with predominant pain, formerly known as pain disorder.
- The diagnosis of conversion disorder requires that the symptom (often deficits involving voluntary motor or sensory function) is not explained by neurological disease, and that there are clinical findings incompatible with neurological disease.
- Factitious disorder involves falsification of medical or psychological symptoms in oneself or others in the absence of external rewards (e.g., deception is done to assume the sick role, not to obtain financial reward as in malingering).
- There is a tremendous cost to the health care system related to somatic symptoms and related disorders, and malingering.

REFERENCES

Access the reference list online at ExpertConsult.com.

CHAPTER 8

Neurophysiologic Testing for Pain

Takashi Nishida, MD ✪ Michael M. Minieka, MD ✪ Leslie Rydberg, MD

Electrophysiologic testing, when properly applied, is a useful tool for the evaluation of patients with pain. Understanding the indications and limitations of each test is absolutely essential for appropriate diagnosis and subsequent treatment.

Electrophysiologic studies are a very sensitive indicator of central and peripheral nervous system involvement but do not indicate underlying disease. For example, testing can diagnose radiculopathy but cannot determine if it is caused by osteophytes, a herniated disc, or diabetes. This chapter describes conventional electrophysiologic tests such as electromyography (EMG), and short latency somatosensory evoked potentials (SSEPs), as well as newer techniques including quantitative sensory testing (QST), laser evoked potentials (LEPs), and contact heat evoked potentials (CHEPs). Invasive testing such as microneurography will not be discussed here.

The role of *sympathetic nervous system* in the production of pain is complex and controversial; nonetheless, testing of the autonomic function is also important for the evaluation of pain complaints because it gives an objective measure of small nerve fiber involvement, as well as evidence of the therapeutic interventions such as sympathetic nerve blocks. The most frequent referrals to the autonomic laboratory are patients with painful peripheral neuropathy such as diabetic polyneuropathy, and so-called complex regional pain syndrome/reflex sympathetic dystrophy (CRPS/RSD). Based on accuracy, reproducibility, and ease of implementation, sudomotor function tests such as sympathetic skin response (SSR) and quantitative sweat test are discussed here. Other quantitative autonomic measures for adrenergic function (Valsalva maneuver, head up tilt) and for cardiovagal function (heart rate variability to deep breathing) are beyond the scope of this discussion.

Finally, although controversial, the value of nociceptive reflexes such as blink reflex, masseter inhibitory reflex (MIR), and flexor reflex for the evaluation of neuropathic pain will be discussed briefly.

ELECTROMYOGRAPHY AND NERVE CONDUCTION STUDIES[1,2]

When strictly defined, EMG indicates only a needle examination of muscles. However, EMG is often used to include both needle studies and nerve conduction studies (NCS). EMG/NCS is extremely useful in the evaluation of the peripheral nervous system. Indeed, the three most common diagnoses in EMG laboratories—peripheral neuropathy, carpal tunnel syndrome, and lumbosacral radiculopathy—all cause pain. EMG/NCS can identify the anatomic site of injury (anterior horn cell, spinal root, plexus, nerve, neuromuscular junction, or muscle), the type of neurons or fibers involved (motor, sensory, or autonomic), the nature of pathologic alteration (demyelination, or axonal degeneration), time course (acute, subacute, or chronic), and severity of injury. This data is clinically relevant for pain management, as it can confirm pathophysiology, assist with prognosis, and guide treatment (optimal site/level for injection).

NERVE CONDUCTION STUDIES

By stimulating peripheral nerve with supramaximal intensity, compound muscle action potential (CMAP) for motor nerve and sensory nerve action potential (SNAP) for sensory nerve are recorded. Amplitude of action potentials as well as the time from stimulation to response is recorded. Latency is the interval between the onset of a stimulus and the onset of a response, expressed in milliseconds. Conduction velocity is obtained by dividing the distance between two stimulation points (mm) of the same nerve by the difference between proximal and distal latencies (ms). This calculated velocity, expressed in meters per seconds (m/s), represents the conduction velocity of the fastest nerve fibers between two points of stimulation. It is important to note that studies may be normal if a disorder is limited to small nerve fibers such as Aδ and C fibers.

The amplitude of CMAP is measured from baseline to negative peak in millivolts, and the amplitude of SNAP is measured from the first positive peak to negative peak in microvolts. Most laboratories have their own normal values for major motor and sensory nerves, with minor differences occurring among laboratories. A lower temperature will prolong distal latencies, reduce conduction velocities, and increase the amplitude of CMAP and SNAP. Age also affects NCSs. Adult values are not attained until 4 years of age, and they decline after age 60 years at a rate of 1–2 m/s per decade. Waveform analyses of CMAP and SNAP help determine normal versus abnormal nerve function (Fig. 8.1). The amplitude of a response should be similar when the same nerve is stimulated proximally and distally. A greater than 20%–50% reduction between distal and proximal stimulation of a motor nerve suggests an abnormal block in conduction between two stimulation points. Many laboratories are now computerized, and the area under an action potential curve can be calculated. Greater than 20%–40% reduction in area also suggests conduction block. A significant reduction in amplitude from proximal to distal stimulation sites without a reduction in area under the response curve, and a significant increase in duration (>15%) suggest temporal dispersion resulting from a relative desynchronization of the components of an action potential that is due to different rates of conduction of each nerve fiber. This also suggests nerve pathology between the proximal and distal stimulation sites.

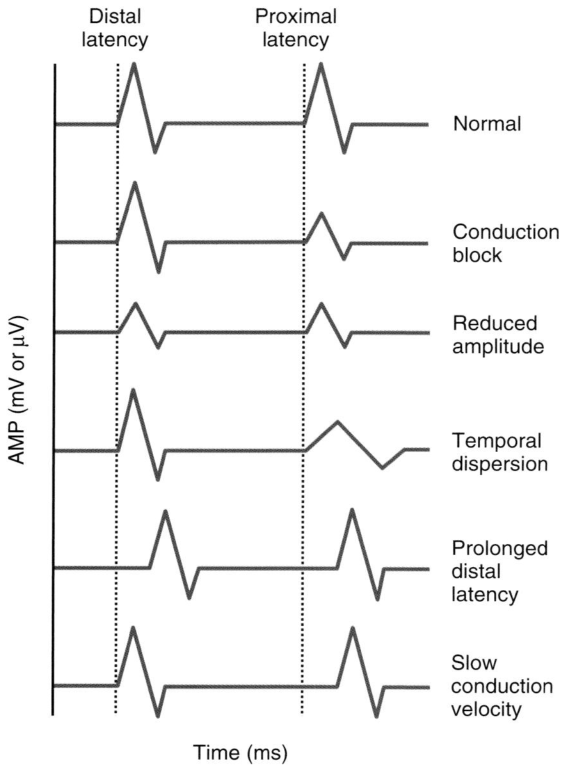

FIG. 8.1 Schematic representation of normal and pathological findings obtained from a nerve conduction velocity study.

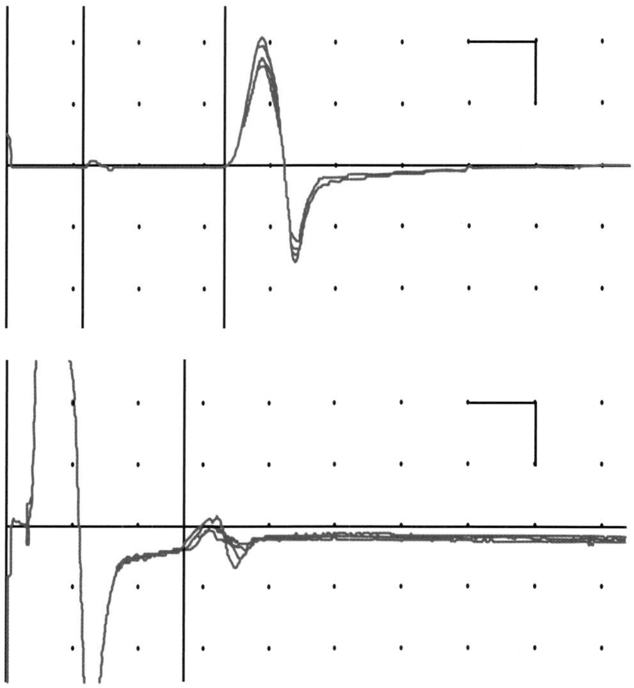

FIG. 8.2 H reflex with tibial nerve stimulation *(top);* time marker 10 ms; amplitude marker 5 mv. F response with median nerve stimulation *(bottom);* time marker 10 ms; amplitude marker 1 mv.

The H reflex is the electrophysiological equivalent of a muscle stretch reflex. A sensory nerve is stimulated with submaximal intensity, and a late motor response is recorded, owing to reflex activation of motor neurons. In adults, H reflexes are easily obtained from soleus muscle and less easily from flexor carpi radialis muscle following the stimulation of tibial and median nerves, respectively. The tibial H reflex is useful in identifying S1 radiculopathy.

F waves are late response recorded from muscle after supramaximal stimulation of a motor nerve. F waves represent a response to a stimulus that travels first to and then from the cord via motor pathways; thus F waves are useful in studying the proximal portion of motor nerves (Fig. 8.2). Unfortunately there is no consensus as to methodology for obtaining responses, and to the patterns of abnormality to be identified.

ELECTROMYOGRAPHY

The electrical activity in a muscle can be measured using disposable needle electrodes. Needle examination is performed in proper steps. An examiner observes activity on insertion of a needle (insertion activity), activity when the needle is maintained in a relaxed muscle (spontaneous activity), and activity during varying degrees of voluntary muscle contraction. The electrical activity is evaluated by sight and sound, as specific activities have specific waveforms and characteristic sounds. Observations are made by the electromyographer during the study; therefore the results of a needle examination are dependent on the experience of the examiner.

Insertion activity, also referred to as injury potential, is caused by movement of the needle electrode, resulting in mechanical damage to the muscle fibers. Increased insertion activity consists of unsustained fibrillation potentials and positive sharp waves. A muscle at rest should be electrically silent. Spontaneous activity in a resting muscle usually suggests a pathologic condition. The type and significance of various spontaneous activities are summarized in Table 8.1, and some examples are shown in Fig. 8.3.

As a muscle contracts, motor unit action potentials (MUAPs) are observed. MUAP represents the summation of muscle fiber action potentials of a given motor unit. With increasing voluntary muscle contraction, individual motor units fire more frequently, and more motor units are recruited to fire. The term *onset frequency* is used to describe the firing rate of a single MUAP maintained at the lowest voluntary muscle contraction (normally less than 10 Hz). Recruitment frequency is defined as the frequency of first MUAP when second MUAP is recruited (normally less than 15 Hz). Reduced number of MUAP (high recruitment frequency) can be seen in neuropathic processes. An increased number of MUAP (low recruitment frequency), however, can be seen in myopathic disorder or defect of neuromuscular junction. During maximum contraction, a full interference pattern consisting of overlapping motor units is seen. MUAPs are analyzed in terms of amplitude, duration, number of phases, and stability. The morphology of the MUAPs is affected by the type of needle electrode used, location of the needle within the motor unit territory, age, temperature, and specific muscle being examined. Large, long duration polyphasic units suggest denervation and re-innervation. Short-duration, small polyphasic units can be seen in myopathic processes. EMG

TABLE 8.1 Potentials Recorded in the Muscle at Rest

Spontaneous Activity	Firing Pattern	Frequency	Waveform	Amplitude	Duration	Significance
Complex repetitive discharge	Regular, abrupt onset and cessation, "motor cycle idling"	5–100 Hz	Polyphasic or serrated, MFAP	100 μV–1 mV	—	Neurogenic (chronic), myopathic (dystrophy)
Cramp discharge	Increase and subside gradually	(1) <150 Hz (2) 4–15 Hz	MUAP	—	—	(1) Ischemic, ↑ Na, (2) ↓ Ca, ↓ Mg, ↑ K
End plate noise	Dense and steady, "sea shell" "hissing"	>150 Hz	Monophasic (negative), MEPP	10–20 μV	0.5–1 ms	Normal
End plate spike	Irregular short burst, "sputtering fat in a frying pan"	50–100 Hz	Biphasic (negative-positive) MFAP	100–300 μV	2–4 ms	Decrease in denervated muscle, increase in reinnervated muscle
Fasciculation potential	Spontaneous, sporadic, "typing on card board"	0.1–10 Hz	MUAP	>1 mv	>5 ms	Normal, neurogenic (motor neuronopathy), myopathic
Fibrillation potential	Regular, "rain on tin roof" "ticking of clock"	1–50 Hz	Biphasic (positive-negative) MFAP	<1 mV	<5 ms	Neurogenic, NMJ defect, myopathic
Myokymic discharge	Semiregular, "marching soldiers"	(1) 2–60 Hz brief (2) 1–5 Hz continuous	MUAP	—	—	Limb (entrapment, radiation), face (MS, brainstem tumor, Bell palsy)
Myotonic discharge	Wax and wane, "dive bomber"	20–80 Hz	(1) Biphasic (positive-negative) (2) Positive MFAP	<1 mV <1 mV	(1) <5 ms (2) 5–20 ms	Myopathic (myotonic syndromes), ↑K, Schwartz-Jampel
Neuromyotonic discharge	Start and stop abruptly, wane, "pinging"	150–300 Hz	MUAP	—	—	Isaac syndrome, stiff-man syndrome, tetany
Positive sharp wave	Regular	1–50 Hz	Biphasic (positive-negative) MFAP	<1 mV	10–100 ms	Same as fibrillation
Neurotonic discharge	Irregular	30–100 Hz	MUAP	—	<200 ms	—

MEPP, *Miniature end plate potential;* MFAP, *muscle fiber action potential;* MUAP, *motor unit action potential;* NMJ, *neuromuscular junction.*

findings in neuropathic and myopathic disorder are summarized in Table 8.2.

While performing an EMG/NCS, several questions must be answered by the examiner.

WHERE IS THE LESION? (LOCALIZATION)

EMG/NCS is very useful in localizing the specific anatomical site of a lesion that is causing pain. For example, a complaint of burning feet can be caused by a diffuse peripheral neuropathy (as in diabetes), by a plexus injury after surgery, or by a lumbosacral radiculopathy due to spinal stenosis. Each of these has different findings and can be localized by EMG/NCS. In general, changes in conduction, either a prolonged distal latency or a slow velocity, suggest a pathologic lesion between the site of stimulation and the recording site. Abnormally small amplitude, however, can occur from an injury anywhere distal to the motor or sensory neuron. A sampling on needle examination of muscles representing different nerves and roots can further localize the site of injury. Using the example of burning feet, let us examine the differential diagnosis and its EMG/NCS findings.

Peripheral Neuropathy: Nerve conduction velocity (NCV) can localize the peripheral neuropathy (classically distal symmetric) as well identify the underlying pathophysiology (axonal and/or demyelinating and motor and/or sensory involvement), which can aid the clinician in diagnosis of the underlying etiology. NCV can also assist with severity (higher degree of motor/axonal involvement and presence of abnormalities in the hand usually signify a more severe process). Needle findings would depend on the severity of motor nerve involvement, are seen in distal muscles before proximal muscles, and are usually normal unless the neuropathy is severe.

Median Mononeuropathy at the Wrist: NCS are useful to localize the abnormality to a specific nerve (median) and to the specific location (wrist). In CTS (carpal tunnel syndrome), the underlying pathophysiology is demyelination

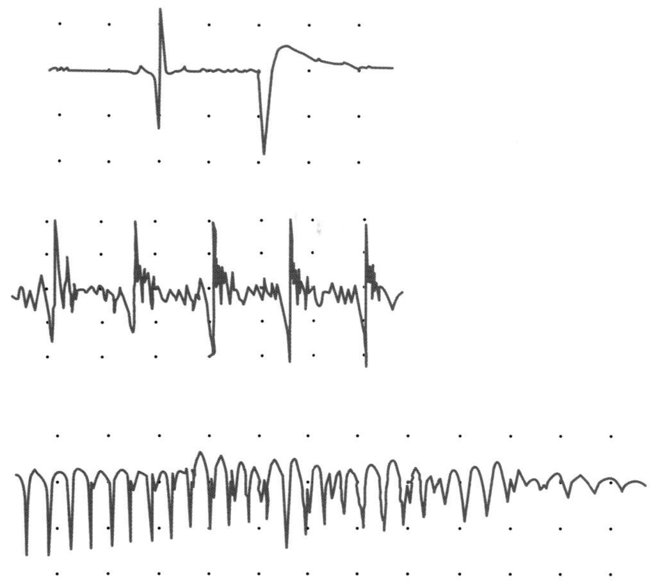

FIG. 8.3 Spontaneous activities. Fibrillation potential and positive wave *(top panel)*, and complex repetitive discharges *(middle panel)*; time marker 10 ms; amplitude marker 100 μv. Myotonic discharges *(bottom panel)*; time marker 20 ms; amplitude marker 200 μv.

TABLE 8.2 EMG Findings in Neurogenic and Myopathic Disorders

EMG	Normal	Neurogenic (Axonal)	NMJ Defect	Myopathic
Insertional activity	N	↑	↑	↑
Spontaneous activity	—	+	+	+
MUAP amplitude	0.1–5 mV	↑	↓	↓
Duration	3–15 ms	↑	↓	↓
Phase	<5	↑	↑	↑
Stability	N	N	Variable	N
Recruitment	N	↓	N	↑

EMG, *Electromyography;* MUAP, *motor unit action potential;* N, *normal;* NMJ, *neuromuscular junction.*

that affects the sensory fibers first. A more severe process will involve the motor fibers and will lead to axonal changes. The combined sensory index described by Robinson can be used improve the sensitivity of diagnosing CTS via NCS.[3]

Radiculopathy: Sensory NCV are critical in localizing a lesion to the root level; the preganglionic location of the root injury means that SNAPs will be normal. This is critical in clinical interpretation of electrodiagnostic studies, because EMG/NCV can only detect radiculopathies that affect the motor fibers (radiculopathies that only cause pain/sensory findings therefore may have normal EMG findings). EMG can localize the lesion to a specific nerve root or roots. A typical pattern of abnormality includes changes in muscles from different peripheral nerves that are innervated by the same nerve root (i.e., L5 radiculopathy with abnormalities in the anterior tibialis and gluteus medius muscles). Paraspinal muscles are innervated by the dorsal rami and are typically abnormal. EMG abnormalities first appear in corresponding paraspinal muscles because of their proximity to the injury site. Abnormalities are next seen in the proximal and then distal muscles within the specific myotomal distribution of the injured nerve root.

Anatomic localization based on EMG/NCS is summarized in Table 8.3.

IS THE LESION AXONAL OR DEMYELINATING? (PATHOPHYSIOLOGY)

Based on the EMG/NCS findings, the distinction can be made with relative ease. If an injury occurs at the cell body or axon, axonal degeneration occurs resulting in low-amplitude CMAPs/SNAPs throughout the nerve being studied. If an injury is directed against the myelin, demyelination ensues resulting in slowed conduction velocity and prolonged latencies.

Conduction block, or a focal failure of transition of the nerve signal, is also seen in demyelinating processes. Another manifestation of focal demyelination can be temporal dispersion. The characteristics of conduction block and temporal dispersion have been described previously.

In the majority of peripheral neuropathy, both demyelination and axonal injury will occur; however, characterizing the primary pathological process is important to establish an etiology and to assess the extent of injury. Demyelinating neuropathies can be further divided into segmental (acquired) and uniform (hereditary) types. In the former, nonuniform slowing in individual myelinated nerve fibers results in conduction block and temporal dispersion. In the latter, prolonged latency and slowing of conduction predominate as a result of uniform involvement of all myelinated fibers. Table 8.4 summarizes the EMG/NCS characteristics of demyelinating and axonal injuries.

IS THE LESION MOTOR, SENSORY, OR AUTONOMIC? (FIBER TYPE SPECIFICITY)

NCS test motor and sensory components separately. Many peripheral nervous system diseases affect both motor and sensory nerves. In a case of distal sensory or motor neuropathies, amplitudes as well as velocities are abnormal. With a dorsal root ganglia lesion or anterior horn cell disease, NCS show small amplitude SNAP or CMAP, respectively, and as a rule normal velocity. Routine EMG/NCS do not test the integrity of the autonomic nervous system. Autonomic tests will be discussed separately.

IS THE LESION FOCAL, MULTIFOCAL, OR DIFFUSE? (DISTRIBUTION)

By determining the distribution of abnormalities, neuropathy for example can be further divided into mononeuropathy, multifocal neuropathy, and polyneuropathy. A focal lesion such as carpal tunnel syndrome will result in abnormalities limited to the distal segment of a median nerve. If the same nerve is affected disproportionately in the opposite limb or one nerve is affected more than the other in the same limb, a multifocal disorder is suggested. In a fully developed polyneuropathy, motor and sensory

TABLE 8.3 Anatomical Localization Based on the EMG and NCV Studies

Lesion	Motor Nerve Conduction	Sensory Nerve Conduction	RNS	EMG
Dorsal root ganglia (sensory neuronopathy)	N	N, ↓ amp	N	N
Anterior horn cell (motor neuronopathy)	N, ↓ amp	N	N/Abn	Abn
Root (radiculopathy)	N, ↓ amp	N	N	Abn
Plexus (plexopathy)	N, ↓ amp	N, ↓ amp	N	Abn
Nerve (neuropathy)	Abn	Abn	N	Abn
NMJ defect	N, ↓ amp	N	Abn	Abn
Muscle (myopathy)	N, ↓ amp	N	N/Abn	Abn

Abn, *Abnormal;* EMG, *electromyography;* N, *normal;* NCV, *nerve conduction velocity;* NMJ, *neuromuscular junction;* RNS, *repetitive nerve stimulation.*

TABLE 8.4 NCV and EMG Characteristics of the Demyelinating and Axonal Injuries

	NCV	EMG
Demyelination	1. Prolonged latency, more than 13% of normal 2. Slow NCV, less than 70% of normal 3. Conduction block 4. Temporal dispersion	1. Normal insertional activity, no spontaneous activity 2. Reduced recruitment with conduction block 3. Normal MUAP morphology
Axonal injury	1. Normal latency 2. Slow NCV, more than 70% of normal 3. Small CMAP/SNAP amplitude	1. Increased insertional activity, spontaneous activity 2. Reduced recruitment 3. Large amplitude, long duration polyphasics with reinnervation 4. Satellite potentials

CMAP, *Compound muscle action potential;* EMG, *Electromyography;* MUAP, *motor unit action potential;* NCV, *nerve conduction velocity;* SNAP, *sensory nerve action potential.*

nerves in both upper and lower extremities are affected in equal and symmetrical fashion; in milder cases, however, the abnormalities will be more significant in distal sensory nerves of the lower extremities (length dependent).

HOW OLD IS THE INJURY? (CHRONICITY)

Following an axonal injury, the nerve distal to the lesion undergoes Wallerian degeneration. For the first 2–3 days, motor conductions distal to a lesion will be normal. Then CMAP amplitude drops progressively, reaching a nadir at about 7 days. SNAP amplitudes distal to a lesion are unaffected for 5–6 days but by day 10–11, the nadir is reached. After an axonal motor nerve injury, EMG findings will change slowly. Initially, insertional activity is increased. Positive sharp waves and fibrillation potentials may not occur for 1–4 weeks following a nerve injury, depending on the length between site of nerve injury and corresponding muscles.[4] The abnormal spontaneous activity can resolve in 3–6 months. Therefore needle studies performed less than 1–4 weeks after injury, or later than 3–6 months after injury, may not detect positive sharp waves or fibrillations. Large-amplitude, long-duration polyphasic MUAPs seen in denervation and re-innervation develop 3–6 months after an injury. Table 8.5 summarizes the chronology of EMG/NCS findings after axonal injury.

HOW BAD IS THE INJURY? (SEVERITY AND PROGNOSIS)[3]

The severity of an injury can be determined if EMG/NCS is done in a timely manner. The amplitude of CMAP and/or SNAP difference between the same nerve on affected and unaffected sides gives an idea of extent of injury and potential recovery if they are determined sequentially. A paucity of spontaneous activity in affected muscles 4 weeks after injury indicates an excellent outcome for the return of muscle function. Markedly reduced recruitment of MUAPs indicates severe lesion except for neurapraxia. In general, axonal injury has a worse prognosis than demyelinating disorders.

QUANTITATIVE SENSORY TESTING[5]

The test provides a quantitative measure to detect large and small fiber dysfunction. Various stimuli at varying intensities are applied to the skin, and a patient is asked to indicate when he or she begins to feel the stimulus. A consensus report defines "sensory detection threshold" as "the smallest stimulus that can be detected at least 50% of the time." By increasing and decreasing stimulus intensity from the predetermined level, "appearance" and "disappearance" thresholds can be determined. Sensory modalities commonly used are vibration and thermal senses—warm, cold, heat pain, and cold pain (Fig. 8.4). Vibration threshold measures large myelinated fiber function, whereas warm, heat pain and cold pain thresholds reflect the function of unmyelinated C fibers. Cold threshold measures small myelinated Aδ fiber function.

QST measures not only peripheral nerve fiber function but also central pathway function. Vibratory sense is carried by the dorsal columns and thermal senses via the spinothalamic tract. Normal values depend on methodology, sensory modality tested, and site of test. Sensory detection threshold increases with age; therefore results should be compared with the age-matched reference values.

TABLE 8.5 Chronology of the NCV and EMG Findings Following Axonal Injury

	NCV	EMG
0–1 week	↓ Amp, proximal	↓ Recruitment
1–2 weeks	↓ Amp, proximal and distal	↓ Recruitment ↑ Insertional activity
2–3 weeks	↓ Amp, proximal and distal	↓ Recruitment ↑ Fibrillation potentials
1–3 months	↑ Amp	↓ Fibrillation potentials ↓ Amp, ↑ duration, ↑ phase
3–6 months	↑ Amp	↑ Recruitment ↑ Amp, ↑ duration, ↑ phase

EMG, *Electromyography;* NCV, *nerve conduction velocity.*

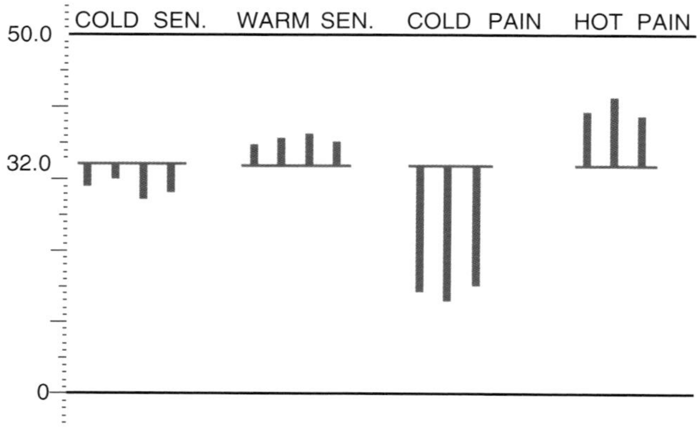

FIG. 8.4 Example of a thermal quantitative sensory testing in a normal subject. Temperature, in degrees centigrade, on vertical scale. *Solid bar* represents each trial. *SEN,* Sensation.

QST can be used to detect subtle sensory changes that may be missed by NCS. Increased or decreased thermal detection threshold (hypoesthesia or hyperesthesia) and thermal pain threshold (hypoalgesia or hyperalgesia) have been reported in many painful neuropathies. Cold or heat hyperalgesia is a feature of RSD. Heat hyperalgesia is common in erythromeralgia, and *a*ngry *b*ackfiring *C* nociceptor (or ABC) syndrome. *C*old hypoesthesia, *c*old hyperalgesia, and *c*old limb are features of the CCC syndrome, whereas thermal hypoesthesia and hyperalgesia (anesthesia dolorosa) are typical manifestations of postherpetic neuralgia.

QST allows early detection of disease. Sequential testing can be used to monitor disease progression and therapeutic efficacy. However, QST is not objective and relies on patient cooperation. QST does not localize a lesion, as it tests the integrity of the entire sensory pathway from nerve ending to cortex.

SHORT LATENCY SOMATOSENSORY EVOKED POTENTIALS[6,7]

Conventional sensory NCS assess a lesion distal to the dorsal root ganglion. SSEPs provide a quantitative measure to study the entire sensory pathway. Typically a mixed nerve, such as median nerve at the wrist or tibial nerve at the ankle, is repeatedly stimulated and responses are recorded along the sensory pathway. Those responses are averaged to improve signal-to-noise ratio. Stimulations of the skin within a dermatome or cutaneous nerve, such as superficial radial or sural nerve, have more limited value because of the low amplitude response. Increased intensity and longer duration of stimulus are required to elicit an optimal response.

Stimulations are mediated by group Ia and II sensory afferents; dorsal root ganglion (neuron I); dorsal columns, gracilis, and cuneatus nuclei (neuron II); contralateral medial lemniscus; ventroposterolateral nucleus of the thalamus (neuron III); and sensory cortex. Clinically, touch-pressure, position-movement senses are affected with the injury to the dorsal column pathway in both the central and peripheral nervous system. Each identifiable component is labeled according to its polarity (negative or positive) and its mean peak latency (in millisecond) following stimulation. Useful obligate potentials after median nerve stimulation include EP (Erb's point), N13 (dorsal column of the cervical cord), P14 (caudal medial lemniscus), N18 (thalamus), and N20 (sensory cortex). Identifiable potentials after tibial nerve stimulation are PF (popliteal fossa), LP (lumbar potential), P31 (caudal medial lemniscus), N34 (thalamus), and P37 (sensory cortex; Fig. 8.5). Knowledge of the generator source of these peaks allows us to localize lesions to parts of the pathway. Age, temperature, limb length, medications, level of attention, and sleep may alter latency and amplitude. Therefore every laboratory has its own normal values. Adult norms are reached at about 8 years of age. Criteria for abnormality include absence of any obligate waves and prolongation of interpeak intervals. For example, absence of N18, N20, or a prolonged P14-N20 interval suggests a lesion between the medulla and sensory cortex. Table 8.6 summarizes some typical SSEP findings and resulting localization. Absolute latency is a less reliable indicator of abnormality because it varies with limb length. A side-to-side amplitude ratio less than half is considered abnormal by some. Application of SSEPs for a patient with pain is limited to the identification of a potential structural or compressive lesion involving peripheral or central sensory pathway.

LASER EVOKED POTENTIALS AND CONTACT HEAT EVOKED POTENTIALS[7,8]

A CO_2 laser can be used to generate pain-related cerebral potentials. Laser stimulator produces radiant heat quickly and activates Aδ and C nociceptors. Twenty to 40 stimuli are delivered at the intervals of 6–10 seconds. Late component, which occurs at approximately 220–340 ms following stimulation of the hand, corresponds to Aδ fiber conduction, and ultra-late component at 800–1000 ms corresponds to C fiber; both components are maximum in amplitude (10–50 μV) at the vertex (C_Z). LEPs provide an objective measure to assess the function of pain and temperature pathways in patients with neuropathic pain. In a lesion involving the spinothalamic tract, including small fiber neuropathy, SSEPs are usually normal but LEPs are abnormal. LEPs are not yet available in most electrophysiological laboratories, because it is technically difficult to

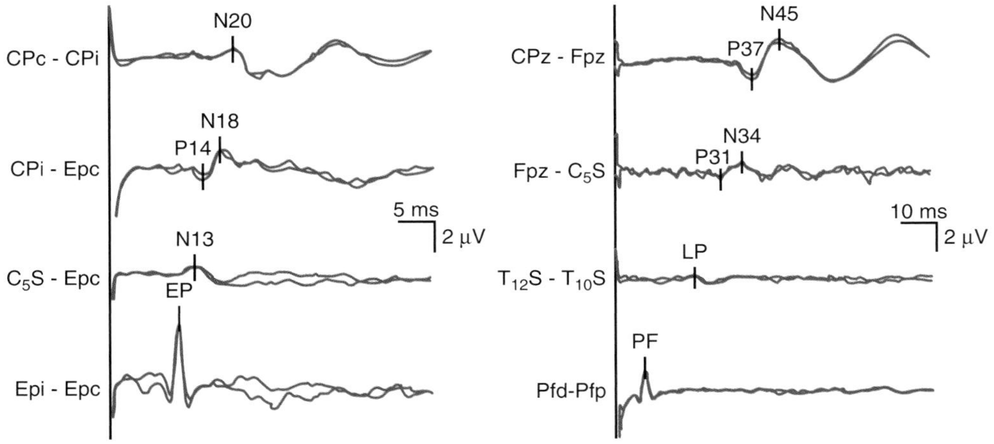

FIG. 8.5 Median *(left)* and tibial *(right)* somatosensory evoked potentials in a normal subject. *CPc,* Contralateral central-parietal; *CPi,* ipsilateral central-parietal; *CPz,* midline central-parietal; *CS,* cervical spine; *EP,* Erb's potential; *EPc,* contralateral Erb's point; *EPi,* ipsilateral Erb's point; *Fpz,* midline frontopolar; *LP,* lumbar potential; *TS,* thoracic spine; *PF,* popliteal fossa; *Pfd,* popliteal fossa, distal; *Pfp,* popliteal fossa, proximal.

TABLE 8.6 Localization by SSEP

SSEPs	Abnormality	Lesion
Median nerve	1. Absent EP	Median nerve—brachial plexus
	P14	Above plexus
	N20	Above medulla
	2. Prolonged EP—P14	Brachial plexus—medulla
	P14—N20	Medulla—sensory cortex
Tibial nerve	1. Absent LP	Tibial nerve—cauda equina
	P37	Above lumbar spinal cord
	2. Prolonged LP—P37	Spinal cord—sensory cortex

EP, *Erb's potential;* LP, *lumbar potential;* SSEPs, *somatosensory evoked potentials.*

perform and causes skin burns and pigmentation. However, recent advances in technology enable us to use natural heat, which goes up quickly at the rate of 50°C/s (CHEPs). Latencies and amplitudes are comparable to those of LEPs. They are easy to perform and cause no side effects. Therefore this testing will eventually become a standard method to assess nociceptive dysfunction.

SYMPATHETIC SKIN RESPONSE[9]

The first report of the galvanic skin response appeared in 1890. Since then, various terminology has been introduced on the basis of different stimulating and recording methods (e.g., electrodermal activity, SSR, peripheral autonomic surface potential, and psychogalvanic reflex). A standard method of obtaining SSR is to place a recording electrode on the palmar and plantar surface, because these recording sites yield higher amplitudes. A stimulator is placed on the median and the tibial nerves of the opposite limb, and the stimulus is given randomly at a rate of no less than one per minute, and with a stimulus intensity that is sufficient to cause mild pain. A minimum of 5–10 responses should be recorded, and SSR responses are obtainable 60%–100% of the time in normal subjects.

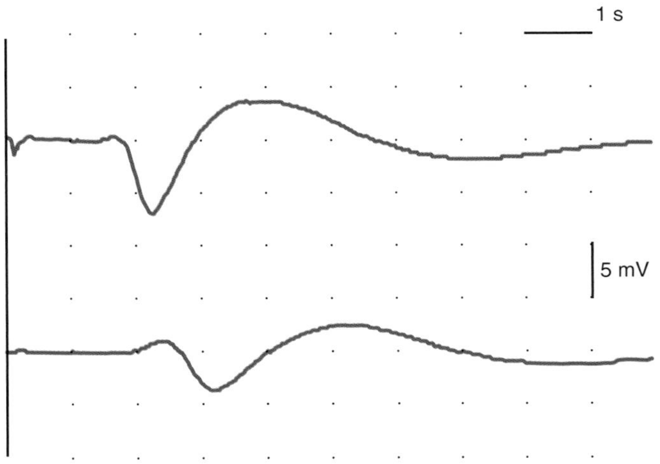

FIG. 8.6 Normal sympathetic skin response recorded simultaneously from the palm of the hand *(top)* and sole of the foot *(bottom)* by electrical stimulation.

Waveforms are usually triphasic, with an initial small negativity followed by a large positive wave, and a subsequent prolonged negative wave (Fig. 8.6). Waveforms can also be monophasic or diphasic with an initial negative or positive peak. Maximal peak-to-peak amplitudes and mean latencies are measured. Amplitude and latency variability can be minimized by reducing stimulus frequency, increasing stimulus intensity, and/or changing stimulus site or mode. Low skin temperature, low level of attention, medication (especially anticholinergics), age, and habituation will also attenuate the response. Normal amplitude is more than 1 mV for hand, and more than 0.2 mV for foot. Mean palmar latency is 1.4 ± 0.1 second and plantar latency is 1.9 ± 0.1 second. SSR measures change of epidermal resistance due to sweat gland activity. The somatic afferent limb depends on the stimulus type (electrical shock, loud noise, visual threat, deep breathing); with the electrical stimulation, the afferent limb occurs via large myelinated fibers. The efferent limb is a sympathetic pathway, originating in the posterior hypothalamus, descending through the spinal cord to the intermediolateral cell column (T1–L2) and paravertebral ganglia, and then to the sweat gland via small unmyelinated fibers. Therefore it is important to note that neuropathy affecting large myelinated fibers exhibits abnormal SSR when electrical stimulation is used.

Low amplitude or absent response indicates abnormal sympathetic reflex arc, and the lesion can be central or peripheral, preganglionic or postganglionic. A side-to-side amplitude difference of more than 50% is considered to be abnormal by some. In studies of diabetic, uremic, and amyloid neuropathies, the result of SSR correlated well with autonomic symptoms. As a rule, SSR is abnormal in axonal neuropathies. An exception is the demyelinating neuropathy with prominent autonomic features, such as Guillain-Barré syndrome. Some studies have reported abnormal SSR test results in patients with CRPS/RSD, and others have not. Immediately following the sympathetic nerve block or sympathectomy, SSR is absent or reduced in amplitude. The SSR is usually normal in entrapment neuropathy, and radiculopathy. SSR evoked by magnetic stimulation in the neck bypasses the afferent limb and directly stimulates postganglionic fibers. This method has less propensity to habituate, and therefore less fluctuation of amplitude and latency occurs.

QUANTITATIVE SWEAT TEST[10]

This is a sensitive, reproducible, and quantitative method to test sudomotor function. A multicompartment plastic "sweat cell" is tightly secured to the skin. The outer compartment is filled with acetylcholine solution, and dry air flows constantly to an inner compartment through an instrument that measures the change of humidity (sudorometer). A direct current is applied, and the water content in the inner compartment is continuously measured before, during, and after the stimulus. The basis of the test is that the axon terminal of the sweat gland under the outer compartment is activated by acetylcholine iontophoresis; the impulse travels centripetally to a branch point and then distally to the axon terminal under the inner compartment, where acetylcholine is released and a sweating response results. Use of the term "axon reflex" should be discouraged, because only the postganglionic sympathetic sudomotor axon is considered to be involved in this setup. With a latency of 1–2 minutes after the induction of the stimulus, sweat output increases rapidly while stimulation continues; then the stimulator is turned off, and sweat output returns to its prestimulus baseline within 5 minutes (Fig. 8.7). The area under the curve represents the total amount of sweat output expressed in microliter per square centimeter, and the normal value varies depending on the site of testing, gender, and age of the subject. Distal limbs, males, and younger subjects tend to sweat more. Reduced or absent response indicates postganglionic disorder. Normal response does not rule out preganglionic involvement. Excessive and persistent sweating is also considered abnormal. Comparison is made between the two limbs, and an asymmetry of more than 25% is considered to be abnormal.

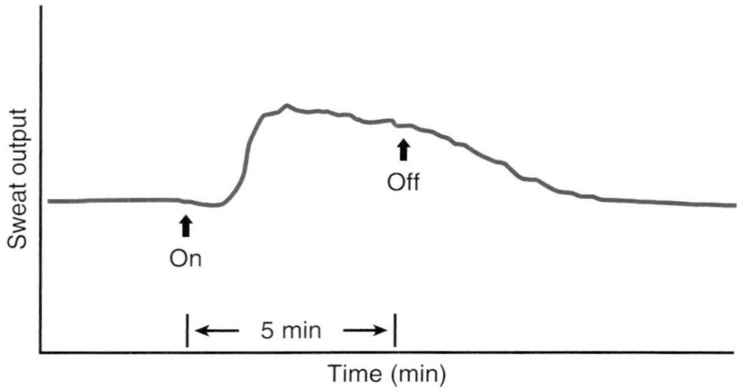

FIG. 8.7 Example of a normal quantitative sudomotor axon reflex test. On, off, stimulator on and off.

Sweat test abnormalities correlate well with the symptoms of CRPS/RSD-related pain, for which the pathophysiologic mechanism is uncertain; perhaps a lower firing threshold, or an increased firing frequency due to denervation hypersensitivity of the sudomotor axons, may produce excitation of the sweat glands.

NOCICEPTIVE REFLEXES[8,11]

Brink reflex is recorded by electrically stimulating the supraorbital branch of the trigeminal nerve. Ipsilateral R1 (10–13 ms) and bilateral R2 potentials (30–41 ms) are obtained from the orbicularis oculi muscles. The MIR is recorded from the masseter muscles bilaterally with stimulation of the mentalis nerve, while the muscle is fully activated by clenching teeth. Ongoing EMG activity is interrupted by two silent periods—early phase with a latency of 10–15 ms and late phase with 40–50 ms. These trigeminal reflexes have been reported normal in tic douloureux, but abnormal in facial pain due to neuropathy, multiple sclerosis, cerebellopontine angle tumor, and so on. However, its afferent path is at least in part mediated by nonnociceptive fibers. Flexion reflex or withdrawal reflex is obtained by painful stimulation of a nerve or skin. RIII flexion reflex (80–90 ms) recorded from the short head of biceps femoris by stimulating the sural nerve has been found useful to assess efficacy of pain medications.

ULTRASONOGRAPHY AS A COMPLEMENTARY TECHNIQUE[12,13]

Due to improvements in technology, increase in physician training, and excellent safety profile, diagnostic ultrasound is being used more frequently in the workup of neuromusculoskeletal pathology. It can be used to directly image muscle and nerve, and has a role in localization of nerve entrapment. It may also have a role as a complimentary technique in EMG/NCV. Ultrasound can theoretically be used to localize the nerve in cases of difficult anatomy such as obesity, history of surgical nerve transposition, or technically challenging NCV. Ultrasound can also assist with accurate muscle localization in deeper muscles, in patients with obesity, in patients who are unresponsive or uncooperative, in muscles that travel near vascular structures, and to assess muscles near the lungs or abdominal organs.

KEY POINTS

- Electrophysiological studies are a very sensitive indicator of central and peripheral nervous system involvement but do not indicate underlying disease.
- EMG/NCS studies can identify the anatomic site of injury, the type of neurons or fibers involved, the nature of the pathologic alteration, and severity of injury.
- In QST, cold threshold measures Aδ fiber function, whereas warm, heat pain, and cold pain thresholds reflect the function of C fibers.
- SSEPs provide a quantitative measure to study the entire sensory pathway, mediated by type Ia and II sensory afferents.
- LEPs and CHEPs measure the function of Aδ and C fibers. CHEPs have a potential to become a standard neurophysiologic method.
- SSR and quantitative sweat test have a limited role but are useful for the evaluation of painful diabetic neuropathy or CRPS/RSD.
- Nociceptive reflexes have an extremely limited role.

REFERENCES

Access the reference list online at ExpertConsult.com.

CHAPTER 9

Anatomy, Imaging, and Common Pain-Generating Degenerative Pathologies of the Spine

Benjamin P. Liu, MD ◦ Matthew T. Walker, MD ◦ Eric M. Spitzer, MD ◦ Murugusundaram Veeramani, MBBS ◦ Eric J. Russell, MD, FACR, FSIR

ANATOMY

OSSEOUS SPINAL COLUMN

The spinal column is typically composed of 7 cervical, 12 thoracic, 5 lumbar, and 5 fused sacral segments. The terminal portion of the osseous spinal column, the coccygeal segments, varies in number, but four segments can typically be visualized. The morphology of the individual vertebrae is quite consistent throughout, except for the first two cervical segments (C1 and C2) and the sacrococcygeal levels.

The C1 level, commonly referred to as the atlas, comprises an anterior arch, posterior arch, and paired lateral masses (Fig. 9.1A). The lateral masses articulate with the occipital condyles superiorly and the body of C2 inferiorly (see Fig. 9.1B). C1 does not have a vertebral body, and it is not separated from adjacent levels by an intervertebral disc. The C2 vertebra, commonly referred to as the axis, has some of the typical features of the remainder of the vertebral segments but is unique in having a superior extension of bone from the vertebral body that articulates with the dorsal margin of the anterior arch of C1: This bony projection is called the odontoid process or dens and allows for head rotation (see Fig. 9.1B). Unique to the segments from C3 through C7 are the uncinate processes that arise from the dorsolateral margins of the superior end plates of the vertebral bodies and articulate with the level above (Fig. 9.2).[1]

The typical cervical, thoracic, and lumbar vertebrae consist of an anterior body, paired pedicles, articular pillars and laminae, and a single dorsal midline spinous process (Fig. 9.3). The pedicles attach the body to the posterior neural elements. The articular pillars are composed of the pars interarticularis and the superior and inferior articular processes. Each level from C3 to L5 has superior and inferior articular processes that serve as the main posterior contact between adjacent levels. The surface of the superior articular process is the inferior facet of the associated zygapophyseal joint, and the surface of the inferior articular process is the superior facet of the joint. The "superior processes" at C1 and C2 and the "inferior process" at C1 are more descriptively referred to as articular surfaces, as they do not have a true morphologic extension away from the vertebral segments. The two laminae extend dorsomedially and connect to form the root of the spinous process. The spinous process projects dorsally and serves as an attachment point for the posterior ligamentous structures. The pedicles, articular pillars, and lamina serve to enclose and protect the spinal canal and contents, particularly the spinal cord and nerve roots. Transverse processes vary in size from short in the cervical spine to long in the lumbar spine. In the mid-cervical spine, the transverse processes help to enclose and form the osseous transverse foramina that transmit the vertebral artery and contents. In the thoracic and lumbar spine, the transverse processes serve as anchoring points for the muscles that help to stabilize and protect the spinal column and its contents.

JOINTS

Six specific types of synovial joints exist from the skull base to the lumbosacral junction, including the atlanto-occipital, atlantoaxial, uncovertebral, costovertebral, costotransverse, and zygapophyseal (facet) joints.[2] The atlanto-occipital joint is formed by the bilateral inferiorly convex occipital condyles and the bilateral concave superior articular surfaces of the C1 lateral masses (see Fig. 9.1B). The main atlantoaxial joint is formed by the inferior articular surfaces of C1 and the superior articular surfaces of C2 (see Fig. 9.1B). A true synovial-lined joint also exists between the ventral dens and the dorsal surface of the C1 anterior arch and the dorsal aspect of the dens and the posterior ligamentous structures. The uncovertebral joints (joints of Luschka) exist only in the cervical spine below C2. The osseous uncinate processes arise from the dorsolateral margin of the superior end plates of the C3–C7 vertebral bodies and articulate with the level above: uncovertebral joints therefore exist from C2–C3 to C6–C7 (see Fig. 9.2). The joints of Luschka have features of both cartilaginous and synovial joints, and when degenerated, they can result in foraminal stenosis and even central stenosis.[1,3] As their names imply, the costovertebral and costotransverse joints are articulations between the ribs (costo-) and the vertebral bodies or transverse processes of the thoracic spine (Fig. 9.4).

The facet joints are the most prevalent joint in the spinal column and are formed by the inferior and superior articular processes of adjacent vertebral bodies. The facet surfaces (named relative to the joint space as described below) are covered with articular cartilage that allows for bending motion and offers some protection to shearing forces. The joints are encapsulated by a true synovial lining and loose capsular ligaments.[4] In the cervical spine, there is a thick fibrous capsule laterally under which a small synovial recess may protrude. In the lumbar spine, a thick fibrous capsule is present

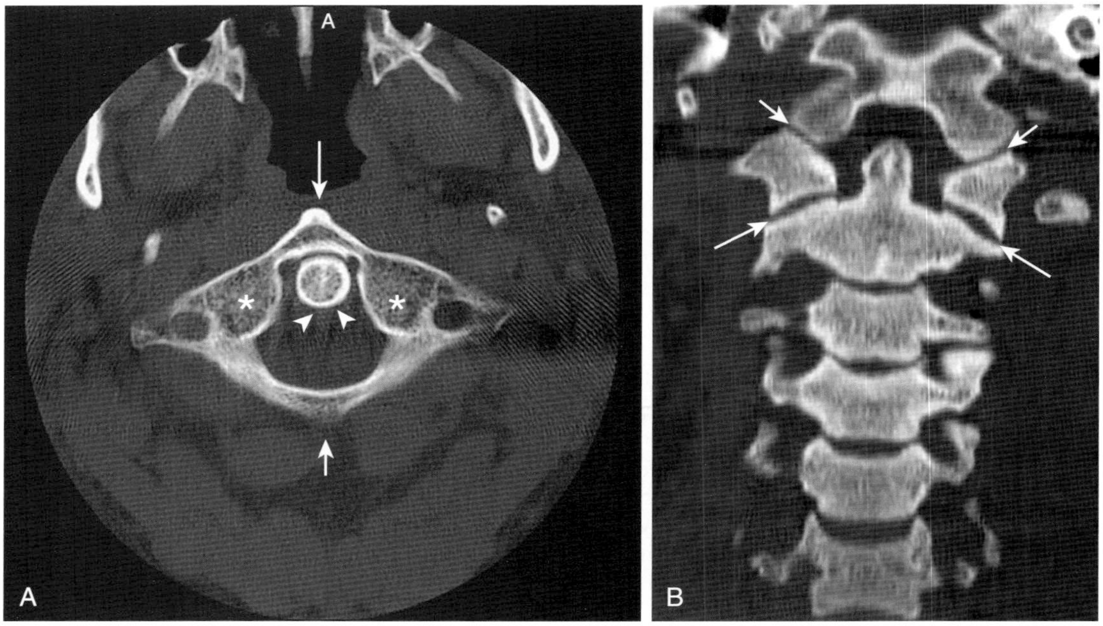

FIG. 9.1 (A) Axial computed tomography (CT) image through the atlas shows the anterior arch *(long arrow)*, posterior arch *(short arrow)*, and paired lateral masses *(asterisks)*. The tip of the odontoid process *(arrowheads)* articulates with the anterior arch of C1. (B) Coronal CT reconstruction through the cervical spine demonstrates the articulations between the occipital condyles and the lateral masses of C1 (atlanto-occipital joints, *small arrows*). Also, note the atlantoaxial joints *(long arrows)* between the lateral masses of C1 and the body of C2.

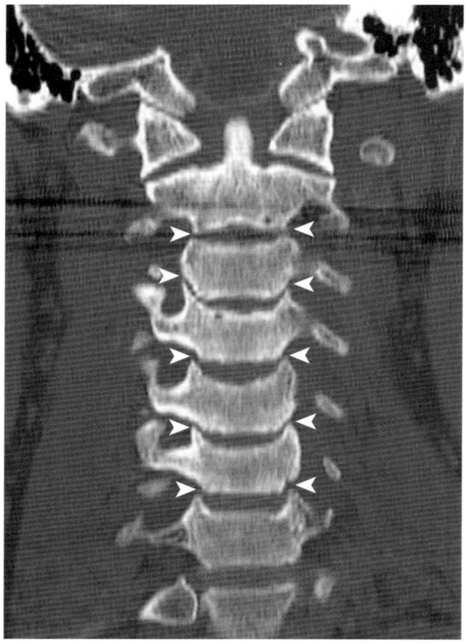

FIG. 9.2 Coronal computed tomography reconstruction through the cervical spine profiles the uncinate processes and uncovertebral joints *(arrowheads)*.

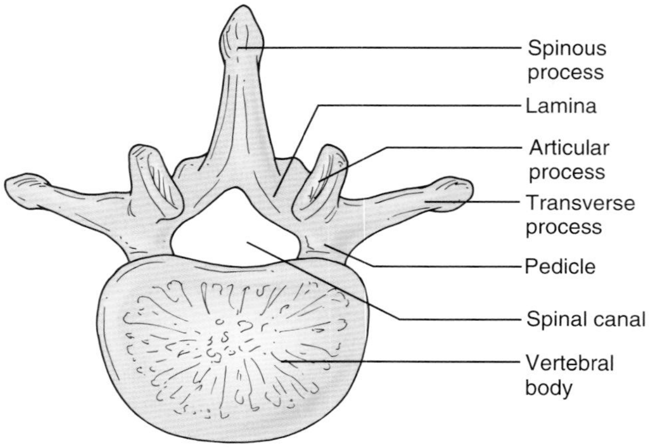

FIG. 9.3 Axial diagram of a typical vertebral body.

along the posterior margin of the facet joint. The inferior synovial recess occurs at the caudal extent of this capsule and is the common location for access to the joint space.[5,6] A complete discussion of the innervation of the facet joints is beyond the scope of this chapter. In general, the facet joints are dually innervated from paired medial branches of the dorsal primary rami.[7,8] This dual innervation explains why complete denervation of a symptomatic facet joint requires treatment of both medial branches. Knowledge of the different facet joint orientations is important when planning facet joint interventions. The cervical facet joints are obliquely oriented from superior to posterior with a ventral to dorsal angle when viewed in the sagittal plane (Fig. 9.5A). The thoracic facet joints are oriented in the coronal plane limiting access for percutaneous procedures (see Fig. 9.5B). The lumbar facet joints have a lunate configuration with the posterior margin oriented in the oblique sagittal plane and the anterior margin oriented in the oblique coronal plane (see Fig. 9.5C). Access to the joint under fluoroscopy is accomplished from a shallow oblique sagittal projection.[9]

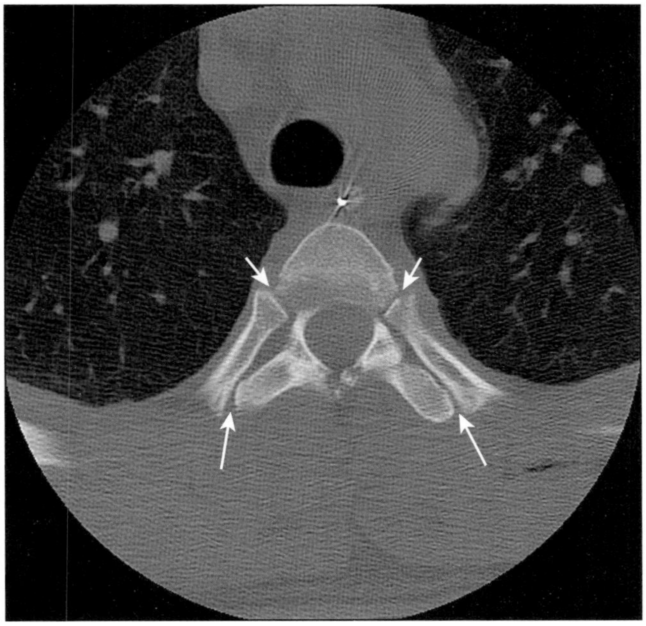

FIG. 9.4 Axial computed tomography image through the mid-thoracic spine identifies the costotransverse *(long arrows)* and costovertebral joints *(short arrows)*.

TRANSVERSE FORAMEN, INTERVERTEBRAL FORAMEN, AND NERVE ROOTS

The transverse foramen, also known as the vertebral foramen or foramen transversarium, occurs in the cervical spine from C1 to C7. The transverse foramina develop when the neural processes posteriorly fuse with the vestigial costal element anteriorly.[10,11] The contents of the transverse foramina include the vertebral artery, vertebral venous plexus, fibers of the sympathetic chain, and fat. Typically round or oval, these foramina vary in size and shape and often reflect the underlying size of the traversing vertebral artery.[12] The vertebral artery typically enters the foramen at C6, but it can enter as high as C3. In the sagittal view, the vertebral artery is a few millimeters ventral to the adjacent exiting nerve root (Fig. 9.6).

In the cervical spine, the intervertebral foramen runs obliquely anterolaterally. It is bounded by the pedicles, uncinate process, vertebral body, and superior articular facet. The exiting cervical nerves are positioned posteroinferiorly in the intervertebral foramina (see Fig. 9.6). Small foraminal veins connecting the epidural venous plexus and the anterior longitudinal intraspinal venous channels with the perivertebral venous plexus within the transverse foramina traverse the intervertebral foramen (Fig. 9.7).[13] There are eight paired cervical nerve roots, the first exiting the spinal canal between the skull base and C1. Therefore, in the cervical spine, the number of the nerve root passing through the foramen is one greater than the number of the pedicle that it passes beneath. For example, the nerve root passing through the intervertebral foramen at C3–C4 is the C4 nerve root.

The thoracic spine intervertebral foramina are rather constant, bounded by the pedicles, vertebral body, disc, and superior articular process of the vertebra below. The thoracic spinal nerves are more closely associated with the superiorly positioned articular process compared to the cervical spine. Small veins run through the intervertebral foramina as in the cervical spine. The exiting nerve roots are designated by the pedicle under which they immediately course. For example, at the T8–T9 level, the T8 spinal nerve root exits.

Much like the thoracic spine, the lumbar spine intervertebral foramina are bounded by the pedicles, vertebral body, disc, and superior articular process. The spinal nerve roots exit at a 45-degree angle inferolaterally and are closely associated with the medial and inferior margins of the pedicle under which they exit (Fig. 9.8). The spinal nerve roots are numbered as in the thoracic spine; the numbered root exits below the same numbered pedicle. For example, at the L4–L5 level, the L4 spinal nerve exits.

Throughout the spine, the exiting nerve roots are composed of a smaller, ventral motor root and a larger, dorsal sensory root. The dorsal root contains a ganglion that can range in size from 5 to 15 mm.[14] This dorsal root ganglion (DRG) lies within the intervertebral foramen and is most apparent in the lumbar and sacral spine. Small arterial branches from the lumbar arteries supply the DRG and have a fenestrated capillary endothelium. This anatomic configuration results in normal enhancement of the DRG on contrast examinations (see Figs. 9.8 and 9.9).[15]

When contemplating a transforaminal or periganglionic intervention in the thoracolumbar region, one must consider the potential complication resulting from damage to the artery of the lumbar enlargement (artery of Adamkiewicz).[16] This artery is the primary supply to the lower two-thirds of the spinal cord and enters the spinal canal via an intervertebral foramen. Although it typically enters on the left from T9–L1, the artery of Adamkiewicz can enter on either side from T5–L4. The artery usually runs in the more superior and ventral aspect of the foramen (Fig. 9.10).[17] Techniques to improve the safety of epidural steroid injections have been recently described.[16]

INTERVERTEBRAL DISCS

Intervertebral discs separate the vertebral bodies and contribute a significant proportion (20%–35%) of the height to the spinal column. The discs are thicker in the cervical and lumbar regions and thicker anteriorly than posteriorly, contributing to the lordotic curvatures of the spine in these regions. The primary function of the disc is to absorb the impact of daily axial loading and confer some flexibility. Discs are composed of three main components: the nucleus pulposus, annulus fibrosis, and the cartilaginous end plate.[18,19] The nucleus pulposus contains type II collagen, hyaluronic acid, and glycosaminoglycans. This composition confers excellent compressive resistance and, when hydrated, has characteristic imaging findings on magnetic resonance imaging (MRI). The annulus fibrosis consists of an outer dense circumferential fibrous band and an inner fibrocartilaginous layer. The outer layer fibers, also known as Sharpey fibers, insert into the ring apophyses. The cartilaginous end plate is composed of hyaline cartilage that tightly adheres to the vertebral end plate. Vascular supply to the disc is primarily via small nutrient channels through this cartilaginous end plate.[20,21]

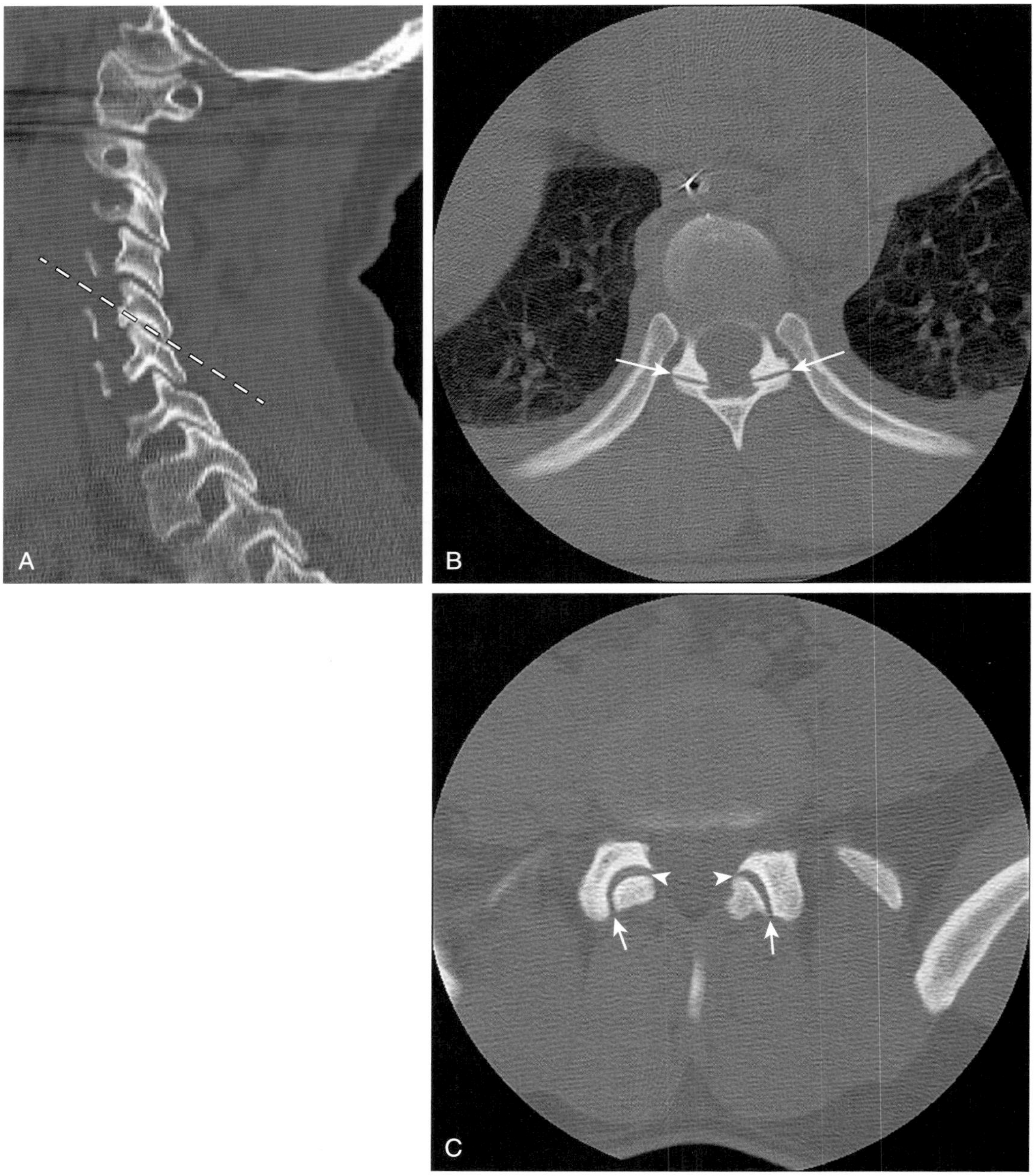

FIG. 9.5 (A) Sagittal computed tomography (CT) reconstruction of the cervical spine. Note the oblique orientation of the cervical facet joints *(dashed line)*. There are several approaches to the cervical facets including anterolateral, direct lateral, and posterolateral obliquities. (B) Axial CT image through the midthoracic spine. The facet joints *(arrows)* are oriented in the oblique coronal plane. Safe and reliable access to these joints is best achieved under CT guidance. (C) Axial CT image through the mid-lumbar spine. Note the lunate configuration of these facet joints. With the patient in the prone position, a shallow oblique projection profiles the dorsal margin *(arrows)* of the joint space, thus allowing safe access to the joint. A steeper oblique projection profiles the ventral component *(arrowheads)* of the joint space, but access to the joint is impeded by the intervening articular process.

LIGAMENTS

Ligaments of the spine provide stability while allowing flexion, extension, and rotation. There are five main ligamentous structures throughout the spinal column: anterior longitudinal ligament (ALL), posterior longitudinal ligament (PLL), ligamentum flavum, interspinous ligaments, and supraspinous ligament. The ALL and PLL run along the anterior and posterior margins of the vertebral bodies, respectively (Fig. 9.11).[22] The ALL adheres to the vertebral body and intervertebral discs. The PLL adheres to the annulus fibrosis of the disc but does not contact the posterior vertebral margin to any significant degree. The ligamentum flavum runs along the length of the spinal canal extending between adjacent laminar segments and defining the dorsolateral margins of the spinal canal. The interspinous ligaments run between adjacent spinous processes, whereas the supraspinous ligament runs along the tips of the spinous processes.

Specialized ligaments are present at the craniocervical junction, including the atlanto-occipital ligament, apical ligament, tectorial membrane, and the cruciate ligaments that form the transverse ligament.[23] These ligaments provide stability and flexibility at the craniocervical junction. Further discussion of these ligaments is beyond the scope of this chapter.

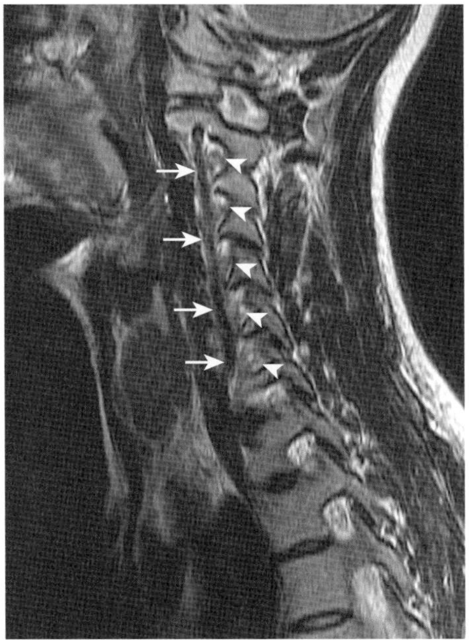

FIG. 9.6 Parasagittal image through the foramen transversaria. The linear dark flow void *(arrows)* is the vertebral artery. Note the position of the vertebral artery immediately ventral to the exiting spinal nerve roots *(arrowheads)*.

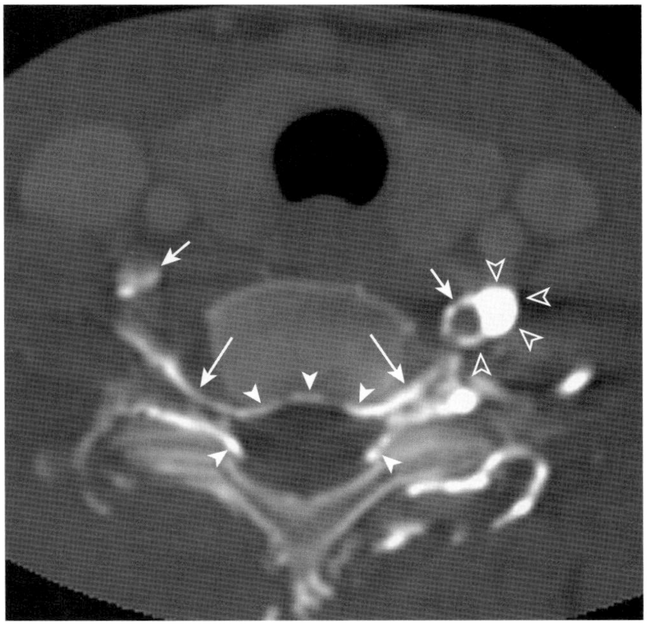

FIG. 9.7 Axial computed tomography (CT) image through the lower cervical spine. Contrast was administered for a neck CT but, as commonly occurs, some contrast filled the venous system in a retrograde fashion. The venous connection between the epidural space *(closed arrowheads)* and the perivertebral venous plexus *(open arrowheads)* via branches through the intervertebral foramina *(long arrows)* are well seen. The vertebral arteries *(short arrows)*, not yet within the vertebral foramina, are encircled with venous opacification particularly on the left.

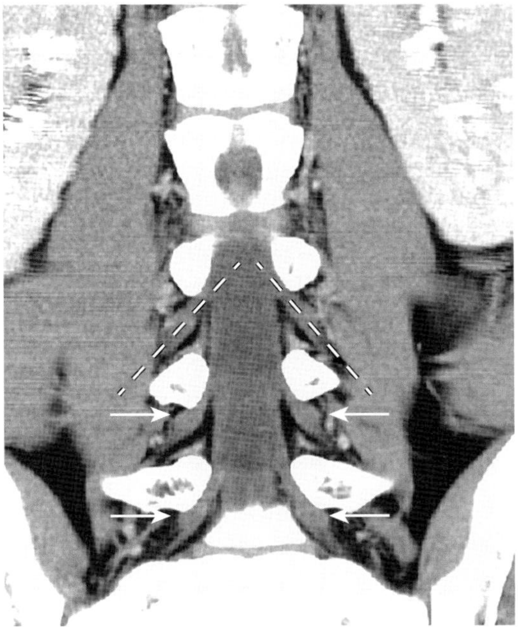

FIG. 9.8 Coronal computed tomography reconstruction after contrast administration. Note the orientation of the exiting lumbar nerve roots *(dashed lines)* relative to the spinal canal and intervertebral foramina. Enhancement of the dorsal root ganglia *(arrows)* is evident.

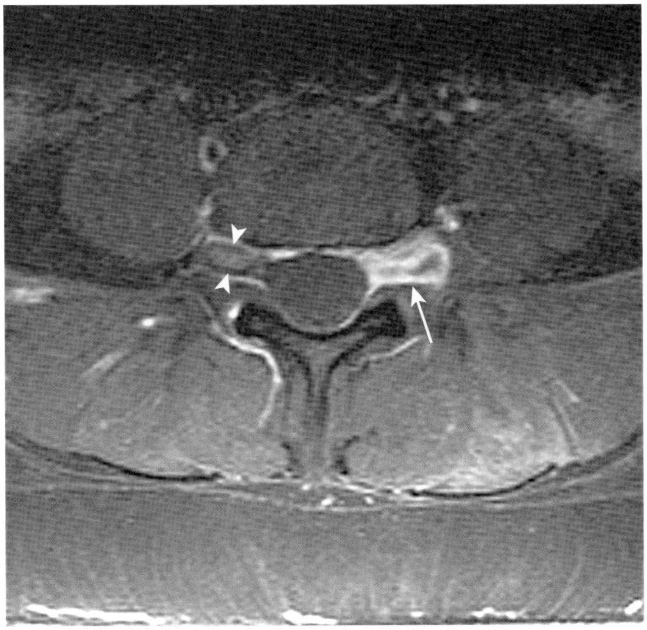

FIG. 9.9 Axial postgadolinium T1-weighted fat-suppressed magnetic resonance image. In the left foramen, the oval peripherally enhancing lesion *(arrow)* is a sequestered disc fragment. In the right foramen, normal enhancement of the dorsal root ganglion *(arrowheads)* is identified.

IMAGING OVERVIEW

CONVENTIONAL RADIOGRAPHS (X-RAYS)

Conventional or plain radiographs record differential attenuation of the x-ray beam by tissues based on their differential densities. For example, the cortical bone is very dense and almost completely attenuates the beam. The heart is soft tissue and partially attenuates the beam, and the lung is mostly air, thus attenuating very little of the beam. Conventional radiographs are quick, inexpensive, and easy to perform and have excellent spatial resolution. Important information about the spine can be obtained

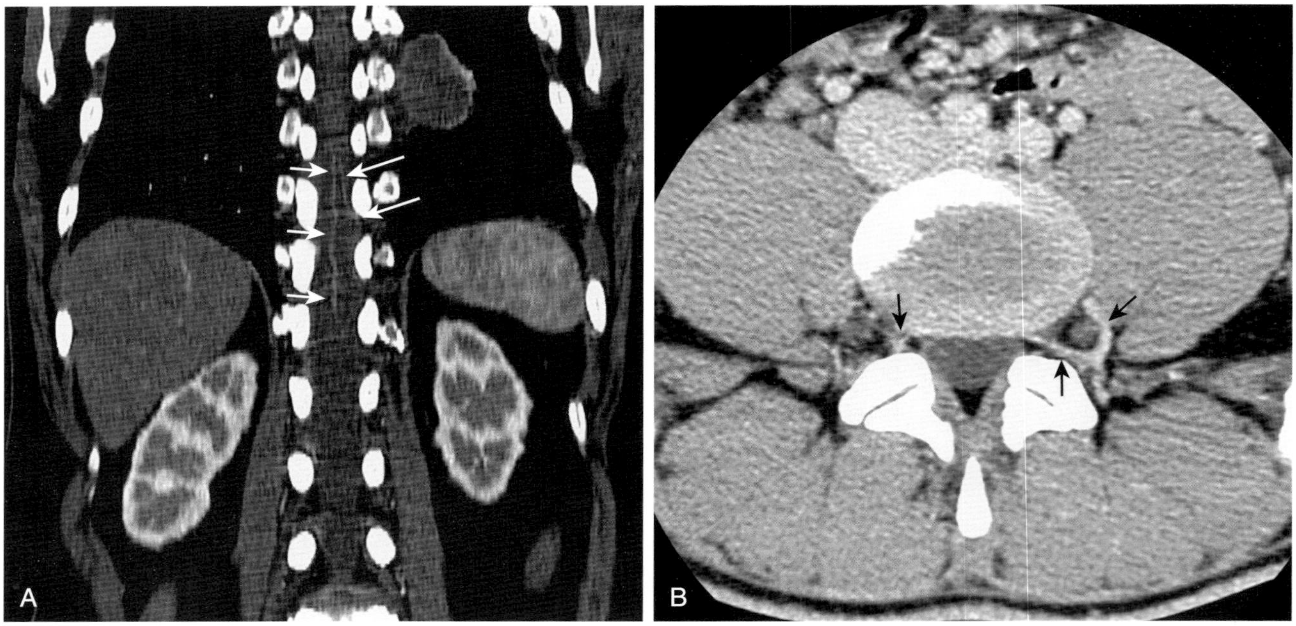

FIG. 9.10 (A) Coronal computed tomography (CT) reconstruction of a contrast-enhanced aorta study. The high-density linear structure on the surface of the spinal cord is the anterior spinal artery *(short arrows)*. The artery of Adamkiewicz *(long arrows)* enters the spinal canal through the left T10–T11 intervertebral foramen. (B) Axial CT image postcontrast through the mid-lumbar spine demonstrates typical venous structures *(arrows)* within and lateral to the intervertebral foramen.

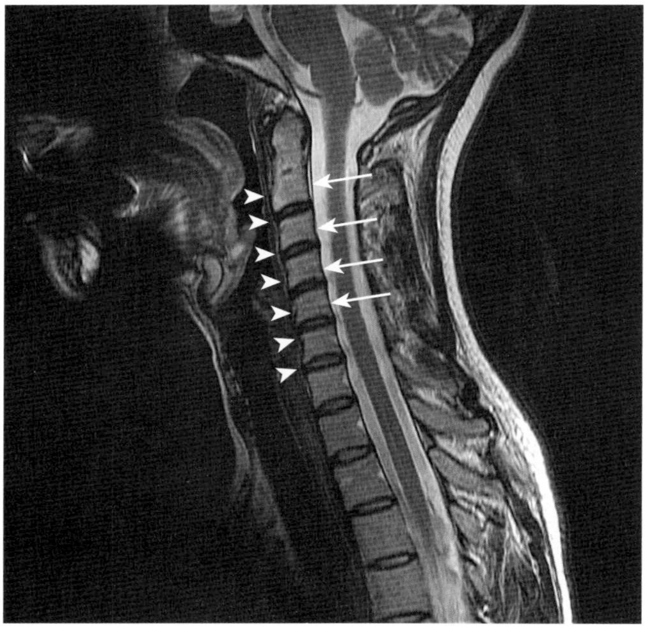

FIG. 9.11 Sagittal T2-weighted image through the cervical spine. The thin linear hypointense signal paralleling the ventral margins of the vertebral bodies and discs represents the anterior longitudinal ligament *(arrowheads)*. The posterior longitudinal ligament *(arrows)* has a similar appearance but runs along the dorsal margin of the intervertebral discs.

with conventional radiographs, including alignment, structure, and mineralization. Dynamic, weight-bearing upright flexion and extension views can reveal a stable or unstable spine in chronic and acute scenarios. This is the most commonly available modality that allows for this type of stress-related imaging. Osseous foraminal stenosis and spondylolysis can be diagnosed with oblique projections. Vertebral fractures and joint dislocations can be detected, although acuity can be difficult to discern and details are not as well characterized as with computed tomography (CT). Although conventional radiographs are far less optimal than CT for soft tissue evaluation, degenerative changes of the disc can be identified such as disc dehydration (air in disc) and disc collapse.

Standard frontal anterior-posterior (AP) (including odontoid view when imaging the cervical spine) and lateral projections are the minimum required for adequate evaluation (Figs. 9.12A–C, 9.13A, B, 9.14A–C). In the cervical and lumbar regions, oblique projections are helpful in evaluating the facet joints, articular processes, and intervertebral foramina (see Figs. 9.12D, E, 9.14D, E). When spondylolisthesis or spondylolysis is present, or with fractures and/or ligamentous disruption, flexion and extension views aid in demonstration of abnormal motion. Flexion and extension views may be supplemented by direct real-time observation using fluoroscopy.

Plain films can detect changes related to systemic diseases such as ankylosing spondylitis and diffuse sclerotic/lytic states (Fig. 9.15). Also, there is no good substitute for plain radiographs to evaluate overall alignment abnormalities in patients with extensive kyphoscoliotic deformities.

Conventional radiography is the easiest and most cost-effective method of assessing alignment and structure of the spine in both traumatic and nontraumatic conditions. On lateral projection, three longitudinal curves may be used to evaluate alignment of the vertebrae (Fig. 9.16). The anterior and posterior spinal lines trace the course of the anterior and posterior longitudinal ligaments, respectively. The spinolaminar line traces the course of the

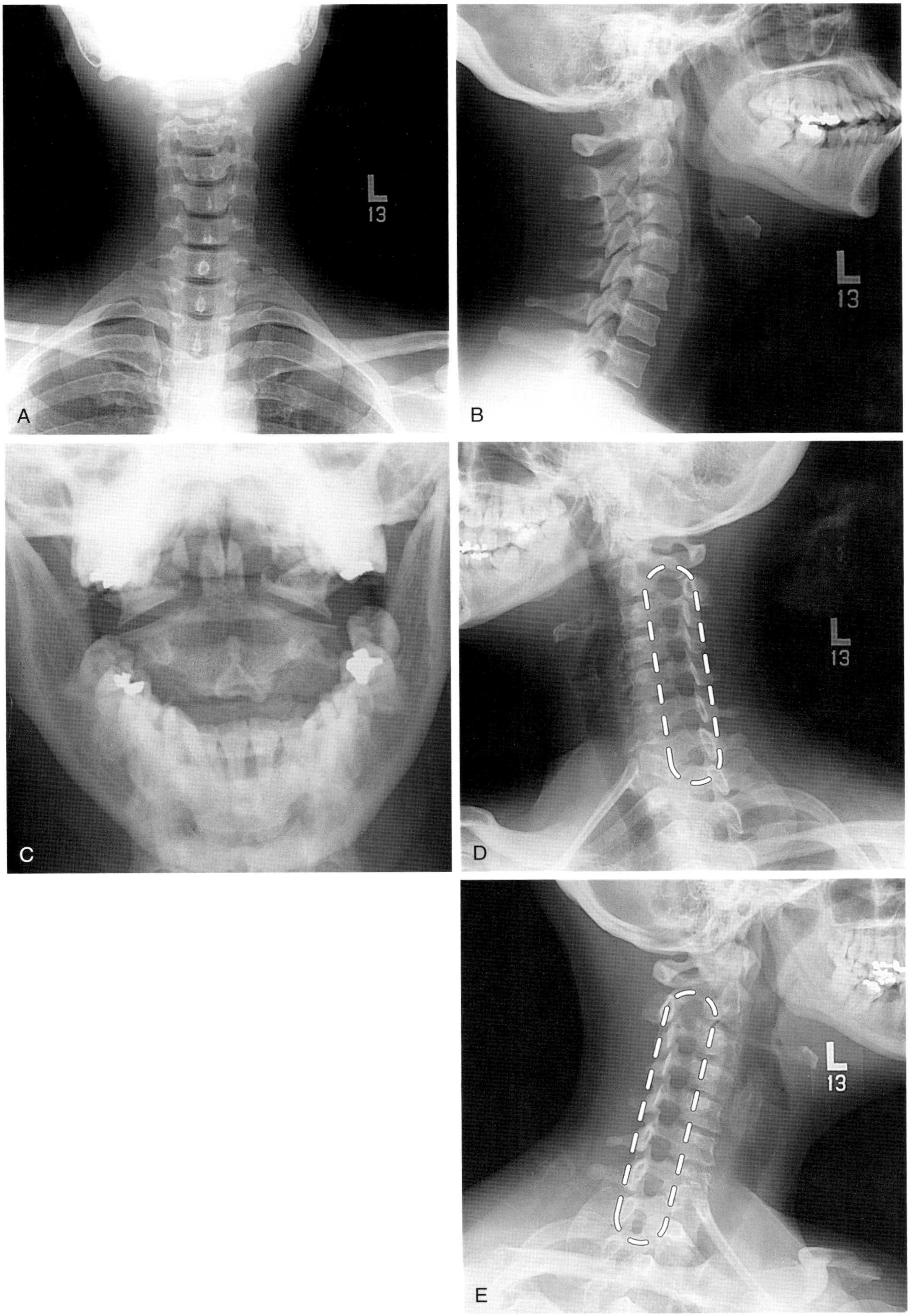

FIG. 9.12 (A–E) Routine five-view cervical spine series. AP, lateral, odontoid, and bilateral oblique views are obtained. Properly positioned oblique views can demonstrate osseous foraminal stenosis. The foramina *(dashed ovals)* in this case are all normal.

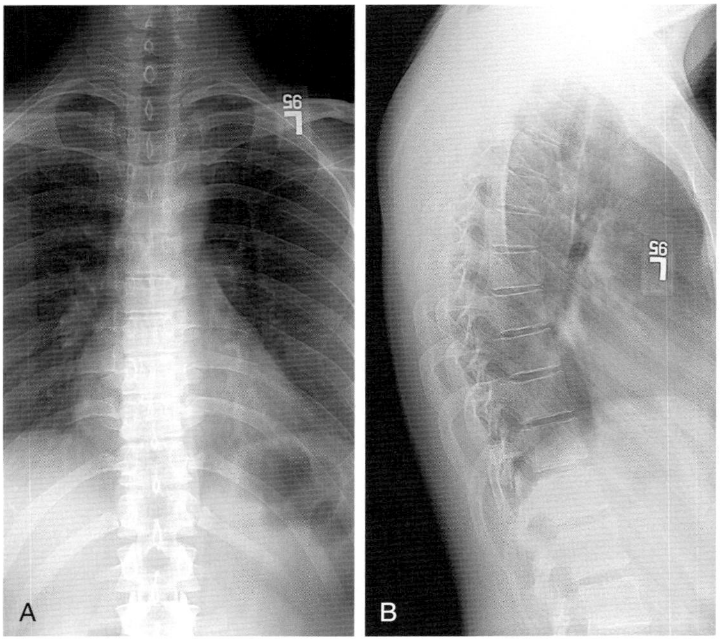

FIG. 9.13 (A and B) Standard images of the thoracic spine include an AP and lateral view.

ligamentum flavum along the deep surface of the laminae. On frontal projection, a vertical line drawn through the tips of the spinous processes serves as a reference for evaluation of lateral curvature (Fig. 9.17). The relationship of this line and the pedicles demonstrates rotational malalignment.

Plain radiographs can easily depict the failure of implanted hardware, such as screw loosening and rod fractures. Even known hardware fractures can be difficult to detect with CT due to beam-hardening artifacts that can obscure large portions of the images.

MYELOGRAPHY AND POSTMYELOGRAPHY COMPUTED TOMOGRAPHY

Myelography is the radiographic technique used to evaluate the contents of the spinal canal by the introduction of a nonionic, water-soluble, radiographically dense iodinated contrast material into the spinal subarachnoid space. This contrast material outlines the spinal cord and nerve roots, which appear as filling defects in the radiodense contrast column on conventional radiographs. Extradural indentations into the contrast column are observed and generally represent disc abnormalities, ligament thickening, or hypertrophic facet degenerative changes. Spinal stenosis can be diagnosed and nerve root impingement can be detected. Redundant thickened nerve roots and arachnoiditis can also be demonstrated (Fig. 9.18). Myelography should always be followed by a postmyelography CT scan to provide better definition of anatomic relationships of the contents of the spinal canal to the surrounding structures.

The use of myelography has decreased significantly due to the relatively invasive nature of the procedure and the availability of other noninvasive imaging tools, including CT and MRI, which provide excellent spatial and contrast resolution. The risks of myelography are directly related to the lumbar puncture (LP) and injection including positional headache, contrast-related seizure, and infection. The most common of these complications is the post-LP positional headache.[24] If this headache does not respond to conservative therapy, an epidural blood patch can be performed for more definitive treatment.[25] Seizures related to intrathecal contrast administration are uncommon, but the seizure threshold decreases with certain medications including numerous antidepressants.[26] In general, patients should be screened for specific medications and rescheduled if they are found to be on any seizure threshold–reducing medications. Myelography is now used mainly as a problem-solving tool when CT or MRI examination cannot be performed due to contraindications, are equivocal, or are limited due to artifacts from surgical hardware.

COMPUTED TOMOGRAPHY

CT is an x-ray technique that is considerably more sensitive to the differential attenuation of the x-ray beam than plain film radiography. CT provides the best possible definition of osseous structures and has excellent spatial resolution. The newest generation of CT scanners employs slip-ring technology (helical acquisition), multidetector systems, high-speed rotation, and dynamic table translation to optimally image the spine. Dose-reduction software now changes the patient dose "on the fly": The current (mA), and therefore the dose, changes in response to the thickness of the individual patient at each slice. Overlapping data sets can be acquired that allow for multiplanar reformatting, and three-dimensional data sets can be acquired for volumetric analysis or volume rendering applications.

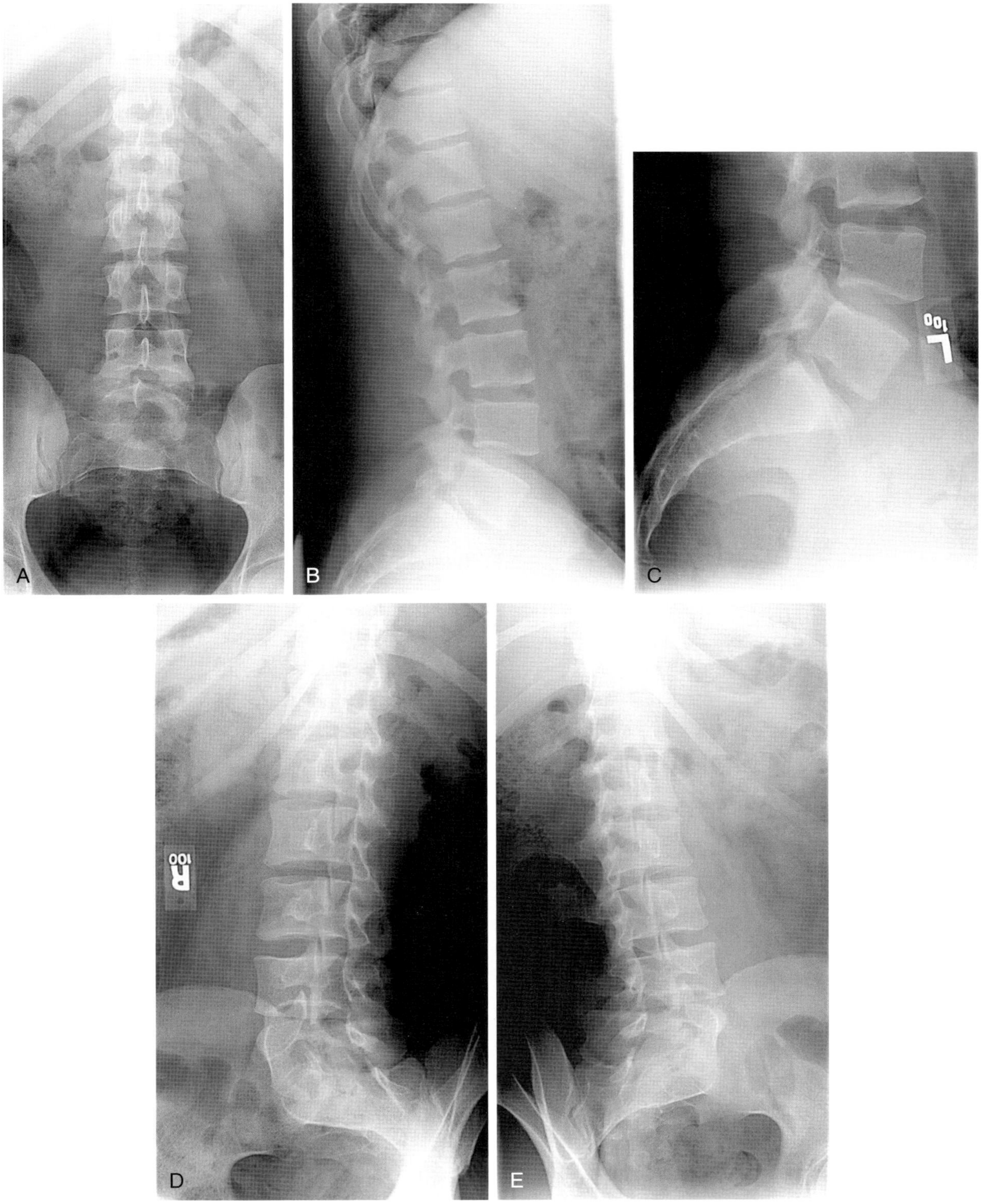

FIG. 9.14 (A–E) Routine five-view lumbar spine series. AP, lateral, coned-down view of the lumbosacral junction, and bilateral oblique views.

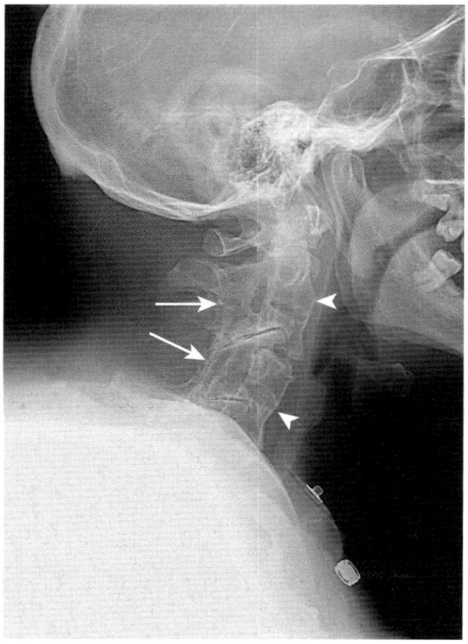

FIG. 9.15 In this single lateral cervical spine film, the findings consistent with ankylosing spondylitis are easily identified, including facet joint ankylosis *(arrows)* and vertebral body fusion *(arrowheads)*.

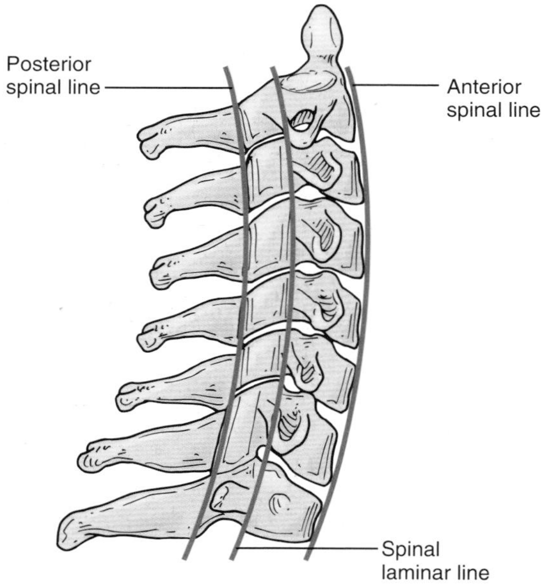

FIG. 9.16 Lateral diagram of the cervical spine demonstrating the spinal laminar, posterior spinal, and anterior spinal lines.

As with conventional radiographs, CT imaging is based on differential attenuation of the x-ray beam but can differentiate not only bone from soft tissue but also between different densities of bone and soft tissue structures. Differences in radiographic density of ligament, disc material, and cerebrospinal fluid (CSF) make identification of disc herniations and ligamentous disorders possible using CT (Fig. 9.19). Subtle areas of bone sclerosis or lysis can easily be displayed with CT. Windowing techniques used in the display of CT images allow optimal viewing of image data depending on the

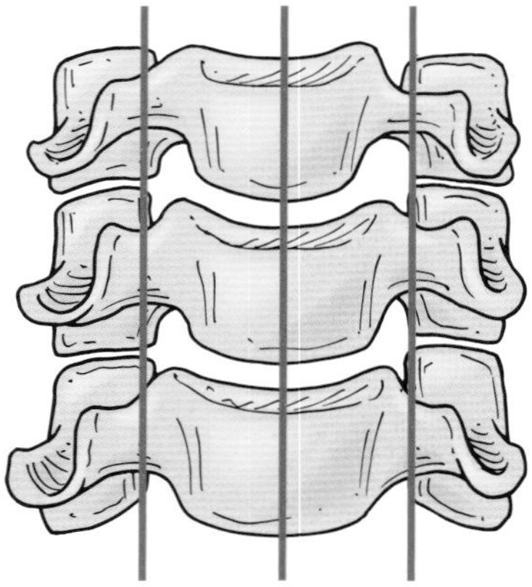

FIG. 9.17 Frontal diagram of the cervical spine showing normal alignment of the spinous processes.

tissue type of interest. The administration of intravenous iodinated contrast material may be valuable in certain circumstances to highlight vascular structures, such as the epidural venous plexus or adjacent arteries, or to demonstrate abnormal soft tissue enhancement (tumor, inflammation, infection).

Artifacts from metallic surgical implants, such as spinal rods, transpedicular screws, laminar wires/hooks, and intervertebral/vertebral body cages, can severely limit the diagnostic value of CT images. In these cases, conventional radiographs and myelography may prove to be the best diagnostic imaging modalities. Even this limitation improves as CT scanners evolve and postprocessing techniques improve, such as CT metal artifact reduction with iterative reconstruction technique.[27] Compared to several years earlier, there are now 256-slice and 320-slice multidetector CT scanners in existence that provide increasingly higher spatial resolution. There are also dual source CT scanners with greater capability for differentiating attenuation among different soft tissue, osseous, and metallic structures. The radiation dose from CT can be several times that of plain radiography, depending on technique and protocols. Hence, appropriate care should be exercised in using it in the more sensitive populations, including children, pregnant females, and other young adults.

MAGNETIC RESONANCE IMAGING

MRI uses strong magnets, gradient fields, and radiofrequency waves to localize and characterize tissues based on the amount and state of the ubiquitously present hydrogen atoms (protons). There is no ionizing radiation employed with MRI, but there are risks including those related to energy deposition, electrical and metal implants, and an unknown/unquantified risk to the fetus.[28–32] The very good soft tissue contrast resolution afforded by MRI and its multiplanar tomographic capability make it the most versatile and useful diagnostic imaging modality for spinal disorders. It provides a wide field of view with excellent definition of tissue types, such as bone marrow, muscle, ligament, disc material, and nerve roots. MRI allows precise definition of extradural, intradural extramedullary, and intramedullary

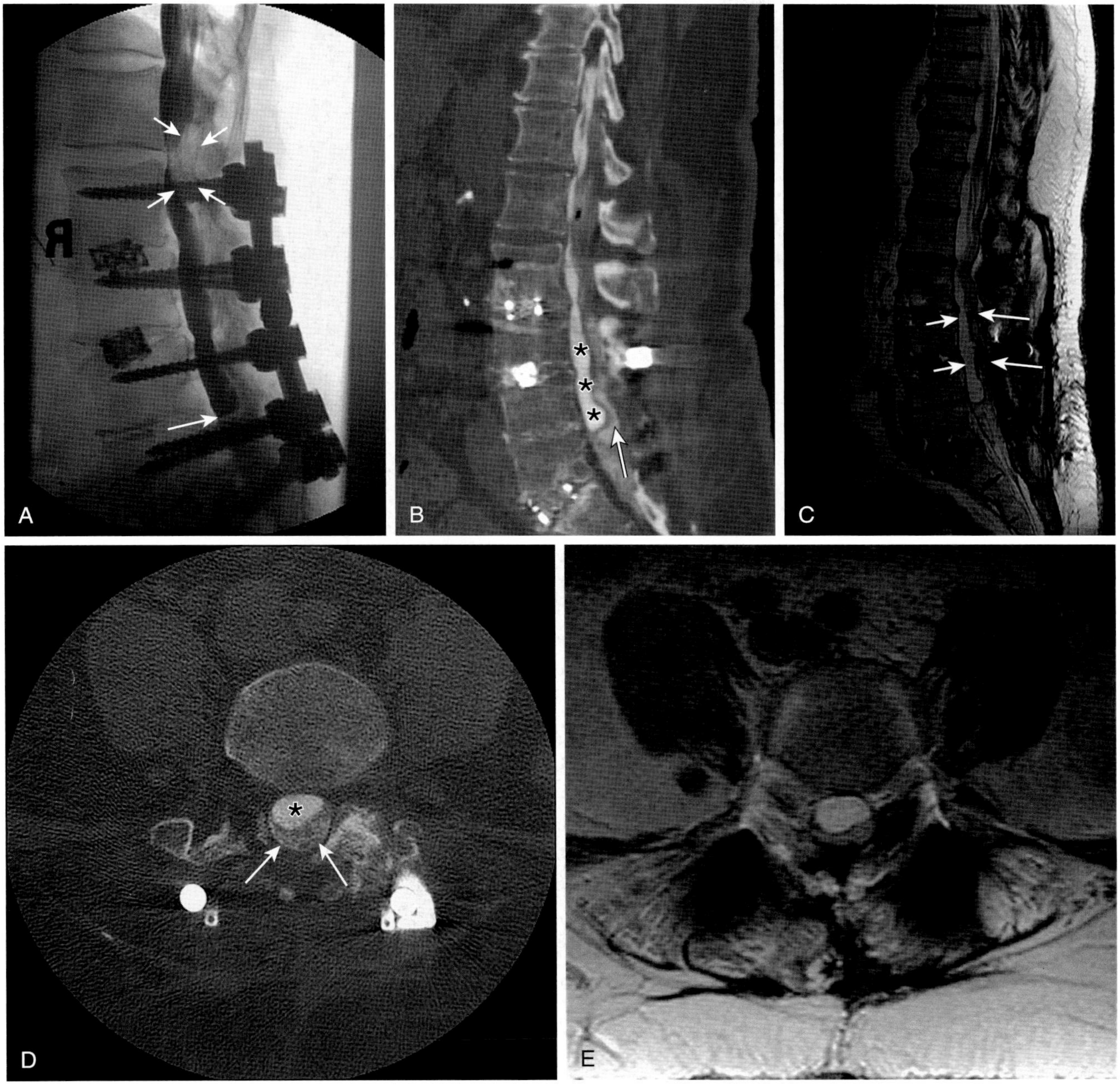

FIG. 9.18 (A) This lateral lumbar spine film was obtained after routine myelography. The patient has undergone posterolateral fusion from L2 to S1. A waist of contrast column attenuation *(short arrows)* is seen at L1–L2 indicating ligamentum flavum thickening. At the L4–L5 level, the intrathecal contrast is compartmentalized *(long arrow)* suggesting arachnoiditis. (B) Sagittal computed tomography (CT) reconstruction demonstrates a dense ventral subarachnoid collection of contrast *(asterisks)* and a less dense collection dorsally *(arrow)*. This appearance is consistent with arachnoiditis. (C) Sagittal T2-weighted magnetic resonance imaging (MRI) identifies the dorsal position of the nerve roots *(long arrows)* in the thecal sac and the compartmentalization of the cerebrospinal fluid spaces *(short arrows)*. (D) This axial CT myelographic image shows clumping and peripheral displacement of the spinal nerve roots *(arrows)* with ventral accumulation of contrast *(asterisk)*. (E) Axial T2-weighted MRI was obtained at the same level as the CT image and demonstrates the same findings.

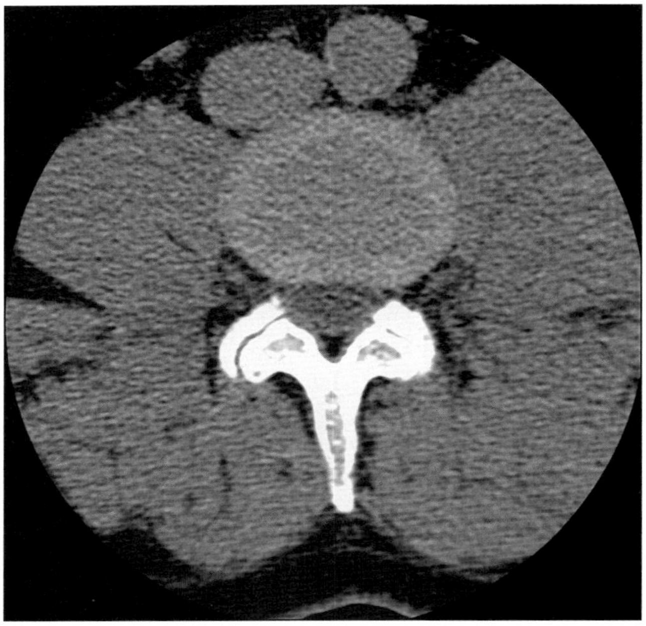

FIG. 9.19 Computed tomography (CT) images represent differential attenuation of the x-ray beam by the bones and soft tissues. Fat is low density and is hypodense on CT. Cerebrospinal fluid is less dense than the ligamenta flava, which are similar in density to the disc and muscles. Cortical bone is generally the densest endogenous structure.

pathology. Evaluation of medullary bone with MRI is excellent, and many osseous conditions resulting in marrow edema or marrow replacement (e.g., metastatic disease and myeloma) are well demonstrated. However, demonstration of dense cortical bone, sclerotic lesions, and osteophytes is less precise than by CT.

Standard MRI protocols usually include sagittal and axial images with T1- and T2-weighted sequences. T1 weighting provides excellent anatomical delineation. In general, high signal intensity on T1 represents fat (such as in fatty bone marrow, subcutaneous fat), whereas low signal intensity represents fluid (such as CSF, bone marrow edema, and normal nucleus pulposus) (Fig. 9.20A). T2 weighting makes fat-containing structures less bright than on T1 and makes fluid-containing structures hyperintense (bright) (see Fig. 9.20B). Soft tissue structures such as muscles and spinal cord have intermediate signal intensities on T1 and T2 sequences. The short-tau inversion recovery (STIR) sequence is a fat-suppressed, T2-weighted sequence that is extremely sensitive to minute amounts of fluid (see Fig. 9.20C). This sequence is particularly useful in detecting edema as can be seen with traumatic injury, malignancy, and infection.[33] Gradient recalled echo (GRE) T2-weighted imaging is sensitive to blood products and calcium and is particularly useful in the setting of spine trauma for evaluating the spinal cord (see Fig. 9.20D).[34,35] When evaluating scoliosis, coronal T1- or T2-weighted imaging may be added to better assess the extent of curvature (see Fig. 9.20E).

In the cervical spine, thin-section axial two- or three-dimensional GRE T2 images are used to further evaluate central canal and intervertebral foraminal stenosis. The degree of stenosis produced by osteophytes may be exaggerated on the GRE T2 sequence because of the sensitivity to susceptibility artifacts. Proton density (intermediate T2) and T2-weighted axial images are used in the lumbar region. Whether using a GRE T2 axial image in the cervical spine or a spin echo T2-weighted axial image in the thoracic or lumbar spine, the effect is the same: a "myelographic" effect is produced with hyperintense CSF within the thecal sac surrounding the intermediate signal intensity of the spinal cord and nerve roots (Fig. 9.21).

When evaluating for infection, multiple sclerosis, intramedullary neoplasm, metastatic disease, or postoperative scarring, sagittal and axial T1-weighted images prior to and following the intravenous administration of gadolinium contrast material are indicated. The addition of fat-suppression techniques can further highlight areas of pathologic enhancement, especially in the bone marrow and the paraspinal region. The combination of contrast administration and fat suppression increases diagnostic sensitivity in cases of osteomyelitis/discitis, epidural abscess or tumor, meningitis, leptomeningeal carcinomatosis, and perineural scarring (Fig. 9.22).

MRI of the spine is usually performed with the patient in supine position due to the configuration of most MRI scanners. Upright MRI scanners are available in very few facilities but allow for upright weight-bearing imaging of the spine, generally at a cost of increased motion artifact and lower resolution. In addition, flexion and extension MRI of the spine can be performed in most modern MR scanners and may demonstrate dynamic changes in stenosis with position (Fig. 9.23).[36,37]

Unfortunately, some patients cannot be examined using MRI. The most common problem encountered is claustrophobia. This is often overcome by light/moderate sedation, but this sometimes requires the services of an anesthesiologist. Another alternative is the "open-magnet" MRI systems, but the tradeoff is lower field strength and therefore poorer spatial resolution, less signal to noise, and fewer sequence options.[38] Modern "closed" scanners have wider and shorter bores, making claustrophobia less of an issue. Strict contraindications for MRI relate to the very strong magnetic field required for imaging. Some patients with cardiac pacemakers, metallic foreign bodies, and specific metallic surgical implants cannot be evaluated using MRI. Some cardiac pacemakers may be disabled or reprogrammed or their leads repositioned by the magnetic field.[39] Metallic foreign bodies or surgical implants, such as older cerebral aneurysm clips and heart valves, may be displaced by the magnetic field with catastrophic outcomes. Comprehensive references are available to determine which implants are safe to be placed into the magnetic field.[40] Specialized MRI centers may be able to scan patients with cardiac pacemakers, metallic foreign bodies, or metallic surgical implants, but this process follows strict conditional guidelines.[41,42] If an implanted cardiac device is involved, often clearance from cardiology is necessary prior to MRI and combined oversight by radiology and cardiology occurs during the scan. Metallic implants may also create severe artifact and distort the images significantly, rendering them nondiagnostic.

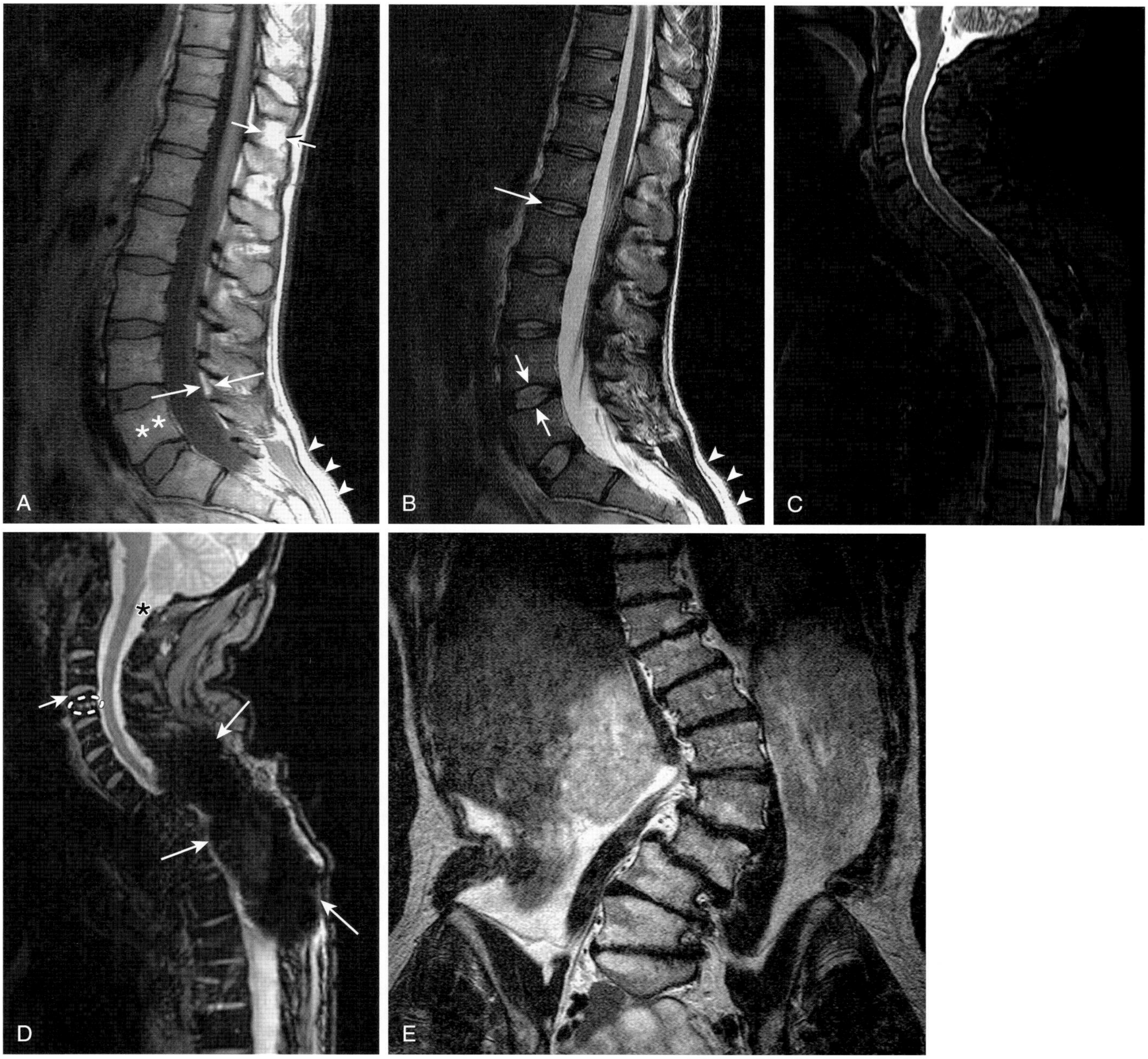

FIG. 9.20 (A) T1-weighted sagittal image through the lumbar spine. Fat is hyperintense on T1 images and is seen in the subcutaneous soft tissues *(arrowheads)*, interspinous regions *(short arrows)*, epidural space *(long arrows)*, and bone marrow *(asterisks)*. The intervertebral discs are mildly hypointense relative to the vertebral marrow. The cerebrospinal fluid (CSF) is hypointense relative to all but cortical bone. (B) T2-weighted sagittal image. In this sequence, the CSF is the most hyperintense *(white)* structure. Fat remains hyperintense *(arrowheads)* but is less bright than on the T1-weighted sequence. Note the high signal intensity within the intervertebral discs indicating normal disc hydration *(short arrows)*. A small, normal hypointense intranuclear cleft is visible in many discs including at L1–L2 *(long arrow)*. (C) The short-tau inversion recovery sequence is a T2-weighted sequence with a fat-suppression technique. The CSF remains hyperintense but the fat has "dropped out" and is now hypointense. Edema is easily depicted in the vertebral bodies or soft tissues using this sequence. (D) The gradient recalled echo sequence is a fast T2-weighted sequence that is particularly susceptible to inhomogeneities in the magnetic field as are produced by blood, calcium, and metal. In this image, the discs *(short arrow)*, CSF *(asterisk)*, and basivertebral plexi *(dashed oval)* are hyperintense whereas the bone and fascial planes are hypointense. Blooming *(long arrows)* is seen dorsal to C7–T5 due to metallic surgical hardware. (E) Any coronal acquisition, in this case, a T2-weighted image, helps the interpreter understand the curves involved in kyphoscoliosis.

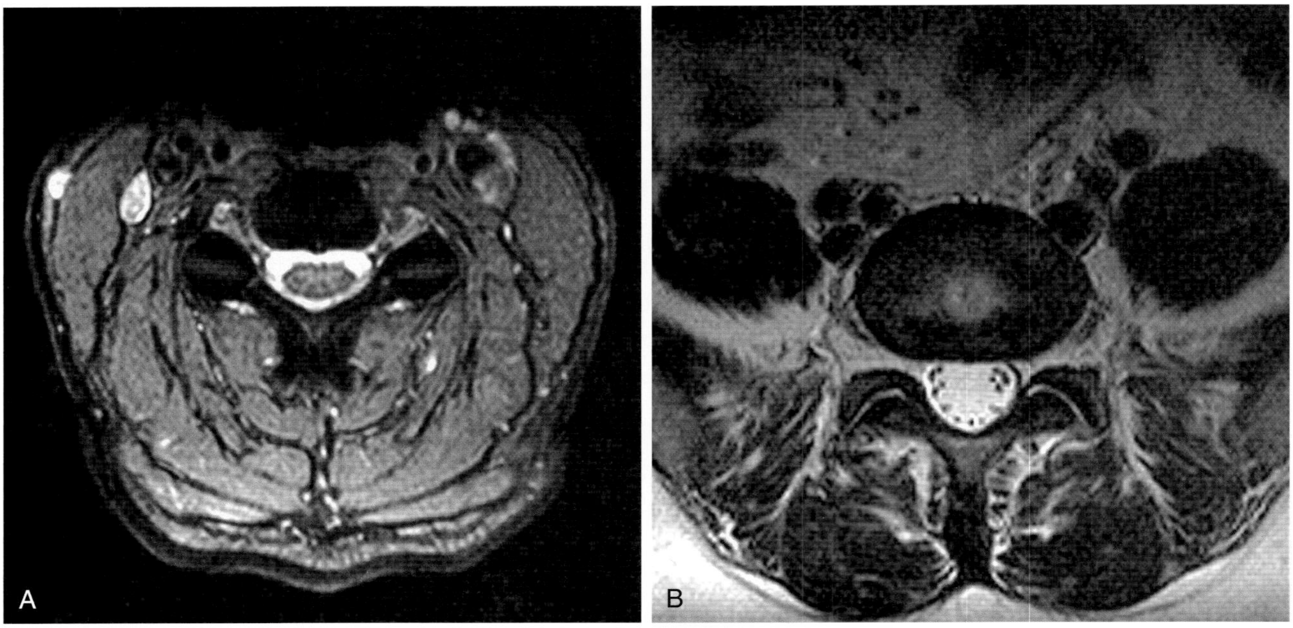

FIG. 9.21 (A) In the cervical spine, the "myelographic effect" is achieved with a T2-weighted gradient recalled echo sequence. This sequence is less susceptible to pulsation artifact but very sensitive to susceptibility artifact. The latter property can lead to overestimation of foraminal or canal stenosis from osteophytes. (B) In the lumbar spine, cerebrospinal fluid pulsation is dampened and typically not an issue. A conventional or fast spin echo T2-weighted technique is used to achieve the "myelographic effect."

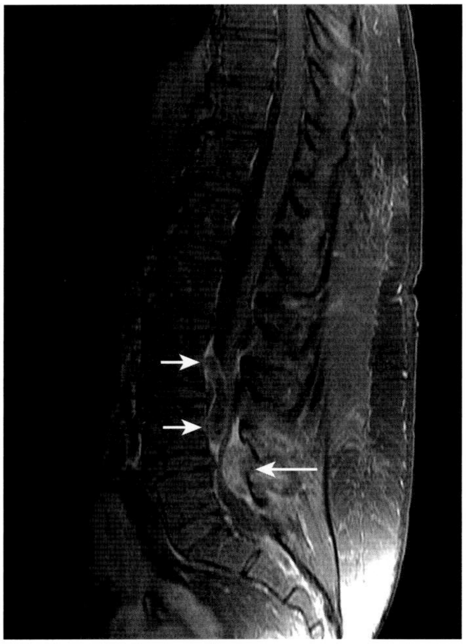

FIG. 9.22 Sagittal postgadolinium T1-weighted fat saturated image. Inflammatory processes are easily identified such as the large ventral *(short arrows)* and dorsal *(long arrow)* epidural abscess seen here.

DEGENERATIVE DISC DISEASE

OVERVIEW

Discogenic pain refers to back pain arising from the disc itself. Degenerative disc disease is a pathologic process, not entirely related to aging, of uncertain etiology that may cause acute or chronic low-back pain.[43,44] However, a recent meta-analysis by Brinjikji et al. showed that imaging findings of spine degeneration are also present in a high proportion of asymptomatic individuals, increasing with age, and therefore these imaging findings must be carefully interpreted in the context of a patient's clinical condition.[45] The conventional radiographic findings in degenerative disc disease include disc-space narrowing, vacuum disc, end-plate sclerosis, and osteophyte formation (Fig. 9.24A).[46,47] CT scans identify these same changes, but they identify these changes earlier in the course of degeneration (see Fig. 9.24B). Due to its excellent soft tissue contrast and multiplanar capabilities, MRI is the modality of choice to evaluate disc degeneration, and much effort has been placed into correlating MRI findings with potentially symptomatic levels. In the right hands, a provocative test, discography, can be used to determine the symptomatic levels of discogenic back pain and correlate clinical symptoms with the imaging features on the post-discography CT. In the evaluation of discogenic back pain, Bartynski found that disc-margin shape correlates with features of internal derangement in significantly painful discs encountered at provocative lumbar discography.[48–50] Although each finding of degenerative disc disease is discussed separately, the imaging findings are most often seen together when degenerative disc disease is present.

DISC DEHYDRATION AND NARROWING

With T1 weighting, the distinction between hydrated and nonhydrated disc is unapparent; therefore, the disc appears homogeneous (Fig. 9.25A). The water content of the intervertebral disc is responsible for the bright

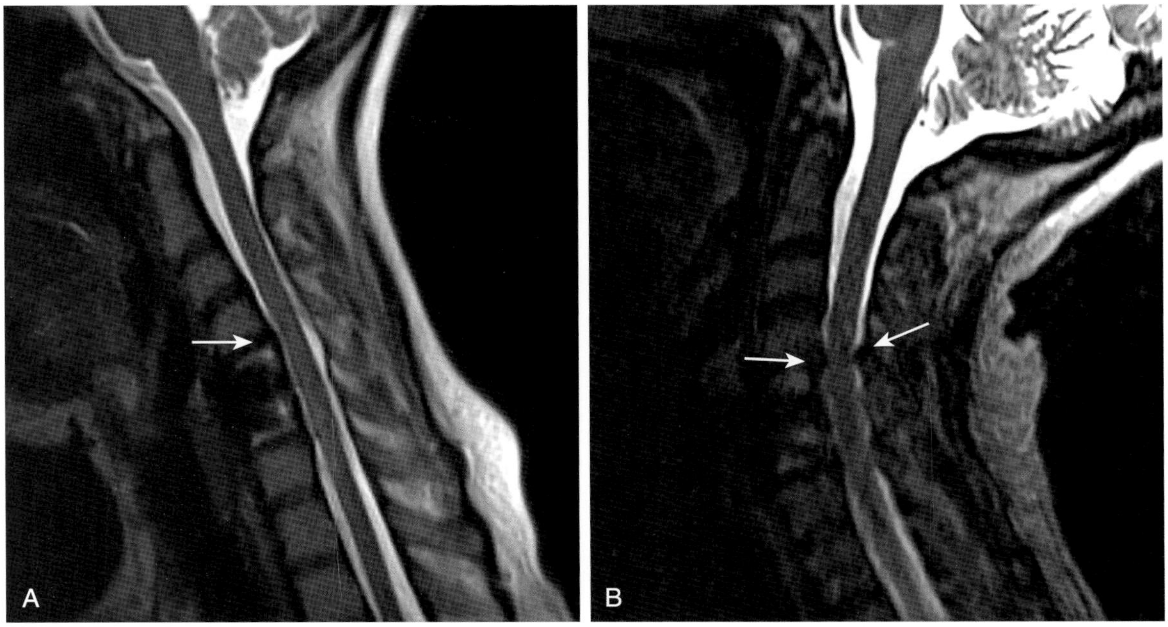

FIG. 9.23 (A) Sagittal T2-weighted magnetic resonance image of the cervical spine in flexion position showing no significant stenosis at the C4–C5 intervertebral disc level *(arrow)* above the C5–C6 anterior spinal fusion; however, dynamic changes in stenosis may occur with position. (B) In extension position, there are increased disc bulging and ligamentum flavum bulging *(arrows)* that cause increased spinal canal stenosis at C4–C5.

signal on T2-weighted MRI (see Fig. 9.25B).[51] The tightly packed annular fibers account for the dark T2 signal surrounding the centrally bright nucleus pulposus. Disc hydration, and therefore T2 disc signal, normally decreases with age, but it should remain brighter than the signal of bone marrow on T2-weighted sequences. The pathologic process of degenerative disease results in accelerated disc desiccation, which results in a more significant decrease in disc signal, and the most severe end of the spectrum of which is complete loss of the signal (see Fig. 9.24B–D). Degenerated discs occasionally demonstrate an accumulation of intradiscal gas (nitrogen) that can be detected on plain film, CT, and MRI.[52] On MRI, this "vacuum disc phenomenon" is typically hypointense on T1- and T2-weighted sequences due to lack of protons. Inexplicably, vacuum discs occasionally fill with fluid and can demonstrate high signal intensity on T2-weighted sequences.

Disc height is interpreted relative to other intervertebral levels in the same patient. Individual disc heights can be categorized as either normal or as mildly, moderately, or severely diminished based on percentage loss of disc height compared to a normal level. In a study comparing the disc heights of young versus middle-aged men, it was found that young, healthy men had narrower disc heights compared with middle-aged men.[53] Taken alone, therefore, disc height is not used as an indicator of disc degeneration. The main importance of loss of disc space height is the concomitant decrease in size of the intervertebral foramina and the related potential for nerve root compression.

ANNULAR FISSURES/TEARS

In 1992 Aprill and Bogduk reported a high-intensity zone within the midline posterior annulus, discontinuous with the central high signal nucleus pulposus, as a strong predictor of positive discography in patients with low back pain.[54] The linear hyperintense signal on T2-weighted images in the posterior or posterolateral disc represents radial and concentric fissuring of the annular fibers extending from the nucleus to the outer one-third of the annulus.[55] An element of inflammation (granulation tissue) is also thought to contribute to the high intensity zone based on enhancement on postcontrast T1-weighted images. Annular degeneration can be divided into three types including concentric fissuring, transverse fissures, and radial fissures.[47,56] Concentric fissuring occurs due to collagen fiber delamination of the annulus fibrosis with deposition of mucoid material.[57] This fissuring is high-signal intensity on T2-weighted sequences and parallels the margins of the disc (Fig. 9.26). Transverse fissures are small foci of T2 hyperintensity at the junction of Sharpey fibers with the vertebral body ring apophyses.[57] Both concentric fissuring and transverse fissures may imply disc degeneration but are not generally symptomatic. Radial fissures are full-thickness disruptions of the annulus and represent primary failure of the annulus (Fig. 9.27).[57] The lateral and posterior margins of the outer third of the annulus fibrosis and the PLL are richly innervated by nociceptive nerve endings and therefore disruption is felt to be a source of discogenic back pain.[19] It is this feature that supports the notion that radial fissures can produce pain, whereas transverse fissures and concentric

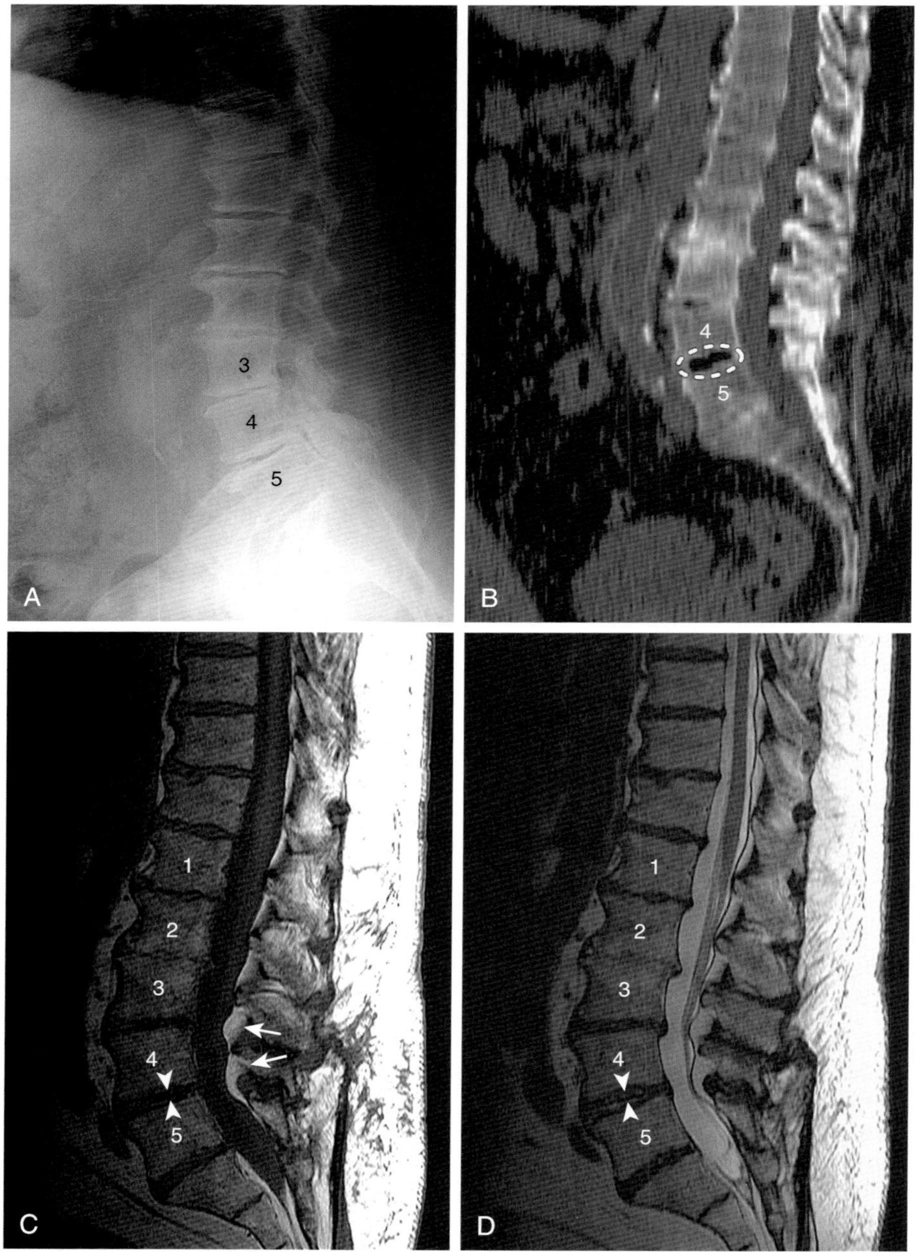

FIG. 9.24 (A) The conventional radiographic findings of disc degenerative changes are seen here including loss of disc space height, vacuum disc phenomenon, end plate sclerosis, and osteophyte formation. (B) This sagittal reconstruction from an abdominal computed tomography (CT) scan easily depicts the same changes. A vacuum disc is particularly well seen at L4–L5 *(dashed oval)*. (C) Sagittal T1-weighted image in the same patient shows classic degenerative changes. The vacuum disc at L4–L5 is hypointense *(arrowheads)*. The dorsal epidural space *(arrows)* behind L3–L4 and L4–L5 is large and would be an easy target for epidural steroid injections. (D) This T2-weighted image shows diffuse disc desiccation and complete loss of disc space height at L2–L3. Multiple disc bulges are seen indenting the ventral subarachnoid space at all levels except L5–S1. The linear hypointense signal representing the vacuum disc *(arrowheads)* at L4–L5 is smaller than would be predicted by the CT image.

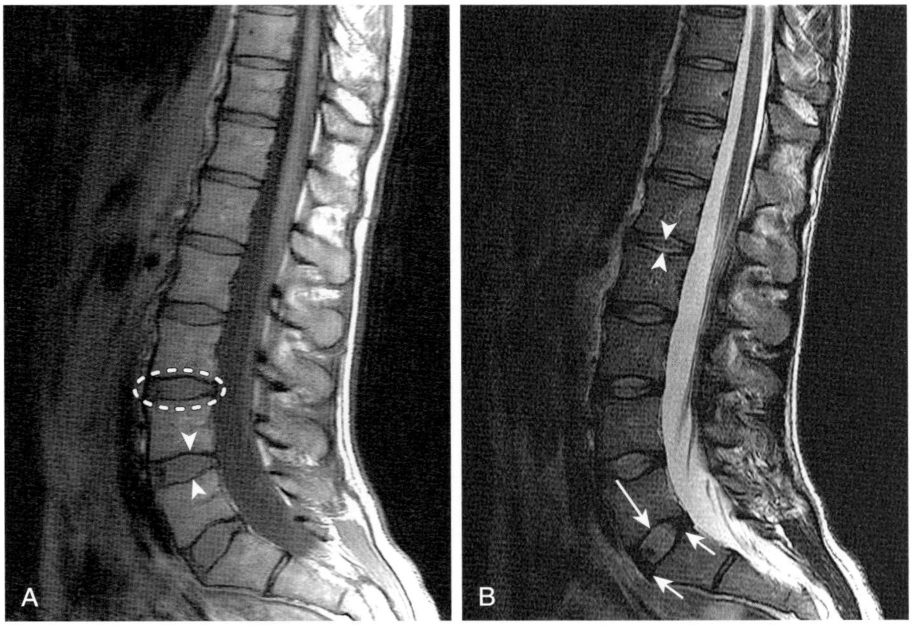

FIG. 9.25 (A) On T1-weighted images, the normal intervertebral disc is homogeneously isointense *(dashed oval)*. The black signal outlining the superior and inferior margins of the disc *(arrowheads)* represents the cortex of the adjacent vertebral bodies. (B) In this T2-weighted image, the tightly packed annular fibers are hypointense *(short arrows)*. The hydrated nucleus *(long arrow)* is hyperintense except for the central linear intranuclear cleft *(arrowheads)*. This intranuclear cleft is a normal finding and should not be misinterpreted as focal desiccation.

fissures should not produce pain. With the publication of the revised "Lumbar disc nomenclature: version 2.0" in 2014, fissure is the term preferred over tear.[56]

SUBCHONDRAL MARROW CHANGES

Degenerative disease in the vertebral end plates and adjacent bone marrow, referred to as Modic-type changes, are classified into three types based on signal characteristics of T1- and T2-weighted signal characteristics.[58] Type I changes refer to low signal in the vertebral end plates and adjacent marrow on T1- and increased signal on T2-weighted images, representing vascularized marrow (Fig. 9.28A, B). Enhancement of Modic changes, particularly Type I, is not uncommon (see Fig. 9.28C).

Type II changes show increased signal intensity on T1- and increased signal or isointensity on T2-weighted images, representing fatty replacement of the bone marrow (Fig. 9.29). Type III changes consist of low signal on both T1- and T2-weighted sequences due to subchondral sclerosis (Fig. 9.30).

It has been suggested that subchondral marrow changes represent chemical inflammation in the vertebral end plates that is a reaction to the diffusion of toxic substances from a degenerated disc.[59,60] Modic changes, therefore, could be a secondary sign of discogenic low back pain. Although Braithwaite et al. found subchondral marrow changes to be very specific, low sensitivity limits the value of Modic changes in detecting the source of a patient's low back pain.[61] One investigator found no relationship between Modic changes and provocative discography.[62]

DISC HERNIATION

OVERVIEW

In an attempt to standardize the reporting of normal and pathologic conditions of the lumbar spine, the North American Spine Society (NASS), the American Society of Neuroradiology (ASNR), and the American Society of Spine Radiology (ASSR) combined task forces to create recommendations that provide a common nomenclature to promote uniform descriptions of pathologic processes affecting the discs.[63] This was first published in 2001, and a subsequent revised "Lumbar disc nomenclature: version 2.0" was released in 2014.[56]

Due to its superior soft tissue resolution, MRI is the imaging modality of choice to evaluate disc herniations. CT is also useful, but is typically relegated to use as a secondary study either to better delineate bony abnormalities or for patients who cannot undergo or tolerate an MRI examination. CT myelography can be added when contraindications preclude the use of MRI and plain CT is inadequate to define the clinical problem.

DISC CONTOUR

Disc herniation has been defined as a localized displacement of disc material beyond the limits of the intervertebral disc space. A "circumferential bulge" describes disc material bulging out beyond 50%–100% of the edges of the vertebral body's ring apophysis and is not considered a disc herniation. Localized herniated disc material, in

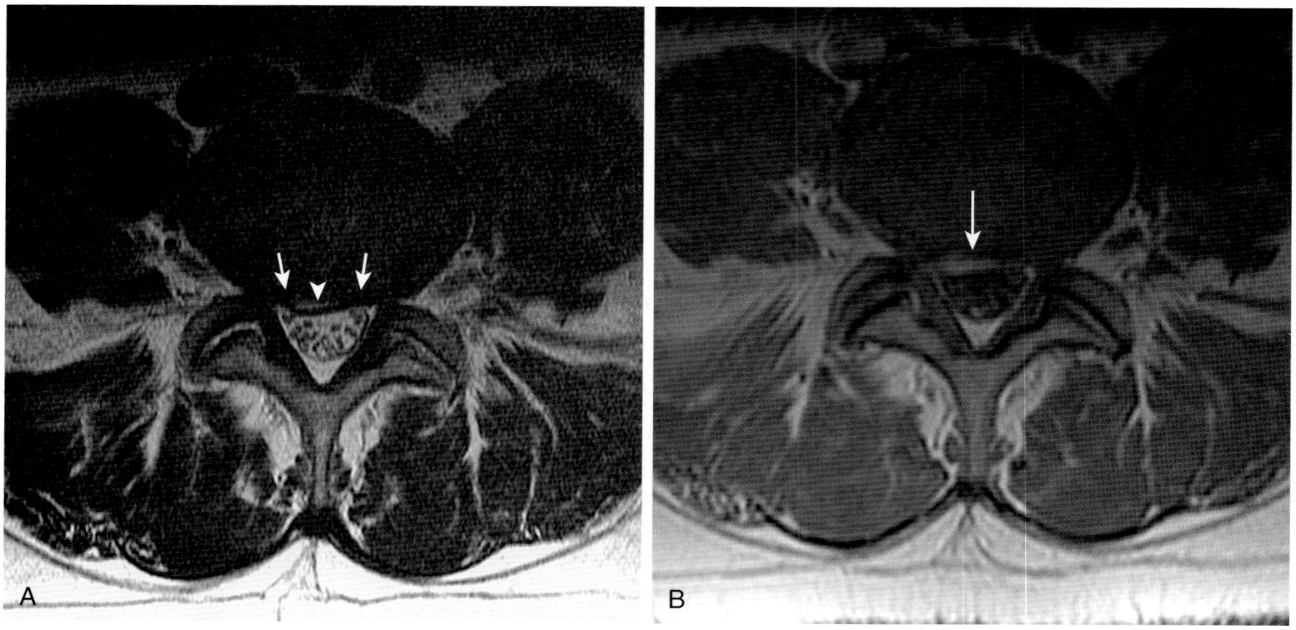

FIG. 9.26 (A) Axial T2-weighted image through the L4–L5 level. There is a right paracentral protrusion *(short arrows)* that indents the ventral thecal sac. Linear hyperintense signal in the central dorsal annulus *(arrowhead)* parallels the disc margin and represents mucoid deposition within a concentric fissure. (B) On postgadolinium T1-weighted imaging, annular fissures of any type can enhance *(long arrow)* as in this case. Enhancement implies nothing other than the likely presence of a reparative process such as granulation tissue.

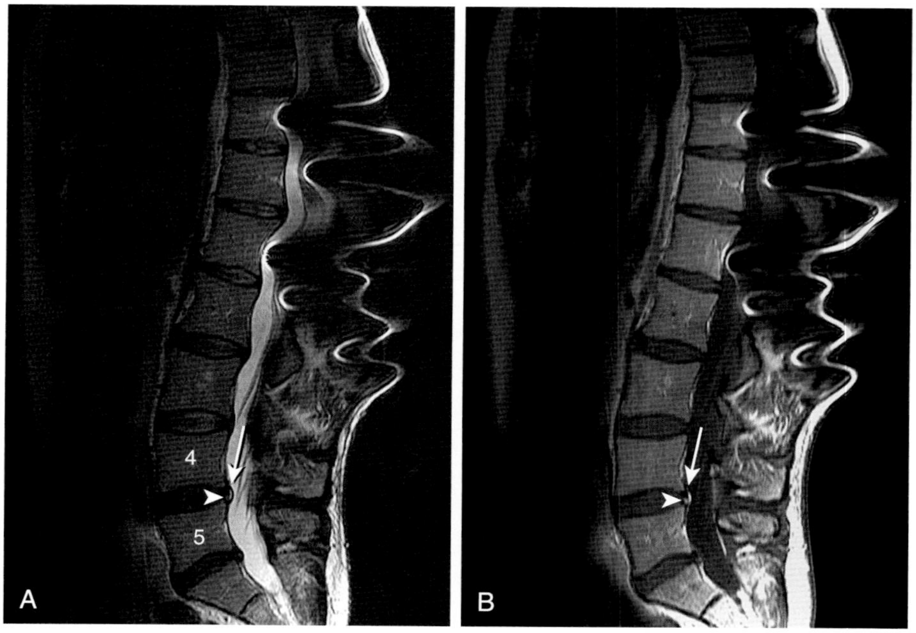

FIG. 9.27 (A and B) At the L4–L5 level, a dorsal concentric annular fissure *(arrow)* and a radial fissure *(arrowhead)* are identified. Both these fissures enhance on the postgadolinium T1-weighted sagittal image.

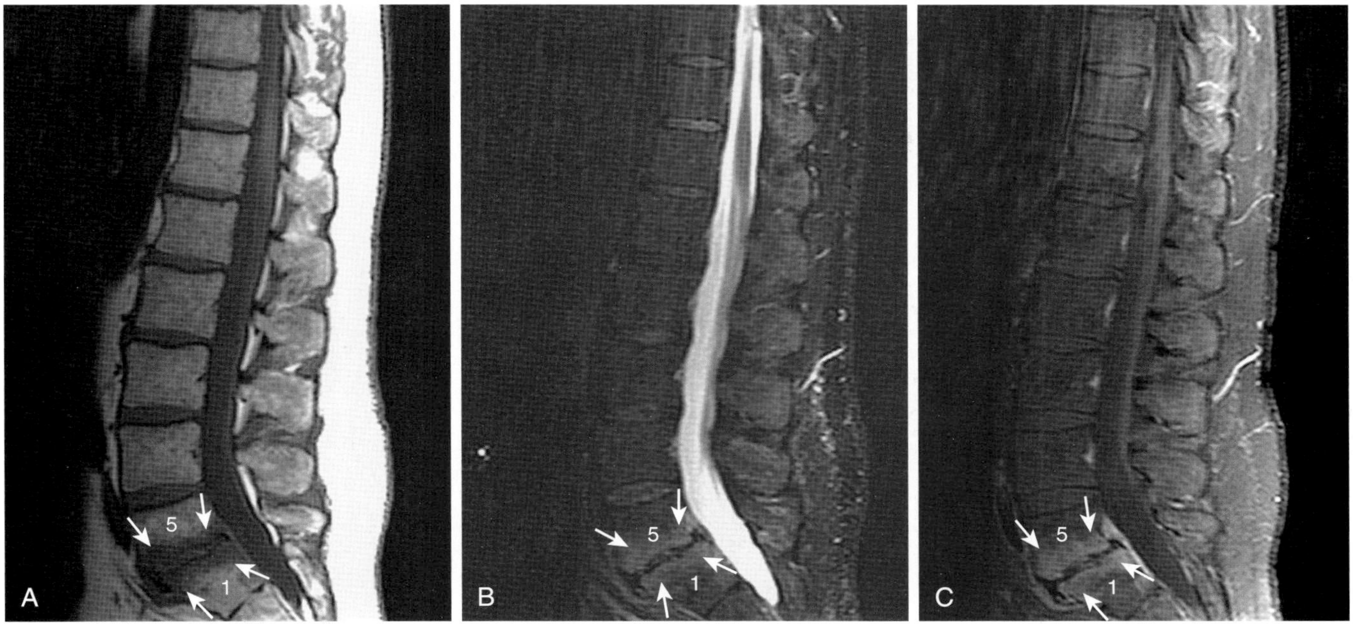

FIG. 9.28 Sagittal (A) T1, (B) short-tau inversion recovery, and (C) postgadolinium T1-weighted fat saturation images show the typical Modic type 1 subchondral marrow changes *(arrows)* at L5–S1. The signal and enhancement resemble that which is seen with early osteomyelitis.

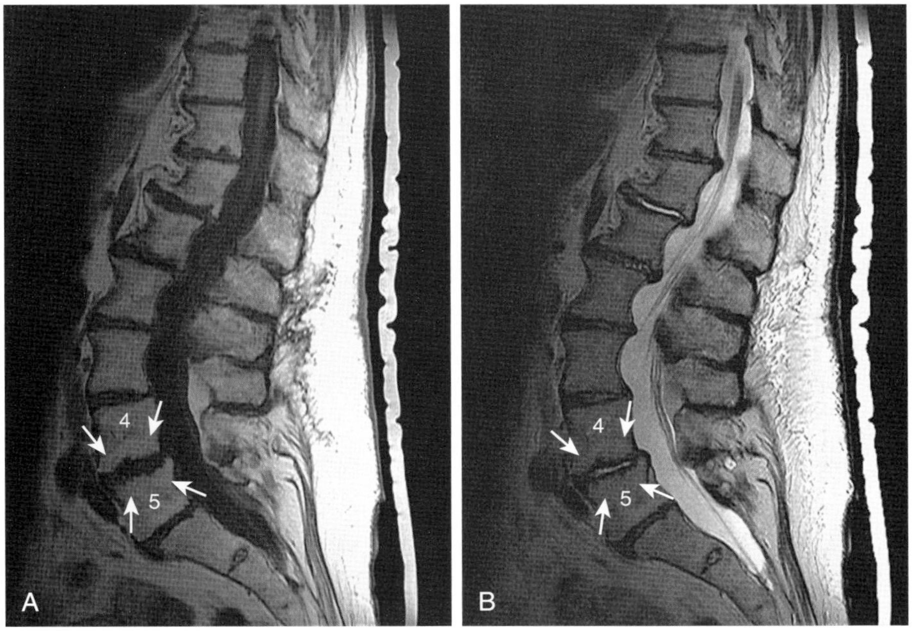

FIG. 9.29 Sagittal (A) T1- and (B) T2-weighted images show classic Modic type 2 changes at L4–L5. The hyperintense end plate signal *(arrows)* on both sequences represents focal fatty replacement of bone marrow.

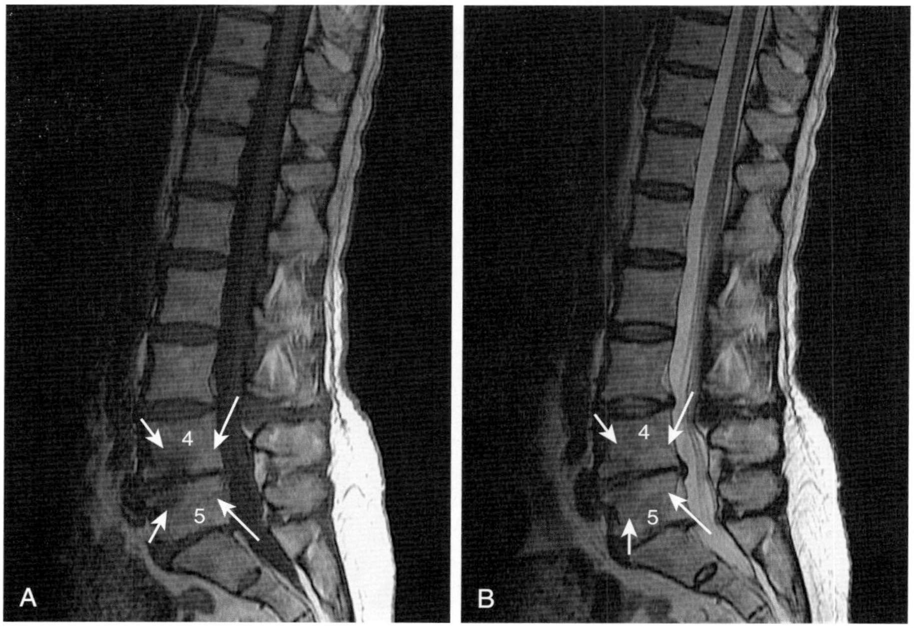

FIG. 9.30 Sagittal (A) T1- and (B) T2-weighted images show Modic type 3 changes *(short arrows)* along the ventral half of the L4–L5 end plates. Interestingly, Modic type 2 changes *(long arrows)* are present at the same level along the dorsal half of the end plates.

other words, disc extending beyond the end plate margin less than 50% of the disc circumference, can be termed "focal" (less than 25%) or "broad-based" (25%–50%). A focal disc herniation can also occur into adjacent vertebral end plates, commonly referred to as a Schmorl node (Fig. 9.31).

The terms "protrusion" and "extrusion" describe disc herniations based on the shape of the herniated disc fragment and its relationship to the parent disc margin. A protrusion describes a localized disc herniation that has its base wider than the furthest extent of the apex of herniated disc material (Fig. 9.32A). An extruded disc is defined by the presence of a herniated disc, where the diameter of the disc fragment from base to apex is wider than the width of the fragment at the base (see Fig. 9.32B). A sequestered or free-fragment disc herniation is disc material that has completely separated from the parent disc. Describing disc herniations using these terms is not meant to imply any significance regarding symptom production or the best method of treatment.

Disc migration in the cranial or caudal directions is best evaluated in the sagittal plane. A posterior disc extrusion may be contained by the PLL and migrate inferiorly or less commonly, superiorly. Such extrusions may appear on axial imaging as a protrusion, but they are easily identified as a migrated extrusion on sagittal imaging. Measurements are taken from the posterior margin of the superior or inferior end plate of the vertebral body, to describe the extent of migration for the surgeon. Migrated fragments are usually paramedian, since the attachment of the PLL to the posterior vertebral body at midline tends to direct the fragment unilaterally. While the majority of sequestered disc fragments are ventral in location, the rare migration of a sequestered disc fragment into the dorsal epidural space[64] (see section "Intraspinal Facet Cysts" for additional discussion) or within the thecal sac have been described.

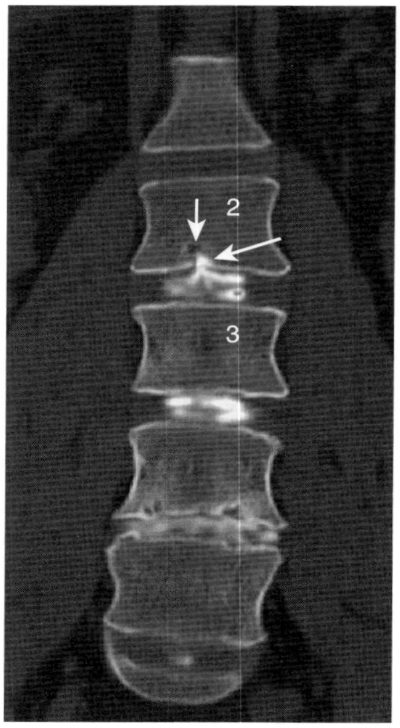

FIG. 9.31 Postdiscography computed tomography (CT). CT coronal reconstruction after lumbar discography from L2 to L5. There is a Schmorl node extending through the inferior end plate of L2. A sclerotic margin *(short arrow)* is present. Contrast *(long arrow)* from the L2 to L3 discogram is seen extending into the Schmorl node (intervertebral disc herniation).

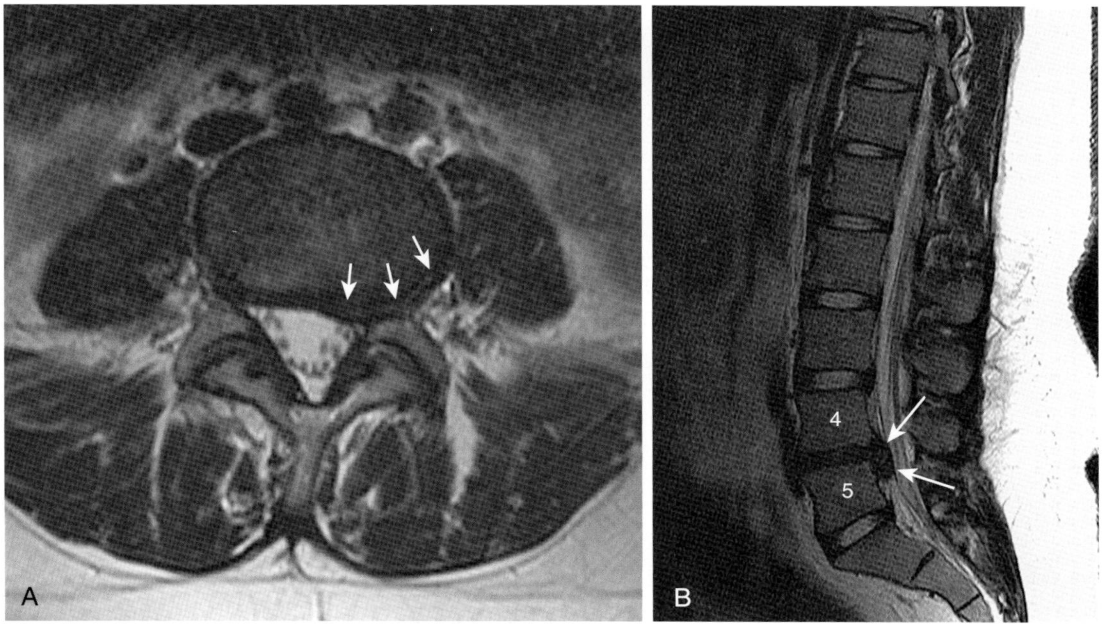

FIG. 9.32 (A) Axial T2-weighted magnetic resonance imaging (MRI) demonstrating a broad-based left parasagittal, foraminal, and far lateral herniation *(short arrows)*. This morphology is consistent with a disc protrusion. (B) Parasagittal T2-weighted MRI shows a large disc extrusion *(long arrows)* at the L4–L5 level. Disc material elevates the posterior longitudinal ligament and has migrated 6 mm caudal to the parent disc.

DISC HERNIATION POSITION

Using anatomic landmarks to describe the location of a disc herniation provides a precise and consistent classification.[65] An axial image at the level of the disc has four "zones" based on arbitrary sagittal and parasagittal lines drawn through specific anatomic landmarks. The term "central" means the posterior midline aspect of the disc, between the medial aspects of the articular facets. Right and left paracentral/paramedian descriptors can be added if the disc favors one side or the other. The "subarticular" zone is between the medial aspect of the articular process and the medial aspect of the ipsilateral pedicle. The "foraminal" zone is between the parasagittal planes defined by the medial and lateral aspects of the pedicle. Finally, the "extraforaminal" zone is beyond the parasagittal line of the lateral aspect of the pedicle.

Of note, the term "lateral recess" describes the area along the medial border of the pedicle, below the level of the disc and the superior vertebral end plate, and is a part of but does not describe the entire subarticular zone (Fig. 9.33). Strictly speaking, disc herniations that protrude directly posteriorly are not in the lateral recess and can only reach the lateral recess by traveling superiorly or inferiorly from the disc. For example, an L3–L4 disc extrusion that projects inferiorly would enter the lateral recess of L4 and encroach on the L4 nerve root as it descends beneath the L4 pedicle.

On sagittal images, the position of a herniated disc in the craniocaudal direction can be separated into levels based on anatomic landmarks. The suprapedicular level extends from just above the pedicle to the superior end plate. The pedicle level is defined by the superior and inferior edges of the pedicle. The infrapedicular level extends from below the inferior edge of the pedicle to the inferior end plate.

Depending on the position of a herniated disc, it can compress adjacent nerve roots. For example, in the cervical spine, a central or paramedian disc herniation affects the descending nerve roots and not the exiting nerve root at that level. For instance, a right paramedian small disc extrusion at C3–C4 most likely compresses the descending right C5 nerve root. A foraminal disc abnormality affects the exiting nerve root at that level. For instance, a right foraminal disc extrusion at C3–C4 likely compresses the right C4 nerve root. In the thoracic and lumbar spine, the nerve roots are numbered differently (exiting root is associated with superior level). In addition, a right paramedian disc extrusion at T3–T4 or L3–L4 likely affects the descending right T4 or right L4 nerve roots, respectively. A right foraminal disc extrusion at T3–T4 or L3–L4 compresses the exiting right T3 or L4 nerve roots.

The degree of neural compression can be graded based on the change in the normal round or oval configuration of the spinal cord, nerve root, or root ganglion produced by the herniated disc. Mild compression is defined as 75%–99% of the normal diameter of the structure being maintained. Similarly, moderate and severe compression is described as 50%–74% and less than 50% of the normal diameter, respectively.

FACET JOINT

OVERVIEW

The facet joint is another potential source of low back pain. Considering the numerous potential causes of low back pain, it can be difficult to isolate the facet joint clinically or by imaging as the primary cause of a

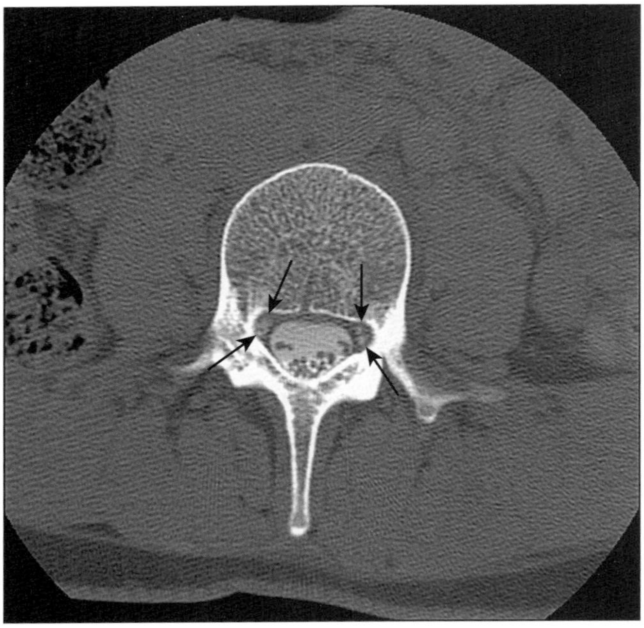

FIG. 9.33 Axial computed tomography (CT) myelogram image in the mid-lumbar spine. The lateral recesses *(arrows)* reside just medial to the medial margin of each pedicle and contain the exiting nerve roots. In this image, the exiting nerve root sleeves are opacified with contrast.

patient's pain. Facet joint syndrome is a controversial diagnosis referring to focal or referred pain arising from or anatomically correlating with a degenerated facet joint.[66,67]

IMAGING

Facet joint arthropathy includes hypertrophic osteophytic overgrowth, subchondral sclerosis, bone marrow edema, joint space narrowing/widening, joint effusions, and periarticular soft tissue edema.[68] Osteophytosis and subchondral sclerosis are hypointense on T1- and T2-weighted imaging. Bone marrow and periarticular soft tissue edema are hypointense on T1- but hyperintense on T2-weighted sequences (Fig. 9.34A, B). A fat-suppressed T2-weighted sequence is particularly sensitive at detecting marrow or soft tissue edema. The joint space can narrow or, if instability and abnormal motion occur, widen. A small amount of synovial fluid exists in the joint space but effusions are commonly seen, particularly in widened facet joints (see Fig. 9.34C). Facet joint arthropathy can result in pain secondary to the intrinsic abnormalities of the bone and joint or can result in extrinsic compression of descending nerve roots in the lateral recess or exiting nerve roots in the intervertebral foramen. Facet joint osteoarthritis can be accurately diagnosed by CT scanning, although the ability to detect bone marrow or periarticular edema is limited. In the cervical spine, subtle sclerotic changes and osteophytes are easily detected on CT, whereas on MRI, the changes are either more difficult to detect or are overestimated, particularly on the GRE sequence images. Plain films can detect some facet degenerative changes, including sclerosis and hypertrophic overgrowth, but are generally the least-sensitive modality.

INTRASPINAL FACET CYSTS

OVERVIEW

Intraspinal facet cysts are fluid-filled, rounded structures with a smooth border that originate from the facet joint. Facet joint arthritic changes and spinal instability are thought to lead to protrusion of articular tissue forming an adjacent cyst.[69,70] The lining of a cyst may contain synovial epithelial cells (synovial cyst) or a fibrous wall surrounding myxoid material (ganglion cyst).[71] Radiologically, both types of cysts appear identical. Treatment and prognosis of synovial and ganglion cysts are the same (decompression) and distinguishing between them is not clinically important. It has been postulated that ganglion cysts represent synovial cysts that have undergone degeneration and lost their communication with the facet joint.[72] For simplicity, the following discussion refers to all facet-related cysts as synovial cysts.

Synovial cysts are almost invariably discovered adjacent to a degenerated facet joint. They can arise off the dorsal surface of the joint, protruding into the posterior soft tissues but not compressing any neural structures. These cysts can also arise off the ventral surface and protrude into the intervertebral foramen, lateral recess, or lateral spinal canal. Depending on the location, a synovial cyst can compress the central spinal canal, an exiting nerve root (in the foramen), or a descending nerve root (in the lateral recess or lateral spinal canal). Synovial cysts can also be intrinsically painful, because they are often lined with a nociceptive synovial lining.

IMAGING

For CT scans, an uncomplicated synovial cyst is isodense to CSF and is located next to a degenerated facet joint and occasionally has a calcified wall (Fig. 9.35A, B).[73] Proteinaceous material or blood within the cyst may be isodense to the adjacent muscle or ligament. CT can also clearly demonstrate gas located within a juxta-articular cystic structure that, when present, almost always represents a synovial cyst. CT myelography may better demonstrate the degree of mass effect or stenosis related to an intraspinal or foraminal synovial cyst, by better defining the spinal subarachnoid space with contrast.

Typical MRI findings for synovial cysts include T1- and T2-prolongation and therefore generally follow CSF signal (see Fig. 9.35C, D).[74] Some synovial cysts contain proteinaceous or hemorrhagic material and can also demonstrate T1 hyperintensity. Acute hemorrhage can cause a rapid increase in the size of the cyst and result in acute pain or radiculopathy. The wall of a synovial cyst is typically composed of tough fibrous material, and it may be partially or completely calcified. The degree of calcification is anecdotally predictive of the potential success of percutaneous decompression. Peripheral enhancement of a synovial cyst is common and should not be mistaken as an aggressive feature (see Fig. 9.35E).

An important consideration in the differential diagnosis of a juxta-articular cyst is an extruded disc fragment.[64] Recognizing that the lesion is juxta-articular, and is related to a degenerated facet joint, is the key to making the correct diagnosis. Alternatively, a short-term follow-up MRI

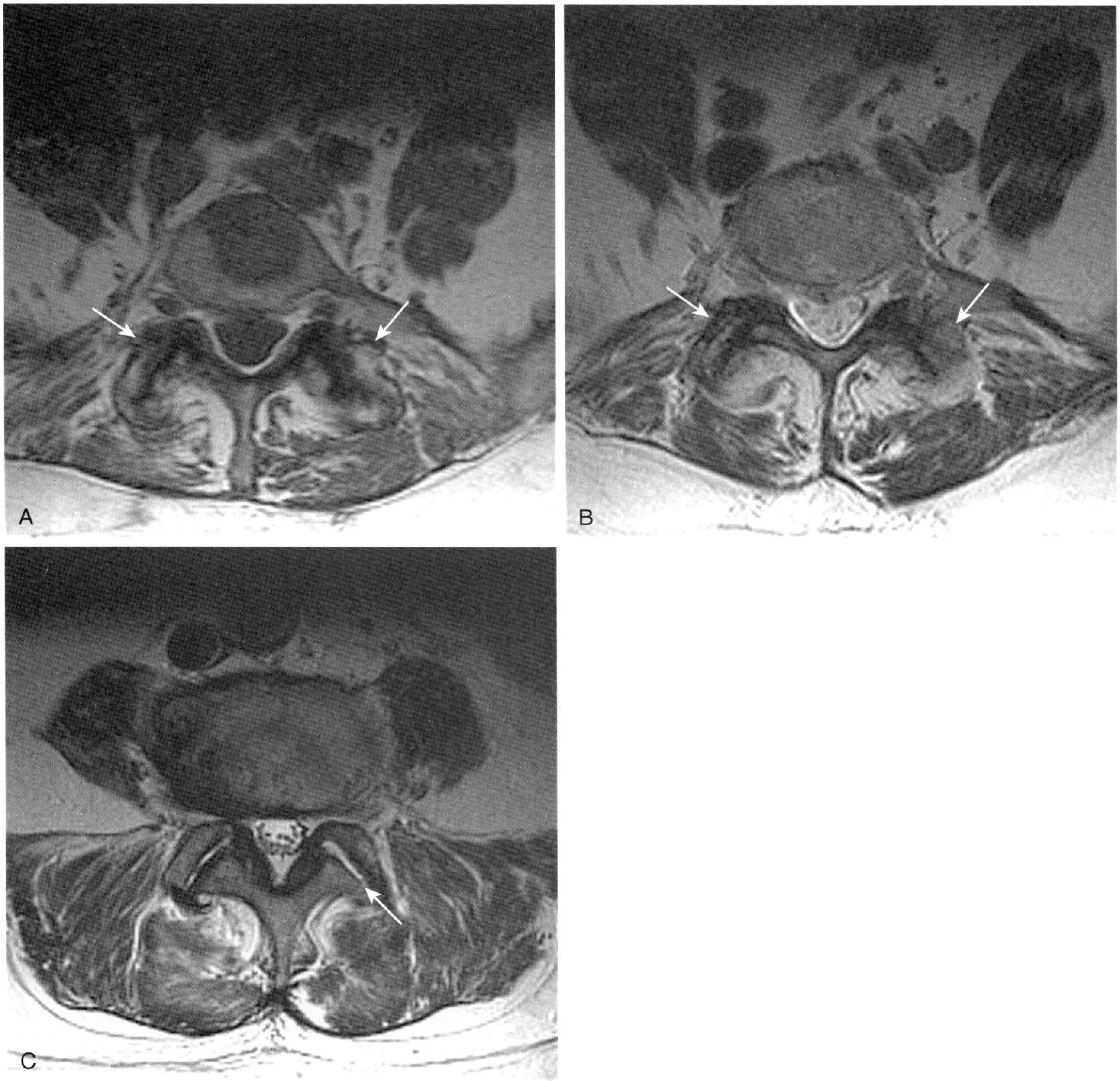

FIG. 9.34 Axial (A) T1-weighted and (B) T2-weighted magnetic resonance imaging (MRI) through the L5–S1 level demonstrate facet degenerative changes *(arrows)* including loss of the joint space, osteophyte overgrowth, and subchondral sclerosis. (C) Axial T2-weighted MRI shows a typical facet joint effusion *(arrow)*.

might show resolution of a disc fragment, but no change in the case of a synovial cyst. Treatment options include conservative management, percutaneous decompression, or surgical removal. Successful outcomes have been reported with all approaches.[75,76]

SPINAL STENOSIS

OVERVIEW

CT effectively evaluates spinal stenosis caused by bony abnormalities of the vertebral column and can show a contributing component of a bulging or herniated disc. CT myelography requires an LP, but this technique has the added benefit of outlining nerve roots and the contour of the thecal sac, particularly, as it relates to disc abnormalities and hypertrophic ligaments. MRI, using axial GRE T2 images in the cervical spine and conventional or fast spin echo T2-weighted images in the thoracic and lumbar spine, provides a noninvasive technique to evaluate the central canal and intervertebral foramen without significant artifact from CSF flow within the canal. If surgical hardware is present, conventional T2-weighted images are used to minimize susceptibility artifact. In some circumstances, axial T1-weighted sequences can be helpful.

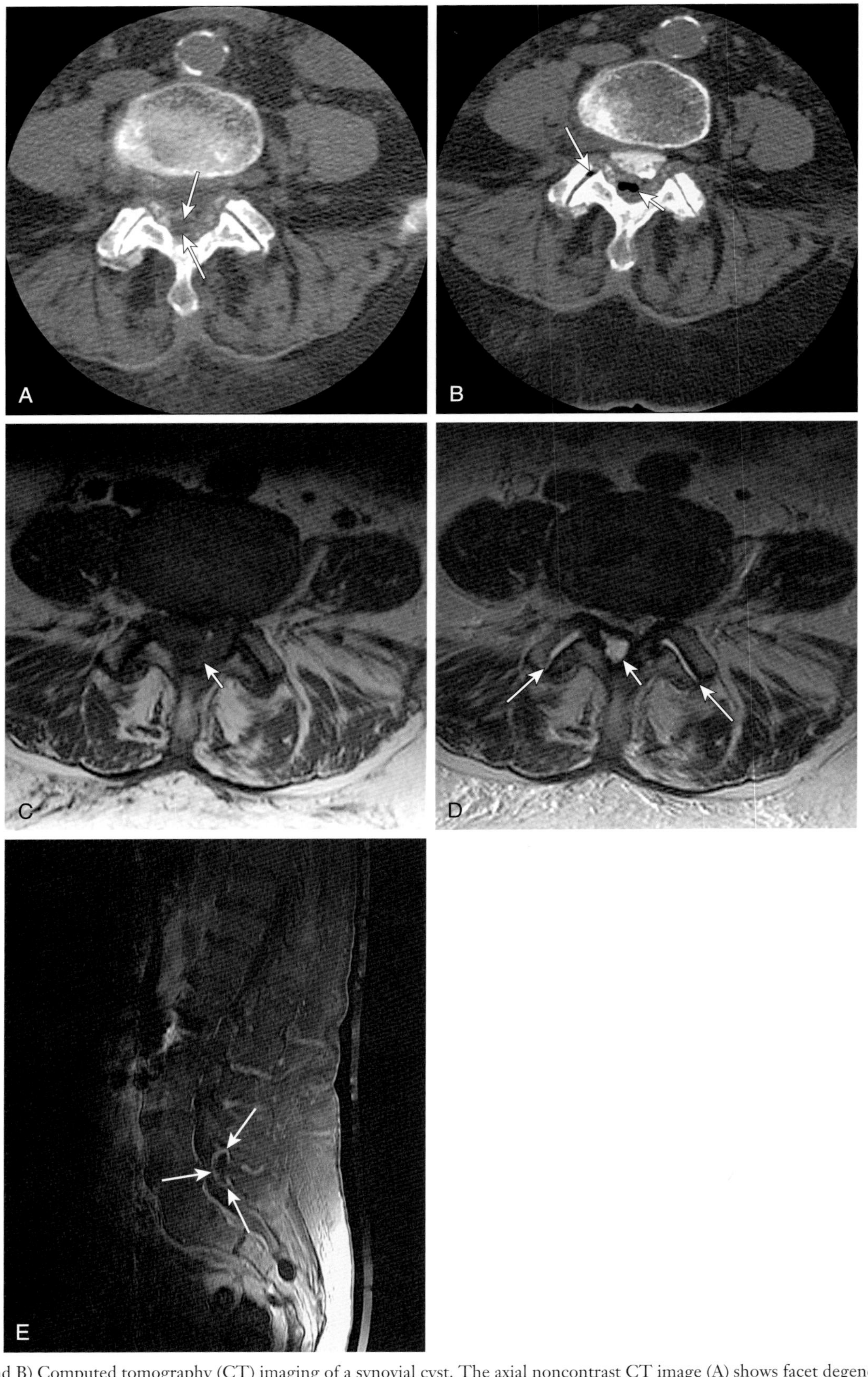

FIG. 9.35 (A and B) Computed tomography (CT) imaging of a synovial cyst. The axial noncontrast CT image (A) shows facet degenerative changes particularly on the patient's right. Ligamentum thickening and calcification are also present. Just deep to the right lamina and partially within the ligamentum flavum, the hypodense synovial cyst *(arrows)* is identified. The patient underwent myelography followed by percutaneous aspiration and steroid injection of the cyst. The postprocedure axial CT image (B) shows persistent mass effect by the partially calcified cyst. Note the presence of air in the cyst *(short arrow)* and the joint *(long arrows)*, which was introduced through the injection and confirms communication between the degenerated facet and the synovial cyst. (C–E) Magnetic resonance imaging of a synovial cyst. On T1-weighted imaging (C), the cyst *(short arrow)* is almost indistinguishable from ligamentum flavum thickening. The T2-weighted image (D) identifies hyperintense fluid within the synovial cyst *(short arrow)* and the joint spaces *(long arrows)*, which is consistent with synovial fluid. Peripheral enhancement *(arrows)* of the synovial cyst wall is common as is demonstrated in the parasagittal postgadolinium T1-weighted fat saturation image (E).

GRADING SPINAL STENOSIS

Although there are various methods to grade spinal stenosis, no single technique has proved reliable in predicting symptoms or favorable surgical outcome. Also, the reliability of grading the severity of lumbar spinal stenosis has been challenged.[77] Consequently, it is difficult to interpret studies examining the efficacy of treatment if there is disagreement on the grading of stenosis.

One grading scheme used by Renfrew in a large spinal imaging practice compares the AP dimension of an abnormal level to an adjacent normal level of the spinal canal in the same patient.[78] The inherent spinal canal diameter is also evaluated to consider the possibility of a developmentally narrow canal.

Mild, moderate, and severe stenoses are assigned relative to the degree of narrowing (Fig. 9.36). Mild stenosis is defined as 75%–99% maintenance of the AP dimension of the normal level, while moderate and severe are 50%–74% and less than 50%, respectively. Using the AP dimension is not absolute, and stenosis can be upgraded or downgraded depending on the developmental size of the canal and the amount of space surrounding the nerve roots.

In a similar manner, the intervertebral foramen can be graded. The foramen is evaluated in the AP and craniocaudad dimension. Stenosis in the foramen can be described as craniocaudal, AP, or combined depending on the site of narrowing. Mild foraminal stenosis usually reflects some narrowing of the inferior part of the foramen by a disc bulge or hypertrophic superior articular process. Moderate narrowing implies loss of fat along a portion of the nerve root and some nerve root displacement. Severe foraminal stenosis is used when little to no fat is visible in the foramen and the nerve root is clearly displaced and/or compressed. These changes are most sensitively detected on a sagittal T1-weighted MRI sequence (Fig. 9.37).

SPONDYLOLYSIS AND SPONDYLOLISTHESIS

OVERVIEW

Spondylolysis refers to a discontinuity in the pars interarticularis of the articular pillar. The etiology is uncertain but likely related to chronic microtrauma leading to a stress-type reaction or fracture, particularly in the lumbar spine.[79] Spondylolysis is usually bilateral, most commonly occurring in the lumbar spine at L5. Spondylolysis can occur in the cervical and thoracic spine, albeit rarely, and may be more related to a developmental abnormality as opposed to trauma in these locations (Fig. 9.38). When bilateral pars fractures are present, the vertebral body can slip forward. This is most apparent in the lumbar spine where axial loading and incompetent pars result in spondylolisthesis. Mild and moderate slips generally do not narrow, but paradoxically enlarge the central canal. Severe spondylolisthesis elongates the spinal canal in the AP direction and narrows the spinal canal in the sagittal plane. All degrees of listhesis tend to result in foraminal stenosis and nerve root compression.

IMAGING

The test of choice to diagnose spondylolysis is CT. Sclerosis and fractures of the pars can be optimally depicted in any plane and the degree of osseous canal or foraminal narrowing can be assessed. MRI can show similar findings, although the actual fracture can sometimes be elusive (Fig. 9.39A, B). MRI exquisitely demonstrates the foraminal stenosis and nerve root compression that are invariably present with spondylolysis and spondylolisthesis (see Fig. 9.39C). MRI also demonstrates cartilaginous overgrowth in the pars fracture that may also contribute to canal and foraminal stenosis. Plain films can easily depict the spondylolisthesis and can demonstrate the pars defect, particularly with an oblique projection. Plain films can be effectively employed to correlate bone detail with an MRI examination, although most imagers prefer CT.

OSTEOPOROTIC COMPRESSION FRACTURES

OVERVIEW

Osteoporotic compression fractures are a major cause of severe back pain in the elderly population, especially women. Benign osteoporotic compression fractures are not always related to a specific trauma and can present with acute onset debilitating back pain, significantly compromising mobility and quality of life. Most compression fractures occur in the mid-thoracic spine and upper lumbar spine, most often affecting the vertebral bodies with the most axial load. Bone pain is generated by irritation of the interosseous and periosteal nociceptive C fibers because of mechanical deformity, altered axial loading, and inflammation.[80] The vertebral body height decreases, often along the anterior column with an anterior wedge appearance. Bone fragments from the superior or inferior end plates can retropulse into the spinal canal causing spinal canal stenosis and sometimes spinal cord compression. The amount of decrease in vertebral body height varies from very mild, just along an end plate, to severe with almost complete loss of vertebral body height. Regardless of the degree of height loss, any acute compression fracture can cause significant pain to the patient. In benign osteoporotic compression fractures, the fracture and edema are usually isolated to the vertebral body and do not extend into the pedicle or posterior elements. Although acute compression fractures can be associated with paravertebral hematomas that can mimic a mass, benign compression fractures are not associated with destructive epidural or paravertebral masses. If there is extension of the edema into the posterior elements or an associated mass, a pathologic compression fracture should be considered. Also, the posterior aspect of the vertebral body is usually straight in benign fractures, while pathologic fractures often have a convex border posteriorly.[81]

Cement augmentation with vertebroplasty or kyphoplasty has been a widely used procedure to treat the patient's pain and improve quality of life. Vertebroplasty involves guiding a trocar needle through the pedicle such that the tip is placed in the anterior third of the fractured vertebral body. Once positioned, polymethylmethacrylate (PMMA) is dispersed within the vertebral body. Kyphoplasty uses a similar technique with the addition of balloon inflation within the vertebral body in an attempt to restore some of the vertebral body height and create

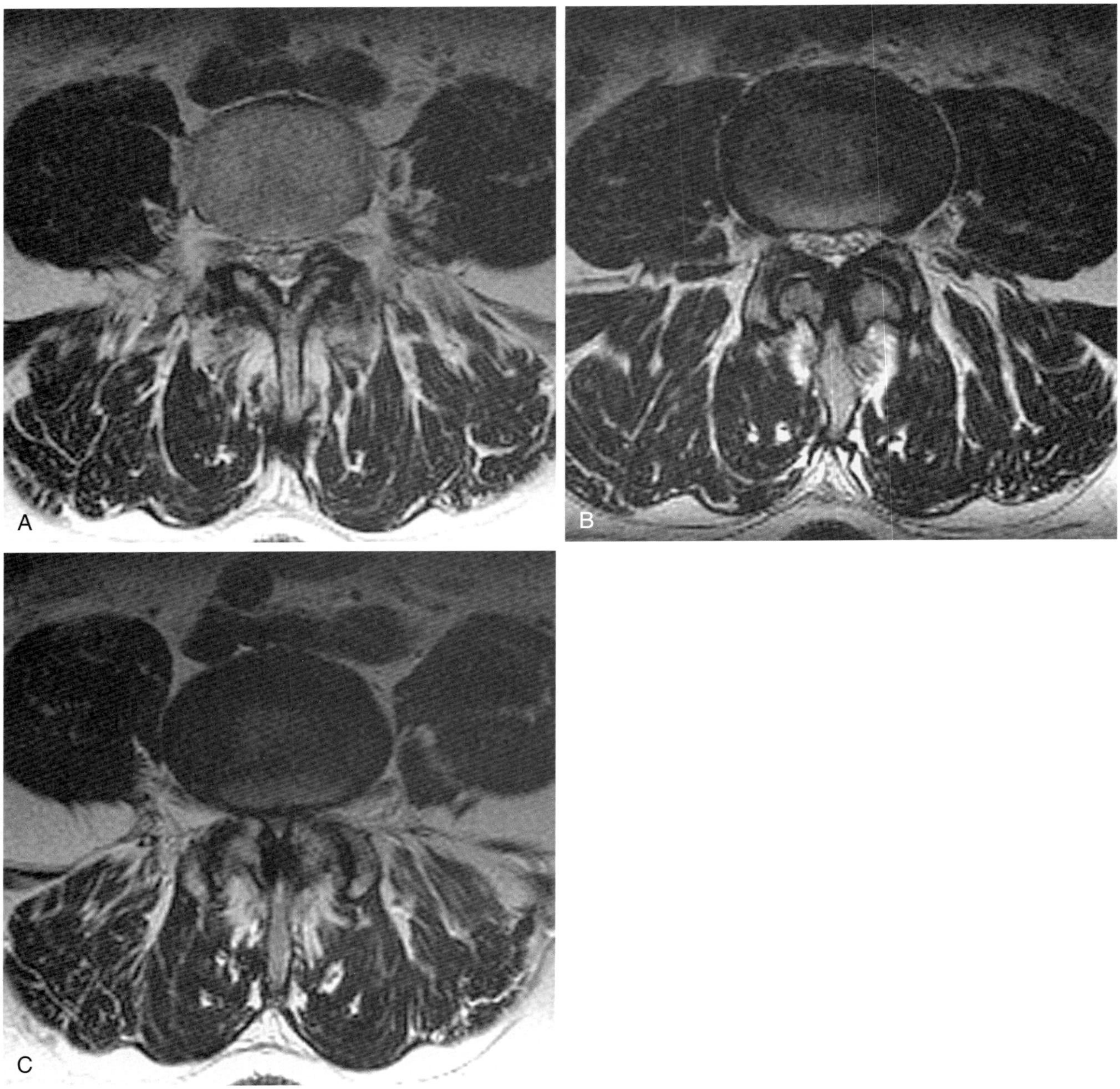

FIG. 9.36 Axial T2-weighted images in the same patient showing (A) mild, (B) moderate, and (C) severe spinal stenosis. In this patient, mild stenosis is produced by subtle facet degenerative changes. Moderate stenosis is produced by the "trifecta" of disc bulging, ligament thickening, and facet degenerative changes. In severe stenosis, the trifecta is again responsible and results in severe compression of the lumbar nerve roots.

a cavity for cement deposition. Both procedures produce significant and equivalent pain relief with similar risk profiles.[82] Studies have shown, however, that the less expensive vertebroplasty procedure can achieve a similar amount of height restoration as kyphoplasty.[83–86] Despite recent controversy of the effectiveness of cement augmentation in pain relief, vertebroplasty and kyphoplasty remain accepted as a treatment for providing immediate pain relief and improved quality of life.[87–90] The most recent masked randomized controlled trial demonstrates the efficacy of vertebroplasty in patients with severe pain and compression fractures of less than 6 weeks' duration.[91]

IMAGING

Plain radiographs identify compression deformities on the lateral view, and a radiograph is most often the initial test performed. CT images with reconstructions

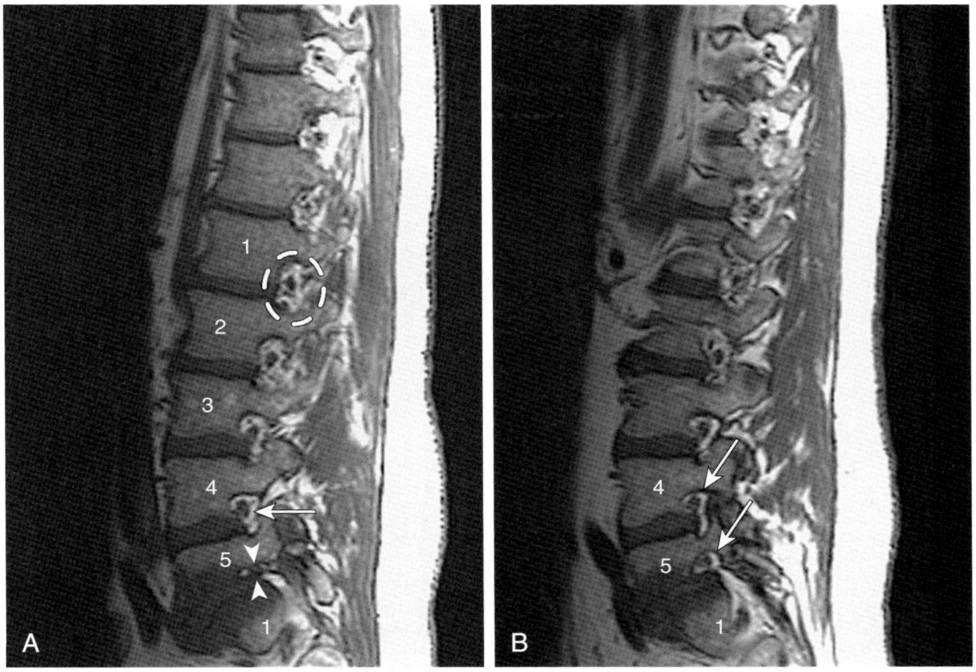

FIG. 9.37 Parasagittal T1-weighted images show (A) mild and severe and (B) moderate foraminal stenosis. In (A) mild stenosis is identified at L4–L5 *(arrow)* and severe stenosis at L5–S1. The severe stenosis is due to loss of disc space height, disc bulging, and osteophyte formation off the vertebral body and superior articular process and results in compression of the exiting nerve root *(arrowheads)*. Note the normal appearance on the foramen at L1–L2 *(dashed oval)*. In (B) moderate stenosis is identified at L4–L5 and L5–S1 secondary to similar degenerative changes *(arrows)*. Note early encroachment on the exiting L4 nerve root at L4–L5.

have excellent resolution of the fracture line(s) within the vertebral body and can help determine the amount of bone fragment retropulsion into the central spinal canal, if any is present. However, x-rays and CT do not provide information on the acuity of the fracture. MRI images, specifically hyperintensity on the STIR (T2-weighted fat suppression) sequence and hypointense signal on the T1-weighted image representing the edematous changes, provide the information needed to diagnose acute compression fractures (Fig. 9.40A, B). Fracture lines also can be seen on MRI images as a hypointense band on T1- and T2-weighted images. Chronic healed compression deformities do not show edematous signal change within a compression deformity. Also, acute compression deformities with only minimal loss of vertebral body height, not readily appreciated on plain films, can be seen on an MRI exam due to the edema from the acute fracture.

CONCLUSION

A radiological image of the spine is an invaluable tool in diagnosing the source of the patient's pain complaint and pinpointing the exact level of spinal pathology. The ability to understand plain x-ray, CT, and MRI of the spine should help the pain medicine physician decide the suitable intervention for his patients. In this chapter, we strived to facilitate such appropriate care.

KEY POINTS

- The artery of Adamkiewicz is the primary supply to the lower two-thirds of the spinal cord and enters the spinal canal via an intervertebral foramen. Although it typically enters on the left from T9–L1, the artery can enter on either side from T5–L4. The T1
- Conventional radiography is the easiest and most cost-effective method of assessing alignment and structure of the spine in both traumatic and nontraumatic conditions. Plain radiographs can easily depict the failure of implanted hardware, such as screw loosening and rod fractures.
- The use of myelography has decreased significantly due to the relatively invasive nature of the procedure and the availability of other noninvasive imaging tools, including CT and MRI, which provide excellent spatial and contrast resolution.
- CT provides the best possible definition of osseous structures and has excellent spatial resolution.
- Disc height is interpreted relative to other intervertebral levels in the same patient.
- A high intensity zone within the midline posterior annulus, discontinuous with the central high signal nucleus pulposus, is a strong predictor of positive discography in patients with back pain.
- Modic-type changes, indicative of degenerative disease in the vertebral end plates and adjacent bone marrow, are classified into three types based on signal characteristics of T1- and T2-weighted signal characteristics.

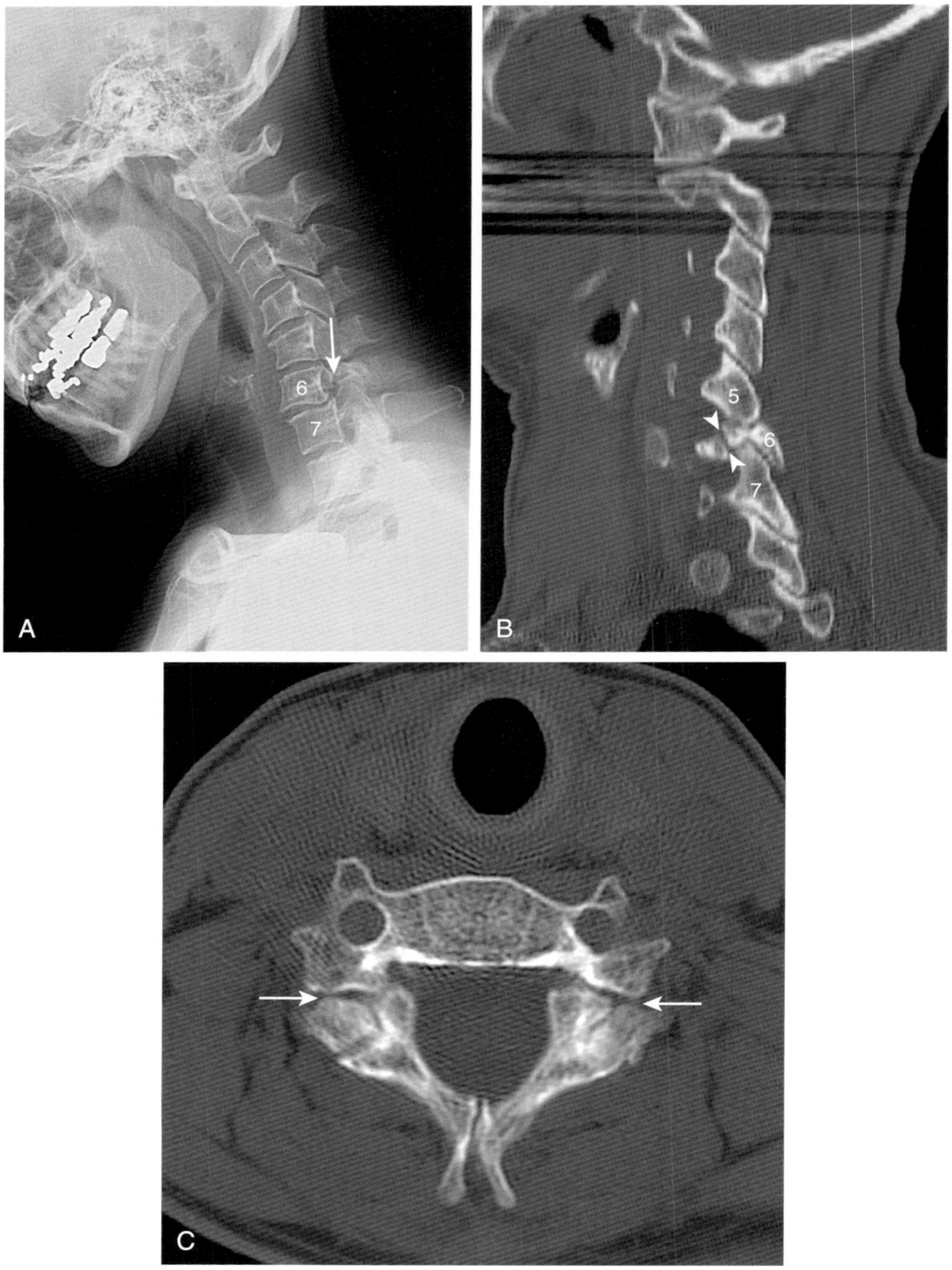

FIG. 9.38 Developmental cervical spondylolysis on (A) lateral plain film, (B) sagittal computed tomography (CT) reconstruction, and (C) axial CT imaging. The plain film reveals a reversed lordosis and anterior subluxation of C6 on C7. Pars deficiencies are suggested *(arrow)*. One of the pars fractures is well profiled on the sagittal CT reconstruction *(arrowheads)*. The axial CT image demonstrates bilateral pars interarticularis fractures *(arrows)*. The sclerotic margins support a chronic process.

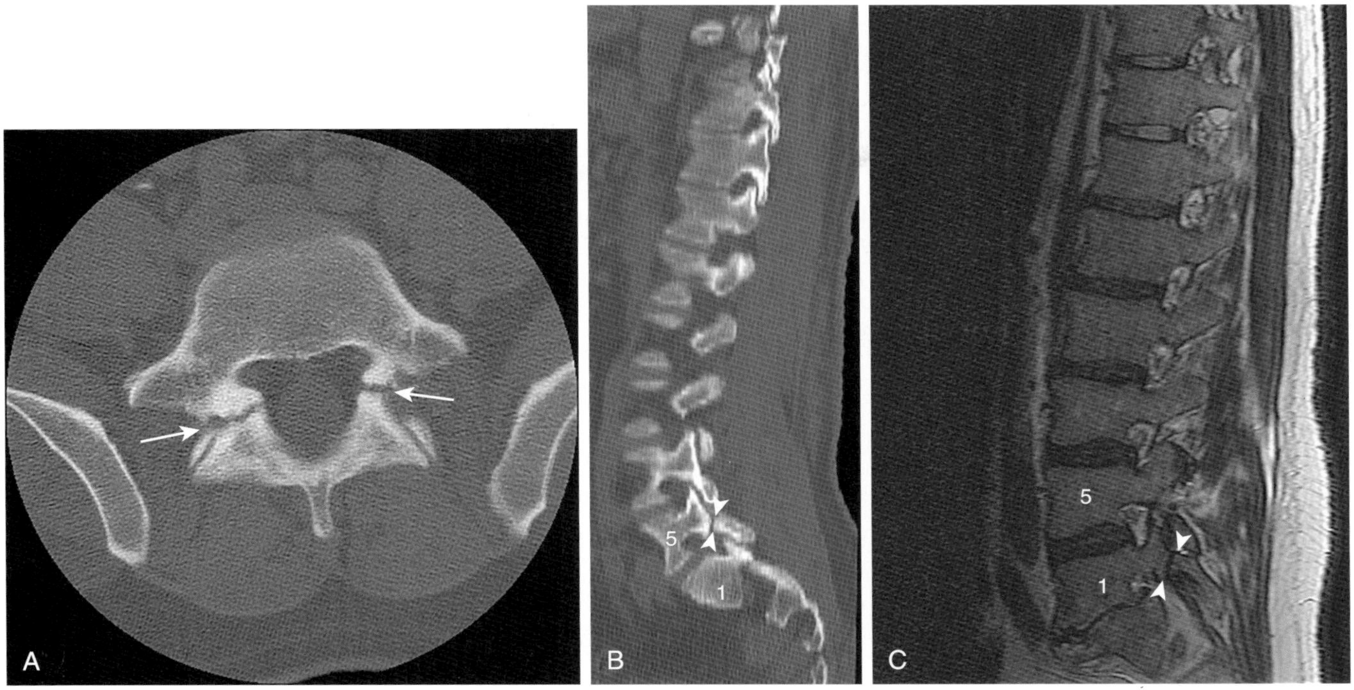

FIG. 9.39 Developmental lumbar spondylolysis on (A) axial computed tomography (CT), (B) sagittal CT reconstruction, and (C) sagittal T2-weighted magnetic resonance imaging (MRI). The axial CT image shows the deficient pars interarticularis *(arrows)* and associated sclerosis. One of the pars defects is easily confirmed on the sagittal CT reconstruction *(arrowheads)* and is identifiable but more subtle on the sagittal MRI *(arrowheads)*.

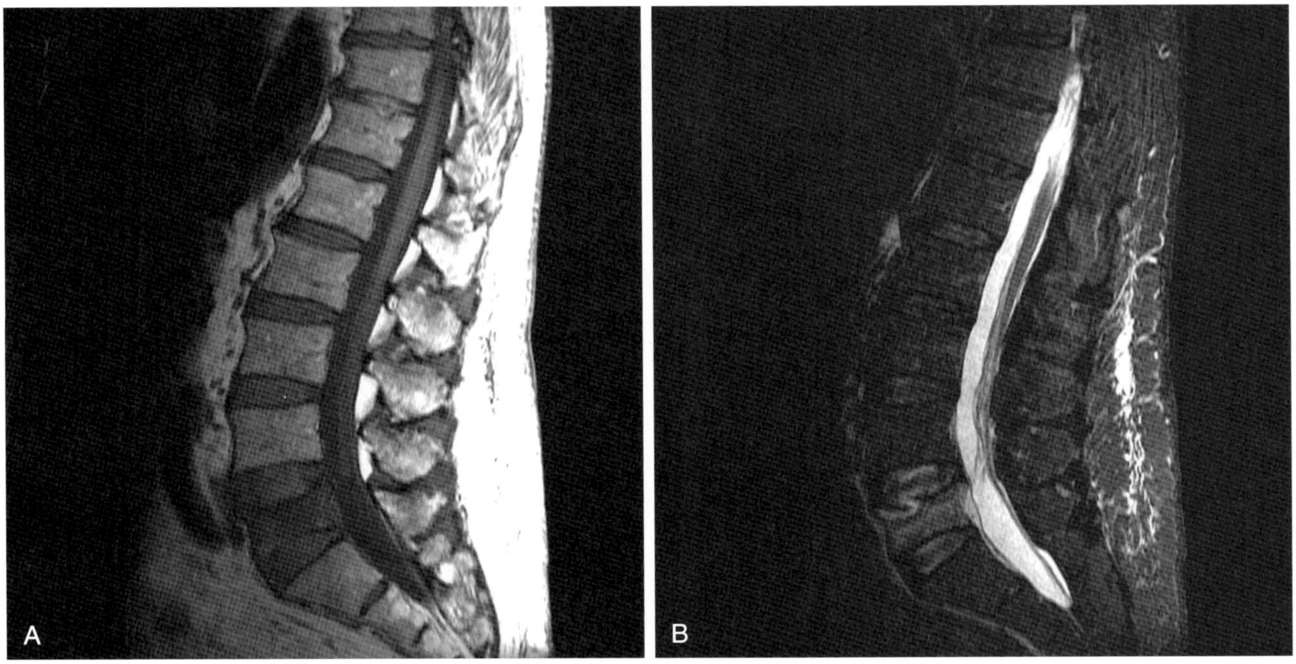

FIG. 9.40 (A) Sagittal T1 and (B) STIR sequences, showing the classic magnetic resonance imaging appearance of an osteoporotic compression fracture at L5. The T1-weighted sequence shows abnormal T1-hypointense signal throughout the L5 vertebral body. There is a mild compression deformity of the L5 superior end plate of approximately 20%. There is mild buckling of the posterior cortical margin of L5. The short-tau inversion recovery sequence (fat suppression T2-weighted image) shows diffuse T2-hyperintensity corresponding to the T1-hypointensity. The marrow signal changes are consistent with edema and relate to inflammation and micromotion of the fractured trabeculae. The curvilinear high T2 signal under the anterior margin of the superior end plate represents fluid within a discrete fracture cleft.

- Using anatomic landmarks to describe the location of a disc herniation provides a precise and consistent classification.
- Although there are various methods to grade spinal stenosis, no single technique has proved reliable in predicting symptoms or favorable surgical outcome.
- Spondylolysis refers to a discontinuity in the pars interarticularis of the articular pillar. It is likely related to chronic microtrauma leading to a stress-type reaction or fracture.
- The posterior aspect of the vertebral body is usually straight in benign fractures, while pathologic fractures often have a convex border posteriorly.
- Despite recent controversy of the effectiveness of cement augmentation in pain relief, vertebroplasty and kyphoplasty remain accepted as a treatment for providing immediate pain relief and improved quality of life.

ACKNOWLEDGMENTS

The authors would like to thank Rita Jarmon and David Botos for help in preparing this chapter.

REFERENCES

Access the reference list online at ExpertConsult.com.

CHAPTER 10

Determination of Disability

David Richard Walega, MD, MSCI

Nearly one in five Americans report a disability, a proportion that increases with age, low literacy, and low education level, according to the Centers for Disease Control and Prevention. Mobility problems related to arthritis, back, or spine problems are the most prevalent causes of self-reported disability in the United States.[1] A growing public health concern with the aging US population, disability-related health care costs exceed $400 billion per year. More than 7 million disability assessments are made each year in the United States, many of which are made by physicians in the field of pain medicine.

Regardless of training, background, or specialty, physicians are asked for assessments, opinions, and expertise regarding disability or impairment in their patients.[2] The process of disability assessment can be fraught with subjective bias, and the role of determining disability can pose ethical issues for treating physicians. As "healers," physicians aim to maximize the health, well-being, and functional potential of patients, but in disability determination, physicians become advocates for patients' financial interests and health care resources, the role which can conflict with the "healer" role. For some physicians, disability determination causes discomfort or unease, especially when opinions between physician and patient differ or when litigation is involved.

Disability determination is not typically a part of medical education, and in most states, no formal training or certification is required for physicians to make these assessments.[3] In turn, many physicians lack experience or training in the methods of assessing disability, how to perform an independent medical evaluation (IME), how to assess a patient's ability to return to work, or how to assess what activities a patient is capable of performing. In theory, disability determination should be a transparent, unprejudiced, and objective process, and impairments, functional limitations, and work restrictions should be associated with objective evidence for tissue damage, organ dysfunction, or cognitive dysfunction. Furthermore, this evidence should be reproducible with high interrater agreement. Knowledge of basic terminology in disability determination is important to the pain specialist.

Disability is an alteration in one's physical or cognitive capacity to perform a specific task, function, or activity and is highly dependent on individuality and context. Disability is greatly influenced by education, age, and social and cultural factors, as well as vocational opportunities and training and is therefore contextual and subjective. There is no universally accepted method for the assessment of disability. In fact, the definition of disability varies widely among government entitlement programs, private disability insurers, state Workers' Compensation Boards, and others.

In contrast, **impairment** is an objective term that defines the loss or loss of use of, or derangement of any body part, organ function or organ system, or cognitive and psychological functioning. Impairment can be temporary or permanent, and can be reproducibly measured through testing or physician assessment. **Handicap** is the legal or social policy term used to describe a disability.

An **impairment rating** or **whole person impairment rating** is an objective assessment of a patient's disablement and should reflect the severity of a particular medical condition and the way one's activities of daily living or vocation are affected. For example, the accidental amputation of a finger in a concert pianist creates a much greater impairment than the same injury in a truck driver. Validated, evidence-based methods for calculating these impairments are important.

Impairment ratings can be calculated using the American Medical Association's (AMA) Guides to the Evaluation of Permanent Impairment, currently in its sixth edition.[4] Previously faulted for lack of validity and reliability, the Guides in its current iteration is meant to be a more accurate tool to measure functional loss as an integral part of the impairment rating and provide a more standardized assessment of activities of daily living and functional limitations from a particular injury or disease process. Overall, the impairment rating defines the impact of injury or disease on one's ability to perform self-care, manual tasks, maintain home and health, manage in an emergency, care for one's children or dependents and to communicate, function independently, travel, and work. The more serious the injury and the more impactful the impairment for an individual, the larger the whole person impairment rating will be. In most cases, impairment is considered permanent if there is no significant change in the condition over a 12-month period. The calculation of impairment ratings using the Guides remains a complicated process when injury or disease severity is high or when multiple injuries or diseases are involved.

This system is meant to be logical, systematic, and fair. In contrast to prior editions of the Guides that used a "tables method" and "range-of-motion method" for calculating impairment rating based on anatomic loss or damage assessed with physical examination or diagnostic findings, the new Guides uses a "diagnosis based impairment model" to provide a more individualized assessment of impairment with a multidimensional approach.[5]

In general, an impairment class for any injury or disease is defined on a scale of 0–4, shown in Table 10.1, and an impairment rating or percentage is calculated (no impairment, minimal impairment, moderate impairment, severe impairment, very severe impairment) using categories or scores defined by a patient's history, clinical presentation, physical examination findings, diagnostic or objective test results, functional history, and burden of treatment compliance. For each organ system or body region, the Guides provide clinical examples and calculations for the clinician to follow.[4]

TABLE 10.1 Sample Impairment Functional Classification From American Medical Association's Guides

Functional Class	Impairment
0	No symptoms with strenuous activity
1	Symptoms with strenuous activity; no symptoms with normal activity; individual is independent
2	Symptoms with normal activity; individual is independent
3	Symptoms with minimal activity; individual is partially dependent
4	Symptoms at rest; individual is totally dependent

From Rondinelli RD, Genovese E, Katz RT, et al. Guides to the Evaluation of Permanent Impairment. *6th ed. American Medical Association; 2008.*

For example, a 20-year-old female with a low back injury incurred while lifting a toddler while working in a day care center, who responds to conservative therapy over the course of 3 weeks but still complains of mild nonradiating low back pain with heavy lifting, and on physical examination has only normal findings, radiographs are normal. Her impairment rating is calculated a 0 because she experienced a minor injury, had a short period of treatment, has no physical examination findings, and demonstrates full physical function because she can still work and take care of herself with complete independence.

In contrast, one with more complicated and serious pain, physical examination findings, and long-term limitations would have a much higher impairment rating. For instance, a 52-year-old male chauffeur is a restrained driver in an auto accident, wherein his car collides with a retaining wall. He suffers L4-5 and L5-S1 disc herniations that required laminectomies at two levels and a two-level posterior spine fusion with implanted hardware. At maximal medical improvement (MMI) 1 year later, he has a foot drop on examination and loss of sensation in the right L4, L5 and S1 dermatomes, and right L5 and S1 radiculopathies are confirmed on electromyelography. Pain and function do not improve with rehabilitation and strength training and after a year of treatment, and he takes multiple medications to control pain at rest and with any activity. He must use an orthotic on the left ankle in addition to a cane to ambulate and he cannot drive a car due to his right leg and foot weakness. A Pain Disability Questionnaire confirms that his function is extremely limited in several domains. Using this patient information and the charts, tables, and equations in The Spine and Pelvis chapter of the Guides, his impairment rating is noted within the class 4 range, which translates to 25%–33% whole person impairment. This impairment rating is then modified with a grade (A, B, C, D, or E; A being the lowest grade, and E being the most severe grade) by considering the functional impairments, physical examination findings, and objective findings in this particular case, within an impairment class. In this case, a net adjustment of 2 is calculated when considering the high severity in the listed domains, which translates to a grade E.

Note that the Pain Disability Questionnaire is used more in research studies.[6] Other questionnaires used in back disability and functional impairments include the Pain Disability Index, Oswestry Low Back Pain Questionnaire, the Roland-Morris Low Back Pain and Disability Questionnaire, Quebec Back pain Disability Scale, and the Waddell Disability Index.[7–11] Although the different questionnaires have been compared,[12] it is beyond the scope of this chapter to detail these comparisons.

The Guides outlines a systematic approach to this rating system, which is increasingly complicated with more impactful injuries and disease processes. In addition, impairments from multiple organ systems or body regions are accounted for by adding impairment values together; however, the complexity of this process is beyond the scope of this chapter. Although the Guides was redeveloped to be accurate, reliable, unbiased, and reproducible, this modification of impairment rating has not been tested or validated in rigorous trials[13] but because it is the only evidence-based and peer-reviewed impairment assessment tool available in the United States, the Guides may be the best reference for calculating impairment ratings.

Impairment ratings are used in calculating damage awards and other monetary compensation packages. It is important to note that an impairment rating should not be assessed until the patient has reached MMI, the state at which all potential healing, repair, and treatment has been completed, and the impairment is permanent and unlikely to change significantly within the ensuing 1-year period.

DISABILITY PROGRAMS

The Social Security Administration (SSA) is a government agency that administers two federally entitlement programs, Title II (Social Security Disability Insurance) and Title XVI (Supplemental Security Income). The Social Security Act defines disability as "the inability to engage in any substantial gainful activity by reason of a medically determinable physical or mental impairment which can be expected to result in death or has lasted or can be expected to last for a continuous period of not less than 12 months."[14] Disability is based on the interplay between vocational and medical issues. In this context, the role of the physician is to document medical findings and define medical impairments and functional limitations of a patient applying for these government-issued benefits. The Blue Book Listing of Impairments (for treating physicians) and the Green Book (for consultant physicians) are published SSA guidelines used for the determination of disability.[14] Physician office notes, diagnostic test results, or written narratives will be requested by the SSA in the disability determination process of a patient. Often, there will be more than one impairment or cause for disability. In those patients without a severe impairment that renders one disabled based on a single particular medical problem, **"medical equivalence"** may be recognized, wherein multiple impairments result in additive functional limitations that equal the severity of a single impairment. Reduced **residual functional capacity** (RFC) may also be assessed. The RFC takes into account the proportion of the typical 8-hour work day an individual can sit, stand, or walk; the number of pounds one can lift and carry; how frequently or infrequently one is capable of performing these tasks; and the cognitive and psychological demands of work, also taking into account one's vision and hearing abilities. An adjudicator assesses whether an individual is capable of sedentary, light, medium, heavy, or very heavy work duties, taking into account the assessments of treating and consulting physicians, and the age, education, and prior work experience of an applicant. For example, sedentary work requires the ability to sit for 6 hours, to stand/walk for 2 hours, and to lift no more than 10 pounds at a time. Light and medium work require the ability to stand/walk for 6 hours and to lift no more than 20 or 50 pounds, respectively.[14]

Workmen's compensation programs are meant to provide the injured worker prompt and appropriate medical treatment and restore a worker to his or her preinjury state and enable the return to work and gainful employment. The funding and administration of these programs vary from state to state. Four categories of work-related disability are possible—temporary partial, temporary total, permanent partial, permanent total—and the work-related injury can be mental or physical. The duration and extent of workmen's compensation benefits are determined by the category into which the claimant falls and may include medical expenses, wages, and a monetary settlement. In general, the injured worker may be provided monetary benefits for lost wages due to an injury, or may be provided with short- or long-term medical care depending on the severity and duration of a work-related injury. A treating physician may play a significant role in coordinating and advocating for the medical care of the injured worker, as well as assessing impairment and disability.

Short- and long-term disability plans are private insurance policies that provide compensation to those with policies who are disabled by injury or illness, under temporary or permanent conditions. These policies are often a part of an employee benefits package but can also be purchased privately. These policies typically do not cover medical expenses. With these private programs, disability is defined as the inability to perform the majority of activities required of a specific occupation. Duration, qualifications for, and restrictions of benefits will vary from policy to policy.

DISABILITY EVALUATIONS

The **IME** is a comprehensive assessment of a patient performed by a trained physician. In contrast to the conventional doctor-patient relationship, the evaluating physician for an IME does not provide medical care and does not initiate a therapeutic relationship with the person undergoing the evaluation. The purpose of the IME is to objectively assess the impact of an injury and subsequent disability in the patients' ability to function in a variety of domains including self-care, work duty, and leisure or recreational activity. The evaluating physician reviews the treatment that has been rendered, performs a comprehensive examination, and reviews pertinent diagnostic tests and procedure reports and then comments on the current clinical status, relevant diagnoses, and whether the patient is at MMI. The IME report should address causation of the injury and the relationship of the injury to the impairment, and any anatomic, physiologic, or psychological impairments should be identified and described in addition to the permanence of these impairments. Functional limitations, defined as the lack of ability to perform activities within the normal human range as a result of a specific impairment, should be specifically addressed in an IME report. Examples would include the inability to lift more than 25 pounds due to a lumbar intervertebral disc herniation or an inability to function independently due to an anoxic brain injury. Significant pain behaviors are often identified during the IME, although evidence shows that malingering is present in 1%–10% of chronic pain patients.[15] The credibility of the patient should be addressed in the IME report. The mechanics of the disability evaluation and impairment rating are found in the AMA Guides to the Evaluation of Permanent Impairment. Table 10.2 lists the important contents of the IME report.

TABLE 10.2 Components of an Independent Medical Evaluation

- Narrative history
- Current clinical status
- Results of physical examination and diagnostic studies
- Causation of injury and relationship to job duties
- Maximal medical improvement assessment
- Pertinent diagnoses
- Impairments and function limitations
- Permanence of impairments and limitations
- Analysis of job tasks
- Assessment of ability to perform specific job tasks

In contrast to an IME, **functional capacity evaluation** (FCE) and **work capacity evaluation** (WCE) are measures of a patient's functional ability and are typically performed by a physical therapist or occupational therapist. Tolerances of sitting, standing, walking bending, reaching, lifting and climbing are typically assessed in real time, preferably by a trained and unbiased evaluator. There is typically specific emphasis on the ability to lift and carry specific weights. The outcome of these evaluations is highly dependent on the patient's motivation and effort and is inherently subjective to the examiner, especially in chronic pain patients. Relatedly, WCE simulates a specific workplace environment, and a person's ability to functional normally within the simulated environment, to predict how well the injured worker can function upon return to the workplace. The WCE is easier to perform for sedentary or light duty jobs as compared with technical labor-intensive jobs, wherein heavy equipment, tools, or vehicles are needed.

MANAGING DISABILITY IN PAIN PRACTICES

Due to the nature of painful or disabling diseases, pain specialists must often balance disability evaluation and assessment with patient and disease management. An emphasis on proactive patient management is important, especially with recurrent pain symptoms.[16] Disability and function should be addressed early in the doctor-patient relationship and continually reassessed when function remains limited. Management should include an assessment of disability risk, patient education, and psychosocial support, in addition to a treatment plan that includes specific expectations for improvement.[17] Red flags for protracted disability include noncompliance with treatment, poor participation in physical therapy or rehabilitation, refusal or inability to return to work, noncompliance with weight loss, exercise, and smoking cessation recommendations, and patient hostility, anger, and disruptive behavior.[18] However, an overemphasis on nonorganic signs as a hallmark of malingering conversion disorder or impending disability has been called into question.[19] **Disability syndrome** is a set of counterproductive and dysfunctional attitudes and beliefs that develop over time as an individual adapts to the role of being a disabled person. The more significant the dysfunction in the patient, the more important a multidisciplinary approach to pain management, with an emphasis on functional restoration and maximizing coping skills is necessary.

When setting treatment and rehabilitation goals for an established patient, physicians are often more lenient regarding recovery time and return to work after an injury. However, when new patients with long-standing disability issues are evaluated, physicians may be more demanding of a higher level of activity or performance. Catastrophizing, fear avoidance beliefs, and other maladaptive behaviors should be identified and addressed by the pain specialist because these are predictors of chronic pain and subsequent protracted disability.

KEY POINTS

- Disability is a vaguely defined term that describes the inability to perform specific tasks or functions.
- Impairment is an objective loss of function due to an injury or disease.
- Pain specialists require an understanding of disability terminology to provide objective ongoing or independent assessment of pain patients with disabilities and impairments.
- Physicians should use validated, evidence-based methods when providing impairment ratings.

REFERENCES

Access the reference list online at ExpertConsult.com.

SECTION III

Perioperative Pain Management

SECTION OUTLINE HEAD

CHAPTER 11

Preventive Analgesia

Christina M. Spofford, MD, PhD ◎ Robert W. Hurley, MD, PhD

One goal of the perioperative physician anesthesiologist is to provide sufficient analgesia during a surgical procedure so that it can be performed at the highest surgical standard with the least possible impact on the patient. This objective includes the prevention of intraoperative pain, as well as short- (acute) and long-term (chronic/persistent) postoperative pain. Over the past 30 years, many strategies have been employed toward this end; unfortunately, the prevalence of postoperative pain remains problematic, with at least half of patients reporting moderate to severe pain at the time of discharge.[1] Despite many postoperative pain studies in basic science labs and clinical trials, there remains no "best" approach. These failures can be attributed to a multitude of factors, including the study design of clinical trials, an incomplete understanding of the basic neurophysiology of the surgical injury, the semantics of the terminology used to describe the phenomena, and understanding the concept of what constitutes postoperative pain.

TERMINOLOGY

Preventive analgesia: Preventive analgesia is generally defined as an antinociceptive treatment that attenuates pain from high-intensity noxious stimuli before, during, and after the insult. The goal of preventive analgesia is to attenuate afferent input produced by the peripheral nervous system that can alter peripheral or central sensory processing. This afferent input, left unchecked, can cause central sensitization and subsequent chronic postsurgical pain. There are two phases to the noxious stimuli: the primary phase during which the noxious stimuli is related to the surgical injury itself (cutting, retracting, stretching, etc.), and the secondary phase during which the ongoing noxious stimuli is produced by the release of chemicals, including inflammatory mediators from damaged tissue (Fig. 11.1). The secondary phase can begin during the intraoperative period and extend long into the postoperative recovery period (see Fig. 11.1). The duration of the postoperative recovery period and severity of pain depends on many factors, including the type and extent of the surgical operation, the immunological and nutritional status of the patient, the baseline psychological profile, as well as the associated medical comorbidities such as preexisting pain and drugs used to treat pain. The importance of addressing and treating the two phases of the injury is borne out in the literature and has prompted the evolution from "pre-emptive" to "preventive" analgesia.

Many advances have been made toward understanding the pathophysiology of nociceptive pathways. Both physicians and basic science researchers have become more knowledgeable about the nociceptive mediators that act in the periphery and activate the primary nociceptive afferent, as well as those that act centrally at the level of the spinal cord and brain. We now appreciate that tissue injury produces changes in the peripheral afferent neuron and in the spinal cord, both contributing to prolonged excitability. This hypersensitive state can persist for days to months, and contributes to acute and chronic postsurgical pain, a process referred to as *peripheral and central sensitization* (see Chapters 1 and 2 for details).

PATHOPHYSIOLOGY OF PREVENTIVE ANALGESIA

POSTINJURY SENSITIZATION

Sensitization can occur in both the peripheral and central nervous systems (CNS) following a surgical injury. The relative contribution of each component is a matter of debate. However, following tissue injury, gene expression is altered[2] and mediators are released to activate the peripheral nociceptive afferent. The continued activation of these afferents enhances the patient's response to further stimuli. The inflammatory mediators can activate and increase the sensitivity of the nociceptors, thereby changing the nociceptive threshold of the afferent. Persistent activation can also lead to alterations in the neurophysiological properties of the primary afferent itself. Peripheral sensitization refers to the summation of these processes.

There are a number of events that occur on the cellular level that are responsible for peripheral sensitization. Transient receptor potential vanilloid (TRPV) receptors on small C fibers are nonselective cation channels. TRPV receptors are known to play an important role in peripheral sensitization and, thus, are prime targets for novel analgesics. They are activated by repeated heat stimulation, acidic environments, and a wide variety of mediators found in postoperative healing tissues (prostaglandin E2, serotonin, bradykinin, epinephrine, adenosine triphosphate, interleukin-1a, interleukin-6, tumor necrosis factor, chemokines, and nerve growth factor). Activation of TRPV channels results in a painful burning sensation.[3] The release of these mediators also increases the magnitude of Na^+ current in sensory neuron voltage-gated sodium channels.[4] The activation of TRPV and these Na^+ channels begin a vicious circle that culminates in increased pain. Both sensory neuron-specific sodium channels and TRPV receptors can be phosphorylated by intracellular kinases (protein kinase C or tyrosine kinase), thereby potentiating the release of excitatory amino acids and peptides from sensory afferents and accentuating the pain. The inflammatory activation of TRPV receptors and sensory neuron-specific sodium channels results in vasodilatation and edema. The neurogenic inflammation is mediated by a calcitonin gene-related peptide, substance P, and neurokinin A, and can further sensitize the nociceptive afferents, leading to allodynia or hyperalgesia.[5,6]

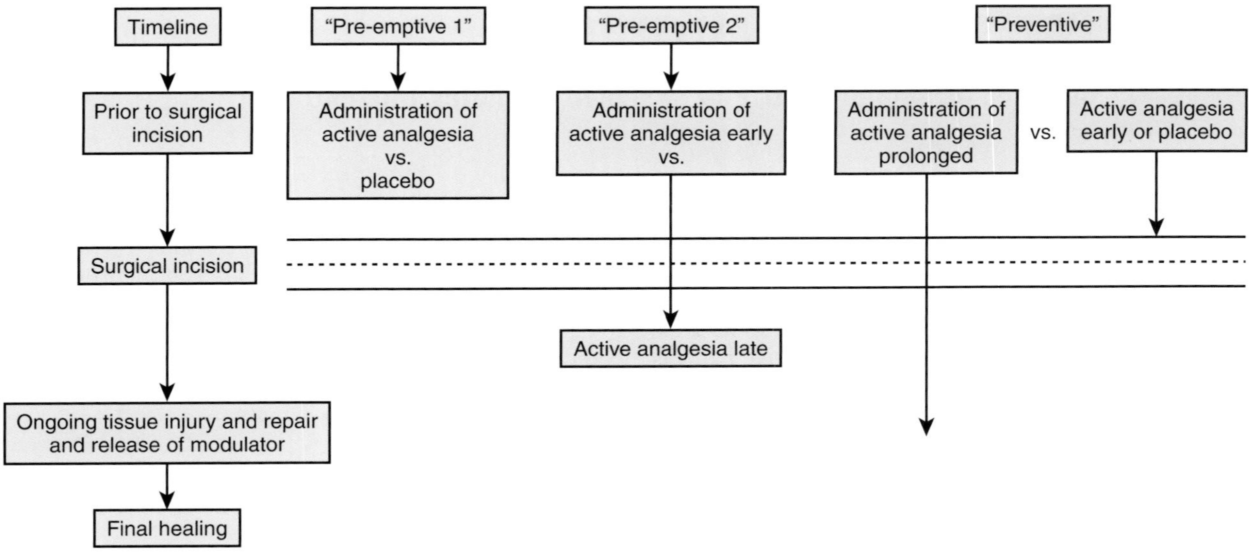

FIG. 11.1 Timeline of surgical injury and recovery on the *y*-axis and timeline of perioperative analgesic interventions on the *x*-axis. Representation of research study design differences of "pre-emptive" versus "preventive" analgesia.

Hypersensitivity and alterations also take place in the CNS, the spinal cord, and supraspinal structures as a result of a surgical injury. Following a tissue injury, such as an incision through the skin, fascia, and muscle, a subset of A-delta and C fibers become spontaneously active[7] and barrage the second-order neurons in the spinal cord. In turn, these neurons release excitatory neurotransmitters, which increase the amplitude of the spinal cord neuron response and lower the response threshold for further stimuli. Therefore the response of the dorsal horn neurons to a particular stimulus—be it noxious (hyperalgesia) and/or innocuous (allodynia)—is altered, and perception of the painful stimulus is increased in intensity as well as duration. The injury also results in alterations of dorsal horn neurons. These neurons react to nonnoxious stimuli as if they were noxious (allodynia) and to noxious stimuli (hyperalgesia) with an exaggerated response, but they also begin to respond to stimuli outside their original receptive field (secondary sites). There is evidence that C fiber input from an injury also causes formation of anatomic connections at the spinal cord level between neurons that respond to A-beta fiber transmission and neurons that respond to A-delta and C fiber transmission. Animal studies have shown that A-beta fibers from injured tissue begin to produce and release substance P, normally found in C fibers, and contribute to pain sensitivity.[8] Central sensitization has two temporally distinct phases. An early phase of hypersensitivity is triggered by changes in glutamate receptor phosphorylation and ion channel properties. The second phase (longer lasting) involves transcriptional changes that result in the formation of new proteins responsible for prolonged pain hypersensitivity.[9]

The development of central and/or peripheral sensitization after traumatic injury or surgical incision can result in amplification of pain, or pain greater than the magnitude anticipated postoperatively. Therefore preventing the establishment of altered central processing by analgesic treatment may, in the short term, reduce postprocedural or traumatic pain and accelerate recovery. In the long term, the benefits may include a reduction in chronic pain and improvement in the patient's quality of recovery and overall function. Theoretically, providing analgesia to block the initial barrage of afferent produced by the surgical incision can result in a reduction of pain from minor or short-duration surgical procedures. However, surgical procedures that produce substantial tissue injury, resulting in the release of inflammatory mediators and peripheral or central sensitization, will require analgesic techniques that are in effect throughout the period of injury and recovery. Crile[10] first discussed this concept at the turn of the century. Woolf[11] established the neurophysiological basis of central sensitization after injury in a series of animal experiments, and Wall, in an editorial, suggested preinjury analgesia for the reduction of postinjury pain.[12]

PREVENTIVE ANALGESIA IN CLINICAL INVESTIGATIONS

Preventive analgesic studies compare the effects of continuous analgesic therapy when administered throughout the perioperative period versus preemptive analgesia, which refers to the administration in the preoperative period only, or when no treatment is provided.

Many studies and meta-analyses have been performed to determine if aggressive analgesia before surgery impacts postoperative pain scores or prevalence of chronic postoperative pain. Interestingly, in one large study,[13] no benefit was noted in the preemptive group that was treated with nonsteroidal antiinflammatory drugs (NSAIDs), intravenous opioids, intravenous ketamine, peripheral local anesthetics, and caudal analgesia for postoperative pain relief. However, an N-methyl-D-aspartate (NMDA) receptor antagonist, dextromethorphan, did demonstrate a preemptive effect. Single-dose epidural studies showed some benefit, although in most of the trials, improvements were insignificant. The administration of continuous epidural infusion produced statistically improved pain scores, but did not support that preemptive analgesia was of greater benefit than applying the analgesic technique after the onset of surgery.[14] Most of these studies do not support the concept of preemptive analgesia, although several do find a role for preventive analgesia.

A more recent meta-analysis, using more stringent inclusion criteria from the Cochrane collaboration, found a pronounced preventive effect with epidural analgesia, local anesthetic wound infiltration, and systemic NSAID administration, but had mixed results for opioids or systemic NMDA receptor antagonists (Fig. 11.2).[15] This was followed by a randomized controlled study, in which the use of perioperative parecoxib in lumbar spine surgery was shown to reduce postoperative opioid consumption, lower pain scores, and increase patient satisfaction with their analgesic regimen.[16] Similar results in plastic, ambulatory, otolaryngologic surgery have been found with celecoxib.[17–19] However, a meta-analysis of randomized controlled trials using perioperative NSAIDs or Cox 2 inhibitors demonstrated a reduction in postoperative pain scores with nonselective NSAIDs, but not with Cox 2 inhibitors alone.[20] Cox 2 inhibitors were found to reduce postoperative morphine consumption, but were also associated with an increased risk of renal failure (number required to harm of 73). Additionally, in the trials that used ketamine and Cox 2 inhibitors, no significant difference was noted; however, three trials that used intravenous or intramuscular dextromethorphan and Cox 2 inhibitors had a reduction in either pain intensity or supplemental analgesic use in the postoperative period.

Despite the findings of Ong and colleagues, the use of the NMDA antagonist, ketamine, has increased in recent years. Its major benefit is probably related to its modulation of opioid-induced hyperalgesia. A decrease in opioid-induced hyperalgesia has been associated with lower postoperative pain scores and opioid consumption.[21,22] Interestingly, in the setting of anesthetics in which no opioids were administered, the preoperative bolus administration of ketamine alone provided no postoperative benefit.[23]

The gabapentinoids have gained popularity for preventive analgesia in the perioperative period.[24] Despite early positive trials with these drugs for a variety of surgeries, new systematic reviews with meta-regression analyses of gabapentin as a prophylactic analgesic have been performed. In the most recent analysis by Doleman and colleagues,[25] 133 randomized controlled trials were included where preoperative gabapentin versus placebo were studied. The finding of this analysis revealed that gabapentin reduced morphine-equivalent consumption by 8.44 mg (7.26–9.62, $P < .001$). The study also noted gabapentin mildly reduced pain scores for the first 24 hours, with the greatest effect at 1 hour postoperatively (mean reduction in pain score by 1.68 points on a 11-point pain scale). These results, although positive, are less robust than previously reported, likely due to underpowered study designs.[25] Although gabapentin and pregabalin have few side effects, their use preoperatively can impact the anesthetic plan, as they have consistently been shown to cause postoperative sedation. One trial that investigated the use of gabapentin for neurosurgery resulted in prolonged endotracheal intubation.[26] Therefore it is important that the anesthesiologist adjust the quantity of commonly administered sedatives and/or general anesthetics given to the patient preoperatively or intraoperatively.

Regional anesthesia is used extensively to provide both intraoperative and postoperative anesthesia and analgesia. Barreveld and colleagues conducted a systematic review from 2005 to 2012 of studies in which local anesthetics were used for analgesia.[27] The review included both peripheral nerve block analgesia and intravenous lidocaine infusions, but not spinal or epidural anesthesia/analgesia. The results of this review support the use of local anesthetics as a preventive analgesic technique. Peripheral nerve blocks provide superior analgesia to intravenous local anesthetic for upper and lower extremity procedures. It is unclear if the robust effect of peripheral block is also related to the systemic uptake of the local anesthetic drugs, with subsequent CNS effects.

The combination of experimental data and positive clinical trials strongly suggests that preventive analgesia is a clinically relevant phenomenon. In a systematic review of clinical trials examining preemptive or preventive analgesic approaches, Katz[28] reported an analgesic benefit of preventive analgesia, with no such benefit when using a preemptive strategy. Maximal clinical benefit is observed when there is complete blockade of noxious stimuli, with extension of the blockade into the postoperative period. Recent preclinical and clinical studies provide substantial evidence that central sensitization and persistent pain after surgical incision is predominantly maintained by the incoming barrage of sensitized peripheral pain fibers throughout the perioperative period[29] and extending into the postsurgical recovery period. By preventing central sensitization and its prolongation by peripheral input, preventive analgesia, along with intensive multimodal analgesic interventions, could theoretically reduce acute postprocedure pain/hyperalgesia and chronic pain after surgery or trauma.[30–32]

CONCEPTUAL CHALLENGES OF PREVENTIVE ANALGESIA

The surgical incision does not produce a single, one-time noxious stimulus, but a continuous barrage of C fiber and A-delta fiber input to the spinal cord. Hence a single, preincisional analgesic intervention is not likely to block this assault throughout the postsurgical recovery period, thereby allowing nociceptive information to reach the spinal cord and resulting in central sensitization. Likewise, the inflammatory processes incited by the surgical incision (either directly released mediators or induced genes in injured tissues that lead to mediator production) also produce central sensitization for a prolonged period following surgery. The difficulty is in predicting the *duration* of the noxious inflammatory state and *which patients* will go on to develop chronic postsurgical pain. Clearly, surgical technique, patient characteristics, and other factors play a role in this phenomenon, making comparative studies difficult.

Confounding the issue of the efficacy of preventive analgesia is the diversity of single intervention versus continuous

PAIN SCORES

Drug	Citation	Effect	Lower	Upper	N total	P value
Epidural analgesia	Aida (1999)	.72	−.28	1.16	88	.00
Epidural analgesia	Aida (2000)	.74	−.21	1.28	60	.00
Epidural analgesia	Dahl (1992)	−.25	−.98	.47	32	.47
Epidural analgesia	Dahl (1994)	−.60	−1.34	.14	32	.09
Epidural analgesia	Esmaoglu (2001)	.00	−.64	.64	40	1.00
Epidural analgesia	Holthusen (1994)	−.35	−1.19	.49	25	.38
Epidural analgesia	Katz (1994)	.96	−.29	1.62	42	.00
Epidural analgesia	Katz (2000)	.38	−.79	.04	94	.07
Epidural analgesia	Kundra (1997)	.73	−.05	1.50	30	.05
Epidural analgesia	Kundra (1998)	.51	−.02	1.04	60	.05
Epidural analgesia	Obata (1999)	.47	−.01	.96	70	.05
Epidural analgesia	Richards (1998)	−.22	−.79	.35	50	.44
Epidural analgesia	Wong (1997)	.73	−.05	1.50	30	.05
Epidural analgesia (13)		**.25**	**.10**	**.41**	**653**	**.00**
Local anesthetics	Altintas (2000)	−.57	−1.15	.02	49	.05
Local anesthetics	Dahl (1993)	.63	−.04	1.21	50	.03
Local anesthetics	Fischer (2000)	.47	−.01	.96	70	.05
Local anesthetics	Gill (2001)	−.43	−1.14	.28	34	.21
Local anesthetics	Hanlon (2000)	−.30	−.76	.17	74	.20
Local anesthetics	Ke (1998)	.64	−.03	1.30	39	.05
Local anesthetics	Kissin (2001)	.73	−.05	1.50	30	.05
Local anesthetics	Molliex (1996)	−.38	−.98	.23	45	.21
Local anesthetics	Orntoft (1994)	−.32	−1.18	.53	24	.42
Local anesthetics	Pasqualucc (1996)	.68	.15	1.21	60	.01
Local anesthetics	Turner (1994)	−.09	−.61	.43	60	.72
Local anesthetics (11)		**.10**	**−.07**	**.27**	**535**	**.26**
NMDA antagonists	Chia (1999)	−.42	−.94	.11	60	.11
NMDA antagonists	Dahl (2000)	−.48	−.98	.07	60	.06
NMDA antagonists	Helmy (2001)	.63	−.03	1.28	40	.05
NMDA antagonists	Mathisen (1999)	−.10	−.74	.54	40	.76
NMDA antagonists	Menigaux (2000)	−.19	−.94	.58	30	.60
NMDA antagonists	Rogers (1995)	−.22	−.57	.13	128	.21
NMDA antagonists	Wu (1999)	1.39	−.81	1.97	60	.00
NMDA antagonists (7)		**.00**	**−.19**	**.20**	**418**	**.97**
NSAIDs	Buggy (1994)	−.17	−.81	.47	40	.58
NSAIDs	Colbert (1998)	.54	−.07	1.00	77	.02
NSAIDs	Fletcher (1995)	.70	−.04	1.36	40	.03
NSAIDs	Hanlon (1996)	.63	−.03	1.28	40	.05
NSAIDs	Nagatsuka (2000)	.00	−.44	.44	82	1.00
NSAIDs	Nelson (1993)	−.19	−.63	.44	41	.53
NSAIDs	Norman (2001)	.67	−.07	1.27	48	.02
NSAIDs	Ong (2003)	.79	.25	1.33	60	.00
NSAIDs	Reuben (2002)	.92	.25	1.60	40	.00
NSAIDs	Romsing (1998)	−.38	−1.06	.29	37	.24
NSAIDs	Sisk (1989)	−.92	−1.60	−.25	40	.01
NSAIDs	Sisk (1990)	−.80	−1.29	−.31	72	.00
NSAIDs (12)		**.14**	**−.02**	**.30**	**617**	**.09**
Systemic opioids	Doyle (1998)	.73	−.05	1.5	30	.05
Systemic opioids	Fassoulaki (1995)	−.05	−.75	.65	34	.88
Systemic opioids	Mansfield (1994)	−.08	−.60	.44	60	.76
Systemic opioids	Millar (1998)	−.09	−.60	.43	60	.74
Systemic opioids	Richmond (1993)	−.93	−1.05	−.36	60	.00
Systemic opioids	Sarantopoulos (1996)	−.30	−.95	.34	40	.34
Systemic opioids	Wilson (1994)	−.63	−1.28	.03	40	.05
Systemic opioids (7)		**−.24**	**−.46**	**−.01**	**324**	**.04**

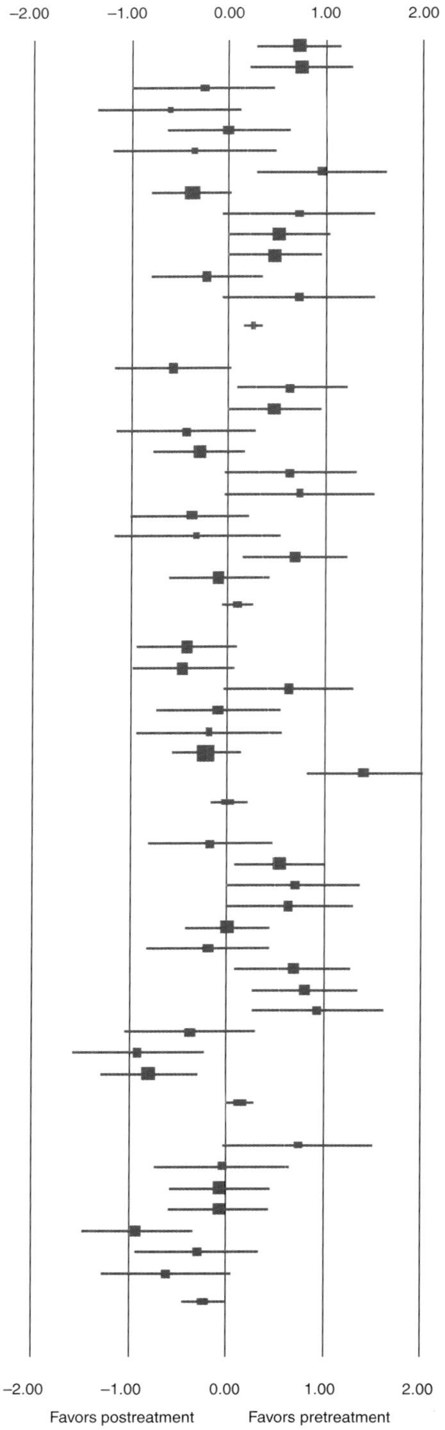

FIG. 11.2 Pain scores. Squares to the left of the centerline represent a study, in which the findings favor posttreatment; those to the right favor pretreatment of preemptive analgesia. *(From Ong CK, Lirk P, Seymour RA, Jenkins BJ. The efficacy of preemptive analgesia for acute postoperative pain management: a meta-analysis.* Anesth Analg *2005;100:757–773.)*

intervention used in these studies. First of all, failure of the medical literature, including the many reviews and meta-analyses, appears to lie in *not* investigating the efficacy of each technique in its own study. Second, many studies included the use of premedications or intraoperative analgesic adjuvants, as well as nitrous oxide, all of which have a well-known analgesic effects that could have made it difficult to detect significant differences between the control and experimental groups. Third, no completely objective standard exists to measure pain. Pain severity measured by visual analogue and numeric rating scales, as well as amount of opioid consumption, is often used in clinical trials as measures of outcome. Pain rating scales, though self-reported, are reliable, and can be used systematically as indices of pain. Opioid consumption is, indeed, a reflection of pain intensity, but it is not a reliable index, as it is profoundly influenced by various psychological factors, including anxiety level, mood, cultural beliefs, prior opioid use, and expectation of recovery. A fourth reason that preventive analgesia is not an obvious phenomenon in clinical trials may be that it is extremely difficult to completely block noxious input from reaching the spinal cord, despite the analgesic technique used. Researchers have used plasma cortisol levels as a determinant of the stress response to determine if complete neural blockade occurs during surgery. Kehlet and colleagues showed that only a block extending from T4 to S5 prevented a rise in cortisol levels following lower abdominal surgery.[33] Finally, suboptimal results in these studies may be related to the lack of comprehensive analysis of subgroups involving medication, method of delivery, *and* type of surgical procedure performed. Although it has been common practice to consider surgical interventions as a homogeneous injury, there is growing evidence that analgesia may need to be procedure-specific.[34] This approach to subgroup analysis, though appropriate, will require the generation of substantially more data to evaluate the efficacy of each medication regimen for each specific surgical intervention.

FUTURE CONSIDERATIONS

Other questions that require further investigation to completely treat postsurgical pain include: What are the components that make up postsurgical pain? What are their respective contributions to that postsurgical pain? Surgical injury, including the lacerating and crushing of nociceptive afferents, is of foremost importance in this regard, followed by the inflammatory response. The secondary effects of the injury, including peripheral and central sensitization, are becoming increasingly evident. However, one component that has not been clearly elucidated is the most commonly administered and intraoperative analgesic: the opioid. Chronic opioid therapy is associated with decreased pain thresholds, and hence requires increased use of analgesics[35]; intraoperative opioids have been associated with postoperative hyperalgesia, a phenomenon known as opioid-induced hyperalgesia.[21] This begs the question, is the preemptive or preventive effect of nonopioid adjuvant analgesics the result of true intrinsic preemptive properties of the intervention, or is it the product of substituting one analgesic without hyperalgesic side effects for one with these side effects? In one study, ketamine was shown to decrease postoperative opioid use following intraoperative opioid administration; this outcome was interpreted to mean that ketamine reduced the opioid-induced hyperalgesia[21]; however, the same result could also be interpreted as a preemptive or preventive effect.

SUMMARY

The management of postoperative pain has improved tremendously with the development of intravenous patient-controlled analgesia and the greater use of peripheral nerve and epidural catheters to deliver local anesthetics. Nevertheless, the more logical approach remains to block the development of pain before it is produced; this is the theoretical promise of preemptive or preventive analgesia. Unfortunately, the optimal medication or delivery technique has not yet been identified. Although advances have been made to help understand which patients are more likely to develop chronic pain after surgery, no clear validated instrument exists to fully predict this. Despite this limitation, programs are being developed to treat high-risk patients throughout the perioperative period with good success.[36] Neuroplasticity is a well-recognized phenomenon, although is not yet fully understood. As we develop a better understanding of this process through more research, additional studies investigating the effects of preemptive analgesia will continue. It is a commonly held belief that completely blocking the afferent input, combined with a multimodal approach, may be most effective. This may very well be true; however, the data do not fully back up this premise. However, until further data emerge, expert panels recommend the use of preoperative patient education and delineation of expectations, intraoperative use of multimodal analgesics including continuous regional anesthesia, acetaminophen, NSAIDs, and gabapentinoids, and postoperative coordination of care with availability of pain specialists.[37] It is because of the potential of preventive analgesia to revolutionize the field of pain medicine that, despite inconsistent data, it continues to be an area of great interest and exploration.

KEY POINTS

- Chronic postoperative pain results from peripheral and central sensitization.
- The NMDA receptor responds to glutamate, an excitatory amino acid.
- The concept of preventive analgesia is using antinociceptive treatment to cover the entire period of high-intensity noxious stimuli (incision) to attenuate peripheral or central sensory processing.
- The primary phase is that during which noxious stimuli are related to the surgical injury, and the secondary phase is that during which ongoing noxious stimuli are related to the release of chemicals, including inflammatory mediators from damaged tissue. The secondary phase can begin intraoperatively and continue long into the postoperative recovery period.
- Although several experimental studies support the concept of preventive analgesia, human clinical studies have demonstrated inconsistent and controversial results.
- Therapies that have been tested in preventive trials include NSAIDs, opioids, ketamine, peripheral local anesthetics, intravenous local anesthetics, caudal and epidural analgesia, dextromethorphan, and gabapentinoids.

REFERENCES

Access the reference list online at ExpertConsult.com.

CHAPTER 12

Perioperative Nonopioid Infusions for Postoperative Pain Management

Hubert A. Benzon, MD, MPH, FAAP ◎ Ravi D. Shah, MD ◎ Honorio T. Benzon, MD

Opioids are the most commonly used medications for perioperative pain control. However, opioid-related side effects such as nausea, vomiting, constipation, and respiratory depression often accompany the use of opioids. Many studies have evaluated the efficacy of perioperative nonopioid pain infusions to decrease postoperative pain and minimize the use of opioids after surgery. These include the use of ketamine, lidocaine, naloxone, and magnesium. In addition, infusions of the short-acting beta-blocker esmolol and the alpha-2 agonist dexmedetomidine have also been investigated as adjuvants to reduce the postoperative opioid requirement. In this chapter, the results of the studies on infusions of ketamine, lidocaine, naloxone, esmolol, alpha-2 agonists, and magnesium will be discussed, and recommendations made on their clinical applicability as part of perioperative pain management.

INTRAVENOUS KETAMINE INFUSION

Ketamine is a noncompetitive N-methyl-D-aspartate (NMDA) glutamate receptor antagonist and a sodium channel blocker.[1] The drug is available as racemic ketamine, which contains the S (+) and R (–) stereoisomers. The S (+) ketamine has 4 times greater affinity for the NMDA receptor than the R (–) ketamine. Ketamine has a half-life of 80–180 minutes. Its metabolite norketamine has a longer half-life and is one-third as potent as the parent compound.[2] Early studies have shown ketamine to have analgesic properties at low, subanesthetic doses.[3–7] The analgesic effects of ketamine occur at plasma concentrations of 100–150 ng/mL.[8]

Ketamine has many qualities as an analgesic and does not have the same side-effect profile as opioids do. Ketamine does not suppress cardiovascular function in the presence of an intact nervous system,[9] does not depress the laryngeal protective reflexes and causes less depression of ventilation compared with opioids,[10] and may even stimulate respiration.[11] However, ketamine does have undesirable characteristics, including postoperative malaise,[12] accumulation of metabolites,[13] development of tolerance,[14] cardiovascular excitation, and the occurrence of psychotomimetic side effects.[15,16] Psychotomimetic effects are the most common feared complication by clinical practitioners, but few studies have formally evaluated these side effects.[4–7]

Randomized controlled clinical studies on perioperative IV ketamine showed beneficial effect. In a study in patients who underwent cervical and lumbar spine surgery, ketamine (1 mg/kg bolus followed by 83 $\mu g.kg^{-1}.h^{-1}$) resulted in less analgesic requirements, lower pain scores, and better satisfaction than patients who had saline infusion or those who had lower dose of ketamine infusion (same 1 mg/kg bolus but at an infusion rate of 42 $\mu g.kg^{-1}.h^{-1}$).[17] The same beneficial effects were seen in patients who had major abdominal surgery. Perioperative ketamine infusion (0.5 mg/kg bolus followed by 2 $\mu g.kg^{-1}.min^{-1}$) for 48 hours after surgery resulted in lower pain scores and less morphine consumption than patients who had saline infusion or those who had the same infusion given intraoperatively.[18] To better evaluate the effect of a ketamine bolus on the infusion, a group of investigators[19] compared ketamine bolus followed by an infusion, versus ketamine bolus alone given either before the surgical incision or at wound closure in patients undergoing gynecologic laparotomy. They noted that the patients who had the ketamine bolus and infusion had lower morphine consumption and lower pain scores. Ketamine infusion also reduced postoperative opioid consumption in subjects who had spinal anesthesia for cesarean section.[20]

In patients who had total intravenous (IV) anesthesia with remifentanil and propofol infusions, no beneficial effect of ketamine infusion was noted.[21] The lack of benefit may be related to the investigators' generous use of intraoperative opioids. A review that evaluated more than 4700 patients demonstrated the efficacy of ketamine in reducing pain and postoperative opioid consumption, especially for upper abdominal, thoracic, and major orthopedic surgical procedures.[22] Despite less opioid use, 25 out of 32 treatment groups (78%) experienced less pain than the placebo groups at some point postoperatively.

Perioperative IV ketamine infusion may not prevent postamputation pain.[23] Ketamine 0.5 mg/kg bolus followed by an infusion of 0.5 $mg.kg^{-1}.h^{-1}$ for 72 hours was not effective in reducing morphine consumption or in decreasing the incidence of stump allodynia. At 6-month follow-up, the incidences of phantom pain and stump pain were 47% in the ketamine group compared with 71% and 35% in the control (saline) group. There was no statistical difference in the incidences, so the investigators concluded that IV ketamine did not significantly reduce acute central sensitization or the incidence and severity of postamputation pain.[23]

The addition of an IV ketamine infusion to epidural analgesia in patients who underwent colorectal surgery resulted in less patient-controlled analgesia (PCA) morphine requirements and reduced areas of hyperalgesia.[24] Another group of investigators noted the salutary effect of adding low-dose IV ketamine (0.05 $mg.kg^{-1}.h^{-1}$, approximately 3 mg/h) to epidural analgesia after thoracotomy.[25] In this study, the patients with a ketamine infusion had less pain and took less analgesics at 3 months after surgery. Ketamine infusion therefore appears to have a beneficial effect on epidural analgesia. This beneficial effect of ketamine in preventing chronic pain after surgery was not confirmed in other studies.[26,27] In one study, a ketamine infusion (1 mg/kg at induction, 1 $mg.kg^{-1}.h^{-1}$ during surgery, and then 1 mg/kg for 24 hours) in addition to intrapleural ropivacaine, improved immediate postoperative pain compared with saline.[26] However, at 4 months after surgery, the analgesic intake and neuropathic pain scores were similar in both groups. In another study, the incidences of moderate and severe postthoracotomy pain syndrome at 3 and 6 months were similar in the ketamine and control groups.[27]

The addition of ketamine infusion appears to be beneficial in opioid tolerant patients. An earlier study by Loftus et al. showed reduced opioid consumption in the first 48 hours after back surgery in patients who had a ketamine bolus ([0.5 mg/kg] and intraoperative infusion [10 μg.kg^{-1}.min^{-1}]).[28] A later study showed that the addition of ketamine infusion (0.2 mg.kg^{-1}.h^{-1}) to hydromorphone IV PCA resulted in a statistically significant reduction of "average" pain scores in opioid-dependent patients.[29] It should be noted that the "least" and "worst" pain scores and postoperative opioid use did not differ between the ketamine and control groups.

Most of the studies showed no increased side effects when low-dose ketamine infusions are used. Zakine et al.[18] did not observe nightmares, delusions, sleep, or psychiatric disorders in their study. Sleep disturbance and psychomotor performances were similar between the ketamine infusion group and control group. In a quantitative systematic review, Laskowski and colleagues detected that hallucinations and nightmares were more common with ketamine, but sedation was not.[22] They noted that when ketamine was efficacious for pain, postoperative nausea and vomiting were diminished.

Studies on ketamine infusion involved a small number of patients, different ketamine regimens, different routes of administration, and large variations in clinical settings.[22,30–34] Most of the randomized controlled studies showed some beneficial effects of a low-dose ketamine infusion. A recent review and meta-analysis by Wang et al.[35] that looked at 36 randomized controlled trials encompassing 2502 eligible patients determined that the addition of ketamine to a morphine or hydromorphine PCA decreased postoperative pain intensity at 6–72 hours postoperatively, morphine consumption at 24–72 hours postoperatively, as well as postoperative nausea and vomiting. There was not enough data to determine any significant adverse events such as hallucinations.

In summary, ketamine infusion appears to improve the efficacy of epidural analgesia. It does not seem to have any effect when the anesthetic technique is total IV anesthesia where moderate or substantial amounts of intraoperative opioid are used. Ketamine also has a beneficial effect when added to PCA postoperatively by decreasing pain intensity, opioid consumption, and side effects. IV ketamine may find its use as an adjunct in opioid-tolerant patients, or in patients with a higher incidence of chronic postsurgical pain such as thoracotomy, inguinal herniorraphies, or mastectomies.

INTRAVENOUS LIDOCAINE INFUSION

Lidocaine has peripheral and central properties that are suitable for pain relief. It decreases albumin extravasation in animal models of chemical peritonitis[36] and inhibits leukocyte migration and metabolic activation.[37] Lidocaine modifies the neuronal responses in the dorsal horn[38] and suppresses synaptic spinal transmission by decreasing C-fiber evoked activity in the spinal cord.[39] Clinically, local anesthetic infusions have been used in the treatment of neuropathic pain[40,41] and pain from burns.[42]

Studies showed the beneficial effects of IV lidocaine in abdominal surgery. In a randomized, double-blind, placebo-controlled study, Cassuto et al.[43] showed the analgesic efficacy of a low-dose lidocaine infusion in patients who underwent cholecystectomy. After an IV bolus of 100 mg of lidocaine, the investigators infused lidocaine at 2 mg/min, starting at 30 minutes before the surgery, and continued for 24 hours after the surgery. Compared with the group who had saline infusions, the patients with lidocaine infusions had significantly lower pain scores during the first day of surgery, and required significantly less meperidine during the first two postoperative days. Other randomized controlled studies showed the technique to result in lower postoperative pain scores, less opioid consumption, faster return of bowel function, and reduced hospital stay.[44–46] Groudine et al.[44] compared lidocaine with saline in patients who had radical retropubic prostatectomy. In the lidocaine group, the patients had 1.5 mg/kg bolus of lidocaine before induction, an intraoperative infusion of either 3 mg/min or 2 mg/min (for patients with weights <70 kg) that was continued until 1 hour postoperatively. The analgesic consumption between the patients in the two groups was the same. However, the patients who had lidocaine infusions had lower pain scores, a shorter return of bowel movement (62 ± 13 hours vs. 74 ± 16 hours), and a shorter hospital stay (4 vs. 5 days). In patients who underwent major abdominal surgery, Koppert et al.[45] gave a 1.5 mg/kg bolus over 10 minutes, followed by 1.5 mg.kg^{-1}.h^{-1} 30 minutes before surgical incision and continued up to 1 hour after the end of surgery. The lidocaine infusion group had lower pain scores, less morphine requirement (130 vs. 159 mg) over a 72-hour period, and bowel movements sooner compared with the control.[45] The opioid-sparing effect was noted to be most pronounced on the third postoperative day. These prompted the investigators to consider that the lidocaine infusion may have a true preventive analgesic effect. In another study in patients who underwent laparoscopic colectomy,[46] patients were given a lidocaine bolus injection of 1.5 mg/kg at the induction of anesthesia followed by a continuous infusion of 2 mg.kg^{-1}.h^{-1} intraoperatively and 1.33 mg.kg^{-1}.h^{-1} postoperatively for 24 hours. The times to first flatus (17 vs. 28 hours), defecation (28 vs. 51 hours), and hospital discharge (2 vs. 3 days) were significantly shorter in the patients who had the lidocaine infusion compared with control. In addition, the lidocaine infusion also significantly reduced postoperative pain and fatigue scores and opioid consumption.

A recent trial by Peng et al.[47] demonstrated a beneficial effect of IV lidocaine in craniotomy procedures. Looking at 94 patients undergoing supratentorial craniotomy, patients received either a lidocaine bolus (1.5 mg/kg) followed by an infusion of 2 mg.kg^{-1}.h^{-1} for the duration of surgery or placebo (normal saline). The incidence of mild pain was lower in the lidocaine group compared with control, and the number of patients leaving the postanesthesia care unit (PACU) with a numerical rating scale (NRS) pain score of 0 was greater in the lidocaine group. They also noted that there were no differences in blood pressure, heart rate, and bispectral index scores, intraoperatively. These data were, however, a secondary finding from a clinical trial whose primary outcome was actually neuropsychological outcome (which interestingly was found to not be different between the two groups). Furthermore, pain scores were only assessed in the PACU and not any further during their hospital stay.

Two studies looked at pain relief and also the effect of the lidocaine infusion on markers of inflammation and immune response. A randomized study in patients who underwent open hysterectomy showed less severe postoperative pain in the first 8 hours after surgery, both at rest and during coughing.[48] However, there was no difference in pain scores for the 12–72 hours after surgery between IV lidocaine and IV saline. The authors noted less ex vivo production of IL-1ra and IL-6, and better maintenance of the lymphocyte proliferation response to phytohemagglutinin-M in the IV saline group, signifying the ability of lidocaine to reduce surgery-induced immune changes. Another study did not notice better pain scores but showed other beneficial effects when lidocaine infusion was employed in patients undergoing colorectal surgery. Another group of investigators[49] gave an IV bolus of lidocaine, 1.5 mg/kg, followed by a continuous infusion of 2 mg/min until 4 hours postoperatively. The pain ratings were the same in the lidocaine and saline control groups. However, the return of bowel function was shorter, and the length of hospital stay was decreased by 1 day in the lidocaine group. The authors also noted significant reduction of the plasma levels of IL6, IL8, complement C3a, and IL-1ra, as well as expression of CD11b, P-selectin, and platelet-leukocyte aggregates. The findings showed the ability of IV lidocaine to modify surgery-induced inflammatory activity.

The beneficial effects of IV lidocaine infusion were not duplicated in patients who had a total hip replacement or coronary artery bypass graft surgery. In a randomized, double-blind, placebo-controlled study, 1.5 mg/kg lidocaine bolus was given over 10 minutes at 30 minutes before surgical incision, followed by an infusion of 1.5 $mg.kg^{-1}.h^{-1}$ until 1 hour after the end of the surgery.[50] There was no difference between the lidocaine and control groups in terms of postoperative pain scores and opioid consumption (17 vs. 15 mg morphine over 24 hours), and no difference in hip flexion. In patients who underwent coronary artery bypass surgery, low-dose lidocaine infusion was also noted to be ineffective in reducing the supplemental fentanyl, midazolam, or propanolol postoperative requirements.[51] In this study, the lidocaine infusion did not reduce the time to extubation, ICU stay, or hospital length of stay. In view of the minimal studies done so far, additional studies are needed to determine if lidocaine infusion is truly ineffective in these surgical settings.

Initial studies on lidocaine infusion (1.5 mg/kg bolus followed by an infusion of 2 $mg.kg^{-1}.h^{-1}$) in patients undergoing ambulatory surgery noted that the infusion resulted in less intraoperative opioid use and less pain scores.[52] De Oliveira et al. determined that perioperative lidocaine not only reduced postoperative pain and opioid consumption but also improved overall quality of postsurgical recovery in patients undergoing outpatient laparoscopic gynecologic surgery. Patients who received lidocaine met discharge criteria faster than the group who received saline.[53]

IV lidocaine infusion is not as effective as perioperative epidural analgesia. IV lidocaine was inferior to thoracic epidural analgesia in terms of pain relief and attenuation of cytokine "surge" in patients who underwent colonic surgery. This was shown by Kuo et al.,[54] who demonstrated that thoracic epidural analgesia resulted in better pain relief, lower opioid consumption, earlier return of bowel function, and lesser production of cytokines than IV lidocaine during the 72-hour observation study period. The patients who received IV lidocaine did experience better pain relief and less cytokine release compared with the control group.

A randomized, unblinded study compared IV lidocaine infusion with epidural analgesia in patients who had open colon resection.[55] The IV lidocaine group had infusions of 1–2 mg/min (1 mg/min in <70 kg patients and 2 mg/min in ≥70 kg patients), while the epidural analgesia group had 10 mL/h of 0.125% bupivacaine and hydromorphone 6 µg/mL. The infusions were started within 1 hour of the end of surgery and continued until return of bowel function or by the fifth day. There were no statistical differences in the average pain scores (VAS of 2.2 in the epidural group vs. 3.1 in the IV lidocaine group) and a trend toward greater opioid consumption in the IV lidocaine group. The return of bowel function or the length of hospital stay was not statistically different between the groups.[55] It is interesting to note that two chronic pain patients in the IV lidocaine group were excluded and an epidural had to be subsequently placed in one of the patients for "further pain treatment."

Two meta-analyses publications showed beneficial effects of a perioperative lidocaine infusion. An earlier meta-analysis of eight trials noted improved rehabilitation and shortened hospital stay when a lidocaine infusion was used.[56] The improved recovery was supported by decreased postoperative pain at 24 hours after surgery, lower incidence of nausea and vomiting, and shorter duration of ileus. The ability of IV lidocaine to shorten the duration of ileus was shown not only clinically (e.g., first passage of gas and feces), but also through radiopaque markers and serial abdominal radiographs.[57] The other meta-analysis evaluated over 1700 patients[58] and showed that at 6 hours postoperatively, IV lidocaine infusion reduced pain at rest (weighted mean difference [WMD] −8.70, 95% confidence intervals [CI] −16.19 to −1.21), during cough (WMD −11.19, 95% CI −17.73 to −4.65), and during movement (WMD −9.56, 95% CI −17.31 to −1.80). IV lidocaine infusion also reduced morphine requirement (WMD −8.44 mg, 95% CI −11.32 to −5.56), time to first flatus (WMD −7.62 hours, 95% CI −10.78 to −4.45), time to first feces (WMD −10.71 hours, 95% CI −16.14 to −5.28), nausea/vomiting (risk ratios = 0.71, 95% CI 0.57–0.90), and hospital length of stay (WMD −0.17 days, 95% CI −0.41 to 0.07). The authors concluded that lidocaine infusions are beneficial in abdominal surgery.

The beneficial effects of a perioperative lidocaine infusion in abdominal surgery may be related to its ability to suppress inflammatory processes from the surgery. IV lidocaine attenuates increased levels of proinflammatory cytokines, preventing the development of peripheral and central nervous system sensitization that leads to clinical hyperalgesia.[59]

Systemic perioperative lidocaine has been shown to reduce the development of postsurgical pain syndrome after mastectomies.[60] The effect was very large, but the study sample size was small (36 subjects). Larger randomized trials

TABLE 12.1 Efficacy of Perioperative Ketamine and Lidocaine Intravenous Infusions

	Ketamine	Lidocaine
Bolus dose	0.5–1 mg/kg	100 mg–1.5 mg/kg
Usual infusion dose	40–100 mg.kg^{-1}.h^{-1}	2–3 mg/min (2 mg/min for patients <70 kg)
Infusion dose with epidural analgesia	0.05 (approximately 3 mg/h) –0.25 mg.kg^{-1}.h^{-1}	
Efficacy		
Abdominal surgery	Beneficial	Beneficial
Pelvic: gynecologic, urologic	Beneficial	Beneficial
Spine surgery	Beneficial	
Total hip replacement		Not beneficial
Coronary artery bypass surgery		Not beneficial
Total intravenous anesthesia (TIVA)	No additional benefit	
Concomitant patient-controlled epidural analgesia (PCEA)	Additional benefit	
Compared with PCEA		Blinded study showed less efficacy,[52] while a randomized but unblinded study showed nonstatistically significant pain scores and a trend toward greater opioid consumption in the IV lidocaine group[53]

Reprinted with permission from Benzon HT. Perioperative non-opioid infusions for postoperative pain management. In: Benzon HT, Raja SN, Liu SS, Fishman FM, Cohen SP, eds. Essentials of Pain Medicine and Regional Anesthesia. *3rd ed. New York: Elsevier Churchill Livingstone; 2011:206-211.*

are needed to refute or confirm the role of lidocaine as an effective intervention in reducing chronic postsurgical pain.

The comparative effects of perioperative IV ketamine and lidocaine infusions are shown in Table 12.1. It can be seen that infusion of either drug is beneficial in abdominal surgery. Ketamine infusion is effective in spine surgery but showed no added benefit when the technique of general anesthesia was total IV anesthesia. Lidocaine infusion appears to have no benefit in patients who undergo total hip replacement or coronary artery bypass surgery. As noted, a randomized blinded study showed less efficacy of IV lidocaine infusion when compared with epidural analgesia.

INTRAVENOUS NALOXONE INFUSION

Naloxone is a pure mu-receptor antagonist. Naloxone infusions have been used to decrease the incidence of nausea, vomiting, respiratory depression, and urinary retention after epidural[61,62] and intrathecal opioids.[63,64] Its use comes with the possibility of reversing analgesia from the opioid.[65] Naloxone infusion at 10 μg.kg^{-1}.h^{-1} reduced the duration and quality of analgesia from epidural morphine or fentanyl.[61,62] The infusion of naloxone at 1 μg.kg^{-1}.h^{-1} attenuated the pain relief in patients who had intrathecal diamorphine after lumbar laminectomy.[64] In a retrospective study patients who had radical prostatectomy and given 0.8–1.7 mg intrathecal morphine, an IV infusion of naloxone at 5 μg.kg^{-1}.h^{-1} provided excellent analgesia with infrequent and minor side effects.[66]

The efficacy of naloxone infusion in decreasing the incidence of side effects from neuraxial opioids led a group of investigators to look at the effect of naloxone infusion on PCA morphine.[67] In a randomized, double-blind study, 60 patients who underwent hysterectomy were assigned into three groups: (1) PCA morphine, 1 mg/mL, with saline infusion; (2) PCA morphine with low-dose naloxone infusion (0.25 μg.kg^{-1}.h^{-1}); and (3) PCA morphine with high-dose naloxone infusion (1 μg.kg^{-1}.h^{-1}).[67] They noted that both naloxone doses were equally effective in reducing the incidence of nausea and vomiting, and pruritus compared with placebo. There was no difference in the pain scores between the three groups, even though the cumulative morphine usage was significantly lower in the low-dose group (42.3 ± 24.1 mg) compared with the placebo (59.1 ± 27.4 mg) or the high-dose group (64.7 ± 33 mg). There was no respiratory depression and no difference in sedation scores, respiratory rate, hemodynamic parameters, or antiemetic use among the three groups.[67] Another group of investigators[68] examined the effect of a 24-hour low-dose naloxone infusion in 90 patients who had hysterectomies. They showed that naloxone significantly reduced morphine consumption over the first 24 postoperative hours compared with the control group (saline). Morphine consumption was also lower, 19.5 (standard deviation [SD] 3.4 mg vs. 27.5 [SD 5.9] mg). In addition, the incidence and severity of nausea and vomiting was significantly reduced in the naloxone group, similar to what was observed in a previous study.[68]

Naloxone's dose-dependent effect on pain leads to its ability to improve postoperative analgesia. Small doses of naloxone produced analgesia in rats, while large doses resulted in hyperalgesia.[69] Naloxone was shown to initially produce analgesia in a dose-dependent manner and then caused hyperalgesia.[70] Other investigators noted this biphasic or dual modulatory effect of naloxone.[71–73] The mechanisms of analgesic effect of naloxone may be related to the release of endorphins or displacement of endorphins from receptor sites not related to analgesia.[74] Augmentation of the activity of opioid receptors is another possibility, although this upregulation phenomenon has been demonstrated after prolonged naloxone infusion (7 days) and in animals.[75,76] At higher doses, naloxone blocks the action of the released or displaced endorphin at the postsynaptic receptor.

There is no added benefit when naloxone is administered via IV PCA.[77–79] The different pharmacokinetics of the drug when given intermittently compared with when given as infusion explain the lack of added benefit. Naloxone has an alpha half-life of 4 minutes and a beta half-life of 55–60 minutes[80,81]; a continuous infusion of the drug therefore results in constant plasma levels resulting in a more consistent effect.

The present indication for IV naloxone infusion is to control the side effects of neuraxial opioids. Few studies such as the one by Gan et al.[67] and the one from Movafegh et al.[68] showed the efficacy of a low-dose naloxone infusion in reducing opioid consumption. Its increased clinical use for postoperative analgesia should await additional controlled studies in different surgical procedures.

MAGNESIUM INFUSION

Magnesium is the second most common intracellular ion, with a crucial role in maintaining the functions of organisms. Magnesium is an essential component for the function of enzymes, neurotransmission, and cell signaling.[82] Animal studies demonstrated that magnesium is an antagonist of NMDA receptors and minimizes the perception and duration of pain.[83] Since dietary intake is the main source of magnesium in humans, long periods of dietary restriction as well as unpredictable operating room schedules are important causes of hypomagnesemia during the perioperative period.[84] The perioperative administration of IV fluids may also contribute to the development of low levels of magnesium.

The effect of systemic magnesium on postoperative analgesia has been examined in a large variety of surgical procedures. Two studies looked at the effect of IV magnesium to minimize postoperative pain in patients undergoing major abdominal surgery.[85–86] Both studies used an initial bolus of magnesium sulfate (50 mg/kg), followed by a postoperative infusion. One study examined only 40 patients, and the authors were not able to detect an opioid-sparing effect of magnesium.[85] In contrast, another study looked at 48 patients and noted that morphine consumption was significantly higher in the control group compared with the magnesium group on the first postoperative day (52 ± 4 mg vs. 30 ± 3 mg).[86]

Lower postoperative pain scores and less cumulative postoperative analgesic consumption were noted in patients who underwent total abdominal hysterectomy and who received magnesium compared with placebo.[87] Spine surgery is another procedure where perioperative magnesium infusion has been confirmed to improve postoperative analgesia.[88] An area that remains to be investigated is the use of systemic magnesium to minimize postoperative pain in ambulatory surgical patients. One study[89] investigated 200 patients who underwent ambulatory ilioinguinal hernia repair or varicose vein operation under general anesthesia, and randomized them to receive magnesium sulfate 4 g IV or normal saline after anesthetic induction. There was no difference in postoperative opioid consumption or pain scores between the study groups. However, the patients in the study received a concomitant multimodal analgesic regimen which consisted of diclofenac 100 mg rectally for the patients who underwent varicose vein surgery and a postoperative ilioinguinal-iliohypogastric nerve block for the patients who had hernia repair. As of this writing, it remains to be determined if perioperative magnesium infusion is a valuable adjunct in minimizing postoperative pain in ambulatory surgical procedures.

De Oliveira et al. performed a meta-analysis to quantitatively assess the effect of perioperative magnesium infusions on postoperative pain outcomes.[90] The authors evaluated 20 randomized clinical trials, and more than 1200 subjects were included in their final analysis. In most of the studies, 30–50 mg/kg bolus was initially given, followed by an intraoperative of infusion of 10–15 $mg.kg^{-1}.h^{-1}$. The overall effect of magnesium on postoperative pain was small for early pain at rest −0.74 (99% CI, −1.08 to −0.48) on a 0–10 numerical rating scale. The overall effect of magnesium compared with saline was also small for late pain (24 hours) at rest, −0.36 (99% CI, −0.63 to −0.09). In contrast, the effect of magnesium on opioid-sparing compared with saline was substantial, −10.52 (99% CI, −13.50 to −7.54) mg morphine IV equivalents. After performing a subgroup analysis, the authors concluded that the intraoperative and postoperative administration of magnesium had greater analgesic effect than a sole intraoperative administration. None of the studies included in the meta-analysis reported signs or symptoms of magnesium toxicity related to high levels of perioperative magnesium.

A recent study looking at IV magnesium in children undergoing tonsillectomy found no benefit to those patients who received magnesium. Benzon et al. performed a double-blind randomized placebo controlled trial in children aged 3–10 years of age undergoing tonsillectomy procedure.[91] They used a loading dose of magnesium 30 mg/kg over 15 minutes, followed by a continuous infusion of 10 $mg.kg^{-1}.h^{-1}$ versus a control group of equivalent volume of normal saline. Looking at Face, Legs, Activity, Cry, Consolability (FLACC) scores and opioid consumption postoperatively, they found no difference in pain scores or narcotic use up to 90 minutes postoperatively.

Overall, magnesium infusion seems to be a promising strategy to minimize postoperative opioid requirement. The lack of reported toxicity also makes it a safe option. However, more studies are still needed to confirm the analgesic effect of systemic magnesium for ambulatory surgical procedures.

ESMOLOL INFUSION

Esmolol is a cardioselective $beta_1$ receptor blocker commonly used in the anesthesia to treat intraoperative tachyarrhythmias or to blunt the adrenergic response caused by various stimuli such as intubation, surgical stimulation, and extubation. The drug has a very rapid onset and short duration of action.[92] Esmolol is rapidly hydrolyzed by plasma esterases at the ester-methyl side chain, which is the basis for the drug's short duration of action. Esmolol's elimination half-life is about 9 minutes.[93]

The effect of esmolol infusions on postoperative pain has been examined by several investigators; most studies demonstrated a favorable analgesic effect. Esmolol was first used as an alternative to opioid analgesics in 1991 in ambulatory arthroscopic procedures.[94] The investigators compared esmolol to alfentanil to supplement propofol-N_2O-atracurium anesthesia and concluded that that esmolol may be used in place of alfentanil to supplement anesthesia in outpatients undergoing arthroscopic procedures. Avoiding alfentanil did not decrease the incidence of postoperative nausea and vomiting in this outpatient population.

The effect of perioperative esmolol administration was compared with saline in patients who underwent hysterectomy.[95] The perioperative esmolol administration reduced the intraoperative use of inhalation anesthetic and fentanyl, decreased hemodynamic responses, and reduced morphine consumption (by 17 mg IV morphine equivalents) for the first 3 postoperative days. Another study compared esmolol with either intermittent fentanyl or continuous remifentanil on postoperative opioid-sparing, side effects, and time of discharge in patients undergoing ambulatory cholecystectomy.[96] Based on the results, the conclusion by the investigators was that an intraoperative IV infusion of esmolol contributes to a significant decrease in postoperative administration of fentanyl and ondansetron and facilitates earlier discharge. The analgesic properties of esmolol in patients undergoing laparoscopic appendectomy were confirmed in another study.[97]

The safety of perioperative esmolol infusions has been examined by a systematic review of 67 randomized controlled trials.[98] Esmolol infusions titrated to a hemodynamic end point was noted to be safe and effective in low-risk patients. However, safety data from studies in higher-risk patients are needed to establish a perioperative safety and efficacy profile of esmolol.

In summary, esmolol infusions appear to be a valid strategy to ameliorate postoperative pain. The results of randomized studies are particularly encouraging in the ambulatory surgical population.

ALPHA-2 AGONISTS

Alpha-2 agonists are often used as anesthetic adjuncts because of their desirable properties, including anxiolysis, sedation, and hypnosis.[99] Alpha-2 agonists have also been found to have analgesic properties. Their analgesic effect is attributed to the stimulation of 2-adrenoreceptors located in the central nervous system and spinal cord. It has also been suggested that systemic alpha-2 agonists potentiate the analgesic effects of opioids.[100] Systemic clonidine is thought to have opioid-sparing and antiemetic properties, but its routine clinical use as an infusion has been limited by the presence of adverse effects such as hypotension and bradycardia.[101] Another alpha-2 agonist commonly used in the perioperative setting is dexmedetomidine. An IV infusion of dexmedetomidine is commonly initiated with a 1 µg/kg loading dose, administered over 10 minutes, followed by a maintenance infusion of 0.2–1.0 $\mu g.kg^{-1}.h^{-1}$.[102]

The initial trial to evaluate the effect of dexmedetomidine infusion on postsurgical pain was performed in patients who had laparoscopic tubal ligation.[103] Based on the results, the authors concluded that IV dexmedetomidine relieves pain and reduces opioid drug requirements. However, it is accompanied with sedation and a high incidence of bradycardia. Another study also detected a beneficial opioid-sparing effect of dexmedetomidine after major inpatient surgery.[104] A later study evaluated dexmedetomidine infusion on pain outcomes in patients undergoing abdominal hysterectomy.[105] In this study, 50 women were randomly assigned to two groups. One group (n = 25) received a loading dose of dexmedetomidine 1 µg/kg IV during induction of anesthesia, followed by a continuous infusion at a rate of 0.5 $\mu g.kg^{-1}.h^{-1}$ throughout the operation. The authors showed that continuous IV dexmedetomidine during abdominal surgery provides effective postoperative analgesia and reduces postoperative morphine requirements without increasing the incidence of side effects.

Blaudszun et al. performed a meta-analysis of randomized trials on 1792 patients and detected an opioid-sparing effect of dexmedetomidine compared with placebo of −4.1 mg IV morphine equivalents (95% CI, −6.0 to −2.2 mg).[106] However, dexmedetomidine increased the risk of postoperative bradycardia (the number needed to harm being three).

In summary, dexmedetomidine appears to be a promising perioperative analgesic, decreasing opioid requirements after surgery. It does not increase the incidence of side effects, although it can result in bradycardia.

CONCLUSION

Several preoperative nonopioid infusions are available to reduce postoperative pain. Ketamine infusions are important adjuncts in opioid-dependent patients, while lidocaine infusions not only decrease perioperative opioid requirements in abdominal surgeries but also shorten bowel recovery. Esmolol and dexmedetomidine infusions have well-documented opioid-sparing effects and offer potential advantages in patients with enhanced cardiovascular responses to surgical stimuli. Systemic magnesium may be a viable alternative, but convincing evidence of improved patient outcomes is still lacking. The widespread use of low-dose naloxone infusions also awaits additional study. Finally, the effect of these perioperative nonopioid infusions on the incidence of chronic postsurgical pain requires additional study.

KEY POINTS

- Ketamine infusions have been noted to be a beneficial adjunct in the control of perioperative pain in opioid-dependent patients.
- Lidocaine infusions are beneficial in abdominal surgeries but not in total hip surgery. It accelerates the postoperative return of bowel function.
- While a low-dose naloxone infusion is effective in reducing postoperative opioid consumption, additional studies are needed to delineate its role in different surgical settings and whether the analgesic effect of concomitant opioid is diminished.
- Intraoperative and postoperative administration of magnesium may have an opioid-sparing effect. Several studies have reported no signs of systemic toxicity.
- Esmolol infusions are an effective adjuvant in reducing the anesthetic requirement and decreasing acute hemodynamic responses to noxious surgical stimuli. Esmolol can also reduce postoperative opioid requirements and can reduce side effects (e.g., postoperative nausea and vomiting) in ambulatory surgery patients.
- The adjunctive use of dexmedetomidine infusions reduces both anesthetic and opioid requirements. However, it may result in bradycardia and sedation.

REFERENCES

Access the reference list online at ExpertConsult.com.

CHAPTER 13

Patient-Controlled Analgesia

Ellen M. Soffin, MD, PhD ⊗ Spencer S. Liu, MD

Patient-controlled analgesia (PCA) has become a standard technique in the clinical treatment of pain. PCA systems allow patients to self-administer predetermined doses of analgesic medication, and to record patient usage information during the previous 1-hour and 24-hour periods. This information can help optimize drug delivery based on the analgesic requirement and pattern of use of the individual patient.

Current PCA models usually include a combination of physician-determined variables, including the initial loading dose, demand (bolus) dose, lockout interval, basal continuous infusions, and 1- to 4-hour maximal dose limits. The patient then controls the timing of the demand dose by pressing a button to trigger administration of the drug via an intravenous line. Newer devices allow for entries in units of μg, mg, and mL, thereby reducing the potential for programming errors. Optimization of efficacy and safety depends on the selection of a demand dose large enough to provide sufficient analgesia but small enough to minimize side effects. A lockout interval is the time during which there will be no drug delivery, even if the patient pushes the demand button. Although no dose will be delivered during the lockout period, the frequency of demand presses is nonetheless collected and can be used to help assess patient comfort. Theoretically, use of a lockout interval which is less than the time to peak effect of the drug may result in inadvertent overdosage due to stacking of analgesic doses. However, lockout intervals between 5 and 10 minutes appear optimal regardless of the opioid used.[1,2]

This chapter details the risks and benefits of PCA, recommended dosing strategies for several PCA modalities, and use of PCA in special clinical populations.

SAFETY AND EFFICACY OF PATIENT-CONTROLLED ANALGESIA

ADVANTAGES OF PATIENT-CONTROLLED ANALGESIA

PCA is one of the most popular methods for providing postoperative analgesia. Data suggest use of PCA is associated with higher patient satisfaction,[3–6] and enhanced perception of control over pain[3,5,6] and recovery after surgery.[7] In several studies, PCA pumps have been shown to be more effective than intermittent intramuscular (IM)[8] or intravenous (IV)[9] injections. Other advantages include avoidance of (painful) IM injections,[10] and rapid treatment of pain due to not having to involve nurses in the administration of analgesia.[11]

Because of the ease with which each demand dose can be provided, small boluses can be given frequently. When used properly, the ability of patients to titrate analgesics to their needs can theoretically generate a steady plasma level of analgesia and avoid the peaks and troughs associated with bolus dosing on a 3- to 4-hour basis. PCA may avoid subtherapeutic opioid concentration troughs, which can be associated with unpleasant recovery, guarding, poor chest expansion, and reluctance to mobilize. PCA may also help avoid excessive peak plasma concentrations, with associated respiratory depression and sedation.[12]

Two early meta-analyses produced somewhat contradictory results regarding analgesic efficacy of PCA compared with IM nurse administered opioids. One[13] indicated significant patient preference and better pain scores for PCA, compared with IM analgesia, but found no differences in total opiate consumption or postoperative length of stay. Although the other study[4] also indicated greater patient satisfaction with PCA, there was no statistically significant difference in pain relief in patients treated by PCA and non-PCA methods. The most recent meta-analyses performed to study the efficacy and safety of PCA[5,6] both concluded that overall there is moderate to low-quality evidence that PCA provides slightly better pain control and increased patient satisfaction compared with nonpatient-controlled methods, but patients used higher total doses of analgesia when treated by PCA. Side effects were similar between the groups, with the exception of pruritus, which occurred significantly more frequently in patients using PCA. Other studies report similar incidences of nausea and vomiting, sedation, pruritus, and bowel function, suggesting that the differences in total opioid dosages between PCA and non-PCA approaches may be relatively unimportant.[9,14,15] Given the continuing popularity of PCA, these results are surprising: It appears that good results can be obtained regardless of delivery method, provided that analgesia can truly be given on demand with appropriate doses and intervals. In many circumstances, PCA is the best way to achieve these goals.

DISADVANTAGES OF PATIENT-CONTROLLED ANALGESIA

Disadvantages of PCA can constrain its use and effectiveness. The most frequent negative perceptions relate to inadequate analgesia and/or presence of side effects, but some patients also report not trusting the PCA pump, fearing overdose or addiction,[10,11] and having difficulty understanding and/or using the PCA.[7] Chumbley et al. reported 22% of patients feared addiction and 30% feared overdose,[10] much higher than the 4% and 11%, respectively, reported by Kluger and Owen.[11] However, 43% of patients in the former study did not receive preoperative education about PCA, whereas all patients in the latter study received education about pain management and PCA prior to surgery. In a recent prospective study,[7] 49% of patients reported not knowing if they would receive a dose of medication when they pushed the PCA button, and of these, 22% believed that this uncertainty exacerbated their pain. These findings were not affected by patient education about using the PCA.

Sedation and respiratory depression can occur as a result of repeated excessive PCA use, mistaking the PCA handset for the nurse-call button, and family, visitor, or unauthorized nurse-activated demand boluses.[16] Operator errors can occur via programming of incorrect bolus dose size, concentration, background infusion, and/or unintended background infusion. Incorrect procedures may lead to use of the wrong syringe or analgesic mixture. Standardization of protocols and drug concentrations within an institution may reduce the chance of program errors.[17,18] Newer PCA pumps have been designed with a human factors approach, which has significantly reduced both programming times and rates of programming errors.[19]

Mechanical malfunctions of a PCA pump can occur, with inadvertent excessive medication delivery.[20,21] Despite this, the safety of PCA is supported by meta-analysis. There is no significant difference in the frequency or severity of oversedation and respiratory depression with PCA than with conventional intramuscular or intravenous dosing.[3]

SAFETY OF PATIENT-CONTROLLED ANALGESIA

Safe use of PCA requires that the patient controls the analgesic delivery. Increasing plasma concentrations of opioid usually cause sedation prior to causing clinically significant respiratory depression. Sedation usually impairs the ability of the patient to activate the PCA. Both nursing personnel and the patient's family members must understand this concept, so that only the patient pushes the demand button. Ideally, patients, nurses, and family members should receive education about PCA use. Not every patient is a good candidate for PCA: Patients must be cooperative, comprehend the concept, and be able to push the PCA button. PCA may not be appropriate for very young children, or for patients with certain mental or physical limitations. Nurse controlled analgesia (NCA) may be used if the patient's age, developmental level, or muscle strength interact with the ability to use the device. NCA is a safe and effective method of analgesic administration in the pediatric ICU setting.[22] Finally, because of pharmacokinetic and pharmacodynamic variability among patients, conventional PCA settings may need to be adjusted for the individual.[12]

Device misconnections leading to wrong-route medication administration have been the subject of at least two Sentinel Event Alerts issued by the Joint Commission. Sentinel Event Alert #36 cites nine cases of tubing misconnections involving seven adults and two infants.[23] Deaths occurred in eight of these instances, and one resulted in permanent loss of function. These cases included instances of epidural infusions misconnected to peripheral IV lines; notably, these incidents are believed to occur more frequently than reported, since patient harm does not always result. Recommendations in the updated Sentinel Event Alert #53 focus on system redesign, rather than clinician practice changes in order to prevent misconnection errors.[24] Specifically, the Joint Commission recommends the adoption of new connector standards in development that will make it virtually impossible to (mis)connect delivery systems with different functions.

IMPORTANCE OF ACUTE PAIN SERVICE

Implementation of an Acute Pain Service (APS), which often consists of a team of physicians and nurses that are well educated about PCA, may also promote PCA safety and efficacy. Comparison of PCA managed by an APS versus PCA managed by the surgical staff indicated that patients with APS-supervised PCA had significantly fewer side effects, were more likely to have adjustments made to the PCA dose in response to inadequate analgesia or side effects, and were more likely to transition to oral opioids rather than IM opioids after PCA.[25] This suggests that an APS is more likely to tailor the PCA to suit individual patients. Some of the benefits ascribed to PCA may be due to an association between PCA use and supervision of the analgesic regimen by concerned and knowledgeable clinicians.

TYPES OF PATIENT-CONTROLLED ANALGESIA

INTRAVENOUS PATIENT-CONTROLLED ANALGESIA

Many opioids have been used effectively for intravenous patient-controlled analgesia (IV PCA). Opioids that are pure μ-receptor agonists tend to be the first choice for IV PCA.[26] The ideal opioid for IV PCA has a rapid onset of action, high efficacy, and intermediate duration of action without significant accumulation of drug or metabolites over time.[12] Morphine, hydromorphone, and fentanyl most closely fulfill these criteria and are widely used for opioid-based IV PCA. Conversely, meperidine is generally considered a poor choice for IV PCA agent because the active metabolite, normeperidine, can accumulate and cause CNS excitation, including delirium, tremors, myoclonus, and seizures.[27] However, there may be occasions when meperidine is a reasonable analgesic option. The most recent study examining the safety and efficacy profile of meperidine PCA[28] indicated a CNS toxicity rate of 2%, and recommended a maximum safe dose of 10 mg/kg per day for no longer than 3 days. Patients should be without comorbid renal or hepatic dysfunction, and require careful evaluation and monitoring. All opioids have a similar spectrum of adverse effects, although qualitative differences are detectable. The patient's clinical history and hospital protocols tend to influence the choice of opioid selected for IV PCA. There are few prominent differences in pain scores and incidence of adverse effects between different opioids.[26,29,30] Consequently, patients tend to be satisfied with PCA regardless of the opioid used. The typical dosing, lockout interval, and basal infusion parameters are indicated in Table 13.1.

For safety reasons, a continuous background infusion with IV PCA should only rarely be prescribed for spontaneously breathing opioid-naïve patients.[31,32] Continuous infusions pose increased risk for respiratory depression.[33–35] If a patient becomes sedated, continuing delivery of opioid at a basal rate may cause respiratory depression. Continuous opioid infusion in association with PCA may provide more constant plasma opioid levels and improve analgesia.[32] However, other investigators found that addition of

TABLE 13.1 Sample Regimens for Opioid Intravenous Patient-Controlled Analgesia

Drug	Bolus (Dose)	Lockout Interval (min)
Fentanyl	15–50 μg	3–10
Hydromorphone	0.1–0.5 mg	5–15
Meperidine	5–15 mg	5–15
Morphine	0.5–3 mg	5–20
Oxymorphone	0.2–0.8 mg	5–15
Remifentanil (labor)	0.5 μg.kg^{-1}	2
Sufentanil	3–10 μg	5–10

a basal infusion rate did not reduce pain, fatigue, or anxiety,[31,36] and failed to improve quality of sleep. The number of patient demands, number of supplemental bolus doses, and total opioid use were also not changed in patients receiving basal infusions of opioids. Additionally, most PCA programming errors that have resulted in adverse side effects occurred during the use of basal infusions.[35] In selected opioid-tolerant patients with high opioid requirements, a background infusion may be used to deliver the equivalent of the usual opioid dose taken by the patient.[12] Use of a background rate of infusion may necessitate higher vigilance and/or increased monitoring of the patient.

The addition of ketamine (an N-methyl-D-aspartate [NMDA] receptor antagonist) to IV PCA solutions may improve analgesia in some, but not all, circumstances. The use of ketamine as a PCA adjunct is biologically attractive for several reasons: NMDA receptor activation is associated with the early development of opioid tolerance, an effect that could be ameliorated by ketamine.[37,38] Additionally, NMDA receptor antagonists are inherently analgesic, providing both a (direct) pain-control benefit and an (indirect) opiate sparing effect. Optimization of postoperative IV PCA after spine and hip surgery indicated the ideal ratio of morphine and ketamine to be 1:1, with a lockout interval of 8 minutes.[39] However, two studies showed that either ketamine as an adjunct for IV PCA did not improve pain, or that the potential usefulness of ketamine was offset by a high incidence of adverse effects and no opioid-sparing.[40,41] One study used a PCA regimen comprising background infusion plus PRN bolus doses of fentanyl/ketamine/ondansetron in patients at high risk of postoperative nausea and vomiting after major spine surgery.[42] Although total fentanyl consumption was reduced in the ketamine-PCA group, the severity of nausea was significantly higher, with similar reported pain scores. It is also important to consider the possibility that ketamine can arouse psychomimetic effects and impair cognition.

Clonidine is an α2-adrenoreceptor agonist with analgesic properties. The addition of clonidine to morphine PCA significantly reduced nausea and vomiting in a female population undergoing lower abdominal surgery.[43] However, other studies fail to show significant benefits from inclusion of clonidine with IV PCA.[44]

Dexmedetomidine is a potent, highly selective α2-adrenoreceptor agonist, with analgesic, anxiolytic, and sedative properties, but without effects on respiratory function.[45] Perioperative infusion is associated with improved analgesia, reductions in opiate consumption, and less postoperative nausea and vomiting.[46] To date, there is one study investigating the analgesic effect of adding dexmedetomidine to morphine IV PCA. Patients received either morphine 1 mg/mL PCA or morphine 1 mg/mL plus dexmedetomidine 5 μg/mL PCA, programmed to deliver 1 mL per demand bolus, with a 5-minute lockout and no background infusion. The addition of dexmedetomidine resulted in superior analgesia, significant morphine sparing, and less nausea. These benefits were achieved without additional sedation or undesired hemodynamic changes.

NONINTRAVENOUS PATIENT-CONTROLLED ANALGESIAS

The defining concept of PCA is patient-demand drug administration. Although IV PCA is the most common and studied route of delivery, the two common alternative routes are patient-controlled epidural analgesia and patient-controlled peripheral nerve catheter analgesia.

Patient-Controlled Epidural Analgesia

In many situations, epidural analgesia is superior to IV PCA. A meta-analysis demonstrated that for all types of surgery and pain assessments, all forms of epidural analgesia, including patient-controlled epidural analgesia (PCEA), provided superior postoperative analgesia compared with IV PCA.[47] This conclusion is corroborated by a systematic review of the analgesic efficacy of epidural analgesia versus systemic opioids.[48]

The beneficial postoperative effects of epidural analgesia are more apparent for high-risk patients or those undergoing higher risk procedures. Epidural analgesia with a local anesthetic combined with an opioid provides better postoperative analgesia than epidural or systemic opioids alone, and may improve postoperative outcome.[49,50] Use of local anesthetic alone may result in excessive motor blockade. Despite numerous investigations, the ideal PCEA epidural analgesic solution or the ideal delivery variables remain controversial. In contrast to IV PCA, a continuous background infusion is routinely used for PCEA. A background infusion can maintain a continuous segmental sensory block, but may increase the incidence of hypotension and motor block. The addition of clonidine (2 μg/mL) to ropivacaine-fentanyl PCEA after total knee arthroplasty reduced the need for opioid rescue without jeopardizing hemodynamics.[51] Similarly, the addition of clonidine (10–20 μg/h) to bupivacaine-fentanyl PCEA produced both dose-dependent improvement in analgesia at rest and dose-dependent decrease in blood pressure and pulse rate, and an increase in vasopressor requirement.[52] PCEA with clonidine plus local anesthetic can also avoid some of the usual opioid-related side effects such as nausea or pruritus. To facilitate transition to oral analgesia, the PCEA settings can be reduced gradually rather than abruptly, terminating the PCEA. This can be done, for example, by eliminating the basal rate 6 hours prior to stopping the PCEA.

TABLE 13.2 Suggested Starting Regimens for Patient-Controlled Epidural Analgesia

Surgical Site	Drug and Concentration	Basal Rate (mL/h)	Demand Dose (mL)	Lockout (min)
Obstetric (Labor)	Bupivacaine 0.025% + Fentanyl 10 µg.mL^{-1}	3	3	10
Obstetric (Labor)	Ropivacaine 0.08% + Fentanyl 2 µg.mL^{-1}	5	5	10
1. Abdomen 2. Lower extremity (lumbar epidural)	Bupivacaine 0.0625% + Fentanyl 5 µg.mL^{-1}	4	4	10
Hysterectomy	Bupivacaine 0.125% + Fentanyl 5 µg.mL^{-1} ± Clonidine 0.75 µg.mL^{-1} (NB: 30 mL limit/4 h)	4	3	10
Hip or knee surgery	Bupivacaine 0.06% + Hydromorphone 10 µg.mL^{-1}	4	4	10
Hip or knee surgery	Bupivacaine 0.06% + Clonidine 1 µg.mL^{-1}	4	4	10

Source: Hospital for Special Surgery, Heitmiller ES, Schwengel DA. Johns Hopkins Anesthesiology Handbook, *Elsevier Heath Sciences, 2009, pp 406–410.*

In addition to providing better pain control, epidural analgesia also has the potential benefits of decreased morbidity, such as fewer cardiopulmonary complications, less thromboembolism, better mental status, earlier restoration of gastrointestinal function, enhanced functional exercise capacity and health-related quality of life, and earlier discharge from the hospital.[53–56] A large database study further suggests mortality is lower for patients who receive neuraxial or combined neuraxial-general anesthesia, and transfusion requirements are lowest for those receiving neuraxial anesthesia compared with all other groups.[57] Cancer recurrence and metastasis may also be lower in patients who receive paravertebral or epidural analgesia compared with conventional systemic opioids after mastectomy[58] or prostatectomy.[59] Finally, a recent meta-analysis of 14 prospective and retrospective studies of a range of cancer types demonstrated a positive association between epidural analgesia and overall survival, but no difference in recurrence-free survival compared with general anesthesia with opioid analgesia.[60]

The potential benefits of PCEA must be weighed against potential risks associated with placement of a catheter, which include epidural hematoma, infection, or neurological injury.[26] In particular, thromboprophylaxis with potent anticoagulants may limit the use of PCEA.[61] Suggested regimens for starting a PCEA by surgical indication are shown in Table 13.2.

Peripheral Nerve Catheter Patient-Controlled Analgesia

Nerve block techniques are increasingly popular for management of postoperative pain, particularly after orthopedic surgery. Many common nerve blocks, including brachial plexus, sciatic, and femoral nerve blocks, are amenable to having peripheral nerve catheters inserted for extended analgesia. Peripheral nerve blockade on both the upper and lower extremities can improve postoperative analgesia and patient satisfaction.[63] Infections and neurological complications, although rare, are possible. In contrast with neuraxial blocks, there is less concern about interaction of anticoagulants and peripheral nerve blocks. Ropivacaine may be associated with reduction of complete motor and sensory block, compared with bupivacaine.[64] Common concentrations of local anesthetic for peripheral nerve catheter patient-controlled analgesia (PNC PCA) include ropivacaine, 0.2%–0.3%, and bupivacaine, 0.12%–0.25% (Table 13.3). Including opioids in PNC PCA solutions is probably unnecessary, as peripheral opioids may increase side effects without improving analgesia.[65,66] The addition of clonidine to ropivacaine for PNC PCA does not improve analgesia.[67]

A continuous infusion of local anesthetics is generally used in PNC PCA, as this improves analgesia compared with bolus dosing only. A low dose continuous infusion (combined with a demand dose) reduces local anesthetic consumption without compromising analgesia, in comparison with continuous infusion alone.[68] For moderately painful shoulder surgery, decreasing an interscalene catheter infusion of ropivacaine 0.2% from a basal rate from 8 to 4 mL/h provided similar analgesia, but the reduction caused a higher incidence of breakthrough pain incidence and sleep disturbance.[69]

SPECIAL CONDITIONS

In addition to management of adult postoperative pain, PCA can also be used for the management of labor pain, pediatric postoperative pain, and cancer pain.

LABOR PAIN

The most common modality for analgesia in labor is epidural. PCEA is a highly effective way of providing safe and superior labor analgesia. A multicenter, randomized controlled trial found that IV PCA and PCEA had the same rates of cesarean delivery or instrumental vaginal delivery.[70] However, patients receiving IV PCA were more likely to receive antiemetic therapy, had more sedation, and more neonates in this group required naloxone and active resuscitation (52% vs. 31%). Patients receiving PCEA had better pain relief and greater satisfaction. The optimal choice of epidural infusion mixture and PCEA regimen is still debated. A meta-analysis comparing continuous epidural infusion (CEI) to PCEA without background infusion concluded that patients in labor receiving PCEA are less likely to require anesthetic interventions, require lower doses of

TABLE 13.3 Sample Peripheral Nerve Catheter Patient-Controlled Analgesia Regimens

Catheter	Surgery	Patient-Controlled Analgesia Solution	Basal Rate (mL/h)	Demand Dose (mL)	Lockout (min)
Interscalene, infraclavicular	Rotator cuff repair; hand surgery	Ropivacaine 0.2%	6–8	2–4	20
Subgluteus or popliteal sciatic	Foot and ankle surgery	Ropivacaine 0.2%	5–8	3–5	20–60

Source: Hospital for Special Surgery.

TABLE 13.4 Sample Regimens for Pediatric Intravenous Patient-Controlled Analgesia

Drug	Bolus (μg/kg)	Lockout (min)
Morphine	10–20	7–15
Hydromorphone	5–15	15
Fentanyl	0.5–2	7–15

All patients should receive an initial loading dose of an analgesic before starting PCA for maintenance. Adjust doses, lockouts, and limits based on required loading dose, age, state of health, and presence of opioid tolerance. Use lower end of dosing range for opioid-naive. Assess patient and pain control at regular intervals and adjust settings if needed.

local anesthetic, and have less motor block than those who received CEI.[62] The addition of a basal rate to PCEA may further improve labor analgesia. Demand-only PCEA was associated with higher incidence of breakthrough pain, higher pain scores, shorter duration of effective analgesia, and lower maternal satisfaction, compared with PCEA with background infusion.[71]

Despite the superiority of PCEA for pain control in labor, some parturients do not want epidural analgesia or have clinical conditions that contraindicate its use. In this situation IV PCA should be considered. Administration of opioids to parturients can cause newborn sedation or impaired respiration. Some practitioners limit exposure of the fetus to opioids by discontinuing IV PCA once the mother's cervix is dilated. Compared with bolus parenteral opioids, IV PCA facilitates titration of analgesia as labor progresses, and can better compensate for interpatient variability in analgesic requirements. For this reason, IV PCA (compared with intermittent IM dosing) may provide better pain relief, and reduce maternal sedation, respiratory depression, and nausea.[57] Compared with IM dosing, IV PCA for labor analgesia reduces umbilical cord blood opioid levels (indicating less placental drug transfer); in most cases IV PCA does not cause significant fetal depression.[72,73] Use of shorter-acting opioids for labor IV PCA (such as fentanyl, alfentanil, and remifentanil) may reduce neonatal respiratory depression.[73,74]

PAIN CONTROL IN PEDIATRIC PATIENTS

PCA can reduce pain effectively and safely for adolescents and children. The critical determinant of successful PCA implementation in the pediatric population is the ability of the patient to understand the basic principles of PCA use. As a result, children younger than 4 years of age are not good candidates for PCA use. Children aged 4–6 years can use PCA pumps with the encouragement of nursing staff and parents. Nonetheless, the success rate in this age group is low. Children older than 7 years of age often can use PCA independently. Parental assistance for PCA use by young children has been advocated by some investigators. Implementation of formal parent education programs along with close observation by nursing staff is necessary if parent-controlled analgesia is to be considered. Parent-controlled analgesia bypasses the basic safety system of PCA and has been discouraged in the postoperative setting. Basal opioid infusions have also been successfully used by some physicians in the pediatric population for postoperative analgesia. However, some studies have shown an increased risk of hypoxemia in children receiving basal narcotic infusions with PCA.[75] In a clinical context where continuous opioid infusions are deemed necessary, methods of detecting opioid-induced respiratory depression, such as pulse-oximetry, should be considered. In addition to the caution required for the use of continuous infusion in the pediatric population, concurrent administration of drugs with respiratory depressant effects should also be viewed with extreme vigilance. Typical PCA dosing for children via IV, epidural, and PNC routes are shown in Tables 13.4–13.6.

PAIN CONTROL IN CANCER PATIENTS

PCA is one of the multimodal methods of effective cancer pain management in the inpatient setting for both adults and pediatric patients. The dosages of narcotics used in treating cancer pain often surpass those used postoperatively. Consequently, the utilization of basal continuous opioid infusions for the management of cancer pain is very valuable, and in contrast to postoperative pain management, should be encouraged.[76] Parenteral narcotics provide a vital route for providing analgesia in patients with moderate to severe cancer pain. One study demonstrated changing the route of opioid administration, including the use of PCA-administered parenteral narcotics, is an important tactic for patients that have refractory cancer pain.[77] Moreover, the use of methadone in PCA pumps, a practice uncommonly advocated for postoperative pain, is also a useful consideration in treating intractable cancer pain.[78]

PAIN CONTROL IN PATIENTS WITH OBSTRUCTIVE SLEEP APNEA

Strategies for pain management in patients with obstructive sleep apnea (OSA) emphasize the use of multimodal analgesia, long-acting local anesthetic infiltration of the surgical wound, regional techniques, and minimizing

TABLE 13.5 Suggested Settings for Pediatric Patient-Controlled Epidural Analgesia

Drug	Basal Rate (mL.kg.h^{-1})	Demand Dose (mL.kg^{-1})	Lockout (min)	One-Hour Limit (mL.kg.h^{-1})
Bupivacaine 0.06% + Hydromorphone 10 µg mL^{-1}	0.1–0.3	0.1	Minimum of 10 min	Max = 0.4

Source: Hospital for Special Surgery.

TABLE 13.6 Suggested Settings for Pediatric Peripheral Nerve Catheter Patient-Controlled Analgesia

Drug	Basal Rate (mL.kg.h^{-1})	One-Hour Limit (mL.kg.h^{-1})
Ropivacaine 0.2%	0.1–0.2	1.25 *Note: the maximum safe dose is equivalent to 2.5 mg.kg.h^{-1}*

Source: Hospital for Special Surgery.

the use of sedatives and opioids.[79] Several studies have demonstrated that opioids exacerbate both central and obstructive events in patients with OSA, placing these patients at higher risk of respiratory depression and respiratory failure.[80,81] This increased sensitivity was also seen in patients on chronic opioid therapy (6 months or longer).[82]

Current recommendations are that IV PCA should be used with caution in patients with known or suspected OSA.[79,83] If an IV PCA is used, a basal infusion is not recommended, because the use of a basal rate is associated with increased risk of respiratory depression.[81,84]

Opiate-containing EPCA is likewise associated with respiratory depression in patients with OSA. A recent meta-analysis including 121 patients suggested an incidence of major cardiorespiratory complications (including three deaths, one cardiorespiratory arrest, and two episodes of severe respiratory depression) of 4.1%.[85] Significantly, five of these major complications occurred in patients receiving continuous fentanyl-based epidural infusions. The authors note that, to date, all studies are small and comprise low-quality evidence, and that the true rate of cardiorespiratory complications in OSA patients receiving neuraxial opiods is difficult to determine from the available data.

Patients with OSA on postoperative opioid PCA therapy should be monitored by continuous pulse oximetry.[79] The appropriate setting for monitoring remains controversial: Although some evidence supports a step down or ICU location,[86] the most recent ASA practice guidelines[79] concluded that the literature is insufficient to offer guidance regarding either the setting or duration of monitoring. Finally, patients should have supplemental oxygen provided for hypoxic events, and home continuous positive airway pressure (CPAP) therapy should be continued for the entire hospital stay.[83]

KEY POINTS

- PCA is a programmable delivery system for self-administration of predetermined doses of analgesic medication at the push of a button. PCA improves satisfaction.
- Safe use of PCA requires the patient to control analgesic delivery. Increasing plasma concentrations of opioids usually causes sedation prior to respiratory depression. Sedation usually impairs the ability of the patient to activate the PCA.
- The ideal opioid for IV PCA has rapid onset of action, high efficacy, and intermediate duration of action. Morphine, fentanyl, and hydromorphone fit these criteria.
- Opioid-naïve patients should not usually receive postoperative basal IV opioid infusions, due to increased risk of respiratory depression without improved analgesia. Basal infusions are often used for cancer and opiate tolerant patients.
- PCEA is recommended for routine use during labor analgesia. IV PCA for labor may be used, but offers inferior analgesia and may depress neonatal ventilation and neurologic status.
- PCEA may provide superior postoperative analgesia and lower morbidity for a variety of surgical procedures when compared with IV PCA. The potential benefits of PCEA must be balanced against the potential risks associated with the placement of the catheter.
- PNC PCA may be the ideal postoperative analgesic modality to facilitate rehabilitation after orthopedic and plastic surgery procedures.
- Most children older than 7 years can understand and safely use PCA. Children under ages 3–5, or patients with mental or physical limitations, may not be able to effectively use PCA.
- Patients with OSA are at elevated risk of respiratory depression from opiate-containing PCA. Basal opiate infusions should be avoided and patients monitored by pulse oximetry. Home CPAP should be continued.

REFERENCES

Access the reference list online at ExpertConsult.com.

CHAPTER 14

Intrathecal Opioids for Postoperative Pain

Nikki Conlin, MD ◎ Michael C. Grant, MD ◎ Christopher L. Wu, MD

Since the first use of intrathecal (IT) morphine in 1979 the use of IT opioids has become commonplace in current clinical anesthetic practice. Multiple published reports and clinical investigations describing the use of IT opioids exist. In addition, human and animal studies have elucidated the mechanism of action of IT opioids, side effect profiles, dose-response pharmacology, interaction with adjuvant agents, and clinical uses for a wide range of surgical cases. IT opioids are commonly used for postoperative analgesia in obstetric and gynecology surgery, orthopedic joint and spine surgery, thoracic surgery, vascular surgery, cardiac surgery, pediatric surgery, urological surgery, and abdominal surgery.

MECHANISM OF ACTION OF INTRATHECAL OPIOIDS

Nociceptive information is transmitted by multiple afferent neurons that play a major role in the transmission of pain. These neurons consist of small-diameter unmyelinated fibers and thinly myelinated fibers (C fibers and Aδ fibers, respectively). Once activated they release excitatory transmitters such as substance P and ultimately contribute to the perception of pain. Central terminals of small unmyelinated fibers are located in Rexed laminae I, II, and III. Opioid receptors exist in Rexed laminae I, II, and V in the dorsal horn of the spinal cord. This location provides the anatomic basis for selective opioid analgesia in the cerebrospinal fluid (CSF). IT morphine injected into the CSF blocks the transmission of substance P and is mediated by gamma-aminobutyric acid (GABA) presynaptically and glycine postsynaptically.

The pharmacologic properties of various opioids determine their speed of onset, duration of action, and side effect profile (Table 14.1). Lipophilicity (vs. hydrophilicity) is the key property affecting the speed of onset and duration of action. Highly lipid-soluble drugs (i.e., fentanyl and sufentanil) have a faster onset but shorter duration of action when used intrathecally. Shortly after injection, CSF levels are barely detectible because the drug is quickly distributed to the spinal cord. This may result in a more segmental spread of analgesia and a lower concentration reaching the brain, decreasing the risk of delayed respiratory depression (e.g., 12–24 hours after injection). In contrast, hydrophilic opioids, such as morphine, have a slower onset of action and longer duration of action and remain detectable in the CSF long after injection. Delayed respiratory depression may be more likely with morphine than with other lipophilic drugs, as morphine remains in the CSF long enough to circulate rostrally to the brainstem and respiratory centers.

An exception to these general rules is IT meperidine, exhibiting both local anesthetic properties and IT opioid receptor–binding properties that allow it to be used as a sole agent for surgery.[1] It produces spinal anesthesia that is qualitatively similar to that achieved with conventional local anesthetics. The onset of action for meperidine is similar to that of fentanyl despite being significantly less lipid soluble; however, its duration is longer than that of fentanyl. In contrast to morphine, meperidine has a shorter duration of action because it dissipates from the CSF four times faster than morphine.[1]

ADVANTAGES OF INTRATHECAL OPIOIDS

There are several advantages inherent to the use of IT opioids compared with other either intravenous (IV)/epidural opioids or neuraxial local anesthetics (Table 14.2). Equianalgesic doses of IT opioids are typically a small fraction of those used for IV or epidural use. The resultant serum levels, especially with morphine, are barely detectable, thus limiting certain systemic effects while maximizing the analgesic properties. The duration of analgesia for a hydrophilic opioid such as morphine is greater compared with IV or epidural administration.[2] A single IT injection of morphine 0.1–0.5 mg will provide up to 15–24 hours of analgesia.[3,4] IT morphine may be of benefit in certain clinical situations. For instance, IT opioids may provide an advantage over epidural catheters in operations where anticoagulation will be started immediately postoperatively, necessitating the removal of the epidural catheter at the conclusion of surgery.

TABLE 14.1 Characteristics of Intrathecal Opioids

Opioid	Oil-Water Partition Coefficient[a]	Typical Adult Intrathecal Dose	Onset of Analgesia (min)	Duration of Analgesia (min)
Morphine	1.4	0.05–0.6 mg	30–60	480–1440
Meperidine	39	10–100 mg	2–12	60–400
Fentanyl	816	10–50 μg	5–10	30–120
Sufentanil	1727	2.5–12.5 μg	3–6	60–180

[a]*A higher number reflects increased lipophilicity.*

TABLE 14.2 Advantages of Intrathecal Opioids

Long duration of action
Small doses required for equianalgesic effect
Almost undetectable vascular absorption
Ease of cannulating the intrathecal space
Minimal hemodynamic changes
No motor blockade
No sensory loss

TABLE 14.3 Side Effects of Intrathecal Opioids

Mild respiratory depression	Respiratory arrest
Pruritus	Generalized muscle rigidity
Sedation	Nystagmus
Nausea	Epileptic seizure
Vomiting	Myoclonus
Urinary retention	Hyperalgesia Neurotoxicity Water retention

Unlike neuraxially administered local anesthetics, opioids do not cause adverse hemodynamic changes when administered intrathecally. In addition, opioids do not cause motor blockade or sensory loss, potentially allowing earlier ambulation.[5] IT opioids do provide a sparing effect for local anesthetics, allowing lower doses to be used intrathecally or epidurally while still maintaining adequate analgesia.[6]

SIDE EFFECTS OF INTRATHECAL OPIOIDS

IT opioid use does come with a number of adverse effects (Table 14.3). Most of these side effects are dose dependent and may be more common for agents administered intrathecally than by other routes. A majority of the side effects are mediated via interactions with opioid receptors.

The most feared complication is respiratory depression. The clinical use of IT morphine began in the 1980s and was accompanied with a high incidence of respiratory depression. Large IT doses of morphine (up to 20 mg) were administered and associated with an alarmingly high rate of respiratory depression.[7] Correlations between dose and respiratory depression were noted as larger doses resulted in higher incidence of respiratory depression. Clinically significant respiratory depression is typically not seen with doses less than 0.4 mg of IT morphine.[6] However, there have been isolated cases in which respiratory depression has occurred with smaller doses than those specified.[8,9]

The incidence of respiratory depression is difficult to quantify; however, from the available literature it appears to be less than 1% for IT opioids.[10] Indeed, the incidence of respiratory depression is less than 1% for opioids regardless of the route of administration. A meta-analysis of IT morphine in spinal anesthesia noted that IT morphine did not increase the overall risk of respiratory compromise; however, higher doses of IT morphine were associated with more episodes of respiratory depression when compared with lower doses.[11] Furthermore, when added to a general anesthetic, IT morphine appears to be associated with an increased risk of respiratory depression (odds ratio = 7.86; 95% confidence interval [CI]: 1.54–40.3).[12]

Respiratory depression typically occurs within minutes to hours for the lipophilic opioids. Early respiratory depression (defined in minutes) is not reported with hydrophilic opioids such as morphine. For morphine, delayed respiratory depression characteristically occurs 6–12 hours after administration but has been reported up to 19 hours after IT injection.[13] Considerable hypoventilation may occur following IT morphine even in the presence of "normal" pulse oximetry and respiratory rate. Sedation may be another indicator of impending respiratory depression; however, only arterial blood gas analysis reliably identifies hypercarbia. Supplemental oxygen may prevent hypoxemia but may not correct the underlying etiology or even worsen hypoventilation and hypercarbia due to the elimination of hypoxic respiratory drive, especially when obstruction of the airway (e.g., obstructive sleep apnea) is implicated.

The risk of respiratory depression increases with the addition of systemic opioids and sedatives, increases with age of patient, increases with lack of opioid tolerance (i.e., opioid-naïve state), increases with obesity, and increases with sleep apnea.[3] Respiratory depression occurs when hydrophilic opioids within the CSF migrate and react with opioid receptors in the ventral medulla. Naloxone has been used effectively to treat respiratory depression. Naloxone will need to be readministered or used as a continuous infusion due to its short half-life. Long-acting opioid antagonists have also been used for treatment and prevention of respiratory depression.

The risk of postoperative respiratory depression after the use of IT opioids has created some debate about whether intensive care unit monitoring is required after patients leave the postanesthesia care unit. Lipid soluble opioids have a low likelihood of delayed respiratory depression. However, hydrophilic opioids have a higher incidence and have prompted some institutions to require admission to a monitored unit for all patients receiving IT morphine. In addition, the requirement for monitored beds may in itself be reason enough to discourage the administration of IT opioids to patients who would otherwise benefit from such therapeutics. Patients with comorbidities such as sleep apnea, sedation, pulmonary disease, and mental status changes should be monitored closely after receiving IT opioids. IT morphine should not be used for ambulatory surgery. A higher dose of IT opioid may be acceptable for opioid-tolerant patients. Practice guidelines for the prevention, detection, and management for respiratory depression associated with neuraxial opioid administration have been published.[14]

The most common side effect of IT opioids is pruritus.[13] Compared with placebo, IT morphine is associated with an increased risk of pruritus, with higher doses being associated with a greater risk than are lower doses (relative risk [RR] = 1.8, 95% CI: 1.4–2.2 for <0.3 mg morphine; and RR = 5.0, 95% CI: 2.9–8.6 for >0.3 mg morphine).[11] Pruritus is usually noted in the facial areas innervated by the trigeminal nerve; however, itching may also be generalized. Although IT opioid-induced pruritus is likely due to cephalad migration of the drug and interaction with opioid receptors in the trigeminal nucleus located superficially in the medulla, the exact etiology is unclear.[13] The incidence has been reported anywhere from 20% to 100% in various studies and may be dose dependent.[5,13,15] It is difficult to determine differences in the incidence of pruritus among the different opioids due to methodologic issues; however, it appears the patients who receive morphine have a higher incidence of pruritus than those who receive fentanyl.[13] The obstetric patient population appears to have one of the highest incidences of pruritus.[13,15] Despite the relatively high incidence of pruritus, very few patients actually request treatment, because the pruritus anecdotally is often noted as a problematic side effect only after clinician prompting. Itching does not appear to be histamine mediated nor is it related to systemic absorption of drug. Antihistamines are minimally effective as treatment; however, their sedating properties may relieve symptoms in some patients. Opioid receptor antagonists, such as naloxone, and opioid agonist-antagonists are effective in the treatment of pruritus.[13,16] Low-dose IV naloxone may be effective in attenuating pruritus but does not generally decrease the analgesic efficacy of IT opioids. Ondansetron may be an effective agent for treating spinal or epidural morphine-induced pruritus.[17] Prophylactic ondansetron 0.1 mg/kg IV has been shown to reduce the incidence of pruritus after IT morphine.[17]

Nausea and vomiting are also common and troublesome side effects after IT opioid injection. Although the incidence is lower than that seen with pruritus, these patients more often require treatment. Nausea occurs in approximately 20%–40% of patients receiving IT opioids.[13] Although the underlying mechanism is not related to systemic absorption, the incidence is comparable with IV and epidural administration. Nausea usually occurs within 4 hours of injection and may be more likely when IT morphine is used.[13] Numerous studies have shown a slight correlation between dose and nausea and vomiting, whereas others have failed to show a connection. The presumed mechanism is the cephalad migration of drug and subsequent interaction with opioid receptors in the area postrema. A meta-analysis suggests that nausea and vomiting induced by IT morphine is not dose dependent. Compared with placebo, low doses of IT morphine (<0.3) were associated with an increased risk of nausea (RR = 1.4; 95% CI: 1.1–1.7) and vomiting (RR = 3.1; 95% CI: 1.5–6.4); however, doses of IT morphine >0.3 mg did not result in an increased risk of either nausea (RR = 1.2; 95% CI: 0.9–1.6) or vomiting (RR = 1.3; 95% CI: 0.9–1.9) compared with lower doses.[11] Naloxone is generally effective in the treatment of nausea and vomiting induced by IT opioids. Long-acting opioid antagonists may not be as effective in treating nausea, but there may be a benefit if given prophylactically.[18,19]

Urinary retention following IT opioids appears to be much more common than after equivalent doses given intravenously. The incidence of urinary retention varies considerably but occurs most frequently in males.[11] Urinary retention induced by IT opioids does not appear to be dose related, may be more frequent when IT morphine is administered, and is likely related to opioid receptor–induced inhibition of sacral parasympathetic nervous system outflow, resulting in detrusor relaxation and an increase in bladder capacity.[13] Naloxone may be effective in treatment, although bladder catheterization may be required.[13]

Sedation is a dose-dependent side effect of IT opioids that occurs with all opioids. Respiratory depression should be suspected when sedation occurs with other opioids.[3,13] The difference in the incidence of sedation from IT, IV, and epidural routes is not well documented but appears to be common regardless of the route of delivery. Opioid receptor antagonists are effective in decreasing the level of sedation. Chronic opioid use and subsequent tolerance may decrease the incidence of sedation.

Numerous, although rare, side effects of IT opioids are present in the literature. Generalized muscle rigidity in a neonate was reported following fentanyl during cesarean delivery.[20] Muscle rigidity and myoclonic movements, not mediated by opioid receptors, are also reported in adults.[13] Nystagmus, double vision, and convulsive movements of the eyelids have been described.[9] Epileptic seizure has also been reported following an IT morphine bolus.[21] Large doses of IT morphine have been linked to hyperalgesia in laboratory animals.[13]

CLINICAL USES OF INTRATHECAL OPIOIDS FOR POSTOPERATIVE ANALGESIA

Numerous case reports, randomized clinical trials, and dose-response studies have been completed over the past two decades related to the use of IT opioids for postoperative pain management in a variety of procedures, including obstetric, orthopedic, abdominal, pediatric, and cardiac surgeries. The great majority of trials have evaluated the use of IT morphine due to its long-lasting analgesic effects. The lipophilic opioids do play a role in postoperative analgesia; however, their relatively short duration may limit their utility for single-dose IT administration in the management of postoperative pain.

There are more studies on the use of IT opioids in postoperative obstetric patients (excluding labor analgesia) than in any other patient population. In general, there has been a trend toward using lower doses of hydrophilic opioids, which provide reasonable levels of postoperative analgesia with a lower incidence of side effects (Table 14.4). Milner et al. demonstrated that 0.1 mg of IT morphine produces analgesia comparable with a dose of 0.2 mg but with significantly less nausea and vomiting.[22] When comparing 0.1-, 0.2-, and 0.3-mg doses of IT morphine, Sarvela et al. concluded that the dose of 0.1 mg of IT morphine provided optimal postoperative analgesia for cesarean section patients.[15] Sufentanil (10 μg) improves and prolongs the duration of surgical analgesia in patients undergoing cesarean section but at the cost of increased hypotension and pruritus. More recent studies have discovered genetic variants in the μ-opioid receptor, which may partially explain the variable responses to IT opioids for labor analgesia.[23]

Lower extremity orthopedic patients are frequently ideal candidates for regional anesthesia and IT opioids due to the presence of significant postoperative pain, which can be difficult to control. The addition of 0.3 mg IT morphine to patients receiving bupivacaine spinal anesthesia significantly reduces pain and IV morphine patient-controlled analgesia (PCA) requirements compared with patients

TABLE 14.4 Dose-Response Studies of Intrathecal Morphine

Study (Author, Year)	Study Population *(n)*	Trial Design	Doses Examined (mg)	Optimal Dose (mg)
Jacobson et al. (1988)	ORTHO (33)	DB, RCT	0, 0.3, 1, 2.5	0.3–1
Boezaart et al. (1999)	ORTHO (60)	DB, RCT	0.2, 0.3, 0.4	0.3
Kirson et al. (1989)	GU (10)	DB, RCT	0, 0.1, 0.2	0.1
Sarma and Bostrom (1993)	GYN (80)	DB, RCT	0, 0.1, 0.3, 0.5	0.3
Yamaguchi et al. (1990)	GI (139)	RCT	0, 0.04, 0.06, 0.08, 0.10, 0.12, 0.15, 0.20	0.06–0.12
Jiang et al. (1991)	OB (63)	RCT	0, 0.025, 0.05, 0.075, 0.1, 0.125	0.075–0.125
Milner et al. (1996)	OB (50)	RCT	0.1, 0.2	0.1
Kelly et al. (1998)[a]	OB (80)	RCT	0, 0.125, 0.25, 0.375	—
Palmer et al. (1999)	OB (108)	DB, RCT	0, 0.025, 0.05, 0.075, 0.1, 0.2, 0.3, 0.4, or 0.5	0.1
Sarvela et al. (2002)	OB (150)	DB, RCT	0.1, 0.2	0.1
Demiraran et al. (2008)	ORTHO (60)	RCT	0, 0.16	0.16

[a]*Diamorphine.*

DB, *Double blind;* GI, *abdominal;* GU, *Urologic;* GYN, *gynecologic;* OB, *obstetric (cesarean section);* ORTHO, *orthopedics;* RCT, *randomized controlled trial.*

Studies: Boezaart AP, Eksteen JA, Spuy GV, Rossouw P, Knipe M. Intrathecal morphine. Double-blind evaluation of optimal dosage for analgesia after major lumbar spinal surgery. Spine *1999;24:1131-1137; Demiraran Y, Yucel I, Akcali GE, et al. Adding intrathecal morphine to unilateral spinal anesthesia results in better pain relief following knee arthroscopy.* J Anesth *2008;22(4):367-372; Jacobson L, Chabal C, Brody MC. A dose–response study of intrathecal morphine: efficacy, duration, optimal dose, and side effects.* Anesth Analg *1988;67:1082-1088; Jiang CJ, Liu CC, Wu TJ, et al. Mini-dose intrathecal morphine for post-cesarean section analgesia.* Ma Zui Xue Za Zhi *1991;29:683-689; Kelly MC, Cara-bine UA, Mirakhur RK. Intrathecal diamorphine for analgesia after caesarean section. A dose finding study and assessment of side-effects.* Anaesthesia *1998;53:231-237; Kirson LE, Goldman JM, Slover RB. Low-dose intrathecal morphine for post-operative pain control in patients undergoing transurethral resection of the prostate.* Anesthesiology *1989;71:192-195; Milner AR, Bogod DG, Harwood RJ. Intrathecal administration of morphine for elective caesarean section. A comparison between 0.1 mg and 0.2 mg.* Anaesthesia *1996;51:871-873; Palmer CM, Emerson S, Volgoropolous D, et al. Dose–response relationship of intrathecal morphine for postcesarean analgesia.* Anesthesiology *1999;90:437-444; Sarma VJ, Bostrom UV. Intrathecal morphine for the relief of post-hysterectomy pain—a double-blind, dose–response study.* Acta Anaesthesiol Scand *1993;37:223-227; Sarvela J, Halonen P, Soikkeli A, et al. A double-blinded, randomized comparison of intrathecal and epidural morphine for elective cesarean delivery.* Anesth Analg *2002;95:436-440; Yamaguchi H, Watanabe S, Motokawa K, et al. Intrathecal morphine dose–response data for pain relief after cholecystectomy.* Anesth Analg *1990;70:168-171.*

receiving bupivacaine spinal anesthesia with placebo following knee arthroplasty, with no significant difference in hypoxemia or apnea between the groups.[24] A dose-response study in patients undergoing major lumbar spinal surgery demonstrated that 0.3–0.4 mg of IT morphine provided superior analgesia compared with a dose of 0.2 mg.[25] The arterial carbon dioxide tension was higher in the group who received 0.4 mg of IT morphine, and no clinical signs of respiratory depression were noted. The use of high-dose morphine (10–20 µg/kg) has been reported to provide excellent analgesia without significant respiratory depression in patients undergoing spinal fusion with instrumentation.[25] Patients who received doses of 20 µg/kg of IT morphine remained pain free longer, required less additional narcotic, and had fewer respiratory complications. Another study also noted that up to 0.2 mg of IT morphine provided effective analgesia for up to 48 hours without any need for additional systemic opioids in many patients undergoing orthopedic surgery.[26] IT morphine is clearly beneficial in reducing additional opioid requirements in patients undergoing orthopedic surgery, but the optimal dose is not clear. For patients who are opioid tolerant, higher doses are probably acceptable, whereas doses of less than 0.3 mg may be ideal for opioid-naïve individuals.

IT opioids have also been used in cardiac surgery. Although IT morphine has been demonstrated to provide pain relief following coronary artery bypass grafting (CABG), the fear of bleeding complications in a patient who is systemically heparinized may have limited the use of this technique. Numerous studies have used IT opioids in patients undergoing heart surgery with CABG without the subsequent development of epidural hematoma. An IT dose of 5 µg/kg morphine produces superior analgesia compared with IV PCA morphine over 24 hours in patients having off-pump CABG, although extubation times were significantly longer in the IT morphine group.[27] Alhashemi et al. also found that larger doses (0.5 mg) of IT morphine prolonged extubation time but improved analgesia.[28] They concluded that 250 µg is the optimal dose of IT morphine to provide significant postoperative analgesia without delaying tracheal extubation. Other data suggest that IT morphine (7 µg/kg) for patients undergoing cardiac surgery may actually result in earlier extubation and possible decrease the length of the intensive care unit stay.[29]

An ample amount of literature now exists describing the use of IT opioids in pediatric patients. It is important to note that the standard doses often used in adults may be excessive in children. In a dose-dependent study using 0, 2, or 5 µg/kg of IT morphine in children 9–19 years of age undergoing a spinal fusion, the two IT opioid groups had superior postoperative analgesia.[30] The 2- and 5-µg/kg doses had a similar effectiveness and side effect profile. Although more dose-response studies are needed in pediatric patients, IT morphine in doses less than 10 µg/kg has been demonstrated to be effective in children 6 months of age or older.

IT opioid combinations will provide superior analgesia versus systemic opioids in patients undergoing vascular and thoracic procedures. Compared with those who received IV PCA morphine, patients who received a mixture of either 20 µg of fentanyl with 0.2 mg of morphine or 50 µg of sufentanil with 0.5 mg of morphine have improved pain control and minimal side effects, with the exception of an increased frequency of urinary retention.[2,4] Although epidural analgesia with local anesthetics and opioids is likely superior to IT opioids in decreasing pulmonary complications after thoracotomy,[31] IT opioids may be a good alternative to epidural analgesia in situations where an epidural catheter cannot be maintained.

IT opioids have been demonstrated to provide excellent analgesia in abdominal procedures. The use of low-dose IT morphine (0.075–0.1 mg) in providing adequate postoperative pain control was confirmed in a subsequent study.[32] At least one study has suggested that morphine (0.3 mg), when combined with IV PCA with opioids in elderly patients undergoing major colorectal surgery, improves immediate postoperative pain and decreased parenteral morphine consumption.[33]

ADJUVANTS TO INTRATHECAL OPIOIDS

Numerous studies have been published that have used other IT agents in combination with IT opioids in an effort to improve analgesia while minimizing side effects. Most of these adjuncts are analgesics that do not interact with opioid receptors. Other adjunct agents are used to alleviate or prevent side effects of IT opioids but may have varying degrees of analgesic properties.

Clonidine, an alpha2 receptor agonist, has been used to improve analgesia in combination with IT opioids, as well as with IT local anesthetics. Clonidine increases the duration of sensory and motor blockade from bupivacaine spinal anesthesia through several mechanisms. Alpha2-adrenergic agonists administered intrathecally may increase the antinociceptive threshold by activating descending noradrenergic pathways in the spinal cord. The clinical data on the analgesic interaction between clonidine and opioid are equivocal. Another study also failed to demonstrate a benefit from the addition of oral clonidine to IT morphine.[34] Most of the evidence indicates that lower doses of 15–30 µg may be equally efficacious as larger doses while decreasing side effects such as sedation, hypotension, and bradycardia. When added to IT morphine, IT clonidine is associated with decreased opioid use and increased time to first analgesic administration but also with increased incidence of hypotension.[35] IT dexmedetomidine has been used to provide analgesia.[36,37] Clonidine and dexmedetomidine may provide antinociceptive synergy at the spinal cord.[38] Finally, magnesium has been used as an IT adjuvant. IT magnesium is associated with an increase duration of spinal anesthesia without any change in blood pressure.[39]

CONCLUSION

IT opioids have been shown to be a safe and effective method of postoperative pain control. The benefit of long-lasting, noncyclic pain relief obtained with IT hydrophilic opioids, along with the lack of hemodynamic effects and motor blockade, makes this an excellent option for some patients. Patients should be assessed for adverse reactions, including nausea, vomiting, pruritus, respiratory depression, urinary retention, and sedation following administration of IT opioids. These can be easily treated with currently available pharmacologic agents. The wide variety of surgical procedures that are conducive to the use of IT opioids offers many opportunities for incorporation of this modality. It is certainly not the ideal technique in many cases, but when used appropriately it may confer significant benefits to patients.

KEY POINTS

- The pharmacologic properties of IT opioids reflect the extent of the hydrophilicity versus lipophilicity of the specific opioid: lipophilic opioids (fentanyl and sufentanil) have a faster onset and shorter duration of action, whereas hydrophilic opioids (morphine) have a delayed onset and prolonged duration of action (and certain side effects such as delayed respiratory depression).
- Like opioids administered by other routes, IT opioids may result in widely recognized opioid-related side effects, such as nausea, vomiting, pruritus, and respiratory depression. The incidence of respiratory depression from clinically relevant doses of IT opioids is no greater than when given by other routes. Frequent monitoring of patients who have received IT opioids is recommended; however, the need for an intensive care unit–like setting for postoperative monitoring of these patients is controversial.
- Delayed respiratory depression is more likely with hydrophilic opioid use; however, it is much less likely with the currently clinically accepted doses, which are lower than those used one to two decades ago. The following factors may contribute to the development of respiratory depression after IT opioid administration: opioid-naïve state, concurrent use of systemic opioids or sedatives, age, and sleep or obstructive sleep apnea.[40]

REFERENCES

Access the reference list online at ExpertConsult.com.

CHAPTER 15

Epidural Opioids for Postoperative Pain

Gabriel A. Hernandez, MD ◎ Michael C. Grant, MD ◎ Christopher L. Wu, MD

Opioids have routinely been used to manage postoperative pain, most commonly via the intravenous (IV) route; however, anesthesiologists may administer opioids epidurally, either as a single injection or a continuous infusion. The anesthesiologist can choose from a variety of available epidural opioids, each with its unique pharmacokinetic profile that gives the clinician freedom to choose the appropriate drug for the clinical scenario. Despite some of the side effects associated with epidural opioid administration, there are many advantages to using epidural opioids for analgesia. Epidural opioids are widely used to facilitate neuraxial blockade and aid in postoperative analgesia.

PHARMACOLOGY OF EPIDURAL OPIOIDS

Opioids administered in the epidural space will diffuse into the surrounding tissues, including epidural fat and veins, and will no longer be available to bind to opioid receptors and produce analgesia. Opioids administered into the epidural space generally produce analgesia via two mechanisms: via the cerebrospinal fluid (CSF) and via supraspinal or systemic analgesia. Some epidural opioids may be absorbed into the plasma and redistributed to the brainstem via the bloodstream to produce supraspinally mediated analgesia, whereas other opioids must diffuse through the spinal meninges into the CSF to produce spinally mediated analgesia. The interactions between the physiochemical properties of the spinal meninges and epidural opioids are complex and the permeability of an opioid through the spinal meninges is dependent on many factors, including its lipid solubility.[1] Once inside the CSF, epidural opioids interact with spinal opioid receptors located in lamina II of the dorsal horn of the spinal cord, resulting in antinociception via presynaptic reduction of afferent neurotransmitter release and postsynaptic hyperpolarization of dorsal horn neurons. The extent of the lipid solubility of the epidural opioid is one of the key pharmacologic properties that determines its analgesic and side effect profile. After single-dose epidural administration, lipophilic opioids (e.g., fentanyl, sufentanil) generally have a quicker onset but shorter duration of action when compared with opioids that are more hydrophilic (e.g., hydromorphone, morphine). In addition, the degree of lipid solubility of the epidural opioid will determine its side effect profile. The more lipid soluble opioids are more rapidly cleared from the CSF, which may limit the presence of delayed respiratory depression (>12–24 hours after administration) which may be more prevalent in hydrophilic opioids.

Epidural opioids do not consistently produce analgesia like intrathecal opioids, which are expected to produce analgesia via a direct effect on the spinal cord and redistribution within the intrathecal space. The degree to which lipophilic opioids produce analgesia via spinal or supraspinal mechanisms is still somewhat controversial.[1,2] It is generally thought that lipophilic opioids will produce analgesia mostly by systemic uptake and redistribution of the opioid to brainstem opioid receptors, although some data suggest that epidural fentanyl for labor analgesia may produce a selective spinal analgesic effect.[1,3] This systemic redistribution of epidurally administered lipophilic opioid is especially obvious when a continuous infusion is used for a long duration of time. Alternatively, hydrophilic opioids are primarily thought to have an analgesic site of action in the intrathecal space.[4,5] After the hydrophilic opioid has penetrated the dura into the CSF after epidural administration, the opioid will remain within the CSF to produce spinal analgesia and spread cephalad or rostral in the CSF to act at the brainstem. The rostral spread of hydrophilic opioid to the brainstem may be associated with facial pruritus, nausea, and sedation.[6]

INJECTION OF SINGLE-DOSE EPIDURAL OPIOIDS

A single-dose injection of neuraxial opioids can provide effective postoperative analgesia as a sole analgesic agent. Although they may be used alone in this regard, multiple studies have shown that analgesia is more effective when they are combined with local anesthetics. However, the analgesic profile (duration of analgesia and side effects) is dependent primarily on the degree of lipophilicity (vs. hydrophilicity), with hydrophilic agents such as morphine and hydromorphone having a longer duration of action versus lipophilic agents such as fentanyl and sufentanil. The clinician should consider choosing an opioid tailored to the surgical procedure to maximize analgesia and minimize the side effects, while taking into account the pharmacokinetic differences between hydrophilic and lipophilic opioids. For example, a single injection of a hydrophilic opioid like morphine typically provides 12 to 18 hours of analgesia and would be advantageous for postoperative analgesia in surgical inpatients with appropriate monitoring. For outpatient surgery, a lipophilic opioid may be more appropriate because its analgesic onset is more rapid and duration of action is shorter.

Both lipophilic and hydrophilic opioids may provide effective postoperative analgesia when administered as a single dose. In comparison to IV fentanyl boluses, epidural fentanyl boluses have been shown to provide adequate pain relief and inhibit physiologic, hormonal, and metabolic responses observed in the postoperative period, as shown by lower blood glucose and plasma cortisol levels for the first 20 hours after surgery. Administering a single epidural bolus of lipophilic opioid like fentanyl may provide a rapid onset (5–10 minutes) but relatively transient postoperative analgesia (up to 4 hours). Diluting the epidural dose of fentanyl (typically 50–100 μg) in at least 10 mL of preservative-free normal saline may hasten onset and

TABLE 15.1 Common Doses of Epidural Opioids[a]

	Single Dose
Fentanyl	50–100 μg
Sufentanil	10–50 μg
Alfentanil	0.5–1 mg
Morphine	1–5 mg
Diamorphine	4–6 mg
Hydromorphone	0.5–1 mg
Meperidine	20–60 mg
Methadone	4–8 mg

[a]*Doses based on use of neuraxial opioid alone. Lower doses may be effective when administered to the elderly or when injected in the cervical or thoracic region.*

prolong analgesia. Administering a single epidural bolus of hydrophilic opioid like morphine may provide a slower onset but provide a relatively longer postoperative analgesia window, which is very useful for certain procedures, including cesarean deliveries and major abdominal vascular surgery. Combining a hydrophilic and lipophilic opioid in a single epidural injection will combine the side effect profile of the short onset time and long duration of analgesia of both a lipophilic and hydrophilic opioid, respectively.

Epidural analgesia is also very convenient because administering analgesia before the onset of surgical nociceptive stimuli may prevent initiation of the feedback loop, which allows for preventive analgesia.[7] If the epidural site is not congruent with the site of surgical incision (e.g., upper thoracic catheter for a lower abdominal surgery), a hydrophilic opioid administered into the epidural space will be very effective (either as a single shot or continuous infusion) in providing analgesia via its action in the CSF. Commonly used dosages for epidural administration of opioids are provided in Table 15.1. The doses of epidural morphine may need to be decreased for elderly patients and thoracic catheter sites, so as to avoid respiratory depression and other side effects.

CONTINUOUS INFUSION OF EPIDURAL OPIOIDS

The main difference between single boluses of epidural opioids and continuous infusions of epidural opioids is that, when epidural opioids are used alone for postoperative pain control, analgesic infusions of epidural opioids will not generally cause motor block or hypotension due to sympathetic blockade, as may be seen with patients receiving local anesthetic via their epidural catheter.[8] Otherwise, the similar principles apply for infusions of lipophilic (fentanyl, sufentanil) and hydrophilic (morphine, hydromorphone) opioids as they do for single-bolus doses. Although the exact site of analgesic action (spinal vs. supraspinal/systemic) for continuous epidural infusions of lipophilic opioids has not yet been well characterized, epidural infusions of lipophilic opioids produce analgesia primarily via a supraspinal/systemic mechanism. In these trials, there were no differences in plasma concentrations, side effects, or pain scores between those receiving either IV or epidural infusions of fentanyl. The overall advantage of administering continuous epidural infusions of lipophilic opioids alone is minimal.[1]

Alternatively, continuous infusions of hydrophilic opioids produce analgesia via opioid receptors in the spinal cord. Epidural infusions of hydrophilic opioids are just as effective as single-bolus doses in providing postoperative pain control in cases in which the epidural catheter is located at a site not ideal for the location of the surgical incision or when side effects (e.g., hypotension, motor block) limit the utility of a local anesthetic-only epidural analgesic solution. A continuous epidural infusion of morphine may provide superior analgesia when compared with systemic opioids or intermittent boluses of epidural morphine.

In common clinical practice, continuous infusions of epidural opioids are administered with a local anesthetic rather than just epidural opioids alone. This combination may provide analgesic advantages over infusions of either opioid or local anesthetic alone, although the incidence of side effects may or may not be diminished.[6,9] The choice of opioid varies among anesthesiologists and clinicians: Many will choose to use a lipophilic opioid (fentanyl 2–5 μg/mL or sufentanil 0.5–1 μg/mL) as part of a patient-controlled epidural analgesia (PCEA) regimen to allow for rapid titration of analgesia; however, use of a hydrophilic opioid (morphine 0.05–0.1 mg/mL or hydromorphone 0.01–0.05 mg/mL) as part of a local anesthetic–opioid epidural analgesic regimen may also provide effective postoperative analgesia.[8]

SIDE EFFECTS OF EPIDURAL OPIOIDS

Epidural opioids exhibit the same side effects of pruritus, respiratory depression, nausea, and vomiting as opioids administered systematically. The side effect profile varies between hydrophilic and lipophilic opioids, and the severity of the side effects is usually dose dependent. Unlike local anesthetics given via the epidural space, epidural opioids are rarely directly responsible for hypotension and have little effect on heart rate or mean arterial blood pressure in comparison with being given systemically.[10] It is essential to consider other etiologies for the side effects, and it is important to have standing orders and nursing protocols for the monitoring of neurologic status (e.g., sensory and motor functions) and side effects with clinician notification of critical parameters.

RESPIRATORY DEPRESSION

The risk of respiratory depression with epidural opioids is not elevated when compared with systemic opioids and is typically reported to be from 0.1% to 0.9%.[11,12] Still, it is one of the side effects that is most concerning, especially in patients who are elderly, have an underlying pulmonary disease or decreased respiratory reserve, have underwent thoracic surgery, and/or are also taking systemic opioids and sedatives.

There are differences in the respiratory depressant profile between epidural lipophilic and hydrophilic opioids. Lipophilic opioids administered in the epidural space are associated with early (typically within 2–4 hours of administration) rather than late (more than 2–4 hours after administration) respiratory depression. Lipophilic opioids are rapidly absorbed systemically from the epidural venous plexus and delivered to the brain and respiratory centers. Hence the onset and resolution of respiratory depression from lipophilic opioids occur relatively quickly. Alternatively, the onset of respiratory depression after epidural administration of hydrophilic opioids is generally slower than that seen with epidural administration of lipophilic opioids. Hydrophilic epidural opioids are primarily delivered to the brain via relatively slower rostral migration in the CSF rather than the more rapid systemic absorption and redistribution of lipophilic opioids. Cephalad spread of hydrophilic opioids typically occurs within 12 hours following injection. Respiratory depression from epidural administration of hydrophilic opioids can therefore occur later, typically within 6–12 hours after injection. Administration of naloxone (increments of 0.1–0.4 mg) is generally effective in reversing respiratory depression; however, a continuous infusion of naloxone (0.5–5 μg/kg per hour) may be needed because the duration of action of naloxone is shorter than the respiratory depressant effect of epidural opioids. Practice guidelines for the prevention, detection, and management of respiratory depression associated with neuraxial opioid administration have been published.[13]

NAUSEA AND VOMITING

The physiology behind nausea and vomiting associated with opioids results from interactions with opioid receptors in the area postrema and chemotactic trigger zone of the medulla.

The occurrence of nausea and vomiting after a single-bolus dose of epidural opioids has been recorded to be between 20% and 50%, and the overall incidence of nausea and vomiting with a continuous epidural infusion appears to be between 45% and 80%.[6,14–16] For epidurally administered hydrophilic opioids, nausea and vomiting may be related to the cephalad migration of opioid within the CSF to the area postrema in the medulla.[6] Common treatment of epidural opioid–induced nausea and vomiting includes naloxone, droperidol, metoclopramide, ondansetron, dexamethasone, transdermal scopolamine, and sometimes even a small dose of propofol.[17]

PRURITUS

The etiology of epidural opioid–induced pruritus is unclear and may be related to activation of an "itch center" in the medulla, interaction with opioid receptors in the trigeminal nucleus or nerve roots, or changes in the sensory modulation of the trigeminal and upper cervical spinal cord due to cephalad migration of the opioid. It is important to note that opioid-induced pruritus does not appear to be associated with peripheral histamine release.[6] Pruritus from epidural opioids occurs in up to 60% of patients exposed, compared with an incidence of 15%–18% in patients exposed to IV opioids.[18,19] Some systematic data show no evidence of a dose-dependent relationship with epidural opioid–induced pruritus, whereas other studies suggest a relationship. It continues to be uncertain whether there is a relationship,[18] but it is certain that naloxone, naltrexone, nalbuphine, and droperidol appear to be effective in managing epidural opioid–induced pruritus.[19] Interestingly, studies have shown that there is a relation between the severity of epidural opioid–induced pruritus and the A118G polymorphisms of the human opioid receptor gene.[20] For patients being managed for postcesarean analgesia with epidural morphine, the severity of epidural opioid–induced pruritus was significantly lower in individuals with the homogenous recessive allele in the A118G polymorphism, in comparison with individuals with the homogenous dominant allele or heterozygous genotype.

URINARY RETENTION

The physiology behind urinary retention associated with administration of epidural opioids stems from activation of spinal opioid receptors leading to an increase in detrusor muscle strength contraction.[6] The incidence of urinary retention with epidurally administered opioids appears to be fairly high (70%–80%), especially in comparison with systematically administered opioids, for which the occurrence of urinary retention is only 18%.[6,21,22] The development of urinary retention does not appear to be dose dependent. Low-dose naloxone may be effective in treating epidural opioid–induced urinary retention but at the risk of reversing analgesia.

PATIENT OUTCOMES AND EPIDURAL MORPHINE

The use of a local anesthetic–based epidural anesthetic–analgesic technique may be associated with a decrease in perioperative morbidity and mortality.[23] The analgesic and physiologic benefits of a local anesthetic–based epidural solution may be attributed in part to the attenuation or even complete suppression of pathophysiologic changes that occur in the perioperative period. Unlike local anesthetics, use of an opioid-based epidural analgesic solution typically can only confer partial attenuation of perioperative pathophysiology despite the superior analgesia provided by epidural morphine versus systemic opioids. Thus the beneficial effect of epidural morphine on patient outcomes may not be as apparent when compared with local anesthetic–based epidural techniques.

Administration of epidural morphine may modify the perioperative stress response, although to a lesser extent when compared with local anesthetics. Unlike what occurs with local anesthetics, use of epidural morphine will still allow transmission of nociceptive information through the central nervous system. Because of the inability to completely suppress the neuroendocrine stress response, epidural opioids do not consistently prevent the perioperative increases in cortisol, epinephrine, or glucose but may attenuate increases in levels of norepinephrine. Despite the fact that epidural morphine can only partially attenuate the perioperative pathophysiologic response, there are data suggesting an improvement in patient outcomes with the perioperative use of epidural morphine compared with systemic opioids (Tables 15.2 and 15.3). Mixtures of local anesthetic and opioid can minimize the risk of respiratory depression, somnolence, and pruritus associated with only opioid use, while also reducing incidence of hypotension and motor block associated with only local anesthetic use.

TABLE 15.2 Outcome Studies of Epidural Morphine Versus Systemic Opioids for Postoperative Analgesia

Study (Author, Year)	Study Population *(n)*	Trial Design	Morbidity (EA vs. SYST)
Ali et al. (2010)	ABD/THOR (60)	RCT	Improved quality of recovery with epidural opioids
Bauer et al. (2008)	THOR (94)	RCT	Improvement in pulmonary FVC and FEV1 postoperatively for TEA ($P < .001$ and $P = .003$)
Steinberg et al. (2002)	ABD (41)	RCT	Improved return of bowel function with EA
Park et al. (2001)	ABD (1021)	RCT	22% vs. 37%[a]
Tsui et al. (1997)	ABD–THOR	RCT	EA improved pulmonary (EA: 13% vs. 25%; $P = .002$) and CV (EA: 21% vs. 43%; $P < .001$) outcomes and LOS (EA: 22 ± 20 vs. 30 ± 37; $P = .005$)
Major et al. (1996)	ABD (65)	OBS	Improvement in EA for CV ($P = .0002$)/pulmonary ($P = .019$) outcomes, LOS ICU ($P = .024$)
Liu et al. (1995)	ABD (54)	RCT	No difference in GI recovery between epidural and systemic opioids
Beattie et al. (1993)	Mixed (55)	RCT	Improvement in EA for CV ischemia (EA: 17.2% vs. 50%; $P = .01$) and tachyarrhythmia (EA: 20.7% vs. 50%; $P < .05$)
Her et al. (1990)	ABD (49)	OBS	Improvement in EA for need for ventilatory support ($P = .0002$), respiratory failure ($P = .018$), and LOS ICU (EA: 2.7 days vs. 3.8 days; $P = .003$)
Hasenbos et al. (1987)	THOR (129)	RCT	Improvement in EA for pulmonary complications (EA: 12.1% vs. 38%)
Rawal (1984)	ABD	RCT	Improvement in EA for pulmonary complications (EA: 13% vs. 40%), GI function (EA: 56.7 ± 3.1 h vs. 75.1 ± 3.1 h; $P < .05$), and LOS (EA: 7 ± 0.5 days vs. 9 ± 0.6 days; $P < .05$)

[a]*Data represented are a subgroup (aortic aneurysm repair) of the study that which showed no overall difference. Morbidity data are combined.*

ABD, *Abdominal surgery;* CV, *cardiovascular;* EA, *epidural morphine analgesia;* FVC, *functional vital capacity;* FEV1, *forced expiratory volume in one second;* GI, *gastrointestinal;* ICU, *intensive care unit;* LOS, *length of stay;* OBS, *observational trial;* RCT, *randomized controlled trial;* SYST, *systemic opioid analgesia;* TEA, *thoracic epidural analgesia;* THOR, *thoracic surgery.*

Studies: Ali M, Winter DC, Hanly AM, O'Hagan C, Keaveny J, Broe P. Prospective, randomized, controlled trial of thoracic epidural or patient-controlled opiate analgesia on perioperative quality of life. Br J Anaesth. *2010;104:292-297; Bauer C, Hentz JG, Ducrocq X, et al. Lung function after lobectomy: a randomized, double-blinded trial comparing thoracic epidural ropivacaine/sufentanil and intravenous morphine for patient-controlled analgesia.* Anesth Analg. *2007;105:238-244; Beattie WS, Buckley DN, Forrest JB. Epidural morphine reduces the risk of postoperative myocardial ischaemia in patients with cardiac risk factors.* Can J Anaesth *1993;40:532-541; Hasenbos M, van Egmond J, Gielen M, Crul JF. Post-operative analgesia by high thoracic epidural versus intramuscular nicomorphine after thoracotomy: III. The effects of pre- and post-operative analgesia on morbidity.* Acta Anaesthesiol Scand *1987;31:608-615; Her C, Kizelshteyn G, Walker V, Hayes D, Lees DE. Combined epidural and general anesthesia for abdominal aortic surgery.* J Cardiothorac Anesth *1990;4:552-557; Liu SS, Carpenter RL, Mackey DC, et al. Effects of perioperative analgesic technique on rate of recovery after colon surgery.* Anesthesiology *1995;83:757-765; Major CP Jr, Greer MS, Russell WL, Roe SM. Postoperative pulmonary complications and morbidity after abdominal aneurysmectomy: a comparison of postoperative epidural versus parenteral opioid analgesia.* Am Surg *1996;62:45-51; Park WY, Thompson JS, Lee KK. Effect of epidural anesthesia and analgesia on perioperative outcome: a randomized, controlled Veterans Affairs cooperative study.* Ann Surg *2001;234:560-569; Rawal N, Sjostrand V, Christoffersson E, Dahlström B, Arvill A, Rydman H. Comparison of intramuscular and epidural morphine for postoperative analgesia in the grossly obese: influence on postoperative ambulation and pulmonary function.* Anesth Analg *1984;63:583-592; Tsui SL, Law S, Fok M, et al. Postoperative analgesia reduces mortality and morbidity after esophagectomy.* Am J Surg *1997;173:472-478.*

TABLE 15.3 Meta-Analyses Analyzing Epidural Opioids

Author, Year	Patient Population	*n*	Major Findings	Comments
Youssef et al. (2014)	Mixed (orthopedic, abdominal, thoracic, C-section)	1513 (24 RCTs)	More PONV (OR = 1.91; 95% CI, 1.14–3.18; $P = .014$) and perhaps pruritus (OR = 1.64; 95% CI, 0.98–2.76; $P = .162$) with morphine compared to fentanyl Total opioid consumption differed only in the trials comparing morphine and fentanyl, where patients in the morphine group required 1.2 mg (of morphine equivalent) less (95% CI, 0.27–2.18)	19 of the 24 studies compare two of the following opioids: morphine, fentanyl, or sufentanil. Analgesic outcome, in terms of VAS pain score, was similar between the epidural opioids studied
Sumida et al. (2009)	Mixed	3 RCTs	Use of EREM was associated with significantly higher odds of respiratory depression when compared with IVPCA (OR = 5.80; 95% CI: 1.05, 31.93, $P = .04$)	—
Mhuircheartaigh RJ et al. (2009)	Mixed (366 orthopedic, 474 abdominopelvic, 73 C-section)	970 (5 RCTs)	Epidural morphine associated with less postoperative IVPCA opioid than epidural placebo. EREM use was strongly associated with lower pain scores with less IVPCA opioid. Moderate or severe pruritus was more common with IVPCA plus epidural morphine, whatever the formulation, compared with IVPCA plus placebo.	Hip surgery studies compared IVPCA plus EREM with IVPCA plus placebo and tended to involve older subjects than abdominal surgery and CS, which used MS 5 mg as a control rather than placebo.

CI, *Confidence interval;* CS, *cesarean section;* EREM, *extended-release epidural morphine;* IV, *intravenous;* OR, *odds ratio;* PCA, *patient-controlled analgesia;* PONV, *postoperative nausea and vomiting;* RCT, *randomized controlled trial;* VAS, *visual analog scale.*

Studies: Youssef N, Orlov D, Alie T, et al. What epidural opioid results in the best analgesia outcomes and fewest side effects after surgery?: a meta-analysis of randomized controlled trials. Anesth Analg *2014;119:965-977; Sumida S, Lesley MR, Hanna MN, Murphy JD, Kumar K, Wu CL. Meta-analysis of the effect of extended-release epidural morphine versus intravenous patient-controlled analgesia on respiratory depression.* J Opioid Manag *2009;5:301-305; Mhuircheartaigh RJ, Moore RA, McQuay HJ. Analysis of individual patient data from clinical trials: epidural morphine for postoperative pain.* Br J Anaesth *2009;103:874-881.*

CONCLUSION

Epidural opioids provide a viable option in treatment of postoperative pain, with analgesic properties and side effects that differ based on the exact epidural opioid administered.[24] The lipid solubility of the specific epidural opioid is the primary factor in determining its analgesic and side effect profile. Single-dose hydrophilic opioids can provide extended analgesia, which is perfect for inpatient surgical populations that can be monitored, whereas lipophilic opioids will provide postoperative analgesia over a relatively shorter period of time. Continuous infusions of hydrophilic opioids alone will provide sufficient postoperative analgesia even when the catheter insertion site is not congruent to the incision site. Continuous infusions of lipophilic opioids alone will not provide a selective spinal site of action, but rather because they can be titrated quickly, lipophilic opioid infusions are commonly used in local anesthetic–opioid mixtures in PCEA. Studies have shown that hydrophilic opioids administered into the epidural space may improve patient outcomes, especially in high-risk patients.

KEY POINTS

- As seen with intrathecal opioids, the pharmacologic properties of epidurally administered opioids reflect the extent of the hydrophilicity versus lipophilicity of the specific opioid: lipophilic opioids (fentanyl and sufentanil) have a shorter onset and duration of action, whereas hydrophilic opioids (morphine, hydromorphone) have a delayed onset and prolonged duration of action (and certain side effects such as delayed respiratory depression).
- Epidural opioids exhibit the same side effects (respiratory depression, pruritus, nausea, and vomiting) as opioids given systemically. Many of these side effects appear to be dose dependent; however, the side effect profile is slightly different between lipophilic and hydrophilic epidural opioids. The incidence of respiratory depression is similar regardless of the route of administration (epidural vs. systemic). Certain groups of patients may be at higher risk for developing respiratory depression after epidural administration of opioids.
- The clinician should consider the analgesic and side effect profile of epidural lipophilic and hydrophilic opioids and tailor these for individual clinical scenarios (e.g., avoiding a long-acting hydrophilic opioid such as morphine for ambulatory surgery).
- The use of epidural morphine can only partially attenuate the perioperative pathophysiologic response, unlike local anesthetics, which can cause complete suppression of pathophysiologic changes during perioperative period. However, several studies have shown that perioperative use of epidural morphine (vs. systemic opioids) may result in an improvement in patient outcomes, such as reductions in cardiovascular-pulmonary complications and even decreased mortality.

REFERENCES

Access the reference list online at ExpertConsult.com.

CHAPTER 16 CONTINUOUS PERIPHERAL NERVE BLOCKS

Brian M. Ilfeld, MD, MS (Clinical Investigation) ✪ Edward R. Mariano, MD, MAS (Clinical Research)

INTRODUCTION

Providing continuous peripheral nerve blocks (CPNB), also called "perineural local anesthetic infusion," involves the percutaneous insertion of a catheter directly adjacent to the peripheral nerve(s) supplying the surgical site (Fig. 16.1), as opposed to a "wound" catheter placed directly at a surgical site. Site-specific, potent analgesia may then be provided with few, if any, side effects. CPNB was first described in 1946 using a cork to stabilize a needle placed adjacent to the brachial plexus divisions to provide a "continuous" supraclavicular block.[1]

INDICATIONS FOR CONTINUOUS PERIPHERAL NERVE BLOCKS

As with all procedures, CPNB is associated with inherent risks (see section on "Potential Risks/Complications"). Therefore, CPNB is usually provided to patients expected to have at least moderate postoperative pain of a duration greater than 24 hours that is not easily managed with oral analgesics. However, opioid requirements and opioid-related side effects may be decreased with the use of CPNB following *mildly* painful procedures. Because not all patients desire, or are capable of accepting, the extra responsibility that comes with the catheter and pump system, appropriate patient selection is crucial for safe CPNB, particularly in the ambulatory environment. Although recommendations for the use of various catheter locations for specific surgical procedures exist,[2] there is little published data specifically illuminating this issue.[3] In general,

- Axillary, infraclavicular, or supraclavicular infusions are used for surgical procedures involving the hand, wrist, forearm, and elbow[4];
- Interscalene catheters are used for surgical procedures involving the shoulder or proximal humerus[5];
- Thoracic paravertebral catheters are used for breast or thorax procedures[6,7];
- Psoas compartment catheters are used for hip surgery[8,9];
- Fascia iliaca, femoral, and psoas compartment catheters are used for knee or thigh procedures[10];
- Popliteal or subgluteal catheters are used for surgical procedures of the leg, ankle, and foot.[11]

The authors recommend using an interscalene catheter for shoulder or proximal humerus procedures,[5] infraclavicular catheter for more distal procedures of the upper extremity,[4] a transversus abdominis plane catheter for inguinal or lower abdominal procedures,[12] a femoral catheter for knee surgery, and a popliteal-sciatic catheter for foot/leg procedures.[13]

EQUIPMENT AND TECHNIQUES

ULTRASOUND-GUIDED CATHETER INSERTION

For ultrasound-guided procedures, the term "long axis" is used when the length of a nerve is within the ultrasound beam, compared with "short axis" when viewed in cross-section.[14,15] A needle inserted with its length within a two-dimensional ultrasound beam is described as "in plane," while a needle inserted across a two-dimensional ultrasound beam is "out of plane."[16]

Needle In-Plane, Nerve in Short-Axis Approach

This is the most frequently published *single*-injection peripheral nerve block orientation because this view allows for easier identification and differentiation from surrounding structures. When the long axis of the needle is inserted within the ultrasound plane, the needle tip location can be more easily identified relative to the target nerve. Local anesthetic spread may be observed if the initial local anesthetic bolus is placed through the needle, and adjustment of the needle tip made when necessary. However, when the perineural catheter is inserted past the needle tip, it has the tendency to bypass the nerve given the perpendicular orientation of the block needle and target nerve,[17] although there are certain anatomic locations that often allow a catheter to be passed and remain perineural.[18,19] Some practitioners have advocated either passing the catheter a minimal distance past the needle tip, or advancing the catheter further initially and then, after needle removal, retracting the catheter such that its orifice(s) lie a minimal distance (<2 cm) past the original needle tip position[20] (although others have suggested this may result in a dislodged catheter tip as the needle is withdrawn over the catheter, especially by trainees). Some advocate using an extremely flexible perineural catheter in an attempt to keep the catheter tip in close proximity to the target nerve if the catheter is inserted more than a minimal distance.[21] Nonetheless, others describe reorienting the needle from an in-plane to a more parallel trajectory and inserting a stimulating catheter to better monitor catheter tip location.[22]

There are multiple benefits of the needle in-plane, nerve in short-axis approach. First, practitioners may learn only one technique since it may be used for both single-injection and catheter insertion procedures. Furthermore, it may be used for nearly all anatomic catheter locations, even for deeper target nerves.[23] If a 17- or 18-gauge needle is used, the needle tip may be more easily identified and remains within the ultrasound plane due to its rigidity compared with smaller gauge needles.[24] While some have speculated that the use of a large needle is more painful, seven prospective studies reported a median catheter-insertion pain score of 0–2 on a 0–10 numeric rating scale (10 = most pain

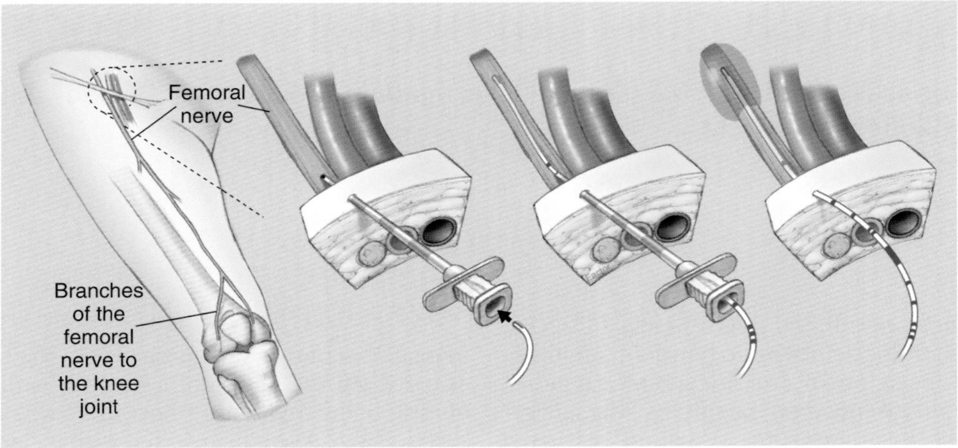

FIG. 16.1 Insertion of a femoral perineural catheter used to provide a continuous peripheral nerve block.

imaginable) when the needle track was first anesthetized with lidocaine via a 25–27-gauge needle.[20,23,25–30] In addition, the potential benefits of using a larger needle gauge (fewer needle passes given the relative ease of keeping a rigid, larger-gauge needle in plane; less risk of undesired tissue contact due to misinterpretation of the needle shaft for the needle tip) must be weighed against the potential risks (increased patient discomfort; increased tissue trauma; increased injury if a vessel is punctured).

There are disadvantages of this approach as well. They include new needle entry sites relative to the nerve compared with more traditional nerve stimulation modalities which typically use a parallel needle-to-nerve insertion; challenges keeping the needle shaft in-plane[31]; difficult needle tip visualization for relatively deep nerves[32,33]; and, as noted above, the catheter tip may bypass the target nerve given the perpendicular orientation of the needle and nerve.[17] If an extremely flexible catheter is used in an attempt to minimize this issue, it is sometimes difficult to thread past the tip of the placement needle.

Needle Out-of-Plane, Nerve in Short-Axis Approach

There are potential benefits of this approach. They include a generally familiar parallel needle-to-nerve trajectory used with traditional nerve stimulation techniques (and also vascular access); and because the needle is parallel to the target nerve, the catheter theoretically may remain in closer proximity to the nerve, even when threaded more than a centimeter past the needle tip.[20,25] However, a disadvantage of this technique is the relative inability to visualize the advancing needle tip,[20,34] which some speculate increases the likelihood of unwanted contact with nerves, vessels, peritoneum, pleura, or even meninges.[35] Practitioners often use a combination of tissue movement and "hydro-location" in which fluid is injected and the resulting expansion infers the needle tip location (either with or without color Doppler flow).[34,36] It has been suggested that for superficial catheters (e.g., interscalene and femoral), the consequent "longitudinal" orientation of needle with nerve makes precise visualization of needle tip less critical, as the needle tip tends to remain relatively close to the nerve if the needle tip is advanced beyond the ultrasound beam. However, for deeper nerves, this technique is not as straightforward as guiding the needle tip to a target nerve as in the in-plane technique described above and may be more difficult to master (and nearly impossible at times).[32,33]

Needle In-Plane and Nerve in Long-Axis Approach

Superficially, this technique appears to have the benefits of both previously described approaches, with few limitations. The nerve can be viewed along with the needle shaft/tip, and the catheter monitored as it exits the needle parallel to the target nerve. The difficulty lies in keeping three structures, the needle, nerve, and catheter, in the ultrasound plane.[37] In addition, to view the nerve in long axis, the nerve itself must be relatively straight; and there can be only one target nerve as opposed to multiple trunks or cords as found within the brachial plexus. Evidence of this technique's difficulties may be found in the scarcity of published reports.[37,38]

Limitations on the length of this chapter precludes a discussion of multiple additional ultrasound-related issues, such as transducer selection, the concomitant use of nerve stimulation (an important tool in a subset of patients),[39] and various methods for catheter tip localization.[40] Overall, little clinical data exists comparing aspects of any one placement technique with another.

STIMULATING VERSUS NONSTIMULATING CATHETERS

Up to 40% of catheters have been reported misplaced upon insertion.[41] There are multiple techniques and equipment available for catheter insertion. One common technique involves locating the target nerve using nerve stimulation via an insulated needle, and then injecting a bolus of local anesthetic via a needle to provide a surgical block, followed by the introduction of a "nonstimulating" catheter.[42] However, when using this technique, it is possible to provide a successful surgical block but inaccurate catheter placement. With the use of ultrasound guidance, the catheter tip may be directly viewed if inserted 1 cm past the needle tip, and then the needle can be withdrawn over the catheter with the operator continuously visualizing the catheter tip location to be certain that it is not dislodged. If ultrasound is not used, some investigators first insert the catheter and then administer a bolus of local anesthetic via the catheter in an effort to avoid catheter tip misplacement, with a reported failure rate of 1%–8%. Alternatively, catheters that deliver current to their tips have been developed in an attempt to improve initial placement success rates.[43] These catheters provide feedback on the positional relationship of the catheter tip to the target nerve prior to local anesthetic dosing. While there is evidence that passing current via the catheter may improve the accuracy of catheter placement with minor benefits in the lower extremity,[44–47] the nonstimulating catheters of these three studies were advanced 4–10 cm past the needle tip, which greatly increases the risk of the catheter tip-to-nerve distance and decreasing the effectiveness of the local anesthetic infusion.[48] Further study is required to identify the optimal equipment for perineural infusion.

INFUSION MANAGEMENT

Currently, there is insufficient information to determine if there is an optimal local anesthetic for CPNB. The majority of perineural infusion publications have involved bupivacaine (0.1%–0.25%) or ropivacaine (0.1%–0.4%),[49] although levobupivacaine and shorter acting agents have been reported.[13] The main determinant of CPNB effects, local anesthetic concentration and volume or simply total drug dose, remains unknown, although there is evidence that for continuous femoral and posterior lumbar plexus blocks, local anesthetic concentration and volume do not influence nerve block characteristics, suggesting that local anesthetic dose (mass) is the primary determinant of perineural infusion effects.[8,50] There are no adjuncts added to local anesthetics that have been demonstrated to provide benefits during CPNB.[51–53] Additionally, epinephrine and opioids have been added to local anesthetic infusions, but there are currently insufficient published data to draw any definitive conclusions regarding the safety of the former or the efficacy of the latter.[54–59]

Many variables probably affect the optimal regimen, including the surgical procedure, catheter location, physical therapy regimen, and the specific local anesthetic infused. For procedures resulting in at least moderate postoperative pain, a basal infusion optimizes benefits such as analgesia and sleep quality.[60–62] Providing patients with the ability to self-administer local anesthetic doses increases perioperative benefits such as improving analgesia, minimizing supplemental opioids, and allowing a decreased basal infusion rate, which minimizes the risk of limb weakness and maximizes the infusion duration for ambulatory patients with a finite local anesthetic infusion pump reservoir volume.[60–62] Unfortunately, insufficient information is available to base recommendations on the optimal basal rate, bolus volume, or lockout period accounting for the many variables that may affect these values (e.g., catheter type, location, surgical procedure). Until recommendations based on prospectively collected data are published, practitioners should be aware that investigators have reported successful analgesia using the following with long-acting local anesthetics: basal rate of 4–8 mL/h, bolus volume of 2–5 mL, and lockout duration of 20–60 minutes.

One relatively new technique is now possible due to the advent of new infusion pumps that can repeatedly administer automated bolus doses. Initial reports suggested improved analgesia using this technique[63,64]; however, subsequent volunteer-based trials do not appear to support using this modality.[65,66] Additional research is required, especially involving adductor canal, supraclavicular, and transversus abdominis plane catheters for which a bolus dose might improve local anesthetic spread with beneficial effects.

The dosing issue has particular importance for lower extremity CPNB. Although inhibition of pain fibers is the primary goal for postoperative CPNB, currently available local anesthetics approved for clinical use decrease other afferent (e.g., nonpain-related sensory and proprioception) and efferent (e.g., motor) nerve fibers as well,[67] resulting in undesirable side effects such as muscular weakness.[49] There is growing evidence that lower extremity CPNB may increase the risk of patient falls,[68,69] although to what degree the perineural local anesthetic infusion was a contributing factor in these cases remains unknown, because the studies were neither designed nor powered to detect such (presumably) rare complications. Nonetheless, patient falls during perineural infusion are now being highlighted in the surgical and anesthesiology literature.[68–72] Until additional data are available, practitioners may want to consider steps that may minimize the risk of falls, including minimizing the dose/mass of local anesthetic; providing limited-volume patient-controlled bolus doses that allow for a decreased basal dose without compromising analgesia in some cases,[73]although not all[60]; using a knee immobilizer and walker/crutches during ambulation,[74] and educating physical therapists, nurses, and surgeons of possible CPNB-induced muscle weakness and necessary fall precautions.

In addition, a perineural infusion into the adductor canal, an aponeurotic tunnel in the midthird of the thigh deep to the sartorius muscle, dramatically reduces quadriceps weakness relative to a catheter inserted adjacent to the femoral nerve.[75] This is most likely due to the fact that there is only one nerve within this canal that serves the quadriceps, as opposed to the femoral that innervates the entire quadriceps muscle. Unfortunately, there is also data that suggests adductor catheters provide somewhat inferior analgesia compared with femoral infusions[76,77]; but considering that a weakened quadriceps muscle probably increases the risk of falling, the risk-benefit ratio might be favorable towards the adductor location.[78]

POTENTIAL RISKS/COMPLICATIONS

Two of the largest prospective investigations to date involving over 2100 patients combined suggest that the incidence of CPNB-related complications is very low—at least as low as,[79] if not lower than, single-injection techniques.[80,81] Other prospective studies suggest a similar incidence of complications.[82,83]

The most commonly reported complication is "secondary block failure" with a range of 0%–50%.[84] The incidence of this complication is presumably dependent upon many factors, including the experience of the practitioner, equipment and technique, and patient factors such as body

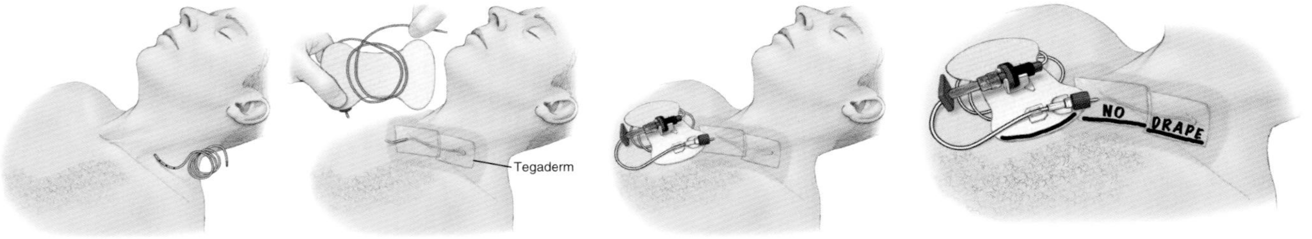

FIG. 16.2 Securing an anteriolateral interscalene perineural catheter used to provide a continuous peripheral nerve block.

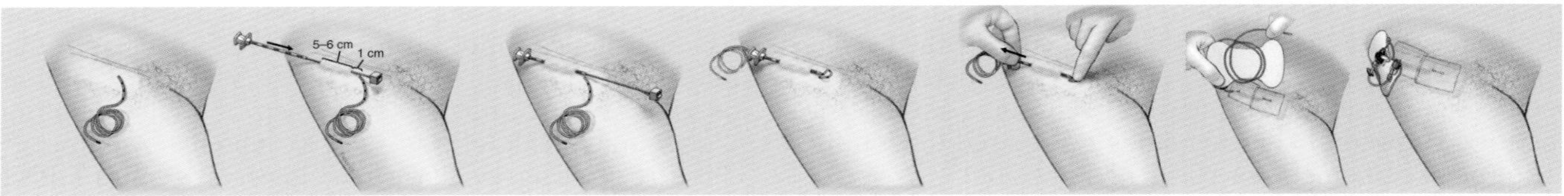

FIG. 16.3 Tunneling a femoral stimulating catheter used to provide a continuous peripheral nerve block.

habitus. Although definitive data is lacking, it is probable that the use of ultrasound improves catheter insertion success rates.[23,27,29,30,85,86] Ultrasound also decreases other risks, such as vascular puncture (reported between 0 and 11% with nerve stimulation),[23,87] peri-neuraxis catheter placement, and intravascular and intraneural catheter insertion.[88] Prolonged Horner syndrome due to neck hematoma is a rare complication, but it has been reported.[89] While a hematoma may require weeks for resolution (months for a Horner syndrome), practitioners and patients should be reassured with the multiple case reports of complete neural recovery following hematoma resolution.

Nerve injury is a recognized complication following placement of both single injection and CPNB, presumably related to needle trauma and/or subsequent local anesthetic/adjuvant neurotoxicity. The prospective clinical evidence from human subjects suggests that the incidence of neural injury from a perineural catheter and ropivacaine (0.2%) infusion is no higher than following single-injection regional blocks.[79,80,90,91] There is also evidence that for patients with diabetes, the risk of local anesthetic-induced nerve injury is increased.[92]

The most common complication during perineural infusion is simply inadvertent catheter dislodgement (0%–50%). Every effort to optimally secure the catheter must be made to maximize patient benefits (Fig. 16.2). Measures have included the use of sterile liquid adhesive (e.g., benzoin), sterile tape (e.g., Steri-Strips), securing of the catheter-hub connection with either tape or specifically designed devices (e.g., Statlock), subcutaneous tunneling of the catheter (Fig. 16.3), and the use of 2-octyl cyanoacrylate glue.[93] Using a combination of these maneuvers, investigators have reported a catheter retention rate of 95%–100% for over 5 days of infusion.[3] Other complications occurring during infusion include phrenic nerve block and ipsilateral diaphragm dysfunction during interscalene CPNB, local anesthetic toxicity (incredibly rare), and infection. While the reported rate of inflammation (3%–4%)[81,94,95] and catheter bacterial colonization (6%–57%) are seemingly high,[96,97] clinically relevant infection is relatively rare (incidence 0%–3%[98,99]; but most reports <1%).[79,80,90,91,96] In all but a few cases, infections completely resolve within 10 days; even in the worst-case scenarios, there has never been a permanent injury due to infection.[81,98,100] There are additional potential CPNB complications, such as catheter knotting (do not pass the catheter >5 cm past the needle tip),[101] retention (on with the Arrow Stimucath),[61] and shearing (do not withdraw the catheter back into the needle unless the design is approved for this maneuver).[90,102]

CONCLUSION

There is a large and growing body of evidence that CPNBs provide a multitude of clinical benefits. However, because of the relatively recent evolution of modern techniques, illuminating data are often unavailable. Future prospective investigation is required to determine the optimal catheter design(s), insertion technique(s), insertion approach(es), infusate(s), delivery regimen, infusion duration, and true incidence of complications. Only by prospectively comparing various approaches will their relative benefits and drawbacks be truly revealed and the science of perineural infusion advanced.

KEY POINTS

- CPNB is usually provided to patients expected to have at least moderate postoperative pain of a duration greater than 24 hours that is not easily managed with oral analgesics.
- The authors recommend using an interscalene catheter for shoulder or proximal humerus procedures; infraclavicular catheter for more distal procedures of the upper extremity; a transversus abdominis plane catheter for inguinal or lower abdominal procedures; a femoral catheter for knee surgery; and a popliteal-sciatic catheter for foot/leg procedures.
- There are multiple benefits of the needle in-plane, nerve in short-axis approach. It may be used for both single-injection and catheter insertion procedures and may be used for nearly all anatomic catheter locations, even for deeper target nerves.

- Disadvantages of the needle in-plane, nerve in short-axis approach include new needle entry sites; challenges keeping the needle shaft in-plane; difficult needle tip visualization for relatively deep nerves; and the catheter tip may bypass the target nerve given the perpendicular orientation of the needle and nerve.
- Currently, there is insufficient information to determine if there is an optimal local anesthetic for CPNB.
- The inhibition of pain fibers is the primary goal for postoperative CPNB. Currently available local anesthetics approved for clinical use decrease other afferent (e.g., nonpain-related sensory and proprioception) and efferent (e.g., motor) nerve fibers, resulting in undesirable side effects such as muscular weakness.
- Practitioners may want to consider steps that may minimize the risk of falls, including minimizing the dose/mass of local anesthetic; providing limited-volume patient-controlled bolus doses; using a knee immobilizer and walker/crutches during ambulation; and educating physical therapists, nurses, and surgeons of possible CPNB-induced muscle weakness and necessary fall precautions.

REFERENCES

Access the reference list online at ExpertConsult.com.

CHAPTER 17

PEDIATRIC POSTOPERATIVE PAIN

David J. Krodel, MD, MS ◎ Patrick K. Birmingham, MD, FAAP

Historically underrecognized and undertreated, pediatric pain management has improved dramatically since the early 1990s. Advances in pain assessment, pharmacologic studies of opioid and nonopioid analgesics in children, and development of physician-directed hospital-based acute pain services have been important factors in this development.[1–4]

ANATOMIC AND PHYSIOLOGIC DIFFERENCES

The rational use of analgesics in pediatric patients, particularly neonates and infants, requires recognition of maturational changes that occur after birth in body composition and core organ function.[5,6]

Total body water represents about 80% of body weight in full-term newborns. This drops to 60% of body weight by 2 years of age with a large proportional decrease in extracellular fluid volume. The larger extracellular and total body water stores in infancy lead to a greater volume of distribution for water-soluble drugs. Newborns have smaller skeletal muscle mass and fat stores, decreasing the amount of drug bound to inactive sites in muscle and fat. These stores increase during infancy.

Cardiac output is relatively higher in infants and children than adults and is preferentially distributed to vessel-rich tissues such as the brain, allowing for rapid equilibration of drug concentrations. Immaturity of the blood-brain barrier in early infancy allows increased passage of more water-soluble medications such as morphine. This combination of increased blood flow to the brain and increased drug passage through the blood-brain barrier can lead to higher central nervous system (CNS) drug concentrations and more side effects at a lower plasma concentration.

Renal and hepatic blood flow is also increased in infants relative to adults. As glomerular filtration, renal tubular function, and hepatic enzyme systems mature, generally reaching adult values within the first year of life, increased blood flow to these organs leads to increased drug metabolism and excretion.

Both the quantity and binding ability of serum albumin and alpha-1-acid glycoprotein (AAG) are decreased in newborns relative to adults. This may result in higher levels of unbound drugs, with greater drug effect and toxicity at lower overall serum levels. This has led to lower local anesthetic dosing recommendations in neonates and young infants, although neonates have shown the ability to acutely increase AAG levels while on continuous local anesthetic infusions. The difference in serum protein quantity and binding ability disappears by approximately 6 months of age.

Neurotransmitters and peripheral and central pathways necessary for pain transmission are intact and functional by late gestation, although opiate receptors may function differently in the newborn than in adults. Cardiorespiratory, hormonal, and metabolic responses to pain in adults have also been well documented to occur in neonates.

The spinal cord and dura mater in the newborn infant extend to approximately the third lumbar (L3) and third sacral (S3) vertebral level, respectively, and reach the adult levels of approximately L1 and S1 by about 1 year of age. The lower-lying spinal cord in young infants is thus theoretically more vulnerable to injury during needle insertion at mid to upper lumbar levels. The intercristal line connecting the posterior superior iliac crests, used as a surface landmark during needle insertion, crosses the spinal column at the S1 level in neonates versus the L4 or L5 level in adults. There is less, and more loosely connected, fat in the epidural space in infants versus adults, explaining in part the relative ease with which epidural catheters inserted at the base of the sacrum can be threaded to lumbar or thoracic levels in infants and small children.

PAIN ASSESSMENT

Depending on developmental age and other factors, the pediatric patient may be unable or unwilling to verbalize or quantify pain similar to his adult counterpart. Nonetheless, a number of developmentally appropriate pain assessment scales have been designed for use in both infants and children. They are based on self-report, behavioral, and/or physiologic measures (Table 17.1) and have been tested, validated, and

TABLE 17.1 Age and Measures of Pain Intensity

Age	Self-Report Measures	Behavior Measures	Physiologic Measures
Birth to 3 years	Not available	Of primary importance	Of secondary importance
3 years–6 years	Specialized developmentally appropriate scales available	Primary if self-report not available	Of secondary importance
>6 year	Of primary importance	Of secondary importance	—

From McGrath PJ, Beyer J, Cleeland C, Eland J, McGrath PA, Portenoy R. American Academy of Pediatrics Report of the subcommittee on assessment and methodologic issues in the management of pain in childhood cancer. Pediatrics *1990;86:816.*

employed in research protocols (Table 17.2). Children over approximately 8–10 years of age may be able to use the standard adult numeric rating or visual analog scale to self-report their pain.[7,8] Specialized self-reporting scales are available for children and can be used in patients as young as 3 years of age (Fig. 17.1).[9] Behavioral or physiologic measures are available for younger ages and for developmentally disabled children (Table 17.3).[10,11]

TABLE 17.2 Measurement Tools for Postoperative Pain Research in Pediatrics

Measurement Tool	Domain Assessed
Behavior Score	Postoperative pain
Beyer Oucher Scoring System	Postoperative pain
CHEOPS	Postoperative pain
CHIPPS	Postoperative pain
COMFORT Scale	Postoperative pain
CRIES Scale	Postoperative pain
FLACC, rFLACC	Postoperative pain, cognitively impaired
NCCPC-PV	Postoperative pain, nonverbal, developmentally delayed
Objective Pain Discomfort Score	Postoperative pain
Objective Pain Score	Postoperative pain
Objective Pediatric Pain Scale	Postoperative pain
Observational Pain Scale	Postoperative pain
PPMS	Postoperative pain
Wong-Baker Faces Scale	Postoperative pain

CHEOPS, *Children's Hospital of Eastern Ontario Pain Scale;* CHIPPS, *children and infants postoperative pain scale;* CRIES, *crying, requires oxygen for saturation less than 95%, increased vital signs, expression, sleepless score scale;* FLACC, *face, legs, activity, cry, and consolability;* NCCPC-PV, *noncommunicating children's pain checklist-postop version;* PPMS, *parents postoperative pain measure scale.*
(Table created with the assistance of Honorio T. Benzon, MD).

NONOPIOID ANALGESICS

ACETAMINOPHEN

Acetaminophen (paracetamol) is very commonly used in pediatric patients, alone or in combination with other analgesics.[12] It can be administered rectally in the perioperative period in infants or children for whom oral intake is not an option. Due to variable and slower adsorption with rectal dosing, a higher initial dose may be needed for rectal administration (Table 17.4).[13] Suppository insertion prior to surgical incision does not appear to significantly alter acetaminophen kinetics and may result in more timely analgesia in the early postoperative period. Higher dose rectal acetaminophen has been shown to be equi-analgesic to intravenous ketorolac following tonsillectomy and to have a significant opioid-sparing effect in children undergoing outpatient surgery. Intravenous acetaminophen is also appropriate in patients in whom oral intake is not an option. Blood levels via this route are more reliable than the rectal form.

Acetaminophen dosing in premature and term neonates is less well defined. Despite age-related differences in elimination pathways, overall elimination in small studies is similar between neonates, children, and adults. Dose-dependent hepatotoxicity is the most serious acute side effect of acetaminophen administration. Acute hepatotoxicity appears to be less common and less likely to be fatal in children than adults.

NONSTEROIDAL ANTIINFLAMMATORY DRUGS

Nonsteroidal antiinflammatory drugs (NSAIDs) are also widely administered to children. Studies of intravenous, intramuscular, and rectal NSAID administration in pediatric surgical patients demonstrate reduced postoperative pain scores and decreased supplemental analgesic requirements. Intravenous ketorolac is used widely in children, with a generally good safety record. The clinical significance of NSAID effects on bleeding remains controversial, leading to its avoidance by some in procedures where postoperative

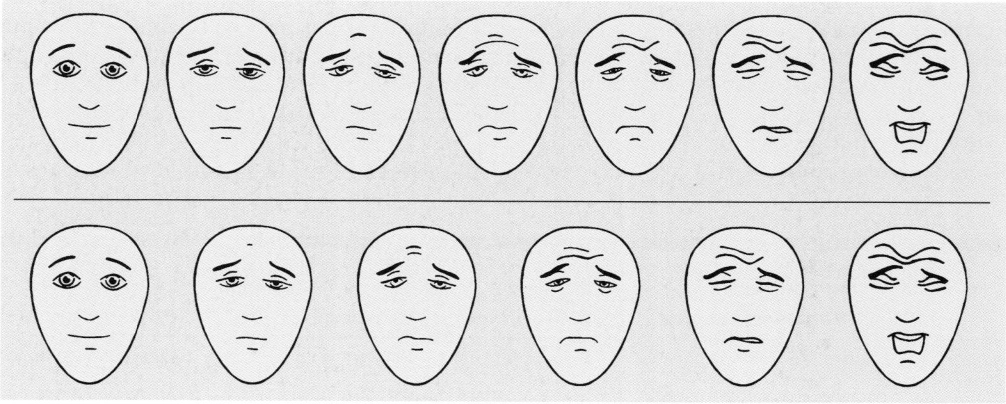

FIG. 17.1 *Top:* Faces Pain Scale (Bieri et al. 1990), scored 0–6. *Bottom:* Faces Pain Scale-Revised, scored 0-2-4-6-8-10 (or 0-1-2-3-4-5). Instructions: "These faces show how much something can hurt. This face [point to left-most face] shows no pain. The faces show more and more pain [point to each from left to right] up to this one [point to right-most face]—it shows very much pain. Point to the face that shows how much you hurt [right now]". *(From Hicks CL, von Baeyer CL, Spafford PA, van Korlaar I, Goodenough B. The faces pain scale—revised: toward a common metric in pediatric pain measurement.* Pain *2001;93:173-183.)*

bleeding is a particular concern. In particular, meta-analysis of bleeding after tonsillectomy showed a significant increased risk of bleeding with ketorolac, but a nonsignificant increased risk with other NSAIDs.[14] NSAIDs reduced the risk of postoperative vomiting after tonsillectomy (presumably due to reduced opioid use). Bleeding, renal damage, and gastritis are more likely to occur with prolonged administration and in the presence of coexisting disease. The clinical significance of NSAID inhibitory effects on osteogenesis following bone surgery, as documented in animal studies, remains unclear, but nonunion following orthopedic surgery in children is less of an issue than in adults. Acetaminophen and NSAIDs are often given in combination, as they work by different mechanisms, and their toxicity does not appear to be additive.

ASPIRIN (ACETYLSALICYLIC ACID)

Aspirin is not used for postoperative pain management in infants and children because of a highly significant association with Reye syndrome.[15] Reye syndrome is an acute, fulminant, and potentially fatal hepatoencephalopathy that occurs in children with influenza-like illness or varicella who ingest aspirin-containing medications.

DEXMEDETOMIDINE

Dexmedetomidine, a potent alpha-2 agonist, has profound sedative and analgesic properties. Its administration as a bolus dose may aid in decreasing emergence agitation in the pediatric population, presumably through its sedative properties, but increased analgesia may play a role as well.[16]

GABAPENTINOIDS

Gabapentin and pregabalin have other antiseizure activity and analgesic properties in neuropathic (e.g., diabetic neuropathy) and other chronic pain conditions (e.g., fibromyalgia). These medications have been shown to reduce opioid consumption after painful surgical procedures in adults and in adolescents with idiopathic scoliosis undergoing spinal fusion; however, the benefit in other adolescent surgical populations has been debated.[17–19]

OPIOID ANALGESIA

Oral, parenteral, and epidural opioids are widely employed in infants and children to optimize postoperative comfort. Oral hydrocodone (usually in combination with

TABLE 17.3 Revised Face, Legs, Activity, Cry, and Consolability Scale

Categories	Scoring 0	Scoring 1	Scoring 2
Face	No particular expression or smile	Occasional grimace or frown, withdrawn, disinterested	Frequent to constant frown, clenched jaw, quivering chin
Legs	Normal position or relaxed	Uneasy, restless, tense	Kicking, or legs drawn up
Activity	Lying quietly, normal position, moves easily	Squirming, shifting back and forth, tense	Arched, rigid, or jerking
Cry	No cry (awake or asleep)	Moans or whimpers, occasional complaint	Crying steadily, screams or sobs, frequent complaints
Consolability	Content, relaxed	Reassured by occasional touching, hugging, being talked to, distractable	Difficult to console or comfort

Each of the five categories is scored from 0 to 2, for a total score range of 0 to 10. 2002, The Regents of the University of Michigan. A revised scale (rFLACC) adds additional descriptors in each of the five categories to aid pain assessment in developmentally disabled children.

TABLE 17.4 Nonopioid Analgesic Dosing

Medication	Dose (mg/kg)	Total Single Dose (mg)	Dosing Interval (h)	Maximum Daily Dose (Pt < 60 kg) (mg/kg)	Maximum Daily dose (Pt ≥ 60 kg) (mg)
Acetaminophen[a] (oral)	10–15 mg/kg	650–1000	4	75–100	4000
Acetaminophen[a,b] (rectal)	35–40 mg/kg loading dose; 20 mg/kg thereafter	Less defined	6	75–100	4000
Acetaminophen[a] (intravenous)	10–15 mg/kg	650–1000	4–6	75–100	4000
Ibuprofen	6–10 mg/kg	400–600 mg	6	40	2400
Naproxen	5–6 mg/kg	250–375 mg	12	24	1000
Ketorolac	0.3–0.5 mg/kg IV	15 mg < 50 kg; 30 mg > 50 kg	6	2 (IV)	120
Tramadol	1–2 mg/kg	100 mg	6	8	400

[a]*Dosing in neonates and young infants is less-defined, but approximately 50% of above recommendation.*
[b]*No evidence of accumulation at 24 hours.*
Dose ranges are approximate and may vary depending on individual patient assessment.

TABLE 17.5 Oral Opioid Analgesic Dosing Guidelines

Medication	Potency Relative to Morphine	Typical Starting Dose (mg/kg)	Typical Dose (mg if >60 kg)	Dosing Interval (h)
Morphine	1	0.3	15–20	3–4
Hydrocodone	1–1.5	0.1–0.2	5–10	4–6
Oxycodone	1–1.5	0.1–0.2	5–10	4–6
Hydromorphone	5–7	0.04–0.08	2–4	3–4
Methadone	1	0.1–0.2	10	6–12

Dose ranges are approximate.

TABLE 17.6 Patient-Controlled Analgesia Parameters

Choice of Opioid	Morphine	Hydromorphone	Fentanyl
Loading dose (over 1–5 minutes)	0.05–0.10 mg/kg	5–10 μg/kg	0.5–2.0 μg/kg
Demand dose	0.01–0.02 mg/kg	2–4 μg/kg	0.2–0.4 μg/kg
Lockout time	5–15 minutes	5–15 minutes	5–15 minutes
1-hour limit (optional)	0.10–0.20 mg/kg	30–40 μg/kg	3–4 μg/kg
Continuous infusion (optional)	0.01–0.02 mg/kg/h	2–3 μg/kg/h	0.2–0.4 μg/kg/h

Dose ranges are approximate; selection of opioid and actual parameters depends on assessment of individual patient.
Adapted from Birmingham PK. Recent advances in acute pain management. Curr Probl Pediatr *1995;25:99-112.*

acetaminophen) is commonly used for postoperative analgesia in children over 6 months of age. Codeine, as a prodrug of morphine metabolized by cytochrome P450 (CYP)2D6, has been associated with poor analgesia in so-called "slow metabolizers" and with lethal respiratory depression in "ultrarapid metabolizers."[20] Due to its unpredictable effects and side effects based on CYP2D6 genotype (and immaturity in the case of infants less than 6 months of age), more predictable opioids may be preferred.[21] Other opioids metabolized by CYP2D6 such as oxycodone, hydrocodone, and tramadol probably should be avoided in known poor or rapid metabolizers and infants less than 6 months of age, although except for tramadol no clinical evidence has shown their efficacy or side effects to vary in these populations. Medications without CYP2D6 metabolism such as morphine, hydromorphone, methadone, fentanyl, buprenorphine, and oxymorphone may be more appropriate in these populations (Table 17.5). Ongoing research in CYP genotyping may better guide prescribing in the future. Intravenous and transdermal fentanyl is also used in appropriate doses in children.

In addition, opioid dosing may need to be adjusted for other patient characteristics, especially the presence of obstructive sleep apnea (OSA) or sleep-disordered breathing (SDB). Opioid dosing in patients with OSA/SDB should be decreased by approximately 50% to avoid apneic/hypoxic events with particular attention to posttonsillectomy patients.[22]

For inpatients, parenteral opioids are still given on an as-needed basis to some patients, but patient-controlled analgesia (PCA) has been increasingly used since the early 1990s. Epidural opioids are also used in pediatric populations.

PATIENT-CONTROLLED ANALGESIA

PCA is used in children as young as 5–6 years of age, with morphine the most commonly used and studied opioid, and hydromorphone and fentanyl more commonly used alternatives (Table 17.6). Compared to as needed, nurse administered intramuscular opioids, PCA has been shown to be safe in children and provide more effective analgesia with greater patient satisfaction.[23] PCA may be used safely with appropriate monitoring with or without a continuous opioid infusion.[24] Continuous opioid infusion with PCA appears to increase sleep, sedation, and total opioid consumption, but this has not been shown to reliably improve pain scores.[25–27]

PARENT/NURSE-ASSISTED ANALGESIA

The concept of PCA has been expanded to allow parent- or nurse-assisted analgesia (authorized PCA-by proxy or PCA-P) in select cases in which the patient is unwilling or unable, because of age, developmental delay, or physical disability, to operate the PCA button. This technique is used with caution as it removes one of the safety features of PCA, in that the patient is theoretically less likely to self-overdose.[28] PCA-P has been safely used for postoperative analgesia and painful oncologic and other medical conditions (e.g., mucositis).[29] Although not as common as PCA-P, parent/nurse controlled epidural analgesia (PCEA-P) has been used to optimize dosing flexibility and pain relief given via the epidural route.

CONTINUOUS INTRAVENOUS INFUSIONS

Continuous intravenous opioid infusions are used alone (or in combination with PCA) to provide pain relief following

TABLE 17.7 Continuous Intravenous Morphine Infusion for Postoperative Analgesia in Infants and Children

Age Range of Subjects (Estimated Gestational Age at Birth)	Infusion (μg/kg/h)	Comments	Number of Subjects
1–18 days (32–40 weeks)	15	Some patients mechanically ventilated	20
1–49 days (35–41 weeks)	6–40	Some patients mechanically ventilated; seizures at 32 and 40 μg/kg/h; recommend rate of 15 μg/kg/h	12
3 months–12 years	14–21	Less total morphine than with time-contingent IM morphine	20
<1–14 years	10–40	Spontaneously ventilating	121
14 months–17 years	10–30	Postoperative cardiac; able to wean from mechanical ventilation	44
1–15 years	20	Superior to IM morphine	20
1–16 years	10–40	Superior to IM morphine	46
3–22 years	20–40	Cerebral palsy patients	55

IM, *Intramuscular*.
Adapted from Birmingham PK, Hall SC. Drug infusions in pediatric anesthesia. In Fragen RF, ed. Drug Infusions in Anesthesiology. *2nd ed. Philadelphia: Lippincott-Raven; 1996:193-224.*

TABLE 17.8 Suggested Pediatric Epidural Dosing Guidelines

Medication	Initial Bolus	Infusion Solution	Infusion Limits
Bupivacaine	≤2.5–3 mg/kg	0.0625%–0.1%	≤0.4–0.5 mg/kg/h
Ropivacaine	≤2.5–3 mg/kg	0.1%–0.2%	≤0.4–0.5 mg/kg/h
Fentanyl	1–2 μg/kg	2–5 μg/mL	0.5–2 μg/kg/h
Morphine	10–30 μg/kg	5–10 μg/mL	1–5 μg/kg/h
Hydromorphone	2–6 μg/kg	2–5 μg/mL	1–2.5 μg/kg/h
Clonidine	1–2 μg/kg	0.5–1 μg/mL	0.1–0.5 μg/kg/h

These are approximate dose ranges. Actual dose selected depends on individual patient assessment. Infants less than 3–6 months of age generally receive a 30%–50% reduction in initial dosing and hourly infusion rates of local anesthetic or opioid.

pediatric surgery. Compared to adults given morphine, neonates and premature infants have a longer elimination half-life, lower plasma clearance and marked interindividual variability in plasma morphine concentration. For a given dose, they achieve a higher plasma concentration for a longer duration. By approximately 6–12 months of age, the kinetics of morphine and fentanyl approach adult values, and children soon thereafter demonstrate increased plasma clearance and a shorter elimination half-life. Continuous morphine infusion rates and patient age ranges are summarized in Table 17.7.

REGIONAL ANALGESIA

"SINGLE SHOT" CAUDALS

One of the most widely used pediatric regional techniques for postoperative analgesia is the "single shot" caudal (SSC). Its popularity stems in part from the readily palpable landmarks and relative ease of caudal block insertion in infants and children versus adults. SSC is used in infants and children up to approximately 8–10 years of age having surgery from lumbosacral to lower-thoracic dermatome levels with anticipated moderate postoperative pain. Bupivacaine in concentrations of 0.125%–0.25% is the most commonly used and studied local anesthetic for SSC. Injection volumes of 0.5–1.5 mL/kg provide upper lumbar to low-thoracic levels, respectively. An upper volume limit of 20 mL is generally used. The maximum recommended bupivacaine dose is 2.5–3.0 mg/kg, with an upper limit of 1.25 mg/kg recommended in early infancy. While its use is considered discretionary by some authors, a test dose of 0.1 mL/kg (maximum 3 mL) of local anesthetic with 1:200,000 epinephrine (5 μg/kg) may be used to ensure correct needle or catheter position. A 25% increase in T-wave amplitude, 10 beats/min increase in heart rate, or 10% increase in systolic blood pressure within 60 seconds of administration is considered a positive test dose. It is unclear whether block placement at the beginning versus the end of the procedure prolongs postoperative analgesia.[30]

Although usually used alone, bupivacaine can be combined epidurally with fentanyl, morphine, the alpha-2-adrenergic agonist clonidine, or other additives to prolong the duration and/or density of analgesia. Delayed respiratory depression up to 22 hours can occur with epidural morphine. Greater risk is seen in children less than 1 year of age and when parenteral opioids have also been given.

CONTINUOUS EPIDURAL INFUSION

Epidural local anesthetic infusions with or without opioids or alpha-2-agonists have been used in infants and children for postoperative analgesia. Bolus and infusion rate recommendations for bupivacaine, fentanyl, morphine, and clonidine are listed in Table 17.8. Lower infusion rates are generally recommended in neonates and infants less than 3–6 months old. This is because of lower protein binding and consequently higher free fractions of drug, and because of pharmacokinetic differences, potentially resulting in higher plasma levels and prolonged drug half-life. Substitution of other opioids, such as those with mixed agonist-antagonist effects, may minimize clinical side effects. As a rule, optimal analgesia is obtained with the catheter tip positioned at or near the dermatomes to be blocked. It is possible in infants and smaller children to thread caudally inserted catheters to lumbar or thoracic levels. Epidural needle and catheter insertion routinely occurs following induction of general anesthesia in infants and children unable or unwilling to cooperate. The safety of both peripheral and neuraxial block placement under general anesthesia in children has been demonstrated.[31] Patient-controlled epidural analgesia has been successively used in children as young as 5 years of age.[32]

PERIPHERAL NERVE BLOCKS

Peripheral and truncal nerve blocks also play an increasing role in pediatric postoperative pain relief.[33] These are largely performed under ultrasound guidance. Ilioinguinal/iliohypogastric, rectus sheath, transverse abdominus plane (TAP), head and neck, and upper and lower extremity blocks and catheters are being done more frequently to provide analgesia in suitable candidates. Multicenter databases have largely demonstrated the safety of performing these blocks under general anesthesia, more commonly with the aid of ultrasound guidance.[30,34]

SUMMARY

The basic tenet of pediatrics that children are not merely small adults holds true for postoperative pain management. It is not only the differences in neural, renal, and hepatic physiology influencing pediatric pharmacology. It is also differences in the psychosocial interpretation of pain by children and their caregivers and differences in the ability of caregivers and medical professionals to assess levels of pain. This necessitates a unique approach to postoperative pain control in children. These challenges highlight certain universal principles of postoperative pain management, such as the use of nonopioid adjuncts and regional anesthesia where appropriate to help minimize the use of opioid pain medications. Other principles of postoperative pain management are altered substantially. One example is the now widely accepted administration of regional anesthesia under general anesthesia to maximize procedural safety. Another is the use of proxies (both nurses and parents) for PCA use in patients who are developmentally disabled. Further research is required to help better understand what adult postoperative pain control therapies can be applied safely and effectively in children.

KEY POINTS

- Anatomic and physiologic differences in neonates and young infants necessitate lower doses of epidural local anesthetics and intravenous opioids up to 4–6 months of life.
- Behavioral or physiologic measures of pain intensity are available for infants and children unable to self-report their pain.
- Aspirin is not routinely used for postoperative pain control in children because of an association with Reye syndrome, a potentially fatal hepatoencephalopathy.
- Epidural analgesia by single injection or following epidural catheter insertion is commonly employed in infants and young children following induction of general anesthesia.
- Intravenous and epidural PCA can be used in children as young as 5–6 years of age.
- Nurse- or parent-assisted analgesia can be used in select circumstances for children unable or unwilling to operate an IV or epidural PCA button.

REFERENCES

Access the reference list online at ExpertConsult.com.

CHAPTER 18

Chronic Pain After Surgery

Colin J.L. McCartney, MBChB, PhD, FRCA, FCARCSI, FRCPC
Steven Tremblay, BScPT, MD, FRCPC

Approximately 40 million surgical procedures take place across North America each year, and by most conservative estimates, 10%–15% of those patients will go on to suffer chronic pain 1 year after surgery.[1] In fact, a recent US national survey of the incidence, patient satisfaction, and perceptions of postsurgical pain by Gan et al.[2] showed that 74% of patients experienced postdischarge moderate to severe pain after surgery. Gan et al.[2] also demonstrated that 80% of the surveyed population were worried about postoperative pain compared with 58% 10 years ago, demonstrating that postoperative pain is a growing concern. This is a silent epidemic of devastating proportions both for those who suffer the pain and the associated emotional costs related to distress and for society as a whole, who bear the financial cost of lost productivity and treatment of pain-related problems. Investigations in recent years have given better definitions of the extent of the problem, some of the factors that may predict the onset of chronic pain after surgery, and methods of preventing chronic pain. In addition, the future will bring us better definitions of the genetic basis of development of chronic pain, allowing us to better counsel patients prior to different types of surgery regarding the risk of chronic pain in relation to surgery and possibly allowing us to better aim the most intensive treatments at those patients to reduce morbidity. This chapter will discuss the extent of the problem of chronic postsurgical pain (CPSP), the factors associated with development, the typical presentation of CPSP, the genetics of CPSP, and possible methods of preventing CPSP.

WHAT IS CHRONIC PAIN AFTER SURGERY?

Without a good definition, it is not possible to estimate the extent of a problem. Very few papers examining the epidemiology of chronic pain after surgery have used a consistent definition. This absence has led to large variability in the estimation of chronic pain across different studies, and has slowed progress in acquisition of knowledge in this area.

Macrae and Crombie, in their original paper on chronic pain after surgery,[1] proposed a working definition as follows:

1. The pain should have developed after a surgical procedure.
2. The pain should be of at least 2 months' duration.
3. Other causes of the pain should be excluded (e.g., recurrence of malignancy or infection).
4. The possibility that the pain is continuing from a preexisting problem should be explored and exclusion attempted.

This was the first worthy attempt to define CPSP, and future studies would benefit from using such a consistent definition. In a recent *British Journal of Anaesthesia* (BJA) editorial, Werner et al.[3] presented revised criteria (Table 18.1) based on more recent data[4,5] that are more in line with the International Association for the Study of Pain (IASP) definition, which states that the pain has to persist "past the normal time of healing." However, an obvious problem with this definition is that some types of CPSP are related to a preexisting preoperative painful condition (e.g., phantom limb pain). Nevertheless, the use of a consistent definition of CPSP in the future will significantly help develop an accurate description of the extent of the problem and allow better focus on the areas of greatest need.

EPIDEMIOLOGY OF CHRONIC PAIN AFTER SURGERY

The incidence of chronic pain after surgery varies significantly by site of surgical procedure (Table 18.2); however, most reports support an incidence of at least 10% of patients having pain 1 year after surgery. Several high quality reviews in the last 10 years have highlighted the problem of chronic pain after surgery. Crombie, Davies, and Macrae[1] highlighted the problem with their survey of greater than 5000 patients presenting to North British pain clinics and found that surgery contributed to pain in 22.5% of those patients. In particular abdominal, anal, perineal, and genital pain were associated with surgical procedures. Perkins and Kehlet[17] reviewed the evidence for chronic pain after surgery and found an incidence of phantom limb pain of 30%–81%, greater than 50% for chronic postthoracotomy pain, postmastectomy pain

TABLE 18.1 Present and Proposed Criteria Regarding Persistent Postsurgical Pain[3]

- Present criteria
  - The pain should have developed after a surgical procedure.
  - The pain should be of at least 2 months' duration.
  - Other causes for the pain should be excluded—for example, continuing malignancy (after surgery for cancer) or chronic infection.
  - In particular, the possibility that the pain is continuing from a preexisting problem should be explored and exclusion attempted.
- Proposed updated criteria
  - The pain develops after a surgical procedure or increases in intensity after the surgical procedures.
  - The pain should be of at least 3–6 months' duration and significantly affect the quality of life.
  - The pain is either a continuation of acute postsurgery pain or develops after an asymptomatic period.
  - The pain is either localized to the surgical field, projected to the innervation territory of a nerve situated in the surgical field, or referred to a dermatome (after surgery in deep somatic or visceral tissues).
  - Other causes of the pain should be excluded—for example, infection or continuing malignancy in cancer surgery.

TABLE 18.2 Incidence of Chronic Pain After Surgery by Surgical Site

Study	Surgical Procedure	Patients With Data	Follow-Up	Incidence of Chronic Pain
Nikolajsen et al.[6]	Amputation	60	1 year	Phantom pain 70%
Richardson et al.[7]	Amputation	52	6 months	Phantom pain 78.8%
Jensen et al.[8]	Amputation	58	2 years	Phantom pain 59%
Tasmuth et al.[9]	Breast surgery	93	1 year	13%–33%
Nikolajsen et al.[6]	Cesarean section	220	1 year	Scar pain 12.3%
Aasvang et al.[10]	Hernia repair	694	1 year	56.6%
Nikolajsen et al.[11]	Hip replacement	1048	12–18-month prevalence	12.1% moderate to very severe pain
Borly et al.[12]	Open cholecystectomy	80	1 year	26%
Meyerson et al.[13]	Sternotomy for cardiac surgery	318	1 year	28%
Katz et al.[14]	Thoracotomy	23	18 months	52%
Perttunen et al.[15]	Thoracotomy	67	1 year	61%
Gotoda et al.[16]	Thoracotomy	91	1 year	41%

syndrome in 11%–57%, phantom breast pain in 13%–24%, and postbreast-surgery arm and shoulder pain in 12%–51%. Chronic pain after cholecystectomy is common (3%–56%), and the overall incidence of chronic pain after inguinal hernia surgery is 11.5%. Joris et al.[18] has also recently shown in a retrospective analysis that the incidence of CPSP after colorectal surgery can be up to 17%.

In the last 15 years, despite improvements in methods of providing acute pain control, there have been no dramatic improvements in the incidence of chronic pain after surgery. Studies examining pain after inguinal hernia repair,[19] breast surgery,[20] thoracic surgery,[21] and hip surgery[11] indicate that a very conservative estimate of approximately 10% of patients continue to suffer chronic pain following many types of surgery. As outlined previously, this number grossly underrepresents the true incidence, as also evidenced in the more current literature, which indicates an incidence closer to 40%.[22]

FACTORS ASSOCIATED WITH CHRONIC PAIN AFTER SURGERY

Factors that are associated with an increased likelihood of developing chronic pain after surgery are summarized in Table 18.3. It is not known at the present time whether all of these factors are causally related (as opposed to associations) to the development of chronic pain. These factors can be divided into preoperative, intraoperative, and postoperative factors. Preoperative factors include moderate to severe preoperative chronic pain, repeat surgery, and psychological factors. Intraoperative factors include surgery in a low volume center, surgical approach (open vs. laparoscopic), and intraoperative nerve injury. Postoperative factors include acute pain (moderate to severe), radiation therapy, and neurotoxic chemotherapy. In a recent multicenter prospective observational trial, multivariate analysis identified orthopedic surgery, preoperative pain, and percentage of time in severe pain as risk factors.[23] In fact, in this study, the authors stated that "a 10% increase in the percentage of time in severe pain was associated with a 30% increase in the incidence of CPSP."[23]

TABLE 18.3 Factors Associated With Development of Chronic Pain After Surgery

Preoperative Factors	Intraoperative Factors	Postoperative Factors
Pain—moderate to severe of greater than 1-month duration	Surgical approach with risk of nerve injury	Acute pain—moderate to severe
Repeat surgery	Nonlaparoscopic technique	Neurotoxic chemotherapy
Psychologic factors	Surgery in low volume center	Radiation therapy to site

Preoperative Factors

Preoperative pain: A consistent factor associated with the development of acute and chronic postsurgical pain across many types of surgery is the presence of preoperative pain. This is of particular relevance to anesthesiologists, because we are often the main advocates for good quality postoperative pain management. The presence of preoperative pain is a risk factor for the development of early acute postoperative pain—pain in the days, weeks, and months following surgery.[24] A further amplifying factor is that the presence of severe acute postoperative pain also is a risk factor for development of chronic postsurgical pain. Kalkman et al.[19] examined preoperative factors predicting severe acute pain after surgery and found independent predictors of severe pain, including preoperative pain, female gender, younger age, incision size, and type of surgery. Thomas et al.[20] examined patients having hip or knee replacement and spinal decompressive surgery, and also found that predictors of severe postoperative pain included preoperative pain, female gender, and younger age. A very consistent factor in the development of CPSP is the presence of either severe preoperative pain, postoperative pain, or both. No other patient factor is as consistently related to the development of CPSP as pain itself.

Several factors may explain the consistent relationship of preoperative and severe acute postoperative pain predicting chronic postsurgical pain,[24] including:

1. Preoperative opioid tolerance leading to underestimation and underdosing of postoperative opioid analgesics
2. Intraoperative nerve damage and the associated central nervous system changes, such a central sensitization and "wind-up"
3. Sensitization of pain nociceptors in the surgical field
4. Postoperative ectopic activity in injured primary afferents and collateral sprouting from intact nociceptive Aδ afferents neighboring the area supplied by injured afferents
5. Central sensitization induced by the surgery and maintained by further input from the surgical site during the healing process
6. Structural changes in the central nervous system (plasticity) induced by nociceptive inputs with consequent reduction in normal inhibitory control systems leading to "centralization" of pain and development of pain memories
7. Heretofore unidentified pain genes that may confer increased risk of developing both severe acute and chronic postsurgical pain
8. Psychological and emotional factors such as emotional numbing and catastrophizing (discussed later)
9. Social and environmental factors such as solicitous responding from significant others and social support (discussed later)
10. Response bias over time—that is, some individuals have a tendency to report more pain than other individuals
11. Publication bias in which findings of a significant relationship between pain before and after surgery are published, whereas negative findings are rejected and do not get published

PSYCHOSOCIAL FACTORS AND CPSP

Several psychosocial predictors of chronic postsurgical pain have been identified including increased preoperative anxiety,[25] an introverted personality, less catastrophizing, social support and solicitous responding in the week after amputation, higher emotional numbing scores at 6 and 9 months,[26] fear of surgery, and "psychic vulnerability."[27] To further support this point, Pinto et al.[28] demonstrated in her prospective study looking at postsurgical pain in women undergoing hysterectomy that presurgical and postsurgical anxiety, pain catastrophizing, and emotional illness revealed a predictive role in CPSP.

Pain catastrophizing relates to unrealistic beliefs that the current situation will lead to the worst possible pain outcome. Lewis et al.[29] demonstrated in their systematic review and meta-analysis that even though preoperative pain was the major contributing factor to patients developing CPSP, catastrophizing and the presence of mental health disorders were also strong predictors of persistent pain after total knee arthroplasty. Consistently in the pain literature, chronic pain patients who do not catastrophize fare better than patients who do. It is therefore somewhat paradoxical that the opposite has been found in the prediction of patients who are at risk of CPSP, and may be an artefact of the method by which data were collected.[30]

Solicitous responding refers to the behaviors on the part of spouses or significant others who unwittingly reinforce patients' negative behaviors and thereby increase their frequency of occurrence. For example, an empathic spouse may reinforce negative behavior by insisting that her partner rest when in fact a more appropriate response would be to encourage activity. Such solicitous behaviors may in fact have the unintended consequence of increasing pain-related behaviors and contributing to pain-related disability. The reader is directed to the comprehensive review by Katz and Seltzer for further information.[24]

INTRAOPERATIVE FACTORS

Three main surgical factors have a possible influence on the incidence of CPSP:

1. Experience of the surgeon.
   The experience of the surgeon can affect morbidity following surgery. Tasmuth et al.[9] studied patients after breast cancer surgery and found that patients who had surgery in low volume units suffered more CPSP than patients in specialist units where higher numbers of patients had surgery. Other studies, however, have shown equivocal results. Courtney et al.[31] demonstrated no correlation between the grade of surgeon and severe pain after hernia repair.
2. Avoidance of intraoperative nerve injury.
   Many basic science studies have successfully demonstrated that intentional nerve injury in animals produces behaviors that resemble symptoms of neuropathic pain in humans. It would therefore make sense during surgical procedures on humans to reduce, as much as possible, any chance of causing intraoperative nerve injury. Many CPSP syndromes occur following surgery around significant nerve structures. Examples include pain after inguinal hernia repair (ilioinguinal and iliohypogastric nerves), axillary dissection (intercostobrachial nerve), and postthoracotomy pain (intercostal nerves). When a nerve is injured, it emits a long-lasting, high frequency burst of activity.[32,33] This activity is transmitted to the central nervous system, where the massive excitatory stimulus activates postsynaptic N-methyl-D-aspartate (NMDA) receptors, leading to excitotoxic destruction of inhibitory interneurons,[30] disinhibition of pain pathways, and increased postoperative pain. The avoidance of intraoperative nerve injury would be a useful preventative measure and should be attempted wherever possible.
3. Use of minimally invasive surgical techniques where possible.
   Although the size of the surgical procedure does not correlate well with incidence of CPSP, the type of procedure and how it is performed can influence CPSP. Wallace and colleagues studied the incidence of

chronic pain after different types of breast surgery and found that mastectomy had a much greater incidence of CPSP (53%) compared with breast reduction surgery (22%).[34] Inguinal hernia repair appears to show significant reductions in CPSP when a laparoscopic technique is used, as compared with an open approach, and these results have been confirmed by several studies.[10,35] The use of lightweight mesh during open incisional hernia repair seems to be associated with less CPSP,[36] without increasing the risk of postoperative complication. Unfortunately, Garcia-Torado et al.,[37] in their review of the literature of studies focusing on the most adequate surgical procedure for prevention of CPSP in thoracotomy patients, demonstrated that there is very little scientific evidence in the prevention of postthoracotomy pain. Further studies looking at surgical techniques and the prevention of CPSP will be helpful in guiding patient therapy.

GENETIC FACTORS

The study of the genetics of pain is in infancy, and there are no current research reports that provide data on genes that may predispose patients to chronic postsurgical pain. There are only a handful of reports that identify polymorphisms in human genes associated with chronic pain, including COMT (encoding catechol-O-methyl transferase), 5-HTTLPR (the gene encoding the serotinin transporter that has been found to associate significantly with severity of migraine),[38] burning mouth syndrome,[39] irritable bowel syndrome, and fibromyalgia. IL1RN (encoding the IL-1 receptor antagonist) and MC1R (encoding the melanocortin-1 receptor) in vulvodynia, IL23R in Crohn disease, and GCH1 (encoding GTP cyclohydrolase, an enzyme catalyzing tetrahydrobiopterin, BH4, an essential cofactor for catecholamine, serotonin, and nitric oxide production) have been implicated in persistent radicular pain following discectomy. Recent work has examined OPRM1 (encoding the mu opioid receptor) including a systematic review[40] that attempted to determine the relationship of this gene to opioid sensitivity, side effects, or pain levels. Only 7% of the overall variance could be explained by genetic factors, and the authors concluded that only a minor degree of variance in the clinical setting could be related to pharmacogenetic factors. Montes et al.[41] demonstrated in their multicenter cohort study looking at patients having inguinal hernia repair, hysterectomy, and thoracotomies that an uncertainty in the knowledge of genetic factors requires us to continue to rely on clinical factors to determine CPSP predisposition. Despite the evidence of association between other genes and chronic pain conditions at this time, any plan to incorporate genotyping information into the ability to predict who will develop chronic pain is premature.[42] In a recent review article, Clarke et al.[43] claim that analyzing patients' DNA sequences, blood, and salivary pain biomarkers, as well as their analgesic responses to medications, will help us better understand CPSP pathophysiology and help develop predictive algorithms to help establish a patient's possibility of acquiring CPSP even before surgery. They go on to state that CPSP is likely 50% influenced by genetic determinants. This knowledge will enable us to develop personalized mechanism-based pain treatments.[43] Genetic factors relating to CPSP bear much promise; however, it is clear that significant amounts of work are required before they become of use in clinical practice.

PREVENTION OF CHRONIC PAIN AFTER SURGERY

In a recent systematic review of randomized trials of the interventions for the prediction and management of CPSP after total knee replacement, Beswick et al.[44] highlighted the lack of evidence about our ability to predict and manage chronic postsurgical pain in this patient population. Given that 10%–34% of patients can experience chronic postsurgical pain, it is imperative that we consider developing evidence-based care for this and other patient populations. Of the factors that we are aware of that are associated with the generation of chronic postoperative pain, several are within the direct control of anesthesiologists and surgeons in the perioperative period. Several studies have now demonstrated that severe acute pain after surgery is associated with an increased incidence of chronic pain. In a landmark study, Katz et al.[14] examined patients who had undergone lateral thoracotomy 18 months prior and found that 52% of patients reported chronic pain. Of many factors, early severe postoperative pain was the only factor that significantly predicted development of long-term pain. In a study of trauma patients undergoing elective surgery, greater acute pain on postoperative day 4 was associated with chronic pain after surgery.[45] Iohom et al.[46] recently examined the effect of a multimodal regimen on patients having breast cancer surgery, and demonstrated a relationship between severe postoperative pain and subsequent CPSP.

The relationship between severe acute pain and subsequent chronic pain is all the more worrying, given that it appears that a high proportion of patients continue to suffer moderate to extreme levels of pain after surgery.[47] Attempts to adequately prevent or treat severe acute pain may reduce the incidence of chronic pain. Puolakka et al.[48] performed a study looking at postoperative pain post knee arthroplasty, and demonstrated that if the patient had moderate to severe pain during the first postoperative week, the risk of progressing to chronic pain was up to 10 times greater compared with patients with mild pain during the same period. In addition, the ability to avoid intraoperative nerve injury and minimally invasive operative techniques both appear to reduce the chances of developing CPSP.

PREVENTIVE ANALGESIA

If severe acute pain after surgery can predispose to CPSP, it follows that prevention of acute pain after surgery may help reduce the incidence. In anesthesia and acute pain management, the practice of treating pain only after it occurs is slowly being replaced by a preventative approach. Although these methods have been developed primarily for reducing acute pain, the secondary aim of reducing transition to chronicity has also been a significant motivation. The theory that acute postoperative pain might be intensified by central sensitization induced by surgery was originally conceived by Crile[49] and later advocated by Wall,[50] who suggested that "pre-emptive preoperative analgesia" would block central sensitization caused by surgical insult and thus reduce the severity of acute postoperative pain. Subsequent attempts to validate this concept of "preemptive analgesia" were limited by an overzealous definition attempting to prove that a preincisional intervention would be superior to the same intervention following incision.[51] This definition was flawed because surgical insult causing sensitization would be expected to occur throughout surgery and for several hours or days afterward. It was therefore really no great surprise that a subsequent meta-analysis[52] demonstrated no benefit of preemptive analgesia according to this definition. More recently, a more clinically relevant term "preventive analgesia" has been developed.[53] Preventive analgesia refers to the attempt to block nociceptive input through the application of several analgesic agents, acting at different sites (multimodal analgesia) starting prior to surgery and continuing for several hours or days following surgery. A successful preventive analgesic intervention would reduce or ablate pain for hours, days, or weeks following surgery and well beyond the duration of action of the initial analgesic intervention.[54] Several studies that have examined best analgesic methods, including preventive analgesia, have demonstrated benefits, and these are described in the following sections according to type of intervention.

LOCAL ANESTHETIC TECHNIQUES

Epidural analgesia provides significant acute pain benefits in the early perioperative period, especially for major abdominal and thoracic surgery, and several large studies have demonstrated these benefits. However, the ability to prevent progression to chronicity has been less effective, with mixed results across several studies. Andreae et al.,[55] in their systematic review and meta-analysis, pooled data from 23 RCTs and strongly favored epidural analgesia and paravertebral block for pain control in patients undergoing thoracotomy and mastectomy. The superior perioperative pain control was attributed to preventing CPSP in one patient out of every four or five patients treated. Lavand'homme et al.[56] compared the epidural or intravenous route using local anesthetic, an opioid, or clonidine in one of four groups for patients undergoing major abdominal surgery. All patients received a bolus and infusion of low dose ketamine started preincision and maintained throughout the procedure. Patients in the intravenous alone group had much higher pain scores at rest and with movement compared with the other groups. The incidence of chronic pain in the intravenous alone group was significantly greater at 6 months (48%) and 12 months (28%) than other groups who had been given an epidural technique.

Gottschalk et al.[57] examined men undergoing radical prostatectomy randomizing either to epidural bupivacaine, fentanyl, or saline, followed by postoperative patient-controlled epidural analgesia. Acute pain in the hospital was greatly reduced for the two groups that had been treated prior to incision, and incidence of pain 9.5 weeks (though not at 3.5 or 5.5 weeks) following surgery was significantly lower in the groups who had been treated in this way.

For patients having thoracotomy, Obata et al.[58] compared patients receiving preincisional epidural mepivacaine compared with the same intervention at completion of surgery. Assessment at 3 and 6 months after surgery found a significant reduction in postthoracotomy pain in patients who received the preincisional epidural mepivacaine. Sentürk et al.[59] demonstrated significant benefits of an epidural compared with intravenous analgesic technique when used for patients having thoracotomy, with patients in the epidural groups having significantly lower incidence and intensity of chronic postthoracotomy pain. However, Ochroch et al.,[60] when randomizing patients to epidural bupivacaine and fentanyl either preincision or after rib approximation, could not demonstrate any differences in chronic pain 48 weeks after surgery.

The use of epidural analgesia for prevention of chronic phantom limb pain has been less effective. Despite early promise of the benefits of epidural analgesia in preventing postamputation pain, a more rigorous study by Nikolajsen et al.[6] failed to demonstrate benefit. Up until recently, peripheral nerve blocks alone have had a disappointing effect on the incidence of CPSP, despite their clear benefits in reducing acute postoperative pain. McCartney et al.[61] randomized 100 patients to either axillary block or general anesthesia for ambulatory upper limb surgery, and despite significantly improved perioperative outcomes, patients had identical incidence of pain 2 weeks following surgery. However, Iohom et al.[46] compared a multimodal analgesic regimen, including both a paravertebral catheter and an intravenous cyclooxygenase-2 (COX2) inhibitor (parecoxib), followed by oral celecoxib with a standard treatment group (including postoperative diclofenac) for patients having breast cancer surgery. Patients in the paravertebral catheter group had significantly less acute pain and also a lower incidence of chronic pain at 2–3 months following surgery (0% vs. 85%).

In a recent commentary, Richebé et al.[62] state that clinical studies have shown that the use of regional anesthesia decreases intraoperative opioid use, acute hyperalgesia, and the risk of chronic pain after surgery.[56,63,64] They commented on a study that looked at the use of sciatic nerve block and the progression to persistent central pain sensitization after surgery.[63] In this study, animals received sciatic nerve blocks before surgery. The animals then had lower extremity surgery, with a continuous infusion of local anesthetic infusion, which decreased the central sensitization. A new experiment included intraoperative fentanyl during the general anesthetic part of the study. Exposure to fentanyl cancelled the decrease in central sensitization (even with the presence of the sciatic nerve block). This model supports the supposition that opioids enhance central pain sensitization.[62] Therefore, peripheral nerve blocks may help prevent central pain sensitization by decreasing opioid use intraoperatively.

N-METHYL-D-ASPARTATE RECEPTOR ANTAGONISTS

NMDA receptors play an important role in acute pain hypersensitivity states and the generation of CPSP. Several studies have demonstrated benefits of NMDA receptor antagonists in the prevention of pain following surgery. McCartney et al. systematically reviewed this area[54] and determined that both ketamine and dextromethorphan provide analgesic benefits beyond the clinical duration of action of either drug (five half-lives). Longer duration benefits are more controversial. Katz et al.[65] examined both short- and long-term effects of preoperative or postincisional intravenous fentanyl, and low dose intravenous ketamine compared with a standard treatment receiving fentanyl but not ketamine on postoperative pain in men undergoing radical prostatectomy under general anesthesia. Pain scores did not differ at any time during the first 3 postoperative days, although by the third day the hourly rate of opioid consumption was significantly less in the pretreated group. Unfortunately, no differences were seen in pain outcomes at 2 weeks and 6 months following surgery. Schley et al.[66] compared two groups of patients undergoing unilateral upper extremity amputation under continuous brachial plexus block. The treatment group also received a daily dose of the NMDA receptor antagonist memantine. In addition to improved acute pain control, the memantine group also had less chronic phantom pain at 4 weeks and 6 months (but not at 12 months) after surgery. Remerand et al.[67] studied patients having total hip arthroplasty under general anesthesia and randomized the treatment group to receive a preoperative bolus and then 24 h continuous infusion of intravenous ketamine. At day 30, postoperatively the ketamine group had less need for two crutches or a walking frame, and from day 30 to 180 decreased the number of patients with persistent pain at rest in the operated hip ($P = 0.008$). However, Sen et al.[68] also compared ketamine, gabapentin, and placebo for patients having hysterectomy, and found that although opioid consumption was reduced in both ketamine and gabapentin groups, only the gabapentin group had reduced incidence of incisional pain scores at the 1-, 3-, and 6-month follow-up visits. In their review of pharmacotherapy for the prevention of chronic pain after surgery in adults, the Cochrane Collaboration identified 40 RCTs of various pharmacological therapies, including intravenous and oral ketamine, oral gabapentin/pregabalin, amitriptyline, nonsteroidal antiinflammatory drugs (NSAIDs), IV steroids, IV fentanyl, IV lidocaine, and inhaled nitrous oxide.[69] The meta-analysis shows a statistically significant reduction in the incidence of chronic pain after surgery, subsequent to treatment with ketamine (Fig. 18.1) but not with gabapentin, pregabalin, NSAIDS, steroids, fentanyl, lidocaine, or mexiletine.

GABAPENTIN AND PREGABALIN

Both gabapentin and pregabalin bind to the $\alpha 2\delta$ unit of the calcium channel, and are useful components of multimodal analgesia, producing opioid-sparing effects and reducing the severity of acute postoperative pain. Gabapentin has been shown to increase inhibitory current in hippocampal neurons.[3] A number of studies have also examined their effect on CPSP. Fassoulaki et al.[70] randomized 50 patients having breast cancer surgery to either multimodal analgesia including gabapentin or placebo control. At 3 months but not 6 months after surgery, patients in the multimodal group had significantly lower incidence of axilla pain (14% vs. 45%), arm pain (23% vs. 59%), and analgesic use (0% vs. 23%) compared with the placebo control patients.

Brogly et al.[71] examined the effect of gabapentin 1200 mg compared with placebo in a randomized study of 50 patients having thyroidectomy under general anesthesia. All patients also received a bilateral superficial cervical plexus block after induction. Although there were no obvious differences in acute pain (possibly masked by the cervical plexus block), patients in the gabapentin group did have a significantly lower incidence of neuropathic pain (4.3% vs. 29.2%) 6 months following surgery.

Buvanendran et al.[72] examined the effects of perioperative oral pregabalin started before total knee arthroplasty and continued for 14 days after surgery. Patients receiving oral pregabalin had less acute pain and also less neuropathic pain at 3 and 6 months following surgery. However, an earlier randomized study by Fassoulaki et al.[73] randomized patients having breast surgery to gabapentin, mexilitine, or placebo, and although they demonstrated better acute pain control, there was no difference in pain at 3 months following surgery. Nonetheless, Humble et al.[74] were able to demonstrate in a systematic review of evidence for perioperative intervention reducing acute and chronic pain associated with amputation, mastectomy, and thoracotomy that appropriate intraoperative and postoperative pain management with gabapentinoids, antidepressants, local anesthetics, and regional anesthesia may potentially reduce the severity of acute and chronic pain.

NSAIDS

Nonsteroidal antiinflammatory drugs have powerful analgesic effects and are effective components of a multimodal analgesic regimen for acute postoperative pain control. It is less certain at this time if they have any impact on the incidence of CPSP.

PREVENTIVE ANALGESIA SUMMARY

It is clear across numerous studies that providing effective acute pain control is best performed using multimodal analgesic techniques, including local anesthetics, opioids, and other agents such as NMDA receptor antagonists and/or gabapentin and associated drugs. Several studies indicate that there is an association between better acute pain control and reduction in CPSP. It would therefore seem wise to strive for best acute pain control for our patients, in the knowledge that for some patients and procedures, this will also translate into better long-term outcomes.

FUTURE STRATEGIES FOR PREVENTING CPSP

Good perioperative analgesia and minimization of surgical tissue injury will remain important goals for both anesthesiologists and surgeons in the perioperative period. The broader and more consistent use of multimodal analgesic techniques remain the simplest current method by which anesthesiologists could have a major impact on the development of CPSP. Screening strategies for psychological risk factors may be an important method in high-risk surgical procedures such as breast and thoracic surgery. Identification of the high-risk patient will allow more effective targeting of such patients with potent analgesic

Study or Subgroup	Ketamine Events	Ketamine Total	Placebo Events	Placebo Total	Weight	Risk Ratio M-H, Fixed, 95% CI
1.5.1 Abdominal and/or pelvic surgery						
De Kock 2001	1	19	3	9	4.9%	0.16 [0.02, 1.31]
De Kock 2001	0	19	2	9	4.0%	0.10 [0.01, 1.89]
Katz 2004a	2	36	4	19	6.3%	0.26 [0.05, 1.31]
Katz 2004a	6	34	3	19	4.6%	1.12 [0.31, 3.97]
Subtotal (95% CI)		**108**		**56**	**19.8%**	**0.40 [0.19, 0.88]**
Total events	9		12			
Heterogeneity: $Chi^2 = 4.37$, df = 3 ($P = 0.22$); $I^2 = 31\%$						
Test for overall effect: $Z = 2.28$ ($P = 0.02$)						
1.5.2 Amputation						
Hayes 2004	7	15	12	17	13.5%	0.66 [0.35, 1.23]
Subtotal (95% CI)		**15**		**17**	**13.5%**	**0.66 [0.35, 1.23]**
Total events	7		12			
Heterogeneity: Not applicable						
Test for overall effect: $Z = 1.30$ ($P = 0.19$)						
1.5.3 Breaset surgery						
Malek 2006	14	46	14	40	18.0%	0.87 [0.47, 1.60]
Subtotal (95% CI)		**46**		**40**	**18.0%**	**0.87 [0.47, 1.60]**
Total events	14		14			
Heterogeneity: Not applicable						
Test for overall effect: $Z = 0.45$ ($P = 0.65$)						
1.5.4 Orthopedic surgery						
Pertin 2009	2	5	5	7	5.0%	0.56 [0.17, 1.81]
Remerand 2009	16	72	24	70	29.3%	0.65 [0.38, 1.11]
Sveticic 2008	1	17	1	19	1.1%	1.12 [0.08, 16.52]
Subtotal (95% CI)		**94**		**96**	**35.4%**	**0.65 [0.40, 1.06]**
Total events	19		30			
Heterogeneity: $Chi^2 = 0.22$, df = 2 ($P = 0.90$); $I^2 = 0\%$						
Test for overall effect: $Z = 1.74$ ($P = 0.08$)						
1.5.5 Thoracotomy						
Suzuki 2006	6	22	11	22	13.2%	0.55 [0.25, 1.21]
Subtotal (95% CI)		**22**		**22**	**13.2%**	**0.55 [0.25, 1.21]**
Total events	6		11			
Heterogeneity: Not applicable						
Test for overall effect: $Z = 1.48$ ($P = 0.14$)						
Total (95% CI)		**285**		**231**	**100.0%**	**0.63 [0.47, 0.83]**
Total events	55		79			
Heterogeneity: $Chi^2 = 6.52$, df = 9 ($P = 0.69$); $I^2 = 0\%$						
Test for overall effect: $Z = 3.23$ ($P = 0.001$)						
Test for subgroup differences: $Chi^2 = 2.49$, df = 4 ($P = 0.65$); $I^2 = 0\%$						

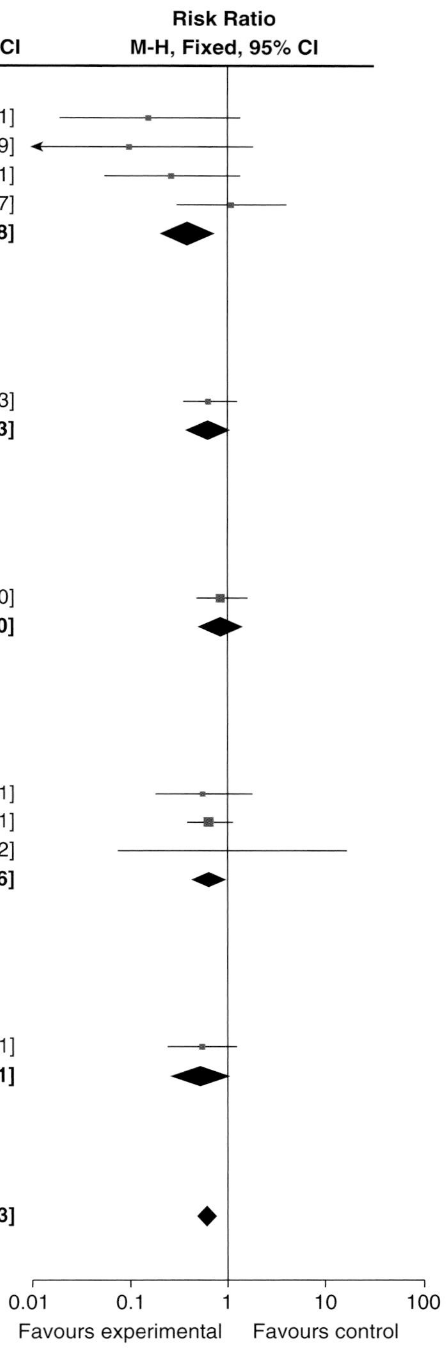

FIG. 18.1 Forest plot of comparison: I Ketamine versus placebo comparisons, outcome: 1.5 incidence of any pain at 6 months (all studies). The *diamond* represents the point estimate and confidence intervals when you combine and average all the individual studies together.

techniques in the perioperative period. The use of genetic screening for patients at risk of CPSP remains elusive, and much more research will be required before this strategy becomes a reality.

Several interesting avenues of research focusing on novel analgesic targets are being developed including glial-cell-line-derived neurotrophic factor (GDNF),[75] neurokinin 1 (NK-1) receptor antagonists,[76] voltage-gated Na channel blockade,[77] and purinergic receptor antagonists.[78]

CONCLUSION

Most people will experience surgery of one sort or another during their lifetime, and for a significant proportion, this will lead to CPSP. The development of chronic postsurgical pain is common and dependent on numerous factors (Fig. 18.2). At the present time, anesthesiologists can make a difference by providing effective treatment of postoperative pain, including at least two modalities of multimodal analgesia, preferably starting before surgical incision. Other factors, including avoidance of intraoperative nerve

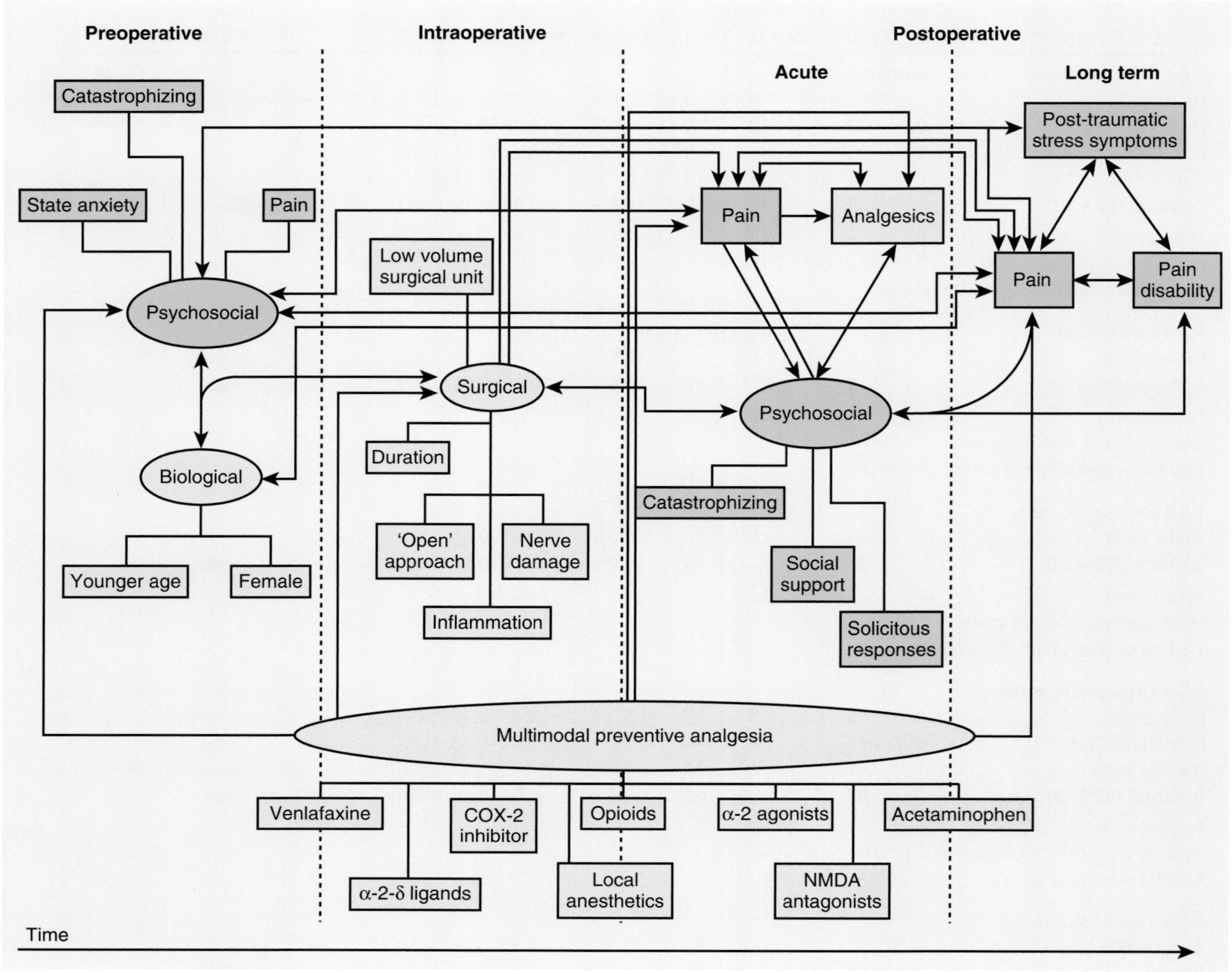

FIG. 18.2 Schematic illustration of the processes involved in the development of chronic postsurgical pain and pain disability showing relationships *(arrows)* among preoperative, intraoperative, and postoperative factors. Lines with double arrows between variables show associative relationships reported in the literature. Lines with a single arrowhead show causal relationships based on randomized controlled trials of preventive analgesia. *COX-2*, Cyclooxygenase-2; *NMDA*, N-methyl-D-aspartate. *(From Katz J, Seltzer Z. Transition from acute to chronic postsurgical pain: risk factors and protective factors.* Expert Rev Neurother *2009;9:723-744.)*

injury and minimally invasive techniques, may also help reduce incidence of CPSP. Factors such as patient psyche and genetic factors are less easy to control; however, better knowledge in the future may allow patients to properly consider the risks of developing CPSP and using aggressive and/or novel treatments to optimally prevent and manage chronic pain after surgery.

KEY POINTS

- Chronic pain after surgery is common.
- Risk factors include patients with preexisting pain, psychosocial factors, age and gender, and possibly genetic susceptibility.
- CPSP can be prevented using good surgical technique (avoiding nerve damage and minimally invasive techniques) and aggressive multimodal analgesia starting immediately prior to surgery.
- Future strategies should include more consistent use of multimodal analgesia across surgical populations and screening for high-risk patients using psychological and genetic factors.

REFERENCES

Access the reference list online at ExpertConsult.com.

SECTION IV

Chronic Pain Syndromes

SECTION OUTLINE HEAD

CHAPTER 19

Migraine Headache and the Trigeminal Autonomic Cephalalgias

Jack M. Rozental, MD, PhD, MBA

MIGRAINE HEADACHE

EPIDEMIOLOGY

Migraine headache represents a very common benign headache syndrome; it is sometimes referred to as a vascular headache. Approximately two-thirds of migraines occur in women. The prevalence in North America, ascertained through epidemiologic studies, is 12%–17.6% in females and 4%–6% in males. Prior to puberty, the prevalence of migraine in boys and girls is similar; during and after adolescence, the incidence increases more rapidly in girls. In females, prevalence increases up to the age of about 40, after which it decreases; the decrease becomes steeper as women approach menopause. Among those with severe migraine, about 25% have four or more migraines per month. More than 80% of patients with severe migraines experience headache-related disability that ranges from decreased productivity to time off work during an attack. The cost in productivity may exceed $20 billion per year in the United States. Although the cause of migraines is unknown, the risk of suffering from migraines is about 50% higher among those who have a first-degree relative with migraines; however, genetic factors appear to account for fewer than 50% of all migraines.[1–4]

PATHOPHYSIOLOGY

The pain-generating structures of the head include the venous sinuses, meningeal and large cerebral arteries, basal meninges, muscles, skin, and cranial nerves V, IX, and X. A plexus of largely unmyelinated fibers arises from the trigeminal ganglion (cranial nerve V) and innervates the cerebral and pial arteries, the venous sinuses, and the dura mater; this plexus is referred to as the trigeminovascular system. A similar plexus arises from the dorsal roots of the upper three cervical nerves and innervates comparable structures in the posterior fossa. The neurons in the trigeminovascular system contain substance P, one of the major nociceptive neurotransmitters of primary sensory neurons; calcitonin gene-related peptide (CGRP), which causes vasodilatation and when infused intravenously into susceptible individuals triggers headache; and neurokinin A, which is similar in structure and function to substance P. When the trigeminal ganglion is stimulated and causes antidromic activation of the trigeminovascular system, these peptide neurotransmitters are released near the blood vessels they innervate; this results in vasodilatation with consequent extravasation of plasma, or so-called sterile neurogenic inflammation. Leakage of plasma proteins from the dilated blood vessels in turn stimulates the trigeminal nerve endings and causes nociceptive orthodromic signals to the trigeminal ganglion; the end result of this sterile neurogenic inflammation is the perception of pain in and around the head. Neurogenic inflammation is blocked by substances that act as agonists on a subset of serotonin (5-hydroxytryptamine [5-HT]) receptors: the 5-HT_{1D} and 5-HT_{1B} receptors. The major drugs used to abort acute migraine attacks are agonists at the $5\text{-HT}_{1D/1B}$ receptors. Drugs that act as agonists at these sites are thought to reduce neurogenic inflammation by inhibiting the trigeminal nerve endings and by their actions on blood vessels; their vasoconstricting action may or may not be necessary for analgesia. Agonists at the $5\text{-HT}_{1D/1B}$ receptors include ergot alkaloids (ergotamine, dihydroergotamine [DHE]) and triptans (sumatriptan and others). Similarly, stimulation of pain-generating structures in the head activates neurons in the trigeminal nucleus caudalis and in the dorsal horn at the upper cervical levels.[5–7]

Thus stimulation of the trigeminal ganglion, through antidromic release of neurotransmitters, results in increased cerebral and extracerebral blood flow. Stimulation of the dorsal raphe nucleus, a serotonergic nucleus in the midbrain, also increases cerebral blood flow. In contrast, stimulation of the nucleus coeruleus, the major source of central noradrenergic input, causes a decrease in cerebral blood flow.

Interneurons in the spinal cord and brainstem that are part of the descending pain modulation system use enkephalins and gamma-aminobutyric acid (GABA) as neurotransmitters. An ascending serotonergic pathway in the midbrain raphe region relays painful stimuli to the ventroposteromedial (VPM) thalamus via the quintothalamic tract. A descending endogenous pain modulating system originates in the periaqueductal gray region of the midbrain, one of whose major relay structures is the nucleus raphe magnus in the medulla. After this relay, the descending pain modulating system connects with the spinal tract of the trigeminal nerve and the dorsal horns of the first through third cervical nerves. Stimulation of the periaqueductal gray region causes headache. The major neurotransmitters of this pain modulating system are norepinephrine, serotonin, and enkephalins.[5,6]

In patients who have migraines with aura, it is thought that the cortex, particularly the occipital cortex, is hyperexcitable. The cause of this hyperexcitability is unknown, but may relate to decreased intracellular magnesium levels, to a dysfunction of brain mitochondria, or to abnormal calcium channels. The aura phase of migraine begins as a wave of cortical neural excitation, accompanied by hyperemia, and is followed by an electrical wave of spreading neural depression and oligemia that advances at a rate of 2–6 mm/min (a rate similar to that of the developing aura). During the oligemic phase, blood flow remains above the ischemic threshold. Neither the spreading neural excitation/hyperemia nor the ensuing spreading depression and oligemia respect vascular territories; they are thus thought to represent neural, not vascular, phenomena.[8] The trigeminovascular system might be activated through polysynaptic pathways from the activated cortex, or directly by the same mechanism that causes the aura.[5] Aura usually precedes but sometimes accompanies the headache phase of migraine. Spreading neural depression and oligemia in the cortex might also occur in migraine without aura.

A growing body of evidence points to the importance of dopamine in the pathophysiology of migraine and its associated symptoms.[9] Dopamine receptor hypersensitivity may be responsible for the nausea, vomiting, hypotension, and dizziness that frequently accompany and sometimes characterize attacks of migraine. These symptoms can be elicited by low doses of dopamine or by dopamine agonists—especially in migraneurs. Antiemetics, most of which are dopamine receptor antagonists (especially at the D2 receptor), are frequently useful, and sometimes effective in and of themselves in treating migraine attacks.

DIAGNOSIS

The diagnosis of migraine is made by a suggestive clinical history and a normal neurologic examination (Table 19.1). The classic description of migraine is that of a recurrent headache lasting 2–72 hours, of moderate to severe intensity, pulsating, aggravated by routine physical activity, and associated with nausea, emesis, photophobia, phonophobia, and/or osmophobia (aversion to odors). The major subtypes of migraine are migraine with aura and migraine without aura. The most frequent migrainous aura consists of visual symptoms such as bright spots, dark spots, tunnel vision, or zigzag lines (fortification spectra). Other common auras include numbness or paresthesias in one arm or on the side of the body. The aura is followed (or sometimes accompanied) by an intense, crescendo head pain, frequently unilateral or retro-ocular; it may be described as pounding, throbbing, pressurelike, exploding, stabbing, or viselike.[10] Migrainous auras, particularly visual ones, occasionally occur independently of pain; these are called migraine equivalents. Typically, the headache phase lasts from 30 minutes to 1 day. Occasionally the headache becomes intractable and lasts a week or longer: this is status migrainosus. There seems to be a slightly increased risk for stroke among migraneurs, particularly in women who have migraine with aura. The absolute number of strokes in this population remains low, and epidemiologically, the increase in risk is most easily defined for women older than age 40 or 50.[11–14]

A migraine whose aura seems to originate in the brainstem or involve both hemispheres is called basilar migraine.[15] A typical aura in basilar migraine might present with bilateral visual loss or blindness. Following, or independent of, the visual phenomena, patients may complain of vertigo, dysarthria, diplopia, tinnitus, ataxia, a decreased level of consciousness, or bilateral sensory (paresthesias) or subjective motor symptoms (there should be no objective weakness); sometimes nausea and emesis are prominent. Some patients present with other types of auras such as a dysphasia, and as such may resemble a transient ischemic attack (TIA), a stroke, or an evolving neurologic catastrophe.

TABLE 19.1 International Headache Society Diagnostic Criteria for Migraine

Migraine Without Aura
At least five headache attacks
Headaches last 4–72 h if untreated
Has at least two of the following, but not weakness: Unilateral pain Pulsating Intensity is moderate to severe Aggravated by routine physical activity
Has at least one of the following: Phonophobia Photophobia Nausea Emesis
Migraine With Aura
At least two headache attacks that also fulfill the characteristics of migraine without aura
Headaches usually follow the aura but may begin with it and last 4–72 h if untreated.
Has at least one of several reversible symptoms (lasting 4 min–60 min), but no weakness
Positive or negative visual symptoms such as scintillating scotomas, blind spot (scotoma), blurred vision, zigzag lines, homonymous hemianopsia
Postive or negative sensory symptoms such as tingling or numbness
Basilar Migraine
At least two attacks of migraine with an aura whose symptoms are reversible and localize to the brainstem or are bihemispheric, but without weakness
Symptoms can include: Dysarthria Dizziness or vertigo Bilateral visual symptoms, including temporary blindness Diplopia Nystagmus Ataxia Decreased level of consciousness Bilateral paresthesiae Tinnitus with or without decreased hearing
Aura Without Headache
At least two attacks of symptoms typical of auras, but not weakness, such as visual, sensory, or speech disturbances that resolve within 1 h and are not followed by a headache
Hemiplegic Migraine
At least two attacks of migraine with a reversible aura of motor weakness that can last 1 h to days
Also includes one of the following: Positive or negative visual symptoms Positive or negative sensory symptoms Dysphasia or dysarthria
Frequently accompanied by symptoms typical of basilar migraine
If at least one first- or second-degree relative has a migrainous aura that includes motor weakness, it is *familial hemiplegic migraine* and is associated with a mutation in the neuronal calcium channel.
If no first- or second-degree relative has a migrainous aura that includes motor weakness, it is *sporadic hemiplegic migraine*.

From Headache Classification Committee of the International Headache Society (IHS). The International Classification of Headache Disorders, *3rd edition.* Cephalalgia *2013;33:629-808.*

Some patients develop severe headache, sometimes described as exploding, related to exertion: These are exertional migraines. Exertional migraines can develop while engaged in heavy work or sports, lifting weights, or during sexual climax (the latter are more frequent in males).[16] On the other hand, a severe ocular headache that presents with ophthalmoplegia (usually of the oculomotor nerve, including a dilated pupil) is no longer considered an "ophthalmoplegic migraine." The ophthalmoplegia can last hours to months and is now believed to represent an inflammatory neuritis or the Tolosa–Hunt syndrome.[10] Painful ophthalmoplegia usually has a dramatic presentation and always warrants a careful evaluation.[17]

Given a typical history and reasonable clinical judgment, a migraine can be recognized and treated as such. Occasionally the clinical circumstance requires that the physician be more circumspect and make an effort to exclude other causes for headache that, if left undiagnosed and untreated, will result in an adverse patient outcome. Some other causes for headache include a cerebral aneurysm with or without subarachnoid hemorrhage, vascular malformations with or without hemorrhage, venous thrombosis, central nervous system infections, space-occupying lesions, increased intracranial pressure, vascular dissection, and arteritis.[10,17,18]

TREATMENT

Migraines can be treated abortively (after they start) or prophylactically (with daily medication aimed at reducing the frequency or intensity of the headaches).

Acute Migraine Headaches (Abortive Treatment)

The following are drugs that are useful for the treatment of acute migraine headaches (abortive treatment).

A. Triptans[19] (Imitrex, Maxalt, Zomig, Frova, Relpax, Amerge, and others) are 5-$HT_{1D/1B}$ receptor agonists. These drugs are available in a variety of forms. For example, Imitrex is available in an autoinjector, as a tablet, as a nasal spray, and as of this year, as a nasal powder; Maxalt and Zomig are available as tablets and as orally disintegrating tablets; and Zomig is also available as a nasal spray. In general, injectable preparations have a quicker onset of action, followed by nasal sprays and orally disintegrating tablets and tablets that must be swallowed. These different formulations allow treatment to be tailored to the patient's needs. Patients whose headaches are accompanied by significant nausea and vomiting, or whose productivity depends on a timely return to work, might prefer an injectable preparation or a nasal spray. Orally disintegrating tablets also are useful in patients with significant nausea and vomiting. Approximately 60%–80% of patients achieve significant relief from a triptan; however, the headache will recur in up to one-third of patients. A second dose of the same preparation, taken 2–24 hours after the first, may again provide significant relief. A triptan should not be used again for at least 24 hours after the second dose. Triptans should not be administered within 24 hours of another substance with vasoconstricting properties (e.g., another triptan, ergotamine, DHE, or isometheptane). Triptans should not be administered within 2 weeks of discontinuation of a monoamine oxidase inhibitor. Triptans should not be prescribed to patients with ischemic or other heart disease or uncontrolled hypertension; they should be avoided in patients with complicated auras such as dysphasias and confusional states and in basilar migraine. The major side effects of triptans include a sensation of chest pressure, flushing, tingling, dizziness, and dysphoria. These usually resolve in less than 1 hour. Vasoconstrictor drugs should be avoided during pregnancy, although several large population-based studies have failed to identify an increase in birth defects or in pregnancy-related complications among women who used triptans (mainly sumatriptan or naraptriptan) during pregnancy. Although each of the triptans has unique pharmacokinetic properties, clinically there is little practical difference between them. That said, the different formulations allow treatment to be individualized, and if a patient does not respond well to or suffers unacceptable side effects from one triptan, they may tolerate or respond better to another. For example, in patients whose pain returns within a few hours of taking a triptan, one with a longer half-life (Frova, Amerge) can be tried instead.

B. Ergotamine tartrate is an older drug with 5-HT agonist activity that also is very effective for migraines.[17,20] One to two tablets are taken at the onset of the headache or aura, followed by 1 tablet every 30 minutes until the headache is gone or until a maximum of 5 tablets per headache or 10 tablets per week have been consumed. If consumed in excess, ergotamine-containing preparations can cause vasospastic complications and are emetogenic.

C. Isometheptane (Midrin) is another older but effective drug with 5-HT agonist and sympathomimetic (vasoconstrictive) activity.[17,20] Midrin also contains dichloralphenazone, a mild sedative-hypnotic drug similar to chloral hydrate. One to two capsules are taken at the onset of the headache or aura, followed by 1 capsule every hour until the headache is gone or until a maximum of 5 capsules per headache or 10 capsules per week have been consumed. Isometheptane has fewer vasospastic complications than ergotamine. Ergots and isometheptane should be avoided during pregnancy and are relatively contraindicated in basilar migraine.

D. Preparations containing butalbital (such as Fioricet, which also contains acetaminophen and caffeine, or Fiorinal, which contains aspirin and caffeine) are effective and can be used alone or together with one of the vasoconstricting abortive drugs (a triptan, ergotamine, or isometheptane). One to two tablets can be taken every 4 hours as needed. Barbiturate-containing preparations cause drowsiness and can be habit forming if used excessively.[17,20]

E. Narcotic-containing preparations, such as those with codeine, hydromorphone, or hydrocodone (in combination with aspirin or acetaminophen), are used too frequently, particularly in the emergency room, and should be used only as drugs of last resort. Narcotics bind opiate receptors and mask pain, but they do not bind serotonin receptors and therefore do not interrupt the putative pathophysiologic mechanism of migraine. The short- and long-term complications associated with the frequent use of narcotics argues that they should be used sparingly at best.[17,20]

F. Antinauseants, such as prochlorperazine, chlorpromazine, or metoclopramide, by virtue of their effect on serotonin receptors, are effective against migraine pain. Their action as antagonists of the D2 dopamine receptor helps control the associated gastrointestinal symptoms, and this makes them excellent adjuvant drugs.[17,20,21]

G. DHE, is generally administered parenterally, but also is available as a 4 mg/mL nasal spray. Administered by the intravenous or intramuscular route, the dose should not exceed 2–3 mg in 24 hours. Administered over 1 day or several days, intravenous DHE remains the drug of choice for treatment of status migrainosus. As a vasoconstrictor, this drug should be avoided during pregnancy and is relatively contraindicated in basilar migraine.[17,20]

H. Nonsteroidal antiinflammatory drugs (NSAIDs) work for some patients with mild to moderate migraine pain. Ketorolac, which can be administered intramuscularly, and indomethacin, which also is available as a suppository, may be particularly useful. Some patients with mild headache or headaches that do not last long respond well to over-the-counter analgesic preparations.[17,20] Aspirin, particularly combined with acetaminophen and caffeine (Excedrin), remains an effective and inexpensive over-the-counter treatment.[22] Cambia (diclofenac combined with potassium bicarbonate) is US Food and Drug Administration (FDA) approved for the treatment of migraine; it likely owes its effectiveness to its rapid gastrointestinal absorption. Cambia is as effective as a triptan in onset of action and control of symptoms, and is worth considering in patients in whom vasoconstricting drugs are contraindicated or who experience intolerable side effects.

I. Corticosteroids are sometimes useful when used for a limited time and under strict medical supervision; in fact, short courses of steroid have been shown to decrease the recurrence and frequency of migraine. They can be used alone or with other abortive medication for the relief of an intractable migraine (status migrainosus). Both short- and long-term use of steroids entails significant potential for morbidity.[17,20]

Chronic Use of Drugs

The chronic use (averaging at least 10 times per month over a prolonged period of time) of any of the triptans, NSAIDs, acetaminophen, butalbital, narcotics, ergotamine, DHE, and isometheptane can lead to development of a medication overuse, or rebound, headache syndrome.[18,23–26] Chronic use of these compounds more than twice per week should be discouraged. Prophylactic regimens generally are not effective in the setting of rebound. The treatment of medication overuse headache is discontinuation of all analgesics (including triptans, ergots, etc.). In patients who take frequent narcotics or barbiturates, these should be discontinued slowly. Painkiller withdrawal frequently results in a temporary but dramatic exacerbation of the pain, which can last several days. The physiologic washout period, during which patients may continue to experience frequent headaches, lasts at least 2 weeks; patients should continue to refrain from analgesic medications for a total of 10–12 weeks, although the physician should use judgment with respect to treatment of an occasional breakthrough migraine during that period. If patients require analgesics at least twice per week, they should be offered a prophylactic regimen.

Prophylactic Treatment

The following are drugs that are useful for prophylactic treatment.

A. Beta-blockers, such as propranolol, metoprolol, atenolol, timolol, and nadolol, are frequently effective first-line prophylactic drugs; propranolol and timolol are FDA approved for migraine prophylaxis.[2,27] In most healthy people, 60–80 mg once per day of a long-acting propranolol preparation can be started, and the dosage can be adjusted as necessary. Side effects include dizziness from bradycardia or hypotension, fatigue, depression, worsening of symptoms in patients with asthma, or chronic obstructive pulmonary disease, gastrointestinal distress, blunting of hypoglycemic symptoms in patients with diabetes, and vivid dreams.

B. Anticonvulsants such as valproic acid (Depakote and Depakote ER) and carbamazepine have been used as prophylaxis against migraine for a long time.[2,28] Depakote and Topamax are FDA approved for migraine prophylaxis; carbamazepine is classified as only "possibly effective" based on the evidence available. The usual starting dose for Depakote ER is 500 mg per day; the dose should be adjusted as necessary at 2–4-week intervals. Valproic acid can cause weight gain, hair loss, tremor, abdominal distress, and easy bruisability. Frequent side effects of Topamax are mental confusion and paresthesiae; another is weight loss, which has made this drug increasingly popular. In addition, Topamax is an inhibitor of carbonic anhydrase, and it has been reported to be useful in treating the syndrome of idiopathic increased intracranial pressure (previously called pseudotumor cerebri).

C. Antidepressants, particularly amitriptyline (at a starting dose of 10–25 mg at bedtime) and venlafaxine (at a starting dose of 37.5 mg in the morning), are active prophylactic drugs.[2,17,20] Most patients who respond to amitriptyline usually do so at doses of 25–200 mg at bedtime; the effectiveness of other tricyclic antidepressants such as nortriptyline, imipramine, or desipramine has not been established. Tricyclics help induce sleep, which may constitute one of the mechanisms by which they help migraneurs. The major side effects from tricyclics relate to their anticholinergic action and include a dry mouth, excessive daytime sleepiness, dizziness, urinary retention, glaucoma, cardiac arrhythmias, and photosensitization. There is inadequate evidence to recommend the specific serotonin reuptake inhibitors (SSRIs) and other serotonin norepinephrine reuptake inhibitors (SNRIs). Antidepressants are relatively contraindicated in patients who use triptans, as they may suffer from excessive serotonin stimulation (serotonin syndrome), although the incidence of this complication is virtually negligible unless the patient is on very high doses of the antidepressant. The association between migraine and depression (depressed patients have more migraines and migraines are a risk factor for depression) make antidepressants a good choice for prophylaxis.

D. Candesartan (an angiotensin receptor blocker) or lisinopril (an angiotensin converting enzyme [ACE] inhibitor) are occasionally useful as prophylactic agents.[2,17,20] There is inadequate evidence to support the use of calcium channel blockers such as verapamil for migraine (although they are of proven use in cluster). Evidence does not support the use of gabapentin, lamotrigine, or oxcarbazepine as migraine preventives.

E. Individualized injections of botulinum toxin A injection (Botox) into the pericranial muscles (31 injections into 7 specific sites) increases the number of headache-free days in some patients with chronic migraine.[29] The drug is approved for treatment in patients who have 15 or more headache days per month, each lasting 4 hours or more. Improvement may be delayed for up to 2 weeks following treatment, and the beneficial effect may last up to 90 days postinjection.

Complementary and Alternative Modalities

Many patients with chronic headaches use some form of complementary and alternative modalities (CAM). There are several reasons they might, including among others, patient dissatisfaction with the efficacy or side effects of more conventional drugs, cost, and availability without a prescription. It should be noted that, as supplements, these compounds have not been through rigorous clinical trials, and their manufacture, quality control, and labeling is not supervised by the FDA. In that regard, some equally uncontrolled studies have found that many preparations may, or may not, contain what is stated on the label. One particular supplement to be aware of is butterbur (Petasites). Butterbur has been through two small Class A trials that demonstrated effectiveness in migraine prevention[30,31]; however, the studies were conducted with a specifically purified preparation that was certified to be free of pirrolizidine alkaloids (PA), highly toxic compounds that are hepatotoxic and may cause cancer. Following the trials, the purification method was changed and the subsequent preparations have not been subject to rigorous analysis for PA. After multiple reports of mild to severe liver toxicity, several European countries have had butterbur removed from their markets. Supplements that might be tried in the right setting include magnesium citrate or oxide, 400 mg/day; riboflavin (vitamin B2), 400 mg/day; co-Q10 150 mg/day to 300 mg/day; and the transcutaneous nerve stimulator (TENS) device.

SELF-HELP STRATEGIES

The following are self-help strategies that can minimize the incidence of migraines.[2]

A. If the patient consumes caffeinated beverages (coffee, tea, soda, cocoa), total caffeine should be limited to less than 400 mg/day (to avoid caffeinism), and the decrease in intake should include weekends, vacations, and holidays (to avoid a caffeine withdrawal headache).

B. If they trigger headaches, foods high in tyramine (a metabolite of tyrosine often a product of fermentation or decay), which are thought to play a role as a migraine trigger, can be avoided. Some foods high in tyramine are chocolate, aged cheeses, yogurt, sour cream, soy sauce, chicken liver, banana, avocado, nuts, and yeast extracts (including beer).

C. Foods high in nitrates can be avoided, as these might precipitate a migraine by virtue of their vasodilating properties. Some foods high in nitrates include processed meats (hot dogs, salami, bacon, sausage, corned beef) and other canned, smoked, or aged meats.

D. Some patients are sensitive to certain food additives. Two examples include monosodium glutamate, frequently used in restaurants and added to cooked, packaged, and canned foods as a flavor enhancer, and aspartame (Nutrasweet). These substances contain glutamate, an excitatory neurotransmitter.

E. Many migraneurs are sensitive to alcoholic beverages, particularly those that are aged, such as beer, wines, and some spirits.[17,20] Alcohol also tends to dilate blood vessels.

F. Miscellaneous, but not unusual, causes of migraine include new medications,[16] stressful situations, post-stress situations, lack of adequate rest or changes in sleep habit, allergies, and noncompliance with a prophylactic regimen. Patients should not allow themselves to become dehydrated, either during a headache or between headaches. If bright light is an irritant during or between headaches, patients should wear optical-quality sunglasses that block at least 85% of incident sunlight (and 100% of ultraviolet light) when outdoors.

G. The trigeminal autonomic cephalalgias (TAC): Cluster headache, paroxysmal hemicrania and short-lasting unilateral neuralgiform headache with conjunctival injection and tearing (SUNCT).

TRIGEMINAL AUTONOMIC CEPHALALGIAS (TAC)

The TAC represent a group of three headache disorders characterized by the occurrence of pain in the distribution of the first division of the trigeminal nerve accompanied by prominent autonomic features in the same distribution. These headaches are cluster, hemicrania (paroxysmal hemicrania and hemicrania continua), and SUNCT. The headaches are distinguished by their predominance in either males or females, their frequency, and their duration (Table 19.2). In addition, all present with some combination of ocular redness, tearing, swelling, miosis, or ptosis; additional symptoms can include forehead sweating and rhinorrhea.[10]

Cluster headache lasts longest and presents with circadian periodicity, but overall, clusters tend to occur relatively infrequently—such as yearly. SUNCT have the shortest duration but a high frequency of attacks. The duration and frequency of paroxysmal hemicrania is intermediate. Hemicrania continua is characterized by continuous pain with exacerbations.[32,33]

TABLE 19.2 Trigeminal Autonomic Cephalalgias

Type	Male:Female	Frequency	Duration
Cluster	5.5:1	1 or several/day	15–90 min
Hemicrania	1:3	Up to 30/day	5–45 min
SUNCT	8:1	Up to 180/day	5–60 s

From Headache Classification Committee of the International Headache Society (IHS). The international classification of headache disorders, 3rd edition. Cephalalgia *2013;33:629-808.*

CLUSTER HEADACHE

Cluster headaches, unlike migraine, affect predominantly males; the prevalence is 0.1%–0.3% of the population. A family history of cluster is not frequent. In the majority of cases, attacks begin between the ages of 20 and 40.

Pathophysiology

The pathophysiologic mechanism of cluster headaches is not known. Some investigators believe that cluster headache lies within a continuum of head pains that include cluster and severe migraine at one extreme and tension-type headache at the other. Thus, at least to some degree, the underlying mechanism of most chronic, recurring headache syndromes would be shared. Some of the clinical features of cluster, which seem to reflect local vasoactive phenomena, support the argument that neurogenic inflammation also plays a role in this headache type.[5,33]

Diagnosis

Cluster headache is diagnosed by a suggestive clinical history and a normal neurologic examination. Typically, severe pain, which lasts between 15 and 90 minutes, awakens the patient. The pain is unilateral and periorbital; it may include the temple, forehead, and cheek (the distribution of the first division of the trigeminal nerve). The syndrome is accompanied by lacrimation, conjunctival injection, nasal stuffiness, ptosis (with or without eyelid edema), and miosis ipsilateral to the pain. During a cluster phase, the headaches, which can be single or multiple in a 24-hour period, occur with circadian predictability and tend to have a similar duration. Unlike patients with migraine, who seek a dark, quiet environment, patients with cluster tend to pace, scream, or appear agitated; nausea and vomiting are uncommon. A bout of cluster may last several days or several months.[10] An attack can be provoked by alcohol.

Treatment

In general, the drugs that are used to treat migraine are useful in cluster, except that the role for treatment aimed at aborting an acute headache is limited because the attack has usually run its course by the time the agent has exerted its effect.[32] Therefore cluster is best treated early on with prophylactic drugs, with the aim of interrupting the cluster. The major limitation of drugs aimed at interrupting the cluster (drugs used in migraine prophylaxis) is their slow onset of action, with most requiring 2–4 weeks to demonstrate activity at the initial dose, and similar intervals for subsequent dose adjustments.

Interrupting the Cluster

The following drugs are useful for interrupting the cluster.

A. Calcium channel blockers, such as verapamil, are frequently prescribed.[34] Verapamil usually requires administration at relatively high doses, 120–480 mg/day, to be effective.
B. Anticonvulsants such as valproic acid (Depakote and Depakote ER) and carbamazepine can be useful to help abort a cluster. The usual starting dose for Depakote ER is 500 mg per day; the dose should be adjusted as necessary at 2–6-week intervals. Valproic acid can cause weight gain, hair loss, tremor, and abdominal distress.
C. Lithium carbonate can be useful in patients with cluster; in fact, cluster remains the major indication for lithium in the treatment of headaches.
D. Antidepressants, particularly amitriptyline at a starting dose of 10–25 mg at bedtime, are sometimes added to an anticluster regimen, but there is no good evidence for their activity. Tricyclics help induce sleep, which may constitute one of the mechanisms by which they help patients with cluster. The major side effects from tricyclics relate to their anticholinergic effects and include a dry mouth, excessive daytime sleepiness, dizziness, urinary retention, glaucoma, cardiac arrhythmias, and photosensitization.
E. Beta-blockers, such as propranolol, metoprolol, atenolol, timolol, and nadolol, are also used frequently for cluster. In most healthy people, 60–80 mg once per day of a long-acting propranolol preparation can be started, and the dosage can be adjusted as necessary. Side effects include dizziness from bradycardia or hypotension, fatigue, depression, worsening of symptoms in patients with asthma or chronic obstructive pulmonary disease, gastrointestinal distress, blunting of hypoglycemic symptoms in patients with diabetes, and vivid dreams.
F. Corticosteroids are useful as adjuvants to other drugs in breaking a cluster. They should be started simultaneously with one of the other prophylactic drugs. Corticosteroids are to be used for a limited time, and under strict medical supervision. Both short- and long-term use of steroids entails significant potential for morbidity.
G. Given the regularity and sometimes circadian predictability of the headache onset during a cluster, ergotamine, isometheptane, a triptan, or an NSAID can be administered up to several hours prior to an anticipated attack (e.g., at bedtime). When used for a limited time, this strategy can be useful to prevent a headache until the prophylactic drugs become effective.
H. Among the NSAIDs, indomethacin appears to be more active than others. It also can be used in anticipation of a headache to block its onset. Indomethacin can be administered in doses up to 150 mg/day but tends to irritate the gastric mucosa. Other NSAIDs might work for some patients with milder headaches. In general, the onset of action of oral formulations tends to occur at about the time the current headache has run its course.

I. In chronic cluster, an ipsilateral occipital nerve block or a sphenopalatine ganglion block can be useful adjuvants to help break the cycle.

Treatment of an Acute Cluster Headache

The following are approaches to the treatment of an acute headache:

- As stated previously, the onset of action of most analgesics tends to occur at about the time the current headache has run its course. However, inhaled oxygen remains the standard for treatment of an acute cluster headache.[35] Oxygen should be administered at 12 L/minute through a nonrebreather mask for 15 minutes, as soon after the onset of the attack as feasible. The treatment can be repeated after a brief interval. Patients should be prescribed oxygen for home use.
- It is not clear if parenteral or nasal formulations of a triptan might be useful in this setting, especially for headaches of longer duration.

PAROXYSMAL HEMICRANIA

Paroxysmal hemicrania occurs more frequently in women. The syndrome consists of frequent, unremitting, unilateral headaches exhibiting a frequency of a few to more than 20 per day; the headaches last 5–45 minutes each. The pain, throbbing or boring, is localized on one side of the head, around the eye and temple (in the distribution of the first division of the trigeminal nerve). As in cluster, the pain is accompanied by autonomic phenomena: redness and tearing of the eye, eyelid swelling, nasal congestion, and/or rhinorrhea.[10,36] Ptosis is sometimes seen. Patients usually sit quietly. The hallmark of hemicrania is its dramatic response to indomethacin, which can be administered in doses up to 150 mg/day and, as long as it is tolerated, can be used for long periods of time. Concurrent use of indomethacin with a proton pump inhibitor might decrease gastric irritation.

SHORT-LASTING UNILATERAL NEURALGIFORM HEADACHE WITH CONJUNCTIVAL INJECTION AND TEARING

SUNCT is a rare headache that occurs almost exclusively in males. The pain, with bursts of stabbing, throbbing, or burning around the eye or temple, lasts 5 seconds to 5 minutes and occurs in paroxysms of up to 30 per hour (with an average of 5–6 per hour). Here, too, the pain is accompanied by autonomic phenomena in the distribution of the first division of the trigeminal nerve: redness and tearing of the eye, eyelid swelling, nasal congestion, and/or rhinorrhea.[10] The headaches tend to not respond well to most treatments, but might be amenable to prophylactic treatment with anticonvulsants including lamotrigine and oxcarbazepine. The presence of autonomic phenomena, as well as its location in the first division of the trigeminal nerve, differentiates it from a trigeminal neuralgia.

KEY POINTS

- The incidence of migraines in females increases into the early 40s.
- Consuming more than about 400 mg of caffeine per day can predispose one to chronic migraines.
- Basilar migraine can present with mental status changes.
- Vasoconstrictor drugs, such as triptans, are contraindicated in basilar migraine.
- Analgesic overuse (use of analgesics 10 days per month or more) can lead to chronic daily migraine.
- The TAC are cluster, hemicrania, and SUNCT.
- Cluster is best treated acutely with oxygen, prophylactically with valproic acid or verapamil.
- Hemicranias—paroxysmal or continua—are singularly responsive to treatment with indomethacin.

REFERENCES

Access the reference list online at ExpertConsult.com.

CHAPTER

20

Tension-Type Headache, Chronic Tension-Type Headache, and Other Chronic Headache Types

Jack M. Rozental, MD, PhD, MBA

EPIDEMIOLOGY

Tension-type headache (TTH) is the most common headache type and also the most difficult to classify.[1] Many different, and equally vague, terms have been applied to this headache or to what probably are variants of the same syndrome. Headaches in general are thought to affect more than 90% of the population at one time or another, with about 15% of those fitting the description of migrainous or vascular headache. This leaves about 70% of the population with some variant of TTH.[2] Moreover, almost all patients with migraine, cluster headache, trigeminal nerve neuralgias, and other recurring cephalgic syndromes have interposed TTH.[3–5]

DIAGNOSIS

TENSION-TYPE HEADACHE AND CHRONIC DAILY HEADACHE

The pain of a TTH tends to be duller, less intense, and less localized than that of a migraine or a cluster attack. The pain usually lasts several hours to a day, but it may continue for days or weeks. During a severe TTH, patients can experience photophobia, phonophobia, nausea, and occasionally emesis. Pain referred to the neck is common; patients also frequently complain of "a knot in the neck," but the neurologic examination is normal.[6]

The major variants of TTH are those with disorder of the pericranial muscles, those without disorder of the pericranial muscles, and chronic TTH (CTTH) (with or without disorder of the pericranial muscles). Those with disorder of the pericranial muscles are characterized by tenderness on palpation of those muscles, increased activity on electromyography (EMG), or both. TTH without disorder of the pericranial muscles lacks those characteristics. CTTH, previously called chronic daily headache, is diagnosed in a patient with a headache frequency of 15 days per month or 180 headaches per year averaged over a 6-month period.[6] Fibromyalgia and the myofascial pain syndrome also are associated with frequent or chronic daily headaches.

ANALGESIC MEDICATION OVERUSE HEADACHE

A common variety of chronic daily headache occurs in patients with headaches of any sort, particularly, tension-type or episodic migraines, in whom these temporarily exacerbate and become more frequent. Patients begin using analgesic preparations (e.g., nonsteroidal antiinflammatory drugs [NSAIDs], acetaminophen, aspirin, butalbital, narcotics, ergot derivatives, triptans) on a regular basis (generally 10 times or more per month) and eventually develop analgesic overuse, or rebound, headaches.[7–10] Thus, patients should be advised against using analgesics more than twice per week over a prolonged period. If they require analgesics at least twice per week, they should be offered a prophylactic regimen.

In adolescents (age 12–14 years at the time of diagnosis), the cause and prognosis of chronic daily headache (CDH) might be distinct from that in adults. Many of these children seem to have personal or family history of migraine. When followed for up to 8 years, 40% continue to experience CDH after 1 year, 25% after 2 years, and 12% after 8 years. Without specific medical intervention, the majority of adolescents with CDH seem to evolve into adults who suffer from episodic migraine and episodic TTH.

The mainstay of treatment for medication overuse headache (MOH) is total withdrawal from analgesics for a period not shorter than 2 months. The patients most likely to be headache-free at the end of that time are migraneurs (67% reduction) and those with mixed TTH and migraines (37% reduction); patients diagnosed with TTH alone are less likely to report large reductions in headache frequency but do report large reductions in pain intensity. The initial several days to 2 weeks following analgesic withdrawal might be the most difficult and are frequently punctuated with a severe rebound headache; antiemetics and maintaining hydration, as well as patience, are effective. Using steroids during this period has no effect on outcome. One additional characteristic of patients with MOH is that drugs administered with prophylactic intent tend to not work (or to not work as well) unless analgesics are discontinued. Patients whose MOH is typified by the regular use of narcotics or barbiturates may require a controlled tapering off the drugs and management of potential withdrawal symptoms.

A particularly severe, persistent, or unusual headache should always prompt consideration of alternative explanations, and, when appropriate, these should be investigated thoroughly.[1,3,6,11] For example, temporal arteritis should be considered in an elderly patient with a persistent headache of recent onset whether other typical elements are present in the history and physical examination. In these patients, an erythrocyte sedimentation rate or a sensitive c-reactive protein (s-CRP) should be ordered immediately, and consideration should be given to treatment with a corticosteroid and to a temporal artery biopsy. Likewise, one would not want to miss an infectious meningitis, the sentinel bleed of an aneurysm, an undiagnosed intracranial vascular malformation, a subdural hematoma, acute hydrocephalus, venous thrombosis, or an arterial dissection. Idiopathic intracranial hypertension (previously called pseudotumor cerebri) usually presents in overweight young women with chronic headaches, a normal examination, a normal scan and papilledema, although a subset of these patients do not have papilledema.[6,12] The diagnosis is made when a lumbar puncture reveals an otherwise normal fluid under high pressure (at least 20–25 cm H_2O). Therefore, when dictated by clinical judgment, imaging, lumbar puncture, or other tests deemed necessary are indicated.

PATHOPHYSIOLOGY OF TENSION-TYPE HEADACHE

The pathophysiologic bases for TTH and CTTH are unknown. Some investigators believe that TTH lies at one end of a physiologic spectrum that includes severe migraine and cluster at one end and TTH at the other. Under this assumption, at least to some degree, the underlying mechanism of most chronic, recurring headache syndromes would be shared.[13–15] The muscle contraction theory of TTH relates pain to prolonged contraction, or spasm, of cervical or pericranial muscles but no objective data support the theory. Most patients with a headache, migrainous or TTH, have pericranial muscle tenderness or sore spots; however, many individuals without headache also have them. During a headache, patients with a more severe headache tend to have more tender pericranial muscles; but the relationship between tenderness of the pericranial muscles and headaches is not straightforward. Increased tenderness during headaches may represent cutaneous allodynia.

The relationship between cervicogenic disorders and headache is similarly unclear, although most painful disorders of the neck are associated with some sort of headache. Cervical pain can be referred to the head from intervertebral discs, interspinous ligaments, zygapophyseal joints, the periosteum, paracervical muscles, carotid and vertebral arteries, and from irritation of the C1, C2, and C3 nerve roots. The dorsal rami of the first three cervical nerve roots supply the sensory innervation to the neck and to the scalp caudal to the innervation of the trigeminal nerve, and to the meninges and arteries of the posterior fossa. Headache also can arise from pathology in the area of the foramen magnum. Some examples include a Chiari I malformation, the Dandy-Walker syndrome, atlantoaxial dislocation (e.g., from rheumatoid arthritis), Paget disease of the bone, and basilar invagination.

TREATMENT

As with other headache types, both abortive and prophylactic treatment strategies are available for the treatment of TTH and CTTH.

Abortive Treatment Strategies

For the occasional TTH, an over-the-counter (OTC) analgesic preparation is all that is required. The number of OTC preparations continues to increase, and although they are generally safe, the lay population has little basis on which to decide how to choose among them or how to use them properly. Most people decide on a preparation either on a trial-and-error basis or are swayed by the marketing (e.g., "for tension headache," "for sinus pain," "multi-symptom relief," and "PM" preparations). Several OTC analgesic preparations involve combinations of drugs (e.g., aspirin plus acetaminophen) and may contain caffeine. Caffeine combined with analgesics such as aspirin, acetaminophen, and ibuprofen enhances their analgesic effectiveness. Stronger headaches may require an analgesic (aspirin, acetaminophen, or ibuprofen) in combination with either codeine or butalbital with or without caffeine. Used infrequently, the additional analgesic effectiveness obtained by adding codeine or butalbital comes with little increase in adverse effects or risk of dependence.

If aspirin or acetaminophen, with or without codeine, butalbital, or caffeine are ineffective in controlling the headache, the choice of an alternative analgesic should proceed in an orderly fashion by testing in turn members of different NSAID chemical categories at adequate doses. Indomethacin is reported to be more effective than alternative NSAIDs for pain of cephalic origin; it is particularly effective in treating hemicrania—see Chapter 19. Occasionally, a patient responds well to stress management modalities or acupuncture (anyone considering acupuncture should ascertain the qualifications of the practitioner and insist on new, not sterilized, needles for every session), but it is impossible to predict accurately in whom these modalities are likely to be beneficial. The major chemical categories of NSAIDs include the following:

Carboxylic acids—this group includes aspirin, which is an acetylated acid, and salsalate and choline magnesium trisalicylate, which are nonacetylated.

Propionic acids—ibuprofen, naproxen, ketoprofen, and fenoprofen.

Aryl and heterocyclic acids—indomethacin, diclofenac, sulindac, and tolmetin.

Fenamic acids—mefenamic acid and meclofenamate.

Enolic acids—piroxicam and phenylbutazone.

Pyrrolo-pyrrole—ketorolac.

Cyclooxygenase 2 (COX-2) inhibitors—celecoxib.

Prophylactic Treatment Strategies

Fortunately, CTTH and TTH that are frequent or otherwise annoying respond to many of the agents used in migraine prophylaxis. It is possible that this reflects on the presumed common mechanism that is felt to underlie both disorders.

A. Antidepressants, particularly amitriptyline or nortriptylene at a starting dose of 10–25 mg at bedtime, are active prophylactic drugs.[16] Most patients who respond to tricyclic antidepressants (amitriptyline, nortriptyline, imipramine, or desipramine) usually do so at doses of 25–200 mg at bedtime; an occasional patient may require more. Tricyclics help induce sleep, which may constitute one of the mechanisms by which they help. The major side effects from tricyclics relate to their anticholinergic effects and include a dry mouth, excessive daytime sleepiness, dizziness, urinary retention, glaucoma, cardiac arrhythmias, and photosensitization;

they can also cause weight gain. The specific serotonin reuptake inhibitors (SSRIs) and specific serotonin-norepinephrine reuptake inhibitors (SNRIs) might be tried in patients who do not respond or who develop intolerable side effects from tricyclic drugs. The major side effects of the SSRIs and SNRIs include jitteriness, tremors, gastrointestinal distress, decreased libido, and occasionally headaches. In addition, these drugs are relatively contraindicated in patients who use triptans, as they may suffer from excessive serotonin stimulation (serotonin syndrome).

B. Beta-blockers, such as propranolol, metoprolol, atenolol, timolol, and nadolol, can be tried and sometimes prove effective.[17] In most healthy people, 60–80 mg once per day of a long-acting propranolol preparation can be started and the dosage can be adjusted as necessary. Side effects include dizziness from bradycardia or hypotension, fatigue, depression, worsening of symptoms in patients with asthma or chronic obstructive pulmonary disease, gastrointestinal distress, blunting of hypoglycemic symptoms in patients with diabetes, and vivid dreams.

C. Anticonvulsants such as valproic acid (Depakote and Depakote extended release preparation [ER]) are sometimes worth a try to prophylax against frequent TTH.[18] The usual starting dose for Depakote ER is 500 mg per day; the dose should be adjusted as necessary at 2–6-week intervals. The author usually adjusts the dose in 500-mg increments and recommends the ER to maintain once per day dosing. Valproic acid can cause weight gain, hair loss, tremor, and abdominal distress.

D. Although still controversial, a botulinum toxin A (Botox) injection into the most tender pericranial muscle(s) or directly into a trigger point has been reported to increase significantly the number of headache-free days in patients with CTTH. This should not be confused with its indication for chronic migraine (see Chapter 19), and patients can expect that insurance rarely, if ever, covers the cost.

The drugs used in TTH and CTTH are in Box 20.1.

BOX 20.1 Drugs Used in Tension-Type Headache and Chronic Tension-Type Headache

RESCUE TREATMENTS

- Over-the-counter analgesics
- Simple analgesics: aspirin, ibuprofen, naproxen, acetaminophen
- Combination analgesics: aspirin with acetaminophen and caffeine

PRESCRIPTION ANALGESICS

- NSAIDs, most commonly: indomethacin, diclofenac, ketorolac
- Preparations containing butalbital (with or without caffeine)
- Preparations containing codeine (with or without caffeine)

PROPHYLACTIC TREATMENTS

- Antidepressants: amitriptyline, nortriptyline, imipramine, desipramine, venlafaxine
- Beta-blockers: propranolol, metoprolol, atenolol, timolol, nadolol
- Anticonvulsants: valproic acid, topiramate
- Botulinum toxin injection

NSAIDs, Nonsteroidal antiinflammatory drugs.

OTHER CHRONIC HEADACHE TYPES

"SINUS" HEADACHE

Patients frequently complain of "sinus headaches."[3–5,19,20] They present after a variety of diagnostic tests have failed to corroborate the diagnosis of chronic sinusitis and after one or more courses of antibiotics, antihistamines, decongestants, nasal steroids, and analgesics have failed to provide significant relief. Those patients almost invariably also self-medicate with a variety of OTC preparations (the hallmark of which is the display of "sinus" and "relief" prominently on the label) that may combine an antihistamine, a decongestant, and an analgesic (with or without caffeine). These are not true sinus headaches, and many of these patients have either some degree of MOH at the time of presentation or an undiagnosed mild to moderate migraine. The diagnostic confusion arises because patients complain of periorbital pain and might also experience some nasal stuffiness; patients thus attribute the origin of the pain to the adjacent sinuses. True sinus pain occurs when the ability of the sinus to drain is impaired by an acute blockage of the osteum (e.g., from an upper respiratory infection or for some anatomic reason), a bacterial infection takes hold, the mucosa becomes inflamed and pressure builds in the sinus; this is accompanied by purulent discharge, fever, and localized tenderness. One caveat is that true sinus or nasal inflammation can be a trigger for migraine. The rest of these "sinus headaches" are likely a multifactorial TTH or CTTH but may represent a mild migraine in which the local parasympathetic activation mediated through the trigeminal nerve causes pain or sinus pressure and nasal discharge.[3–5,19,20] The care of these patients needs to be coordinated so that the various potential components of the headache are adequately addressed and treated.

SLEEP DISORDERS

Habitual snoring is increasingly being recognized as a cause of chronic daily headache.[21] Sleep-disordered breathing from, for example, sleep apnea may precipitate headaches from the resultant hypoxemia and hypercapnia (which causes cerebral vasodilation). Snoring, with or without sleep apnea, can disrupt sleep architecture or interrupt sleep, either of which can result in headaches. If a history suggestive of snoring, repeated nocturnal arousals, or paroxysmal leg movements during sleep is obtained, a diagnostic polysomnogram will provide invaluable information. A history suggestive of paroxysmal leg movements should also prompt a ferritin level, which should be at least 40 ng/mL or the patient should be prescribed an iron supplement. Treatment of the sleep disorder might not provide complete headache relief but it usually provides some. Hypnic headaches represent another syndrome of recurring head pain that awakens patients from REM sleep.[22] The headache most commonly has its onset after the age of 50, is about twice as frequent in women as in men, has its onset about 2–4 hours after falling asleep, and lasts about 30–60 minutes. This headache responds best to treatment with either indomethacin or lithium, or caffeine before bed.

POSTTRAUMATIC

Posttraumatic headache occurs frequently following mild to moderate closed head injury or a whiplash injury (rapid flexion and extension trauma of the neck); loss of consciousness need not have occurred. In addition to headache, the syndrome may include pain in the neck or shoulders, dizziness, cognitive complaints and disturbances of sleep, mood, and/or personality. The syndrome should begin within 2 weeks of the injury; it is considered acute if it lasts 8 weeks or less and chronic if it lasts longer, although this distinction is arbitrary. These sequelae may reflect underlying brain injury relating to the trauma and injury to the head, face, jaw, and neck. This headache is treated in accord with the general principles mentioned above but with additional consideration being given to addition of physical therapy and to identification and treatment of a possible contributing occipital or supraorbital nerve neuralgia. An occipital neuralgia (also called "cervicogenic" headache) can arise from injury around the area of the C2–3 zygapophyseal joint, which is common in whiplash; the pain, paresthesiae or dysesthesiae usually are referred to the occipital scalp. On examination, the nerve is tender to palpation or percussion along the course of the dorsal ramus of C2, particularly around the cranial insertion of the trapezius muscle, lateral to the occipital protuberance. Treatment of occipital neuralgia is a nerve block with or without adding a drug useful in the treatment of neuropathic pain such as gabapentin.

Trauma can also result in a chronic cerebrospinal fluid (CSF) leak with consequent CSF hypotension and a chronic low-pressure headache (see Chapter 21). This headache, usually associated with an opening CSF pressure of 90 mm of water or less, typically manifests when the patient assumes a sitting or standing position and improves when the patient lies down. Most posttraumatic leaks arise around the cervico-thoracic junction. Treatment is similar to that of a post lumbar puncture headache.

KEY POINTS

- Chronic daily headaches are frequently caused by analgesic overuse—using analgesic medication 10 or more times per month.
- Prophylactic medication usually does not work in the setting of analgesic overuse headache.
- "Sinus headaches" are rarely that they usually represent analgesic overuse or parasympathetic symptoms of a milder migraine.
- Sleep-disordered breathing can cause headaches, particularly those patients that wake with a headache.
- Posttraumatic headaches can include occipital neuralgia and CSF hypotension from a chronic CSF leak.

REFERENCES

Access the reference list online at ExpertConsult.com.

CHAPTER 21

Postmeningeal Puncture Headache and Spontaneous Intracranial Hypotension

Samer Abdel-Aziz, MD ◎ Honorio T. Benzon, MD ◎ Robert W. Hurley, MD, PhD

POSTMENINGEAL PUNCTURE HEADACHE

Postdural puncture headache (PDPH) was first described in 1898 by August Bier, after a spinal anesthetic, as a severe headache worsened by standing or sitting and alleviated in the recumbent position. Bier hypothesized that the headache was caused by the loss of cerebrospinal fluid (CSF) during the spinal anesthetic placement.[1] Given that the CSF is encased by both the meningeal layer of the arachnoid mater and the dura mater, a more correct term for PDPH, as described by Harrington and Schmitt, is meningeal puncture headache (MPH); however, the most commonly used term remains PDPH.[2] An orthostatic bilateral headache following meningeal puncture is the pathognomonic symptom of MPH. The absence of an orthostatic component should lead to a search for other causes, leaving MPH as a diagnosis of exclusion. The headache is characteristically occipital and/or frontal and is always bilateral. Symptoms associated with MPH can include neck stiffness, nausea, vomiting, photophobia, diplopia, scalp paresthesia, upper and lower limb pain, auditory changes including tinnitus, hypoacusia, and mental status changes.[3,4] Noninfectious arachnoiditis has been described with associated urinary and fecal incontinence, blindness, subdural hematomas, intracerebral hemorrhage, and seizures.[5,6] Headache commonly presents within the first 24–48 hours following a meningeal puncture; however, there have been many reports of headache presenting as late as 7 days after the meningeal puncture. Additionally, Reamy reports an MPH presenting at 12 days after the meningeal puncture in a parturient.[7] Most headaches resolve within 7 days, but in rare cases, they can persist for several months.[8] Few cases of atypical postmeningeal puncture symptoms have been reported. Liu et al. reported two cases of MPH that were worse in the recumbent position and improved when standing.[9] McGrady and Freshwater reported a case of posterior neck pain without headache after spinal anesthesia.[10]

PATHOPHYSIOLOGY

The pathophysiology of the MPH is not completely understood, but there are several proposed hypotheses. One is based on the Monro–Kellie rule and another is based on mechanical traction. Both hypotheses accept that CSF escapes through a known or probable meningeal puncture at a rate that exceeds CSF production. The Monro–Kellie rule states that in an intact skull, the sum of the volumes of brain, CSF, and intracranial blood are constant; therefore, with CSF volume loss, compensatory vasodilatation and venous hypervolemia occur, which may contribute to the headache.[8,9] The average CSF production rate is 500 mL/day with an average adult intrathecal volume of 150 mL.[8] CSF leakage from a meningeal puncture, leading to a loss of CSF pressure, contributes to a loss of the buoyancy support of the brain and is one theory that contributes to the headache.[11] A higher level of lumbar puncture reduces the hydrostatic pressure at the meningeal puncture site, which may explain why MPHs are not commonly associated with cervical punctures.[8] The uncompensated loss of CSF leads to a subarachnoid deficit of CSF and often a reduction in the subarachnoid pressure. The normal CSF opening pressure in the horizontal position is 70–180 mm H_2O.[9] Although CSF hypotension (CSF pressure < 60 mm H_2O) is often noted, the significance of the reduction in subarachnoid pressure is unclear, because it does not consistently correlate with the presentation of headache.[12,13] The development of an MPH does not seem to be related to the amount of CSF leaked.[14] It is probable that the headache is related to sudden alterations in CSF volume, as proposed by Raskin, who theorized that the sudden loss of CSF volume and the change in pressure differential between the inside and outside of the intracranial venous structures result in venous dilatation.[15,16] The direct traction hypothesis states that the reduction in CSF total volume, especially in the spinal region, allows the brain to shift caudally, placing traction on the pain-sensitive intracranial structures and causing cerebral vasodilatation that produces the classic headache symptoms. Pain-sensitive intracranial structures include the dura, cranial nerves, and bridging veins. The ophthalmic branch of the trigeminal nerve, which refers pain to the frontal region, innervates the bridging veins and the dura. In addition to causing pain, traction on bridging veins can cause a tear in the dura, thus leading to a potential subdural hemorrhage.[17] The posterior fossa structures are innervated by the glossopharyngeal and vagus nerves that refer pain to the occipital region. Traction of the vagus nerve can also stimulate the chemoreceptor regions of the medulla causing nausea and vomiting. Finally, traction on the upper cervical nerves can present as occipital, cervical, and shoulder pain and stiffness. Schabel et al. reported one case of arm pain following meningeal puncture that resolved with an epidural blood patch (EBP).[18] In addition to generating pain, traction or pressure on the abducens nerve (CN VI) can cause nerve palsy with paralysis of the lateral rectus muscle; this can manifest as diplopia. Diplopia usually occurs 4–10 days after meningeal puncture but can persist for up to 3 weeks. Full recovery can generally be expected in 2 weeks to 8 months, although permanent cases have rarely been reported.[19] Another proposed mechanism for the visual changes is secondary to crowding of the optic chiasm, which is observed on the magnetic resonance imaging (MRI) of patients with intracranial hypotension.[20] Finally, oculomotor nerve (CN III) and trochlear nerve (CN IV) palsies have been attributed to intracranial hypotension due to brainstem compression and ischemia.[21] In contrast, the Monro–Kellie hypothesis proposes that a reduction in intracranial CSF volume is compensated by increased intracranial blood volume, because the sum of the brain, CSF, and blood volumes is constant. In accordance with the Monro–Kellie rule, the increase in blood volume causes cerebral vasodilatation, which activates the trigeminovascular system, similar to what occurs in migraine attacks. The input reaches the thalamus through the quintothalamic tract and refers pain to the ophthalmic branch and the first three cervical roots. This hypothesis is supported by MRI observations of contrast enhancement of the thickened meninges in MPH secondary to dural venous dilation.[22] Decreased intracranial pressure is probably a secondary cause, because not all patients with classic MPH have intracranial hypotension.[12]

THE ROLE OF ARACHNOID MATER IN THE PATHOGENESIS OF CEREBROSPINAL FLUID LEAK

Reina et al. demonstrated that the dura mater is composed of 78–82 overlapping layers in multiple orientations, therefore making a hole exclusively parallel or across the fibers impossible.[23] Furthermore, as early as 1938, Weed postulated that the arachnoid might be the barrier between the dura and the CSF.[24] In 1967, Waggener and Beggs, based on electron microscopy observations, labeled the arachnoid membrane as a physiologic barrier impermeable to CSF.[25] However, Nabeshima et al. demonstrated by electron microscopy that tight junctions exist only in the outer layer of the arachnoid, similar to those found in capillary endothelium of the brain. The cells of the dura do not contain tight junctions.[24] Because of these anatomical observations, the concept of exclusive dural puncture to access the CSF and cause a CSF leak is not correct. In a study to differentiate the comparative permeability of the three meningeal layers, Bernards and Hill found the arachnoid mater to be the principal diffusion barrier to CSF.[26] Although anesthesiologists probably intend to include puncture of the arachnoid when they refer to a post-"dural" puncture headache, the importance of arachnoid puncture for CSF access should be emphasized.

MENINGES AND RESPONSE TO TRAUMA

In neurosurgical experience, often-minor meningeal perforations need to be closed either directly or through the application of synthetic or biological meningeal graft material. Failure to close a meningeal perforation may lead to adhesions, a continuous CSF leak, and increased risk of infection. It was initially thought that meningeal closure was facilitated by fibroblastic proliferation from the cut edge of the dura mater. However, in 1959, Keener showed that meningeal repair was facilitated by fibroblastic proliferation from surrounding tissue and blood clots. His study also showed that dura mater repair was promoted by damage to the pia or arachnoid mater and the presence of blood clots.[27] It is therefore possible that a spinal needle carefully placed in the subarachnoid space may not promote substantial dural healing, as trauma to adjacent tissue is minimal.

DIAGNOSIS

The diagnosis of an MPH is described according to the International Classification of Headache Disorders. It is primarily based on the history of a meningeal puncture or possible meningeal puncture with the headache worsening within 15 minutes after sitting or standing; improving within 15 minutes after lying down; and accompanied by the presence of at least one symptom among neck stiffness, tinnitus, hypoacusia, photophobia, and nausea. The time period within which the headache appears is debatable, and it can occur within a day or take as long as 12 days to develop. This differentiates it from pneumocephalus-related headache that is most often present immediately following an inadvertent meningeal puncture and injection of air.[28] These factors will largely establish the diagnosis of MPH that can be accompanied by a multitude of signs and symptoms as illustrated above. Because the diagnosis of MPH is largely based on a thorough history and physical examination, it is important to note that certain critical signs and symptoms may indicate concomitant intracranial pathology. The most important of these signs is a changing pattern of the headache. For example, if the headache is no longer postural, if it becomes constant, if it becomes localized unilaterally, or if there is new-onset nausea and vomiting, then further investigation is warranted.[29] Another critical change is increasing neurological alterations, which include sedation, seizures, and new-onset motor and/or sensory deficits. The presence of these signs and symptoms necessitates neurology consultation and additional diagnostic studies. Based on case reports, the differential diagnosis of MPH with changing symptomatology should include intracerebral hemorrhage, infection, eclampsia, and cerebral venous thrombosis.

INCIDENCE

The incidence of MPH has a very wide range, from 1% to 63%.[30] The determinants of this difference in incidence include the needle size, the design of the needle tip, and the orientation of the needle bevel during meningeal puncture.[31] Smaller needle diameters correlate with a lower incidence of MPH. A study on cadaver dural samples found a sixfold greater mean leak when using 22-gauge needles compared to 25-gauge needles.[32] Another study showed that with a 22-gauge Quincke, the rate of MPH was 11% compared to an incidence of 7% using a 25-gauge pencil point needle, although an obvious flaw in this study was the presence of two independent variables.[33] It is important to realize that most unintentional meningeal punctures during epidural anesthesia occur with a 17- or 18-gauge Tuohy needle, which is a cutting needle. In an in vitro study comparing epidural needle diameter and CSF leakage, Angle et al. found reduced CSF leakage with a 20-gauge versus a 17-gauge Tuohy needle puncture.[34] The effect of needle tip design may be more important for lowering incidence of MPH.[35] Spinal needles are designed with cutting bevels, as in the Quincke-type, or pencil point tips, as in the Whitacre-type. Many studies have shown that noncutting pencil point needles (Whitacre-type) are associated with a lower incidence of MPH.[32,36–38] The incidence of MPH with a 20- to 22-gauge cutting needle is estimated to be 36% compared to an incidence of less than

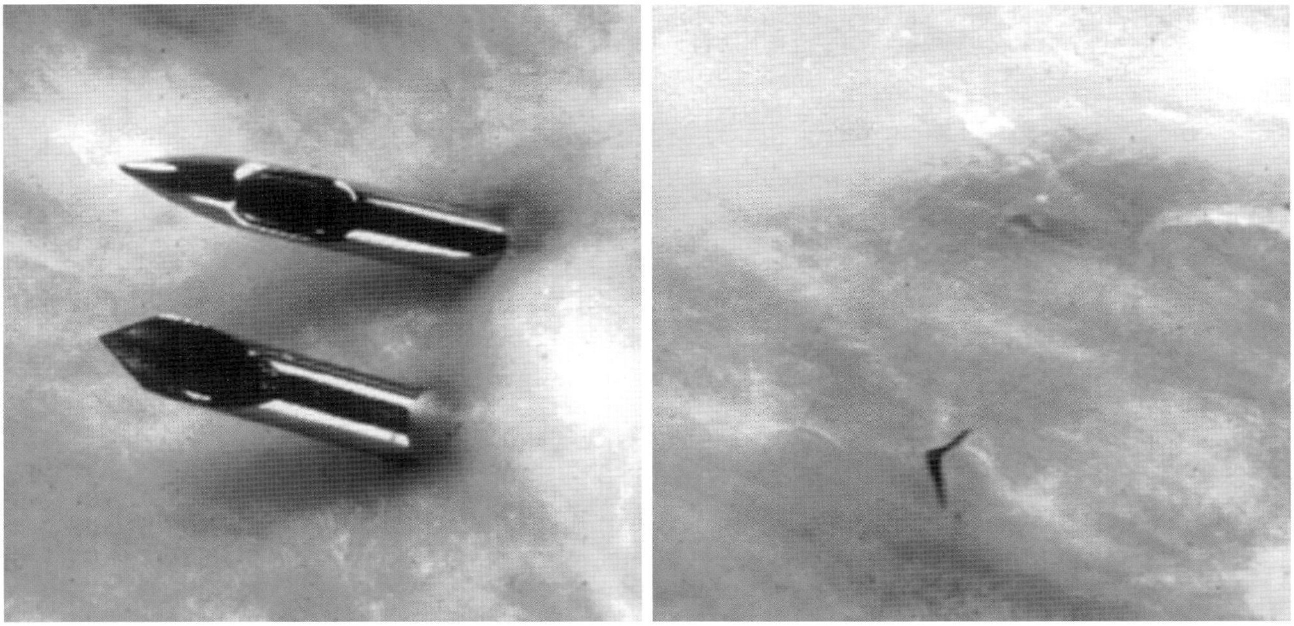

FIG. 21.1 Two types of spinal needle tips: "Atraumatic Sprotte needle" *(upper)* and "traumatic Quincke needle" *(lower)* of the same diameter *(left)*. As shown on the right, the atraumatic needle causes a smaller dural defect *(upper)* than the traumatic needle *(lower)*. The smaller defect should theoretically result in a lower incidence of postlumbar puncture headache. *(From Strupp M, Schueler O, Straube A, Von Stuckrad-Barre S, Brandt T: "Atraumatic" Sprotte needle reduces the incidence of postlumbar puncture headaches.* Neurology. *57(12):2310-2312, 2001.)*

2% with a 22-gauge noncutting needle.[35] There appears to be an even lower incidence of MPH with a larger-diameter blunt tip needle compared to a smaller-diameter cutting needle. One study showed a 2.7% incidence of MPH with a 27-gauge Quincke needle versus 1.2% incidence with a 25-gauge Whitacre needle.[39] The proposed mechanism behind this difference is that a blunt tip needle divides but does not disturb the continuity of the meningeal fibers, whereas a cutting tip needle cuts the meningeal fibers. Electron microscopy studies show that a blunt tip needle produces an irregular hole in the dura versus a clean cut puncture observed with a cutting needle.[35] (Figs. 21.1 and 21.2). As discussed earlier, this may result in an increased inflammatory reaction with the blunt tip needle, which promotes hole closure. The orientation of the bevel to the dura during meningeal puncture has been proposed as a factor affecting the amount of CSF leakage and the incidence of MPH. In an in vitro study, Cruickshank and Hopkinson showed a 21% reduction in the leakage of CSF if the bevel was parallel to the long axis of the spinal cord.[40] In a study by Norris et al. performed in 1558 parturients, the authors compared the incidence of meningeal puncture and MPH between orienting the epidural needle parallel or perpendicular to the long axis of the spinal cord during epidural catheter placement. Although both groups had a similar incidence of meningeal puncture, patients in the parallel orientation group reported significantly less MPH intensity and required fewer EBPs.[41] Richman et al. also found that parallel, rather than perpendicular, insertion of the needle resulted in a statistically significant lower incidence of MPH, 10.9% versus 25.8%, respectively.[31] We know from electron microscopy that the dura mater is a meshwork of collagen, and that these elastic fibers lack a specific orientation. However, the cells of the arachnoid mater are oriented parallel to the long axis of the spinal cord, which may explain the reduction in the rate of MPH when using a parallel insertion technique.

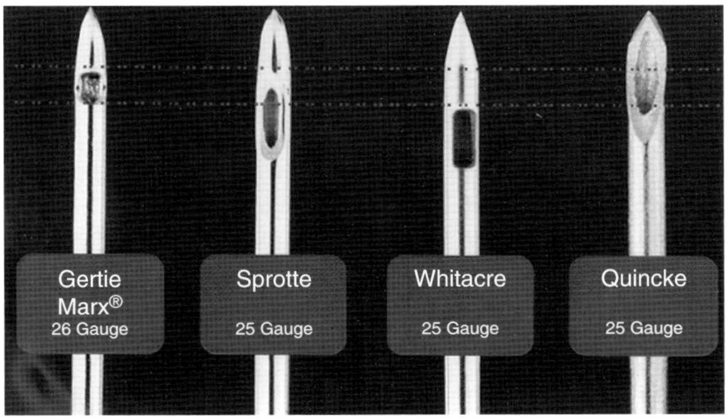

FIG. 21.2 Four types of spinal needle tips. Gertie Marx, Sprotte, and Whitacre are noncutting needles, while Quincke is a cutting needle. *(From Arendt K, Demaerschalk BM, Wingerchuk DM, Camann W: Atraumatic lumbar puncture needles: after all these years, are we still missing the point?* Neurologist. *15(1):17-20, 2009.)*

RISK FACTORS

Independent risk factors of MPH include the female gender, pregnancy, falling in the age group of 20–50 years of age, and a having a low body mass index.[42] The decreased incidence in obese patients is due to the increase in intraabdominal pressure, which may act as an abdominal binder that helps in sealing the defect in the meninges and decreasing the loss of CSF. On the other hand, younger women may be at a greater risk because of increased dural fibers elasticity, which tends to maintain a patent meningeal defect when compared to the less elastic dura in older patients.[43] It was previously thought that MPHs were rare in younger children, but it has been demonstrated to occur with equal frequency in children of all ages.[33,44] Vercauteren et al. reported a higher incidence of MPH after diagnostic meningeal punctures performed by neurologists and neuroradiologists.[45] This is most likely due to the use of larger-gauge needles and less experience performing the procedure. Diagnostic lumbar meningeal punctures require a 20- or 22-gauge needle to facilitate measurement of opening pressure and withdrawal of CSF over a reasonably brief time period. With needles smaller than 22 gauge, collection of 2 mL of CSF may take 6 minutes or longer and measurement of CSF pressure may be less accurate.[46] There is also a higher incidence of MPH in patients with a headache prior to the meningeal puncture and a history of prior MPH. Singh et al. performed a 5-year audit of accidental meningeal punctures and PDPHs in obstetric anesthesia. Of 40,894 consecutive parturients, they found a rate of 0.73% accidental meningeal puncture and a 0.49% incidence of MPH.[47] However, higher rates, ranging between 1% and 2.6%, have been quoted.[39] Choi et al. showed that in parturients who experienced an unintentional meningeal puncture while receiving a labor epidural, more than 50% developed an MPH.[48]

PREVENTION

Prevention of MPH depends on needle size, needle tip, and bevel orientation during meningeal puncture. The smallest needle with a noncutting tip oriented parallel to the long axis of the spinal cord will reduce the incidence of MPH the most. In the case of accidental meningeal puncture while placing an epidural catheter, placing the catheter intrathecally has been shown to decrease the incidence of MPH. In a comparative outcome study of known subarachnoid punctures with 18-gauge Tuohy needles, Ayad et al. reported that intrathecal catheter placement after accidental meningeal puncture in obstetric patients reduced the MPH incidence from 81% in the group that had an epidural catheter placed to 31% in the group that had an intrathecal catheter placed and removed right after delivery and to 3% in the group that had an intrathecal catheter placed and left in place for 24 hours after delivery. The authors therefore recommended intrathecal catheterization for 24 hours to reduce the rate of MPH.[49] Van de Velde et al. summarized results from a large number of studies and noted that the incidence of MPH was 51% when an intrathecal catheter was used and 66% when an epidural catheter was used and that the incidence of EBP was 33% and 59%, respectively. However, this analysis combined data from both retrospective and prospective studies, many of which were underpowered and not randomized.[50] A survey among obstetric anesthesiologists practicing in North America reported that 75% of respondents place the catheter epidurally after accidental meningeal puncture and that 25% place it intrathecally; however, 76% believed leaving an intrathecal catheter in place for 24 hours would reduce the incidence of headache.[51] Another survey among Australian obstetric anesthetists showed that 64% would remove the Tuohy needle and re-site it in the case of accidental meningeal puncture during the placement of a labor epidural. The most common reason behind this decision was concern regarding the safety of intrathecal catheters, particularly the risk of misuse.[52]

Other proposed preventive procedures include prophylactic EBPs and epidural saline injections and infusions. In a small study, Charsley and Abram found that intrathecal injection of 10 mL normal saline reduced the incidence of MPH.[53] Little evidence exists for prophylactic EBPs, though they are commonly done.[54] Existing studies regarding prophylactic EBP are limited by small patient numbers.[55,56] Other limitations include the small volumes of blood injected according to some reviews.[57] In a quantitative systemic review, Apfel et al. found that the relative risk (RR) for headache after prophylactic EBP was 0.48 in five nonrandomized controlled trials (non-RCTs) and 0.32 in four randomized controlled trials (RCTs), but due to heterogeneity between the studies and publication bias from small non-RCTs with positive results, a large multi-center RCT to determine the best practice was recommended.[58]

TREATMENT

Treatment of MPH should be initiated once the diagnosis has been clearly established based on history, physical examination, and appropriate diagnostic tests. Treatment options should be balanced by the understanding that 85% of MPHs last less than 5 days and that MPHs are rarely associated with significant morbidity.[59] Treatment of MPH should start with conservative therapy. Recumbent bed rest relieves the symptoms of MPH but has no therapeutic benefit. A meta-analysis by Thoennissen et al. failed to show that bed rest after meningeal puncture was better than immediate mobilization in reducing the incidence of MPH.[60] Aggressive hydration is a common therapy despite the fact that there are no studies to support its effectiveness. Medications reported to be beneficial in the treatment of MPH include methylxanthines, caffeine, theophylline, sumatriptan, adrenocorticotropic hormone, and corticosteroids.[2] Caffeine, a potent central nervous system stimulant, causes cerebral vasoconstriction and is the most widely used pharmacologic therapy for MPH. Caffeine is administered as an oral dose of 300 mg or an intravenous dose of 500 mg in 500 or 1000 mL of normal saline infused over 2 hours; the intravenous dose can be repeated in 2–4 hours if needed.[61] Although caffeine is safe and effective, there have been reports of seizures, anxiety, and arrhythmias associated with its use. The existing literature does not seem to support caffeine as a therapeutic agent to treat MPH.[2] Caffeine is contraindicated in patients with a history of seizure disorder and in patients with pregnancy-induced hypertension. The effect of caffeine is transient and the dose must be repeated, because it does not address the underlying pathology.[62] Theophylline, another cerebral vasoconstrictor effective in the treatment of MPH, is not widely used or supported by the literature. Other pharmacologic agents such as serotonin agonists (sumatriptan) and corticotrophin are infrequently used and have been found to be ineffective in the treatment of severe MPH. However, Bussone et al. found in a nonrandomized study that frovatriptan was useful in the prevention of MPH in patients undergoing diagnostic lumbar punctures.[3] Recent studies suggest that drugs such as pregabalin and gabapentin might be useful in the management of MPH. One RCT compared the use of pregabalin for 5 days with placebo in 40 patients who developed MPH after spinal anesthesia or lumbar puncture and found that the group that received pregabalin had significantly lower pain scores after the second day of treatment and lower diclofenac requirements.[63] Another RCT comparing the use of gabapentin with the use of ergotamine/caffeine in 42 patients with MPH found that gabapentin significantly reduced pain, nausea, and vomiting compared to ergotamine/caffeine.[64] However, more studies are needed to confirm the usefulness of these drugs.

Once pharmacologic and other noninvasive options have been exhausted without relief and the patient is unable to wait for the natural resolution of the headache, more invasive options may be considered. Epidural treatments for MPH include the administration of saline, colloids, fibrin glue, and blood.[2] The gold standard treatment for MPH is an EBP. There are numerous variations of the EBP; however, the standard and most common treatment remains the epidural autologous blood patch. This treatment offers complete resolution of symptoms in a large proportion of patients. In the remaining patients, it reduces headache severity and allows them to return to their everyday activities.[65] Contraindications to an EBP are similar to those for any spinal or epidural procedure.[3] The first is patient refusal in general or for a specific reason. For a Jehovah's Witness patient concerned about blood transfusions, alternative patching materials are available.[42] Second, the patient's coagulation status must be assessed to reduce the risk of an epidural hematoma.[66] Finally, it is not recommended to place an EBP in a septic patient, a febrile patient, or through a localized infection site due to the obvious concern of introducing bacteria into the epidural space. Concerns about an EBP in HIV-positive patients are unfounded, because HIV crosses the blood–brain barrier early in the course of the disease.[67] The mechanism of EBP is controversial; however, it is generally believed to exert its effect via two separate mechanisms. There is an initial early effect, which occurs within minutes, secondary to compression of the dura toward the spinal cord and reduction in intradural volume. The EBP blood spreads both longitudinally and circumferentially, thus enveloping the entire dural sac. The reduction in the spinal intradural volume shifts the CSF cephalad, thus resuspending the brain and reducing traction. In agreement with the Monro–Kellie rule, this intracranial shift in CSF also reduces cerebral vasodilation and intracranial blood volume. Due to this early effect, patients often report rapid relief following an EBP. However, by utilizing post-EBP MRI, Beards et al. demonstrated that the compressive mass effect of a blood patch disappeared by 7 hours post patching. A second more lasting effect is due to sealing of the dural/arachnoid tear with a gelatinous plug. This sealing of the dural/arachnoid hole prevents further loss of CSF and allows for regeneration and restoration of the CSF volume. The plug acts as a bridge until permanent repair of the dural/arachnoid hole occurs. The occurrence of this second effect is more variable and can account for the failure of an EBP despite initial relief. Dubost et al. measured optic nerve sheet diameter (ONSD), which is a marker of intracranial pressure (ICP), in patients with MPH after receiving EBPs. They found that an EBP was followed by ONSD enlargement in subjects with a successful EBP but not in subjects with EBP failure. Since ONSD is a surrogate marker of ICP, this suggests that sustained increase in ICP is associated with successful EBP.[68]

Risk factors for EBP failure include placement earlier than 24 hours after meningeal puncture, using too small of a volume of autologous blood, and performance of the procedure with residual local anesthetic in the epidural space. Ong et al. and Blanche et al. were unable to find any conclusive impact of an EBP on the efficacy of future epidural anesthetics.[69,70]

The technique of an EBP, first described by Gormley in 1960, is straightforward based on the placement of a single-shot epidural.[71] It usually requires two people, one to locate the epidural space and the other to draw the blood. Sterility is of great importance, both during epidural space localization and during blood collection. The patient can be either sitting or in the lateral decubitus position during the procedure depending on the difficulty in locating the epidural space and the patient's ability to tolerate the upright position. Selection of the level of placement should be guided by the observation that 15 mL of blood preferentially spreads cephalad six segments and caudad three segments, or one spinal segment per 1.6 mL of blood.[72] It is therefore common to select a site caudad to the suspected meningeal tear. Colonna-Romano and Linton reported that a lumbar EBP was successfully used to treat an MPH due to a C6–C7 cervical meningeal puncture.[73] This may be due to the increase in the subarachnoid pressure and the resultant cerebral vasoconstriction and deactivation of the brain adenosine receptors. More caudad levels are also associated with a reduced risk of direct cord compression. Although historically different volumes of blood have been used, the ideal target volume is 20 mL.[74] This is the most widely accepted and cited volume if the patient tolerates placement. If the patient complains of excessive back or leg pain or pressure during injection, a lower volume can be placed. Chen et al. found that a volume of 7.5 mL of autologous blood in the epidural space was comparable to 15 mL of blood in its analgesic effect on MPH but with less nerve root irritation pain during injection.[75] After the EBP, the patient should remain supine with the legs slightly elevated. Intravenous fluids can be administered during this time. In a small study, Martin et al. found that 2 hours in the supine position, post-EBP provided 100% relief versus 60% relief in patients who remained supine for 30 minutes only.[76] Although initial relief has been reported in the overwhelming majority of patients, the overall long-term relief of MPH from an initial EBP is between 61% and 75%.[77] Alternative meningeal patching materials include epidural fibrin glue and epidural Dextran-40.[78] Although both of these materials have been successfully employed, they are not widely used due to cost and safety concerns, especially when compared to autologous blood. Dextran-40 may be an alternative in Jehovah's Witnesses. Another alternative to EBP is epidural saline boluses or infusions. Epidural saline boluses or infusions have not been shown to be effective alternatives and often require more interventions with lower success rates, as saline is absorbed from the epidural space faster than blood. In an RCT, Al-metwalli studied the effect of epidural morphine in the prevention of MPH after inadvertent meningeal puncture. One group received an epidural injection of 3 mg of morphine in 10 mL of saline, that was repeated in 24 hours, while the control group received an epidural injection of 10 mL of saline repeated in 24 hours. The incidence of headache was 12% in the morphine group and 48% in the saline group. The need for a therapeutic EBP was also less in the morphine group.[79] As a last resort, surgical repair of a meningeal tear may be considered, although it is a more invasive procedure generally reserved for severe cases of chronic MPHs that have not responded to EBPs.

Complications of an EBP are rare. The most common complication is mild low back and radicular pain following the procedure that resolves spontaneously in a few days and can be treated with nonsteroidal antiinflammatory drugs (NSAIDs).[80] Other possible complications include epidural hematoma, infection, and arachnoiditis due to unintentional subdural or subarachnoid injection of the blood. There are two reported cases of facial nerve paralysis following EBP, which resolved spontaneously.[81] Mokri reported a case of symptomatic intracranial hypertension following an EBP.[82]

MENINGEAL PUNCTURE HEADACHE SUMMARY

MPH and its management is a well-known and widely accepted entity in the anesthesia community. A postural headache is the cardinal sign that indicates an MPH. In the setting of a meningeal puncture or possible meningeal puncture with pathognomonic symptoms, the diagnosis of MPH should be straightforward. Although it is nonfatal, it can have significant morbidity and should be treated seriously. Treatment should start with conservative therapy, as the headache usually subsides in 5–7 days. An EBP is the gold standard in treating MPH not responding to conservative management. Surgical repair is rarely required in patients with chronic MPH.

SPONTANEOUS INTRACRANIAL HYPOTENSION

Spontaneous intracranial hypotension (SIH) was initially described in the early 1900s. It is a syndrome with symptoms similar to MPH, but the patient has no previous history of meningeal puncture. The incidence is approximately 5 in 100,000 person-years. Women are affected twice as often as men, and the peak incidence is in the fourth or fifth decade of life.[83]

CLINICAL SYMPTOMS OF SPONTANEOUS INTRACRANIAL HYPOTENSION

This syndrome is usually suspected in a patient with postural headache that occurs after a fall, trauma, whiplash, exercise, or violent coughing. Although classically postural, the headache can be nonpositional or even paradoxical (worse when lying down).[84] The headache can be gradual or thunderclap in onset and has also been described as exertional, intermittent, or mainly occurring at the end of the day. The headache results from the downward displacement of the brain from loss of buoyancy with traction on the pain-sensitive structures, including the meninges. Another mechanism is from compensatory dilation of the intracranial venous structures, which are pain-sensitive. The next most common symptoms are neck pain or stiffness, nausea, and vomiting. Other symptoms include blurred vision, tinnitus, vertigo, and photophobia. Tinnitus is secondary to the transmission of the abnormal CSF pressure to the perilymph,[85] while the vision and balance abnormalities are due to stretching of the optic and vestibulocochlear nerves. Hyperprolactinemia and galactorrhea are a result of distortion of the pituitary stalk.[86] Symptoms referable to the spine include back pain and radiculopathy, presumably from compression of the nerve roots or spinal cord by the leaked CSF. The International Classification of Headache Disorders has published diagnostic criteria for SIH (Table 21.1),[87] although some experts consider the criteria to be too restrictive.[88] The differential diagnoses of SIH include primary and secondary headache disorders. Secondary headaches to be considered are subarachnoid hemorrhage, carotid/vertebral artery dissection, cerebral venous sinus thrombosis, benign intracranial hypotension, posttraumatic headache, and meningitis.[83]

TABLE 21.1 Diagnostic Criteria for Spontaneous Intracranial Hypotension, From the International Headache Society

A. Diffuse and/or dull headache that worsens within 15 min after sitting or standing, fulfilling criterion D, and with one of the following:
   1. Neck stiffness
   2. Tinnitus
   3. Hypacusia
   4. Photophobia
   5. Nausea
B. At least one of the following:
   1. Evidence of low CSF pressure on MRI (e.g., pachymeningeal enhancement)
   2. Evidence of CSF leakage on conventional myelography, CTM, or cisternography
   3. CSF opening pressure < 60 mm H_2O in sitting position
C. No history of meningeal puncture or other cause of CSF fistula
D. Headache resolves within 72 h after epimeningeal blood patching

CSF, *Cerebrospinal fluid;* CTM, *CT myelography;* MRI, *magnetic resonance imaging.*
From Headache Classification Subcommittee of the International Headache Society. The International Classification of Headache Disorders, 2nd ed. Cephalalgia. *24(Suppl 1):1-160, 2004.*

The most commonly accepted etiology of SIH is leakage of the CSF through a weakness of the spinal meninges such as meningeal diverticulum or small tears in the root sleeves or perineural cysts (Tarlov cysts). Other anatomic abnormalities include vertebral osteophytic spur[89,90] and herniated or degenerative disc disease piercing the dura.[91] The onset of symptoms is usually precipitated by a fall, trauma, or exercise. SIH appears to be associated with generalized connective tissue disorders.[83,92] These include Marfan syndrome, Ehlers-Danlos syndrome type II, autosomal dominant polycystic kidney disease, isolated joint hypermobility, joint hypermobility with fascial thinning, and spontaneous retinal detachment.

DIAGNOSIS OF SPONTANEOUS INTRACRANIAL HYPOTENSION

The diagnosis of SIH is confirmed by low CSF pressure on diagnostic lumbar puncture and meningeal enhancement on MRI of the cranium. Diagnostic lumbar puncture usually shows a low CSF pressure (below 60 mm H_2O; reference range, 65–195 mm H_2O). Occasionally, there is no spontaneous flow and the CSF must be aspirated. CSF protein, red cell and white cell counts are usually increased. Head MRI shows meningeal enhancement, subdural fluid collection, caudal displacement of the cerebellar tonsils, and pituitary abnormalities (enlargement or hyperemia).[83,89] Schievink noted five characteristic features of SIH: (1) subdural fluid collections; (2) enhancement of the pachymeninges; (3) engorgement of venous structures; (4) pituitary hyperemia; and (5) sagging of the brain (mnemonic: SEEPS).[83] Meningeal enhancement is usually thickest in patients with low intracranial pressure and subdural fluid collections. A relationship between SIH, subdural fluid collection, and subdural hematoma has been noted.[93–95] Spine MRI of patients with SIH usually shows epidural or paraspinal fluid collections and collapse of the dural sac.[96] It is interesting to note that the meningeal enhancement slowly decreases even after the patient improves with treatment, and it may take 3–5 months for the meningeal changes to resolve.

Radionuclide cisternography (RC) was once considered to be the confirmatory test in the diagnosis of SIH. However, the site of the CSF leak is rarely demonstrated with this diagnostic procedure. The presence of SIH is indirectly proven by the lack of ascent of the injected dye, rapid disappearance of the radioisotope from the CSF (within 4 hours), and the early appearance of the radioisotope in the urinary bladder. The radioisotope is presumed to leak through a meningeal rent into the epidural space, subsequently absorbed by the epidural vessels, carried into the systemic circulation, and excreted by the kidneys. Early appearance of the radioisotope in the bladder within 2.5 hours is considered early filling, and reports have shown the appearance of the radioisotope as early as 45–90 minutes after injection. However, the site of leak is often not demonstrated in cisternography. This is because the patient is brought back to the radiology department after injection of the radioisotope, and images are taken at several time intervals; hence, the leak of the radioisotope may have occurred between images. Other disadvantages of RC include poor spatial resolution, its invasiveness, and possible radioisotope extravasation through the needle tract, resulting in inaccuracy in its interpretation. For these reasons, RC is now considered of limited usefulness in the diagnosis of SIH.[97,98]

Computed tomography myelography (CTM) and intrathecal gadolinium magnetic resonance myelography (Gd-MRM) localize spinal CSF leaks. CTM is now considered the diagnostic procedure of choice to show the location and extent of CSF leak in SIH.[83] It has better localizing power and gives finer details compared with RC. Standard CTM is used to localize slow CSF leaks wherein the CSF is confined to one or two vertebral levels, while dynamic CTM, whereby the contrast is injected intermittently followed by immediate scanning after each injection, is utilized when the leak is suspected to be rapid and spread over several vertebral levels.[99] The location of the leak can be in the cervicothoracic,[83] thoracic,[100] thoracolumbar level,[101] or lumbosacral levels.[97] Gd-MRM has higher sensitivity than CTM for small, slow leaks but is more complex to perform.[98,102]

TREATMENT OF SPONTANEOUS INTRACRANIAL HYPOTENSION

Many patients respond to conservative measures alone including bed rest, oral hydration, steroids, oral or intravenous caffeine, and applying an abdominal binder. EBP is considered when conservative treatment fails. It is the treatment of choice for SIH, although it is less effective in SIH than in PDPH. The lower success rate may be related to the injection of the blood away from the site of the CSF leak, the presence of multiple CSF leaks, and the rare occurrence of CSF leaks at the anterior aspect of the spinal cord or the nerve root sleeves.

In the absence of CTM demonstrating the exact location of CSF leak, most pain medicine practitioners inject the blood at the thoracolumbar area to cover the upper lumbar and the lower thoracic levels. The patient is then placed in a Trendelenburg position for 30–60 minutes.[83] If not effective, then a second injection can be performed in the lumbar region. Ferrante et al.[103] reported excellent results with blind lumbar EBPs in 42 patients with the following protocol: (1) maintain a 30-degree Trendelenburg position 1 hour before, during, and 24 hours after EBP; (2) premedicate with acetazolamide 250 mg 18 and 6 hours before EBP; and (3) refrain from strenuous exercise for 2 weeks after the procedure. The prolonged Trendelenburg position promotes rostral spread of the EBP; maintaining this position for 24 hours after the procedure is probably not necessary. Acetazolamide is a carbonic anhydrase inhibitor that decreases the rate of CSF production. This decreases the rate of CSF leak and favors closure of the meningeal rent. The use of acetazolamide is purely theoretical, as its clinical benefit has not been proven.

There have been reports of multiple EBPs to cover multiple sites of CSF leaks.[104] Ihara et al.[105] performed four EBPs, two at the upper thoracic, one at the lower thoracic, and one at the lumbar area. Benzon et al.[106] performed three EBPs at the thoracic region; the first two blood patches were injected through a midline approach, while the third one was injected through a left paramedian approach since several sites of leak were noted on that side. Performing more than two EBPs is probably not necessary. If one or two EBPs are not effective, then a CTM should preferably be performed before another EBP is attempted to delineate the vertebral level and the side of the CSF leak.[106] The use of a transforaminal EBP, although reported to be successful,[107] should be done as a last resort. This is because of possible compression/occlusion of the radicular artery accompanying the nerve root leading to segmental ischemia of the spinal cord and possible paralysis.[108]

Epidural patches done with fibrin glue alone[109] or with autologous blood[110] have been described. Fibrin glue has been associated with allergic reactions and viral infections.[111,112] Surgical intervention is warranted if multiple EBPs are ineffective and the patient's condition deteriorates.[83,89] Surgery for SIH is challenging and close follow-up is recommended since some patients may develop recurrent CSF leaks.

Recurrence of headache after successful treatment may be due to leak recurrence. If the character of the headache changes, then rebound transient intracranial hypertension[82] or dural venous sinus thrombosis[113] are possibilities.

SPONTANEOUS INTRACRANIAL HYPOTENSION SUMMARY

SIH is characterized by the same symptoms as MPH although without the patient having previous history of meningeal puncture. The CSF pressure is low on diagnostic lumbar puncture and there is meningeal enhancement on the MRI. CTM confirms the diagnosis and helps determine the exact site of CSF leak. If conservative measures are not effective, several EBPs may be required to treat the headache.

KEY POINTS

POSTMENINGEAL PUNCTURE HEADACHE

- The crucial components of MPH are a history of meningeal (dural/arachnoid) puncture and a postural bilateral headache.
- The occurrence of headache after dural/arachnoid puncture is not directly related to the amount of CSF leaked or the subarachnoid pressure. The headache may be secondary to a sudden alteration in CSF volume and subsequent cerebral vasodilatation.
- Concomitant intracranial pathology may be present in patients with MPH. The signs and symptoms include the presence of a significant nonpostural component of the headache, a changing pattern of the headache, and severe nausea and vomiting.
- Prevention of MPH depends mainly on the size of the needle and the design of the needle tip. The smallest practical needle diameter with a noncutting tip is associated with the lowest risk of MPH.
- Initial therapy of MPH in the first 24 hours should be conservative, relying mainly on medications. Approximately 85% of MPHs resolve spontaneously in 5 days.
- The initial and rapid relief from an EBP is secondary to circumferential compression of the dura and reduction of the intradural volume. This shifting of the vertebral subarachnoid CSF cephalad causes resuspension of the cerebral structures and reduction of the traction on pain-sensitive intracranial structures and decreased cerebral vasodilatation. The lasting relief from an EBP is related to sealing of the dural/arachnoid hole.
- Caffeine and theophylline block brain adenosine receptors causing cerebral vasoconstriction. The acute increase in the subarachnoid pressure after an EBP may deactivate adenosine receptors and relieve the headache.

SPONTANEOUS INTRACRANIAL HYPOTENSION

- SIH is characterized by symptoms similar to MPH in a patient with no history of meningeal puncture.
- The etiology of SIH is leakage of the CSF through a weakness of the spinal meninges such as meningeal diverticulum or small tears in the root sleeves or cysts. Other associated anatomical abnormalities are herniated disc and vertebral spurs.
- The hallmarks of SIH consist of postural headache (without a previous history of meningeal puncture), low CSF pressure on diagnostic lumbar puncture, and meningeal enhancement on MRI.
- The symptoms include postural headache; neck stiffness; visual, hearing, and balance disturbances; back pain; and even radiculopathy.
- Although the headache is classically postural, it can be nonpositional or intermittent. It can be gradual or sudden in onset.
- CTM is the diagnostic procedure of choice in SIH because it has a better chance of showing the location of the CSF leak and gives finer details than RC. Gd-MRM is more sensitive than CTM but is also more complex to perform.
- EBP is the treatment of choice for SIH and several EBPs may be required if there are multiple sites of leakage.
- Although fibrin glue can be injected into the epidural space, there are not enough publications or experience to support its routine use.
- If conservative measures and EBPs are not effective, surgical repair can be employed if structural abnormalities or focal CSF leaks are identified.

REFERENCES

Access the reference list online at ExpertConsult.com.

CHAPTER 22

Cervicogenic Headache

Samer Narouze, MD, PhD

INTRODUCTION

Cervicogenic headache was initially defined as unilateral headache that is provoked by neck movement or pressure over tender points in the neck with associated reduced range of movement of the cervical spine. The headache occurs in nonclustering episodes and is usually nonthrobbing in nature, originating from the neck and spreading over the occipital, temporal, and frontal regions.[1–3] However, these clinical criteria are not enough to make a definite diagnosis of cervicogenic headache, as it is sometimes difficult to differentiate clinically between cervicogenic headache, migraine, and tension-type headache.[4–6]

Response to diagnostic block of the nerve supply of these cervical structures or intraarticular injection of local anesthetic into the culprit joint is now considered the major criterion in the diagnosis of cervicogenic headache.[7] Also, cervicogenic headache can be unilateral or bilateral.[7] These clinical characteristics prompted the development of new diagnostic criteria for the diagnosis of cervicogenic headache by the International Headache Society (IHS). More recently, the International Classification of Headache Disorders, 3rd edition (ICHD-3) was released.[8]

DIAGNOSTIC CRITERIA

1. Any headache fulfilling criterion C
2. Clinical, laboratory and/or imaging evidence of a disorder or lesion within the cervical spine or soft tissues of the neck known to be able to cause headache
3. Evidence of causation demonstrated by at least two of the following:
   a. Headache has developed in temporal relation to the onset of the cervical disorder or appearance of the lesion
   b. Headache has significantly improved or resolved in parallel with improvement in or resolution of the cervical disorder or lesion
   c. Cervical range of motion is reduced and headache is made significantly worse by provocative maneuvers
   d. Headache is abolished following diagnostic blockade of a cervical structure or its nerve supply
4. Not better accounted for by another ICHD-3 diagnosis

ETIOLOGY

Cervicogenic headache is referred pain from cervical structures innervated by the upper three cervical spinal nerves. Thus possible sources and differential diagnoses of cervicogenic headache are: atlanto-occipital joint, median and lateral atlanto-axial joints, C2–C3 intervertebral disc, C2–C3 zygapophyseal joint, upper posterior neck and paravertebral muscles, the trapezius and the sternocleidomastoid muscles, spinal and posterior cranial fossa dura matter, cervical spinal nerves and roots, and the vertebral artery.[9]

NEUROANATOMY AND NEUROPHYSIOLOGY

The spinal nucleus of the trigeminal nerve extends caudally to the outer lamina of the dorsal horn of the upper three to four cervical spinal segments. This is known as the trigeminocervical nucleus, which receives afferents from the trigeminal nerve and the upper three cervical spinal nerves. Convergence between these afferents accounts for the cervical-trigeminal pain referral. Therefore, pain originating from cervical structures supplied by the upper cervical spinal nerves could be perceived in areas innervated by the trigeminal nerves such as the orbit and the frontotemporoparietal region. Bartsch and Goadsby showed that noxious stimulation of the greater occipital nerve induces increased central excitability of supratentorial afferents,[10] and vice versa, stimulation of the dura mater increases trigeminocervical neuron's responsiveness to cervical input.[11]

COMMON SOURCES OF CERVICOGENIC HEADACHE

In this chapter, I discuss the clinical presentations of the common causes of cervicogenic headache and how to come up with an accurate diagnosis and a plan of care (Fig. 22.1).[12]

ATLANTO-AXIAL JOINT

The lateral atlanto-axial joint, which is innervated by the C2 ventral ramus, is not an uncommon cause of cervicogenic headache. It may account for 16% of patients with occipital headache.[13] In human volunteers, distending the lateral atlanto-axial joint with contrast agent produces occipital pain.[13]

Clinical presentations suggestive of pain originating from the lateral atlanto-axial joint include occipital or suboccipital pain, focal tenderness over the suboccipital area or over the transverse process of C1, restricted painful rotation of C1 on C2, and pain provocation by passive rotation of C1. These clinical presentations merely indicate that the lateral atlanto-axial joint could be a possible source of occipital headache; however, they are not specific and therefore cannot be used alone to establish the diagnosis.[9] The only means of establishing a definite diagnosis is a diagnostic block with intraarticular injection of local anesthetic.[12]

The pathology of lateral atlanto-axial joint pain is usually osteoarthritis or posttraumatic in nature.[14,15] However, the presence of osteoarthritic changes in imaging

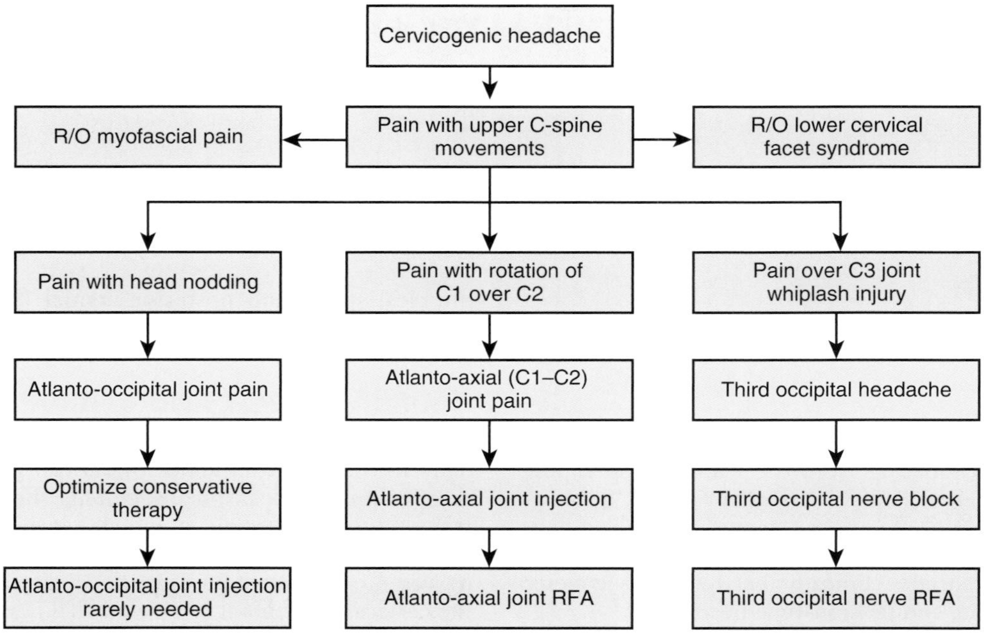

FIG. 22.1 Algorithm for the diagnosis and management of cervicogenic headache. *RFA*, Radiofrequency ablation. *(Reprinted with permission from Narouze S, editor:* Interventional Management of Head and Face Pain: Nerve Blocks and Beyond, *New York: Springer, 2014.)*

studies does not mean that the joint is necessary painful; also, the absence of abnormal findings does not preclude the joint from being painful.

There is no conservative treatment for lateral atlanto-axial joint pain. However, intraarticular steroids are effective in short-term relief of pain originating from the lateral atlanto-axial joint.[16,17] Long-lasting pain relief may require arthrodesis of the lateral atlanto-axial joint.[18,19]

Atlanto-axial joint intraarticular injection has the potential for serious complications, so it is imperative to be familiar with the anatomy of the joint in relation to the surrounding vascular and neural structures (Fig. 22.2). The vertebral artery lies lateral to the atlanto-axial joint as it courses through the C2 and C1 foramina. Then it curves medially to go through the foramen magnum, crossing the medial posterior aspect of the atlanto-occipital joint (see Fig. 22.2). The C2 dorsal root ganglion and nerve root with its surrounding dural sleeve crosses the posterior aspect of the middle of the joint. Therefore during atlanto-axial joint injection, the needle should be directed toward the posterolateral aspect of the joint. This avoids injury to the C2 nerve root medially or the vertebral artery laterally (Figs. 22.3 to 22.5).[12,17] Meticulous attention should be observed to avoid intravascular injection, as the anatomy may be variable. Injection of a contrast agent should be performed under real time fluoroscopy preferably with digital subtraction prior to injection of the local anesthetic, as negative aspiration is not reliable. Inadvertent puncture of the C2 dural sleeve with cerebrospinal fluid (CSF) leak or high spinal spread of the local anesthetic may occur with atlanto-axial joint injection if the needle is directed only a few millimeters medially. Spinal cord injury and syringomyelia are potential serious complications if the needle is directed further medially.

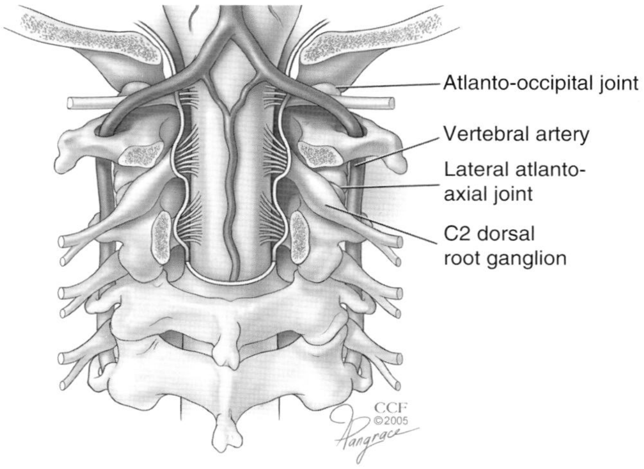

FIG. 22.2 Illustration showing the relationship of the atlanto-axial and atlanto-occipital joints to the vertebral artery. *(Reprinted with permission from Cleveland Clinic.)*

C2–C3 ZYGAPOPHYSIAL JOINT AND THIRD OCCIPITAL HEADACHE

C2–C3 zygapophyseal joint is innervated by the third occipital nerve, which is the superficial medial branch of the dorsal ramus of C3.[20] Pain stemming from this joint (named third occipital headache) was seen in 27% of patients presenting with cervicogenic headache after whiplash injury.[21] Tenderness over the C2–C3 joint is only suggestive, and controlled diagnostic third occipital nerve block (ONB) is mandatory to confirm the diagnosis.

Earlier reports showed that radiofrequency neurotomy of the third occipital nerve was not effective[22]; however, with improved radiofrequency technique, complete relief

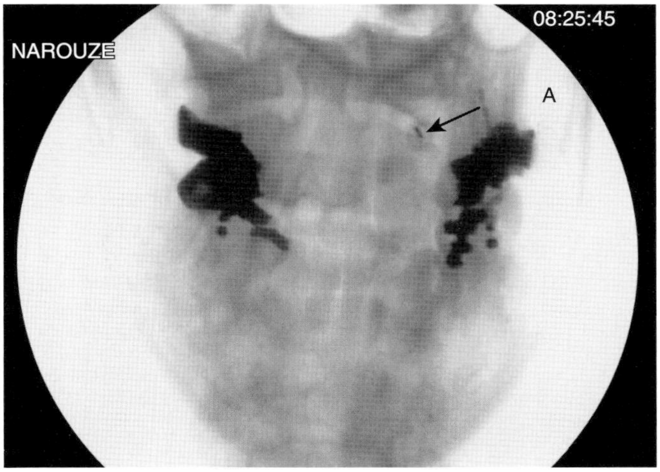

FIG. 22.3 Anteroposterior view showing the needle in a tunnel view inside the lateral part of the lateral AA joint. *(Reprinted with permission from Ohio Pain and Headache Institute.)*

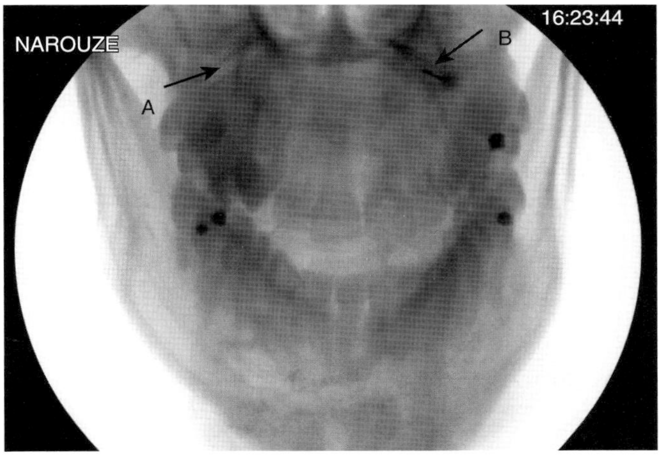

FIG. 22.4 (A) The lateral atlanto-axial joint. (B) The tip of the needle and the contrast agent within the lateral AA joint. *(Reprinted with permission from Ohio Pain and Headache Institute.)*

was obtained in 88% of patients with third occipital headache (Fig. 22.6).[23] The C2–C3 zygapophyseal joint intraarticular steroid injection was effective in one study.[24] On the other hand, Barnsley et al. reported a lack of efficacy of intraarticular steroids for chronic pain stemming from the cervical zygapophyseal joints.[25]

THIRD OCCIPITAL NERVE NEUROLYSIS

The third occipital nerve is the superficial medial branch of C3 dorsal ramus. It supplies the C2–C3 zygapophysial joint while crossing the joint laterally. Also, it supplies part of the semispinalis capitis muscle and its cutaneous branch supplies a small area of skin below the occiput.[20]

Third occipital radiofrequency neurolysis was shown to be effective in the treatment of headache stemming from the C2–C3 joint. The most common side effect is incomplete lesioning of the third occipital nerve because of its variable anatomy.[22] Using the three-needle-technique accommodates all variation in the anatomy of the third occipital nerve from just lateral to the joint line to above or

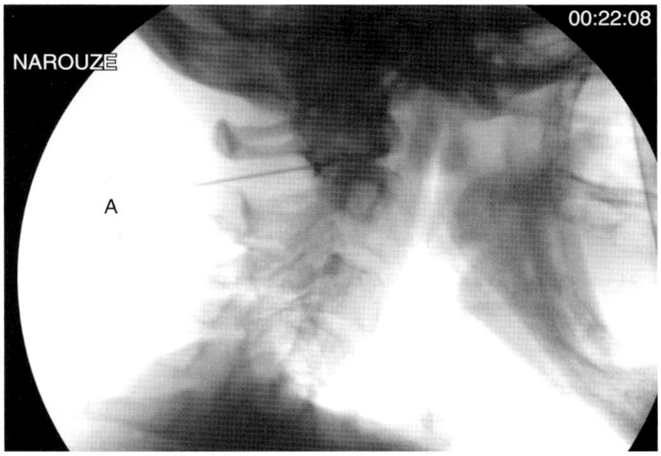

FIG. 22.5 Lateral view showing the tip of the needle and the contrast agent within the lateral AA joint. *(Reprinted with permission from Ohio Pain and Headache Institute.)*

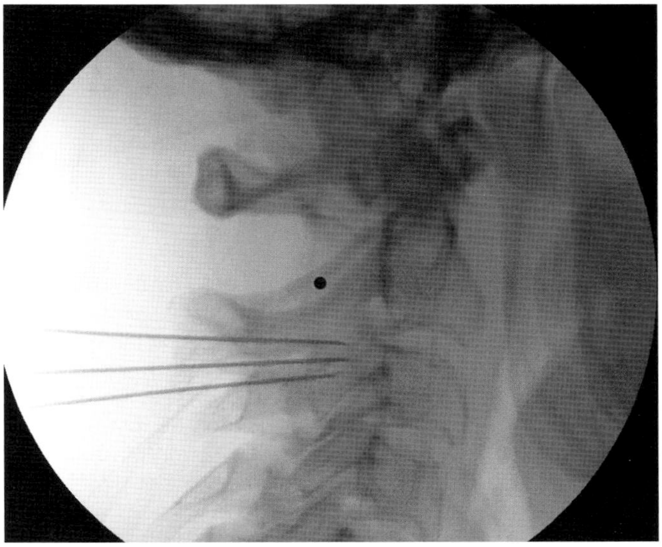

FIG. 22.6 Lateral view showing three radiofrequency needles appropriately placed at the equator of the C2–C3 joint and above and below the joint line. *(Reprinted with permission from Ohio Pain and Headache Institute.)*

below the joint, and creating consecutive lesions no more than one electrode width from adjacent lesion markedly improved the results (see Fig. 22.6).[23]

Anesthesia dolorosa has not been reported with this particular block. However, numbness in the cutaneous distribution of the nerve is very common, whereas dysesthesia and hypersensitivity typically at the border of the area of numbness occur in up to 50% of cases; however, these are temporary complications that usually persist only for few days to weeks.[22,23] Temporary ataxia has been reported in most patients, as third occipital neurotomy partially denervates the semispinalis capitis muscles with the resultant interference of the tonic neck reflexes. Most patients can overcome this sensation by relying on visual cues.[22,23] Other possible complications that are not specific to third ONB, as they may occur with cervical medial branch blocks at lower levels, include infection, hematoma formation, and injury to the vertebral artery or the cervical nerve root if the needle is not positioned appropriately.

TABLE 22.1 Results of Prospective Studies on Pulsed Radiofrequency in Occipital Neuralgia

Authors	Study, Number of Patients	Outcome Measures	Results	Comments
Vanelderen et al.[33]	Prospective; 19 patients; PRF after positive response to nerve; 6-month F/U	VAS for pain, Quality of life, Medication Quantification Scale	Mean pain score and medication scale decreased by 3.6 and 8 units, respectively	PRF is a promising treatment of ON
Choi et al.[34]	Prospective; 10 patients; PRF after response to block; mean F/U 7.5 months	VAS for pain, total pain index	Mean VAS and mean total pain index declined by 6 and 192 units, respectively	PRF is an effective treatment for ON
Huang et al.[35]	Retrospective; 102 patients; PRF after positive response to block	50% or greater relief of pain lasting at least 3 months	52 (51%) had ≥50% relief	Five patients had temporary worsening of pain; one patient developed new pain behind ear and cheek, which resolved within 3 weeks

ON, *Occipital neuralgia;* PRF, *pulsed radiofrequency;* VAS, *visual analog score.*
No complications noted in the studies.

OCCIPITAL NEURALGIA

According to the ICHD, occipital neuralgia is coded separately under cranial neuralgias.[8] It is discussed because of its relevance to cervicogenic headaches.

The diagnostic criteria include the following:

1. Paroxysmal stabbing pain, with or without persistent aching between paroxysms, in the distribution(s) of the greater, lesser, and/or third occipital nerves
2. Tenderness over the affected nerve
3. Pain is eased temporarily by local anesthetic block of the nerve

Occipital neuralgia was long thought to be the result of entrapment of the greater occipital nerve as it emerges from the trapezius muscle. However, surgical nerve release gives only short-term relief in about 80% of cases, while nerve excision provides short-term relief in about 70% of patients.[26,27] Occipital neuralgia must be distinguished from occipital referral of pain from the atlanto-axial or upper zygapophyseal joints or from tender trigger points in neck muscles or their insertions.[8]

The greater occipital nerve is the terminal branch of the dorsal ramus of C2 with contribution from C3, while the lesser occipital nerve is a branch of the dorsal ramus of C3 with contributions from C2. Segmental nerve blocks at C2 and C3 may be necessary to make the diagnosis in some cases.[28]

Cryoneurolysis, radiofrequency ablation, and more permanent neuroablative approaches such as dorsal rhizotomy at C1–C3 and partial posterior rhizotomy at C1–C3 showed variable responses.[29–32] Recently, there has been a growing interest in pulsed radiofrequency (PRF) for the treatment of intractable occipital neuralgia. To date, there are two prospective studies and one retrospective multicenter study with promising results (Table 22.1).[33–35] However, the lack of randomized controlled studies and the variation in the technique with landmark versus imaging guidance limit the wide application of this treatment modality.

OCCIPITAL NEUROSTIMULATION

Percutaneous occipital nerve stimulation (ONS), unlike neuroablative techniques, offer the potential for a minimally invasive, low risk, and reversible approach to managing occipital neuralgia, chronic migraine, cluster headaches,

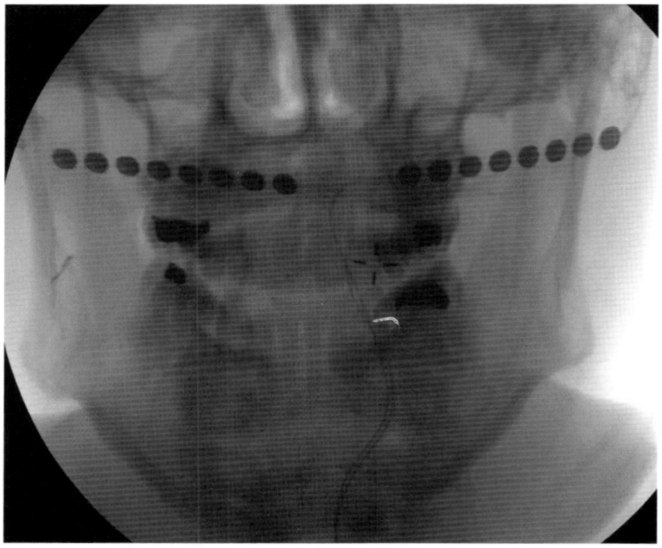

FIG. 22.7 Anteroposterior view showing bilateral occipital surgical leads. *(Reprinted with permission from Ohio Pain and Headache Institute.)*

and other types of intractable primary headaches.[36–38] PET scan studies showed increased regional cerebral blood flow in areas involved in central neuromodulation in chronic migraine patients treated with occipital nerve electrical stimulation.[39] A percutaneous trial of peripheral nerve stimulation is performed using subcutaneous electrodes placed superficial to the cervical muscular fascia at the level of the C1 or the nuchal line. If effective, a permanent implant may be performed using the same electrode lead type or paddle-type surgical lead and attached to a pulse generator implanted in the infraclavicular area, abdomen, flank, or upper buttock (Figs. 22.7 to 22.9).

The occipital nerve stimulation for the treatment of intractable migraine (ONSTIM) trial, examined the safety and efficacy of ONS (Table 22.2).[40] It is a multicenter prospective randomized single-blind controlled feasibility study. Patients who responded favorably to ONB were randomized (2:1:1) into three groups: adjustable stimulation (AS), preset stimulation (PS), or medical management (MM). Those who did not respond to ONB formed an

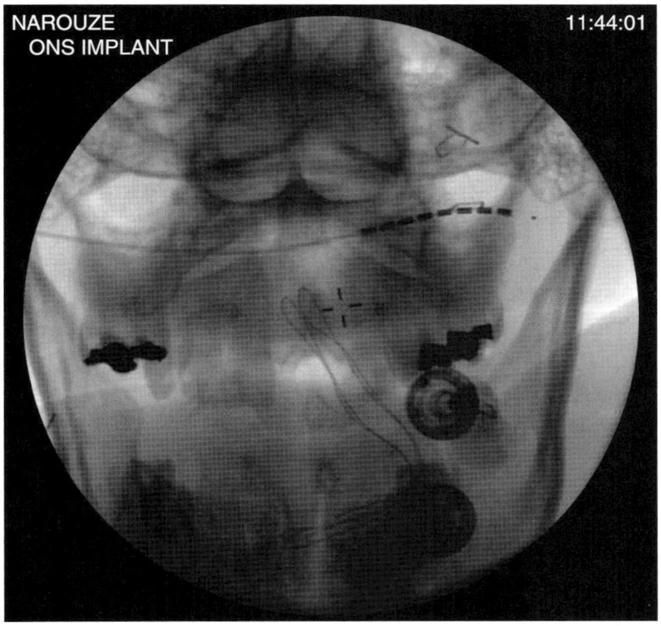

FIG. 22.8 Anteroposterior view showing right occipital percutaneous lead. *(Reprinted with permission from Ohio Pain and Headache Institute.)*

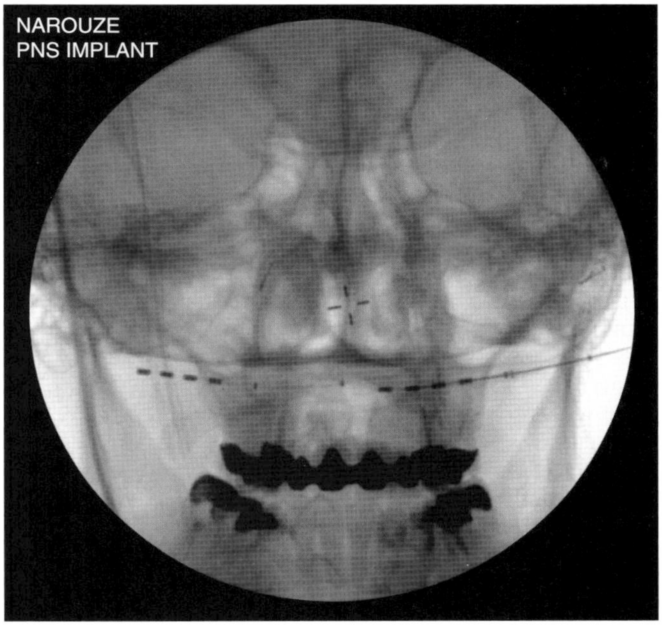

FIG. 22.9 Anteroposterior view showing bilateral occipital self-anchoring leads. *(Reprinted with permission from Ohio Pain and Headache Institute.)*

TABLE 22.2 Randomized Studies on Occipital Nerve Stimulation for Chronic Migraine

Authors	Study, Number of Patients	Outcome Measures	Results	Comments
Saper et al.[40]	Randomized, blinded, controlled, multicenter, feasibility study; (AS-28 patients), (PS-16 patients), or (MM-17 patients) groups.	Responder defined as ≥50% reduction in number of days per month, ≥3-point decrease in average overall pain intensity compared with baseline. POMS and SF-36 also used.	Three-month responder rates were 39% for AS, 6% for PS, and 0% for MM groups, respectively. 66% in AS and 25% in PS groups reported satisfaction with treatment.	Feasibility offers promise for ONS for chronic migraine.
Silberstein et al.[41]	Randomized, blinded, controlled, multicenter study (active, n = 105 or sham, n = 52)	Percent of responders (≥50% relief) at 12 weeks.	No difference in the percent of responders; significant difference in the % of patients who had 30% relief; significant difference in number of headache days, migraine-related disability, and direct reports of pain relief.	Significant reduction in pain, headache days, and migraine-related disability. Most adverse event was implant site pain.

AS, *Adjustable stimulation;* MM, *medical management;* ONS, *occipital nerve stimulation;* POMS, *profile of mood states;* PS, *preset stimulation.*

ancillary group (AG). There were 110 patients enrolled from 9 centers, and 66 subjects completed diary data during 3-month follow-up. At 3 months, percent reduction in headache days/month was 27.0% (AS), 8.8% (PS) (P = .132), 4.4% (MM) (P = .058), 39.9% (AG) (P = .566). Responder rate was 39% (AS), 6% (PS) (P = .032), 0% (MM) (P = .003), and 40% (AG) (P = 1.000).

More recently, another prospective, multicenter, double-blind, controlled study of ONS in patients with chronic migraine (CM) was conducted.[41] There were 157 patients from 15 centers enrolled and randomized (2:1) to either a stimulation trial followed by device implantation and active stimulation for 12 weeks (n = 105) or a stimulation trial followed by device implantation but sham stimulation for 12 weeks (n = 52). After 12 weeks, subjects were unblinded, but patients were followed up for 1 year (see Table 22.2). There was a significant difference in the percentage of patients that achieved a 30% reduction in daily visual analog scale scores (P = .01). There were significant group differences for all assessments at 12 weeks ($P < .01$).

The most frequent complication of the ONS is lead migration. Various anchoring techniques were described to improve lead stability; however, the problem persists.[38]

In one review, lead migration was found to be 33% and 60% 6 months and 1 year postimplant, respectively.[42] The ONSTIM study reported lead migration in 24% of subjects.[40] The use of self-anchoring leads (e.g., tined leads) looks promising.[37] In a series of 12 patients, only one patient had lead migration of a few millimeters with little change in the stimulation pattern, and there was no loss of efficacy.[43] None of 12 patients required a surgical revision for lead migration during a mean follow-up period of 13 months. Unlike spinal cord stimulation, wound dehiscence and infection carry a lower morbidity risk, although this usually requires total system explant.

C2 NEURALGIA

C2 neuralgia is a distinctive type of occipital neuralgia and it is caused by lesions affecting the C2 nerve root or dorsal ganglion such as neuroma, meningioma, or anomalous vessels.[44,45] The C2 root lies posterior to the lateral atlanto-axial joint; thus, disorders or inflammation of this joint may lead to irritation or entrapment of the nerve root.[46] C2 neuralgia manifests as intermittent lancinating occipital pain that is associated with lacrimation, ciliary injection, and rhinorrhea. Abolition of pain by selective C2 nerve root block is essential to make the diagnosis. C2 neuralgia that responds poorly to pharmacotherapy and/or thermocoagulation, decompression, or C2 ganglionectomy may be indicated.[9]

CERVICAL MYOFASCIAL PAIN

Trigger points in the posterior neck muscles, especially the trapezius, sternocleidomastoid, and splenius capitis, have been proposed as a cause of headaches.[47,48] According to the 3rd edition of the ICHD, headache causally associated with cervical myofascial tender spots is coded as episodic or chronic tension-type headache associated with pericranial tenderness.[8]

Moreover, these tender points usually overlie the zygapophyseal joints, so it is difficult to be distinguished from underlying painful joints.[9] Needling therapies in the management of myofascial pain showed no efficacy beyond that of placebo.[49] The use of botulinum toxin is controversial. It might be effective in the management of migraine and chronic daily headaches; however, its efficacy in myofascial pain and cervicogenic headaches is still debated.[50–52]

CERVICAL DISCOGENIC PAIN

C2–C3 provocative discography, but not at the lower levels, can reproduce cervicogenic headache.[53] Radiofrequency lesioning was shown to be effective in obtaining some pain relief for a few months in one study.[54] However, cervical disc interventions are not commonly performed because of the potential for serious complications.

SUMMARY

Cervicogenic headache is one of the most debatable and challenging areas in headache medicine. Patients usually benefit the most from a multidisciplinary approach incorporating physical therapy, pharmacotherapy, psychotherapy (biofeedback and relaxation therapy), alternative medicine (acupuncture), and the judicious utilization of interventional pain management modalities.

KEY POINTS

- Cervicogenic headache is referred pain from cervical structures innervated by the upper cervical spinal nerves.
- The lateral atlanto-axial joint, which is innervated by the C2 ventral ramus, is not an uncommon cause of cervicogenic headache. It may account for 16% of patients with occipital headache.
- C2–C3 zygapophyseal joint is innervated by the third occipital nerve. Pain stemming from this joint (named third occipital headache) was seen in 27% of patients presenting with cervicogenic headache after whiplash injury.
- Third occipital radiofrequency neurolysis is effective in the treatment of headache stemming from the C2–C3 joint
- Occipital neuralgia is a paroxysmal stabbing pain, with or without persistent aching between paroxysms, in the distribution(s) of the greater, lesser, and/or third occipital nerves
- Occipital neuralgia must be distinguished from occipital referral of pain from the atlanto-axial or upper zygapophyseal joints or from tender trigger points in neck muscles or their insertions.
- ONS showed promising results in the treatment of intractable headaches.

REFERENCES

Access the reference list online at ExpertConsult.com.

CHAPTER 23

OROFACIAL PAIN

Samer Narouze, MD, PhD ✪ Jason E. Pope, MD

INTRODUCTION

The incidence and prevalence of orofacial pain in the general population is very high. Care and emphasis should be placed on correct diagnosis and treatment rather than on symptomatic management. Each disorder is described according to the International Classification of Headache Disorders, 3rd edition (ICHD-3) classification and diagnostic criteria. The pathophysiology of the disorder, the clinical picture, and the management (both medical and interventional if applicable) are reviewed.

The ICHD-3 criteria provide a systematic classification for headache and orofacial pain and are divided into three parts: the primary headaches, the secondary headaches, and cranial neuralgias central and primary facial pain (Table 23.1).[1]

We largely discuss sections 11 and 13 of the ICHD-3. However, before considering the diagnoses that are commonly attributed to orofacial pain, it is relevant to provide a brief comment on eliciting the key components of the history and physical examination in the evaluation of headache and orofacial pain. It is important to take a stepwise, systematic approach to the patient's pain. This requires a fundamental knowledge of the ICHD-3 criteria. It should be noted that in one series of 97 consecutive patients presenting to a tertiary care neurologic facility, 29% were not classifiable using the ICHD criteria.[2]

An appropriate physical examination includes a thorough neurologic assessment (including gait, pronator drift, Romberg sign, reflex testing; Hoffman and Babinski signs), heart and carotid auscultation, fundoscopic examination, cervical range of motion (ROM including atlanto-axial and atlanto-occiptial joint), a musculoskeletal evaluation with careful detail to myofascial tenderness and trigger points, maneuvers that provoke radicular signs (Spurling test), cervical facet examination, and Waddell signs of nonorganic pain (tenderness to palpation, stimulation, distraction, regional disturbance in function, and overreaction). Tables 23.2 and 23.3 list the ominous findings and characteristics indicating the need for neuroimaging evaluation, respectively.[3]

ANATOMY AND PATHOPHYSIOLOGY

The trigeminal system provides the relay system for pain and touch sensation to the face and motor function to the muscles of mastication. The trigeminal system is a bilateral structure that spans from the midbrain to the medulla and is composed of four nuclei: the mesencephalic nucleus, the main sensory nucleus, a spinal nucleus of cranial nerve (CN) V, and the motor nucleus. The caudal portion of the trigeminal system nucleus is referred to as the spinal nucleus of CN V and is composed of three regions, in cephalad to caudal order: the subnucleus oralis, the subnucleus interplaris, and the subnucleus caudalis. The subnucleus caudalis is very similar in structure and function to the dorsal horn and extends down to the second or third cervical level. The primary afferent synapses ipsilaterally in the nucleus caudalis and the second order neuron crosses to join the contralateral spinothalamic tract. The trigeminal pathway is termed the ventral trigeminothalamic tract and terminates in the ventral posteromedial (VPM) nucleus of the thalamus.

Activation of nuclei near the trigeminocervical complex may explain the associated aura and symptoms attributed to different headache disorders by either activation of wide dynamic neurons, ephaptic transmission, or by sheer proximity to the complex (solitary nucleus, nucleus ambiguous, or dorsal nucleus of vagus nerve).

Goadsby demonstrated the trigeminocervical convergence mechanism. He electrically stimulated the superior sagittal sinus of adult monkeys, and C-fos was expressed in the superficial laminae of the dorsal horn of C1 and C2 but not in C3.[4]

Anthony examined patients with occipital headache, and he summarized that "projection of pain…overlap between trigeminal nucleus and upper cervical cord…form a column of cells forming the posterior horn…to C4."[5] Consequently, the trigeminocervical complex with the hypothesized reciprocal interactions described by Goadsby

TABLE 23.1 International Classification of Headache Disorders, 3rd Edition Classification Headings

Part I: The Primary Headaches
1. Migraine
2. Tension-type headache
3. Cluster headache and other trigeminal autonomic cephalalgias
4. Other primary headaches
Part II: The Secondary Headaches
5. Headache attributed to trauma or injury to the head and/or neck
6. Headache attributed to cranial or cervical vascular disorder
7. Headache attributed to nonvascular intracranial disorder
8. Headache attributed to a substance or its withdrawal
9. Headache attributed to infection
10. Headache attributed to disorder of homoeostasis
11. Headache or facial pain attributed to disorder of cranium, neck, eyes, ears, nose, sinuses, teeth, mouth or other facial or cranial structure
12. Headache attributed to psychiatric disorder
Part III: Painful Cranial Neuropathies, Other Facial Pains and Other Headaches
13. Painful cranial neuropathies and other facial pains
14. Other headache disorders

TABLE 23.2 Headache With "Red Flag" Symptoms and Signs That Require Further Work-Up

Sudden onset of headache (thunderclap headache)
Fever, rash, and/or stiff neck associated with the headache
Papilledema (optic nerve head swelling)
Dizziness, unsteadiness, dysarthria, weakness, or changes in sensation (numbness or tingling) especially if profound, static, and occurring for the first time
Migraine auras or other previously experienced neurologic migraine accompaniments lasting longer than 1 h
Presence of confusion, drowsiness, or loss of consciousness
Headache is triggered by exertion, coughing, bending, or sexual activity
Headache is progressively worsening and/or resistant to treatment
Previously experienced headache characteristics or accompaniments have substantially changed
Persistent or severe vomiting accompanies the headache
Headaches beginning after age of 50 are associated with a higher risk of arteritis or intracranial tumors. Inquire about unexplained weight loss, sweats, fevers, myalgia, arthralgia, and jaw claudication, which are typical accompaniments of giant cell (temporal) arteritis
Headache occurring in a patient with human immunodeficiency virus or cancer
Frequent emergency department or acute care use
Daily or near-daily use of pain relievers or the need to take more than the recommended dosage of pain relievers to control headache symptoms

TABLE 23.3 Indications for Neuroimaging in Headaches

Urgent
Thunderclap headache with neurologic deficit
Headache with altered mental status or seizure
Prior intervention (if suspect reduced intracranial compliance focal defects, meningismus)
Routine
Thunderclap headache without focal neurologic deficit
Change in headache characteristics (severity, side-shift, worsening)
Headache accompanied by neurologic deficit or abnormality (disequilibrium, pronator drift, weakness, papilledema)
Headache in immunocompromised patients, cancer patients

appear to introduce potential neuromodulatory/ablative sites for a variety of headache disorders in contrast to the accepted headache generator foci (Table 23.4).

HEADACHE ATTRIBUTED TO DISORDER OF CRANIAL BONE

The diagnostic criteria include pain in one or more regions in the head and face with clinical, laboratory, or imaging evidence of a lesion within the cranial bone known to be a valid evidence of generating headache. The source of the pain must be in close temporal association

TABLE 23.4 Secondary Headaches or Facial Pain Attributed to Disorder of Facial and Cranial Structures

ICHD-3	Diagnosis
11	Headache or facial pain attributed to disorder of the cranium, neck, eyes, ears, nose, sinuses, teeth, mouth or other facial or cervical structure
11.1	*Headache attributed to disorder of cranial bone*
11.2	*Headache attributed to disorder of neck*
11.2.1	Cervicogenic headache
11.2.2	Headache attributed to retropharyngeal tendonitis
11.2.3	Headache attributed to craniocervical dystonia
11.3	*Headache attributed to disorder of eyes*
11.3.1	Headache attributed to acute glaucoma
11.3.2	Headache attributed to refractive errors
11.3.3	Headache attributed to heterophoria or heterotropia (latent or manifest squint)
11.3.4	Headache attributed to ocular inflammatory disorder
11.4	*Headache attributed to disorder of ears*
11.5	*Headache attributed to disorder of the nose or paranasal sinuses*
11.6	*Headache attributed to disorder of teeth or jaw*
11.7	*Headache or facial pain attributed to temporomandibular disorder (TMD)*
11.8	*Head or facial pain attributed to inflammation of the stylohyoid ligament*
11.9	*Headache or facial pain attributed to other disorder of cranium, neck, eyes, ears, nose, sinuses, teeth, mouth or other facial or cervical structure*

to and be maximal over the bone lesion and with resolution of the pain after successful treatment of the bone lesion. Most disorders of the skull are not painful with the exception of osteomyelitis, multiple myeloma, and Paget disease.

HEADACHE ATTRIBUTED TO DISORDER OF NECK

These constellations of disorders involve pain referral from neck structures to the head/and or face. The diagnostic criteria hinges on what is excepted as "being generally accepted as a valid cause of headache."

CERVICOGENIC HEADACHE

Cervicogenic headache is pain attributed to a disorder or lesion within the cervical spine or soft tissues that is generally accepted to cause headache or facial pain (see Chapter 22).

RETROPHARYNGEAL TENDONITIS

Retropharyngeal tendonitis (also called longus colli tendonitis) is described as either unilateral or bilateral nonpulsatile pain in the posterior neck radiating to the occiput or entire head accompanied by swollen prevertebral soft tissue measuring greater than 7 mm in adults anterior to the upper cervical vertebral bodies. The pain is exacerbated by neck extension and less commonly with neck rotation and swallowing. The transverse process of the upper three vertebral bodies is tender to palpation. The pain is alleviated within 2 weeks of treatment with antiinflammatory medications. Imaging studies are needed to exclude carotid dissection and in some cases CT aspiration of amorphous calcific material from the swollen periverterbal tissues.[6]

Acute retropharyngeal tendinitis typically occurs in the third through sixth decade of life and presents as a triad of neck pain, odynophagia, and fever. Treatment is usually conservative and includes nonsteroidal antiinflammatory drugs (NSAIDs) or a short course of corticosteroids and it is self-limited in most cases.[7,8]

CRANIOCERVICAL DYSTONIA

Craniocervical dystonia (CCD) is characterized by crampy or "tension-type pain" in the posterior neck radiating to the occiput or entire head accompanied by defective posture of the head or neck due to muscular hyperactivity. The pain is exacerbated by muscle contraction, movement, external pressure, or sustained posture. The pain resolves within 3 months of successful treatment of the underlying muscle hyperactivity. These dystonias include pharyngeal dystonia, spasmodic torticollis, mandibular dystonia, or lingual dystonia.[9]

The prevalence of CCD was estimated to be 1.1–6.1 per 100,000 people with an incidence of 1.1 per 100,000 per year.[10,11] Studies on the pathophysiology of CCD suggest functional defects in dopamine signaling.[12] Treatment involves physical therapy, muscle relaxants, and botulinum toxin injections.

HEADACHE ATTRIBUTED TO RHINOSINUSITIS

This is a secondary cause of frontal headache and pain in one or more region of the face, ears, or teeth that is accompanied by clinical, radiographic, endoscopic, or laboratory evidence of acute rhinosinusitis (Fig. 23.1). Clinical causes include purulence within the nasal cavity, nasal obstruction, new-onset hyposmia/anosmia, and/or fever. The headache/facial pain onset must be congruent with the acute rhinosinusitis and must resolve within 7 days after remission or successful treatment. Conditions that are not considered as causing this headache include deviated septum, nasal turbinate hypertrophy, and sinus membrane atrophy. Chronic sinusitis is not validated as a cause of headache or facial pain unless there is an underlying acute exacerbation.

HEADACHE ATTRIBUTED TO DISORDER OF TEETH, JAWS, OR RELATED STRUCTURES

Disorders of the teeth, jaws, or related structures typically cause toothache and facial pain, and less commonly headache. Pain from the teeth may be referred and cause diffuse headache, as in periodontitis or pericoronitis because of infection or traumatic irritation around the wisdom teeth. The pain is both temporally and structurally related to a disorder of the teeth and/or jaw and is relieved within 3 months of successful treatment of the underlying pathology.

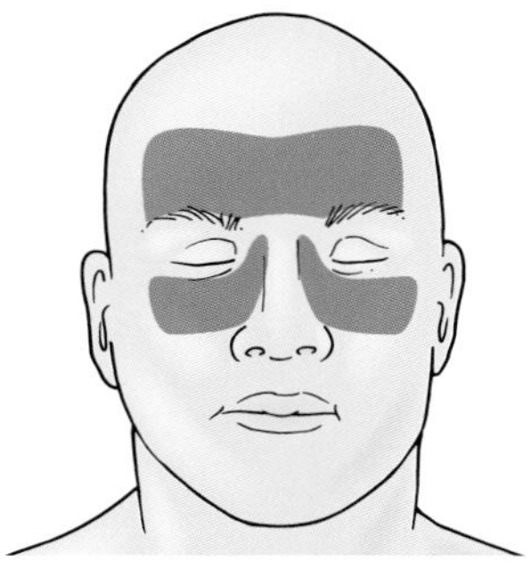

FIG. 23.1 Paranasal sinus.

Acute periodontal nociceptive pain is treated with rest (reduced mechanical stimulation), NSAIDs, topical local anesthetics, and analgesics. Chronic periodontal disease is an immune-mediated inflammatory process that results in destruction of the teeth and the surrounding anchoring bone.[13]

Typically, intraoral lesions are self-limited and resolve within a few weeks. If symptoms persist, dental, or ENT referral is warranted. Some common painful mucosal conditions are listed in Table 23.5.

HEADACHE OR FACIAL PAIN ATTRIBUTED TO TEMPOROMANDIBULAR DISORDER

This is characterized by recurrent pain in one or more regions of the head/face from the temporomandibular joint (TMJ). It is precipitated by jaw movements, chewing, decreased or irregular range of motion, and TMJ tenderness that resolves within 3 months after successful treatment of TMJ disorder. These disorders include disc displacements, osteoarthritis, or joint hypermobility, rheumatoid arthritis, and can be associated with myofascial pain and headache.

The TMJ is a bicondylar joint that contributes to the important functions of mastication and speech. The joint is unique in that the articular surface is covered by fibrocartilage instead of hyaline cartilage. A fibrocartilaginous disc is located between the condyle and the articular fossa and separates the joint cavity into the superior and inferior compartment.[15]

Intracapsular disorders include rheumatoid arthritis, osteoarthritis, and articular disc displacement (Fig. 23.2), while extracapsular disorders include myofascial masticatory pain (Fig. 23.3). Bruxism is hypothesized to contribute to TMJ pain secondary to myofascial strain, tooth attrition, capsulitis, and adhesion formation.

Radiographic examination is usually not helpful. However, when severe symptoms persist after failure of conservative management (splints), periapical radiographs, CT, or MRI is warranted. MRI should not dictate therapy, as asymptomatic individuals have evidence of disc displacement.

Treatment includes management of any secondary causes such as infection, relief of somatization component (stress,

TABLE 23.5 Common Intraoral Causes of Oral Pain[14]

Category	Condition
Infections	Herpetic stomatitis Varicella zoster Candidiasis Acute necrotizing gingivostomatitis
Immune/autoimmune	Allergic reactions (toothpaste, mouthwashes, topical medications) Erosive lichen planus Benign mucous membrane pemphigoid Aphthous stomatitis and aphthous lesions Erythema multiforme Graft-versus-host disease
Traumatic and iatrogenic injuries	Factitial, accidental (burns: chemical, solar, thermal) Self-destructive behaviors (rituals, obsessive behaviors) Iatrogenic (chemotherapy, radiation)
Neoplasia	Squamous cell carcinoma Mucoepidermoid carcinoma Adenocystic carcinoma Intracranial tumors
Neurologic	Burning mouth syndrome and glossodynia Neuralgias Postviral neuralgias Posttraumatic neuropathies Dyskinesias and dystonias
Nutritional and metabolic	Vitamin deficiencies (B_{12}, folate) Mineral deficiencies (iron) Diabetic neuropathy Malabsorption syndromes
Miscellaneous	Xerostomia, secondary to intrinsic or extrinsic conditions Referred pain from esophageal or oropharyngeal malignancy Mucositis secondary to esophageal reflux Angioedema

Adapted from Mehta NR, Scrivani SJ, Maciewicz R: Dental and facial pain. In Benzon HT, Rathmell JP, Wu CL, Turk DC, Argoff CE, editors: Raj's Practical Management of Pain, *ed 4, Philadelphia: Mosby/Elsevier, 2008, pp 505-528.*

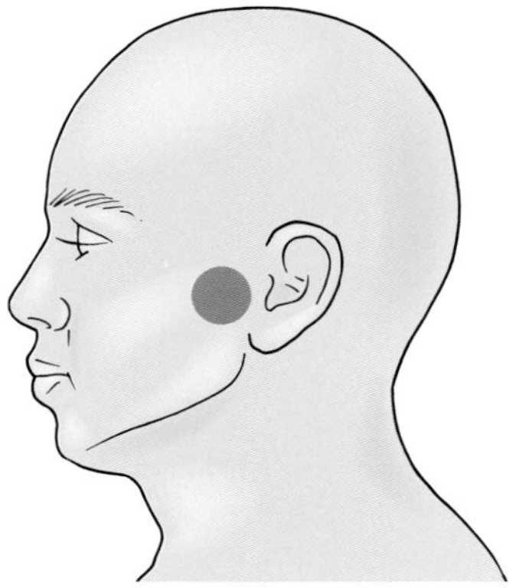

FIG. 23.2 Temporomandibular joint articular disorders.

anxiety), elimination of nocturnal clinching, jaw exercises, and pharmacologic therapy (muscle relaxants, neuropathic pain medications, and antiinflammatory medications). Local anesthetic/steroid and/or botulinum toxin injections

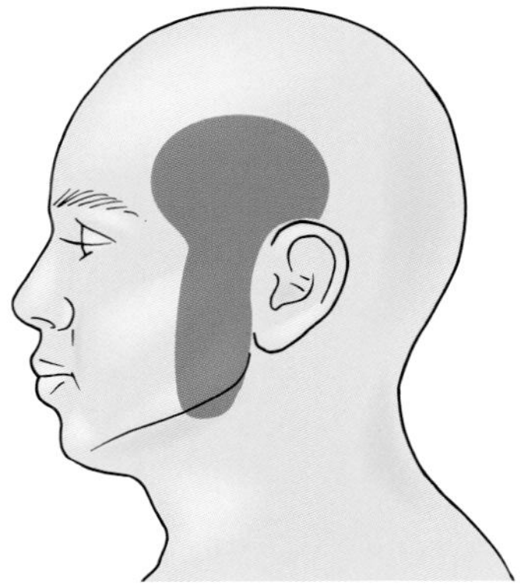

FIG. 23.3 Temporomandibular muscle disorders.

may be indicated in selected cases.[16–18] Surgery should be considered in patients who do not respond to conservative treatment if anatomic disruption is noted.[15] The procedures include total and partial meniscectomy, disc repair, lysis of adhesions, lavage, and in rare instances total joint arthroplasty.[15,19] Total TMJ replacement has a poor outcome.

CRANIAL NEURALGIAS AND CENTRAL CAUSES OF FACIAL PAIN AND OTHER HEADACHES

These headache and facial pain disorders are the most recognized causes of severe morbidity and none more so than trigeminal neuralgia. Table 23.6 allows for a coherent approach to the cranial neuralgias, and we focus on the disorders that can elicit oral and facial pain.

TRIGEMINAL NEURALGIA

Trigeminal neuralgia is the most common form of facial neuropathic pain in elderly people. The incidence of trigeminal neuralgia is 4–5/100,000 people, with approximately 15,000 new cases annually in the United States. Females are 1.5 times more likely to have trigeminal neuralgia then men.[20,21]

The ICHD-3 beta version describes trigeminal neuralgia as either "classical trigeminal neuralgia" or "painful trigeminal neuropathy" (see Table 23.6).

CLASSIC TRIGEMINAL NEURALGIA

This type was previously termed Tic douloureux, primary trigeminal neuralgia, and idiopathic trigeminal neuralgia.

Pathophysiology

Classical trigeminal neuralgia is caused by neurovascular compression, most frequently by the superior cerebellar artery. Most patients have compression of the trigeminal root by tortuous or aberrant vessels as evident by posterior fossa exploration and magnetic resonance imaging (MRI). Imaging should be done to exclude secondary causes. If there is a causative lesion identified, outside of vascular compression, then trigeminal neuralgia is secondary, or "painful trigeminal neuropathy."

TABLE 23.6 Secondary Headaches Attributed to Cranial Neuralgias and Central Causes of Facial Pain

ICHD-3	Diagnosis
13	Painful cranial neuropathies and other facial pains
13.1	*Trigeminal neuralgia*
13.1.1	Classical trigeminal neuralgia
13.1.1.1	Classical trigeminal neuralgia, purely paroxysmal
13.1.1.2	Classical trigeminal neuralgia with concomitant persistent facial pain
13.1.2	Painful trigeminal neuropathy
13.1.2.1	Painful trigeminal neuropathy attributed to acute Herpes zoster
13.1.2.2	Postherpetic trigeminal neuropathy
13.1.2.3	Painful posttraumatic trigeminal neuropathy
13.1.2.4	Painful trigeminal neuropathy attributed to multiple sclerosis (MS) plaque
13.1.2.5	Painful trigeminal neuropathy attributed to space-occupying lesion
13.1.2.6	Painful trigeminal neuropathy attributed to other disorder
13.2	*Glossopharyngeal neuralgia*
13.3	*Nervus intermedius (facial nerve) neuralgia*
13.4	*Occipital neuralgia*
13.5	*Optic neuritis*
13.6	*Headache attributed to ischaemic ocular motor nerve palsy*
13.7	*Tolosa-Hunt syndrome*
13.8	*Paratrigeminal oculosympathetic (Raeder) syndrome*
13.9	*Recurrent painful ophthalmoplegic neuropathy*
13.10	*Burning mouth syndrome (BMS)*
13.11	*Persistent idiopathic facial pain (PIFP)*
13.12	*Central neuropathic pain*
13.12.1	*Central neuropathic pain attributed to multiple sclerosis (MS)*
13.12.2	*Central poststroke pain (CPSP)*

Description

Classic trigeminal neuralgia is a unilateral disorder characterized by brief electric shocklike pains, abrupt in onset and termination, and limited to the distribution of one or more divisions of the trigeminal nerve. Pain is commonly evoked by trivial stimuli including washing, shaving, smoking, talking, and teeth brushing (trigger factors). Small areas in the nasolabial fold and/or chin may be particularly susceptible to the precipitation of pain (trigger areas). It also frequently occurs spontaneously. The pain usually remits for variable periods.

Diagnostic Criteria

A. At least three attacks of unilateral facial pain fulfilling criteria B and C
B. Occurring in one or more divisions of the trigeminal nerve, with no radiation beyond the trigeminal distribution.
C. Pain has at least three of the following four characteristics:
   1. Recurring in paroxysmal attacks lasting from a fraction of a second to 2 minutes
   2. Severe intensity
   3. Electric shocklike, shooting, stabbing, or sharp in quality
   4. Precipitated by innocuous stimuli to the affected side of the face
D. No clinically evident neurological deficits
E. Not better accounted for by another ICHD-3 diagnosis.

Clinical Presentation

- Classic trigeminal neuralgia usually starts in the second or third divisions (V2–V3), affecting the cheek or the chin. In less than 5% of patients, the first division (V1) is affected. Involvement of the V1 hints towards a postherpetic neuralgia
- The pain is strictly unilateral, with right side more than the left at a ratio of 3:2. It may rarely occur bilaterally, in which case, a central cause such as *multiple sclerosis* must be considered, especially in young females.
- Following a painful paroxysm, there is usually a refractory period during which pain cannot be triggered. The pain often evokes spasm of the muscle of the face on the affected side *(tic douloureux)*.
- Neurological examination is essentially normal in patients with classic trigeminal neuralgia. This is different from patients with secondary trigeminal neuralgia where there are some neurological deficits. In such cases, trigeminal neuralgia is a symptom of another disease, for example, multiple sclerosis or cerebellopontine angle neoplasm.
- Mild autonomic symptoms such as lacrimation and/or redness of the eye may be present.
- Between paroxysms, most patients are asymptomatic. However, in a subtype of the classical trigeminal neuralgia with concomitant persistent facial pain, there is prolonged background pain in the affected area. This has been referred to as "atypical trigeminal neuralgia" or "trigeminal neuralgia type 2." This type of trigeminal neuralgia (TN) responds poorly to conservative treatment and to neurosurgical interventions.

Management of Classic Trigeminal Neuralgia

Treatment centers on prevention and abortive therapy. There have been few systematic reviews describing treatment approaches.[22–24] Trigeminal neuralgia usually responds to pharmacotherapy and should be employed before interventions are attempted. Generally, after patients fail conservative treatment, young patients with MRI evidence of vascular compression should be considered for microvascular decompression. Elderly patients or those with no evidence of vascular compression may be a candidate for gamma knife or radiofrequency thermoablation. Conservative treatment strategies include antidepressants and antiepileptics. First-line therapy is carbamazepine or oxycarbamazepine, while second-line treatment is baclofen. Other neuropathic pain medications have been trialed in treatment, but there has been no clear evidence

TABLE 23.7 Interventional Approaches to Trigeminal Neuralgia

A. Surgical Approaches	
Microvascular decompression (MVD)	The vessels in contact with the trigeminal root entry zone are coagulated or separated from the nerve using an inert sponge[25]
B. Percutaneous Approaches	
Gamma knife	Stereotactic radiation therapy: high-dose irradiation of a small section of the trigeminal nerve leading to nonselective damage[26]
Percutaneous balloon microcompression	Pressure-induced ischemia. The technique may be more suitable for treatment of V1 trigeminal neuralgia of the first branch as the corneal reflex tends to remain intact[27,28]
Percutaneous glycerol rhizolysis	Under fluoroscopy, predetermined volume of glycerol is injected for neurolysis[29]
Percutaneous radiofrequency thermocoagulation	This is usually considered for the elderly patient who is high risk for surgical MVD. The outcome may be less favorable than MVD, but it is less invasive with lower morbidity and mortality rates[22]
Pulsed radiofrequency ablation	Although it would seem a safer alternative than the commonly used thermal RFA, its efficacy is questioned in a randomized controlled study[30]
C. Neuromodulation	
Gasserian ganglion Neuromodulation	Stimulation was reported either via a subtemporal craniotomy,[31] or a percutaneous approach[32]

for efficacy.[22] The interventional modalities of treatment include decompressive, ablative, and neuromodulatory strategies using surgical and percutaneous routes (Table 23.7).

GLOSSOPHARYNGEAL NEURALGIA

Glossopharyngeal neuralgia is an uncommon facial pain syndrome characterized by transient severe, sharp, stabbing pain experienced in the ear, base of tongue, tonsillar fossa, or beneath the angle of the jaw. It is unilateral in presentation, lasts for seconds to 2 minutes, and may be precipitated by swallowing, talking, coughing, chewing, or yawning. The incidence is between 0.2% and 1.3% of trigeminal neuralgia and typically begins after the sixth decade.[20] The pain is transmitted via the auricular and pharyngeal branches of the glossopharyngeal nerve, along with the auricular and pharyngeal branches of the vagus nerve. Approximately 2% of patients lose consciousness during the pain paroxysms. If a causative lesion is identified, then the neuralgia is secondary and becomes "symptomatic glossopharyngeal neuralgia."[33]

The glossopharyngeal nerve exits the brain stem and descends through the base of the skull through the jugular foramen. It has contributions from the solitary nucleus, the nucleus ambiguous, and the inferior salivatory nucleus. Its branches include the tympanic, stylopharyngeal, tonsillar, carotid sinus, lingual branches, and communicating branches to the vagus nerve.

Vascular impingement of the nerve roots has been implicated in the pathophysiology of glossopharyngeal neuralgia, commonly microvascular compression by the posterior cerebellar artery.[34] Treatment is primarily conservative medical management with anticonvulsants and analgesics. Refractory cases to conservative management are candidates for surgical or percutaneous treatments, including lesioning and nerve blocks.

NERVUS INTERMEDIUS NEURALGIA (GENICULATE NEURALGIA, RAMSAY-HUNT SYNDROME)

This is a rare disorder characterized by transient bouts of pain in the internal auditory canal, not attributed to any structural lesion, and is intermittent in onset and may last for seconds to minutes. Disorders of salivation, lacrimation, or taste can accompany the pain and are commonly associated with herpes zoster. Typical cases of Ramsay-Hunt Syndrome (RHS) demonstrate the triad of auricular vesicles, ipsilateral facial palsy, and vestibular/cochlear symptoms. Nervus intermedius neuralgia typically occurs after the fifth decade.[34]

The nervus intermedius is part of the facial nerve (cranial nerve VII) and is located between the motor component of the facial nerve and the vestibulocochlear nerve (cranial nerve VIII). It contains sensory branches to external auditory meatus, floor of mouth and palate, and mucosa of nose, and provides taste to the anterior two-thirds of tongue and parasympathetic fibers (superior salivatory nucleus) of the facial nerve. It joins the motor root of the facial nerve in the facial canal at the geniculate ganglion.

Conservative treatment involves the use of neuropathic pain medications, treatment of herpes zoster if RHS is suspected, or surgical decompression.[35]

SUPERIOR LARYNGEAL NEURALGIA

This is characterized by severe pain paroxysms, lasting seconds to minutes, in the lateral aspect of the throat and submandibular region and underneath the ear, precipitated by swallowing, shouting, or turning of the head. A trigger point is identified along the lateral aspect of the ipsilateral hyoid bone or hyothyroid membrane that is relieved by superior laryngeal nerve block, ablation, and/or resection of the superior laryngeal nerve.

The superior laryngeal nerve is a terminal branch of the vagus nerve (cranial nerve X) and receives sympathetic input from the superior cervical ganglion. It divides into the internal and external superior laryngeal nerve (which innervates the cricothyroid muscle). The recurrent laryngeal nerve innervates all other laryngeal muscles, particularly the abductors, and can cause vocal cord paralysis when damaged (injury results in unilateral adduction of vocal cord) and bilaterally can cause airway obstruction.

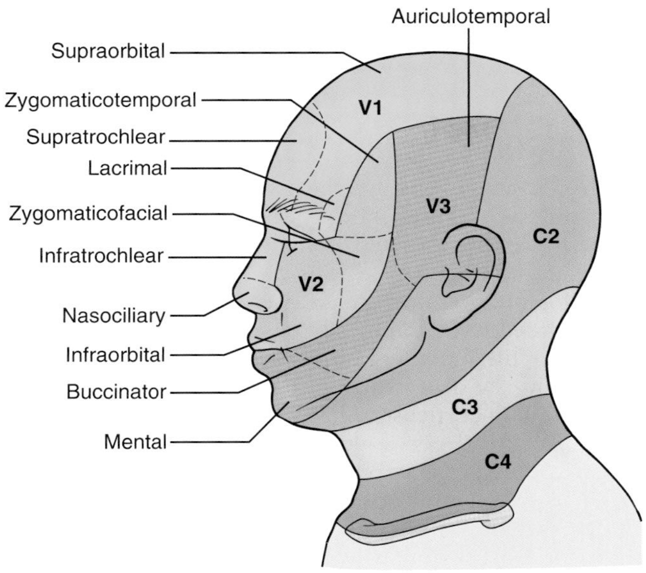

FIG. 23.4 Dermatomes head and neck lateral.

NASOCILIARY NEURALGIA (CHARLIN NEURALGIA)

This is a transient, lancinating pain in the nostril that radiates to medial/frontal region. It lasts seconds to hours. It is precipitated by touching the ipsilateral nostril and abolished by blockade of the nasocilliary nerve.

The nasocilliary nerve is a branch of the ophthalmic nerve (V1) and enters the orbit between the lateral rectus muscles and continues obliquely beneath the superior rectus and superior oblique muscle to the medial wall of the orbital cavity. The terminal branches include the posterior ethmoidal nerve, the long ciliary nerves, the infratrochlear nerve, the communicating branch of the ciliary ganglion, and the anterior ethmoidal nerve.

SUPRAORBITAL NEURALGIA

This pain disorder is characterized by transient or constant pain in the forehead and supraorbital area supplied by the supraorbital nerve (terminal branch of the ophthalmic nerve V1). The pain can be precipitated or reproduced by pressure over the nerve in the supraorbital notch and the diagnosis is confirmed by pain relief with local anesthetic blockade.

OTHER TERMINAL BRANCH NEURALGIAS

These causes of facial pain are usually caused by neuritis of terminal peripheral branches of the trigeminal nerve, exclusive to the nasociliary and supraorbital nerves. Pain is characterized by constant or transient pain in an area innervated by the trigeminal terminal branches. There is tenderness over the affected nerve that is abolished by local anesthetic blockade. The terminal branches of the trigeminal nerve include the infraorbital, lingual, alveolar, or mental nerves (Fig. 23.4).

OCCIPITAL NEURALGIA

Occipital neuralgia is described as paroxysmal stabbing, sharp pain in the distribution of the greater or lesser occipital nerves or third occipital nerve, sometimes accompanied by paresthesia or dysesthesia or tenderness overlying the nerve that is involved. This is discussed in Chapter 22.

CONSTANT PAIN CAUSED BY COMPRESSION, IRRITATION, OR DISTORTION OF CRANIAL NERVES OR UPPER CERVICAL ROOTS BY STRUCTURAL LESIONS

This is described as facial pain or headache attributed to a lesion that directly compromises the afferent nerve fibers mediating pain. The pain is often constant or jabbing in nature and located within the territory supplied by a cranial sensory nerve. There is resolution of the symptoms after decompression or relief of the irritation or distortion of the involved nerve. Anecdotally, facial pain around the ear may represent invasion of lung cancer around the vagus nerve.

OPTIC NEURITIS

Optic neuritis is described as pain behind one or both eyes accompanied by central vision impairment due to a central or paracentral scotoma. It is not caused by compressive lesion but is thought to be due to optic nerve (CNII) inflammation. The onset of pain and visual impairment is separated by less than 1 month, and the pain is self-limited with resolution within 4 weeks. If pain precedes the visual impairment by greater than 4 weeks, then it is classified as "probable optic neuritis." Optic neuritis is often a presenting manifestation of multiple sclerosis.

OCULAR DIABETIC NEUROPATHY

This condition is described as pain around the eye and forehead with paresis of one or more ocular cranial nerves in a patient with diabetes mellitus. Usually, the pain is centered on one eye with pain developing over approximately 2 hours. The cranial nerve paresis is most commonly the third cranial nerve (Oculomotor) and less commonly, the fourth (Trochlear) and sixth (Abducens) cranial nerve. The neuropathy typically develops within 7 days of onset of pain and is not attributed to another disorder. It is important to exclude other causes of cranial nerve palsies, including infection, infarction, hemorrhage, or neoplasm. Consequently, appropriate neuroimaging and perhaps biopsy is warranted.

HEAD OR FACIAL PAIN ATTRIBUTED TO HERPES ZOSTER

Head or facial pain can be caused by herpes zoster. The pain usually precedes the herpetic eruption by less than 7 days, and the pain is congruent with herpetic nerve eruption. Typically, then pain resolves within 3 months. The herpetic zoster affects the trigeminal nerve in approximately

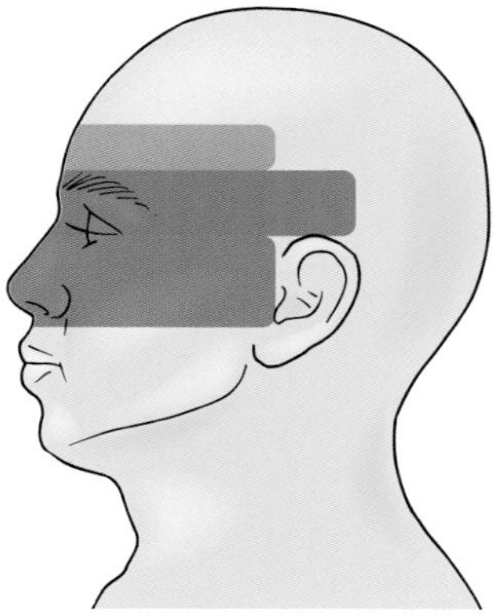

FIG. 23.5 Acute and postherpetic neuralgia.

10% of patients, with the V1 or ophthalmic division most commonly affected (80% of the time) (Fig. 23.5). In contrast, idiopathic trigeminal neuralgia usually affects the V2/3 distribution. Herpetic lesions of the face are not confined to the trigeminal system; it can also involve the geniculate ganglion (causing an eruption near the external auditory meatus). Consequently, ophthalmic herpes can be associated with third, fourth, and six cranial nerve palsies. Zoster can be a harbinger for a more insidious disease process, as it occurs in 10% of patients with lymphoma and 25% of patients with Hodgkin disease.

Postherpetic neuralgia (PHN) is facial pain in the distribution of the affected nerve that persists three months after the skin eruptions. Herpes zoster infection increases with age, with an incidence of 3.4/1000 people per year overall, with greater than 10/1000 in elderly patients over the age of 65.[36] Similarly, it afflicts 50% of patients that have contracted zoster over the age of 60 years and the incidence continues to increase with advanced age.[37]

The pathophysiology of acute herpes zoster correlates with the replication of varicella zoster virus and spread within the dorsal root or ganglion and along the peripheral sensory nerve. It may disseminate locally to adjacent structures, including the spinal cord. The characteristic dermatomal distribution is related to the anatomical or functional disruption of the nervous system. Necrosis of the dorsal root ganglion, the presence of the virus within the nerve elements, and atrophy of the dorsal horn characterize PHN. The exact underlying mechanism remains unclear despite the identified pathological changes, although deafferentation, adrenergic receptor activation, and reduction in presynaptic inhibition may contribute to central sensitization.[38–40]

Management of herpetic pain includes antiviral medications. The more bioavailable medications valaciclovir and famciclovir are more effective than acyclovir[41] in treating acute herpes zoster. The efficacy of steroid use is equivocal. Neuropathic pain medications include anticonvulsants (gabapentin, pregabalin) and antidepressants (amitriptyline, nortriptyline). Other medications commonly employed include topical agents (lidocaine patch), capsacin, opioids, and NMDA antagonists. For a more detailed discussion of the subject, refer to Chapters 28 and 49.

Sympathetic blockade (e.g., stellate ganglion blockade) may be helpful, especially if performed within the first year.[42] In extreme cases, some patients may resort to surgery, including cordotomy, rhizotomy, sympathetcomy, trigeminal tractomy, mesencephalotomy, retrogasserian rhizotomy, or superficial greater petrosal neurotomy.[43]

TOLOSA-HUNT SYNDROME

This syndrome is characterized by episodic orbital pain with paralysis of one or more of the third, fourth, and sixth cranial nerve that resolves spontaneously. Usually, it has a waxing and waning course. The unilateral orbital pain can persist for weeks if untreated. There may be a granuloma demonstrated radiographically or noted via a biopsy. It is a painful ophthalmoplegia, and the pain and paresis occur within 2 weeks of onset and resolve within 72 hours of treatment with corticosteroids. It can also involve divisions of the trigeminal nerve along with the facial, optic, and acoustic nerves. It is important to carefully exclude other causes of the painful ophthalmoplegia including inflammatory (vasculitis, sarcoid), infectious (meningitis), and endocrinologic (diabetes mellitus) causes. It may also be due to cancer (pain is due to a mass effect) or to a primary headache (migraine).

BURNING MOUTH SYNDROME

Pain characterized by an intraoral burning sensation wherein no medical or dental etiology is demonstrated. The mouth pain is daily, persistent for most of the day. Associated symptoms include subjective dryness, mouth, paresthesia, and altered taste.[44] This condition predominately affects woman, and 30%–50% of patients improve spontaneously.

PERSISTENT IDIOPATHIC FACIAL PAIN (ATYPICAL FACE PAIN)

This is facial pain that is present daily and persists for the majority of the day, but does not have features attributed to any of the other cranial neuralgias. It is confined to a poorly defined area of the face and is "deep" in location and not associated with sensory loss or other physical signs. It is not attributed to any other disorder. The pain is commonly in the nasolabial fold or side of the chin and may spread to the upper or lower jaw with a more generalized distribution. It may be triggered by surgery or injury to the face, cheek, or gums. Similar to ophthalmoplegias, atypical face pain can be a harbinger of a disease. Ipsilateral lung carcinoma can be preceded by referred ear, facial, or temple pain secondary to invasion of the vagus nerve.

Education, counseling, and support are essential components of the management strategy. Few reports suggest a role for sphenopalatine ganglion (SPG) block and radiofrequency ablation (RFA) in intractable cases.[45]

CENTRAL NEUROPATHIC FACIAL PAIN

Central causes of facial pain include anesthesia dolorosa, central poststroke pain, facial pain secondary to multiple sclerosis, persistent idiopathic facial pain, and burning mouth syndrome. The pathophysiology is poorly elucidated; however, two processes have been implicated: neuritis with reduction in nerve threshold for a given painful stimulus or a reduction in inhibition from loss of "inhibition."

Characteristically, the pain complaint can vary significantly. The pain may be cramping, constricting, crushing, or shooting/lancinating in character. There may be pins and needles sensation or dysesthesia. Physical examination may show allodynia. Triggering stimuli include extreme temperatures and emotional distress.

ANESTHESIA DOLOROSA

Anesthesia dolorosa is a painful anesthesia or hypesthesia in the distribution of the trigeminal, one of its divisions, or occipital nerve. It is caused by a lesion of the relevant nerve or its central connections and is characterized as persistent pain with diminished sensory loss in the distribution of the nerve. It is often related to surgical trauma via rhizotomy or thermocoagulation of the occipital nerve or the trigeminal ganglion. Anesthesia dolorosa was reported in up to 1.6% and 3% of cases after glycerol rhizotomy and radiofrequency rhizotomy, respectively, in the treatment of trigeminal neuralgia.[22,46,47]

FACIAL PAIN ATTRIBUTED TO MULTIPLE SCLEROSIS

This is characterized by unilateral or bilateral facial pain with or without an associated dysesthesia attributed to a demyelinating lesion in the pons or trigeminothalamic pathway in patients who had multiple sclerosis. In young people with trigeminal neuralgia with side-switch, one needs to be suspicious of multiple sclerosis. Trigeminal neuralgia occurs in 1%–2% of patients with multiple sclerosis (MS).[48]

CENTRAL POSTSTROKE PAIN

Central poststroke pain is a unilateral pain and dysesthesia associated with loss of sensation to pinprick, touch, and temperature of the ipsilateral face. There is usually a history of symptoms suggestive of stroke with a lesion demonstrated radiographically. The pain and dysesthesia develop within 6 months after the stroke, are usually persistent, and are usually attributed to a lesion of the trigeminothalamic pathway, thalamus, or thalamocortical projection. It may affect the trunk and limbs on the ipsilateral or contralateral side. Some estimate prevalence of 8%–11% in patients who had stroke.[49]

CONCLUSION

Oral and facial pain can be an overwhelming complex diagnostic exercise. However, with a careful history and detailed examination, an appropriate treatment plan can be employed. The etiology and complex interrelationships affect the clinical presentation, and the need for a multidisciplinary approach, with the appropriate subspecialty referrals, is crucial for successful treatment.

KEY POINTS

- Diagnosis guides management; an algorithmic approach is necessary to treat patients with headache and facial pain. Accurate diagnosis requires knowledge of the ICHD-3 criteria, and stepwise elimination of primary and secondary headaches.
- Red flags in the history and physical exam require further investigation.
- Treatment centers on preventative and abortive strategies. The appropriate timing for interventional treatment needs to be measured against the severity of impact the pain has on the patient.

REFERENCES

Access the reference list online at ExpertConsult.com.

CHAPTER 24

Overview of Low Back Pain Disorders

Khalid Malik, MD, FRCS ◎ Ariana Nelson, MD

EPIDEMIOLOGY

Low back pain (LBP) is the leading cause of years lived with disability worldwide.[1] In the United States, LBP is the most common reason for lost productivity, workers' compensation claims, and early social security disability benefits. Annually, nearly 50% of adults will have an episode of significant and disabling LBP, which will be protracted in a majority of cases.[2] As a result, poorly controlled LBP is one of the most common motivations for visits to emergency departments and primary care physicians. The economic impact of LBP is exorbitant and consists of direct costs of treatment and indirect costs from lost wages, disability benefits, and litigation fees. The overall annual cost of LBP amounts to over 100 billion dollars in the United States alone.[3,4] Moreover, costs related to LBP have increased immensely in recent decades, mainly due to the availability of new and expensive treatments and an exponential rise in litigation costs and disability benefits paid. Despite the wide availability of treatment options and the enormous cost incurred by this prevalent and disabling health issue, LBP is often poorly controlled and thus remains a significant source of frustration for both sufferers and treating providers. A main contributor to this dissatisfaction is the often concurrent presentation of the various syndromes causing LBP, making diagnosis of a particular or group of etiologies very challenging for the treating physician. Physical exam and imaging studies employed to diagnose LBP syndromes have low sensitivity and specificity and are often incapable of determining the precise source of pain. Additionally, although a wide array of treatments for LBP are available, they are not consistently effective and rarely alter progression of the disease process.

ANATOMY

The majority of LBP originates from the spine and contiguous paraspinal musculature; a basic understanding of spinal anatomy, mechanics, and physiology is therefore crucial to the pain physician. The vertebral column is composed of 7 cervical, 12 thoracic, 5 lumbar, 5 sacral, and 3–5 coccygeal vertebrae. With the exception of the sacral and coccygeal vertebrae, which are ordinarily fused, the two adjacent vertebral bodies (VBs) and the intervening intervertebral disc (IVD) comprise a *vertebral motion segment.* Anteriorly, the linear arrangement of the adjacent vertebral motion segments forms the continuum of the spinal column. The remainder of the spinal column consists of the neural arch, which includes the spinous processes, laminae and the ligamenta flava posteriorly and pedicles, facet joints, and intervertebral foraminae laterally. The neural arch forms the spinal canal, which houses the thecal sac, the layer of fused dura, and arachnoid mater that envelops the spinal cord and nerve roots of the cauda equina. At the most inferior portion of the spinal cord, the conus medullaris, lies the origin of the fibrous filum terminale, which extends to insert on the caudal dura and anchor the cord in the aqueous thecal sac. The spinal cord characteristically ends at the L1–L2 vertebral level, but the thecal sac extends more inferiorly, normally terminating at the S2–S4 level. In addition to the linkage of the VBs by IVDs, each adjacent VB articulates dorsally by way of a pair of synovial joints known as the zygapophysial (facet) joints. The various components of the spinal column also enable attachment of the powerful trunk muscles and spinal ligaments: the ligamentum flavum and the anterior and posterior longitudinal ligaments. A pair of large synovial-fibrous joints, the sacroiliac joints, absorb the tremendous forces transmitted from the spinal column and distribute the pressure equally to the bilateral lower extremities.

The VBs are composed largely of cancellous bone, but this is sheathed in a thin layer of cortical bone. An IVD consists of the outer annulus fibrosus (AF), the inner nucleus pulposus (NP), and vertebral endplates. The distinction between the AF and NP is more pronounced in lower levels of the spinal column but diminishes in cephalad regions and also loses definition with advancing age. Both the NP and the AF consist mainly of an abundant intercellular matrix that is only sparsely populated by cells. The cells contained in the NP are found in clusters and are reminiscent of chondrocytes, whereas cells found in the AF have fibrocytic characteristics.[5] The intercellular matrix composition of the two disc compartments also differs significantly. The NP matrix is gelatinous and has a high concentration of water and proteoglycans, whereas the AF is collagenous and is arranged in interlacing lamellae. These lamellae have increased density in the anterior portion of the disc and are firmly attached to the entire border of each adjacent VB. Although the cancellous VBs and all spinal canal contents are highly vascular, the NP and inner two-thirds of the AF are nearly avascular. The VB endplate cartilage is also avascular and acts as a barrier to separate VB vasculature from the IVDs.

IVDs and the neural canal contents are primarily innervated by nerve plexuses that lie along the anterior longitudinal ligament (ALL) and posterior longitudinal ligament (PLL; Fig. 24.1).[6] The nerve plexus along the ALL receives contributions mainly from the gray rami communicans, while the plexus along the PLL receives the majority of its input from the sinuvertebral nerve with only minimal contributions from the gray rami communicans. At each level, the sinuvertebral nerve originates from the segmental spinal nerve as it exits the intervertebral foramen, reenters the vertebral canal, and receives contributions from the gray rami communicans. The posterior longitudinal ligament plexus innervates the anterior dura and the posterior IVDs. The gray rami communicans emerges from

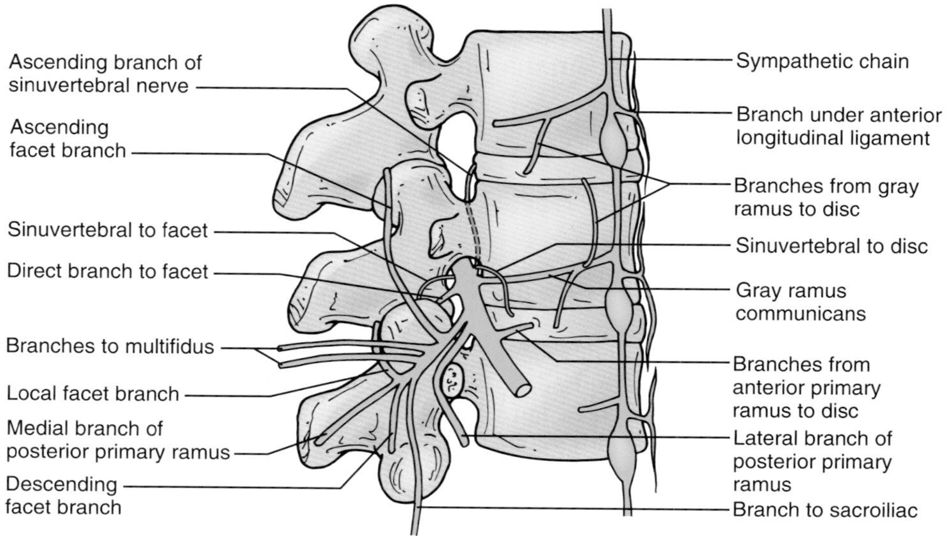

FIG. 24.1 Segmental innervation of the lumbar spine. *(From Paris SV: Anatomy as related to function and pain. Symposium on evaluation and care of lumbar spine problems.* Orthop Clin North Am. *14:475-489, 1983.)*

the sympathetic chain and joins the spinal segmental nerve soon after it exits the intervertebral foramina and runs anteriorly along the inferior third of the VB. It connects to the sympathetic trunk before separating into lateral and anterior branches to innervate the lateral and anterior disc annulus of the disc levels above and below the trunk. The posterior primary ramus, soon after its division from the anterior primary ramus, branches into medial and lateral branches. The medial branch of the posterior primary ramus supplies most dorsal spinal column components including the facet joints, posterior neural arch components, and spinous processes. The AF of the IVD therefore has complex innervation from several sources and includes contributions from sinuvertebral nerves, segmental spinal nerves, gray ramus communicans nerves, and the sympathetic trunk. The efferent nerves carrying information from spinal components rarely follow a single pathway but instead branch extensively and undergo interneuronal convergence within the spinal cord.[7] This, when coupled with the rich autonomic connections present in the spinal column, results in the poor topographical localization of pain of spinal origin, particularly pain originating from the IVD. Although all components of a spinal motion segment have been implicated in generating pain, the majority of pain receptors are found in spinal ligaments, paraspinal muscles, VB periosteum, facet joints, and the outer third of the AF.[8]

SPINAL MECHANICS

The flexibility and remarkable range of motion (ROM) exhibited by an active spine depends almost entirely on the cumulative plasticity exhibited by the IVDs. An individual IVD, however, is only moderately plastic in isolation and the NP is almost incompressible. Forces applied to the spine are substantial and are borne directly by the VBs and IVDs.[9] Extreme compressive forces applied to a healthy IVD can be endured without traumatic injury due to the incompressibility of the NP and equal distribution of tensile force to the AF.[10] Pathophysiologic changes within the degenerated IVD alter the biomechanical properties, causing it to shrink and lose plasticity. These changes in the disc dynamics increase stress on the adjacent vertebral motion segments and propagate dysfunction, hypertrophy, and degenerative changes in several contiguous structures: facet joints, sacroiliac joints, and paraspinal muscles or ligaments.[11] Hypertrophy of the facet joints and ligamenta flava along with bulging of the IVDs leads to narrowing of the spinal canal and the intervertebral foraminae, which can cause pain due to compression of the neural elements.[12] Degenerative changes in one disc can also cause accelerated degenerative changes in the adjacent IVDs. Although the spinal degenerative changes mentioned above are common, their presence or absence correlates poorly to patients' reported symptoms.[13]

PATHOPHYSIOLOGY

The incompressibility exhibited by the NP is a product of its water content, which is the result of osmotic pressure generated by matrix proteoglycans that are synthesized by sparsely present NP cells.[14] Due to its avascularity, the IVD meets its metabolic requirements exclusively through diffusion from capillary beds in adjacent VBs and the outer AF. Matrix metalloproteinases (MMPs) facilitate discal catabolic activities, which exist in delicate balance with anabolic activities.[15] As the IVD lacks scavenger cells, the end products of macromolecular metabolism accumulate within the disc over time.[16] These factors result in a precarious anaerobic environment for the IVD, leaving it vulnerable to a host of hereditary and environmental insults.[17] Lack of nutrition, enhanced MMP activity, and an increase in disc cytokines and proinflammatory mediator concentration all contribute to dysfunction and the decline in the viable NP cell population.[18,19] Reduced NP cellular anabolic activities can lead to reduced NP proteoglycans, osmotic pressure, and water content, which can lead to reduced NP hydrostatic pressure. Factors analogous to those affecting the NP can affect the AF wherein cellular dysfunction and loss can result in the loss of AF collagen. Loss of hydrostatic pressure results in NP laxity and exposes the AF to direct compressive forces. This, along with loss of collagen, may eventually lead to AF failure and the development of tears and fissures extending from the periphery to the NP.[20] These AF tears are gradually infiltrated by granulation tissue, which is highly vascularized, richly innervated, and is abundant in mononuclear cell infiltrates. These cells then release nerve growth factors, which contribute to nerve in-growth and accelerated IVD degeneration. These nerve fibers include vasoregulatory nerves, which accompany the neovascularization, and free nerve endings, which are high in substance P and are likely nociceptive in nature. The high concentrations of proinflammatory mediators within the disrupted discs can also sensitize the neonociceptive nerve endings, maintaining a state of pain and hyperalgesia within the disrupted disc. Overt disc herniation or occult leakage of disc material through the AF tears can cause inflammation of contiguous structures, especially the spinal nerve roots. This may increase local or, more frequently, remote pain in the distribution of the affected nerve root, causing pain in a dermatomal distribution that is known as radicular pain. Leakage of the inflammatory mediators across the vertebral endplates into the VB may cause inflammation followed by hypertrophic new bone formation and sclerosis in the adjacent VB. These inflammatory changes are visible on imaging and as a whole are termed Modic changes. It is unclear if Modic changes are a true etiology of pain or if they are simply a visible manifestation of a degenerating spinal column's maladaptive modulation.[21]

ETIOLOGY

The majority of LBP originates from the various spinal components such as the spinal nerve roots, facet joints, the contiguous paraspinal muscles and ligaments, sacroiliac joints, and the IVDs and VBs. LBP of spinal origin typically is not life-threatening and is due to self-limiting degenerative conditions that seldom cause neurologic compromise. LBP emanating from benign spinal degenerative conditions has been termed lumbago, mechanical LBP, or spondylosis. The common spinal syndromes causing benign LBP include:

- Musculoligamentous strain or sprain
- Herniated disc
- Foraminal stenosis causing symptoms from nerve root compression
- Spinal canal stenosis causing neurogenic claudication or myelopathic symptoms
- Facet joint dysfunction and arthropathy
- Sacroiliac joint dysfunction and arthropathy
- Myofascial pain syndrome
- Degenerative disc disease, discogenic pain, internal disc disruption
- Spondylolisthesis (displacement of a VB compared to the adjacent)
- Spondylolysis (defect in pars interarticularis without vertebral slippage)
- Spinal instability (anomalous movement between the contiguous VBs)
- Spinal conditions causing misalignment such as kyphosis or scoliosis

Infrequently, LBP of spinal origin is from nondegenerative conditions. Such nonmechanical LBP may result from widely diverse pathologic conditions such as:

- Primary or metastatic neoplasm of the spine or its neural contents
- Infections, such as osteomyelitis of the VBs, septic discitis, paraspinal, or epidural abscess
- Noninfectious inflammatory spinal disorders such as ankylosing spondylitis, Reiter syndrome, psoriatic spondylitis, inflammatory bowel disease
- Traumatic or pathologic fractures such as VB compression fractures and dislocations
- Metabolic disorders of the spine such as Paget disease
- Miscellaneous conditions such as Scheuermann disease, osteochondrosis and hemangiomas

LBP can also be referred from adjacent or even distant organs, particularly retroperitoneal structures. Chronic LBP of extraspinal and visceral etiology, however, is uncommon, and is easily distinguished from the common spinal sources of LBP by other associated symptoms related to the various disease processes and lack of local tenderness or pain with active ROM of the spine. The diverse etiology of LBP of visceral origin includes:

- Pelvic visceral disorders such as prostatitis, endometriosis, or pelvic inflammatory disease
- Renal disease such as nephrolithiasis, pyelonephritis, or perinephric abscess
- Vascular disease such as abdominal aortic aneurysm
- Gastrointestinal disease such as pancreatitis, cholecystitis, or perforated bowel

Overall, the relatively less common causes of LBP that are nondegenerative and nonspinal, also referred to as secondary or nonmechanical LBP, are typically rapidly progressive, often cause neurologic compromise, and may be life-threatening.

LBP has also conventionally been labeled as either specific or nonspecific LBP (Table 24.1). As one might infer, specific LBP can be attributed to a definite cause, but nonspecific LBP lacks a clear etiology. Unfortunately, approximately 90% of all LBP patients have at times been diagnosed with nonspecific LBP.[22] Reasons for this elevated incidence include concomitant presence of various LBP syndromes, similar and vague topographic localization of the pain originating from spinal structures and diagnostic imaging techniques that may demonstrate similar abnormalities in symptomatic and asymptomatic individuals.

LBP is divided into three categories based on duration of symptoms. LBP is classified as acute when present for less than 4 weeks, subacute when it persists for over 12 weeks, and chronic when the patient is symptomatic for greater than 3 months. The majority of acute LBP episodes are self-limited and resolve spontaneously within a few days to weeks. Subacute LBP is also generally caused by degenerative conditions such as disc herniations or exacerbations of facet arthropathy, which also tend to be self-limiting but may require treatment to ease symptoms. Chronic LBP, however, can be further categorized as persistent or recurrent and is often refractory to treatment.[23,24] By some

TABLE 24.1 Etiology of Low Back Pain

Mechanical Spinal Pain

1. Musculoligamentous strain or sprain
2. Herniated disc
3. Foraminal stenosis causing symptoms from nerve root compression
4. Spinal canal stenosis causing neurogenic claudication or myelopathic symptoms
5. Facet joint dysfunction and arthropathy
6. Sacroiliac joint dysfunction and arthropathy
7. Myofascial pain syndrome
8. Degenerative disc disease, discogenic pain, internal disc disruption
9. Spondylolisthesis (displacement of a vertebral body compared to the adjacent)
10. Spondylolysis (defect in pars interarticularis without vertebral slippage)
11. Spinal instability (anomalous movement between the contiguous vertebral bodies)
12. Spinal conditions causing misalignment such as kyphosis or scoliosis

Nonmechanical Spinal Pain

1. Primary or metastatic neoplasm of the spine or its neural contents
2. Infections, such as osteomyelitis of the vertebral bodies, septic discitis, paraspinal, or epidural abscess
3. Noninfectious inflammatory spinal disorders such as ankylosing spondylitis, Reiter syndrome, psoriatic spondylitis, inflammatory bowel disease
4. Traumatic or pathologic fractures such as vertebral bodies compression fractures and dislocations
5. Metabolic disorders of the spine such as Paget disease
6. Miscellaneous conditions such as Scheuermann disease or osteochondrosis and hemangiomas

Referred or Visceral Spinal Pain

1. Pelvic visceral disorders such as prostatitis, endometriosis, or pelvic inflammatory disease
2. Renal disease such as nephrolithiasis, pyelonephritis, or perinephric abscess
3. Vascular disease such as abdominal aortic aneurysm
4. Gastrointestinal disease such as pancreatitis, cholecystitis, or perforated bowel

estimates, almost 30% of patients with acute LBP progress to develop chronic LBP. In addition, chronic LBP may be accompanied by a myriad of comorbidities such as depression, behavioral disorders, substance abuse, disability, and secondary gain issues, which can make chronic LBP difficult to treat. The likelihood of return to work diminishes with increased duration of LBP. Patients on medical leave for greater than 6 months due to LBP had lifetime return to work rate of only 50%; this rate decreased to 25% if leave was over a year in duration and to less than 5% if they were off work for greater than 2 years.[25] Chronic LBP, therefore, poses substantial challenges to suffering individuals, their families, and the community as a whole.

RISK FACTORS

The risk factors associated with LBP have been classified into three broad categories: biomechanical, psychosocial, and personal. Biomechanical risk factors are determined by spinal loading, and typically include parameters such as physical stress and the asymmetry of physical tasks the patient is required to perform.[26,27] The psychosocial risk factors pertain to psychogenic stress and are often related to job satisfaction, responsibility, and variety.[28,29] Personal risk factors have been acknowledged as physical, familial, psychologic, anthropometric (e.g., obesity), and gender-related.[30,31] The following risk factors have also been associated with the development of LBP:

- An occupation with elevated physical or emotional stress[32]
- Cigarette smoking[33,34]
- Spinal deformities[35]
- VB endplate injury[36]
- Genetic predisposition[37]
- Peripheral vascular disease[38]
- Obesity[39]

TABLE 24.2 Symptom Evaluation of Patients With Low Back Pain

- Location and radiation of pain:
  - Axial (truncal) pain
  - Dermatomal pain
    - Termed radiculopathy or radiculitis
    - Typically in the lower extremities
- Quality of pain
  - May ask patient to describe pain without guidance
    - "What does the pain feel like?"
  - May formally assess using a standardized assessment tool
    - The Short-Form McGill Pain Questionnaire[41] is commonly used in clinical settings due to its brevity
- Natural history of the pain, e.g., constant, waxing and waning, and progressive over time
- Circumstances of onset of pain such as a history of trauma
- Factors that aggravate or relieve the pain
- Presence of any constitutional symptoms such as fever, malaise, or weight loss
- "Red flag" pain features such as nocturnal pain, bony tenderness, morning stiffness, and history of claudication
- Neurologic symptoms such as numbness, tingling, and weakness
- Bowel or bladder dysfunction
  - Urinary retention
  - Urinary or fecal incontinence
- History of any previous treatments and their efficacy
- Patient's age
- Past medical and surgical history
- Assessment of social and psychological factors that may affect patient's pain
- Impact of the pain on the patient's activities of daily living and ability to sleep, which are more reliable indicators of disability than a subjective pain score.

CLINICAL EVALUATION

Despite the diagnostic complexities and the daunting list of causal conditions, the majority of LBP is caused by benign self-limiting conditions and symptoms typically resolve in 1–3 months.[40] A comprehensive history and physical examination are important components in the diagnosis of various LBP syndromes.

HISTORY

A detailed history of the LBP patient should note the following (Table 24.2):

- Location and radiation of pain:
  - Axial (truncal) pain

- Dermatomal pain
  - Termed radiculopathy or radiculitis
  - Typically in the lower extremities
- Quality of pain
  - May ask patient to describe pain without guidance
    - "What does the pain feel like?"
  - May formally assess using a standardized assessment tool
    - The Short-Form McGill Pain Questionnaire[41] is commonly used in clinical settings due to its brevity
- Natural history of the pain, for example, constant, waxing and waning, progressive over time
- Circumstances of onset of pain such as a history of trauma
- Factors that aggravate or relieve the pain
- Presence of any constitutional symptoms such as fever, malaise, or weight loss
- "Red flag" pain features such as nocturnal pain, bony tenderness, morning stiffness, and history of claudication
- Neurologic symptoms such as numbness, tingling, and weakness
- Bowel or bladder dysfunction
  - Urinary retention
  - Urinary or fecal incontinence
- History of any previous treatments and their efficacy
- Patient age
- Past medical and surgical history
- Assessment of social and psychological factors that may affect patient's pain
- Impact of the pain on the patient's activities of daily living (ADLs) and ability to sleep, which are more reliable indicators of disability than a subjective pain score.

PHYSICAL EXAMINATION

A comprehensive general physical and a detailed neurologic examination should be performed in all patients with LBP. Specific spinal examination should include:

- Assessment of gait
- Range of spinal motion and degree, if any, at which patient experiences pain
- Palpation to assess local spinal and paraspinal tenderness
- Specific tests for the clinical diagnosis of various LBP syndromes, including those for nerve root irritation, facet syndrome, and sacroiliac joint dysfunction, which are discussed in this book in the various chapters dedicated to these syndromes

"RED FLAGS" IN PATIENT'S CLINICAL EVALUATION (TABLE 24.3)

Due to the high prevalence of LBP, its frequent spontaneous resolution, the rarity of serious causes, and the frequent presence of abnormal findings in asymptomatic individuals, performing exhaustive diagnostic testing is not recommended. This practice would lead to inappropriate diagnosis, excessive fiscal impact, and poor treatment results.[42] Therefore, in the United States, the Agency for Health Care Policy and Research (AHCPR) developed guidelines to recognize clinical features that would signify the presence of conditions such as fractures, tumors, and infections that can pose significant threat to life or neurologic function and termed these "red flags." Recognition of these notable clinical signs is essential, as their existence would require further diagnostic testing to either exclude a serious condition or confirm the presence of a benign diagnosis. However, it is possible that a malignant spinal condition may go undetected despite a careful appraisal for these characteristic "red flags." In general, patients with benign mechanical LBP should have pain mainly with spinal movements such as sitting, bending, lifting, or twisting, and the pain should improve while lying down and at night and it should diminish over the course of days to weeks. Benign diagnoses of exclusion, such as muscle sprain or ligamentous strain, should be made with caution in the presence of "red flags." If the clinician hastily arrives at a benign diagnosis, this could delay appropriate workup of LBP due to malignant etiology, leading to increased morbidity and mortality. The characteristic "red flags" are as follows:

- *Age:* Patients less than 20 or over 50 years of age. Younger patients have a higher incidence of congenital and developmental anomalies, while older patients have a greater likelihood of neoplasms, pathologic fractures, serious infections, and life-threatening extraspinal pathologic conditions.
- *Duration of symptoms:* Symptoms lasting over 3 months without any other associated red flag symptoms arising indicate a less serious etiology.

TABLE 24.3 "Red Flags" in Patient's Clinical Evaluation

Age	Less than 20 or over 50 years of age are suspect.
Duration of symptoms	Symptoms of over 3-month duration indicate a less serious etiology.
History of trauma	History of significant traumatic injury or mild trauma in an elderly patient or in a patient with a serious medical condition.
Presence of constitutional symptoms	Such as fever, chills, malaise, night sweats, and unexplained weight loss.
Presence of systemic illness	A history of cancer, recent bacterial infections, intravenous drug abuse, immunosuppression, organ transplantation, and corticosteroid use.
Unrelenting pain	Pain not relieved with rest, supine position, analgesics and night pain.
Presence of cauda equina syndrome	Caused by massive midline disc herniation or rarely by spinal metastases, hematoma, epidural abscess, traumatic compression, acute transverse myelitis, and abdominal aortic dissection. Symptoms include bilateral, but often unequal, lower extremity radicular pains and weakness, gait disturbances, abdominal discomfort and overflow incontinence. Physical examination exhibits neurological dysfunction, saddle anesthesia, diminished anal sphincter tone, and urinary bladder retention. Diagnosis must be made by imaging the entire spine. The treatment is by urgent decompressive surgery.

- *History of trauma:* History of significant traumatic injury or mild trauma in an elderly patient or in a patient with a serious medical condition may indicate traumatic spinal injury.
- *Presence of constitutional symptoms:* Examples such as a history of fever, chills, malaise, night sweats, and unexplained weight loss indicate a more ominous etiology of LBP.
- *Presence of systemic illness:* Patients with a history of cancer, recent bacterial infections, intravenous drug abuse, immunosuppression, organ transplantation, and corticosteroid use are at higher risk for pathologic fractures, epidural and VB abscesses, and spinal metastasis.
- *Unrelenting pain:* Pain of a benign etiology is typically relieved with rest and supine position, especially at night, while pain from a serious pathologic condition is typically unrelenting, may worsen at night, and is not responsive to rest and analgesics.
- *Presence of cauda equina syndrome (CES):* This syndrome is caused by acute compression of the spinal cord or the nerve roots of the cauda equina. CES is characteristically caused by a massive midline IVD herniation or a smaller disc herniation in a patient with preexisting spinal stenosis.[43,44] Rarely, CES may be caused by spinal metastases, hematoma, epidural abscess, traumatic compression, acute transverse myelitis, or abdominal aortic dissection.[45] Typical symptoms include bilateral, but often unequal, lower extremity radicular pain and weakness, gait disturbances, and urinary retention causing abdominal pain or overflow incontinence. In addition to the positive findings on neurologic examination, the patient's physical examination typically reveals saddle anesthesia, diminished sensation in the buttocks and perineum, diminished anal sphincter tone, and evidence of urinary retention. Given the similar constellation of symptoms regardless of the vertebral level of insult, CES must be evaluated by imaging the entire spine.[46] CES is one of the rare neurosurgical emergencies that may require urgent decompressive surgery to reduce permanent neurologic disability.

DIAGNOSTIC TESTING

The most commonly used tests for the diagnosis of LBP syndromes are imaging studies, which typically reveal abnormal findings in both symptomatic and asymptomatic individuals.[47,48] It is therefore necessary to correlate imaging studies with a patient's clinical findings. As previously mentioned, if diagnostic testing is ordered indiscriminately, then the diagnosis may not correspond to the patient's actual clinical presentation. Additionally, as LBP syndromes are commonly self-limiting and benign in the absence of "red flags" in the clinical history, diagnostic testing is not recommended for LBP of less than 4–6 weeks' duration.[49] Ordering these tests selectively should prevent poor outcomes by avoiding inappropriate diagnosis and treatment. In addition to the diagnosis of specific LBP syndromes, diagnostic tests are also used to determine the site of surgical or minimally invasive intervention for LBP.

The following are the diagnostic modalities frequently used for the diagnosis of LBP:

Plain Radiography: Plain radiography allows evaluation of the bony spinal anatomy. It can reliably diagnose certain spinal pathologic lesions such as fractures, deformities, transitional vertebra, spondylolisthesis, and spondylolysis. Subtle spinal abnormalities seen on plain radiography, such as straightening of lumbar lordosis, disc space narrowing, arthritic changes, ossification of the vertebral endplates, and abnormal range of spinal movements or spinal instability are frequently encountered in asymptomatic individuals.[50,51] Spinal radiography therefore exhibits a high rate of abnormal findings in asymptomatic individuals.[52] Major drawbacks of plain spinal radiography include its inability to visualize the soft tissue structures and their abnormalities, such as herniated disc, neural element compression, and soft tissue neoplasms. Spinal x-rays may therefore appear normal even in the presence of significant spinal soft tissue pathology. Spinal roentgenograms have traditionally been the earliest imaging test performed in the evaluation of patients with LBP, chiefly because they are widely available, easy to perform, and are relatively inexpensive. Therefore, even though the routine use of spinal radiography has been discouraged,[53] in the presence of "red flags" in the clinical history, spinal roentgenograms are often the initial screening tests performed.

Traditional plain radiography sequences include anteroposterior (AP), lateral, and oblique views. In the AP view, indicators of normal spinal morphology include vertical alignment of the spinous processes, smooth undulating borders created by lateral masses, and uniformity among the disc spaces. Misalignment of the spinous processes suggests a rotational abnormality such as unilateral facet dislocation or scoliosis. The AP view of the lumbar spine should include the entire pelvis to allow the assessment of acetabula, femoral heads, and the lower portion of the thoracic spine due to the high occurrence of vertebral fracture between T12 and L2 spinal levels. The lateral view provides a superior image of the VBs, facet joints, lordotic spinal curvature, disc space height, and spondylolisthesis. Decreased disc space height is a relatively nonspecific change and may indicate disc degeneration, disc space infection, or postsurgical changes. Oblique views are those taken with the x-ray tube rotated laterally and provide enhanced views of the neural foraminae and pars interarticularis. These views best demonstrate foraminal abnormalities and spondylolysis. Flexion-extension views are typically used to assess for spinal instability as a cause of chronic pain, especially after spinal fusion surgery. The latter views can also be used in trauma patients to assess ligamentous injury. When used to diagnose ligamentous injury, the flexion-extension views should be used exclusively in patients with otherwise normal radiographs and who are neurologically intact, cooperative, and able to recognize early onset of pain or neurologic symptoms with spinal movement. If patients do not satisfy these criteria, then significant neurologic damage cannot be safely avoided.

Bone Scintigraphy: Bone scintigraphy creates images by scanning for the presence of radiographic compounds such as technetium-99m phosphate or gallium-67 citrate. Hence, whereas plain radiography, computerized tomography (CT), and magnetic resonance imaging (MRI) reveal the morphologic changes, bone scintigraphy detects biochemical osseous processes. It is therefore valuable when clinical findings are suspicious for spinal osteomyelitis, neoplasms, or occult fracture. Typically benign primary spinal tumors, such as osteoid osteoma, osteoblastoma, aneurysmal bone cyst, and osteochondroma show as active lesions on bone scintigraphy. Osseous spinal metastases usually appear as asymmetrically scattered multiple foci of increased tracer uptake. Occasionally, aggressive bony tumors, such as myeloma, may not invoke an osteoblastic response and may result in a negative bone scan. In rare cases of severe spinal metastases, diffusely increased tracer uptake may result in a falsely negative bone scan. Anatomically, over half (52%) of spinal metastases will occur in the lumbar region, whereas 36% will occur in the thoracic region and only 12% occur in the cervical region.[54] Topographic location of spinal osseous tumors is also significant; lesions affecting the pedicles are typically malignant, lesions in facet joints tend to be benign and lesions in VBs and spinous processes are equally as likely to be benign or malignant. Bone scintigraphy with the addition of single-photon emission computed tomography (SPECT) provides a three-dimensional spinal image and enhances topographic tumor location. SPECT has been used to distinguish between benign and malignant osseous neoplasms.[55,56]

Computed Tomography: CT uses radiologic data to generate contiguous, overlapping axial images of the scanned area. The imaging data can also be reformatted to construct views in any desired plane. Spinal CT is most useful in evaluating osseous details of the spine in an axial plane, particularly the facet joints and the lateral recesses. It is most valuable in diagnosing fractures, tumors involving the spine, and in showing the relative position of one osseous structure to another, such as partial or complete dislocation and spondylolisthesis. The resolution of the soft tissue structures on spinal CT is inferior to MRI. Spinal CT cannot reliably distinguish between herniated IVD and epidural scar tissue and amongst various spinal canal lesions such as neoplasms of the spinal cord or the nerve roots. Routine use of spinal CT for diagnosis of soft tissue intraspinal canal lesions is therefore discouraged.[57] However, the image is comparable to MRI in diagnostic quality when CT is combined with myelography, and this modality can be used as a substitute when MRI is contraindicated (Fig. 24.2). Radiation exposure is a significant hazard with spinal CT, which limits the frequency with which it may be employed. Spiral CT reduces exposure time, radiation hazard, and motion artifact compared to conventional CT.

MRI: The powerful magnetic field generated in the MRI scanner aligns water molecules, or protons, which constitute the bulk of human body mass, in the direction of the magnetic field applied. Brief bursts of radiofrequency (RF) waves are then transmitted to the tissue and the electromagnetic fields generated alter the proton alignment. Cessation of the RF pulse results in the proton spin decaying to the original state, releasing energy in the form of photons, which are detected and interpreted by the MRI scanner. The protons in the various tissues return to the equilibrium state at dissimilar rates and an image of various soft tissues is created. By changing the timing of scanner sequences, such as the echo time (T_E) and the repetition time (T_R), the contrast between body tissues can be altered. T_2 weighted images use a spin echo (SE) sequence, with long T_E and long T_R intervals, and the water-containing tissues appear white, whereas the fat-rich or water-deprived tissues appear dark (Fig. 24.3). T_1 weighted images, in contrast, use a gradient echo (GRE) sequence, with short T_E and short T_R sequencing, and the tissue contrast on T_1 weighted images is the opposite of the T_2 weighted images. The cerebrospinal fluid appears dark on T_1 weighted images, and it appears white on T_2

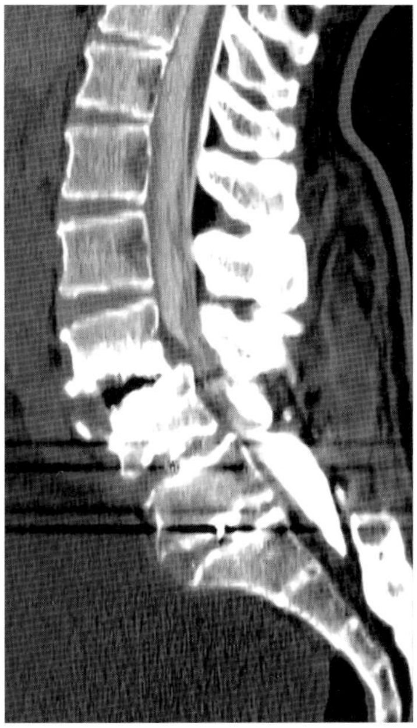

FIG. 24.2 Computerized tomography myelogram sagittal view showing extensive disc degeneration and thecal sac indentation at L4–L5 and L5–S1 levels.

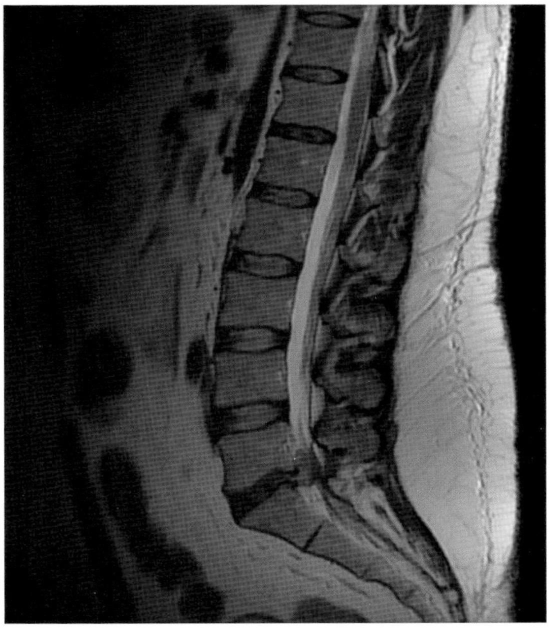

FIG. 24.3 T_2 weighted sagittal magnetic resonance imaging (MRI) scan showing L5–S1 disc degeneration and disc extrusion. Same patient with axial T_2 weighted MRI image showing disc extrusion.

weighted images. On T_2 weighted images, a healthy IVD has high water content and thus appears brighter than the AF.

MRI is currently considered the gold standard in spinal imaging. It provides sharper distinction between different varieties of soft tissues, and the overall resolution is superior. MRI offers excellent images of the spinal canal, the neural foraminae, nerve roots, and the size and shape of the IVD. MRI also allows evaluation of the complete spine in various planes. Contrast medium for MRI, such as gadolinium and manganese, are higher atomic weight elements and possess paramagnetic properties, which enhance tissue resolution. Paramagnetism is a convenient quality of these elements in that an internal magnetic field will be induced in the material when it is placed in an externally applied magnetic field, such as the MRI machine. A contrast enhanced MRI may be performed when greater distinction between various soft tissues is required, such as diagnosis of malignancy or differentiation between scar tissue and recurrent IVD herniation in patients with a history of spine surgery. The addition of contrast permits greater differentiation between structures and permits improved diagnosis of malignancies. Radiopaque contrast agents used for CT include substances such as iodine or barium. The sensitivity and specificity of MRI for identification of bone metastases is 95% and 90%,[54] respectively, which is exponentially superior to plain radiographs, in which 50%–70% of bone must be destroyed for reliable detection.[58]

MRI has no known biological effects and is therefore extremely safe but does have several limitations. MRI requires a more lengthy examination time compared to CT or x-ray (XR) imaging and may be relatively contraindicated in patients that experience claustrophobia. Sedation may be used to ensure that patients will remain comfortable and motionless during the exam. Alternatively, "open" MRI scanners now exist. These diminish claustrophobia symptoms but the image quality is significantly reduced compared to conventional MRI. MRI is absolutely contraindicated in the presence of ferromagnetic implants, such as cardiac pacemakers, intracranial aneurysm clips, mechanical heart valves, intraocular foreign bodies, or the leads of many spinal cord stimulators. The effect of the magnet may violently shift any implanted metal, causing a potentially lethal injury. Stabilization devices used in spinal surgery may cast artifact that can render spinal MRI useless, but are not absolutely contraindicated. Similar to other spinal imaging modalities, spinal MRI may frequently detect findings in asymptomatic individuals.

ELECTRODIAGNOSTIC STUDIES

Electrodiagnostic studies encompass the following:

Electromyography (EMG): Examines spontaneous or evoked skeletal muscle electrical activity.

Nerve conduction velocity (NCV): Evaluates conductive abilities of motor and sensory nerves.

Evoked potentials: Study of brain electrical activity evoked from various nervous system locations, such as somatosensory-evoked potentials (SSEPs) and motor-evoked potentials (MEPs).

The electrodiagnostic studies are useful in localizing the pathologic lesion, determining the extent of the neural injury, predicting the course of recovery, and determining whether the radiologic abnormalities observed are the likely source of a patient's symptoms.[59] These tests are useful in distinguishing between radicular and peripheral neuropathic symptoms when the clinical evaluation is inconclusive. EMG or NCVs, however, provide scant information regarding symptom etiology, and abnormal test results may take several weeks to evolve after an injury. The use of SSEPs and MEPs is generally limited to identifying intraoperative nerve injury during spinal surgery. Compared to spinal imaging, electrodiagnostic studies are less sensitive but have greater specificity.[60]

PSYCHOSOCIAL TESTING

Screening for nonphysical factors is a key component in the management of LBP patients. Psychological, occupational, and socioeconomic factors can complicate both the assessment and the treatment of chronic LBP patients. For example, patients with preexisting dissatisfaction with their occupation are at a greater risk for LBP and a worsened natural history of the pain syndrome.[61] Similarly, patients with an affective disorder, such as depression, and those with a history of substance abuse are also more prone to acquire a chronic pain disorder. Pending litigation and disability issues may also adversely affect the treatment and outlook of chronic LBP patients.

OTHER DIAGNOSTIC TESTS

A variety of other diagnostic and laboratory tests are useful when nondegenerative conditions, such as tumors, infections, and rheumatologic disorders, are considered a cause of LBP. A few such examples include complete blood count, urine analysis, erythrocyte sedimentation rate (ESR), C-reactive protein (CRP), rheumatoid factor (RH-factor), antinuclear antibodies (ANA), and human leukocyte antigen, HLA-B27.

MANAGEMENT

NONINVASIVE TREATMENTS

The following are common noninvasive treatments employed in the treatment of LBP (Table 24.4).

Res

Strict bed rest was historically the mainstay of acute LBP treatment. The current evidence, however, suggests that prolonged bed rest is harmful in patients afflicted with LBP,[62] and bed rest of more than 1 week is not recommended.[63] Furthermore, continuation of daily activities and early return to work is associated with a decrease in chronic disability and cumulative duration of absence from work.[64,65]

Pharmacologic Therapy

- *Nonsteroidal antiinflammatory drugs (NSAIDs):* These drugs are considered moderately effective for the short-term relief of acute LBP,[66] but data regarding the most

TABLE 24.4 Treatments for Low Back Pain

Noninvasive Treatments for Spinal Pain	
Rest	
Pharmacologic therapy	1. Nonsteroidal antiinflammatory drugs 2. Opioids 3. Muscle relaxants 4. Corticosteroids 5. Calcitonin
Physical therapy	1. Body mechanics, ergonomics, posture awareness, and activities of daily living training 2. Strengthening and stretching exercises 3. Organized functional training programs 4. Therapeutic massage 5. Joint mobilizations and manipulations 6. Mechanical traction 7. Electrical muscle stimulation 8. Transcutaneous electrical nerve stimulation 9. Application of superficial and deep thermal modalities 10. Cryotherapy 11. Work hardening
Acupuncture	—
Spinal manipulation	—
Biofeedback	—
Minimally Invasive Treatments for Spinal Pain	
Injection therapy	1. Epidural steroid injections 2. Facet joint injections 3. Sacroiliac joint injection 4. Trigger pain injections
Neuroablative procedures	1. Radiofrequency ablation 2. Chemical neurolysis 3. Cryoablation
Intradiscal procedure	1. Percutaneous disc decompression 2. Intradiscal electrothermal therapy 3. Intradiscal bioculoplasty 4. Stem cell based therapies
Spinal surgery	
Decompression surgery	1. Discectomy 2. Microdiscectomy 3. Endoscopic discectomy 4. Decompression for fixed osseous stenosis
Fusion	1. Anterior fusion 2. Posterior fusion 3. Circumferential fusion 4. Transforaminal lumbar interbody fusion
Disc arthroplasty	1. SB Charite III 2. ProDisc 3. Maverick 4. Flexcore

effective NSAID in treatment of LBP is inconclusive.[67] Support for the use of NSAIDs in the treatment of chronic LBP is lacking, despite pervasive recommendations to use these as a first-line treatment given their perceived benignity. NSAIDs reversibly inhibit COX1 and COX 2 and therefore the production of protective renal prostaglandins, which causes clinically appreciable acute kidney injury in susceptible patients. Chronic NSAID use is also associated with a 1.80-fold increase in the risk of venous thromboembolism, although a pathophysiologic explanation for this phenomenon has not been elucidated.[68]

- *Opioids:* Short-term use of opioid medications may be considered for the relief of acute LBP or severe exacerbations of chronic LBP.[69] A need for prolonged narcotic therapy should prompt reevaluation given that opioids are no more effective than acetaminophen or NSAIDs in the treatment of chronic LBP.[70] Long-term use of opioid medications leads to development of tolerance and addiction and is also associated with increased morbidity and mortality. In recent years, the worldwide death rate from prescription opioid use has steadily increased, which cannot be attributed to improved reporting given that the same sources have noted a decrease in unintentional deaths from illicit drugs.[71]
- *Muscle relaxants:* The use of muscle relaxants has been shown to modestly reduce pain, muscle tension, and immobility in patients with LBP.[72]
- *Corticosteroids:* These are frequently prescribed orally, or even parenterally, for the treatment of acute disc herniation. Evidence to support this practice in the literature is scant.[73,74]
- *Calcitonin:* This drug has shown benefit in pain due to spinal stenosis caused by Paget disease.[75]

Physical Therapy

Physical therapy and rehabilitation interventions used in the management of LBP include the following[76]:

- Training in body mechanics, ergonomics, postural awareness, and ADLs
- Strengthening and stretching exercises
- Organized functional training programs
- Therapeutic massage
- Joint mobilization and manipulations
- Mechanical traction
- Biofeedback
- Electrical muscle stimulation
- Transcutaneous electrical nerve stimulation (TENS)
- Application of superficial and deep thermal modalities
- Cryotherapy
- Work hardening therapy

The treatment goals of various physical therapy modalities include the following:

- Pain relief
- Reduction in muscle spasm
- Improved ROM in the spine
- Improved strength
- Postural correction
- Improvement in functional status

Although the precise role of the various physical therapy modalities in the treatment of LBP is not entirely clear, the evidence is suggestive of beneficial effects of general exercise programs. Strengthening exercise programs that target the paraspinal musculature, and general exercise programs that promote weight loss are considered most beneficial in alleviating LBP, promoting return to work, resuming normal daily activities, and reducing the need for surgical intervention.[77] Many patients will report therapeutic benefit during the time period that passive physical therapy (PT) techniques such as thermotherapy, therapeutic massage, mechanical traction, therapeutic ultrasound, and TENS are physically being applied. However, there is no evidence that enduring clinical improvement results from these modalities beyond the time of application in patients with LBP.[78]

Acupuncture

An analysis of 11 randomized controlled trials (RCTs) on the use of acupuncture in patients with nonspecific LBP led to the following conclusions: (1) overall methodological quality of the RCTs was low; (2) none of the trials clearly evaluated acupuncture; (3) although moderate evidence for efficacy of acupuncture was demonstrated, it was comparable to trigger-point injection and TENS therapy; (4) evidence for the efficacy of acupuncture was lacking when compared to no treatment; and (5) there was limited evidence that acupuncture was more effective than placebo or sham treatment. Routine use of acupuncture for the treatment of LBP is therefore not recommended.[79,80]

Spinal Manipulation

The efficacy of spinal manipulations for the treatment of both acute and chronic LBP has been evaluated by several RCTs and several meta-analyses. Overall, the results of these studies demonstrate that although there may be some advantage to manipulative therapy in the treatment of acute LBP, no statistical or clinical advantage of spinal manipulations exist over conventional treatments for chronic LBP.[81–83]

Biofeedback

Biofeedback, broadly, is a process in which a patient may learn to control autonomic processes, such as heart rate or the perception of noxious stimuli, through conditioning during exposure to external stimuli. In chronic pain, the most common method involves monitoring the physiologic muscle activity of the patient (often using EMG) and communicating the state of contraction or relaxation to the patient via visual or auditory signals. In this manner, the patient can train painful or spastic muscle groups to relax on command. Studies examining biofeedback in the treatment of acute LBP are scarce, but those that exist show limited benefit in chronic LBP patients.[84]

MINIMALLY INVASIVE TREATMENTS

A variety of minimally invasive treatments exist for the treatment of LBP (see Table 24.4), including a range of diagnostic and therapeutic local anesthetics and steroid injections (Fig. 24.4), which may target spinal nerve roots, facet joints, sacroiliac joints, and the various muscles and ligaments. If diagnostic injections of these neural components result in short-term relief of pain, a nerve ablation technique may be employed to achieve longer-lasting results. Nerve ablation is currently most commonly achieved through thermal RF but may also be performed using chemical neurolysis or cryoablation. These neuroablative modalities characteristically target medial and lateral branches of the dorsal rami of the segmental spinal nerves for the treatment of facet and sacroiliac joint mediated pain and, less frequently, dorsal root ganglia are targeted to treat radicular pain. Several minimally invasive techniques to treat herniated/degenerated discs and spinal stenosis have been developed in recent years. The level of support for these from clinicians varies depending on the asserted

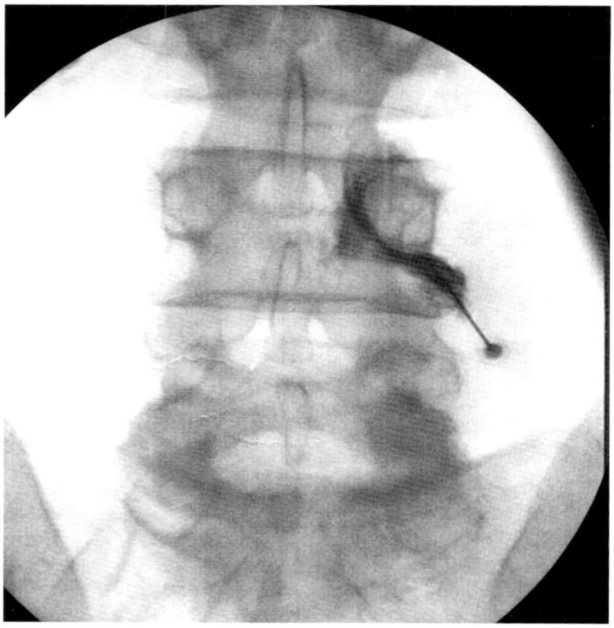

FIG. 24.4 Fluoroscopic image of right-sided L4–L5 transforaminal steroid injection. Dye injection prior to steroid demonstrating proper position and backflow along L4 nerve root sheath.

and demonstrated efficacy of each procedure. These techniques include heating of the IVDs by a variety of proprietary techniques such as intradiscal electrothermal therapy (IDET) and disc biacuplasty. Percutaneous decompression of the herniated disc has been performed by using thermal (either RF or laser) or mechanical nucleotomy. Typically, thermal techniques achieve better pain control outcomes, as they also purportedly eradicate the sensory fibers that innervate the disc.[85] Stem cell-based therapies have shown promising results in early translational studies. Although they are unlikely to be capable of completely repairing the anatomic structure of an IVD, cell-based therapies alone possess the potential for any restoration of biologic functionality. Therefore, IVD regeneration is a rapidly expanding area of research with enormous potential as a completely novel management technique for degenerative disc disease.[86]

SURGICAL TREATMENTS

The majority of surgical treatments employed to relieve LBP incorporate an element of neurologic decompression and/or fusion. However, artificial disc replacement surgery is a recently developed and increasingly popular alternative.

Spinal Decompression

Disc decompression surgery is typically reserved for patients with a herniated disc with distinctive symptoms of persistent radicular pain, positive straight leg raise test, and imaging studies confirming the presence of a herniated IVD. The target for surgical decompression is determined by careful correlation of patient's symptoms and lesions evident on imaging studies. Discectomy became widespread after Mixter and Barr's classic report in 1934[87] and has remained the most commonly performed spine surgery procedure. With some minimal variation, the procedure involves laminectomy or laminotomy, release of ligamentum flavum, removal of the herniated disc fragments, and a vertical annulotomy for the removal of nonherniated disc material. Microdiscectomy was popularized in the late 1970s as a less invasive technique that permits faster recovery and earlier return to work for the patient.[88] More recently, minimally invasive endoscopic discectomy has been performed, which involves limited exposure through a tubular retractor. In older patients, the nerve root compressive symptoms are often the result of local degenerative changes involving the disc, facet joints, and the local ligaments. Such changes may include disc bulges and herniations, facet and ligamentous hypertrophy, osteochondral spurs, and spondylolisthesis. Surgical decompression for these patients characteristically involves osseous decompression of the neural foraminae, central canal, and the lateral recess. In many such patients, especially in the presence of spondylolisthesis and when greater than 50% of the facet joint is resected, a supplemental fusion procedure may be required to impart stability to the spine.

Spinal Fusion

Spinal fusion has been performed for over a century and despite varying results, the number of fusion surgeries performed in the United States more than doubled from 1997 to 2010.[89] Common indications for spinal fusion include spinal deformities, spondylolisthesis, spondylolysis, spinal instability resulting from decompressive surgery, and several diverse causes of mechanical LBP such as degenerative disc disease and discogenic pain. During spinal fusion, the dysfunctional spinal motion segments may be resected and the spine rigidly stabilized with mechanical fusion devices such as pedicular screws, interpedicular fixation plates, and intervertebral spacers (Fig. 24.5). Osseous spinal fusion is attained by the use of bone grafts in the vascularized tissue bed. The key elements required for spinal osteogenesis include precursor cells capable of transformation into bone-forming osteoblasts, osteoconductive materials that serve as scaffolds for the formation of new bone, and osteoinductive growth factors that promote differentiation of progenitor cells into osteoblasts.[90] Autologous bone graft remains the gold standard of osteogenetic material, because it contains all three essential elements. Limitations of autologous bone graft, however, include the morbidity associated with harvest and the limited amount of available graft material. These limitations have led to the use of other osteogenetic materials including bone graft extenders, demineralized bone matrix, calcium carbonate, hydroxyapatite-tricalcium phosphate, bone graft substitutes and osteoinductive substitutes, such as recombinant human bone morphogenic protein (BMP).[91] Spinal fusion can be performed by either posterior, postero-lateral, anterior, or combined circumferential (360 degrees) approach. More recently, transforaminal lumbar interbody fusion (TLIF) technique is used, which provides the advantages of a circumferential fusion through a lower-risk posterior approach.[92] The actual fusion rates after surgery vary from 80% for posterolateral fusions to 97% for circumferential fusions.[93] The results of the spinal fusion vary vastly depending on the condition for which the surgery is performed. When performed for spinal deformities and spondylolisthesis, the results reported are generally favorable.[94,95] However, treatment of degenerative disc disease and discogenic pain with spinal fusion has remained controversial and the success rate is modest.[96] Patients with discogenic pain tend to have greater clinical benefits when the damaged disc is removed. Despite its popularity, spinal fusion remains a salvage procedure, as it reduces spinal mobility and increases stress and consequently degeneration at adjacent spinal levels.

Disc Arthroplasty

Disc arthroplasty was conceived to avert the shortcomings of spinal fusion surgery. During disc arthroplasty, the biologic disc is surgically removed and is replaced by an artificial disc. When compared to spinal fusion, the major benefit of disc replacement surgery includes preservation of spinal ROM and decreased adjacent spinal segment degeneration. The primary indication for disc arthroplasty is recalcitrant disabling LBP secondary to discogenic disc disease confirmed by MRI and discography. The exclusion criteria include evidence of nerve root compression and facet or sacroiliac joint arthropathy. In contrast to the prolonged rehabilitation that typically follows spinal fusion, early and progressive spinal motion is characteristically encouraged after disc arthroplasty to improve functional recovery. Although disc replacement surgery has been advocated since the 1950s, it was not until the early 1980s that a viable design with encouraging results was introduced. Several types of artificial discs are currently marketed; these include SB Charite III, ProDisc, Maverick, and Flexcore. The Link SB Charite III is currently the most commonly used prosthesis, which consists of two cobalt-chrome endplates with a sliding polyethylene core. The endplates are anchored to the VBs at the time of surgery, and the fusion eventually hardens due to bony ingrowth. The biomechanical studies of artificial disc replacement demonstrate increased ROM in flexion, extension, and torsion, whereas relative immobility was seen in lateral bending. Strong evidence now exists in the form of RCTs and well-conducted multicenter prospective trials that total disc replacement is valuable in patients meeting strict selection criteria. Disc replacement prostheses are durable, decrease adjacent segment degeneration, and have a lower incidence of revision than fusion apparatuses.[97]

CONCLUSION

Patients with LBP frequently have pain originating from multiple coexisting pain generators. The diagnosis of a specific pain syndrome consequently is often uncertain. In addition, given the incidence of positive results in asymptomatic individuals and relatively unimpressive findings in many patients with LBP, the available diagnostic tests are frequently unable to precisely diagnose the origin of a patient's pain. The available treatments for LBP also often lack both specificity and efficacy, and therefore do not assist in diagnosis. The root cause of the majority of LBP is the degenerative process within the disc, but disc replacement therapies are not yet available for clinical application. It is therefore not surprising that with lack of explanation for their symptoms and poor treatment results, chronic LBP

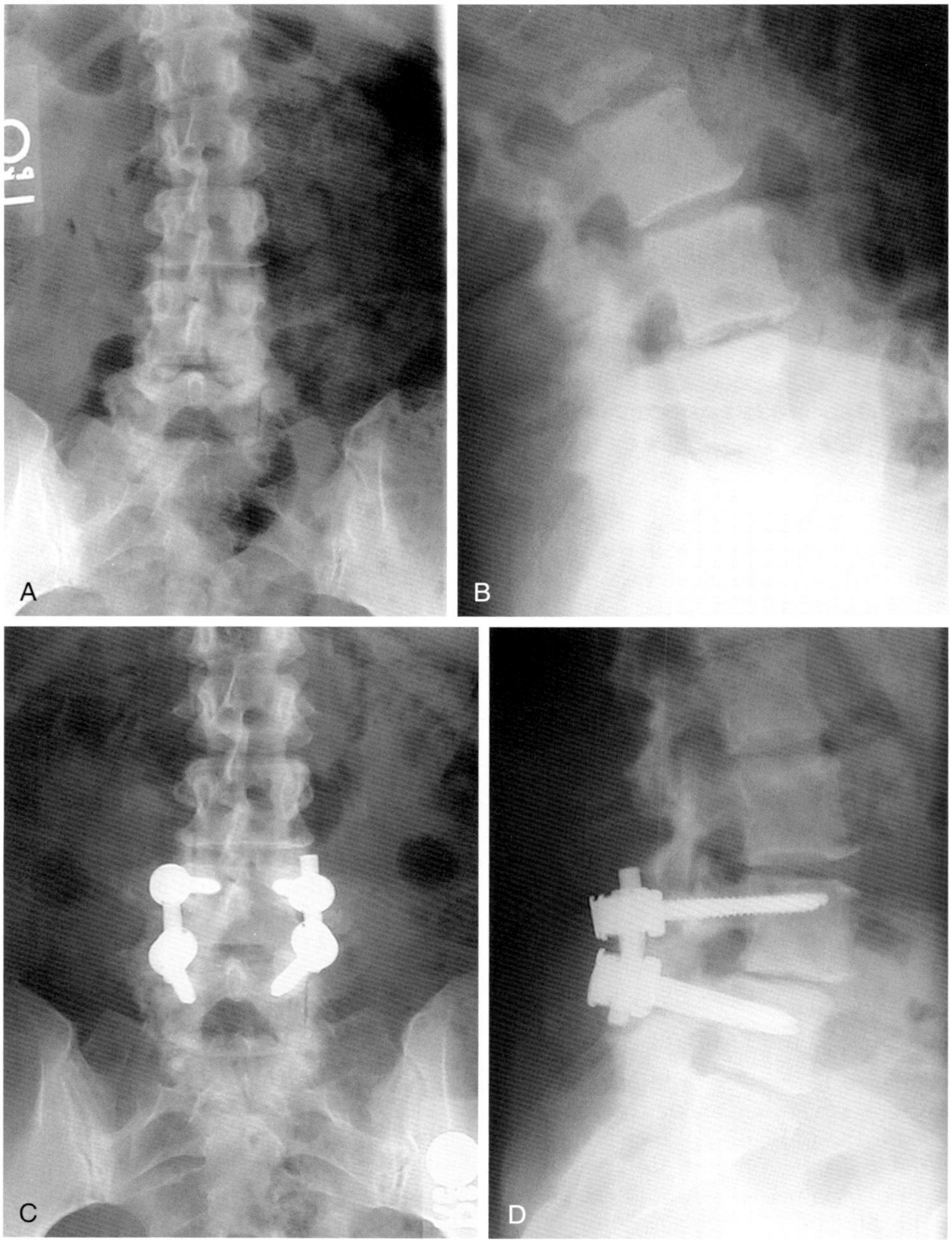

FIG. 24.5 (A) Anteroposterior and (B) lateral lumbar spine radiographs demonstrating grade 1 spondylolisthesis in a 47-year-old woman with disabling back and leg pain refractory to nonoperative treatment. (C and D) Postoperative radiographs demonstrating stable fusion 1 year following posterior decompression and fusion with supplemental instrumentation. Note the robust fusion mass bridging transverse processes laterally. The patient is pain free and has returned to full level of activity including triathlons and skiing.

patients often develop a variety of psychosocial issues. It is therefore vital that the patients with chronic LBP have a clear understanding of the nature of their pain and have realistic expectations of treatment. Because acute LBP frequently has a favorable natural history, in the absence of "red flags," an expectant and symptomatic treatment may be sufficient. This may include a short period of rest and analgesics, but providers should absolutely emphasize early return to normal activities to preserve functional status. Similarly, for many LBP syndromes, invasive spinal procedures are best suited for patients who have failed to improve with more conservative treatments. Due to the significant risks, exorbitant expense, and relatively high incidence of poor outcome, the decision to proceed with invasive spinal procedures must be carefully weighed against any potential benefit. Each patient must be uniquely evaluated before a specific treatment option is recommended. Additionally, as chronic LBP is often accompanied by psychosocial issues, it may best be treated by adopting a multidisciplinary approach and the addition of psychosocial, rehabilitative, and functional restorative modalities. An exercise program directed to increase spinal strength and flexibility may be introduced in all patients to minimize the risk of recurrent LBP. Given the lack of regenerative therapies, it is imperative to identify the behaviors and vocations that accelerate disc degeneration and can lead to chronic LBP. Patients should also be educated in methods of preventing spinal injury and minimizing continued deterioration. Some of the general preventative measures that may be readily adopted may include weight loss, regular exercise, discontinuation of tobacco products, avoidance of excessive or repetitive spinal stress, and maintaining appropriate posture while sitting, driving, and lifting. Future research must be encouraged to facilitate early detection of disc disease and develop therapies that will allow disc regeneration.

KEY POINTS

- Spinal pain is prevalent in the general population and is the most common medical reason for lost productivity, workers' compensation claims, and early social security disability.
- Acute spinal pain is typically self-limited, whereas chronic spinal pain is persistent or episodic and is frequently associated with psychosocial, behavioral, and substance abuse disorders.
- IVD cells exist in a precarious anaerobic environment in which they are vulnerable to a host of deleterious hereditary and environmental factors.
- Structural changes within the disc can alter disc dynamics, which may lead to degenerative changes within the spinal motion segment and the contiguous spinal structures, such as the facet joint.
- Spinal pain may originate from one or multiple spinal column components or structures adjacent to the spine.
- The innervation of the various spinal components is complex and topographic localization of spinal pain is often vague.
- The ubiquitous spinal pain caused by benign degenerative conditions must be differentiated from numerous uncommon but often perilous pathologic conditions.
- The diagnosis of the various spinal pain syndromes is often made arduous by diagnostic tests that lack both sensitivity and specificity.
- Due to its high prevalence and frequent spontaneous resolution, spinal pain should be further characterized by diagnostic tests only when red flags are identified during clinical evaluation of the patient.
- In the absence of progressive neurologic deficits or red flags, acute spinal pain should be treated symptomatically, whereas chronic spinal pain is best treated by implementing a multidisciplinary approach.
- Invasive spinal procedures are best suited for a small group of patients with unrelenting chronic spinal pain that has failed to improve with conservative treatments.

REFERENCES

Access the reference list online at ExpertConsult.com.

CHAPTER 25

Myofascial Pain Syndrome

Andrea L. Nicol, MD, MSc ◎ Matthew Crooks, MD ◎ Eric S. Hsu, MD ◎ F. Michael Ferrante, MD

Myofascial pain (MP) is a soft tissue pain syndrome (STP) with local and referred pain arising from trigger points (TrPs). The term *muscular rheumatism* of Sir William Osler's time gradually gave way to the term *nonarticular rheumatism*, and more recently, to the newer term *soft tissue pain syndromes*, which can be abbreviated as STP.[1] Local STPs include bursitis (subacromial, olecranon, trochanteric, prepatellar, and pes anserine), tenosynovitis (biceps, supraspinatus, infrapatellar, and achilles), and enthesopathies (lateral epicondylitis and medial epicondylitis). Regional STPs include myofascial pain syndrome (MPS) (MPS involving muscles of the trunk and extremities), myofascial pain dysfunction syndrome (MPS involving facial muscles), and complex regional pain syndrome (types I and II). Generalized STPs involve fibromyalgia syndrome (FMS), chronic fatigue syndrome (FMS-like when widespread body pain present), and hypermobility syndromes. Regional STPs such as MP are limited in anatomic distribution over a specific region or quadrant of the body.

TrPs generating MP are localized painful areas of skeletal muscle containing taut bands that can be exquisitely sensitive to digital pressure. TrPs may be active or latent. Active TrPs are present in patients with painful regional conditions. Latent TrPs are asymptomatic but may be revealed by deep palpation on physical examination. Latent TrPs have been found in the shoulder girdle muscles of 45% to 55% of healthy young adults.[2]

MP can occur independent of other pain generators (primary MP).[3] Alternatively, MP often coexists with or is secondary to other acute and chronic painful musculoskeletal conditions including (1) head and neck pain (temporomandibular disorders, cervical degenerative disc disease, cervical facet arthropathy, neck pain after whiplash injury, cervicobrachial syndrome, cervicogenic and chronic tension-type headache), (2) thoracolumbar back pain (degenerative disc disease, kyphosis, scoliosis, lumbar facet arthropathy), (3) pelvic pain, and (4) upper and lower extremity pain. MP is most effectively treated with a multimodal therapeutic regimen including injection, physical therapy, postural or ergonomic correction, and treatment of underlying musculoskeletal pain generators.

PREVALENCE

Reliably establishing the prevalence of MPS proves to be challenging, as there are no widely accepted diagnostic criteria. Few epidemiologic studies have been published, however, and the reported prevalence of MPS ranges from 20% to 95% of patients presenting with musculoskeletal pain at general medical clinics and pain management centers. One study designed to evaluate the prevalence of MPS in an academic internal medicine practice was performed by Skootsky and colleagues.[4] Of 201 patients initially screened, 54 patients had initial complaints of musculoskeletal pain and were studied further. Those that had pain conditions potentially related to MPS had a careful TrP examination performed. MPS was diagnosed when digital pressure on the TrPs for a standardized time period intensified regional pain, and the pain referral pattern corresponded with established referral maps. Ultimately, 16 patients were diagnosed with MPS, representing 30% of patients with musculoskeletal pain and 8% of the 201 originally screened patients. More recently, a study by Chen and Nizar[5] reported an MPS prevalence of 63.5% ($n = 80/126$) among chronic back pain patients, wherein MPS was diagnosed using the following criteria: the presence of a trigger point, reproducible pain, taut band, referred pain, and jump sign. Interestingly, they report that the majority of MPS (81.2%) in their population was secondary to other musculoskeletal or medical causes as opposed to primary MPS.

MPS can be commonly found in select patient populations. MPS is more commonly seen in patients with chronic tension-type headache,[6] temporomandibular disorders, pain in the face–jaw region,[7,8] and in postwhiplash syndrome[9] than in the general patient population. One cross-sectional study surveyed 111 older adults with chronic low back pain versus twenty who were pain free.[10] They were assessed by clinical history and physical examination. Biomechanical and soft tissue pathologies were significantly more common in older adults with chronic low back pain (90%) than in pain-free patients with MPS (10%). Limited data are available regarding risk factors for MPS; however, MPS has been reported to be more prevalent in female patients than male patients.[5,11]

PATHOPHYSIOLOGY

While much remains to be discovered about the etiology of MPS, several theories regarding its pathophysiology have been advanced in recent years. Underlying biomechanical and postural factors may interact with neurologic factors (e.g., radiculopathy), psychological elements including depression and anxiety, and hormonal and nutritional imbalances. These factors (in sum or in part) may create an autonomic dysregulation and, ultimately, central spinal cord sensitization which can amplify the experience of MPS. Vasoactive mediators, algogenic neurotransmitters and inflammatory mediators including bradykinin, norepinephrine, serotonin, calcitonin gene–related peptide, substance P, tumor necrosis factor alpha, and interleukin 1-B have been identified in the hyperirritable loci of TrPs.[12–14] These substances sensitize nociceptors and are responsible for the sensory experience of MP, including referred pain and the local twitch response (LTR).

The motor phenomena of MP have been hypothesized to be caused by excessive acetylcholine (ACh) leakage, which creates dysfunctional endplates that are responsible for taut muscle band formation. Excessive ACh release causes sustained muscle contraction by increased depolarization of the postjunctional endplate. Evidence of maximal sarcomere shortening in TrPs has been found in canine and human subjects.[15] A positive feedback cycle may be created by the interplay of increased ACh release, sarcomere shortening, and the release of sensitizing substances. In a study investigating the hypothalamus-pituitary-adrenocortical and sympathetic-adrenal-medullary system responses to experimentally induced stress in patients with MP, plasma concentrations of cortisol, epinephrine, and norepinephrine were found to be significantly higher in MP patients than in healthy controls.[16]

The taut muscle band present in MPS has a higher resting tension and contains hypercontracted muscle fibers. Chronicity may increase local energy consumption and cause areas of tissue hypoperfusion and ischemia. Vasoactive mediators are released in the setting of muscle ischemia, causing increased ACh release, exacerbation of local ischemia, and sensitization of peripheral nociceptors, thereby causing pain. Abnormal spontaneous electrical activity is present at the site of TrPs, with excessive ACh release creating endplate noise seen on electrophysiological studies at the neuromuscular junction.[17] Spontaneous electrical activity is observed as having two components: a constant, low amplitude background activity of approximately 50 μV and intermittent higher amplitude spikes of 100–700 μV. Spontaneous electrical activity occurs more often in TrPs than in normal tissue and displays aberrant patterns in TrPs. Therefore, this spontaneous electrical activity is distinct from normal miniature endplate potentials. The abnormal electrical activity observed in TrPs is thought to be directly related to excessive ACh release.

The clinical manifestation of abnormal electrical activity in the TrP is an LTR and thought to be mediated by a segmental spinal reflex.[18] Snapping palpation or needling the TrP causes a brisk muscle contraction in the taut band. The location of the LTR is called the "sensory locus," which has been correlated histologically with sensory receptors.[19] The "active locus" is the site where spontaneous electrical activity is recorded, the waveforms of which correspond to published reports of motor endplate noise. According to this model, the sensory locus and the active locus act as the nociceptor and the motor endplate and are distributed throughout muscle. Where these align and are highly concentrated, we observe myofascial TrPs (Box 25.1).

Vasoactive mediators such as those released in the taut bands of MP have been known to sensitize peripheral nociceptive nerve fibers such as those found in skeletal muscle. In a sensitized state, nociceptors spontaneously discharge with a lower threshold to painful stimulation and also exhibit discharge to nonpainful stimuli.[20] Over time, this heightened abnormal peripheral sensory input creates a state of central neuronal sensitization.[21]

DIAGNOSIS

In a survey of 403 responding clinician members of the American Pain Society, 88.5% considered MPS to be a valid clinical disorder and 81% believed it was distinct from FMS.[22] A careful history and physical exam remain the cornerstone of effective diagnosis. The most common presentation of MPS includes the following diagnostic criteria: regional body pain and stiffness, limited range of motion of the affected muscle, twitch response produced from a taut band, referred pain from a TrP to a zone of reference, and resolution of the symptoms with local anesthesia applied to the TrP.[23] MPS may occur after injury, chronic strain with repetitive microtrauma, or without clear precipitating event. Aberrant body mechanics or postural abnormality may initiate or perpetuate the problem. The quality of pain tends to be a deep "aching" of variable intensity, and the pain is confined to a specific anatomic region. Characteristic referred pain patterns are associated with specific muscles, although these referral patterns are often unreliable.[24]

It is essential to have hands-on formal training in the physical examination of MP and TrPs to achieve a reliable result.[1] Musculoskeletal examination should be performed with the objective of identifying orthopedic or neurologic dysfunction that may play a role in generating secondary MPS. Although there are no universally accepted diagnostic criteria for MP, physical findings may be helpful in establishing a diagnosis. A distinct pattern of TrP findings may reveal itself in MPS after a given insult.[9] Active TrPs may be identified by palpation with gentle digital pressure oriented across and perpendicular to the muscle fibers. TrPs are present as a taut muscle bands within skeletal muscle, and palpation of these points may elicit involuntary muscle contraction, the twitch response or "jump" sign. These painful TrPs limit full range of passive motion in the afflicted muscle group. Although these findings have been suggested as diagnostic criteria,[25–27] investigators have found it problematic to demonstrate consistent agreement in the presence or absence of TrPs among examiners in blinded studies with control groups.[28–30] Inconsistencies may be attributed in part to a lack of standardized examination technique and variability in the interpretation of examination findings. Variability in muscle anatomy, physical conditioning, and deconditioning pose obstacles as well. The most

BOX 25.1 Commonly Accepted Diagnostic Characteristics of Myofascial Trigger Points

DIAGNOSTIC HISTORY

- Regional pain
- Onset with sudden muscle overload
- Onset with sustained muscular contraction in shortened position
- Onset with repetitive activity (symptoms increase with increasing stressfulness)

DIAGNOSTIC PHYSICAL EXAMINATION

- Taut band
- Focal spot muscle tenderness
- Pressure-elicited referred pain pattern
- If active, pressure elicits pain recognized as familiar

OTHER CLINICAL CHARACTERISTICS

- Local twitch response—confirmatory, difficult to elicit
- Prompt release of taut-band tension by specific myofascial trigger-point therapy
- Central/attachment myofascial trigger points

Simons DG: Review of enigmatic MTrPs as a common cause of enigmatic musculoskeletal pain and dysfunction. *J Electromyogr Kinesiol.* 14:95-107, 2004.

TABLE 25.1 Clinical Distinctions Between Myofascial Pain Syndrome and Fibromyalgia Syndrome

Clinical Feature	Myofascial Pain	Fibromyalgia
Pain pattern	Local or regional	Generalized
Least distribution	A single muscle	11 tender points
Muscle spasm	+++	++
Trigger points	Local, regional	Not a feature
Tender points	Not a feature	Common, widespread
Taut band	++	—
Twitch response	++	—
Referred pain	+++	—
Fatigue	+	++++
Sleep disturbance	+++	++++
Paresthesias	Regional	Distal
Headaches	Referred head pain	Occipital origin
Irritable bowel	Not a feature	+++
Swelling sensation	+	++

Note: The number of plus signs reflects the significance of correlation and implication in clinical feature.
Source: McMahon SB, Koltzenburg M, editors: Wall and Melzack's Textbook of Pain, *ed. 5, Philadelphia: Elsevier, 2006, pp 669-681.*

reproducible diagnostic findings on physical examination include observation of a TrP in an affected muscle, referral of pain to a zone of reference, and reproduction of the patient's usual pain on physical exam.

Differential diagnosis of MP should include (1) musculoskeletal and neuropathic disorders such as arthritis, degenerative disc disease, radiculopathy, bursitis, and tendonitis; (2) autoimmune or infectious etiologies; (3) metabolic and endocrine dysfunction including hypothyroidism; (4) psychiatric disorders including depression and anxiety; and (5) fibromyalgia. It has been postulated that MPS may be an evolving component of FMS. While on the surface there are similarities, several well-documented findings argue against the connection between MPS and FMS (Table 25.1). Patients with MPS do not exhibit widespread tender point hypersensitivity as in those with FMS. Additionally, FMS tender points do not refer pain to a zone of reference as do the TrPs in MPS. The common TrPs in MPS can coexist with the widespread tender points of FMS.

Common muscle groups associated with MPS can be categorized by the regions in which the muscles anatomically exist or where the muscles can refer pain to. The common regions for MPS include head and neck, shoulder, chest, abdomen, low back, pelvis/hip, knee, and ankle/foot. Box 25.2 describes the muscles that can contribute to pain in each of these regions.

TREATMENT

PHYSICAL MODALITIES

A comprehensive multimodal therapeutic approach is optimal in the treatment of MPS, with the goal of patient education, reduction of pain, and restoration of function. This requires an informed and understanding clinician to coordinate care in a systematic fashion. As the pathogenesis of MP frequently involves postural defect, repetitive microtrauma, and muscle fiber shortening, it is logical that guided physical modalities play a significant role in treatment. On the other hand, ergonomic and behavioral modifications are commonly employed in treatment plans, although there is little clinical evidence of significant outcomes.

Guided stretching has been well documented as successful in reducing MP. This fits mechanistically with the model of shortened sarcomeres in MPS. Travell and Simons described passive stretching of the muscle groups after application of sprayed vapocoolant.[2] The sudden cooling of the vapocoolant in a defined area reduces discomfort from stretching, allowing more vigorous stretch. Noting significant improvement with this method, Travell and Simons termed this the "single most effective treatment" for TrP pain. Structured physical therapy with a well-trained professional can incorporate these techniques along with strengthening, postural realignment, relaxation techniques, and massage.

A randomized controlled trial (RCT) by Gam et al. studied the effects of ultrasound, massage, and exercises on patients with MP in the neck and shoulders.[31] While there was no relative difference in pain reduction within the ultrasound group, there was a reduction in the number of TrPs, although this reduction was characterized as weak. In an RCT of ultrasound applied to myofascial TrPs, Srbely et al. demonstrated significant antinociceptive effects on both infraspinatus and gluteus medius pain pressure threshold at 1, 3, and 5 minutes, but not at 10 and 15 minutes.[32]

There is some evidence of benefit from complementary, manual, and exercise therapies, but the methodologic quality of these studies tends to be flawed.[33] Acupuncture, transcutaneous electrical nerve stimulation (TENS), and laser therapy may be of benefit as part of a comprehensive strategy in refractory cases. It is noted (somewhat

BOX 25.2 Muscles Involved in Regional Myofascial Pain Syndromes

HEAD AND NECK
- Posterior cervical
  - Splenius capitus and cervicis, semispinalis capitus and cervicis
- Sternocleidomastoid
- Upper trapezius
- Levator scapulae
- Facial muscles
  - Temporalis
  - Masseter

SHOULDER
- Trapezius
- Supraspinatus
- Infraspinatus
- Subscapularis
- Teres major and minor
- Latissimus dorsi
- Levator scapulae
- Posterior serratus
- Deltoid
- Pectoralis major and minor

CHEST
- Pectoralis major and minor
- Abdominal obliques
- Intercostal muscles
- Serratus anterior

ABDOMEN
- Serratus anterior
- Abdominal obliques
- Rectus abdominus

LOW BACK
- Psoas
- Quadratus lumborum
- Paraspinal muscles
  - Iliocostalis
  - Longimus thoracis
  - Multifidi
- Abdominal obliques

PELVIS/HIP
- Abdominal muscles
- Psoas
- Quadratus lumborum
- Gluteal muscles
- Piriformis
- Pectineus
- Semitendinosis
- Obturators
- Gemellae

KNEE
- Vastus medius and lateralis
- Hamstrings
- Gastrocnemius

ANKLE/FOOT
- Gastrocnemius
- Soleus
- Tibialis anterior
- Fibularis longus and brevis
- Long flexor and extensor muscles of the leg
- Intrinsic foot muscles

controversially) that classical acupuncture points may show clinical correspondence to the location of TrPs.[34] Melzack et al. reported 100% anatomic and 71% clinical pain correspondence of myofascial TrPs with classical acupuncture points.[35] More studies are needed (particularly RCTs) to draw definitive conclusions about the roles of acupuncture, TENS, and laser therapy in the treatment of MPS. At present, the sum of the evidence is contradictory or inadequate.[36]

PHARMACOTHERAPY

Systemic medications are often useful additions to a comprehensive treatment plan. Although few RCTs exist to support their efficacy, nonsteroidal antiinflammatory drugs (NSAIDs) and antidepressants have been employed to relieve pain associated with TrPs. NSAIDs provide symptomatic relief but at the price of long-term side effects. These effects include cardiovascular morbidity and mortality, gastritis, and renal dysfunction. There is a paucity of RCTs detailing evidence of the effectiveness of NSAIDs in MPS. Rather, data from studies of other pain syndromes (arthritis and fibromyalgia) are used to guide treatment of MPS. Ibuprofen has been shown to be effective in acute myofascial strain, significantly reducing pain in a study of 77 emergency department patients. These effects were not significantly improved with the addition of the muscle relaxant cyclobenzaprine.[37] The tricyclic antidepressant amitriptyline has been studied in patients with chronic tension-type headache in a double-blind, placebo-controlled crossover study and significantly reduced myofascial tenderness and headache intensity more than placebo.[38]

Muscle relaxants are widely used in MP to reduce muscle spasm, to relieve pain, and to improve sleep disturbance related to MPS pain. The alpha-2 adrenergic agonist tizanidine has been cited as helpful in patients with chronic neck or low back pain in a review of the literature. However, RCTs are needed to assess the risk–benefit ratio of muscle relaxant therapy.[39]

Systemic opioids (including mixed opioid analgesics such as tramadol) have been widely used, especially when the patient has failed more conservative medications. Tramadol has demonstrated reduction in pain and core symptoms in clinical trials with fibromyalgia patients but not in patients with regional pain syndromes such as MPS.[40] As there is little evidence of the efficacy of opioids in MPS, the side effects and consequences of longer-term opioid use are concerning. The occurrence of tolerance, presenting as a loss of analgesic efficacy occurring over time, frequently leads to dose escalation. With long-term use and dose escalation comes the risk of opioid-induced hyperalgesia (an *N*-methyl-D-aspartate [NMDA]–mediated central sensitization phenomenon) that is characterized by escalating pain (often insidiously) in response to increasing opioid analgesic dose.[41] In addition to side effects of gastrointestinal slowing, nausea, sedation, respiratory depression, pruritus, and dysphoria, opioids can cause hormonal changes and lead to osteopenia by influencing the hypothalamic-pituitary-adrenal axis and the hypothalamic-pituitary-gonadal axis. Inappropriate use of opioids, including abuse, addiction, and diversion, has emerged as a major societal problem in recent years and demands responsible physician prescribing and monitoring practices within the guidelines of an informed-consent opioid agreement.

Lidocaine patches may be an effective noninvasive therapy for MP in an appropriately selected patient population. In an RCT of patients with MPS, a total of 60 subjects received lidocaine patch, placebo patch, or local anesthetic TrP injection.[42] Subjective pain-related symptoms significantly decreased for the lidocaine patch and injection groups. Similarly, pain thresholds increased significantly. Pain-related symptoms and thresholds did not change for the placebo group. Patients in the lidocaine patch group noted less discomfort from therapy than the injection group.

TRIGGER POINT INJECTION

Trigger point injection (TPI) is a widely used invasive therapy wherein a needle is guided directly into a TrP that has been previously identified on physical examination. TPI is best utilized in a series of injections and as part of a comprehensive treatment plan that includes guided, structured, physical therapy. This strategy can be particularly beneficial when TPI is initially employed to reduce pain in patients otherwise intolerant of physical therapy or stretching, allowing the physical modalities to be more effective.[43] Saline, corticosteroids, a variety of local anesthetics including lidocaine and bupivacaine, botulinum toxin serotype A (BoNT-A), and dry needling have all been used and studied. Stimulation of the LTR in direct needling of the TrP is valuable in achieving immediate effect.[44] There is good evidence to suggest that there is no advantage of one injection therapy over another or of any drug injectate over dry needling.[45] In a systemic review of 23 RCTs, Cummings and White concluded that any effect derived from TPI is likely derived from the needle itself, rather than any specific substance injected, as there was no difference in therapeutic benefit of "wet" needling versus "dry" needling.[45] Their review also suggested that pain reduction with saline TPI is equal to pain reduction with local anesthetic TPI, both being significant. Although adding corticosteroid preparation to local anesthetic is a common practice, it has not been reliably shown to reduce pain more than TPI with local anesthetic alone. Despite the widespread practice of TPI for MP, there is no consensus regarding the number of injection points, frequency of administration, and volume or type of injectate. Controlled studies are needed to evaluate the comparative efficacy of TPIs and their potential benefits in long-term pain reduction, if any.

BOTULINUM TOXIN

BoNT-A produces sustained and prolonged relaxation of muscles by inhibiting release of Ach at the motor endplate and is itself an analgesic inhibiting central sensitization.[46] Commercially prepared BoNT-A is expensive and should be employed with care by a well-trained physician. Although this therapy is promising, the results of RCTs have been mixed, and multiple systematic reviews have concluded that the current clinical evidence to support the use of BoNT in the treatment of MPS is inconclusive. Ferrante et al. found no statistically significant improvement compared to placebo with BoNT-A injection when injected directly into painful TrPs for cervicothoracic MP.[47] They concluded that although it is intuitive for the clinician to consider therapeutic injection of BoNT-A as a treatment for MP (given its *a priori* similarity to TPI), peculiarities inherent to the use of toxin in lieu of dry needling or local anesthetic must be accounted for (i.e., toxin spread through fascial planes), including the effects of dosing of toxin, volume of injectate, muscles chosen to inject, postural relations and abnormalities, and injection technique. Harden et al.[48] were able to identify a short-term (12-week) reduction in MP of chronic tension-type headache with BoNT-A injection as compared with placebo. Graboski et al.[49] found no significant difference in BoNT-A versus 0.5% bupivacaine injected into TrPs of patients with MPS, although both were effective in reducing pain below baseline level. Venancio et al.[50] studied 45 MP patients who were assigned randomly to one of three groups: dry needling, 0.25% lidocaine TPI, and BoNT–A TPI, and assessed over a 12-week period. While all three groups showed favorable response to treatment, the BoNT-A group demonstrated less use of rescue medication and less postinjection local sensitivity.[50] In a recent study, Nicol et al.[51] reported that BoNT-A injected directly into painful muscle groups using a "follow the pain" and pattern injection technique in lieu of TrPs led to reduced average numerical pain scores, reduced number of headaches per week, and improvement in general activity and sleep quality of life measures. Similar positive findings were seen in studies by Benecke et al.[52] and Miller et al.[53] wherein patients with cervical MP received BoNT-A using a fixed-location injection technique.

New theories regarding the use of botulinum toxin for the treatment of MPS de-emphasize injection into the TrP per se but focus upon selection of patients with significant features of overlap among cervical MPS, headache syndromes, and spasmodic torticollis. It is hypothesized that patients with cervicobrachial MPS reminiscent of spasmodic torticollis (with and without headache) may benefit from institution of botulinum toxin therapy. It is hypothesized that botulinum toxin's role is to help restore aberrant biomechanics and postural abnormalities in conjunction with restorative and rehabilitative physical therapy.[54]

CONCLUSION

MP is widely prevalent in many patients with regional musculoskeletal pain. The challenging nature of MPS with its complex interaction of underlying biomechanical, neurologic, and psychological factors requires an astute, well-trained clinician for early diagnosis and effective treatment. Current data suggest that patients with MPS tend to do worse than patients with discreet musculoskeletal pathology such as disc herniation.[55] MPS can often be refractory to treatment. If the patient is unable to participate in an active functional rehabilitation program due to the limitations of pain, then a comprehensive approach should be considered. A multidisciplinary approach may include psychological counseling for coping strategies, relaxation techniques and biofeedback, cognitive behavioral therapy, and complementary and alternative medicine in addition to standard medical evaluation and management. When a comprehensive program is employed early in the disease course, functional improvement in measures of decreased sick time, improved coping skills, and increased life satisfaction can be demonstrated in patients with whiplash trauma and other MPSs.[56] Should pain persist, it is important to assess the potential contribution of coexisting musculoskeletal or neurologic pathology to MPS. The meticulous clinician should seek to identify and eliminate any underlying source of pain generation. However, despite an abundance of clinical experience and successful outcomes, we need better designed, short- and long-term outcome studies on MP to assess the efficacy and efficiency of traditional and emerging therapies.

KEY POINTS

- MPS is a type of regional STP involving muscles of the trunk and extremities.
- Although MP may generalize, it remains distinct from fibromyalgia.
- Hyperirritable loci of TrPs have been found to contain vasoactive mediators, algogenic neurotransmitters, and inflammatory mediators.
- Excessive ACh leakage has been hypothesized to contribute to dysfunctional motor endplates, creating the sustained muscle contraction responsible for taut bands.
- The clinical manifestation of abnormal electrical activity in the trigger point is an LTR that is thought to be mediated by a segmental spinal reflex. Snapping palpation or needling the trigger point causes a brisk muscle contraction in the taut band.
- Diagnostic findings in the physical examination include observation of TrPs in an affected muscle, referral of pain to a zone of reference, and reproduction of the patient's usual pain.
- Early diagnosis and treatment with a comprehensive multimodal approach is optimal.
- Passive stretching after application of sprayed vapocoolant is a well-documented treatment.
- While there is evidence of the efficacy of TPI for MP, there is no evidence of the advantage of one injection technique over another or the injection of any substance versus dry needling.
- Injection of botulinum toxin is an emerging therapy that may be considered in refractory cases of MP, although evidence of its efficacy is limited at present.

REFERENCES

Access the reference list online at ExpertConsult.com.

CHAPTER 26

FIBROMYALGIA AND CENTRALIZED PAIN STATES

Chad Brummett, MD ⊛ Daniel J. Clauw, MD

EPIDEMIOLOGY

When considered to be a discrete disorder, fibromyalgia (FM) is generally considered to be the second-most common "rheumatic" disease, behind osteoarthritis. Depending on the diagnostic criteria used, the prevalence of FM ranges from 2% to 8% of the population.[1–3] It can develop at any age, including in childhood. It occurs in relatively equal frequency in different countries, cultures, and ethnic groups; there is no evidence that this condition at increased rates in "industrialized" countries and cultures.[2]

Individuals who develop fibromyalgia nearly always have a lifelong history of chronic pain in various regions of the body. Most individuals who eventually develop fibromyalgia have pain in multiple body regions beginning earlier in life. The prevalence of any (regional or widespread) chronic musculoskeletal pain in the population is about 30%; thus, if a single individual has had chronic pain in multiple bodily regions over the course of their lifetime, he or she is exhibiting a "pain prone phenotype" that is an important part of the history in a chronic pain patient. Often beginning in childhood or adolescence, individuals who eventually go on to develop fibromyalgia are more likely to experience headaches, dysmenorrhea, temporomandibular joint disorder (TMJD), chronic fatigue, irritable bowel syndrome (IBS) and other functional gastrointestinal (GI) disorders, interstitial cystitis/painful bladder syndrome, endometriosis, and other regional pain syndromes (especially back and neck pain).[4,5] In fact, what often looks to one healthcare provider as a new episode of acute or subacute pain is in fact simply the latest region of the body experiencing pain.[6] Consequently, many experts in the pain field have begun to feel that especially these "centralized" pain states are best thought of as a single lifelong disease that merely tends to manifest in different bodily regions over time.[7–9]

In addition to fibromyalgia patients having a high personal lifetime history of chronic pain, there is often a strong family history of chronic pain identifiable. The first degree relatives of fibromyalgia patients are 8 times as likely to have this condition as the family members of controls, and they have very high rates of other chronic pain states.[10] The strong familial predisposition to FM is shared by many chronic pain conditions, and there has been an explosion of knowledge recently regarding the strong role of genetic factors in chronic pain states.[9,11] Many of the genes that have been identified to date in leading to increases or decreases in the frequency of chronic pain states, or of pain sensitivity, are mostly involved in regulating the breakdown or binding of neurotransmitters that generally increase pain sensitivity (e.g., glutamate) or decrease pain sensitivity (serotonin, norepinephrine, gamma-aminobutyric acid [GABA]). The fact that pain sensitivity is polygenic and that different individuals develop increased pain sensitivity because of imbalances or altered activity of many different neurotransmitters likely partly explains the "U-shaped curve" seen with many analgesics, wherein they either work fairly well or not at all. Twin studies suggest that approximately 50% of the risk of developing FM or related pain conditions such as IBS and headache is genetic and 50% environmental.[12]

The environmental factors that are most likely to trigger the development of FM are various types of "stressors," typically those that involve acute pain for at least a few weeks. Psychological stress is but one such stressor. FM or similar illnesses can be triggered by certain types of infections[13] (e.g., Epstein-Barr virus, Lyme disease, Q fever, viral hepatitis), trauma[14] (motor vehicle collisions), and deployment to war.[15]

FM also is commonly seen as a comorbidity in other chronic pain conditions such as osteoarthritis, rheumatoid arthritis, and lupus. Approximately 20% to 30% of individuals with these established rheumatic disorders will meet the criteria for FM. This phenomenon had previously been termed "secondary fibromyalgia," but since this is so common and might occur in a subset of nearly any chronic pain cohort, a more popular term we prefer to use for this phenomenon is that these individuals have "centralized" their pain. Thus, although peripheral nociceptive input might be responsible for some or even much of that individual's pain, superimposed central nervous system (CNS) factors also likely amplify pain and lead to other comorbid symptoms such as fatigue, memory problems, and disturbances of sleep and mood.[16] The term "central sensitization" is also sometimes used to describe this phenomenon, but many feel that this particular term should be reserved for the original spinal mechanism that was identified and called by this name rather than the more general phenomenon we now believe can result via a multitude of different spinal and supraspinal mechanisms.[9,17] Regardless of what term an individual uses to describe this phenomenon, it is becoming increasingly important to identify it. Because emerging evidence suggests that therapies that work best for peripheral, nociceptive pain (e.g., NSAIDs, opioids, injections, and surgical procedures) are less likely to be effective in these individuals.[18,19]

FM, especially the "primary" form, is also very comorbid with early life and current stress, and many if not most individuals will have a lifetime history of a psychiatric disorder such as depression or anxiety.[20] There is typically more psychiatric and psychological comorbidity seen in tertiary care settings or in individuals who are refractory to treatment. This bidirectional relationship between FM and psychiatric conditions is likely due in part to the fact that there are common triggers to both sets of conditions (e.g., early life stress or trauma), as well as shared pathophysiology (i.e., most of the same neurotransmitters that affect pain transmission also affect mood, memory, fatigue, sleep). Other potentially modifiable risk factors for developing FM include poor sleep, obesity, physical inactivity, or poor job or life satisfaction. Similarly, cognitive factors such as catastrophizing (the feeling that pain is very bad and associated with a poor prognosis for recovery) or fear of movement have been shown to be poor prognostic factors in FM and other chronic pain states.

PATHOPHYSIOLOGY

The physiological hallmark of centralized pain, central sensitization, or FM is augmented central pain processing. This was originally identified in FM (and still can be clinically) by noting that an individual is diffusely tender to palpation. The scientific terms for this phenomenon are diffuse hyperalgesia (increased pain to normally painful stimuli) and/or allodynia (pain in response to normally nonpainful stimuli). In the absence of an identifiable diffuse "peripheral" inflammatory process involving the body tissues, this strongly suggests that the CNS (i.e., spinal cord and brain) is causing augmented pain processing. In 1990 when the original criteria for FM were first published, this feature of diffuse tenderness was incorporated into the diagnostic criteria by requiring that an individual had a certain number of tender points (11 or greater) in addition to chronic widespread pain in order to qualify for this diagnosis.[21] Subsequent studies using more sophisticated measures of experimental pain testing showed that individuals with FM are more tender everywhere in the body, not just in the 18 regions considered to be "tender points."[22,23] Subsequent experimental pain testing studies have identified multiple potential mechanisms that may be responsible for pain amplification in FM, including a decrease in the activity of descending analgesic pathways,[24,25] as well as a diffuse increase in the processing of all sensory stimuli (not just pain).[26,27]

These initial observations that individuals with FM were diffusely tender led to subsequent functional, chemical, and structural brain neuroimaging studies that have been amongst the best "objective" evidence that the pain in FM and related pain amplification syndrome is "real."[28] These methods such as functional magnetic resonance imaging (fMRI) clearly demonstrate that when individuals with FM are given a mild pressure or heat stimuli that most individuals would feel as "touch" rather than "pain," they experience pain, and similar brain activation patterns in brain areas involved in pain processing.[29,30] fMRI has also proved useful in determining how comorbid psychological factors influence pain processing in FM. For example, in FM patients with variable degrees of comorbid depression, the authors found that the anterior insula and amygdala activations were correlated with depressive symptoms, consistent with these "medial" and prefrontal brain regions being involved with affective or motivational aspects of pain processing (and being more closely related to unpleasantness rather than the sensory intensity of pain).[31] However, the degree of neuronal activation in more lateral structures generally thought to be associated with the "sensory" processing of pain (i.e., where the pain is localized and how intense it is) were not associated with levels of depressive symptoms, or the presence or absence of major depression, consistent with a plethora of evidence in the pain field that pain and depression are largely independent but overlapping physiological processes.

A more recent advance in the use of fMRI is to look at the extent brain regions are "connected" to each other, that is, simultaneously activated (or deactivated).[32] The advantage of resting state analysis is that it is a window into brain changes associated with chronic, ongoing spontaneous pain. Studies have shown that individuals with FM have increased connectivity between brain regions involved in increasing pain transmission and neural networks not normally involved in pain such as the default mode network, and the degree of this hyperconnectedness is related to the severity of ongoing pain.[33,34] A different group has shown that during a painful stimulus, connectivity is decreased between key antinociceptive regions (e.g., the brainstem—the origin of descending analgesic pathways) and a region they had previously identified to be a potential source of dysfunctional pain inhibition in FM.[35,36]

Other imaging techniques have been used to identify the neurotransmitter abnormalities that may be "driving" the pain amplification seen in FM and other chronic pain disorders. Wood and colleagues used positron emission tomography (PET) to show that attenuated dopaminergic activity may be playing a role in pain transmission in FM, and Harris and colleagues showed evidence of decreased *mu* opioid receptor availability (possibly due to increased release of endogenous *mu* opioids) in FM.[37,38] This latter finding as well as previous studies showing increases in endogenous opioids in the cerebrospinal fluid (CSF) of FM patients has been suggested as evidence of why opioid analgesics appear to not be efficacious in FM.

Other groups have used proton spectroscopy (proton magnetic resonance spectroscopy [H-MRS]) to probe other neurotransmitters. Several groups have shown there are increases in brain concentrations of the body's major excitatory neurotransmitter, glutamate, in pain processing regions such as the insula in FM.[39] This finding has also been noted in the CSF in FM.[40] Drugs such as pregabalin and gabapentin are likely working in part in FM by reducing glutamatergic activity.[41] This has been nicely demonstrated by Harris and colleagues who showed that individuals with FM that had the highest pretreatment levels of glutamate in the posterior insula were those most likely to respond to pregabalin.[42] When pregabalin led to improvement in symptoms in these individuals, there was normalization of fMRI and connectivity findings, all suggesting that this neurotransmitter is playing a critical role in the pathogenesis of FM in some individuals. An even more important finding from this study was the fact that individuals with FM with normal or low baseline levels of glutamate in their posterior insula did not respond to pregabalin, even though this drug further lowered glutamate levels in these individuals as well. This helps us understand why no single class of CNS analgesic is likely to work in every patient with pain of CNS origin.

Conversely, H-MRS has recently been used to demonstrate low levels of one of the body's major inhibitory neurotransmitters, GABA.[43] This likely accounts for the efficacy of drugs such as gamma-hydroxybutyrate in FM.[44] This finding may also suggest biological plausibility for the finding that FM patients that have low alcohol consumption (compared to none or high) and have less symptoms and better functionality.[45] Alcohol is known to be a GABA agonist and analgesic, likely showing a U-shaped curve for analgesic effects just as for some beneficial cardiovascular effects. The fact that these imbalances between excitatory and inhibitory neurotransmitters are not diffusely noted in brain structures and seem to be confined to brain regions such as the insula that are known to be involved in polysensory processing[46,47] is concordant with the notion that there is a global problem with sensory hyperresponsiveness that is partly responsible for the pathophysiology of FM and related conditions.[48,49]

Although most agree that the core symptoms of FM are likely due to changes in the CNS, peripheral factors also play an important role in both the pathogenesis and treatment of FM. For example, some elements of the processes of central sensitization can be worsened or driven by ongoing nociceptive input. Thus, it is possible or likely that the many individuals with FM that also have comorbid conditions causing ongoing peripheral nociceptive input (e.g., myofascial pain, osteoarthritis, obesity) would potentially benefit from therapies aimed at reducing peripheral drive of central sensitization. This was suggested in a short-term study by Affaitati et al., which showed that treating these common comorbid conditions could lead to improvement in the widespread pain and tenderness seen in FM.[50]

There is also a current ongoing controversy regarding the meaning of finding decreased intraepidermal nerve fiber density (i.e., small fiber neuropathy) in FM. There is no question that this has been shown by many groups,[51–53] but these authors feel that this is a nonspecific finding seen in many other pain and nonpain conditions, so at present it is not clear whether this plays any role in the pathogenesis of FM or whether doing such testing helps at all in treatment.[54]

DIAGNOSIS OF FIBROMYALGIA

The 1990 American College of Rheumatology criteria for FM were never intended to be used as strict diagnostic criteria for use in clinical practice. Many individuals who clearly have FM do not have pain throughout their entire body, or do not have 11 tender points. Moreover, pain and tenderness occur across a continuum in the population, and it is impossible to know how to distinguish between an individual with symptoms and someone with an "illness."[55]

For this and many other reasons, the alternative 2010 (which need to be administered by a healthcare provider) and 2011 (which are entirely self-report) FM criteria may represent a preferred manner of diagnosing, or thinking about, FM.[56–58] The survey version of these criteria are entirely patient self-reported and can be administered on a single piece of paper. There is a body map with 19 areas (each counted as one point towards a total possible score of 31),[59] a symptom survey that asks about the presence and severity of fatigue, sleep disturbances, memory difficulties (each scored 0–3 for the presence and severity), and irritable bowel, headaches and mood problems (one point each). When used as a dichotomous measure with a variety of "cut points" that can be used, this measure roughly identifies most of the same individuals as the old criteria (except many more males).[57,58] However, when FM is considered

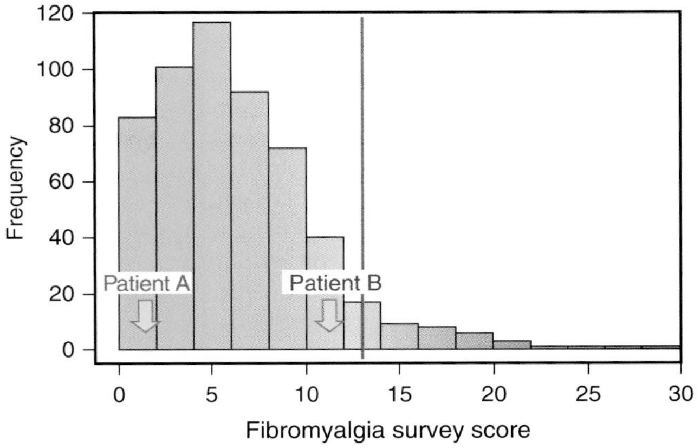

FIG. 26.1 Distribution of fibromyalgianess. After adjustment, compared to Patient A with localized pain and no somatic symptoms, Patient B would need 80 mg more oral morphine equivalents (OME) during first 48 hours of hospitalization and would be 5 times less likely to have improvements in pain at 6 months.[18,61] *(Brummett CM, Urquhart AG, Hassett AL, et al: Characteristics of fibromyalgia independently predict poorer long-term analgesic outcomes following total knee and hip arthroplasty.* Arthritis Rheumatol. *67(5):1386-1394, 2015; Brummett CM, Janda AM, Schueller CM, et al. Survey criteria for fibromyalgia independently predict increased postoperative opioid consumption after lower-extremity joint arthroplasty: a prospective, observational cohort study.* Anesthesiology. *119(6):1434-1443, 2013.)*

more as a physiological construct to determine the location of an individual on the continuum of pain sensitivity, then this can be used as a continuous measure (i.e., degree of "fibromyalgia-ness" or the degree to which pain is centralized) that can be useful in the diagnosis and treatment of virtually any patient with a rheumatic disorder who is experiencing pain.[60]

In several recent studies, this concept of fibromyalgianess or subsyndromal FM has been shown to be very clinically important. In these studies by Brummett and colleagues, individuals who were scheduled for either lower extremity joint replacement or hysterectomy completed a broad self-report battery prior to their surgery. The group hypothesized that individuals with higher FM scores on the 2011 FM Survey Criteria would predict decreased responsiveness to opioids given in the perioperative period and to surgery, ultimately relieving pain. Again, this measure is scored from 0 to 31, with a level of 13 being typically used as the diagnostic cut point of FM. These studies demonstrated that for each one-point increase in this measure from 0 to 31, individuals needed an adjusted 7–9 mg more oral morphine equivalents to control their pain in the first 24–48 hours following surgery and were 15%–20% less likely to improve following arthroplasty.[18,19,61] These findings were independent of a number of preoperative characteristics, including age, sex, anxiety, depression, catastrophizing, and opioid use. More importantly, these findings were linear and the same incremental increase in opioid and surgery nonresponsiveness was seen in individuals well below the threshold used to diagnose FM and extending well into the range of individuals exceeding this threshold. Fig. 26.1 shows two different individuals with osteoarthritis, but neither of whom meet the criteria for FM and are at different portions of the FM continuum; the figure also shows the marked difference in opioid responsiveness and improvement in pain following arthroplasty that these two individuals experience. These data suggest that this measure of fibromyalgianess might serve as the degree of pain centralization that an individual is experiencing and help identify individuals in perioperative or other settings who are less likely to respond to peripherally directed analgesics such as surgery or opioids.

In clinical practice, the clinician should suspect FM in individuals with multifocal pain that cannot be fully explained based on damage or inflammation in those regions of the body. In most cases, musculoskeletal pain is the most prominent feature, but because pain pathways throughout the body are amplified, pain can occur anywhere. Thus, chronic headaches, sore throats, and visceral pain and sensory symptoms are very common in individuals with FM. As previously noted, it is especially helpful to take a lifetime history of chronic pain, since a patient new to a given clinician often arrive with their most recent location of pain. If the clinician recognizes that this same individual has had chronic pain most of their lives in different bodily regions, they (hopefully) are less likely to perform surgery or injections that will solve this individual's problems.

Because pain is a defining feature of FM, it is helpful to focus on the features of the pain that can help distinguish it from other disorders. The pain of FM is typically diffuse or multifocal, often waxes and wanes, and is frequently migratory in nature. These characteristics of "centralized pain" are quite different from "peripheral" pain, where both the location and triggers of pain are typically more constant and predictable. Patients with FM or pain from neural origin may complain of discomfort when they are touched or when wearing tight clothing, and they may experience dysesthesias or paresthesias that accompany the pain.

Another defining characteristic of "centralized" pain is the company it keeps. In addition to pain, individuals typically experience a number of other somatic symptoms. These symptoms can generally be broken into two categories: (1) symptoms of CNS origin that are controlled by the same neurotransmitters that control pain processing and (2) symptoms due to generalized sensory hyperresponsiveness. In the first category, fatigue, memory difficulties, and sleep and mood disturbances are all very common in FM and other centralized pain states. These symptoms are at least partially due to some of the same neurotransmitter abnormalities that contribute to the pathophysiology of as FM, because several of these symptoms typically improve along with pain when an individual is successfully treated with drugs that alter these neurotransmitters. The second type of symptom due to generalized hyperresponsiveness often challenges clinicians to doubt the veracity of an FM patient's complaints. This is often responsible for the "pan-positive review of symptoms" that has often characterized these individuals as "somatizers." The biology of somatization is becoming increasingly understood as a biology of sensory hyperresponsiveness.[62] These sensory symptoms throughout the body can be better understood by clinicians if they realize that all sensory experiences are interpreted by brain regions such as the insula, which are known to be hyperactive in FM and other centralized pain states.

Although the physical examination is generally unremarkable in individuals with FM, it is helpful to assess for diffuse tenderness, and there are many ways that this can be done clinically other than performing a tender point count. For example, individuals with FM are more sensitive to the inflation of a blood pressure cuff.[63] Another way to assess overall pain threshold while also getting other valuable diagnostic information is to assess pain thresholds in the hands and arms of all chronic pain patients. A rapid examination is performed by applying firm pressure over several interphalangeal (IP) joints of each hand and over the adjacent phalanges and then more proximally to include firm palpation of the muscles of the forearm including the lateral epicondyle region. This is one way to assess overall pain threshold and obtain additional diagnostic information about the patient. If the individual is tender in many of these areas, or in just the muscles of the forearm, then they are likely diffusely tender (i.e., have a low central pain threshold). However, if the individual is only tender over the IP joints and not the other regions, and especially if there is any swelling over these joints, one should be more concerned about a systemic autoimmune disorder, whereas if tenderness is confined to just the bones, then this is a symptom of metabolic bone disease or condition causing periostitis (e.g., hyperparathyroidism).

Laboratory testing is generally not useful, except for the purpose of differential diagnosis. The intensity of the diagnostic work-up can be partially guided by the length of time the patient has had symptoms. If the patient's symptoms have persisted for several years, minimal testing is required, whereas a more aggressive strategy should be employed for acute or subacute onset of symptoms. Simple testing should be limited to complete blood count and routine serum chemistries, along with thyroid-stimulating hormone (TSH) and erythrocyte sedimentation rate (ESR) and/or C-reactive protein. Serologic studies such as antinuclear antibody (ANA) and rheumatoid factor assays should generally be avoided unless there are historical features not seen in FM or abnormalities on physical examination.

Once a clinician excludes other potential disorders, an important and at times controversial step in the management of FM is asserting the diagnosis. Despite some assumptions that being "labeled" with FM may adversely affect patients, all existing studies suggest that this is not the case and that the diagnosis of FM is often a tremendous source of relief for the patient and leads to decreased healthcare utilization because of a reduction in referrals and diagnostic testing, or "looking for the cause of the pain."[64]

GENERAL TREATMENT APPROACH

All individuals diagnosed with a condition such as FM should first receive some basic education regarding this disorder. Clinicians can do this in the context of their practice (e.g., with nurse educators or other allied health professionals) or electronically using websites and videos (see below). This education should emphasize that it is important that the patient plays an active role in their management and that some of the most effective therapies are nondrug therapies such as exercise, improving sleep, and reducing stress. Most patients need some combination of pharmacological and nonpharmacological therapies to have meaningful improvement in symptoms and function. Table 26.1 outlines all the evidence-based treatments for individuals with FM.

TABLE 26.1 Evidence-Based Treatments for Fibromyalgia

Treatment	Cost	Specifics	Evidence Level	Side Effects	Clinical Pearls
General Recommendations					
Patient education[107]	Low	Incorporate principles of self-management including a multimodal approach	1, A		Following initial diagnosis spend several visits (or use separate educational sessions) to explain the condition and set treatment expectations.
Nonpharmacological Therapies					
Graded exercise[108]	Low	Aerobic exercise has been best studied but strengthening and stretching have also been shown to be of value	1, A	Worsening of symptoms when program is begun too rapidly	• Counsel patients to "start low, go slow." • For many patients focusing first on increasing daily "activity" is more helpful before starting exercise
Cognitive-behavioral therapy (CBT)[109]	Low	Pain-based CBT programs have been shown to be effective in one-on-one settings, small groups, and via internet	1, A	No significant side effects of CBT *per se* but patient acceptance is often poor when they view this as a "psychological" intervention	• Internet-based programs are gaining acceptance and are more convenient for working patients
Complementary and alternative medicine (CAM) therapies[110]	Variable	Most CAM therapies have not been rigorously studied	1, A	Generally safe	• There is emerging evidence that CAM treatments such as Tai Chi, yoga, balneotherapy, and acupuncture might be effective • Allowing patients to choose which CAM therapies to incorporate into an active treatment program can increase self-efficacy
CNS neurostimulatory therapies[111]		Several different types of CNS neurostimulatory therapies have been shown to be effective in FM and other chronic pain states		Headache	These treatments continue to be refined as we learn about optimal stimulation targets and "dosing."
Pharmacological therapies		Pharmacological therapy is best chosen based on the predominant symptoms, and initiated in low dose with slow dose escalation	Level 5, Consensus		• Some practitioners find that getting patients on a drug regimen that helps improve symptoms prior to initiating nonpharmacological therapies can help improve compliance
Tricyclic compounds[66,112]		• Nortriptyline 10–70 mg qhs • Cyclobenzaprine 5–20 mg qhs	1, A	Dry mouth, weight gain, constipation, "groggy" or drugged feeling	• When effective, they can improve a wide range of symptoms including pain, sleep, bowel, and bladder symptoms • Taking these drugs several hours prior to bedtime improves side effect profile
Serotonin norepinephrine reuptake inhibitors[112]	Doluxetine is generic, milnacipran not	• Duloxetine, 30–120 mg daily • Milnacipran, 100–200 mg daily	1, A	Nausea, palpitations, headache, fatigue, tachycardia, hypertension	• Warning patients about transient nausea, taking with food, and slowly increasing dose can increase tolerability • Milnacipran might be slightly more noradrenergic than duloxetine and thus potentially more helpful for fatigue and memory problems, but it is also more likely to cause HTN
Gabapentinoids[113]	Gabapentin is generic, pregabalin not	• Gabapentin, 800–2400 mg/day in divided doses • Pregabalin up to 600 mg/day in divided doses	1, A	Sedation, weight gain, dizziness	• Giving most or all the dose at bedtime can increase tolerability

Continued

TABLE 26.1 Evidence-Based Treatments for Fibromyalgia—cont'd

Treatment	Cost	Specifics	Evidence Level	Side Effects	Clinical Pearls
Gamma-hydroxybutyrate[44]	Available for treating narcolepsy, cataplexy	GHB 4.5–6.0 g per night in divided doses	1, A	Sedation, respiratory depression and death	• Shown to be efficacious but not approved by US FDA because of safety concerns
Low-dose naltrexone[94]	Low	4.5 mg/day	2 small single-center RCTs		
Cannabinoids[89]	NA	Nabilone 0.5 mg po qhs–1.0 mg bid	1, A	Sedation, dizziness dry mouth	• No synthetic cannabinoid is approved in US for treatment of pain
Tizanidine[92]	Low	Tizanidine 4–8 mg every 6–6 h	One small RCT	Sedation, dizziness	• No long-term safety data
Esreboxetine[78]	NA	Esreboxetine 4 or 8 mg/day	Two RCTs	Hypertension, tachycardia, urinary retention	• Not available in US
Selective serotonin reuptake inhibitors (SSRIs)[112]	SSRIs that should be used in FM (see Pearls) are all generic	Fluoxetine, sertraline, paroxetine	1, A	Nausea, sexual dysfunction, weight gain, sleep disturbance	• Older, less selective SSRIs may have some efficacy in improving pain, especially at higher doses that have more prominent noradrenergic effects • Newer SSRIs (citalopram, escitalopran, desvenlafaxine) are less effective or ineffective as analgesics
NSAIDs		• No evidence of efficacy • Can be helpful to treat comorbid "peripheral pain generators"	5, D	Gastrointestinal, renal, and cardiac side effects	• Use the lowest dose for the shortest period of time to reduce side effects
Opioids		• Tramadol with or without acetaminophen, 50–100 mg every 6 h • No evidence of efficacy for stronger opioids	5, D	Sedation, addiction, tolerance, opioid-induced hyperalgesia	• There is increasing evidence that opioids are less effective for treating chronic pain than previously thought and their risk:benefit profile is worse than other classes of analgesics

CNS, *Central nervous system;* GHB, *gamma hydroxybutyrate;* HTN, *hypertension;* NSAIDs, *nonsteroidal antiinflammatory drugs.*
From Clauw DJ: Fibromyalgia: a clinical review. J Am Med Assoc. *311(15):1547-1555, 2014.*

PHARMACOLOGIC THERAPY

The majority of FM clinical trials have involved antidepressants of one class or another. Trials studying the oldest class of agents, tricyclic antidepressants (TCAs), are most abundant, though several recent studies have focused on selective serotonin reuptake inhibitors (SSRIs) and "atypical antidepressants," a class that includes dual reuptake inhibitors and monoamine oxidase inhibitors (MAOIs).[65]

Tricyclic Antidepressants

The most frequently studied pharmacologic therapy for FM is low doses of tricyclic compounds. Most TCAs increase the concentrations of serotonin and/or norepinephrine (noradrenaline) by directly blocking their respective reuptake. The effectiveness of TCAs, particularly amitriptyline and cyclobenzaprine, in treating the symptoms of pain, poor sleep, and fatigue associated with FM is supported by several randomized, controlled trials.[66] Tolerability can be a problem but can be improved by beginning at very low doses (e.g., 10 mg of amitriptyline or 5 mg of cyclobenzaprine), giving the dose a few hours before bedtime, and very slowly escalating the dose. Very low-dose cyclobenzaprine has recently shown to be quite effective in a subset of individuals with FM with a specific sleep architecture, seemingly with less side effects than seen in some of the earlier studies of higher doses.[67]

Serotonin and Norepinephrine Reuptake Inhibitors

Because of a better side effect profile, newer antidepressants, specifically, SSRIs, are frequently used in FM. The SSRIs fluoxetine, citalopram, and paroxetine have each been evaluated in randomized, placebo controlled trials.[68–72] In general, the results of studies of SSRIs in FM have paralleled the experience in other pain conditions. The newer "highly selective" serotonin reuptake inhibitors, for example, citalopram, seem to be less efficacious than the older SSRIs, which have some noradrenergic activity at higher doses.[73]

Since TCAs and high doses of certain "SSRIs" such as fluoxetine and sertraline that have the most balanced reuptake inhibition are the most effective analgesics, many have concluded that dual receptor inhibitors such as serotonin-NE and NE-serotonin reuptake inhibitors (serotonin norepinephrine reuptake inhibitors [SNRIs] and norepinephrine-selective reuptake inhibitors [NSRIs]) may be of more benefit than pure serotonergic drugs.[73] These drugs are pharmacologically similar to some TCAs in their ability to inhibit the reuptake of both serotonin and NE, but they differ from TCAs in being generally devoid of significant activity at other receptor systems. This selectivity results in diminished side effects and enhanced tolerability. The first available SNRI, venlafaxine, has data to support its use in the management of neuropathic pain, and retrospective trial data demonstrate that this compound is also effective in the prophylaxis of migraine and tension headaches.[74] Two studies in FM have had conflicting results, with the one using a higher dose showing efficacy.[75]

Two newer SNRIs, duloxetine and milnacipran, have undergone more recent multicenter trials and were shown to be effective in several outcome variables, and they are both now approved in the United States for the treatment of FM.[76,77] These drugs seem roughly comparable in the overall efficacy profile, with studies generally noting modest improvement (although not reaching statistical significance in all studies) in domains such as pain, overall improvement, physical functioning, level of fatigue, and degree of reported physical impairment. For both compounds, these effects seemed to be independent of the drug effect on mood, thus suggesting that the analgesic and other positive effects of this class of drugs in FM is not simply due to their antidepressant effects. Both these drugs are better tolerated if taken with food, and patients are warned about likely initial nausea and counseled that this typically resolves in a week or so, and if not, then they should discontinue the drug. The maximum approved dose of duloxetine is 60 mg/day, but it was studied in trials at doses up to 120 mg and shown to be safe; similarly, the initial dose of milnacipran is 100 mg, but some patients will benefit from increasing the dose as high as 200 mg. Hypertension is more likely to be a problem with milnacipran, since it appears to be more noradrenergic; in addition, it might be slightly more likely to help with symptoms such as fatigue.

Esreboxetine, a selective norepinephrine reuptake inhibitor, was also tested and shown to be efficacious in FM.[78] This adds to emerging evidence by suggesting that norepinephrine reuptake activity may be much more important than serotinergic reuptake for analgesic effects.

Anticonvulsants

A few classes of antiepileptic drugs have been shown to be effective in the treatment of various chronic pain conditions, including postherpetic neuralgia and painful diabetic neuropathy.[79] Pregabalin and gabapentin have the same mechanism of action and bind to the alpha-2-delta subunit of calcium channels, and both are approved for the treatment of neuropathic pain and several other indications. Several studies have shown the efficacy of pregabalin against pain, sleep disturbances, and fatigue as compared to placebo in FM, leading to this being the first drug approved in the United States for use in this condition.[80] Gabapentin has been shown to have very similar efficacy and side effect profile in FM.[81] The tolerability of these drugs can be dramatically enhanced by beginning at a low dose and giving either two-thirds of the dose or the entire dose at bedtime. The maximally approved dose of pregabalin is 450 mg, but in trials, it was studied at doses as high as 600 mg and shown to be safe and efficacious. For most patients, the dose of gabapentin needed for analgesic is often 1800–2400 mg/day. Another antiepileptic compound, clonazepam, has demonstrated efficacy in treating temporomandibular disorder and associated jaw pain, and it is useful in the treatment of restless legs syndrome[79] and may be of value in FM. The risks associated with chronic benzodiazepine use likely outweigh the potential benefit. However, two other drugs that are likely working by counteracting the effects of increased glutamatergic activity in FM are memantine and ketamine, both of which have some evidence of efficacy.[82,83]

Combination Therapy

Combinations of multiple classes of adjunctive pain medications have been common practice for many years. A recent study demonstrated that the combination of duloxetine and pregabalin was superior to either drug alone in treating FM.[84] The combination improved pain, as well as Fibromyalgia Impact Questionnaire, SF-36, and Medical Outcome Study (MOS) sleep scores, which is consistent with previous data demonstrating that combinations of therapies with differing mechanisms of action are effective in neuropathic pain.[85]

Other Central Nervous System–Acting Drugs

Sedative-hypnotic compounds are widely used by FM patients. A handful of studies have been published on the use of certain nonbenzodiazepine hypnotics in FM, such as zopiclone and zolpidem. These reports have suggested that these agents can improve the sleep and, perhaps, fatigue of FM patients, although they had no significant effects upon pain.

On the other hand, gamma-hydroxybutyrate (also known as sodium oxybate), a precursor of GABA with powerful sedative properties, was recently shown to be very efficacious in improving fatigue, pain, and sleep architecture in patients with FM.[86] Note, however, that this agent is a scheduled substance due to its abuse potential, and was not approved by the US Food and Drug Administration (FDA) because of safety concerns. Nonetheless, these studies along with the H-MRS showing low GABA suggest that other less toxic GABA agonists may have an important role in treating FM.

Cannabanoids are another class of drugs where there is renewed interest in chronic pain states. There have been two randomized controlled trials (RCTs) of synthetic cannabinoids in FM (both with nabilone), and both studies concluded that the drug was efficacious (in one study for both pain and sleep, in the other study at lower dose for just sleep).[87,88] This is not surprising as there is increased recognition that this class of drugs may have utility in pain of neural origin.[89]

Pramipexole is a dopamine agonist indicated for Parkinson's disease that has shown utility in the treatment of periodic leg movement disorder.[90] One study suggested that this compound may improve both pain and sleep in FM patients, but these results have not been replicated with this or other dopamine agonists.[91] Because of this, this class of drug may be best reserved for individuals with other indications, such as comorbid restless legs syndrome.

Tizanidine is a centrally acting alpha-2 adrenergic agonist approved by the FDA for the treatment of muscle spasticity associated with multiple sclerosis and stroke. Literature suggests that this agent is a useful adjunct in treating several chronic pain conditions, including chronic daily headaches and low back pain. A recent trial reported significant improvements in several parameters in FM, including sleep, pain, and measures of quality of life.[92]

Classic Analgesics

There have been no adequate, randomized controlled clinical trials of opiates in FM, and most in the field (including the authors) have not found this class of compounds to be effective in anecdotal experience. Tramadol is a compound that has some opioid activity (weak mu agonist activity) combined with serotonin/NE reuptake inhibition. This compound does appear to be somewhat efficacious in the management of FM, as both an isolated compound and as fixed-dose combination with acetaminophen.[90]

In addition to the previous studies cited, mechanistic studies suggest why opioids might not be effective in FM (i.e., PET evidence of decrease opioid receptor availability, and high CSF levels of endorphins); recent functional and chemical imaging studies by this same group suggest an even more important potential problem. In these studies, the native state of FM may be akin to that of opioid-induced hyperalgesia, in that the regions with the lowest receptor occupancy are the most hyperalgesic. Thus, it is possible that at least in a subset of individuals, opioids may make these individual's hyperaglesia worse rather than better.[93] This notion is also supported by previously noted clinical studies suggesting that opioid *antagonists* such as naltrexone may be effective in FM.[94] If opioids are used for refractory patients, it is possible that those opioids with mixed opioid antagonist effects (e.g., buprenorphine), norepinephrine reuptake inhibition (tapentadol) or *N*-methyl-D-aspartate (NMDA) receptor blockade (methadone) might be better than pure mu agonists, but this is entirely conjecture. Even though opioids are not recommended for the treatment of FM, studies demonstrate that many FM patients are prescribed opioids.[95]

Many FM patients use nonsteroidal antiinflammatory drugs (NSAIDs) and acetaminophen. Although numerous studies have failed to confirm their effectiveness as analgesics in FM, there is limited evidence that patients may experience enhanced analgesia when treated with combinations of NSAIDs and other agents. This phenomenon may be a result of concurrent "peripheral" pain (i.e., due to damage or inflammation of tissues; e.g., osteoarthritis, rheumatoid arthritis) conditions that may be present, and/or that these comorbid peripheral pain generators might lead to worsening of "central" pain.

NEUROSTIMULATORY THERAPIES

A variety of neurostimulatory therapies can be effective in treating musculoskeletal pain. For some time, transcutaneous electrical nerve stimulation (TENS) has been used to treat musculoskeletal pain.[96,97] Conventional TENS (C-TENS) is given at high stimulation frequency with low intensity. Pain relief is immediate, but short-lived, when it occurs. Acupuncture-like TENS (often abbreviated Al-TENS) is given at a lower frequency and higher intensity (which is sometimes uncomfortable), and when it works generally has a longer lasting effect than C-TENS. These neurostimulatory therapies would be expected to be most helpful for pain of peripheral/nociceptive origin.

A new set of neurostimulatory therapies is emerging that would be expected to be more effective for "centralized" pain, since these therapies all aim to stimulate the CNS and, in doing so, modulate CNS pain transmission. Many such therapies have been developed and tested, with many showing some efficacy in several pain states. These include noninvasive techniques such as repetitive transcranial magnetic stimulation (rTMS), transcranial direct current stimulation (tDCS), and newer ways of noninvasively stimulating brain structures.[98,99] Although the studies to date with these therapies have yielded somewhat inconsistent results, a trend is emerging suggesting that these treatments might be most effective in centralized rather than purely peripheral pain states, and with stimulation parameters that enable signals to travel into deeper cortical tissues than occurs with typical delivery of rTMS and tDCS. Other more invasive techniques have also shown promise in patients with more refractory pain states, such as spinal cord stimulation, deep brain stimulation, and vagal nerve stimulation.

NONPHARMACOLOGIC THERAPIES

The two best-studied nonpharmacological therapies are cognitive-behavioral therapy and exercise. Both therapies have been shown to be efficacious in the treatment of FM, as well as a plethora of other medical conditions.[100,101] Both treatments can lead to sustained (e.g., >1 year) improvements, and are very effective when an individual complies with therapy.

For exercise, it is important to "start low, go slow." Many FM and other chronic pain patients are quite sedentary, and in these individuals, it is important to focus on becoming more active rather than classic "exercise." With respect to exercise, nearly any type (aerobic, stretching, strengthening) can be helpful. It is most important that patients understand that they must become more active and then eventually start very mild exercise (e.g., walking).

There are many elements to cognitive-behavioral therapy, but one that has had increased attention recently has been a focus on using behavioral measures to treat the sleep disorders seen in conditions such as FM.[102] This increased focus on improving sleep is concordant with more and preclinical and clinical research showing how important sleep is in pain transmission.

There is a free website for patients (www.fibroguide.com) that allows patients to access these behavioral interventions over the internet rather than in person, and this website was tested in an RCT and was shown to be effective.[103] "Lighter" options such as this will work well in many patients, whereas in other individuals with more severe psychological or psychiatric comorbidity will benefit from more intensive (i.e., group or one-on-one) treatments. A recent study suggested that adding emotional disclosure to standard cognitive behavioral therapy (CBT) may be of benefit to a subset of patients who receive significant improvement.[104]

Complementary and alternative therapies have been explored by patients managing their own illness and healthcare providers. As with other diseases, there are few controlled trials to advocate their general use. Trigger-point injections, chiropractic manipulation, acupuncture, and myofascial release therapy are among the more commonly used modalities, which achieve varying levels of success. Two randomized, sham-controlled trials of acupuncture showed no difference between the two groups.[105,106] A usual-care comparison group was not studied. There is some evidence that the use of alternative therapies gives patients a greater sense of control over their illness. In instances where this sense of control is accompanied by an improved clinical state, the decision to use these therapies is between physicians and patients themselves.

CONCLUSION

FM is one of a number of centralized pain disorders characterized by widespread body pain and comorbid symptoms, such as trouble thinking and headaches. While the diagnosis has been controversial in the medical community for some time, it is among the best studied pain conditions with overwhelming evidence demonstrating altered CNS pain processing. Treatment should include patient education and a combination of medications, behavioral therapies, lifestyle changes, and complementary treatments, as appropriate.

KEY POINTS

- FM is the prototypical centralized pain condition, which is characterized by widespread body pain and comorbid symptoms, such as fatigue, sleep, and memory problems.
- FM patients have higher levels of CNS neurotransmitters that upregulate pain (e.g., glutamate) and lower levels of those that downregulate pain (e.g., norepinephrine and GABA), with a paradoxical increase in endogenous opioids (which may explain why this condition does not appear to be responsive to opioids).
- Psychological comorbidities are more common in FM patients but do not explain the sensory abnormalities or pain complaints.
- Rather than considering FM as a binary diagnosis, one can consider the degree of "fibromyalgia-ness" as a means of placing patients on the continuum of more peripheral confined pain to more centralized or widespread pain. Individuals with higher degrees of fibromyalgianess are going to be less responsive to therapies that work well for acute or nociceptive pain (i.e., surgery, opioids) and more responsive to drug and nondrug therapies that work in the CNS.
- Opioids are not recommended in treating FM.
- Medications that address the known CNS pathology are preferred, such as tricyclics, serotonin norepinephrine reuptake inhibitors, and gabapentinoids.
- Nonpharmacological therapies can be very effective, especially promoting activity/exercise and improving sleep using sleep hygiene or cognitive-behavioral therapy.
- Although pain and comorbid symptoms may be persistent, many patients appropriately treated for FM can lead normal, functional lives.

REFERENCES

Access the reference list online at ExpertConsult.com.

CHAPTER 27

Complex Regional Pain Syndrome

Kayode Williams, MD, MBA, FFARCSI ◎ **Anthony Guarino, MD** ◎ **Srinivasa N. Raja, MD**

The literature is replete with accounts of the history of the early description of complex regional pain syndrome (CRPS) as part of any publication on the subject. A brief reiteration of this history helps underscore the magnitude of the discovery and highlight the challenges faced by clinicians and researchers alike in moving the discovery forward. CRPS types 1 and 2 (formerly known as reflex sympathetic dystrophy [RSD] and causalgia, respectively) was first reported by Weir Mitchell over a century ago following his observations that Civil War soldiers with peripheral nerve damage from gunshot wounds developed a constant burning pain, which he called *causalgia*. Almost half a century after Mitchell's observation, Sudeck in 1900 observed muscle atrophy and bony demineralization as a complication of infection in the limbs. The radiographic changes started as a "patchy osteoporosis of the small bones of the hands or feet and the distal metaphysis of the forearm or tibial bones"; hence, the name *Sudeck dystrophy*, due to the presence of patchy osteoporosis. Almost five decades later in 1947, the term *reflex sympathetic dystrophy* was coined by Evans to reflect the assumption that the sympathetic nervous system was involved in the abnormal activity observed in the periphery.

In 1994, the Special Consensus Group of the International Association for the Study of Pain (IASP) met in Orlando to review the criteria for the clinical diagnosis of patients presenting with CRPS/RSD. The need for such a consensus among physicians charged with the care of these patients arose from the recognition of the presence of an inhomogeneous set of signs and symptoms that were hitherto used to diagnose the disease with the resultant difficulty in confirming that all practitioners were treating the same condition. In addition, there was lack of evidence for a reflex mechanism and the variable presence of dystrophy. The term *CRPS* was therefore considered broad enough to allow the inclusion of patients who may show varying levels of sympathetic nervous system involvement in maintaining pain through the course of the disease process, hence the term *sympathetically mediated pain* (SMP) or *sympathetically independent pain* (SIP) (Table 27.1).

In 2004, a group of researchers met in Budapest to develop the diagnostic criteria for CRPS (table-Budapest Consensus group criteria). The group endorsed the subtype grouping of CRPS (1 and 2), and in addition approved a codified criteria developed from an empirically based research modification of the earlier IASP diagnostic criteria.[1] The IASP Taxonomy Committee approved the Budapest or "new" IASP criteria in 2012 to help promote further research, recognizing the paucity of strong evidence for efficacy of treatments for CRPS as articulated in rigorous systematic reviews.[2,3]

EPIDEMIOLOGY

There is a paucity of epidemiologic data or outcome studies on CRPS, reflecting the absence of a universal agreement on the set of signs and symptoms that should be present to make the diagnosis in this group of patients. There is growing interest in characterizing the factors that determine the role of inflammatory mediators in the development of the peripheral clinical manifestations of CRPS. An epidemiologic study demonstrated that patients with CRPS also tend to have a history of asthma and migraine headaches.[4,5] In both these disorders, neuropeptides may play a significant role in the pathophysiology of the disease process.[6] Although the true incidence of CRPS is unknown, results of two epidemiologic studies indicate that the incidence per person-years at risk of the disease ranges from 5.46 to 26.6/100,000 person-years at risk.[7,8] It occurs more commonly in females than males, with a ratio of 2:3 to 3:1, and with increasing age. Veldman et al. in a prospective study of 829 patients, 76% of whom were female, found that the age ranged from 9 to 85 years (median age 42 years) with only 12 patients younger than 14 years.[9] Allen and colleagues reviewed epidemiologic data from a tertiary pain center on 134 patients.[10] They found that the CRPS symptoms had existed for a mean duration of 30 months prior to presentation, most patients had seen on average 4.8 physicians before referral to the tertiary center, 17% had pending lawsuits, and 54% had a workers' compensation claim related to CRPS. This study also examined the types of occupation held by CRPS patients at the time of injury. People in the service industries, such as restaurant workers and police officers, suffered almost twice as much as people in other professions, possibly related to the physical activity related to the job. Other associated features that have been identified include the presence of social stressors at the time of development of the condition.[11] In spite of this finding, no specific psychological factors or personality trait has been found to predispose an individual to developing CRPS.

In a web-based epidemiologic survey of CRPS, Sharma and colleagues surveyed 1359 subjects to examine multiple variables (risk factors), including sociodemographic factors.[12] The authors concluded that CRPS commonly occurs among younger females and often results from work-related injuries or surgery. The study also revealed that CRPS is associated with sleep disturbance, functional impairment, and suicidal ideation. de Mos et al. examined outcomes of the disease with regard to the extent of long-lasting impairments.[13] In a retrospective analysis for an average of 5.8 years, 102 patients with CRPS were compared with matched reference patients with similar injuries without CRPS. Sixteen percent of the CRPS patients reported the CRPS to be still progressive, 31% were

TABLE 27.1 International Association for the Study of Pain Diagnostic Criteria for CRPS 1 and CRPS 2

CRPS 1 (Reflex Sympathetic Dystrophy)[a]	CRPS 2 (Causalgia)[b]
1. The presence of an initiating noxious event or a cause of immobilization.	1. The presence of continuing pain, allodynia, or hyperalgesia after a nerve injury, not necessarily limited to the distribution of the injured nerve.
2. Continuing pain, allodynia, or hyperalgesia with which the pain is disproportionate to any inciting event.	2. Evidence at some time of edema, changes in skin blood flow, or abnormal sudomotor activity in the region of the pain.
3. Evidence at some time of edema, changes in skin blood flow, or abnormal sudomotor activity in the region of the pain.	3. This diagnosis is excluded by the existence of conditions that would otherwise account for the degree of pain and dysfunction.
4. This diagnosis is excluded by the existence of conditions that would otherwise account for the degree of pain and dysfunction.	—

[a]*Criteria 2 through 4 must be satisfied.*
[b]*All three criteria must be satisfied.*
CRPS, *Complex regional pain syndrome.*
Source: Stanton-Hicks M: Complex regional pain syndrome. Anesthesiol Clin North Am. *21:733-744, 2003.*

incapable of working, and the patients with poorest outcomes were those with upper extremity involvement. The authors concluded that although severe outcomes were rare, the majority of CRPS patients experience persistent impairment at 2 years or more after onset of the condition.

Given the paucity of information on the long-term prognosis of CRPS patients, a web-based CRPS-UK Registry has been developed and made accessible to centers experienced in diagnosing and managing patients with CRPS.[14] Such registries are likely to provide additional insight on the long-term outcome of patients with CRPS.

PATHOPHYSIOLOGY

CRPS types 1 and 2 differ only by the presence (type 2) or absence (type 1) of evidence of nerve injury. Pain is the hallmark of the condition, and commonly manifests as spontaneous pain, with hyperalgesia and allodynia. Associated signs include vasomotor and sudomotor disturbances, active and passive movement disorders, and trophic changes. CRPS type 2 develops after defined nerve injury, whereas CRPS type 1 develops following minor or major injuries with little or no obvious damage to the nerves in the involved extremity.

There continues to be considerable debate in the literature vis-à-vis the pathophysiology of CRPS. The existing framework focuses on the neurobiological changes, peripherally and centrally. This conceptual compartmentalization allows for examination of the changes in cutaneous innervation, ensuing peripheral sensitization associated with release of inflammatory mediators, involvement of the sympathetic system, and ultimately central sensitization with cortical reorganization.[15]

PERIPHERAL/AFFERENT MECHANISMS

There is evidence that inflammation plays an important role in the elaboration and maintenance of CRPS. Recent studies have demonstrated the presence of increased levels of two neuropeptides associated with inflammatory processes; these include calcitonin gene-related peptide and substance P in patients with CRPS.[16] This line of reasoning is supported by observations that the current use of angiotensin-converting enzyme inhibitors is associated with an increased risk of CRPS, given that angiotensin-converting enzyme is involved in the metabolism of neuropeptides.[17] Furthermore, the role of cytokines in the generation of the peripheral manifestations continues to stimulate the interest of investigators. Independent lines of research have demonstrated that, in patients with CRPS, levels of proinflammatory cytokines such as tumor necrosis factor alpha (TNF-α) and interleukin 6 (IL-6) are increased in skin blisters and biopsies in affected limbs compared with unaffected limbs in patients with CRPS post limb fractures.[18,19] In addition, there is evidence that there is an associated increase in the level of soluble receptors to the proinflammatory cytokines TNF-α, IL-1 and IL-8, during the early stages of CRPS (within 3 months). Conversely, antiinflammatory cytokines, including IL-4, IL-10 and transforming growth factor beta 1 (TGFβ1), are lower.[20–22] Interestingly, it was established that the cutaneous blisters in affected limbs of CRPS patients contain more tryptase compared with unaffected limbs. Given that tryptase is a marker of mast cell activity, it is thought that mast cells may be involved in the release of cytokines.[23]

Another line of investigation aimed at elucidating the peripheral mechanisms includes the imbalance between peripheral vasodilators such as nitric oxide and vasoconstrictors such as endothelin-1. Groeneweg et al. demonstrated that, in artificial blisters in the affected limbs of patients with CRPS, the levels of nitric oxide were lower and the level of endothelin-1 was higher than in the unaffected limb. This imbalance is thought to be due to cytokine-induced inhibition of endothelial nitric oxide, and induction of the transcription of preproendothelin-1.[24] Cytokines also stimulate smooth muscle inducible nitric oxide synthase, leading to production of nitric oxide in muscle and ultimate formation of peroxynitrite (ONOO–) which affects the integrity of the endothelium. A combination of the release of inflammatory cytokines, associated hypoxia due to imbalance of peripheral vasoconstrictors and vasodilators, and formation of free radicals serve as profound peripheral nociceptive stimuli. This potent chronic activation of peripheral nociceptors may account for the sensitization and sensory changes associated with CRPS.

ALTERED CUTANEOUS INNERVATION FOLLOWING INJURY

Current evidence favors the hypothesis that some degree of nerve injury is required, however trivial, to initiate the cascade of events associated with CRPS.[25] Oaklander et al. in 2006 demonstrated that persistent minimal distal nerve injury (MDNI), specifically distal degeneration of small-diameter axons, which subserve pain and autonomic function, were responsible for the symptoms reported in

CRPS 1. The authors found that significantly lower densities of epidermal neuritis (on average 29% lower) were observed in CRPS-affected extremities as compared with the contralateral unaffected limb. Similar changes in neurite density were not seen in non-CRPS conditions such as osteoarthritis. In a study to determine if objective evidence for the presence of nerve damage in CRPS 1 exists,[26] Albrecht et al. in 2006 examined the skin samples from amputated upper and lower extremities from two CRPS patients to detect evidence of nerve injury, using immunofluorescence techniques. They found a reduction in C and A-delta fiber density in the CRPS-affected limbs compared with the nonaffected sites on the same limb, as well as compared with healthy controls. In addition, abnormalities in the innervations around hair follicles and sweat glands were also observed. The causal relationship of these changes relative to the onset of CRPS is unclear.[26]

PERIPHERAL SENSITIZATION

Peripheral sensitization resulting from the persistent nociceptive afferent activity as a result of the initial tissue trauma is thought to occur. Following tissue injury, primary afferent fibers in the traumatized area release neuropeptides such as bradykinin and substance P. The peptides sensitize nociceptors, increase their response to noxious stimuli, and reduce their threshold to mechanical and thermal stimuli. These neurophysiologic changes may account for the hyperalgesia and allodynia pathognomonic of CRPS. Furthermore, the local hyperalgesia is limited to the affected limb and not seen in the contralateral unaffected limb.[27] Examination of the extent of sensory impairment in 24 patients with CRPS 1 revealed that up to half of the patients with chronic CRPS 1 develop hyperesthesia to pinprick and temperature on the affected side or in the upper quadrant of the ipsilateral side.[28] The patients also demonstrated a higher incidence of hyperalgesia and mechanical allodynia in addition to motor impairment. These changes suggested a more widespread alteration of sensory perception in the pathophysiology of CRPS in this group of patients.

The motor system may also be affected as evidenced by a reduction in range of motion, commonly seen in patients with CRPS, that is not explained by the presence of pain-induced kinesiophobia. The presence of severe dystonia in affected and unaffected limbs has also been documented, manifesting as flexion of the fingers, wrists, elbows, and plantar flexion of the toes.[29] The fact that the dystonia responds to intrathecal baclofen indicates that gamma-aminobutyric acid (GABA)-mediated mechanisms may play a role in the development of dystonia in CRPS.

CENTRAL SENSITIZATION

The mechanism by which central sensitization occurs is akin to that described in peripheral sensitization. Persistent nociceptive input associated with nerve injury from tissue trauma results in increased activity of nociceptive neurons in the spinal cord.[30] The central sensitization is mediated by the induced release of neuropeptides such as bradykinin and substance P, and the excitatory neurotransmitter glutamate acting at the spinal receptors for *N*-methyl-D-aspartic acid (NMDA), α-amino-3-hydroxy-5 methyl-4-isoxazole propionic acid (AMPA) and neurokinin-1. This activity results in enhanced response to nonnoxious stimuli (allodynia) and noxious stimuli (hyperalgesia). CRPS patients demonstrate significantly increased wind-up to repeated stimuli applied to the affected limb compared with the unaffected contralateral limb or other limbs.[31] These findings suggest the possibility of central sensitization as a mechanism of persistence of the symptoms associated with CRPS.

Reports suggest that cortical reorganization, manifesting as changes in sensory mapping and activation patterns, might ensue.[32–34] These changes have been observed, using functional magnetic resonance imaging, and can account for some of the sensory disturbances noted. These include changes in tactile discrimination and referred sensations and alteration in the perception of body habitus (see below Cortical Reorganization).[35–39]

SYMPATHETICALLY MEDIATED PAIN

There has been an indication of an interaction between the sympathetic noradrenergic neurons in the periphery and the primary afferent neurons as part of the underlying mechanism of SMP in patients with CRPS 1. Intradermal injection of epinephrine in CRPS patients results in the return of allodynia and spontaneous pain that had previously been relieved by sympathetic blockade, suggesting a peripheral adrenoceptor mediated mechanism in some patients.[40] Spontaneous pain may also be relieved by an infusion of the α-adrenergic blocker phentolamine.[41] It has also been suggested that sympathetic innervations of deep somatic tissues may be as important as cutaneous innervations as a determinant of the sympatho-afferent coupling that occurs particularly in the acute phase of CRPS.[42]

INFLAMMATORY MEDIATORS

As outlined earlier, elaboration of inflammatory mechanisms may be responsible for the peripheral changes seen in the acute phase of CRPS. This may occur either through the classic cascade of release of proinflammatory cytokines (interleukin-1β, IL-2, IL-6, and tumor necrosis factor-α) from mast cells and lymphocytes following tissue trauma or secondary to neurogenic inflammation causing the release of cytokines and neuropeptides (including substance P and calcitonin gene–related peptide [CGRP]).[15] The neuropeptides can increase tissue permeability and cause vasodilatation, giving rise to the "warm CRPS" with edema. Substance P and TNF-α can engender osteoclastic activity, which may contribute to the osteoporosis seen in CRPS. In addition, CGRP can cause an increase in hair growth and sudomotor activity observed in CRPS patients.[16,43]

CORTICAL REORGANIZATION

In recent years, imaging studies, such as functional MRI (fMRI) and single-photon emission CT (SPECT), and mapping techniques based on electroencephalography (EEG) and magnetoencephalography (MEG) have indicated an important role of the central nervous system (CNS) in the pathogenesis of CRPS[44,45] (see Schwenkreis et al.[44] and Bailey et al.[45] for reviews). Cortical reorganization in central somatosensory and motor networks that may result in altered central processing of tactile and nociceptive stimuli and cerebral organization of movement have been reported.[46] For example, Maihofner et al.[47] observed increased strength of magnetic fields and reduced distance between thumb and little finger representation in contralateral S1 cortex after tactile stimulation of the affected hand. Moreover, they observed a shift of the cortical S1 representation of the affected hand toward the lip representation and reported a correlation between the amount of cortical reorganization and the intensity of CRPS pain and the extent of mechanical hyperalgesia. In a follow-up study in the same group of patients a year or more after therapy, Maihofner et al. found a reversal of cortical reorganization with clinical improvement, suggesting a relationship between S1 reorganization and chronic pain.[48] The changes in cortical representations may explain not only the pain, but also a number of the other clinical features occurring in the course of the disease. Neurorehabilitative strategies that are targeted at restoring this impaired sensorimotor function, using strategies such as mirror therapies, are being investigated.

TABLE 27.2 Proposed Clinical Diagnostic Criteria for CRPS

General definition of the syndrome: CRPS describes an array of painful conditions that are characterized by a continuing (spontaneous and/or evoked) regional pain that is seemingly disproportionate in time or degree to the usual course of any known trauma or other lesion. The pain is regional (not in a specific nerve territory or dermatome) and usually has a distal predominance of abnormal sensory, motor, sudomotor, vasomotor, and/or trophic findings. The syndrome shows variable progression over time.

To make the *clinical* diagnosis, the following criteria must be met:

1. Continuing pain, which is disproportionate to any inciting event
2. Must report at least one symptom in *three of the four* following categories:
   Sensory: Reports of hyperesthesia and/or allodynia
   Vasomotor: Reports of temperature asymmetry and/or skin color changes and/or skin color asymmetry
   Sudomotor/edema: Evidence of edema and/or sweating changes and/or sweating asymmetry
   Motor/trophic: Reports of decreased range of motion and/or motor dysfunction (weakness, tremor, dystonia) and/or trophic changes (hair, nail, skin)
3. Must display at least one sign **at time of evaluation** in *two or more* of the following categories:
   Sensory: Evidence of hyperalgesia (to pinprick) and/or allodynia (to light touch and/or temperature sensation and/or deep somatic pressure and/or joint movement)
   Vasomotor: Evidence of temperature asymmetry (<1°C) and/or skin color changes and/or asymmetry
   Sudomotor/edema: Evidence of edema and/or sweating changes and/or sweating asymmetry
   Motor/trophic: Evidence of decreased range of motion and/or motor dysfunction (weakness, tremor, dystonia) and/or trophic changes (hair, nail, skin)
4. There is no other diagnosis that better explains the signs and symptoms

Note: For research purposes, *diagnostic decision rule should be at least one symptom* in all four *symptom categories and at least one sign (observed at evaluation) in two or more sign categories.*

CLINICAL FEATURES

Since the publication of the diagnostic criteria for CRPS by IASP in 1994 (see Table 27.1), major strides have been made to further refine the diagnostic criteria based on internal and external validation studies. This culminated in the Budapest Consensus in 2007 in which the diagnostic criteria was refined to include stricter criteria for clinical diagnosis and research studies.[49,50] The inclusion of "motor and trophic signs and symptoms" in addition to separating vasomotor signs and symptoms from sudomotor category improved specificity without losing sensitivity (Tables 27.2 and 27.3).[50]

The difference between CRPS 1 and 2 is the presence of a definable nerve injury (in CRPS 2 only). The signs and symptoms of both conditions are clinically indistinguishable and include sensory changes, edema, and vasomotor and sudomotor abnormalities. Pain is the key feature for both CRPS 1 and 2 with up to 81% of patients meeting the criteria for CRPS having pain. With CRPS 1, the pain and associated clinical signs and symptoms are typically out of proportion to the inciting event. The pain is typically described as a burning, deep-seated ache with a shooting quality and associated allodynia or hyperalgesia. Symptoms indicative of vasomotor abnormalities occurs in 86.9%, and sudomotor changes including hyperhidrosis/hypohidrosis occur in 52.9% of patients with CRPS. Kinesiophobia and motor weakness have been reported in 74.6% and edema in 79.7%.[51]

DIAGNOSIS

The diagnostic criteria for CRPS types 1 and 2 continue to be based on the patient's symptoms and signs (see Table 27.2). The current revised diagnostic criteria were

TABLE 27.3 Summary of Decision Rules

Criteria/Decision Rule for Proposed Criteria	Sensitivity	Specificity
2+ sign categories and 2+ symptom categories	0.94	0.36
2+ sign categories and 3+ symptom categories	0.85	0.69
2+ sign categories and 4+ symptom categories	0.70	0.94
3+ sign categories and 2+ symptom categories	0.76	0.81
3+ sign categories and 3+ symptom categories	0.70	0.83
3+ sign categories and 4+ symptom categories	0.86	0.75

Source: Harden N, Bruehl S, Stanton-Hicks M, et al: Proposed new diagnostic criteria for complex regional pain syndrome. Pain Med. *8:326-331, 2007.*

developed to enhance the specificity and sensitivity of the previous diagnostic criteria.[50] Studies on the external and internal validation of the IASP criteria suggest that patients should demonstrate at least one symptom in each of the following categories: sensory (hyperesthesia—increased sensitivity to sensory stimulation), vasomotor changes (temperature abnormalities, including skin and color changes), sudomotor (fluid retention—sweating abnormalities, edema), or motor (decreased range of motion, weakness, tremor, dyskinesia, or neglect). In addition, signs in at least two of the four categories indicated above should be noted on physical examination of the patient. A complete history and physical examination, including a through neurologic and vascular examination, will help differentiate from more common conditions that may mimic CRPS. These include neurologic conditions such as painful diabetic neuropathy, entrapment syndromes, discogenic disease, and thoracic outlet syndrome. In addition, vascular conditions should be considered as possible causes in the differential diagnosis, including deep venous thrombosis, cellulitis, vascular insufficiency, lymphedema, and erythromelalgia.[11]

Currently, there is no diagnostic test considered to be a gold standard or objective test that is specific for CRPS. The following tests have been found to help make the diagnosis even though a negative result may not necessarily rule out the possibility of CRPS.

QUANTITATIVE SENSORY TESTING

This involves the use of standardized psychophysical tests of thermal, thermal pain, and vibratory thresholds to assess the function of large fiber, myelinated small fiber, and unmyelinated small afferent fibers. Static and dynamic allodynia, allodynia associated with pinprick, hyperalgesia related to mechanical and heat stimuli, and temporal summation (increased pain to repeated stimuli) may be abnormal in patients with CRPS. Since no specific sensory pattern has been recognized with CRPS, assessment of the signs and changes over time may provide a tool to track response to treatment.

AUTONOMIC FUNCTION TESTS

This includes infrared thermometry and thermography, quantitative sudomotor axon reflex test (QSART), thermoregulatory sweat test (TST), and laser Doppler flowmetry. The limitation of these tests is that most require special equipment and a setup that make clinical applications less viable. In addition, the specificity of abnormalities in these tests in the diagnosis of CRPS or their role as predictors of treatment success is unclear.

TEMPERATURE MEASUREMENT

The use of infrared thermometry and infrared thermography to assess small skin temperature differences between the sides of the body is reported to achieve sensitivity in the order of 76% and specificity of 100%.[52] The utility of this test clinically is dependent on maintaining controlled thermoregulation during measurements. This is difficult to achieve in most clinical situations. Therefore the measurements should be made under conditions where thermoregulation can be controlled to detect differences on both sides for enhanced accuracy of the test. The direction of the temperature difference is dependent on the duration of the disease. Earlier in the disease process the affected limb may demonstrate elevated temperatures, while later on in the more chronic phase of the disease the affected side may show lower temperature compared to the unaffected side.[52]

VASCULAR ABNORMALITIES

In patients with the disease of less than 4 months' duration, vascular reflex responses may be assessed using Doppler flowmetry. The affected extremity may demonstrate higher perfusion.[53] In patients with duration of disease less than 15 months, skin perfusion was found to be either higher or lower, while in patients with a mean duration of 28 months the affected limb demonstrated a lower perfusion and ultimately lower temperatures.

TROPHIC CHANGES

The value of a three-phase bone scintigraphy is in the ability to detect pathologic delayed uptake in the distal bones, such as metacarpophalangeal or metacarpal bones. This is thought to be highly sensitive, although the specificity for CRPS has been questioned. X-ray bone densitometry has also been reported to have a high sensitivity and specificity for CRPS. The ease with which these tests may be performed in clinical practice increases its potential usefulness. Most of these changes have been reported to occur within the first year of the disease.

TREATMENT

Improvements in diagnostic criteria and increased understanding of the pathophysiology of CRPS will help develop clinical trials of mechanism-based treatment modalities. Currently, only a few evidence-based treatment modalities are available; thus, treatment typically involves therapies based on evidence accrued from other neuropathic pain conditions. The treatment philosophy still centers on a multimodal pharmacologic therapy (Table 27.4) and multidisciplinary team approach, with effective pain control, functional restoration, and enhancement of psychological well-being as the key elements (Fig. 27.1).[15,54]

PHARMACOLOGIC THERAPY

Nonsteroidal antiinflammatory drugs (NSAIDs): Although NSAIDs have not been widely studied in the treatment of CRPS, clinical experience demonstrates that NSAIDs can provide mild to moderate pain relief. NSAIDs have been demonstrated to be of value in a retrospective study that examined the utility of intravenous regional anesthesia (IVRA) containing ketorolac; this study revealed that up to 69% of patients experienced partial to complete resolution of their pain.[55]

Antidepressants

Antidepressants have been used widely for the treatment of neuropathic pain. Norepinephrine and serotonin blockers

TABLE 27.4 Overview of Pharmacologic Agents Used in CRPS

Agent	Dose Range	Frequency	Common Side Effects
Antidepressants			
Amitriptyline	10–75 mg/day	Once a day (at night)	Sedation, anticholinergic effects
Nortriptyline	10–75 mg	Once a day (at night)	Sedation, anticholinergic effects
Desipramine	10–75 mg/day	Once a day (at night)	Least sedative/anticholinergic effects
Venlafaxine	37.5–340 mg/day	BID–TID	—
Anticonvulsants			
Gabapentin	900–3600 mg/day	TID	Somnolence, memory impairment, tremors
Pregabalin	150–600 mg/day	BID–TID	Dizziness, somnolence, peripheral edema
Carbamazepine	100–1000 mg/day	BID–QID	Ataxia, sedation, nausea, liver damage, skin rash, bone marrow
Opioids			
Morphine (extended release)	15–60 mg	BID–TID	Nausea, vomiting, constipation, sedation, pruritus
Oxycodone (extended release)	10–60 mg	BID–TID	As for morphine
Methadone	5–20 mg	BID–TID	As for morphine

CRPS, *Complex regional pain syndrome.*
Source: Williams KA, Hurley RW, Lin EE, et al: Neuropathic pain syndromes (CRPS, PHN, PDN). In Benzon HT, Rathmell JP, Wu CL, Turk DC, Argoff CE, editors: Raj's Practical Management of Pain, *ed 4, New York: Mosby, 2008, pp 427-431.*

and selective norepinephrine blockers such as amitriptyline and desipramine, respectively, may exert their influence by modulating the noradrenergic and serotonergic descending pathways. The usual dose range for these drugs is about 10–75 mg by mouth at nighttime.[56] More selective serotonin reuptake inhibitors have not been demonstrated to be as effective as the above. The selective serotonin and norepinephrine reuptake inhibitor duloxetine has been shown to be effective in painful diabetic neuropathy.[57] These drugs have the added value of providing some mood elevation and sedation with improved sleep hygiene when taken at night. Caution is exercised with the use of tricyclic antidepressants in patients older than 65 years due to the potential for cardiac side effects.

Anticonvulsants

Gabapentin and pregabalin have been shown to be effective in diabetic neuropathy and postherpetic neuralgia (PHN).[58,59] Studies in patients with CRPS have also demonstrated analgesic effect of gabapentin. The Food and Drug Administration (FDA) has approved carbamazepine for trigeminal neuralgia and may be considered as a second-tier option for CRPS. The analog of carbamazepine, oxcarbazepine, which does not exhibit the side effects of liver and bone marrow toxicity, may be used as an alternative drug.

Opioids

There is a paucity of long-term studies on oral opioids in the treatment of CRPS or other neuropathic pain conditions. In a randomized placebo-controlled trial, Raja et al. demonstrated that patients with PHN preferred opioids (54%) over tricyclic antidepressants (30%), although the opioids offered only marginally greater pain relief.[56] Opioids are presently considered as third-line drugs for neuropathic pain because of the potential adverse effects and should therefore only be used as part of a multimodal pharmacologic treatment regimen, particularly if other single agents do not provide optimum analgesia.[60]

Ketamine

The NMDA antagonist, ketamine, has been used by anesthesiologists for decades. Other presumed mechanisms of action of ketamine include enhancement of central inhibitory descending tracts and an antiinflammatory CNS effect.[61] Recently, there have been many promising reports of successful treatment of patients considered refractory to traditional CRPS treatments with low-dose ketamine infusions. A randomized placebo-controlled trial showed that i.v. ketamine (0.35 $mgkg^{-1}h^{-1}$, up to 25 mg/h over 4 hours for 10 days) resulted in significant reductions in pain.[62] Some studies report potent analgesia of transient duration,[63] while other studies of longer infusions (4–14 days) have shown analgesia for up to 3 months.[64,65] Use of benzodiazepines during the infusion is recommended to counteract the expected psychotropic side effects. Systematic reviews suggest that the studies are of moderate quality and that the overall evidence is weak for the efficacy of ketamine. A Cochrane review found, based on three randomized trials and a meta-analysis, low-quality evidence to suggest that a course of i.v. ketamine may be effective for CRPS-related pain.[2] A separate meta-analysis concluded that no significant pain relief could be established,[66] while a recent systematic review determined that there was only a weak evidence for the efficacy of ketamine in CRPS. These reports indicate the need for more definitive studies.[67,68]

Bone Targeting Drugs: Calcitonin and Bishphosphonates

Calcitonin

Although the mechanism of action of calcium regulating drugs such as calcitonin is unknown in CRPS, intranasal

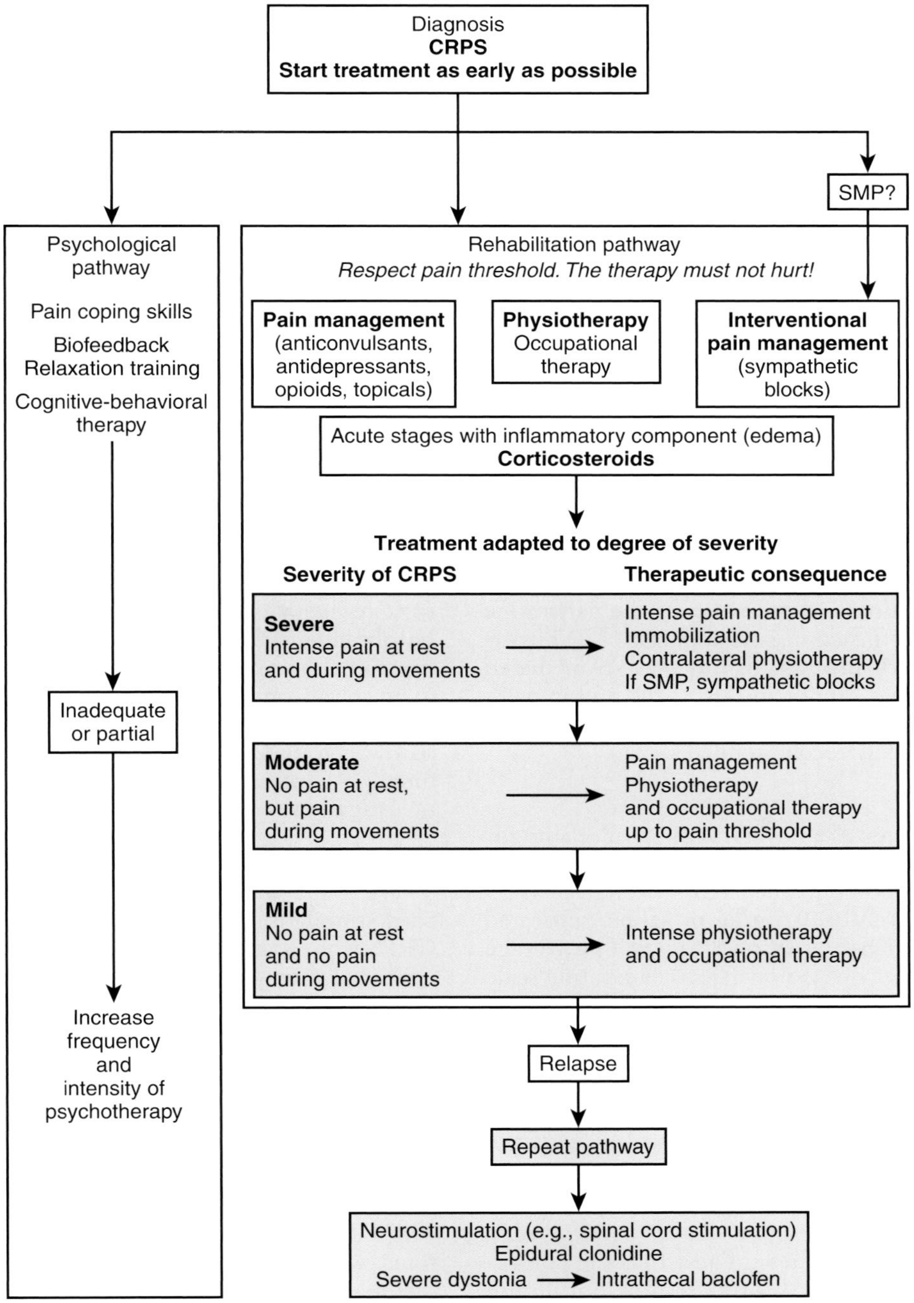

FIG. 27.1 Treatment algorithm. *CRPS*, Complex regional pain syndrome; *SMP*, sympathetically mediated pain. (*Modified from Stanton-Hicks M: Complex regional pain syndrome,* Anesthesiol Clin North Am. *21:733-744, 2003.)*

calcitonin has been suggested to provide pain relief in patients with CRPS. Calcitonin has also received considerable interest because its analgesic properties are derived from the release of β-endorphins. However, in blinded trials involving calcitonin in CRPS, there was no benefit associated with its administration.[69,70]

Bisphosphonates

Five randomized, controlled trials, along with several open label studies, provide evidence for efficacy of i.v. infusions of bisphosphonates (e.g., clodronate, alendronate, pamidronate, neridronate) in decreasing pain and swelling in addition to enhancing range of motion in patients with CRPS.[68,71] Meta-analysis of studies recommend that bisphosphonates should be considered in early CRPS 1.[72] Bisphosphonates decrease pain in bone diseases, such as Paget disease, myeloma and metastatic disease, by their antiosteoclastic properties. Since enhanced osteoclast-mediated bone resorption has not been clearly demonstrated in CRPS, its mechanism of action in this syndrome is unclear. It has been postulated that bisphosphonates may reduce tissue acidosis and lower neuropeptide release from primary afferents and macrophages.[71]

OTHER POTENTIAL THERAPIES

Free radical scavengers have been explored as possible treatment options. In a placebo-controlled trial, both topically applied dimethyl sulfoxide (DMSO) 50%, and oral *N*-acetylcysteine (NAC) were found to be effective in CRPS type 1.[73] The naturally occurring antioxidant, vitamin C, has been suggested to be associated with a lower incidence of CRPS when administered prophylactically to patients with closed radius fractures requiring internal fixation as compared with patients who did not receive vitamin C prophylactically.[74]

Intravenous magnesium administration has also been studied. Although a preliminary open-label study in acute stage CRPS 1 was promising, a subsequent placebo-controlled trial failed to demonstrate significant difference between magnesium and placebo.[75]

Naltrexone

This glial cell modulator antagonizes the Toll-like Receptor 4 pathway and attenuates activated microglia. It is a centrally active immune modulator which at low dose does not antagonize the mu-opioid receptors. Low-dose naltrexone (4.5 mg) has shown efficacy in case reports.[76,77] Naltrexone has already shown promise in other CNS-mediated diseases.[78] Clinical data supporting its use is preliminary; therefore more studies need to be performed before this medication can be widely recommended.

Immunoglobulin IV

IVIG has been suggested as a novel treatment modality for refractory CRPS patients.[79,80] The best evidence is from a double-blind, placebo-controlled cross-over trial in 13 patients who received IVIG 0.5 g/kg or saline, separated by a washout period of greater than 28 days.[81] The average pain intensity was lower by 1.55 on a 0–10 pain rating scale in the IVIG group.

INTERVENTIONAL THERAPIES

Intravenous Regional Anesthesia

There is no strong evidence to support the use of IVRA for sympatholysis in CRPS. Several agents, including guanethidine, reserpine, droperidol, ketanserin, atropine, and lidocaine-methylprednisolone, have been used.[70] The results of two small studies suggest that the combination of local anesthetics with bretylium or botulinum toxin can increase the analgesic duration of IVRA and lumbar sympathetic blocks, respectively. When prilocaine and guanethidine were compared to placebo, no difference was shown after four blocks, whereas stellate ganglion blocks with bupivacaine and regional blocks with guanethidine demonstrated a significant improvement compared to baseline; both treatments showed comparable benefits.

Sympathetic Nerve Blocks

Sympathetic blocks have been utilized as a diagnostic tool to determine if neuropathic pain is SMP or SIP. Price et al. evaluated the diagnostic and therapeutic value of local anesthetics compared to saline in sympathetic blocks. They demonstrated that effects on pain and mechanical allodynia (lasting hours) was similar in both groups; however, the local anesthetic group showed a persistence of benefit beyond the duration of action of the local anesthetic (3–5 days).[82] They concluded that the immediate beneficial effect may be due to a nonspecific mechanism. Sympatholysis is associated with prolonged pain relief in patients who respond to the sympathetic block, and helps to differentiate between SMP and SIP. Ultimately, the clinical benefit of sympathetic ganglion blocks arises from the analgesia provided that allows for the implementation of intense physical therapy with modalities, such as desensitization, that help engender functional restoration in the affected limb.

Intrathecal Baclofen

CRPS can lead to dystonia often refractory to standard treatment, and baclofen a GABA (type B) receptor agonist that inhibits sensory input into the spinal cord has been shown to be effective in some patients with dystonia. Baclofen has therefore been tried as a treatment option in CRPS associated with dystonia. Intrathecal baclofen was successfully used in seven patients with CRPS refractory to benzodiazepines, levodopa, antiepileptic drugs, botulinum toxin, mannitol, surgical/chemical sympathectomy, and oral baclofen. While long-term improvement in dystonia was observed, significant improvements in global intense pain, sharp pain, dull pain, and deep pain was found mainly during the first 6 months of treatment.[83,84] Intrathecal therapy in CRPS requires further investigation.

Spinal Cord Stimulation

There is increasing evidence to support the value of spinal cord stimulation (SCS) in the treatment of patients with CRPS who have experienced suboptimal benefit from conventional therapy.[85–89] As with the challenges of defining the pathophysiology of CRPS, the mechanism by which SCS provides pain control continues to be elusive. Several other questions that remain unanswered include the specifics of stimulation parameters, stimulation patterns, the criteria for a "successful" SCS trial, and the effects of SCS on the natural course of the disease. There has been one case report in an adult and a case series in adolescent girls aged 11–14 years, in which the use of SCS in a patient with CRPS resulted in complete resolution of the symptoms, with symptoms remaining abated at 1–8 years after the intervention.[90,91] In a 5-year follow-up on patients with CRPS type 1, Kemler et al. reported results of a randomized controlled trial in which patients received either SCS plus physical therapy (PT) or PT alone. The authors found that during the first 2 years following implantation, the SCS-plus-PT patients reported greater reduction in pain. However, at the 3-year follow-ups and subsequent time points, the SCS-plus-PT group had similar results to the PT group regarding reduction in pain relief and all other variables measured.[92] However, in a subgroup analysis the SCS-plus-PT group demonstrated a significantly greater global perceived effect to the treatment than the PT group alone. In a systematic review of the clinical and cost-effectiveness literature, Taylor et al. found that SCS appears to be an efficacious and cost-effective treatment for CRPS type 1 (level of evidence A) and type 2 (level of evidence D).[93]

Functional Restoration

Functional restoration is the hallmark of successful treatment of CRPS. This is best achieved in a multidisciplinary setting with the occupational therapist initiating the early desensitization process and the physical therapist addressing muscle strength, flexibility, gait training, and overcoming the kinesiophobia typically associated with advanced CRPS. A recreational therapist may be involved in the later stages of restoration to help the patient return to socialization and engagement in recreational activities that may have been neglected in the course of the disease.[89,94]

Motor Imagery Program

A motor imagery program (MIP) incorporates recognition of the limb laterality, imagined movements, and mirrored movements using a mirror box device. In a randomized controlled study involving patients with CRPS of the upper extremity after a wrist fracture, the patients received conventional treatment or MIP. At 6 and 12 weeks after completion of the six treatments, the patients in the MIP group had significantly less pain and decreased swelling. This treatment modality is promising but requires further investigation.[95,96] A recent Cochrane review concluded that graduated motor imagery and mirror therapy may provide clinically meaningful improvements in pain and function in patients with CRPS 1; however, the quality of the supporting evidence was considered to be very low.[97]

Psychotherapy

Depression and anxiety commonly occur in patients with chronic pain. This is amplified in CRPS because of the uncertainty associated with the cause, course, and treatment of the disorder. The risk of developing posttraumatic stress disorder is present in this patient population amid fears that the disease may progress or recur without warning. Instituting cognitive-behavioral therapy is the most effective psychological intervention found to produce long-lasting reduction in psychological symptoms in both children and adults with CRPS.

KEY POINTS

- The term CRPS has replaced the earlier terms RSD and causalgia as it better represents the varied clinical presentation and diverse pathophysiology. Patients may have varying levels of sympathetic nervous system involvement in maintaining pain through the course of the disease process; hence the terms SMP or SIP are used to describe the mechanisms of pain.
- There is a paucity of epidemiologic data and longitudinal outcome studies on CRPS, reflecting the absence of evidence-based predictors of the time course of the disease.
- CRPS types 1 and 2 differ etiologically by the presence (type 2) or absence (type 1) of evidence of nerve injury. Pain is the hallmark of the condition, and commonly manifests as spontaneous pain, with hyperalgesia and allodynia. Associated signs include vasomotor and sudomotor disturbances, active and/or passive movement deficits and trophic changes.
- The pathophysiology of CRPS is still not well understood. Peripheral and central sensitization and neuroimmune mechanisms are thought to play important roles in CRPS.
- Consensus-based diagnostic criteria for CRPS types 1 and 2 have been developed based on four different clusters of symptoms and signs (see Table 27.2). CRPS is a clinical diagnosis and there is no objective diagnostic test that is considered to be a gold standard for CRPS.
- The treatment paradigm still centers on a multidisciplinary multimodal team approach that includes key elements such as pharmacologic, interventional and neuromodulation therapy for effective pain control (Table 27.4), functional rehabilitation and enhancement of psychological well-being (Fig. 27.1).

REFERENCES

Access the reference list online at ExpertConsult.com.

CHAPTER

28

HERPES ZOSTER AND POSTHERPETIC NEURALGIA

Kenneth Schmader, MD ✪ Robert H. Dworkin, PhD

The objective of this chapter is to provide an overview of the epidemiology, natural history, pathophysiology, treatment, and prevention of herpes zoster and postherpetic neuralgia (PHN). Herpes zoster ("shingles") is a viral infection that is accompanied by acute pain in the majority of patients. The pain associated with herpes zoster does not resolve in a substantial number of patients, which results in a chronic peripheral neuropathic pain condition called PHN.

HERPES ZOSTER

EPIDEMIOLOGY OF HERPES ZOSTER

Following a primary chicken pox infection, the varicella-zoster virus (VZV) establishes latency in sensory ganglia throughout the nervous system. Herpes zoster (shingles) is the reactivation of the virus and its spread from a single dorsal root or cranial nerve ganglion to the corresponding dermatome and neural tissue of the same segment. Herpes zoster has the highest incidence of all neurologic diseases, occurring annually in approximately 1 million people in the United States, during the lifetimes of as much as 20%–30% of the population and in as many as 50% of those living until age 85.[1,2] The likelihood of recurrent zoster in immunocompetent persons was reported to be 5.7% after 8 years from the initial zoster episode.[3]

A fundamental epidemiologic feature of zoster is a marked increase in incidence with aging. The increase in the likelihood of herpes zoster with aging starts around 50–60 years of age and increases markedly into late life in individuals older than 80 years of age. For example, the incidence of herpes zoster per 1000 person-years in a US retrospective database study was 2.1 for persons aged 40–49 years, 4.2 for 50–59, 6.0 for 60–69, 8.6 for 70–79, and 10.7 for 80 and older.[2]

The incidence of herpes zoster is also significantly increased in patients with suppressed cell-mediated immunity. Immunocompromised patients at risk for herpes zoster include persons with Hodgkin disease, non-Hodgkin lymphomas, leukemia, bone marrow and other organ transplants, human immunodeficiency virus (HIV) infection, systemic lupus erythematosus, rheumatoid arthritis, and those individuals taking immunosuppressive medications, including tumor necrosis factor inhibitors.[4,5] White race, female sex, and physical trauma are other risk factors for herpes zoster.[4,6,7]

Patients with herpes zoster who have a vesicular rash may transmit VZV via direct contact, airborne or droplet nuclei to seronegative, nonimmune individuals, such as children who have not received the varicella vaccine or who have had an insufficient response to the vaccine, and susceptible health care workers and staff in hospital or in nursing homes. These individuals may then develop varicella. The exposure of an individual who is latently infected with VZV to herpes zoster does not cause herpes zoster or varicella.

NATURAL HISTORY OF HERPES ZOSTER

The presentation of pain in herpes zoster is variable. In the majority of patients, a prodrome of dermatomal pain precedes the appearance of the characteristic unilateral rash.[8,9] This prodrome begins several days before rash onset in almost all cases, but a series of patients with prodromal pain preceding the appearance of the rash by 7 to more than 100 days has been reported.[10] Thoracic dermatomes are the most commonly affected sites in herpes zoster and account for 50%–70% of all cases; cranial (especially the ophthalmic division of the trigeminal nerve), cervical, and lumbar dermatomes each account for 10%–20% of cases, and sacral dermatomes are affected in 2%–8% of cases. The rash becomes vesicular after several days, then forms a crust, and loss of all scabs usually occurs within 2–4 weeks.[4]

Pain in the affected dermatome accompanies the rash in most patients. Those who did not have a painful prodrome typically begin to experience pain at rash onset or shortly afterwards (Fig. 28.1). VZV-induced acute neuritis is described as burning, deep aching, tingling, itching, or stabbing. A subset of patients may develop severe pain, especially those with trigeminal nerve involvement. Acute herpetic neuralgia has a profound negative impact on functional status and quality of life and usually results in substantial health service utilization.[11,12]

Dermatomal pain without a rash, referred to as *zoster sine herpete*, has also been described, and the finding of VZV DNA in the cerebrospinal fluid of patients with prolonged radicular pain and no rash provides evidence of this syndrome.[13]

In addition to acute pain, the morbidity of herpes zoster includes neurologic disorders and ophthalmologic, cutaneous, and visceral complications. The types of neurologic complications include motor neuropathy, cranial polyneuritis, transverse myelitis, meningoencephalitis, and cerebral angiitis and stroke after ophthalmic zoster. Ophthalmologic complications include keratitis, uveitis, iridocyclitis, panophthalmitis, and glaucoma. Elderly and especially immunosuppressed patients are at greater risk for most of the complications of herpes zoster.

TREATMENT OF HERPES ZOSTER

The main goals of the treatment of herpes zoster are to relieve acute pain and prevent PHN. Treatment of herpes

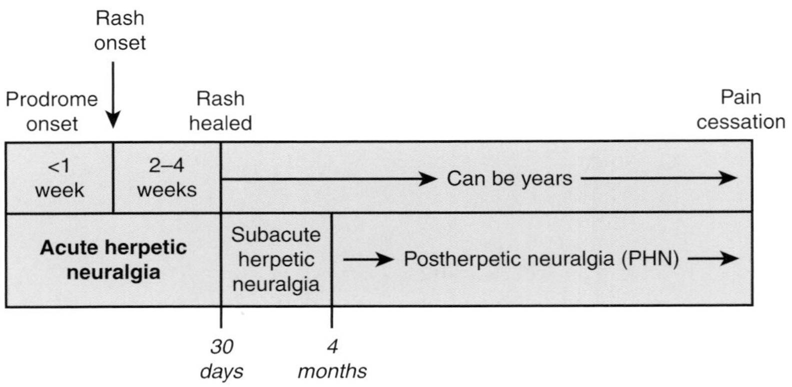

FIG. 28.1 Timeline of pain experienced by herpes zoster patients.

zoster patients with the antiviral agents acyclovir, brivudine, famciclovir, or valacyclovir inhibits viral replication and has been shown to reduce the duration of viral shedding, hasten rash healing, and decrease the severity and duration of acute pain.[5] The results of randomized controlled trials and meta-analyses are conflicting as to whether antiviral agents prevent PHN, partly because of heterogeneity in definitions of PHN and study design, although the duration of pain is decreased in some of these trials. Therefore, based on reduction in acute pain and the potential for reduction in pain duration, antiviral therapy is recommended as first-line treatment in herpes zoster patients who are aged 50 years and older.[14] Famciclovir (500 mg every 8 hours for 7 days), valacyclovir (1 g 3 times daily for 7 days), and brivudine (125 mg daily for 7 days) offer more convenient dosing and higher and more reliable blood levels of antiviral activity compared with acyclovir (800 mg 5 times a day for 7–10 days).

Some patients do not have their acute pain adequately controlled with antiviral therapy and simple analgesics. How then can acute pain and the risk of chronic pain be further reduced beyond that currently achieved by antiviral therapy? Corticosteroids, opioids, gabapentin, and neural blockade have been investigated or considered as strategies to achieve these goals.

Randomized clinical trials (RCTs) demonstrated that the addition of a corticosteroid reduced acute pain but did not contribute significantly beyond the benefits achieved by antiviral therapy alone in reducing prolonged pain.[15,16] The evidence from these trials indicated that corticosteroids do not prevent PHN.

An RCT of oxycodone, gabapentin, or placebo in older adults with herpes zoster showed that oxycodone but not gabapentin provided significantly greater pain relief than placebo.[17] This trial was not powered to analyze PHN, and there are no other controlled trials of the effect of opioids or gabapentin on PHN when used during the acute phase of herpes zoster, except for a crossover study that showed greater pain relief with a single dose of 900 mg of gabapentin versus placebo.[18]

Regarding neural blockade, the results of a randomized controlled trial in patients with herpes zoster treated with oral antiviral therapy showed that a single epidural injection of steroids and local anesthetics relieved acute pain within the first month after rash onset significantly better than usual care but did not reduce the risk of developing PHN.[19] RCTs of multiple epidural injections, continuous epidural infusions, or repetitive paravertebral injections of anesthetics and steroids during herpes zoster reduced PHN or time to complete cessation of pain. Although treatment of herpes zoster patients with multiple epidural injections or continuous epidural infusions is unlikely to be feasible in most settings, these data suggest that aggressive analgesia can be effective in patients with herpes zoster and ongoing moderate to severe pain.[20]

Even if the risk of developing PHN is not reduced by combining antiviral therapy with analgesic or corticosteroid treatment in patients with herpes zoster, effective relief of acute pain is a critical treatment goal. For patients with moderate to severe pain, treatment with a strong opioid analgesic (e.g., oxycodone) is recommended in combination with antiviral therapy. If moderate to severe pain in patients with herpes zoster has not responded rapidly to treatment with an opioid analgesic and antiviral therapy, then the addition of a corticosteroid can be considered. For patients with pain that is inadequately controlled by antiviral agents in combination with oral analgesic medications and/or corticosteroids, referral to a pain specialist or pain center is recommended to evaluate eligibility for neural blockade.[14]

PREVENTION OF HERPES ZOSTER

The Advisory Committee on Immunization Practices (ACIP) of the Centers for Disease Control and Prevention (CDC) recommends the live attenuated zoster vaccine for the prevention of herpes zoster and PHN in immunocompetent adults 60 years of age and older.[4] The recommendation is based on the results of the Shingles Prevention Study, a large placebo controlled trial in persons 60 years and older.[21] In this study, the vaccine reduced incidence of herpes zoster from 11.12 to 5.42 cases (51.3%) per 1000 person-years, reduced the incidence PHN from 1.38 to 0.46 cases (66.5%) per 1000 person years, and reduced the pain burden of illness (a pain severity by duration measure) caused by herpes zoster by 61.1%. The exact duration of the protection against herpes zoster by the zoster vaccine is unknown, but recent studies suggest that the live vaccine efficacy for herpes zoster and pain burden persists through year 8 after vaccination but probably not beyond 10 years.[22,23] In a large randomized placebo controlled trial of the live zoster vaccine in individuals 50–59 years old, vaccine efficacy for prevention of herpes zoster was 69.8%.[24] The US Food and Drug Administration (FDA) licensed the live vaccine for use in immunocompetent adults 50 years of age. However, the ACIP retained the recommendation to vaccinate at 60 years of age and over because zoster vaccine administration should be timed to achieve the greatest reduction in burden of herpes zoster and its complications, which is in persons over 60 years old.[25]

A recently developed subunit zoster vaccine containing VZV glycoprotein E and the AS01b adjuvant system was tested for efficacy against herpes zoster in a multisite randomized placebo controlled trial called the Zoster Efficacy Study in Adults 50 Years of Age or Older (ZOE-50). The intervention was two intramuscular doses of the vaccine or placebo 2 months apart. The results showed that the subunit adjuvanted vaccine reduced the incidence of herpes zoster in this age group by 97.2% with an adequate safety profile.[26] This vaccine is not yet licensed by the FDA but looks to be an exciting addition to our interventions against herpes zoster.

POSTHERPETIC NEURALGIA

EPIDEMIOLOGY AND NATURAL HISTORY

A variety of definitions of PHN have been used by clinicians and investigators, ranging from any pain persisting after rash healing to pain that has persisted at least 6 months after rash onset. The results of studies suggest that the pain associated with herpes zoster has three phases—an acute herpetic neuralgia that accompanies the rash and lasts for approximately 30 days after rash onset, a subacute herpetic neuralgia that lasts from 30 to 120 days after rash onset, and PHN, defined as pain that persists for at least 120 days after rash onset (see Fig. 28.1).[27–29] Although this provides a validated definition for research on PHN, it is probably unnecessary to distinguish between subacute herpetic neuralgia and PHN when treating patients with pain persisting after rash healing.

Because the proportion of herpes zoster patients with pain declines with time, estimates of the percentage of patients who develop PHN depend on its definition. In an analysis of a cohort of 27,225 herpes zoster (HZ) patients in the UK General Practice Research Database, 13.7% of patients developed PHN at least 3 months after HZ diagnosis.[30] Of those patients, 58.5% had moderate to severe pain. In an analysis of 1669 HZ patients in a population-based study of adult residents of Olmsted County, Minnesota, 18% of patients developed PHN, defined as zoster-associated pain persisting at least 90 days.[2] PHN occurred in 33% of individuals aged 79 years and older. Estimates of the number of prevalent cases of PHN have ranged from 500,000 to 1 million in the United States.

PHN is a chronic pain syndrome that can last for years and cause substantial suffering and reduction in quality of life. As is true of other chronic pain syndromes, patients develop depression and other types of psychological distress as well as physical, occupational, and social disability as a consequence of their unremitting pain. There is evidence that pain in PHN can be discontinuous, with pain-free intervals of varying durations occurring.[31] Indeed, PHN can develop even in herpes zoster patients who have not had acute pain.[32]

The quality of pain in PHN compared to herpes zoster has been examined in several studies.[33–35] Sharp, stabbing pain was found to be more common in patients with zoster than in patients with PHN, whereas burning pain was more common in PHN patients and much less likely to be reported by patients with zoster. The investigators noted that the word *tender* was chosen by both groups of patients to describe allodynia (i.e., pain in response to a stimulus that does not normally provoke pain). These adjectives reflect the three different types of pain that have been distinguished in research on PHN—a steady throbbing or burning pain, an intermittent sharp or shooting pain, and allodynia.

Older age is the most well-established risk factor for PHN. In the UK General Practice Research Database study, not only did the incidence of PHN increase with age, but the prevalence of moderate-severe pain also increased with age, from 46% in 50–54-years-olds to 68% in 80–85-year-olds.[30] Furthermore, the duration of PHN increased with pain severity. For individuals with severe pain 3 months after rash onset, the average duration of PHN was 12.5 months. Many independent studies have reported that patients with more severe acute pain are at greater risk for PHN.[29] As noted above, the majority of herpes zoster patients have a painful prodrome before their rash appears, and several studies have found that these patients have a greater risk of PHN than patients who did not have a prodrome. Greater severity and duration of the herpes zoster rash are additional risk factors for the development of PHN that have been identified in multiple studies.

PATHOPHYSIOLOGY

Except for age and psychosocial factors, the risk factors for PHN that have been identified can all be considered concomitants of a more severe infection. More severe zoster infections are accompanied by greater neural damage, and it has been proposed that this neural damage contributes prominently to the development of PHN.[36] However, the nature of this damage and the specific mechanisms by which it causes the persisting pain of PHN remain unclear. What limited knowledge there is of the pathophysiology of PHN derives from studies of neuropathology, sensory dysfunction, and pharmacologic response. There is considerable agreement currently that different peripheral and central mechanisms contribute to PHN and that the qualitatively different types of pain that characterize PHN probably have different underlying mechanisms. This suggests that there may be pathophysiologically distinct subgroups of patients with PHN or that more than one mechanism may be involved in individual patients or both.[37,38]

Watson and his colleagues have conducted an elegant series of postmortem studies of patients of who were suffering from PHN at the time of death and of patients with a history of herpes zoster whose pain did not persist beyond rash healing.[31] In these studies, dorsal horn atrophy and pathologic changes in the sensory ganglion were found on the affected side (and not on the unaffected side) in patients with PHN but not in patients with a history of herpes zoster whose pain did not persist. In a set of studies using punch-skin biopsy, reductions in epidermal nerve fiber density were found in the affected dermatome but not on the contralateral unaffected side in patients with PHN.[39,40] Notably, in both the postmortem studies and the punch-skin biopsy studies, the pathologic features were characteristic of only the affected side in patients with PHN and were not found in patients with a history of zoster whose pain did not persist.

Rowbotham, Fields, and Petersen have conducted an important series of studies of sensory dysfunction and pharmacologic response that address the pathophysiology of PHN.[37,38,41,42] PHN patients with prominent allodynia were found to have relatively normal sensory function as assessed by thermal thresholds and were also more likely to report pain relief following local anesthetic infiltration with lidocaine than patients with primarily constant pain. These authors conclude that at least two different mechanisms may contribute to PHN and propose that the mechanism of allodynia in PHN is abnormal activity in preserved primary afferent nociceptors that have been damaged by the VZV but that remain in continuity with their central targets. Activity in these "irritable" nociceptors may initiate and then maintain a state of central sensitization in which input from large fiber afferents that respond to nonpainful mechanical stimuli causes allodynia.

As opposed to patients with prominent allodynia, PHN patients with predominantly continuous pain were found to have sensory loss in the areas where they have the most pain. This suggests that continuous pain in PHN is caused by a different mechanism than allodynia, possibly involving central structural and functional changes accompanying deafferentation. These may include a structural reorganization of the spinal cord that involves abnormal synaptic connections, as well as functional abnormalities resulting from deafferentation involving hyperexcitability of dorsal horn neurons. A clinical trial that compared oxcarbazepine to placebo in neuropathic pain (including PHN) patients stratified participants by irritable versus nonirritable pain phenotypes. The results showed that the number needed to treat to obtain one patient with more than 50% neuropathic pain relief was 3.9 (95% confidence interval [CI] 2.3–12) in the irritable and 13 (95% CI 5.3–∞) in the nonirritable nociceptor phenotype.[43]

TREATMENT

The efficacy of lidocaine patch 5%, gabapentin, pregabalin, tricyclic antidepressants (TCAs), opioid analgesics, tramadol, and high-concentration capsaicin patch has been demonstrated by the results of randomized controlled trials in patients with PHN,[44–51] although a recent meta-analysis has called the benefits of opioids into question.[52] Depending on the study, in general, these agents produce clinically significant reduction in pain in about 30%–60% of patients. The initial choice of these medications should be guided by the adverse event profiles, potential for drug interactions, and patient comorbidities and treatment preferences, especially because there are no replicated data demonstrating superior effectiveness of one drug over another.[44] In general, the lidocaine patch 5%, gabapentin, and pregabalin can be considered first-line treatments for PHN. TCAs, opioid analgesics, tramadol, and high-dose capsaicin patch require greater caution and/or specialized expertise in the often elderly patient with PHN.

Lidocaine Patch 5%

Treatment with the lidocaine patch 5% consists of the application of up to three patches daily for a maximum of 12 hours applied directly to the area of maximal PHN pain and allodynia, which typically overlaps the affected dermatome.[53,54] The lidocaine patch 5% is not approved for patients with herpes zoster, and it should not be used in patients with open lesions because the available formulation is not sterile. Importantly, whether the patient obtains satisfactory relief from lidocaine patch 5% will usually be apparent within 2–3 weeks and time-consuming dose escalation is not required. The only adverse effects involve skin reactions (e.g., erythema, rash). Systemic absorption is minimal but must be considered in patients receiving oral class I antiarrythmic drugs.

Gabapentin

To reduce the likelihood of adverse effects and increase patient compliance with treatment, gabapentin should be initiated at low dosages—100–300 mg in a single dose at bedtime or 100 mg 3 times daily—and then titrated by 100 mg 3 times daily as tolerated. Because of variability in gabapentin absorption, the final dosage should be determined either by acceptable levels of pain relief or by unacceptable adverse effects that do not resolve over a few weeks. Adverse effects of gabapentin include somnolence, dizziness, and mild peripheral edema, which requires monitoring and possibly dosage adjustment but usually not treatment discontinuation.[55,56] Gabapentin may cause or exacerbate gait and balance problems and cognitive impairment in the elderly. Dosage adjustment is necessary in patients with renal insufficiency, but its generally excellent tolerability, safety, and lack of drug interactions distinguish gabapentin from the other oral medications used in the treatment of PHN.

Pregabalin

Pregabalin is similar in structure to gabapentin.[57] Pregabalin should be initiated at 100–150 mg/day in two or three divided doses. Frail older patients may require lower starting doses. The dose may be increased to 300 mg/day in two or three divided doses within 1 week depending on clinical response and any adverse effects. The maximum dose of 600 mg/day in two or three divided doses can be considered if the patient does not have adequate pain relief at the risk of significantly higher frequency of adverse effects. Dizziness, somnolence, peripheral edema, amblyopia, dry mouth, and gait disturbances are the most common adverse effects of the medication.[57]

Tricyclic Antidepressants

To decrease the likelihood of adverse effects, all TCAs should be initiated at low dosages—10–25 mg in a single dose at bedtime—and should then be slowly titrated as tolerated. It is often claimed that the analgesic effect of

TCAs occurs at lower dosages than their antidepressant effect, but there is no controlled evidence of this. Consequently, TCAs should be titrated to dosages of at least 75–150 mg daily. For titration above 100–150 mg daily, blood levels and the electrocardiogram (EKG) should be monitored. Irrespective of the TCA chosen, it is imperative that patients understand the rationale for treatment, specifically, that TCAs have an analgesic effect that has been demonstrated to be independent of their antidepressant effect. Amitriptyline is widely used for PHN. However, amitriptyline is poorly tolerated and contraindicated in elderly patients.[58] In one of the few randomized, double-blind trials that have compared two different treatments in elderly PHN patients, nortriptyline demonstrated equivalent efficacy to amitriptyline but was better tolerated.[59] Based on the results of this study, nortriptyline should now be considered the preferred TCA for the treatment of PHN in older adults.

Despite the efficacy of TCAs in the treatment of PHN, their cardiac toxicity and side effect profile require considerable caution when treating older patients with PHN.[60] Dry mouth is the most common side effect, and constipation, sweating, dizziness, disturbed vision, and drowsiness also occur frequently. All TCAs must be used very cautiously in patients with a history of cardiovascular disease, glaucoma, urinary retention, and autonomic neuropathy, and a screening EKG to check for cardiac conduction abnormalities is recommended before beginning TCA treatment, especially in patients over 40 years of age. TCAs must be used cautiously when there is a risk of suicide or accidental death from overdose, and TCAs may cause balance problems and cognitive impairment in the elderly. TCAs can block the effects of certain antihypertensive drugs and interact with drugs metabolized by P450 2D6 (e.g., type 1C antiarrythmics). Because all SSRIs inhibit P450 D26, caution is necessary in the concomitant administration of TCAs and SSRIs to prevent toxic TCA plasma concentrations.

In addition, there are no published RCTs of either selective serotonin reuptake inhibitors (e.g., fluoxetine, paroxetine) or selective serotonin and norepinephrine reuptake inhibitors (e.g., duloxetine, venlafaxine) in PHN; thus, it is unknown whether these classes of antidepressant medications are efficacious in PHN. However, considering that TCAs inhibit the reuptake of serotonin and norepinephrine and have well-established efficacy in PHN, it can be predicted that selective serotonin and norepinephrine reuptake inhibitors would also have efficacy in PHN.

Opioid Analgesics

There are numerous short- and long-acting opioid analgesics available, and treatment can begin with a short-acting medication at morphine oral equianalgesic dosages of 5–15 mg every 4 hours as needed.[61,62] After 1–2 weeks of treatment, the total daily dosage can be converted to an equianalgesic dosage of one of the available long-acting opioid analgesics (e.g., controlled-release morphine oxycodone, oxymorphone, or tapentadol, and transdermal fentanyl, levorphanol, and methadone) while the patient continues taking the short-acting medication on an as-needed basis. Evaluation by a pain specialist should be considered when contemplating the use of opioids for PHN especially for daily dosages greater than 100 mg morphine or its equivalent given increasing concerns about the risk/benefit ratio with long-term use of opioids.

The most common adverse effects of opioid analgesics are constipation, sedation, and nausea; in addition, cognitive impairment, and problems with mobility can occur in elderly patients. Opioid analgesics must be used very cautiously in patients with a history of substance abuse or suicide attempts, since accidental death or suicide can occur with overdose. Patients treated with opioid analgesics may develop analgesic tolerance (i.e., a reduction in analgesic benefit over time), although a stable dosage can often be achieved. All patients develop physical dependence (i.e., withdrawal symptoms develop with abrupt discontinuation or rapid dose reduction), and must be advised that they should not abruptly discontinue their medication. The risk of substance abuse developing in patients who do not have a history of substance abuse is not known.

Tramadol

Tramadol is a norepinephrine and serotonin reuptake inhibitor with a major metabolite that is a *mu* opioid agonist.[63] Tramadol should be initiated at low dosages—50 mg once or twice daily—and then titrated every 3–7 days by 50–100 mg/day in divided doses as tolerated. The maximum dosage of tramadol is 400 mg daily; in patients aged over 75, the maximum dosage of tramadol is reduced, for example, to 300 mg daily in divided doses.

The adverse effects of tramadol include dizziness, nausea, constipation, somnolence, and orthostatic hypotension. These occur more frequently when the dosage is escalated rapidly and with concurrent administration of other drugs with similar side effect profiles. There is an increased risk of seizures in patients treated with tramadol who have a history of seizures or who are also receiving antidepressants, opioids, or other drugs that can reduce the seizure threshold. Serotonin syndrome may occur if tramadol is used concurrently with other serotonergic medications, especially selective serotonin reuptake inhibitors (SSRIs) and monoamine oxidase inhibitors. Tramadol may cause or exacerbate cognitive impairment in the elderly, and dosage adjustment is necessary in patients with renal or hepatic disease. Abuse of tramadol is relatively uncommon but does occur.

High-Concentration Capsaicin Patch

Application of the high-concentration capsaicin patch should be performed in specialist clinics by personnel trained in the proper application of the patch.[64] Because of the high concentration, capsaicin can be aerosolized and inhaled, resulting in coughing or sneezing, or get into mucous membranes or the eyes, resulting in irritation. After application of a topical anesthetic, the patch is applied to the most painful area for an hour and then removed. The application can be repeated every 3 months depending on the analgesic response to the patch. Adverse events include acute pain during the procedure, which is usually transient, application-site skin reactions (e.g., erythema), and transient increases in blood pressure.

Sequential and Combination Pharmacologic Treatment

There have been a few clinical trials in which medications have been directly compared with one another in patients with PHN.[59,62,65–67] Such comparisons not only make it possible to directly determine whether treatments vary in their efficacy, safety, and tolerability, but when conducted in the same patients, it also enables evaluating the extent to which treatment response to one medication predicts response to another. For example, treatment responses to opioid analgesics and TCAs were uncorrelated in a recent three-period, placebo-controlled crossover trial, which suggests that when patients have not responded to one of these types of medication, they may still respond to the other.[62]

The prescription of combination pharmacotherapy for PHN is common in clinical practice. The efficacy of this practice has been the subject of recent studies of additive or synergistic benefits of combination treatment. In a 5-week double-blind crossover trial, patients with diabetic polyneuropathy or PHN were randomized to daily active placebo (lorazepam), sustained-release morphine, gabapentin, and a combination of gabapentin and morphine.[65] Baseline mean daily pain (0–10) was 5.72. At maximum tolerated dose, pain was rated at 4.49 with placebo, 4.15 with gabapentin, 3.70 with morphine, and 3.06 with the gabapentin–morphine combination ($P < .05$ for the combination vs. placebo, gabapentin, and morphine). Results for PHN alone were not reported. Constipation, sedation, and dry mouth were the most common adverse effects. In a 6-week double-blind crossover trial, patients with diabetic polyneuropathy or PHN were randomized to receive one of three sequences of daily oral gabapentin, nortriptyline, and their combination.[66] Baseline mean pain intensity was 5.4 (0–10 scale). For patients with PHN, pain with combination treatment (mean 2.5, CI 1.4–3.6) was lower than with nortriptyline (mean 2.9, CI 1.7–4.0) or gabapentin alone (mean 3.4, CI 2.2–4.5), but the overall effect of drug treatment was not significant ($P = .054$), possibly because of small sample size. The most common adverse event was dry mouth secondary to nortriptyline. In an evaluation of a nortriptyline-morphine combination, compared with each drug alone, patients with neuropathic pain, including PHN, were randomized to receive oral nortriptyline, morphine, and their combination in a double-blind crossover trial during 6-week periods.[67] Average daily pain (0–10) at baseline was 5.3. At maximum tolerated dose of the drugs, the average daily pain was 2.6 for combination versus 3.1 for nortriptyline ($P = .046$) and 3.4 for morphine ($P = .002$). Combination treatment resulted in moderate-severe constipation in 43% versus 46% with morphine ($P = .82$) and 5% with nortriptyline ($P < .0001$). Combination treatment resulted in moderate-severe dry mouth in 58% versus 49% with nortriptyline ($P = .84$) and 13% with morphine ($P < .0001$). Somnolence was also among the most frequent adverse effects.

These results suggest that combination therapy may provide additional pain relief in some individuals with PHN who have responded to one or another agent. Disadvantages of combination therapy include an increased risk of adverse effects as the number of medications is increased.

Alternatives to Topical and Oral Medications

A considerable percentage of PHN patients will not respond to medications when used alone and in combination. For these patients, there are a large number of alternative treatments that deserve consideration, and referral to a pain management center should be contemplated sooner rather than later.

Noninvasive treatments include cold application, transcutaneous electrical nerve stimulation (TENS), percutaneous electrical nerve stimulation (PENS), psychological treatments, and acupuncture. These interventions have little risk and may be useful in some patients, but whether they are effective in a population of patients with PHN is unknown and needs to be tested in controlled clinical trials. Some PHN patients may have associated myofascial pain in addition to neuropathic pain.[68] The presence of myofascial pathology is indicated by taut muscle bands (i.e., a group of tense muscle fibers extending from a trigger point to the muscle attachments) and trigger point(s) (i.e., a hyperirritable spot in skeletal muscle that is painful on compression) in the affected dermatome. These patients are good candidates for a trial of PENS.

Invasive treatments may be considered when patients have failed to obtain adequate relief from noninvasive treatment approaches. Invasive treatments include peripheral and central neural blockade, central nervous system (CNS) drug delivery, spinal cord stimulation, and neurosurgical techniques.[20] Neural blockade techniques include sensory nerve, plexus, and sympathetic nerve blocks and epidural and intrathecal blockade with lidocaine-like drugs and/or corticosteroids. Many PHN patients note initial relief of pain with nerve blocks, but few experience long-lasting relief. A study examining intrathecal administration of methylprednisolone in patients with PHN received considerable attention because of the dramatic benefits that were described.[69] However, attempts to replicate these results have not been successful, and intrathecal administration of methylprednisolone is not approved by the FDA, and the well-known risks of intrathecal steroids include neurologic complications and adhesive arachnoiditis.[70,71] CNS drug delivery attempts to place the drug (e.g., morphine) as close as possible to central pain receptors in the spinal cord corresponding to the affected dermatome(s). Spinal cord stimulation requires implantation of an electrode in the thoracic or lumbar epidural space and the placement of a percutaneous electrical stimulator. These interventions represent rational approaches to pain relief but they have not been proven effective in controlled trials, partly because the design and conduct of such trials are difficult, and they carry procedural risks, especially in older patients. In general, these interventions have a limited role in PHN treatment and should be contemplated in patients who have failed all other treatments and continue to have disabling pain.

It is important to conclude by emphasizing that the medications and invasive treatments that are currently available are rarely associated with the complete relief of PHN and evidence of their beneficial effects on quality of life is limited. Medical and invasive management of the patient with PHN should therefore be considered components of a more comprehensive treatment approach, which may include various nonpharmacologic treatments such as psychological counseling.[72]

KEY POINTS

- Herpes zoster (shingles) is caused by reactivation of the VZV, which establishes latency in sensory ganglia after primary infection (chicken pox).
- The characteristic unilateral dermatomal vesicular rash of herpes zoster heals within 2–4 weeks and is accompanied by pain in the majority of patients.
- Older age is associated with an increased risk of herpes zoster because of an age-associated decline in VZV-specific cell-mediated immunity.
- Antiviral therapy with acyclovir, brivudine, famciclovir, or valacyclovir in patients with herpes zoster inhibits viral replication and has been shown to reduce the duration of viral shedding, hasten rash healing, and decrease the duration of pain.
- The supplementation of antiviral therapy with opioids or corticosteroids may provide additional pain relief in herpes zoster patients with moderate to severe acute pain.
- Peripheral, sympathetic, and epidural nerve blocks with local anesthetics and/or corticosteroids appear to relieve acute pain in patients with herpes zoster, but their role in preventing PHN is uncertain because there are few randomized placebo-controlled trials.
- PHN refers to pain that continues after healing of the herpes zoster rash. This peripheral neuropathic pain condition causes substantial distress and disability and can last for years.
- Well-established risk factors for PHN in patients with herpes zoster include older age, more intense acute pain, more severe rash, and a prodrome of dermatomal pain before the rash appears.
- It is likely that different peripheral and central mechanisms contribute to PHN and that the qualitatively different types of pain that characterize PHN have different underlying mechanisms and may respond differently to treatment.
- The efficacy of gabapentin, high-concentration capsaicin patch, lidocaine patch 5%, pregabalin, tramadol, TCAs, and opioid analgesics has been demonstrated by the results of RCTs in patients with PHN, and these medications provide an evidence-based approach to treatment. Combination therapy with opioids-gabapentin, nortriptyline-gabapentin, and opioid-nortriptyline may be more effective than either drug alone.

REFERENCES

Access the reference list online at ExpertConsult.com.

CHAPTER 29

POSTAMPUTATION PAIN

Michael B. Jacobs, MD, MPH ◌ Srinivasa N. Raja, MD ◌ Steven P. Cohen, MD

Amputation of a limb can lead to painful and nonpainful sequelae, such as phantom sensations, telescoping, phantom pain, and residual limb (or "stump") pain. Although the phenomena of abnormal sensations and pain in amputated limbs were reported earlier by several physicians, Weir Mitchell is generally credited with coining the term "phantom limb" to describe the symptoms he observed in American Civil War soldiers.[1] These phenomena occur in the majority of patients after limb amputation, although the nature, frequency, intensity, and duration of symptoms may vary considerably. As with the treatment of most chronic pain conditions, management of the pain-related complications of amputees often necessitates an individualized and interdisciplinary approach due to the multifactorial nature of the causes and variable comorbidities observed in these patients.

DEFINITIONS AND EPIDEMIOLOGY

As of 2005, the prevalence of limb loss in the United States was at least 1.6 million, or 1 in 190; it is expected to rise to 3.6 million, or 1 in 120, by 2050.[2] Forty-two percent of limb loss is considered "major" (i.e., not limited to fingers or toes). Vascular disease (82%) and trauma (16%) are the most frequent causes of amputation, with vascular disease predominating for major limb amputations involving the lower extremities, and industrial accidents, especially involving digits, comprising the leading cause of upper extremity amputations. Other etiologies—including primary and metastatic tumors and congenital abnormalities—constitute much less frequent causes (<2%).[3] The prevalence of multiple limb loss is estimated to be 7.3% of trauma-related amputees, and vascular insufficiency amputees have a 27%–44% risk of contralateral limb amputation after 4 years.[4] The most common sources of postamputation pain (PAP) more than 6 months after amputation are phantom pain and residual limb pain (RLP).[5,6] In addition, those with lower extremity amputation are also at high risk for back pain and other musculoskeletal conditions (e.g., arthralgia and bursitis).[5]

PHANTOM SENSATIONS

Phantom sensations are nonpainful perceptions that occur in the region of the missing body part after a traumatic or surgical amputation. Phantom sensations are common after limb amputation surgery, with an incidence of 90% during the first 6 months.[7] One third of patients experience phantom sensations within 24 hours after their surgery. Excision of a body part, however, is not essential for phantom sensations. Phantom sensations of the arm have been reported after avulsion of the brachial plexus without amputation of the limb.[8] Excision of other body parts—such as the tongue, bladder, rectum, breast, or genitalia—may also present with phantom sensations.

Phantom sensations may present with various manifestations including kinetic sensations and kinesthetic and exteroceptive perceptions. Kinetic sensations are exemplified by perception of movements in the amputated body region, such as flexion/extension of the toes. Kinesthetic perceptions are characterized by distorted representations in size or position of the missing body part (e.g., feeling that the hand or foot is twisted). Exteroceptive perceptions can include paresthesias, tingling, touch, pressure, itching, heat, cold, and wetness. Complete paraplegic and quadriplegic patients can also have phantom sensations. Phantom sensations are commonly experienced in the distal portion of the limbs—hands and feet—possibly due to the rich innervation of these regions and the disproportionately large cortical representation of these regions in the homunculus.

TELESCOPING

Phantom limbs are also associated with a phenomenon called "telescoping": the perception of progressive shortening of the phantom body part resulting in the sensation that the distal part of the limb is becoming more proximal. At the start of the phenomenon, the phantom sensation can feel so real that the patient may actually reach for objects or attempt to ambulate with a phantom leg. However, over time, phantom sensations of the distal extremities may change and become less distinct so that the patient may feel a hand close to the end of the residual limb but not feel the proximal arm or forearm. This phenomenon is common, occurring in up to two thirds of limb amputees.[9]

PHANTOM PAIN

Phantom pain, often referred to as phantom limb pain (PLP), is the perception of dysesthesias, or unpleasant sensations, in the distribution of the missing or deafferentated body part. PLP has been reported to occur in up to 79% of postamputation patients 6 months after surgery,[9] with about 60% of patients still reporting significant PLP 2 years after surgery.[6] The pain can vary in character, duration, frequency, and intensity. It can present as sharp, dull, burning, squeezing, cramping, shooting, or as a shocklike electrical sensation. Patients may occasionally complain of intermittent tremors or painful muscle spasms in the stump associated with paroxysms of PLP.

In a prospective study by Jensen and colleagues of 58 patients undergoing limb amputation, the authors found that PLP often changed in presentation within the first 6 months after amputation.[7] The characteristic of the phantom pain changed from a mainly exteroceptive-like pain (knifelike or sticking) localized in the entire limb or at least involving proximal parts of the lost limb to a mainly proprioceptive type of pain (squeezing or burning) localized in the distal parts of the amputated limb. Forty-seven percent of patients experienced phantom pain within 24 hours after the amputation and 83% within the first 4 days. The study also demonstrated that the frequency, duration, and severity of PLP decreased during the first 6 months, after which the characteristics did not change significantly. Sometimes PLP can resolve spontaneously without treatment. Similar to other neuropathic conditions, PLP persisting longer than 6 months is extremely difficult to treat.

The incidence of PLP seems to be independent of the patient's age, sex, previous health status, and cause of amputation. One factor that appears to increase its incidence after amputation is the presence of pain in the limb before the amputation. In a prospective study of 56 patients who had amputation of a lower limb, Nikolajsen and colleagues[10] noted that the presence of preamputation pain significantly increased the incidence of both residual limb pain (RLP) and PLP after 1 week and the incidence of PLP after 3 months. Approximately 42% of the patients reported that their PLP at 3 months resembled the pain they had experienced at the time of amputation.[10] Associations of PLP with phantom sensations and between PLP and RLP have also been demonstrated for upper limb amputees.

RESIDUAL LIMB PAIN

RLP, classically referred to as "stump pain," is pain localized to the residual body part following amputation. Longitudinal studies previously reported an incidence of RLP of about 20% 2 years after amputation.[6] However, more recent studies with longer duration of follow-up report an incidence of 56%–74%.[5,11] RLP is often secondary to local pathologic processes such as infection; lesions of the skin, soft tissue, or bone; heterotopic ossification (>50% in traumatic amputations); and local ischemia. These processes can generally be classified into the following categories: postsurgical nociceptive, neurogenic, prosthogenic, arthrogenic, ischemic, referred (usually from the spine or joints), sympathetically maintained, and abnormal residual limb tissue (e.g., adhesive scar tissue).[12] RLP can be superficial (localized to the scar region of the incision), felt deep in the distal residual limb, or encompassing the whole residual limb. RLP can frequently be differentiated from PLP based on the fact that it is classically provoked or exacerbated by traction or pressure, which often occurs during the use of a prosthesis. This factor can greatly limit function in lower extremity amputees. The management of RLP entails a detailed history and physical examination that includes ensuring a properly fitting prosthesis. Arthrogenic RLP is usually secondary to abnormal gait and asymmetrically distributed weight bearing, resulting in excessive stress on adjacent joints and/or lumbosacral spine structures. This can lead to bursitis, accelerated arthritis, sacroiliac joint disease, discogenic and facetogenic pain, and lumbosacral radiculopathy.

SPECIAL POPULATIONS

PHANTOM PHENOMENA AFTER MASTECTOMY

Well over 100,000 mastectomies are performed each year in the United States. Recent studies indicate that phantom sensations are felt by 14%–48% of patients who underwent mastectomy.[13,14] Most of these phantom sensations are felt intermittently, occurring once every 2 or 4 weeks. The incidence of phantom pain after mastectomy appears to be lower than that after limb amputation, ranging from 0% to 23%.[13] This lower incidence may be related to the smaller cortical representation of breasts and the fact that breasts do not mediate kinesthetic sensory impulses. The onset of phantom sensation often appears within 3–6 months of surgery and begins to dissipate after 1 year.[14] The phantom pain usually localizes to the entire breast or around the nipple. The relationship between preamputation pain and phantom pain or phantom sensations appears to be less after mastectomy than after limb amputation. There is, however, a striking similarity in the location and character of the pain before and after mastectomy, a phenomenon seen after other amputations. The relationship between phantom pain and preamputation pain is more significant within the first month after mastectomy. In view of the high incidence of pain after breast surgery in general, the only way to distinguish between true "phantom" pain and other sources of postmastectomy pain (e.g., intercostal brachial neuralgia, neuroma) may be via a detailed history and physical examination.

WOUNDED WARRIORS

The US military conflicts since 9/11 have placed more emphasis on the management of traumatic amputation and its complications. As of June 2015, the Department of Defense reports that 1645 individuals have suffered major limb loss since September 2001, including approximately 17% with upper extremity amputations and 30% with multiple limb loss.[4,15] A majority of these injuries are related to blast exposures; therefore many have concomitant comorbidities including traumatic brain injury, posttraumatic stress disorder, peripheral nerve injuries, fractures, and soft tissue injuries. Studies have shown a higher prevalence of chronic pain among individuals with posttraumatic stress and traumatic brain injury than in similar cohorts without these conditions.

The unique mechanisms of injury and related comorbidities associated with amputations in military service members present management challenges that may not be similar to those in other patient populations with PAP. In a study of traumatic amputations in sustained by 30 military personnel during combat or training, the prevalence of PLP was similar (77%), but RLP was higher (87%) than previously reported. In addition, the average (3.3) and worst (5.4) pain intensity as measured on a numerical rating scale was less than in other amputee populations.[16]

PATHOPHYSIOLOGY AND MECHANISMS OF POSTAMPUTATION PAIN

Evidence suggests that phantom phenomena are the result of interactions between altered peripheral, spinal, and supraspinal mechanisms.

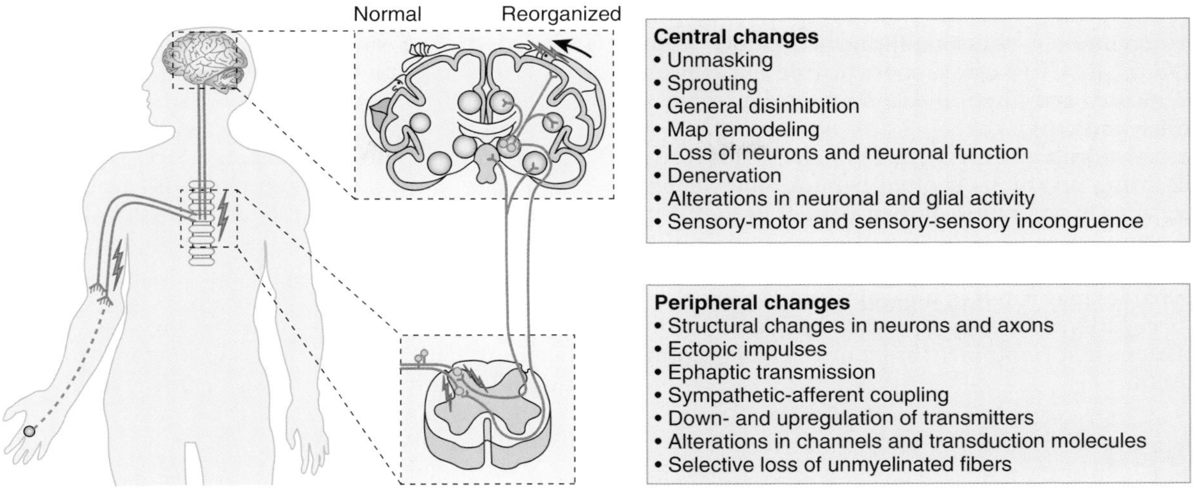

FIG. 29.1 Potential mechanisms of postamputation pain. *(Source: Flor H, Nikolajsen L, Staehelin Jensen T: Phantom limb pain: a case of maladaptive CNS plasticity?* Nat Rev Neurosci. *7:873-881, 2006.)*

Supraspinal mechanisms of phantom phenomena involve the reorganization of the somatosensory cortex following amputation. Ramachandran and coworkers have reported that in upper limb amputees, sensations in the phantom limb could be elicited by brushing the face.[17] Functional magnetic resonance imaging (MRI) studies, also in upper extremity amputees, demonstrate a shift of mouth representation in the somatosensory cortex to the zone previously represented by the arm and hand (i.e., cortical reorganization).[18] A strong correlation was also demonstrated between the size of the deafferentated area and intensity of PLP.[19]

Spinal mechanisms for phantom phenomena likely center on functional changes in the dorsal horn of the spinal cord following a deafferentation injury. The loss of afferent input leads to decreased impulses from brainstem reticular areas, which normally exert inhibitory effects on sensory transmission.[20] The absence of inhibitory effects of sensory input from the missing peripheral body part causes increased autonomous activity of dorsal horn neurons, in effect becoming "sensory epileptic discharges."[6,12] In addition, similar to the process of cortical reorganization, a "spinal reorganization" process may also occur in which adjacent nerve fibers establish connections in regions of the spinal cord that no longer receive afferent input.[21] Several lines of evidence support a spinal mechanism for phantom phenomena. These include the observations that: (1) anticonvulsants and lesions in the substantia gelatinosa of the spinal cord are effective in treating phantom pain[21]; (2) phantom pain develops in lower extremity amputees following new lumbar disc herniation and in upper limb amputees after herpes zoster infection, both of which were successfully treated with epidural steroid injection[22]; (3) phantom pain can be induced with spinal analgesia[23]; (4) in an unusual case, long-standing phantom pain resolved with the development of a cauda equine syndrome from a spinal tumor and recurred following decompression.[24]

Evidence supporting peripheral mechanisms of phantom phenomena includes the demonstration of spontaneous neuronal activity at the proximal ends of cut nerves, the presence of residual limb pathology in some patients with phantom pain, and the relief of phantom pain after the injection of local anesthetic into the painful residual limb.[7,25] Peripheral nerve transection during an amputation initiates axonal regeneration, eventually resulting in a neuroma or a collection of nerve fibers near the end of the residual limb. Afferent fibers in a neuroma may develop ectopic activity, mechanical sensitivity, and chemosensitivity to catecholamines. Upregulation of voltage-sensitive sodium channels, downregulation of potassium channels, and expression of novel receptors in the neuroma can alter the excitability of the affected neurons and increase afferent input.[26] A positive Tinel's sign (tapping on the injured nerve or neuroma, leading to pain in the phantom or residual limb) represents a classic feature of a symptomatic neuroma on physical examination. Injured neurons can also generate new, nonfunctional connections (ephapses), resulting in increased afferent input to the spinal cord. These changes may lead to spontaneous pain; they help explain the amplification in pain caused by emotional distress and/or exposure to cold that leads to increased sympathetic discharge and circulating catecholamines.[27]

PAP is likely caused by a combination of the mechanisms already described as well as others that have yet to be elucidated, since treatments to date have yielded only modest relief of PAP. However, our understanding of the interactions between peripheral, spinal, and supraspinal physiology are the basis for a mechanistic approach to treatment. A summary of the factors thought to be relevant in the development of phantom pain is depicted in Fig. 29.1.

EVALUATION

The first step in the management of PAP is to attempt to identify a specific etiology that can be the target for developing a treatment strategy. The residual limb should be inspected and palpated for skin breakdown, pressure sores, infection, bony abnormalities (e.g., spurs, heterotopic ossification), ischemia (e.g., choke syndrome, changes in color or temperature), or masses. Localized soft tissue tenderness, particularly in the presence of a positive Tinel's sign, which reproduces pain symptoms, may indicate a neuroma.

Imaging (e.g., x-rays, computed tomography [CT], MRI, and more commonly ultrasound) and laboratory testing (e.g., CBC, ESR, CRP) can support or rule out concerns from the history and physical examination, but these are not routinely indicated.

Consultation with an experienced prosthetist for rectifying an ill-fitting prosthesis is often helpful, since patients may experience exaggeration of their pain or even precipitation of phantom pain and/or sensations from use of the prosthetic limb. In addition, changes in gait and altered body mechanics may result in musculoskeletal pain. Physical and occupational therapy to correct gait and postural compensations that result in arthritic or referred pain may also be useful.

TREATMENT

Amputation of a limb affects not only the physical functioning of the individual but may also have significant psychological, social, and societal consequences. Therefore the treatment of PAP is more likely to be successful with an individualized and interdisciplinary approach. Since few controlled trials specifically focus on PAP, treatment strategies often need to be extrapolated from related conditions. After an appropriate evaluation narrows the differential diagnosis, treatments may include pharmacotherapy, physiotherapy and modalities, complementary and alternative therapies, psychological therapies, interventional therapies, and surgery.

PHARMACOTHERAPY

Most medication options for PAP require extrapolation from the treatment of other conditions. For somatic pain, acetaminophen, nonsteroidal antiinflammatory drugs, and/or opioids may be indicated. Neuropathic pain is more likely to respond to adjuvant analgesics such as tricyclic antidepressants (e.g., nortriptyline), anticonvulsants (e.g., gabapentin), or selective norepinephrine reuptake inhibitors (e.g., duloxetine). The results of available randomized controlled trials specifically for the pharmacologic treatment of PAP are summarized in Table 29.1, and some are discussed here.

Tricyclic antidepressants act primarily by inhibiting serotonin and norepinephrine reuptake and partly through sodium channel, alpha adrenergic, *N*-methyl-D-aspartate (NMDA), and acetylcholinergic blockade. Tramadol, a partial mu opioid agonist, has serotonergic and noradrenergic effects similar to those of TCAs. A randomized controlled crossover trial of amitriptyline (average 55 mg daily) or tramadol (average 450 mg daily) versus placebo found that both drugs were effective in the treatment of PLP and RLP.[28] However, a study by Robinson comparing amitriptyline to an active placebo (benztropine mesylate) for the treatment of PLP found no difference in outcomes.[29]

The anticonvulsants gabapentin and pregabalin are believed to work through inhibition of the alpha-2 delta subunit of voltage-gated calcium channels, leading to the decreased release of excitatory neurotransmitters and reduced nerve signal transmission at the dorsal horn. In a randomized controlled crossover trial of gabapentin versus placebo, gabapentin was well tolerated and associated with a significant decrease in PLP but no change in sleep, mood, or activity.[30] A similar randomized controlled crossover trial of gabapentin versus placebo for treatment of PLP or RLP found no significant difference in the primary outcome of pain scores.[31] However, in this study participants reported a statistically significant decrease in "meaningful pain" during the gabapentin phase of treatment compared with placebo, and they noted that benefits outweighed side effects. In another randomized, placebo-controlled trial by Nikolajsen, gabapentin given for 30 days postamputation did not reduce the incidence of short- or long-term PAP.[32] Controlled studies conducted for neuropathic pain have demonstrated that combination therapy with gabapentin and nortriptyline and gabapentin and morphine, may result in supra-additive analgesia than with either agent used alone, but this has not been studied for PAP.[33]

NMDA antagonists block a series of events leading to sensitization of wide dynamic range neurons in the dorsal horn. A study of PAP in cancer patients demonstrated a significant decrease in pain intensity, windup pain, and pressure-pain thresholds following a 45-minute low-dose ketamine infusion compared with a saline infusion.[34] A more recent study found that 1-hour ketamine (0.4 mg/kg) infusions were more effective over 48 hours than placebo in patients with PAP of various etiologies; ketamine plus calcitonin was no better than ketamine alone.[35] Additionally, oral dextromethorphan was shown to be effective in a small placebo-controlled crossover study,[36] but memantine was not found to be effective in the treatment of PLP.[37–39] In summary, the evidence for ketamine is stronger than for the other NMDA antagonists, but the short duration of benefit and high incidence of adverse effects (e.g., hallucinations, alterations of consciousness, mood changes) limit its usefulness.

Calcitonin acts centrally to inhibit neuronal firing in response to peripheral stimulation, which has generated interest in its use for PAP. Unfortunately studies have been equivocal. A controlled study showed that a single infusion of calcitonin led to a reduction in pain intensity in 8 of 13 patients at 1 year.[40] However, a subsequent, similarly designed study referenced in the discussion on NMDA antagonists found calcitonin to be ineffective compared with placebo.[35]

Sodium channel blockers have been studied for both neuropathic and somatic pain. In a double-blinded study by Wu et al., intravenous morphine was found to be more effective than placebo for PLP and RLP, but intravenous lidocaine was superior only for RLP.[41] In a follow-up study of 60 of these patients, oral morphine but not mexiletine (an oral lidocaine analogue) provided significant pain relief at 6 weeks.[42]

Opioids may be beneficial in the treatment of PAP due to their multiple sites of action, including inhibition of pain signaling pathways at the dorsal horn and diminishing the degree of cortical reorganization associated with pain at the supraspinal level. Both intravenous and oral opioids administered for up to 6 weeks have been shown to be effective for PAP, but opioids have not been convincingly shown to reduce long-term pain, improve function, and provide increased benefit as compared with nonopioid treatment for noncancer pain. Moreover, the risk of opioid therapy is increased in individuals with psychopathology,

TABLE 29.1 Randomized Controlled Trials Evaluating Pharmacologic Treatments for Postamputation Pain

Study	N	Treatment/Placebo	Chronicity[a]	Adverse Events	Follow-Up	Effect[b]
Antidepressants						
Robinson et al.[29]	39	1. Oral amitriptyline 10 mg/day titrated to max 125 mg/day 2. Oral benztropine 0.5 mg/day	>3 months	Dry mouth, dizziness	6 weeks	–
Wilder-Smith et al.[28]	94	1. Oral amitriptyline (avg 55 mg/day) 2. Oral tramadol (avg 200 mg/day) 3. Placebo	10–16 years	Nausea, tiredness, dizziness, constipation, headache (all more common with tramadol)	1 month	+
Anticonvulsants						
Bone et al.[30]	19	1. Oral gabapentin titrated to 2400 mg/day 2. Placebo	>6 months	Somnolence, dizziness, headache, nausea	6 weeks	+
Smith et al.[31]	24	1. Oral gabapentin titrated to 3600 mg/day 2. Placebo	>6 months	Not described	6 weeks	–
Nikolajsen et al.[32]	46	1. Oral gabapentin 2400 mg/day 2. Placebo	POD #1 (prevention)	Nausea, stomachache, fatigue, confusion, nightmares, itching, ataxia	6 months	–
NMDA Antagonists						
Nikolajsen et al.[34]	11	1. IV ketamine 0.5 mg/kg infusion ×45 min 2. Placebo	Avg. 4 years	Insobriety, mood elevation, discomfort	45 min	+
Eichenberger et al.[35]	20	1. IV ketamine 0.4 mg/kg infusion ×1 h 2. IV calcitonin 200 IU infusion ×1 h 3. Combo ketamine/calcitonin 4. Placebo	Avg. 12 years	Loss of consciousness, light visual hallucination, hearing impairment (all with ketamine); facial flushing (calcitonin)	48 h	+
Ben Abraham et al.[36]	10	1. Oral dextromethorphan 120 mg/day ×10 days 2. Oral dextromethorphan 180 mg/day ×10 days 3. Placebo	Avg. 4.8 months	None reported	10 days	+
Maier et al.[37]	36	1. Oral memantine 30 mg/day ×3 weeks 2. Placebo	>12 months	Vertigo, fatigue, headache, nausea, restlessness, excitation, cramps	3 weeks	–
Schwenkreis et al.[85]	16	1. Oral memantine 30 mg/day 2. Placebo	>12 months	Not described	3 weeks	–
Wiech et al.[39]	8	1. Oral memantine 30 mg/day ×4 weeks 2. Placebo	Chronic	Fatigue, agitation, dizziness, nausea, headache	30 days	–
Calcitonin						
Jaeger and Maier[40]	21	1. IV calcitonin 200 IU ×20 min infusion 2. Saline infusion	0–7 days post-amputation	Headache, vertigo, nausea, vomiting, augmented phantom sensations, drowsiness, hot flashes	1 year	+
Eichenberger et al.[35]	20	1. IV ketamine 0.4 mg/kg infusion ×1 h 2. IV calcitonin 200 IU infusion ×1 h 3. Combo ketamine/calcitonin 4. Placebo	Avg. 12 years	Loss of consciousness, light visual hallucination, hearing impairment (all with ketamine); facial flushing (calcitonin)	48 h	+
Opioids						
Huse et al.[43]	12	1. Oral morphine up to 300 mg/day 2. Placebo	Chronic	Constipation	4 weeks	+
Wu et al.[41]	32	1. IV morphine 0.2 mg/kg infusion ×40 min 2. IV lidocaine 4 mg/kg infusion ×40 min 3. IV diphenhydramine 40 mg infusion (placebo)	>6 months	Sedation	30 min	+
Wilder-Smith et al.[28]	94	1. Oral amitriptyline (avg. 55 mg/day) 2. Oral tramadol (avg 200 mg/day) 3. Placebo	10–16 years	Nausea, tiredness, dizziness, constipation, headache (all more common with tramadol)	1 month	+

Continued

TABLE 29.1 Randomized Controlled Trials Evaluating Pharmacologic Treatments for Postamputation Pain—cont'd

Study	N	Treatment/Placebo	Chronicity[a]	Adverse Events	Follow-Up	Effect[b]
Wu et al.[42]	56	1. Oral morphine (180 mg/day) 2. Oral mexiletine (1200 mg/day) 3. Placebo	>6 months	Constipation, nausea, drowsiness, dizziness (all more common with morphine)	6 weeks	+ (morphine only)

[a]*Time since amputation or development of postamputation pain.*
[b]*Studies show statistically significant study effect (+) or not (–) of study drug compared with control.*
IV, *Intravenous;* NMDA, N-*methyl-*D-*aspartate.*

which frequently accompanies major limb loss. In a small case series, the investigators showed that cortical reorganization was reduced in two of three participants with PLP who received oral morphine, suggesting that some well-selected candidates may derive benefit.[43]

PREVENTIVE ANALGESIA

The role of preoperative epidural anesthesia is unclear, with conflicting results from several studies. Table 29.2 provides the results of prospective controlled studies for the prevention of PAP. Preoperative epidural anesthesia with bupivacaine and morphine, administered 72 hours preoperatively, was reported to decrease the incidence of phantom pain for up to a year following lower extremity amputation.[44] Similar results were reported when epidural infusions of bupivacaine, diamorphine, and clonidine were started 24–48 hours before a lower limb amputation and continued for 72 hours postoperatively reduced the incidence of phantom pain for up to 1 year.[45] However, a larger randomized double-blind, placebo-controlled study of epidural bupivacaine-morphine anesthesia started 18 hours preoperatively compared with oral or intramuscular morphine failed to corroborate the previous findings.[46] Additionally, a randomized controlled study comparing epidural ketamine-bupivacaine to epidural bupivacaine-saline also failed to demonstrate a significant difference between the two groups.[47]

More recently, there has been a randomized, double-blind, placebo-controlled trial of various epidural and patient-controlled analgesia (PCA) regimens.[48] In that study, epidural infusions of bupivacaine and fentanyl started 48 hours before amputation and continued 48 hours postoperatively significantly reduced PLP at 6 months; the results for opioid PCA were less clear. Collectively, the studies on perioperative analgesia suggest that timing may be critical for any preventive effect on PLP, with those studies in which anesthesia was instituted over 24 hours in advance of amputation, and those in whom the comparative group received suboptimal postoperative pain management, being more likely to yield positive results.

For perineural anesthesia, there is also limited evidence of its preemptive effects. A systematic review and meta-analysis of seven studies with a total of 416 patients showed that perineural anesthesia reduced postoperative opioid consumption but did not improve postoperative pain scores, in-hospital mortality, PLP, or RLP.[49]

PHYSICAL AND OCCUPATIONAL THERAPY

A comprehensive physical and/or occupational therapy program preamputation and postamputation creates a foundation for functional restoration and prevention of complications, including pain. Ideally, the educated patient will develop self-treatment strategies, such as compression garments for the residual limb to control edema, range-of-motion exercises to prevent joint contractures, and adaptation strategies to perform activities of daily living. Proper use of a prosthesis can be important for the prevention and management of PLP, so close consultation with a prosthetist as part of the rehabilitation team can help with the normalization of gait and limb movements. In particular, use of a myoelectric prosthesis reduces cortical reorganization for upper limb amputees[50]; in lower limb amputees, the ability to stand and ambulate while wearing a prosthesis may normalize sensory and motor input and therefore also lead to decreased cortical reorganization.[51]

COMPLEMENTARY AND ALTERNATIVE MEDICINE THERAPIES AND MODALITIES

Various types of therapy techniques and modalities have been studied for the treatment of PAP. Reports suggest that transcutaneous electrical nerve stimulation (TENS), which is thought to rely on the gate-control theory by stimulating large nerve fibers and thereby "closing the gate" on pain signals sent from smaller fibers, may reduce PAP but without long-term benefit.[52] A study of noninvasive limb covers, which are thought to block high-frequency electromagnetic fields that could increase PLP, did not show efficacy in a randomized placebo-controlled trial.[53]

Acupuncture, which may work by modulating the cognitive and affective perceptions of pain, has been shown to be effective for many chronic pain conditions, including neuropathic pain.[54] Traditional Chinese medicine suggests that PLP is the result of stagnation of energy circulating in the body, leading to a disorder of "Qi." Nonrandomized studies using acupuncture showed improvement in PLP compared with usual care.

Mirror therapy was introduced by Ramachandran and coworkers in 1996, and multiple studies have shown its ability to alleviate phantom pain by exploiting the brain's predilection for prioritizing visual stimuli over proprioceptive and somatosensory input.[55,56] It involves strategically placing a mirror adjacent to the intact limb to give the illusion that the missing body part is present and can be purposefully moved. Because sensory experiences can be

TABLE 29.2 Prospective Studies Evaluating Effect of Epidural Anesthesia on Preventing Phantom Limb Pain

Study	N	Treatments	Randomization[a]	Blinding[a]	Preoperative[b]	Hours Preoperative	Intraoperative[b]	Postoperative[b]	Effectiveness[c]
Bach et al.[44]	25	1. Epidural bupivacaine, morphine 2. Opioids, paracetamol, dextropropoxiphen, acetylsalicylic acid	–	–	+	72	+	–	+
Jahangiri et al.[45]	24	1. Perioperative epidural bupivacaine, clonidine, diamorphine 2. On-demand opioids	–	–	+	24–48	+	+	+
Schug et al.[86]	23	1. Perioperative epidural bupivacaine, fentanyl 2. Intraoperative epidural bupivacaine, fentanyl 3. General anesthesia with postoperative systemic opioids	–	–	+	24	+	+	+ (#1 vs. #3 only)
Nikolajsen et al.[46]	60	1. Epidural bupivacaine, morphine 2. Epidural saline, oral or IM morphine	+	+	+	18	+	+	–
Lambert et al.[87]	30	1. Epidural bupivacaine and diamorphine 2. Perineural bupivacaine	+	–	+	24	+	+	–
Wilson et al.[47]	53	1. Epidural ketamine/bupivacaine 2. Epidural bupivacaine	+	+	–	0	+	+	–
Karanikolas et al.[48]	65	1. Epidural anesthesia and analgesia 2. Preoperative IV PCA, postoperative epidural anesthesia and analgesia 3. Perioperative IV PCA and epidural anesthesia 4. Perioperative IV PCA and general anesthesia 5. Conventional anesthesia and analgesia	+	+	+	48	+	+	+

[a]*Randomization and blinding of study patients employed (+) or not employed (–).*
[b]*Preoperative/intraoperative/postoperative epidural infusions started (+) or not (–).*
[c]*Studies show statistically significant study effect (+) or not (–) of study drug compared with control.*
IM, *Intramuscular;* IV, *intravenous;* PCA, *patient-controlled analgesia.*

evoked by visual stimuli, mirror therapy increases spinal motor and cortical excitability (Fig. 29.2). In a randomized crossover study by Chan et al., 22 patients with lower limb PLP were allocated to receive either mirror therapy, covered mirror therapy, or mental visualization. After 4 weeks of therapy for 15 minutes daily, all patients in the mirror therapy group reported a decrease in pain, which was significantly greater than the pain relief experienced by the other groups.[55] In addition, 89% of those who crossed over to mirror therapy also reported a significant decrease in PLP. The simplicity and noninvasiveness of this treatment modality has led to its application not only following limb loss but also in the prevention of PAP.[57]

Mental imagery and phantom exercises are two therapy techniques that attempt to modify and reverse cortical reorganization. With mental imagery, the therapist guides the patient in a series of imagined exercises that treat the phantom limb as a real part of the body. Phantom exercise techniques involve movements of both the intact and phantom limbs. Sometimes these techniques are also combined with muscle relaxation as part of a protocol known as the SantaLucia Alleviation Intervention for Phantom in Amputees' Neurorehabilitation (SAIPAN). A recent randomized controlled trial including 51 patients with PLP and/or RLP compared 4 weeks of physical therapy with mental imagery, phantom exercises, and muscle relaxation with physical therapy alone.[58] After 1 month, the combined therapy techniques showed significant reductions in average and worst pain compared with the control.

Neurostimulation methods targeting the primary motor cortex have been shown to be effective in the treatment of chronic neuropathic pain conditions. The mechanism of action involves motor cortex stimulation (MCS), which may modulate pain through activation of thalamic and subthalamic nuclei. Repetitive transcranial magnetic stimulation (rTMS) involves the use of a time-varying current applied to the scalp to create a magnetic field, which in turn induces an electric field that can generate a secondary current within brain tissue. Randomized controlled trials show that high-frequency rTMS is effective for the treatment of neuropathic pain.[59] A controlled trial showed that 5 days of rTMS was effective at reducing PLP for up to 2 months in 27 upper and lower extremity amputees.[60] Transcranial direct current stimulation (tDCS) is similar to rTMS, but this technique provides lower spatial resolution and a more diffuse spread of stimulation. A randomized double-blind crossover trial evaluated tDCS in eight patients with PLP.[61] The study showed that a 5-day treatment of tDCS compared with sham treatment provided significant improvement of PLP after 1 week.

PSYCHOLOGICAL THERAPIES

Psychological interventions for phantom pain include cognitive and behavioral therapies, hypnosis, biofeedback, and support groups. These interventions may facilitate adaptation to a change in body image, adaptation to chronic pain, and relief of pain-inducing stress, grief, and anger.

Cognitive-behavioral therapy (CBT) is useful in the treatment of chronic pain, although there are no controlled trials for the treatment of PAP. For hypnosis, a randomized controlled trial of 20 patients with 6 months of PLP or RLP showed that three sessions of hypnosis reduced overall pain scores.[62] Evidence for other psychological therapies, such as guided imagery (creating mental images that help promote relaxation and healing) and biofeedback (learned control over autonomic physiologic processes) are lacking.

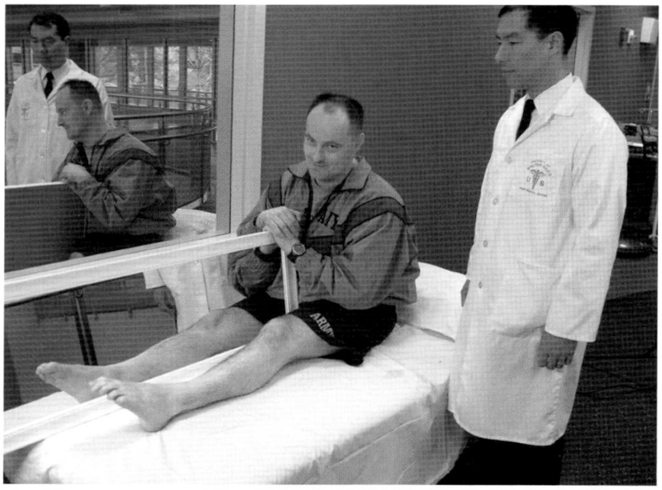

FIG. 29.2 Mirror therapy. *(Photograph courtesy Steven P. Cohen, MD. Permission for publication obtained from patient and physician.)*

Despite the lack of rigorous studies demonstrating the effectiveness of psychological therapies for PAP, a mental health provider can be invaluable in assisting the efforts to care for patients suffering with amputation-related complications, including pain.

INTERVENTIONAL THERAPIES

If conservative measures fail, interventional treatment options may be considered. Local injection therapy is commonly used for diagnostic and potentially therapeutic benefit for PAP. Regional nerve blocks or injections of a local anesthetic may provide immediate pain relief, but the effects are often temporary. In a small randomized controlled pilot trial, patients with PAP received injections of onabotulinumtoxin A (250–300 units) or lidocaine with depomedrol into areas of tenderness in the residual limb.[63] Both treatments significantly improved RLP but not PLP at 6-month follow-up. A small case series found that perineuromal injection of etanercept, a tumor necrosis factor inhibitor, was effective in patients with RLP of less than 1 year in duration.[64]

Autonomic dysfunction is frequently observed in chronic pain, and conditions that are alleviated by sympathetic nerve blockade are classified with sympathetically maintained pain (SMP). In an observational study, sympathetic blocks were performed on 17 amputees.[27] As a result, 50% of patients experienced significant pain relief postprocedure, suggesting that SMP plays a role in PLP and to a lesser extent RLP, but long-term benefits were uncommon.

PLP or RLP arising from amputation neuromas, as evidenced by a concordant reduction in symptoms in response to the injection of a local anesthetic, has been treated with radiofrequency or cryoneurolysis, although evidence is limited to case series.[65,66] Conventional radiofrequency

(CRF) therapy causes thermal coagulation to denature nerve fibers and is effective for treatment of conditions such as facet- or sacroiliac-mediated back pain, but there is a theoretical risk of neuritis and neuroma formation with the treatment of peripheral nerves. Pulsed radiofrequency (PRF) treatment is an alternative treatment using a lower temperature and pulse of electromagnetic radiation to disrupt nerve signaling without denaturing the fibers, thereby reducing the risks associated with CRF. A case series described four patients with upper or lower extremity RLP and PLP that improved significantly with PRF (following successful diagnostic local anesthetic blocks), including average pain, medication requirements, and mobility/prosthesis use.[66] Other case series also document improvement of PAP with PRF of the dorsal root ganglion (e.g., L5 or S1 in patients with lower extremity amputations).[67,68] Cryoneurolysis also denatures nerve fibers but through a cold application. In a case series involving five patients with PLP, three reported over 90% pain relief and two reported 20%–40% pain relief more than 2 years after treatment.[65]

Spinal cord stimulators (SCSs) may function at spinal and supraspinal levels to replace lost afferent input at the dorsal horn and enhance descending pain inhibition. There are no controlled trials in patients with PAP, but case series have documented improvement of RLP and PLP. Broggi et al. reported that 23 of 26 patients were satisfied with SCS for the treatment of PAP.[69] In 2001, a series of 19 patients reported 80% improvement in PLP postimplant, although only 6 patients obtained satisfactory long-term results.[70] A more recent case series found that of four patients with PLP implanted with SCS between 2003 and 2006, three were satisfied with the results at 15- to 66-month follow-up.[71]

Other forms neuromodulation therapies targeting peripheral pain mechanisms have also been utilized. Peripheral nerve stimulation (PNS) involves placement of a stimulator lead at or near the site of peripheral nerve injury. Rauck et al. reported on the use of percutaneously placed PNS for PAP in the lower extremity.[72] Of 14 patients, 9 completed a home trial; after 4 weeks, they reported a decrease in PAP and an "improved" quality of life. Eldabe et al. reported eight patients with an average of 50% pain reduction of PLP at 14 months following dorsal root ganglion stimulation.[73]

SURGERY

Typically, surgical therapies are indicated only when a specific rectifiable pathology is identified. Protruding bone, bony exostosis, wound infection, and poorly healed wounds are clear indications for surgery. A neuroma under constant pressure or near a joint resulting in repeated traction may be treated by excision of the neuroma and repositioning the nerve endings in bone or muscle. Similarly, surgical treatment of heterotopic ossification, which has been reported to occur in up to 63% of traumatic major limb amputations, may be helpful.[74] Selective nerve blocks of peripheral nerves may be useful as a prognostic indicator of the success of excision of a neuroma.

An emerging option for the treatment of neuromas and other peripherally generated PAP is high-frequency electrical nerve block. The foundation for this treatment is based on animal studies demonstrating that the application of a continuous, high-frequency alternating current to nerves results in a conduction block of motor, sensory, and autonomic fibers, making PAP an ideal condition to study.[75] Practically, a surgically implanted electrode is attached to a targeted nerve proximal to the neuroma and powered by an implantable pulse generator that generates high-frequency current to block pain signals. In a pilot case series of 10 patients with RLP, this modality demonstrated significant pain relief, functional improvement, and decreased medication use 90 days after treatment.[76]

A retrospective study of patients undergoing targeted muscle reinnervation (TMR), in which the proximal healthy ends of amputated nerves are connected to other muscles that can be repurposed to allow for control of a myoelectric prosthesis, showed that 14 of 15 patients with RLP had resolution of symptoms after surgery.[77] Further studies are needed to examine the long-term potential of TMR as a treatment option for amputation neuromas.

Intracranial neurostimulation has been used primarily for the treatment of movement disorders but also off label for the treatment of other conditions, including chronic pain.[78] Deep brain stimulation (DBS) of the sensory thalamus or periaqueductal and periventricular gray matter has demonstrated some benefit in PAP. Boccard et al. followed 85 patients who received DBS for neuropathic pain, including 9 amputees.[79] In this cohort, 68% reported significant pain improvement after approximately 28 months of follow-up, including 89% in the amputation group. In another case series, 12 patients (including 5 amputees and 7 with brachial plexus avulsion) were treated with DBS.[80] After 1 year, pain scores decreased 69%, but the amputation group showed the most benefit, with a 90% decrease in pain as well as functional improvements. A meta-analysis noted that patients with peripheral neuropathy or PLP experienced 60%–75% pain relief with DBS.[81]

Another type of intracranial neuromodulation, MCS, has been successfully utilized for the treatment of facial neuropathic pain and central pain states such as spinal cord injury and poststroke pain, but the results are less convincing for PAP. Carroll et al. followed 10 patients with chronic neuropathic pain, 3 of whom had PAP[82]; two of these three patients reported significant improvement of their PLP with MCS lasting through 23 months of follow-up. Complications reported with DBS and MCS include intracranial bleeding, infection, permanent neurologic deficits, seizure disorder, and death.[78]

Dorsal root entry zone (DREZ) lesioning, which has been helpful in patients with avulsion injuries, has not been well studied in patients with PAP.[83,84]

CONCLUSION

The management of PAP remains a challenging endeavor that is only likely to increase in importance as the life expectancy of vascular and cancer amputees and the survival rate of traumatic amputees continue to rise. Persistent pain following major limb amputation occurs in a significant percentage of patients, with the most recent statistics suggesting cumulative prevalence rates exceeding 50% for both residual limb and phantom pain. There are many reasons for the modest results in the treatment of PAP; these include the high incidence of concomitant psychopathology that accompanies limb loss, the inherent difficulties involved in identifying specific pathophysiologic mechanisms that can be pharmacologically targeted, the relative paucity of clinical trials, and the low success rates in general for pain conditions that involve central mechanisms. At present, the optimal treatment of PAP entails a multimodal approach that includes preemptive analgesia when possible, psychotherapy, education and rehabilitation, polypharmacy, and, if indicated, procedural interventions.

KEY POINTS

- The prevalence of limb loss in the United States is expected to rise from 1.6 million in 2005 to 3.6 million by 2050. The most common etiologies are vascular (82%) and traumatic (16%).
- The most common sources of PAP are phantom pain and RLP.
- Phantom phenomena are not fully understood but are thought to result from a combination of reorganization of the somatosensory cortex following amputation (supraspinal mechanisms), functional changes in the dorsal horn of the spinal cord after deafferentation (spinal mechanisms), and spontaneous neuronal activity at the ends of cut nerves (peripheral mechanisms). These form a basis for the mechanistic approach to treatment.
- Results of randomized controlled trials show mixed results for the pharmacologic management of PAP, but common neuropathic pain medications are generally used in these patients.
- Studies on perioperative analgesia suggest that timing may be critical for any preventive effect on phantom pain, with those starting treatment more than 24 hours prior to amputation showing the most benefit.
- Complementary therapies such as mirror therapy, mental imagery, and noninvasive MCS may be beneficial for PAP.
- Psychological therapies are known to be helpful in the management of chronic pain but are not well studied for PAP. Involvement of mental health providers can be invaluable for the interdisciplinary care of complicated patients.
- Interventional treatments such as neuroma injections, radiofrequency, cryoneurolysis, PNS, and spinal cord stimulation are reportedly beneficial for PAP, but evidence is limited to case series.
- Surgical therapies for PAP may include intracranial neurostimulation, peripheral neuromodulation therapies, or resection of neuromas and heterotopic ossification.

REFERENCES

Access the reference list online at ExpertConsult.com.

CHAPTER 30

CENTRAL PAIN STATES

Julie H. Huang-Lionnet, MD, MBA ◎ Chad Brummett, MD ◎ Srinivasa N. Raja, MD

Central pain is a term used to describe the pain associated with a wide range of disorders of the central nervous system (CNS). Whereas the disorders themselves are heterogeneous in nature, there is a great deal of overlap in the central mechanisms precipitating pain and the treatment algorithms. The International Association for the Study of Pain (IASP) defines central pain as "pain initiated or caused by a primary lesion or dysfunction of the CNS." Classically studied disorders of central pain include poststroke, spinal cord injury (SCI), traumatic brain injury, and multiple sclerosis (MS).[1] Central pain is often refractory to treatments, and complete pain relief is rare. In this chapter, we discuss the clinical presentations, pathophysiology, and therapeutic options for central pain of brain and spinal cord origin.

EPIDEMIOLOGY OF CENTRAL PAIN

The leading cause of central pain originating in the brain is stroke. Poststroke pain according to IASP has several pain subtypes with the most common types including central poststroke pain (CPSP), pain secondary to spasticity, shoulder pain, complex regional pain syndrome (CRPS), and headache.[2] Except for MS patients, classically described central pain disorders (stroke, SCI, etc.) are more commonly seen in men. The elderly are more affected in the cases of poststroke pain, while SCI and MS pain tend to affect younger patients.[3] Poststroke pain is generally thought to be underdiagnosed and undertreated. Recent reports suggest that the prevalence varies widely across studies, ranging from 10% to 55% of stroke victims.[2]

In 1906, two French neurologists first described this poststroke "thalamic pain syndrome," also known as the "Dejerine-Roussy syndrome" in their honor.[4] This syndrome can account for one third of CPSP cases. The first postmortem studies of Dejerine-Roussy syndrome revealed that many of its victims had extrathalamic lesions, and modern imaging methods have confirmed and extended these findings. These pain-generating lesions extend from the first synapse of the dorsal horn, or trigeminal nuclei, to the cerebral cortex. The predominant etiology is vascular in origin, accounting for 90% of brain central pain (supratentorial 78% and infratentorial 12%) (Fig. 30.1). Poststroke pain is associated more frequently with ischemic stroke than hemorrhagic stroke.[5] Extrathalamic sites are involved in 50%–75% of cases.[6,7] Chronic poststroke pain more commonly occurs in the presence of thalamic and brainstem lesions.[5] In addition to stroke type and localization, other reported risk factors for development of CPSP include female sex, older age at stroke onset, alcohol use, peripheral vascular disease, statin use, depression, increased muscle tone and spasticity, reduced upper extremity movement, and sensory deficits.[5]

SCI pain has many subtypes of central pain that have been organized under the International Spinal Cord Injury Pain (ISCIP) Classification with Tier 1 organized by pain type (nociceptive, neuropathic, and other pain [i.e., fibromyalgia]); Tier 2 organized by pain subtypes (musculoskeletal pain, visceral pain, other nociceptive pain, SCI-related pain, at-level SCI pain, below-level SCI pain, other neuropathic pain); and Tier 3 organized by primary source if known (i.e., cauda equine lesion, syringomyelia, spinal cord lesion, postthoracotomy pain, spasm-related pain, constipation, pressure ulcer).[8–10] This new pain taxonomy has been incorporated into the International Spinal Cord Injury Pain Basic Data Sets (ISCIPBDS) for standardization in the collection and reporting of SCI pain worldwide.[11] Central pain of spinal origin is predominantly the result of trauma (see Fig. 30.1). Pain can also result from spinal cord tumors and demyelinating lesions. The incidence is reported to vary from 34% to 94% in patients with SCI[12,13] and about 29% in MS patients.[14,15]

Central pain is also prevalent in patients with chronic degenerative diseases of the CNS. For example, almost 10% of patients with Parkinson disease may have sensory complications, including pain[16,17]; and epilepsy can manifest as painful seizures. Also, in contrast to most pathologic processes affecting the CNS, clinicians cannot predict the development of central pain based on the location of a lesion. Many central pain patients maintain their ability to sense touch, vibration, and joint movements. This supports the belief that central pain involves the spinothalamic tract (STT) and its thalamocortical projections. The highest prevalence of central pain is reported in cases of lesions in the spinal cord, medulla, and ventroposterior part of the thalamus.

TAXONOMY

The ISCIP Classification was developed from a task force for the IASP (Table 30.1).[9,10,18,19] As described earlier, SCI pain is broadly divided into nociceptive and neuropathic with subclassification into second and third tiers based on the anatomic structures involved, site of pain, and etiology. Nociceptive pain may be musculoskeletal or visceral in nature. The former may be secondary to overuse of certain parts of the body to compensate for regions of paresis or result from secondary changes in bone or joints. Neuropathic pain is usually seen in areas of sensory abnormalities. Neuropathic pain has been subdivided based on region into at-level (radicular or central), above-level, and below-level pain to indicate the presumed site of the lesion responsible for pain generation.[20] Following SCI, it is reported that 91% of patients have pain 2 weeks after injury. This decreased to 64% at 6 months. Neuropathic at-level pain was present in

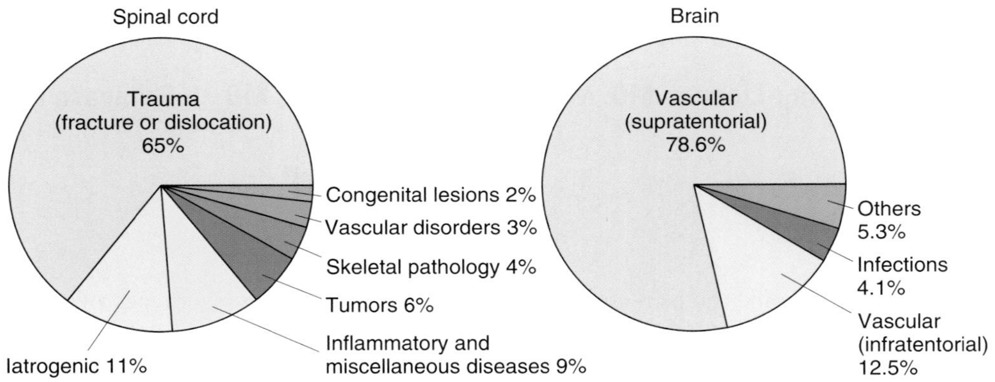

FIG. 30.1 Etiology of central pain states.

TABLE 30.1 Taxonomy of Spinal Cord Injury Pain

Broad Type (Tier One)	Broad System (Tier Two)	Specific Structures and Pathology (Tier Three)
Nociceptive	Musculoskeletal	Bone, joint, muscle trauma, or inflammation Mechanical instability Muscle spasm Secondary overuse syndromes
	Visceral	Renal calculus, bowel dysfunction, and sphincter dysfunction Dysreflexic headache
Neuropathic	Above level	Compressive mononeuropathies Complex regional pain syndromes
	At level	Nerve root compression (including cauda equina) Syringomyelia Spinal cord trauma/ischemia Dual level cord and root trauma
	Below level	Spinal cord trauma/ischemia

Taxonomy of Spinal Cord Injury Pain Spinal Cord Injury Pain: Assessment, Mechanisms, Management, Yezierski, Burchiel, Taxonomy and Epidemiology of Spinal Cord Injury Pain, Siddal, Yezierski, Loeser. 2002 IASP Press. This table has been reproduced with permission of the International Association for the Study of Pain® (IASP). The table may not be reproduced for any other purpose without permission.

38% at 2 weeks and remained the same at 6 months. Neuropathic below-level pain occurred in 14% of subjects at 2 weeks and increased to 19% at 6 months. The prevalence and type of pain described following SCI over a 1-year period are shown in Fig. 30.2.[21] The pain can be spontaneous or stimulus evoked. Longitudinal studies indicate that at-level pain has an early onset, while the below-level pain develops months to years after the spinal injury.[21,22]

Central pain disorders are one of several types of "neuropathic pain," and the definition and diagnosis of neuropathic pain have been discussed at length by researchers throughout the world. The definition outlined by the IASP was "pain caused by a lesion or disease of the somatosensory nervous system." Some experts now believe that central neuropathic pain should be distinguished from peripheral neuropathic pain.[23] A new grading system for neuropathic pain is shown in Table 30.2.[23,24] Although a number of questionnaires and standardized self-report measures have been developed to detect neuropathic pain, the described grading system requires a physical examination.

PATHOPHYSIOLOGIC MECHANISMS

Central pain states likely result from pathophysiologic changes caused by irritation of, or damage to, central pain pathways. The possible pathophysiologic mechanisms that cause and maintain central pain are complex and not well understood (for reviews, see Finnerup[1,8]) Injury to the CNS may result in anatomic, neurochemical, inflammatory, and excitotoxic changes that result in a sensitized and hyperexcitable CNS.

Several neurotransmitters, such as glutamate, gamma-aminobutyric acid (GABA), norepinephrine, serotonin, histamine, and acetylcholine, are involved in the processing of noxious input along the pain pathway. The shift in firing from a rhythmic burst to a single spike is determined by noradrenergic, serotonergic, and cholinergic input to the reticular and relay cells of the thalamus. Similarly, excitatory amino acids, such as glutamate, are released in the region of SCI and may lead to neuronal hyperexcitability. At the spinal cord level, substance P and cholecystokinin (CCK) might play an additional role by influencing the voltage-gated sodium and calcium channels. Potassium channels play a critical role in setting the resting membrane potential and controlling the excitability of neurons.

Central pain in SCI may result from a combination of deafferentation-induced plastic changes in supraspinal areas along with abnormal input from a pain generator in the spinal cord (Fig. 30.3).[25,26] The changes in the CNS may include neuronal hyperexcitability. In SCI, *N*-methyl-D-aspartate receptor (NMDA) activation

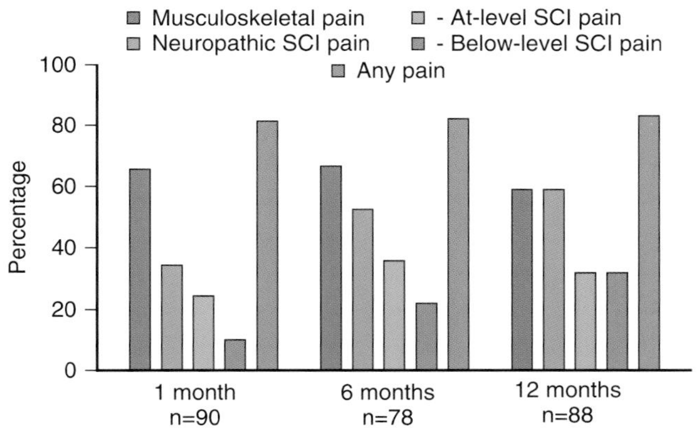

FIG. 30.2 Pain following spinal cord injury. Acute and chronic pain is common following spinal cord injury. The type of pain reported does appear to change with time; however, musculoskeletal pain remains the most common complaint. The prevalence of neuropathic pain increased over time and can be seen at or below the level of the injury. *(From Finnerup NB, Norrbrink C, Trok K, et al. Phenotypes and predictors of pain following traumatic spinal cord injury: a prospective study.* J Pain *2014; 15(1): 40-48.)*

TABLE 30.2 Grading System for Neuropathic Pain

Criteria to be evaluated for each patient
1. Pain with a distinct neuroanatomically plausible distribution[a]
2. A history suggestive of a relevant lesion or disease affecting the peripheral or central somatosensory system[b]
3. Demonstration of the distinct neuroanatomically plausible distribution by at least one confirmatory test[c]
4. Demonstration of the relevant lesion or disease by at least one confirmatory test[d]

[a]*A region corresponding to a peripheral innervation territory or to the topographic representation of a body part in the central nervous system.*
[b]*The suspected lesion or disease is reported to be associated with pain, including a temporal relationship typical for the condition.*
[c]*As part of the neurologic examination, these tests confirm the presence of negative or positive neurologic signs concordant with the distribution of pain. Clinical sensory examination may be supplemented by laboratory and objective tests to uncover subclinical abnormalities.*
[d]*As part of the neurologic examination, these tests confirm the diagnosis of the suspected lesion or disease. These confirmatory tests depend on which lesion or disease is causing neuropathic pain.*
Grading of certainty for the presence of neuropathic pain: definite neuropathic pain: all (1–4); probable neuropathic pain: 1 and 2, plus either 3 or 4; possible neuropathic pain: 1 and 2, without confirmatory evidence from 3 or 4.

might trigger the intracellular cascade leading to the upregulation of neuronal activity/excitability that results in spontaneous and evoked neuronal hyperactivity/hyperexcitability and causes abnormal pain perception. Changes in voltage-sensitive sodium channels can also contribute to changes in nerve membrane excitability. Other important mechanisms might be a loss of endogenous inhibition, including reduced GABA-ergic, opioid, and monoaminergic inhibition. Wide dynamic range (WDR) neuronal hypersensitivity in excitotoxic or ischemic SCI models reveals changes similar to central sensitization following peripheral nerve injury. Analogous to epilepsy, SCI causes one neuronal population to generate hyperactivity and another to respond to this chaotic activity. It appears that a critical threshold in the size of this population must be reached before a patient will experience spontaneous pain.[27]

Advances in functional imaging have increased our understanding of the changes in the brain that are associated with many pain conditions.[28] Central glutamate levels are known to increase in response to pain in healthy humans,[29] and patients with fibromyalgia are known to have elevated central glutamate levels that directly correlate with response to painful stimuli.[30] Decreased opioid binding has also been demonstrated in the pain-processing regions of patients with poststroke pain.[31] The authors go on to suggest that the imbalance of excitatory to inhibitory mechanisms explain, in part, the reason for central pain. Interestingly, gray matter decreased in patients with chronic pain.[32] Whether the change in gray matter is premorbid or due to degeneration from an insult or inflammation from excitatory neurotransmitters (i.e., glutamate) is not known; however, a rat model of peripheral nerve injury was found to be associated with decreased size of the frontal cortex and comorbid anxiety. Patients with complete SCI are known to have a postinjury reorganization of the somatosensory cortex that correlates with pain intensity,[33] a finding previously demonstrated in amputees.[34]

Alterations of the sensory pathways and impaired descending inhibitory mechanism are associated with many pain conditions, including central pain. Craig and coworkers showed that, under normal conditions, the cool-sensitive pathway in the STT might suppress the forebrain's response to nociceptive STT activity.[35] Damage to this pathway may thus explain some of the phenomena seen in a central pain state. They hypothesize that, for central pain to occur, a lateral lamina I spinothalamocortical pathway lesion must be sufficiently large to produce contralateral sensory symptoms. This assumes that central pain is a release phenomenon resulting from the disruption of the normal integrative controls of sensory processing. The disruption of thermal sensibility results in a loss of the cold-induced inhibition of pain with a resultant disinhibition of cold-evoked burning pain. Craig and coworkers suggested that the ventromedial posterior (VMPo) nucleus of the thalamus plays a critical role. Investigations in primates, however, strongly support the existence of a spinothalamocortical pathway from lamina I and the deep layers of the dorsal horn to the contralateral ventral posterior lateral (VPL) nucleus, which extends to area 1 of the S1 somatosensory cortex. A similar pathway might activate neurons of the SII cortex, because direct projections connect the VPL and VPI (inferior) to SII and SI to SII.[36]

Lesions in the spinothalamocortical pathways can cause ectopic discharges in various neurons of the spinal cord and brain. Such ectopic neuronal discharges create an illusion of noxious input because of the imbalance between the lateral (inhibitory) and medial (excitatory) STT. This might explain why pain occurs more often in patients with partial lesions than in those with complete cord and thalamic injuries. It appears that severe CNS lesions, with total destruction of ascending sensory systems, do not lead to a central pain syndrome and that mild, moderate, or severe disruption of the anterolateral ascending system, with partial or complete preservation of the dorsal column/medial lemniscus functions, is most frequently associated with central pain syndrome. Furthermore, even during remission, dysesthesias and pain could be triggered by additional afferent input to the large fiber/dorsal column/medial lemniscus

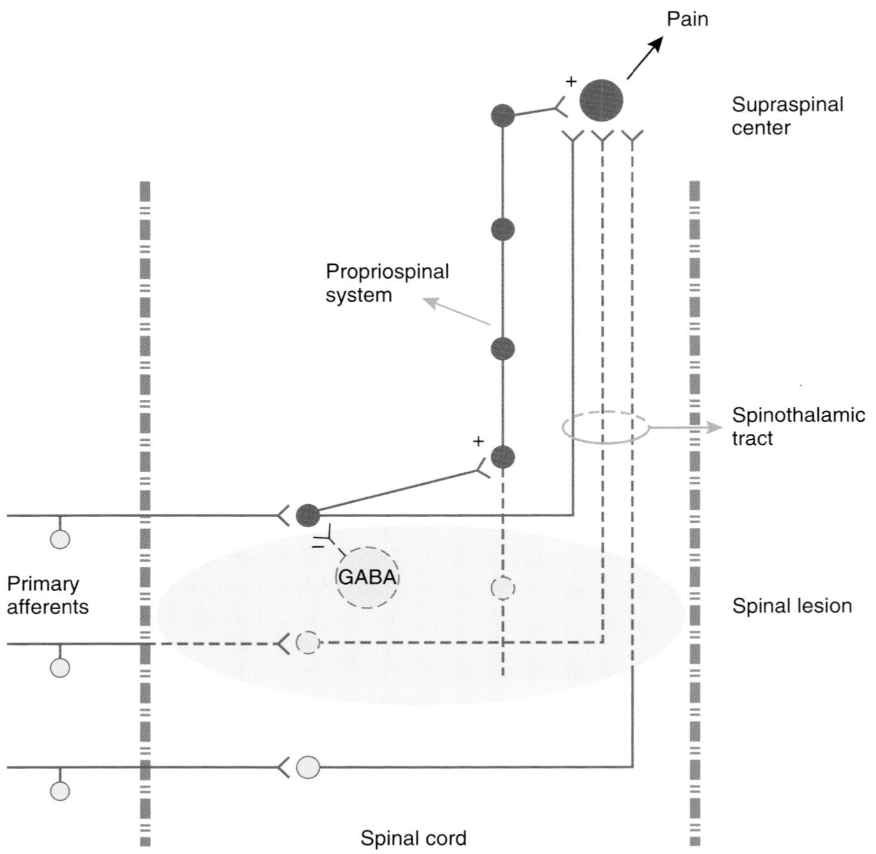

FIG. 30.3 Proposed mechanism of central pain in spinal cord injury. Input from primary afferents can be distorted by two mechanisms. The spinothalamic tract projection neurons from below the spinal injury may be lesioned and give rise to deafferentation hyperexcitability in higher-order neurons including the thalamus. Second-order neurons in the dorsal horn at the rostral end of the spinal lesion may become hyperexcitable because of excitotoxic changes and disinhibition from damaged GABA-ergic neurons at the level of injury. Abnormal input from these second-order neurons in the rostral end of the spinal cord lesion may propagate via the propriospinal system to the deafferentated thalamic neurons resulting in pain referred to areas below injury level. *(Source: Finnerup NB, Jensen TS: Spinal cord injury pain—mechanisms and treatment.* Eur J Neurol. *11:73-82, 2004.)*

system and, once established, might not be abolished by additional deafferentation.

Sensory stimuli act on neural systems that have been modified by previous inputs, and the "memory" of which significantly influences pain behavior. The fact that a memory is not activated by the development of a lesion might explain the long delay in the onset of central pain in some patients. The long-term potentiation that is important for this memory might be mediated by NMDA receptors and their influence on calcium conductance. Thus, central pain frequently develops weeks or months after development of the lesion and is associated with sensory changes involving the spinothalamic pathways, especially changes in temperature perception.

The role of microglia in central pain is an area of great interest. Microglia are the macrophages of the brain and spinal cord that release inflammatory mediators in the event of injury or infection. The activation of microglia and subsequent inflammation is thought to precipitate a cycle of further inflammation and activation of astrocytes.[1] Therapies targeting the cytokines, chemokines, and inflammatory mediators involved in this microglial and astrocytic activation are being increasingly explored.[26]

CLINICAL PRESENTATIONS

The neuropathic component of central pain is often reported starting days to weeks after the CNS lesion and presents as a steady dysesthesia or neuralgia and may also have an evoked component. Although many tools and tests have been proposed to diagnose central pain, the wide range of types and presentations of central pain disorders makes no single measure completely sensitive or specific. The quality of the pain may be burning, aching, shooting, pricking, and tingling. The discomfort is generally constant but may wax and wane and often has a deep and/or a superficial component. In a minority of patients, the pain is intermittent and daily. Nonpainful tactile, thermal, vibratory, auditory, visual, olfactory, and visceral stimuli can provoke or exacerbate spontaneous pain. Anxiety and/or fear can also exacerbate symptoms. Some patients with central pain exhibit the most striking symptoms seen in clinical practice. Patients with classic Dejerine-Roussy syndrome have a rapidly regressing hemiparesis and a sensory deficit to touch, temperature, and pain. Allodynia, hyperalgesia, and spontaneous severe paroxysmal pain on the hemiparetic side also often occur. These patients can exhibit hemiataxia, hemiastereognosia, and choreoathetoid movements. Patients with central pain may have any or all these features depending on the location of the underlying lesion. Organic signs on sensory examination of patients with thalamic lesions include the so-called thalamic midline split for sensory loss and pain. The fact that central pain of any cause is accompanied by delayed hyperalgesia supports the hypothesis of a polysynaptic response. Pain intensity for brainstem and suprathalamic lesions are moderate in intensity, averaging 61 and 50 mm, respectively (on a 100-mm visual analog scale), while pain in thalamic lesions can be severe (average = 79 mm).[37] Many standardized measures have been developed to assess the different aspects of neuropathic pain to develop specific treatment algorithms and further research efforts.

Patients with a history of spontaneous or evoked dysesthesia, hyperesthesia, or paresthesia should undergo specific but simple bedside testing, which may help distinguish different phenotypes of central neuropathic pain. A prospective study that utilized the ISCIPBDS framework showed that early hypersensitivity by sensory testing was a predictor for later onset of below-level (not at-level) central neuropathic pain.[38] Sensory testing in the region where the pain is localized usually shows a paradoxic hypoalgesia (decreased sensitivity to painful stimulus). The region where the patient feels the pain often has decreased sensitivity to thermal stimuli, especially to cold. In fact, the intensity of the pain seems to be related to the magnitude of loss of thermal sensation. Testing for disturbed temperature sensation can be accomplished with a cold metal instrument, ice, or ethyl chloride spray. Touch can be tested with cotton wool, while pinprick sensation should be assessed using the contralateral side as a control. Chronic poststroke pain patients have an intact vibration sensation. Patients may exhibit *mitempfindung* (with sympathy), a phenomenon in which stimulation in one area of the body results in a simultaneous sense of the provoked sensation in another part of the body. These patients may also experience alloesthesia, in which a sensory stimulus on one side of the body is perceived on the other side. A subset of patients who experience burning pain lose the sensation of cold, warmth, and sharpness. In another subgroup of patients who experience shooting/pricking/aching pain, tactile allodynia is predominant. Although some disturbance of sensory function is almost always present on physical examination, clinical findings are few or subtle in many patients. Quantitative sensory testing might reveal side-to-side asymmetries in cooling, warmth, and heat-pain sensation thresholds.

Testing for autonomic dysfunction may be important in patients with SCI. Lesions above the sixth thoracic level (splanchnic outflow) are often associated with autonomic dysreflexia. The dysreflexia is characterized by sudden dramatic increases in blood pressure, high or low heart rate, and headache after sensory input, such as a full bladder. This point becomes especially important in SCI patients having surgery below the level of their lesion, including minor operations of the urinary (i.e., cystoscopy) or gastrointestinal (i.e., colonoscopy) systems where the viscera will be stimulated. Even though patients may lack sensation in the area to which they are having surgery, intense stimulation can precipitate major hemodynamic instability. Complications may include seizures and cerebral hemorrhage.

EXPERIMENTAL MODELS OF CENTRAL PAIN SECONDARY TO SPINAL CORD INJURY

Interesting insights about the mechanisms of central pain following SCI and the potential effects of drugs on pain behavior have been gained from experimental models in rats. The Stockholm group led by Wiesenfeld-Hallin developed a model of photochemically induced spinal cord ischemia,[39] while Yezierski et al. developed a model of excitotoxic SCI.[13] Rats with lesions involving both white and gray matter develop instantaneous morphine-resistant tactile allodynia, which responds to the systemic GABA-B agonist baclofen, and this can be prevented by pretreatment with the NMDA antagonist, MK-801. Intrathecal morphine and clonidine reduced the allodynia. Injections of a CCK-B antagonist decreased allodynia.

THERAPEUTIC OPTIONS

The treatment of central pain is complicated and requires a complete evaluation of the patient's pain and goals for therapy. An important aspect of treating patients with central pain is to define and continuously review the goals of treatment. Patients must be told and periodically reminded that complete cessation of pain is unlikely. Hence, a reasonable goal of therapy is to improve function and reduce pain without creating intolerable side effects. In addition, including treatment strategies for each of the multiple components of the central pain syndrome is of paramount importance. Thus, the various psychological symptoms that come with most types of chronic pain and loss of physical function must be treated. The options available for managing central pain include pharmacotherapy, behavioral therapy, physical therapy, neuromodulation, other interventional therapies, and ablative neurosurgery. Table 30.3 shows a treatment algorithm modified from that which was proposed by Que et al.[40] for the treatment of SCI.

PHARMACOTHERAPY

Antidepressants

The pharmacologic approach is based on a strategy of stepwise combination therapy. The mainstay of this therapy is antidepressants that possibly act by modulating the thalamic burst firing activity via its actions on locus coeruleus noradrenergic neurons and the serotoninergic cells in the dorsal raphe.[41] Amitriptyline is often effective in central poststroke and SCI pain,[42] while some studies have not shown benefit.[43] Amitriptyline's benefit derives, in part, from its ability to prevent reuptake of noradrenaline and serotonin. Tricyclic antidepressants (TCAs) should be titrated to 50–100 mg/day. Insufficient plasma levels at this dose might indicate the need for higher doses. A small pilot study found that amitriptyline given at the time of a thalamic stroke failed to alter the time to, or the potential for developing, chronic poststroke pain.[44] Similarly, findings in a controlled trial failed to support the use of amitriptyline in the treatment of chronic central pain of spinal cord origin.[43] Although amitriptyline is the most studied TCA in central pain, the analgesic efficacy of nortriptyline has been demonstrated to be similar to amitriptyline with less side effects.[45] Simple analgesics, such as, nonsteroidal antiinflammatory drugs (NSAIDs), paracetamol,[26] and spasmolytics (e.g., benzodiazepine) in

TABLE 30.3 Central Pain Treatment Algorithm

Step 1. Identify Problems

Determine existing problems and potential adverse sequelae.

Identify biologic and psychological contributors to pain and their influence on the individual's pain experience.

Determine the impact of pain on the patient's function.

Determine how well the patient has adjusted to the disorder causing their central pain (SCI, stroke, MS).

Determine the risk of and/or presence of additional consequences of pain and the disorder underlying the central pain (i.e., pressure sores, contractures, adverse drug effects).

Step 2. Determine Reasonable Objectives/Goals for Patient and Treating Physician

Pain relief/reduction.

Treatment of spasm—decrease frequency and/or severity.

Increase exercise tolerance and improve function.

Achieve independent living.

Return to work.

Step 3. Create Multidisciplinary Approach

Pharmacologic	Interventional	Physical and Occupational Therapy	Psychosocial
First line	Specific to condition	Structured therapy and home exercises	Psychiatric therapy
AEDs (gabapentin and pregabalin)	Limited evidence	Postural reeducation	Pharmacologic
Second line	Mainly for refractory cases	Spasticity treatment	Counseling
TCAs	Neuromodulation	Bowel/bladder management	CBT
SNRIs	SCS	Braces and devices to assist in home and work function	Pain coping skills
Combinations with AED	DBS	Home/work remodeling	Relaxation
Third line	MCS	Speech therapy	Family support and education
Opioids	Intrathecal therapy		
SSRI	Baclofen		
Fourth line	Morphine		
Ketamine infusion	Clonidine		
Lidocaine infusion	Ziconotide		
	Acupuncture		
	Ablative therapies (DREZ, cordotomy)		

Note: The treatment of central pain requires a careful assessment of the pain and problems associated with the patient's underlying disorder. Understanding goals and setting expectations are essential to creating an appropriate multidisciplinary treatment plan.

AEDs, Antiepileptic drugs; CBT, cognitive-behavioral therapy; DBS, deep brain stimulation; DREZ, dorsal reentry zone lesioning; MCS, motor cortex stimulation; MS, multiple sclerosis; SCI, spinal cord injury; SCS, spinal cord stimulation; SNRIs, serotonin-norepinephrine reuptake inhibitors; SSRIs, selective serotonin reuptake inhibitors; TCAs, tricyclic antidepressants.

Adapted from Que JC, Siddall PJ, Cousins MJ: Pain management in a patient with intractable spinal cord injury pain: a case report and literature review. Anesth Analg. *105:1462-1473, 2007.*

combination with a TCA (e.g., amitriptyline) are reportedly a good regimen to control the common, steady, burning, dysesthetic component of this syndrome.[46]

There have been a few randomized double-blind placebo-controlled studies on serotonin-norepinephrine reuptake inhibitors (SNRIs) in the treatment of central pain. One study looking at the efficacy of duloxetine for the treatment of poststroke or SCI patients showed trends towards decrease in mean pain score after 8 weeks with significantly better relief of the dynamic and cold allodynia components of pain compared to placebo. However, no significant effect on pain intensity, tactile and pressure-related pain, or other domains (SF-36, the Pain Disability Index, and the EQ-5D)[47] was observed. Another study that examined the efficacy of duloxetine for the treatment of central pain in MS patients showed statistically greater improvement in pain, compared to placebo, although greater discontinuation rates secondary to adverse events were reported.[48] A study was done on the efficacy of extended-release venlafaxine for the treatment of central pain with SCI and depression and found clinically relevant reductions in nociceptive pain intensity and interference, although no significant effect on neuropathic pain was observed.[49] These initial studies indicate that SNRIs would likely be useful adjuncts in the treatment of central pain.

Antiepileptic Drugs

Antiepileptic drugs (AEDs) are useful for the treatment of neuropathic pain. Currently, the most commonly prescribed AEDs are gabapentin and pregabalin. Both gabapentin and pregabalin appear to be effective in treating central pain, and there are no studies that allow for direct comparison between the two.[50] Parsons et al. performed a pooled analysis of placebo controlled trials of pregabalin in patients with neuropathic pain secondary to SCI that showed significant reductions in neuropathic pain over a 12–16-week treatment period compared to placebo.[51] In a randomized, placebo-controlled trial, Cardenas et al. showed class I evidence for effectiveness of pregabalin in reducing duration-adjusted average change in pain compared to placebo over a 16-week period in the treatment of central neuropathic pain after SCI.[52] A randomized, double-blind placebo-controlled, multicenter study on the treatment of pregabalin for poststroke central pain failed to show a significant reduction in primary efficacy endpoint (mean pain score on the Daily Pain Rating Scale) in the pregabalin group compared with placebo. However, the pregabalin-treated group showed significant improvements in the secondary endpoints of sleep, anxiety, and clinician global impression of change (CGIC).[53]

A study by Gilron et al.[54] demonstrated that the combination of a TCA and gabapentin was superior for the treatment of neuropathic pain associated with diabetic neuropathy and postherpetic neuralgia when compared to either alone. In a controlled study, pain scores decreased from 7 to 5 (10-point numeric rating scale) in patients with poststroke pain who were given 200 mg/day of lamotrigine.[55] In patients with incomplete SCI, lamotrigine titrated to 400 mg/day significantly reduced pain at or below the injury level. Patients with brush-evoked allodynia and wind-up–like pain near the maximal pain were more likely to have a beneficial effect with lamotrigine than patients without these evoked pains. This trial, however, showed no significant effect of lamotrigine on spontaneous and evoked pain in patients with complete SCI.[56] Chiou-Tan and colleagues found mexiletine of no use in the treatment of central pain states of spinal cord origin.[57]

Two recent randomized, double-blind, placebo-controlled trials that examined the efficacy of levetiracetam have failed to demonstrate a significant benefit of this drug for central pain. One study on central pain in MS patients showed no difference in outcomes over a 6-week treatment period.[58] A second study in poststroke patients with central pain (CPSP) also showed no analgesic effect with more frequent withdrawals and side effects compared to placebo.[59]

Opioids

Opioids may benefit some patients; however, it is not a first-line therapy. Patients who respond to a trial of opioid infusion may be prescribed long-acting opioids, such as the slow-release formulations or the transdermal preparation. In a controlled study, the reduction in the intensity of neuropathic pain was significantly greater during treatment with a high dose (0.75 mg) than it was with lower doses of the μ-agonist levorphanol.[60] Patients with central pain after stroke, however, were the least likely to report benefit. Another controlled trial revealed that intravenous morphine induces analgesic effects on some components of central neuropathic pain syndromes, but only a minority of patients may benefit from long-term opioid treatment.[61] Morphine significantly reduced the intensity of brush-induced allodynia but had no effect on other evoked pains (i.e., static mechanical and thermal allodynia/hyperalgesia).

Na Channel Blockers

The efficacy of systemic lidocaine (5 mg/kg IV over 30 minutes) was evaluated in a double-blind, placebo-controlled, crossover trial on spontaneous and evoked pains (allodynia and hyperalgesia) in 16 patients with chronic poststroke (n = 6) or SCI (n = 10) pain.[62] Systemic lidocaine induced a significant and selective reduction of several components of pain caused by CNS injuries. The observed preferential antihyperalgesic and antiallodynic effects of lidocaine suggest a selective central action on the mechanisms underlying these evoked pains.

N-Methyl-D-Aspartate Receptor Antagonists

There are other less traditional drugs that have been studied in central pain and other neuropathic pain states that may have limited clinical utility but can be used to drive future research. Ketamine has been available since the 1960s but has found limited use outside of the perioperative setting due to its side effects and potential for abuse.[63] Some studies and reports note that ketamine may have a role in central pain, likely due to its unique NMDA antagonist properties, which is believed to be important in the manifestation of central neuropathic pain.[64,65] The optimal route of delivery, dosage, duration, and practicality are still not clearly defined.

Cannabinoids

Another area of interest in refractory central pain is the use of cannabinoids.[66] While cannabis remains a controlled substance, some states have initiated programs for medical marijuana. In a randomized, double-blind, controlled study, an oral spray version of an oromucosal spray, cannabis-based medication was found to improve pain and sleep disturbance when compared with placebo.[67] In the first phase III placebo-controlled study of the efficacy of the Tetrahydrocannabinol/Cannabidiol (THC/CBD) oromucosal spray for treatment of MS-induced neuropathic pain, the primary endpoint (time to treatment failure) was equivocal with a large number of placebo responders in this first phase double-blind period. During the second randomized-withdrawal phase, the primary endpoint and secondary endpoints (NRS and sleep quality) were statistically significant for the THC/CBD spray group compared to placebo. Conflicting findings in the two phases of the study indicate further studies are needed to explore efficacy of the THC/CBD spray in treatment of central neuropathic pain.[68] Research is currently focused on selective cannabanoid receptor agonists that may offer less of the adverse psychoactive properties.

BEHAVIORAL THERAPY

Activities that promote general mental activity, including distraction techniques and physical therapy, seem to play a role in reducing the pain in central pain states. Peripheral sensory input and activation of fronto-orbital brain areas inhibit specific and nonspecific pain pathways. Based on an examination of a series of case reports, Haythornthwaite and colleagues suggest that biofeedback, hypnosis, and cognitive-behavioral interventions all have a beneficial impact on neuropathic pain.[69]

PHYSICAL AND OCCUPATIONAL THERAPY

Physiotherapy may be beneficial, but treatments such as acupuncture, ultrasound, and massage are not effective for long-term treatment of central pain states. Transcutaneous electrical nerve stimulation (TENS) provides long-term benefits to patients with central poststroke pain and those with incomplete SCI.[70] Patients with functional changes or limitations due to the disorder associated with their central pain can greatly benefit from occupational therapy to allow patients to function better in their home or work environments.[40] Some patients will require braces or assist devices. These measures can allow for more independence and benefit the patient psychologically.

NEUROMODULATION

Neuromodulation is a more invasive and expensive modality for the treatment of central pain, which can be effective in well-selected patients. Electroacupuncture has been shown to provide potential benefit in the treatment of chronic pain, while further studies are needed to elucidate the underlying mechanisms of action. A randomized study looking at electroacupuncture in relapsing-remitting MS patients found significant reduction in pain, depression, and quality of life.[71]

Spinal cord stimulation (SCS, also known as dorsal column stimulation) is often a better option than deep brain or motor cortex stimulation (MCS) in patients with SCI, as SCS trials are safe, easy, and reversible. Dorsal columns should be functional above the level of injury to produce paresthesia. Patients with anesthesia dolorosa (pain in an anesthetic area) and patients with incomplete lesions are poor candidates. Patients who experience more than 50% pain relief during trial stimulation are potential candidates for an implant. In patients with treatment failure, deep brain stimulation (DBS) of the tactile relay nucleus of the thalamus or the lemniscal radiations offers hope. Data from Bendok and Levy suggest that paresthesia-producing DBS alleviates steady neuropathic pain.[72] Periventricular/periaqueductal gray (PVG/PAG) DBS is appropriate for nociceptive pain.

For brain-origin central pain, data from Tasker and colleagues show that brain stimulation relieves the steady dysesthetic component in 53% of patients and the evoked component in 25% of patients, but brain stimulation offers no help for the neuralgic component.[73] The neuralgic component is the component sometimes responsive to ablative neurosurgery. In addition, SCS is of no benefit for brain-origin central pain, although patients might report relief during a trial. Paresthesia-producing DBS and MCS are appropriate for the steady component of the pain. For those with allodynia or hyperpathia, PVG/PAG DBS seems to be beneficial. A randomized, controlled, crossover DBS trial showed significantly increased subjective heat pain threshold and reduced pain-induced cerebral activity in the somatosensory cortex in patients with Parkinson disease.[74]

Stimulating the motor cortex offers a new target for the neuromodulation of central pain. Yamamoto and colleagues concluded that patients whose pain was diminished by thiamylal and ketamine, but not by morphine, respond best to MCS.[75] Canavero and colleagues concluded that MCS controls spontaneous and evoked pain but not the nonpainful paresthesias.[76] Patients who might respond well to MCS (MCS) also respond to transcranial magnetic stimulation. Raslan et al. conducted a retrospective study of 11 patients with trigeminal neuropathic or trigeminal deafferentation pain who underwent MCS system implantation that showed satisfactory pain control (>50% pain relief) at 6 months in 8 of the 11 patients with continued long-term pain control in 5 patients, followed up to 33 months.[77]

OTHER INTERVENTIONAL THERAPIES

INTRATHECAL PUMPS

Intrathecal pumps have been used to treat a wide variety of pain conditions and spasticity.[78] The use of intrathecal medications poses issues of time and cost along with additional potential for serious complications.[78,79] The most commonly administered medications are opioids (morphine, hydromorphone, and fentanyl), clonidine, and bupivacaine. The addition of clonidine to morphine was shown to be superior to either drug delivered alone in SCI.[80] Ziconotide, a nonopioid intrathecal medication, is a synthetic form of the cone snail toxin that is approved by the US Food and Drug Administration for the treatment of chronic pain. Ziconotide is one of the few intrathecal medications that has demonstrated efficacy in a randomized, controlled trial[81]; however, its side-effect profile is significant,[82] and some practitioners question its role in pain management.

Baclofen, a GABA agonist, has antinociceptive effects, and its intrathecal administration reduces allodynic responses in animal models of neurogenic central pain.[83] Well-designed clinical studies have demonstrated efficacy with intrathecal baclofen in the treatment of CRPS, which shares many of the attributes of the central pains discussed in this chapter.[84] Intrathecal baclofen can be helpful in treating pain and spasticity as well as multiple types of central pain, including poststroke, SCI, and MS pain.[84,85] Trials range from a single shot of intrathecal baclofen to a multiple-day intrathecal catheter trial. Once implanted, the daily dosing can be slowly increased to effect. As with all intrathecal pumps, there is potential for pump complications independent of the medication infused, thereby necessitating intensive monitoring and regular follow-up.[84]

ABLATIVE NEUROSURGERY

Ablative neurosurgery plays a role in the treatment of the neuralgic component of central pain. Percutaneous radiofrequency dorsal rhizotomy is an option for monoradicular pain syndromes. Ablative surgery includes cordotomy, cordectomy, and dorsal root entry zone (DREZ) lesioning. The goal of cordotomy and cordectomy is interruption of STTs. Cordectomy, the simplest destructive procedure, can benefit patients with complete lesions. It is not acceptable to most patients, because it obviates their hope for eventual restoration of spinal cord function. Percutaneous/open cordotomy achieves the same results as cordectomy and is offered to patients with incomplete lesions, but it carries the risk of aggravating bladder dysfunction and inducing ipsilateral limb paresis. DREZ is equally effective for the neuralgic and the evoked elements of spinal-origin central pain. Nashold and colleagues found this procedure most useful for the relief of end-zone pain (pain starting at the level of injury and extending distally).[86] Pain extending diffusely, often sacrally distributed, and remotely distributed pain, described as phantom or diffuse burning pain, do not respond well to DREZ. Although the procedure preserves the hope for future spinal cord function and avoids risk of limb paresis, it can interfere with residual bladder function and requires a laminectomy and considerable skill.

In the past, surgeons attempted to relieve central pain of cerebral origin with cordotomy, trigeminal DREZ, medial thalamotomy, and mesencephalic tractotomy. Destructive procedures on the cerebral cortex are of historic note only.

FUTURE DIRECTIONS

Ongoing and future research will help to understand the pathophysiology of pain as a disease, including central pain. In the immediate future, neuromodulation seems to hold great promise. New nonopioid analgesics targeting the associated neurotransmitter changes in chronic pain will likely have benefit. Medications specifically altering central glutamate levels and microglia activation may be particularly effective in patients with neuropathic pain. Advances in the study of the genetic factors associated with pain will also hopefully allow for the early detection of patients at risk for chronic central pain after an injury (i.e., SCI). Whether early detection and aggressive therapy will improve outcomes is not known. Nonetheless, the field of pharmacogenomics is rapidly advancing and may offer "personalized analgesia" for patients based on their genetic make-up and pain condition.

KEY POINTS

- Central pain states are common sequelae of SCI and stroke.
- The pathophysiology of central pain is not well understood. Alterations in several neurotransmitters occur, including glutamate, GABA, norepinephrine.
- Involvement of the spinothalamocortical pathway is strongly supported by animal models, but the precise pathway in humans is unknown.
- Preclinical research has helped identify a range of cellular and molecular mechanisms underlying neuronal hyperexcitability, which may serve as potential treatment targets for central pain states.
- The three components of central pain (steady dysesthetic, intermittent neuralgic, and evoked) must all be treated. In central pain of brain origin, steady and evoked components predominate, while in central pain of spinal cord origin steady and neuralgic components predominate.
- A multidisciplinary approach is recommended. Poorly controlled central pain carries a high suicide risk, hence psychosocial support is crucial.
- Pharmacotherapy should begin with a tricyclic antidepressant.
- Membrane stabilizers should be considered for combination with TCAs as a second step.
- Opioids in small doses may be of benefit in a subset of patients but are not first-line agents.
- More involved therapies can be considered in refractory cases, including neuromodulation, intrathecal therapy, and neuroablative procedures.

REFERENCES

Access the reference list online at ExpertConsult.com.

CHAPTER 31

Pelvic Pain

Karina Gritsenko, MD ✪ Marc Samuel Cohen, MS, MD

Chronic pelvic pain (CPP) is a major cause of morbidity and is defined as nonmenstrual-related pain below the umbilicus in men or women that has continued for greater than 6 months and creates a functional disability or requires long-term medical or interventional treatment.[1]

CPP represents a different kind of pain, a different kind of patient, and a problem that is not necessarily straightforward or easy to fix. Due to the chronic nature of illness, the instigator for the pain may be gone but changes in the nervous system continue; thus, pain itself becomes the disease. It is the management of this pain faced by every pain physician that becomes the bulk of pelvic pain issues.

EPIDEMIOLOGY

CPP is an epidemic, and it represents approximately 2%–25% of the general population of women and is estimated to cost $881.5 million in the United States each year.[2–5]

In the United States, primary care practices show a prevalence of one in seven women affected by some form of CPP.[6] In one recent study by Jamieson, women of a reproductive age presenting to primary care practices with pelvic pain issues were shown to represent 39% of patients evaluated in that practice setting.[7] Women in reproductive years in all settings were shown to represent 14.7%–24% of patients[6] with the greatest incidence of pelvic pain found to be in women ages 26–30.[8,9] Of all referrals to gynecologists, 10% are for pelvic pain.[8,10] Of the 10% of gynecologic referrals, these patients are expected to undergo up to approximately 20% of hysterectomies and 40% of laparoscopies in the general population.[11,12] The majority of women with chronic pain indicate chronic pain for 1–5 years, but CPP can be a life-long difficulty.[13]

Although most pelvic pain concerns usually surround women, men also may be diagnosed with CPP issues. Most commonly, causes of CPP in men include chronic (nonbacterial) prostatitis, chronic orchalgia, and prostatodynia.[14] Although men may have chronic pain issues from many disorders such as urinary dysfunction and irritable bowel syndrome (IBS), those listed above represent male-specific causes of pelvic pain. Chronic prostatitis/chronic pelvic pain syndrome (CP/CPPS) is a significant problem, accounting for 9% of all urological visits and 1% of primary care visits with 2 million office visits per year, which corresponds to a large health care burden to the United States.[15,16] One study with a cohort of 51,529 men found 3.2% prevalence of CP/CPPS in men under the age of 50.[15]

On an international level, a similar prevalence of CPP has been described in other countries regarding men and women. In the United Kingdom, incidence of CPP is similar to that of migraine, back pain, and asthma.[17] These numbers extend to beyond medical conditions and personal consequences to pure economics. Epidemiologic studies show that CPP conditions affect the regular person and can seriously impact the day-to-day quality of life and quality of productivity in the workforce.[6,17]

DEMOGRAPHICS

In recently compiled clinical data from the Weill Cornell New York Presbyterian pelvic pain population, it has been shown that the majority of patients with pelvic pain are members of the working force: 22% are professional, 18% are clerical, 9% manual, and 4% are students.[13] At the same time, it has been noted that 15% of working women between the ages of 18 and 50 reported time lost from paid work related to pelvic pain.[6] In a breakdown of the social status of women affected with CPP at Weill Cornell New York Presbyterian, 48% of women are married, 23% are single, 9% divorced, 9% cohabitating, 4% separated, 2% widowed.[13]

While similar data are not readily available for men, CPP has shown to be a significant psychosocial component. Patients commonly report decreased quality of life measures, depression, anxiety compared to spouses, and catastrophizing.[18]

CANCER PAIN

Patients with cancer represent a unique category of pelvic pain patients who deserve special consideration. They can suffer from pain related to tumor burden, radiation, chemotherapy, and surgery. They can experience pain from all available modalities including somatic, sympathetic, visceral, and neuropathic etiologies. Sympathetic and neuropathic pain symptoms are both less responsive to opioid therapy than nociceptive and visceral pain. Consequently, these patients become increasingly complex to treat.

In 1986, the World Health Organization (WHO) established a step-ladder approach specifically for cancer pain patients that revolutionized analgesic care for 70%–90% of patients with cancer pain.[19] This approach emphasized a stepwise approach beginning with nonopioid agents and progression to stronger agents as indicated by patients' clinical condition, with adjuvant agents incorporated including antidepressants, anticonvulsants, topical agents, nonsteroidal antiinflammatory drugs (NSAIDs), anxiolytics, and corticosteroids. Further approaches involved injection therapy, spinal anesthesia, neuroaugmentation, and more permanent, long-lasting neurolytic blocks. This category of patients will be mentioned only briefly, as the typical treatment pathway and goals of treatment are different for cancer patients and are often influenced by life expectancy, tolerance, and tumor growth.

PELVIC PAIN DIFFERENTIAL AND ETIOLOGY

The diagnosis of CPP can be challenging, and 30%–50% of patients with CPP are classified as having "chronic pelvic pain without obvious pathology."[20] For example, referred pain patterns in CPP can be very difficult to identify even with experienced clinicians, and up to one-third of women who undergo diagnostic laparoscopy remain undiagnosed.[21,22] Thus, a diagnosis and subsequent appropriate treatment is not always a straightforward algorithm.

When assessing the pelvic pain patient, it is important to approach these patients in a multidisciplinary fashion. Both diagnosis and management of these patients require good integration and knowledge of all pelvic organ systems and other systems including musculoskeletal, neurological, and psychiatric systems. A significant number of these patients may have various associated problems including bladder or bowel dysfunction, sexual dysfunction, and other systemic or constitutional symptoms. Other associated problems, such as depression, anxiety, and drug addiction, may also coexist.

ETIOLOGY

As CPP is an unclear diagnosis, pain can originate from any organ system and thus a thorough review of systems is essential to a proper assessment of a patient's pain. These assessments can be organized in a system-based review and a gender-specific review (Tables 31.1 and 31.2).

THEORY

As shown by the broad differential of CPP, the pathophysiologic explanation of each disease is outside the scope of this chapter; however, below are some examples of well-known mechanisms.

VASCULAR HYPOTHESIS

A vascular hypothesis, first postulated by Taylor in 1949 and more recently by Beard in 1984, may offer a clue into the mechanism of CPP. It has been noted that pain may be related to dilated pelvic veins in which blood flow is markedly reduced.[23–25] Pelvic venous incompetence is likely seen in 10% of women, and up to 60% of patients with this abnormality develop pelvic congestion syndrome (PCS). These patients can find relief when the dilation is treated with foam sclerotherapy followed by coil embolization to within a centimeter of vein origin.[26,27] Positive results have also been documented with medroxyprogesterone acetate therapy.[28,29] Further studies by Foong in 2000 demonstrated that pelvic vein congestion shows a change in peripheral vascular reactivity that returned to normal after suppression of ovarian activity as compared to controls.[30] Additional observation studies showed a reduction in pain for those patients whom congestion was diminished by hormonal therapy.[29] It seems that some alteration of normal ovarian function was responsible for the observed changes in peripheral blood flow in response to a rise in venous pressure in women with pelvic congestion.

TABLE 31.1 Gender-Specific Causes for Pelvic Pain

Women	Men
Infection, endometriosis, dysmenorrhea (primary—menstruation, middleshmurtz, secondary—fibroids, adenolysis, IUD), dyspareunia, mononeuropathies, myofascial pain, vulvitis, cystitis, ovarian remnant syndrome, sympathetically mediated pain, pelvic congestion, pelvic fibrosis, pelvis neurodystonia, pelvagia, birthing pain	Prostatitis, chronic orchalgia, and prostatodynia, interstitial cystitis, ureteral obstruction
IBS and other GI disorders	IBS and other GI disorders
Sexual/physical abuse	Sexual/physical abuse
Cancer pain	Cancer pain
Psychiatric disorders	Psychiatric disorders
Surgical procedures (adhesions)	Surgical procedures (adhesions)

GI, *Gastrointestinal;* IBS, *irritable bowel syndrome;* IUD, *intrauterine devices.*

TABLE 31.2 Organ-Specific Causes for Pelvic Pain

Reproductive	Visceral: uterus, ovaries, bladder, urethra Somatic: skin, vulva, clitoris, vaginal canal
Vascular	Dilated pelvic vein theory
Musculocutaneous	Ligamentous structures, muscular (iliopsoas, piriformis, quadrates lumborum, sacro-iliac joint, obturator internus, pubococcygeus) Skeletal (referred pain) from spinal lesions
Spinal	Degenerative joint disease, disk herniation, spondylosis, neoplasm of spinal cord/ sacral nerve
Neurologic	Neuralgia/cutaneous nerve entrapment (surgical scar in the lower part of the abdomen), iliohypogastric, ilioinguinal, genitofemoral, lat femoral cutaneous nerves), shingles (herpes zoster infection), spine-related nerve compressions
Gastrointestinal	Irritable bowel syndrome, abdominal epilepsy, abdominal migraine, constipation
Urologic	Bladder dysfunction, chronic (nonbacterial) prostatitis, chronic orchalgia, and prostatodynia
Psychological (psychosocial/ sexual)	Anxiety, depression, somatization, physical or sexual abuse, drug addiction, dependence, family problems, sexual dysfunction

ALTERATION OF STIMULI PROCESSING OR ORGAN FUNCTIONING

It has also been hypothesized that there is a rewiring of stimuli processing or a reorganization of organ function. A separate study by Rapkin in 1995 suggested an alteration in processing of stimuli by the spinal cord and further brain processing of stimuli could occur in women with CPP, a feature also shared by other chronic painful conditions.[31,32] For example, undetected IBS presents in up to half of women referred for gynecological investigation.[17] There is potential that visceral afferents may undergo a change in function similar to those of somatic nociceptors.[33] This begs the question, does CPP represent complex regional painlike syndrome of the pelvis? Further research must be continued before conclusions can be made.

TABLE 31.3 History Assessment

Pattern of onset	Efficacy and toxicity of previous medications
Inciting event	Association with menstrual cycle
Quality (burning, aching, dull, sharp, cramping)	Incontinence
Duration and progression of complaints	Pregnancy
Constant or intermittent nature	Sexual activity
Exacerbating factors (position, eating, urination, defecation, Valsalva)	Sudden weight loss or weight gain
Alleviating factors	Breast or endocrine difficulties
	Family history of ovarian, uterine, or breast cancer

HISTORY AND PHYSICAL EXAM

There are many potential sources of CPP in all organ systems. A thorough history and physical exam are essential for assessment, diagnosis, and treatment of pelvic pain issues.

HISTORY

A history must be conducted consisting of a systematic review of systems-based assessments including gastrointestinal, skeletal, muscular, vascular, reproductive, urinary, neurologic, and psychiatric assessment (Table 31.3).

PHYSICAL EXAM

A physical exam must be tuned towards the specific needs of the patient, specifically, the abdominal exam, pelvic exam, musculoskeletal exam, neurologic exam, and a psychiatric assessment. This review focuses on more in-depth musculoskeletal and neurologic evaluations with the understanding that the abdominal and pelvic examinations are components of any basic physical exam.

Abdominal Assessment

The focused abdominal exam is a core component of any physical exam and especially important in the assessment of pelvic pain. Auscultation for breath sounds, bruits, organomegaly, and palpations in four quadrants are all components of an abdominal exam.

Pelvic Assessment

A pelvic exam is an obvious component in the assessment of pelvic pain. An experienced physician should participate in a thorough examination of gynecologic, urologic, and overall pelvic health.

Musculoskeletal Assessment

All organ systems are important to assess, but, as per Baker in 1993, "musculoskeletal dysfunctions contribute to signs and symptoms of CPP and in many cases may be the primary factor."[34] In addition, "…coordination between the pelvic musculature and the pelvic visceral organs is essential for the proper functioning and integrity of the latter. The pelvic muscular element, which could well be the source of pain, must be evaluated."[35] Several maneuvers exist that can help identify pathology. A select few are listed as follows:

Trendelenburg sign: During single leg standing, the contralateral hip drops indicate hip muscle weakness. This may indicate gluteus medius or core muscle weakness.

Forced Faber test: Pain reported during abduction, flexion, and outward rotation of the hip while supine indicates pain originating from the pelvic girdle or hip joints. The examiner applies pressure to the knee and opposite anterior superior iliac spine during the maneuver.

Posterior pelvic pain provocation Test (P4 Test): Patients hip is flexed to 90 degrees while supine, a positive test in the ipsilateral hip, which is indicative of pain originating from the pelvic girdle or hip joints.

Pelvic floor muscle tenderness: Pain elicited during digital palpation of the lateral vaginal walls is indicative of myofascial pain.

Pelvic floor muscular strength: Positive test for weakness if patient is unable to lift and maintain contraction of the pelvic floor during a digital vaginal exam for at least 5 seconds is indicative of weakness of the internal pelvic core.

Pace maneuver: The patient abducts legs against resistance while seated is indicative of piriformis syndrome

Freiberg maneuver: With the patient supine, forcefully internally rotating the leg causing pain is indicative of priformis syndrome

It was found that examiners achieved 100% specificity in identification of CPP using pelvic floor muscle palpation and forced Faber test.[36]

Neurologic Assessment

The neurologic exam is a natural counterpart to a thorough evaluation and differential of pelvic pain assessment. Below is a clearly stated chart that can allow the practitioner to conduct, assess, and interpret a good physical exam and its neurologic correlations in the lower thoracic, lumbar, and sacral regions (see Table 31.4 for neuromusculoskeletal examination).

Psychiatric Assessment

An often overlooked but essential organ system is the psychiatric component of a patient's physique. A good psychosocial or psychosexual history is needed when organic diseases are excluded or when coexisting psychiatric disorders are suggested. Sufficient history must be obtained to evaluate depression, anxiety disorder, somatization, physical or sexual abuse, drug abuse or dependence, and family problems, marital problems, or sexual problems. A high incidence of physical or sexual abuse is found in 30%–50% of patients with CPP of unknown etiology, and sexual abuse in patients before 15 years of age is associated with later development of CPP.[35,37]

MODALITIES OF CHRONIC PELVIC PAIN

CPP is a common problem and presents a major challenge to health care providers because of its unclear etiology, complex natural history, and poor response to therapy. To treat patients effectively, the identification of the type of pain is absolutely necessary.

TABLE 31.4 Neuromusculoskeletal Examination

Muscle	Innervation	Referral Pattern	Symptoms
Iliopsoas	L1–L4	Lower abdomen, groin, anterior thigh, low back, and lateral trunk	Pain with hip extension and weight-bearing, especially at heel strike
Piriformis	L5–S3	Buttock, pelvic floor, and low back	Pain with standing, walking, and sitting
Quadratus lumborum	T12–L3	Lower abdomen, anterior lateral trunk, anterior thigh, buttock, and sacro-iliac joint	Pain in lateral low back with standing and walking
Sacro-iliac joint	L4–S3	Posterior thigh buttock, pelvic floor, low back	Pain with standing, walking, and a possible "catch" on one side with bending
Obturator internus	L3–S2	Pelvic floor, buttock, posterior thigh, and coccyx	Includes "pressure" in pelvic floor
Pubococcygeus	S1–S4	Pelvic floor, vagina, rectum, buttock	Pain in sitting, dyspareunia

TABLE 31.5 Types of Pain

Pain Category	Description
Nociceptive/somatic	Afferent A delta and C fibers
Nociceptive/visceral	Solid or hollow organs
Sympathetic	After a nerve or limb injury, diffuse burning, allodynia, hyperpathia, sudomotor dysfunction, impaired blood flow
Neuropathic	Sharp lancelike pain

Nociceptive pain: Arises from stimulation of specific pain receptors that can respond to heat, cold, vibration, stretch, and chemical stimuli released from damaged cells and responds well to opioid treatment. An example would include pain experienced in an abrasion.

Somatic: Musculoskeletal system, sharp and well-localized pain, can often be reproduced; for example, pelvic floor dysfunction.

Visceral: Internal organs of main body cavities are usually dull and vague in location and radiating away from the affected organ. Chronic pancreatitis falls into this type.

Nonnociceptive pain: Arises from within the peripheral and central nervous system with no specific receptors existing. Pain is specifically generated by the nerve cell dysfunction and responds less to opioid, and more to antidepressants, anticonvulsants, *N*-methyl-D-aspartate (NMDA) antagonists, and topical capsaicin.

Neuropathic: From within nerve typified by hypersensitivity, tingling, numbness, weakness, burning, shooting. Diabetic neuropathy or lumbar radiculopathy are typical examples.

Sympathetic: Overactive sympathetic nervous system. Chronic regional pain syndrome is a prime example. In addition, pain mechanisms can overlap, and patients may present with complicated overlapping pain. Viscerosomatic convergence (referred pain from the viscera) is based on a principle that visceral innervations that converge terminally in the spinal cord at the same level as overlying somatic structures make it difficult to distinguish between somatic and visceral origins of "referred pain" (see Table 31.5 for categories of pain and their description).[38,39]

MEDICAL TREATMENT

As the causes of pelvic pain can be quite varied, the treatment modalities can also vary. Different genres of medications approach the treatment of pelvic pain using different mechanisms, and, in addition, combination therapy may provide synergistic analgesic options to contribute to the success of pain management control for another subset of the CPP population. As with any diagnosis and treatment in patient care, medical treatment must combine an art and science of medicine, as well as a balance of efficacy, and patient satisfaction, with appropriate side effect profiling.

NONSTEROIDAL ANTIINFLAMMATORY DRUGS

NSAIDs (i.e., ibuprofen and naproxen) have been frequently used for pain control in CPP. These medications inhibit the release of prostaglandins via cyclooxygenase (COX) inhibition, and have been implicated as inflammatory mediators in the pathophysiology of common etiologies of CPP such as dysmenorrhea and endometriosis. There are several consensus statements recommending their use as part of an empiric pain regimen, and they may also be useful at the initiation of a workup.[40–43] Their use is limited by patient comorbidities, drug interactions, and contraindications. For example, NSAIDs should be avoided in patients with clotting or platelet dysfunction, peptic ulcer disease, or renal insufficiency.

ACETAMINOPHEN

Acetaminophen is an antipyretic with a central mechanism of analgesia. While it is reasonable to use with mild pain, there is a paucity evidence supporting its use in CPP, and support is largely anecdotal.[42,44]

OPIOIDS

Opioids are a common therapeutic modality in pain medicine; however, they have many side effects including nausea, vomiting, respiratory depression, tolerance, and a high potential for abuse. Opioids have little evidence for use in chronic pain. When possible, narcotics should be avoided and all other treatments should have been tried and failed.[45–47] Opioids are likely to be beneficial for specific populations such as palliative and acute pain patients; thus, their discussion in this chapter is limited.

ORAL CONTRACEPTIVES, GONADOTROPIN-RELEASING HORMONE ANALOGUES, DANAZOL

Oral contraceptives (OCPs) such as estrogen and progesterone or progesterone only are indicated for both birth control, hormonal regulation, and for CPP. OCPs address cyclic pelvic pain related to ovulation, endometriosis, and premenstrual dysphoric disorder (PMDD). By using hormonal regulation to block ovulation, these etiologies of CPP can be treated, especially in conjunction with NSAIDs; however, several studies have reported progestin alone can result in over 80% reduction or resolution of endometriosis-associated pain.[45] OCPs may be advantageous given they can be continued indefinitely as opposed to most other hormonal interventions, and intrauterine devices (IUDs) have the added benefit of preserved bone density (with levonorgestrel in particular), a life span of up to 5 years, and a reduction in the regularity of menstruations.[48–50]

Use of gonadotropin-releasing hormone (GnRH) analogues result in ovarian suppression and a hypoestrogenic environment for the endometrial stroma, thus inhibiting inflammatory cascades associated with endometrial proliferation. GnRH analogues have been studied regarding endometriosis, one of the most common etiologies of CPP. Benefit in reduction of symptoms when compared to danazol and OCP was similar. There are some findings that show if used in conjunction with aromatase inhibitors, efficacy is increased.[51,52] GnRH analogues are still used as a second-line regimen due to side effects associated with ovarian suppression and higher incidence of CPP after termination of therapy.[40,48]

Danazol is an oral androgen, a derivative of 19-nortestosterone. It decreases the release of gonadotropins from the pituitary, thus blunting the luteinizing hormone surge and preventing endometrial proliferation in a similar way to GnRH agonists. Additionally, danazol functions to increase circulating levels of testosterone, which can lead to undesirable side effects. GnRH analogues have largely replaced its use due to a more favorable side-effect profile. In addition, its use is not recommended beyond 6 months.[41]

ANTIDEPRESSANTS

The role of antidepressants has been well supported in the treatment of chronic pain. As with other medications used in CPP treatment, these agents provide not only analgesia, but other potential psychological mechanism for the treatment of chronic pain.

The analgesic effect of antidepressants are thought to be mediated by inhibition of serotonin (5HT) and norepinephrine (NE) reuptake, leading to increased tone of descending inhibitory spinal pathways with concomitant decrease in ascending nociceptive transmission.[53–57] The pathophysiology behind these mechanisms is still not fully elucidated. It is unclear whether an increase in 5HT or NE is the dominant force behind analgesia. Recent studies show that tricyclic antidepressants (TCAs) and venlafaxine (a 5HT and NE reuptake inhibitor, serotonin–norepinephrine reuptake inhibitor [SNRI]) are equally efficacious; however, there is limited evidence for the efficacy of selective serotonin reuptake inhibitors (SSRIs).[54,58–61] These agents may also augment effects of opioid analgesics.[62] While research does exist showing the role of TCAs in neuropathic pain, there is a lack of research specifically demonstrating its role in CPP.[42] Given that most of the research focuses on neuropathic pain rather than anatomic location or particular etiology, these findings are likely generalizable. The analgesic effect occurs in the absence of depression, at doses lower than those used for depression, and with an earlier onset (i.e., within one week) than that required for an antidepressant effect, suggesting that the mechanisms are different.[53,54]

The following question has been raised: Is there a difference in the analgesic efficacy of antidepressants on the depressed versus the nondepressed population? Trials have addressed depression as a confounding factor through multiple studies. In fact, when using antidepressants for analgesic-oriented trials, depressed patients have been excluded and results have still shown a robust analgesic effect. On the other hand, trials that include depressed patients rarely, if ever, show a higher response rate in depressed patients. Analysis suggests that 50%–90% of the observed improvement in pain is due to a direct analgesic effect rather than an indirect effect of improving mood.[53–57]

Multiple mechanisms may explain some overlap between chronic pain and depression. 5HT and NE play an important role in both disorders. For depression, drugs that act on 5HT or NE alone are equally effective. For pain, drugs using both 5HT and NE are superior to selective agents. A bidirectional relationship between chronic pain and depression does exist, and most evidence supports that chronic pain leads to depression. The latter plays little role in the responsiveness to pain processing and response to pharmacologic therapy.[53–57] Tramadol and tapentadol, opioid agonists with 5HT and NE reuptake inhibition, respectively, show promise especially given the recent findings of monoamine systems in analgesia; however, these agents are too new to make formal recommendations.[42]

ANTICONVULSANTS

Originally synthesized in 1960 by chemist Walter Schindler in Basel, Switzerland, carbamazepine (CBZ) became the prototypic antiepileptic. It was first marketed as a drug to treat trigeminal neuralgia in 1962 and was later approved as an anticonvulsant in 1965. Noted similarities in the pathophysiology of epilepsy and neuropathic pain models justified the use of anticonvulsant drugs in the symptomatic management of neuropathic pain disorders as early as the 1960s.[55,56]

CBZ changes the conductance of sodium ions. While evidence for its role in neuropathic pain exists, this agent has largely fallen out of favor for newer drugs with less severe side-effect profiles.[63,64] The most recent systematic review on this topic has questioned the efficacy of CBZ in neuropathic pain.[56]

More recently, the gamma-aminobutyric acid (GABA) analogues gabapentin (Neurontin) and pregabalin (Lyrica), which modulate voltage gated calcium channels, have been systematically reviewed and found to be effective for neuropathic pain.[42,65] Gabapentin is well tolerated, easily titratable, has fewer interactions than CBZ, has a favorable side-effect profile, and is considered an excellent treatment for neuropathic pain. A study in 2005 provided a comparative prospective randomized controlled trial over 2 years, comparing gabapentin to amitriptyline and to combination therapy. Results from this trial showed that gabapentin alone or in combination with amitriptyline is better than amitriptyline alone in the treatment of female CPP using visual analogue scores as a primary outcome. This evidence has been reconfirmed in a recent Cochrane Review.[66,67] Side effects were also lower in the group with anticonvulsants alone.[67] New evidence posits gabapentin may have increased efficacy if used in conjunction with donepezil (Aricept).[68,69]

Recently, a 2010 systematic review of anticonvulsant therapy does not indicate that anticonvulsants can be considered an evidence-based first-line therapy for pain syndromes outside of trigeminal neuralgia.[70] Surprisingly, the Cochrane Collaboration recently retracted this article; however, the most recent version still upholds this conclusion.[56] Anticonvulsant therapy may be appropriately withheld until other interventions have been tried.[42,56,71]

Other anticonvulsant agents, for example, lamotrigine, oxcarbazepine, topiramate, lacosamide, clonazepam, phenytoin, and valproate, have also been investigated with little benefit noted.[56]

PROMISING THERAPIES

Randomized controlled trials have been performed to evaluate the efficacy of other potential medical therapies in CPP. Overall, the literature is limited but promising with many new potential interventions on the horizon.

Ziconotide is an N-type calcium channel inhibitor derived from conotoxin, a peptide produced by the snail *Conus Magnus*. It is a novel agent that prevents the release of substance P and other nociceptive mediators.[72] It was recently approved for intrathecal administration in the management of chronic pain. EMA401 is a competitive antagonist of the angiotensin 2 type 2 receptor, a site known to mediate nociception with a role in neuropathic pain. It is currently in phase II clinical trials for its role in chronic pain.[73,74] The $Na_v1.7$ channel is a sodium channel known to be present in nociceptive neurons. They are not found in the myocardium or central nervous system (CNS); thus, their potential safety margin is much higher than traditional local anesthetics. In addition, several selective $Na_v1.7$ blockers are in phase II clinical development including funapide, raxatrigine, and ralfinamide.[75–77] These agents show clear evidence of efficacy in chronic pain, and may have a role in CPP; however, this specific indication has yet to be explored.

Tanezumab is a monoclonal antibody directed against nerve growth factor developed as a pain adjunct. It has undergone phase II trials, specifically investigating its use in CPP conditions. One trial investigating its role in chronic abacterial prostatitis will need a larger population to demonstrate efficacy, but preliminary evidence is promising. A second study looking at interstitial cystitis was terminated early due to safety concerns; however, several phase III trials have been completed, showing its safety profile in patients with arthritis. This agent is an exciting possibility given its potential role specific to CPP.[78,79]

PROCEDURAL PAIN MEDICINE

INTERVENTIONAL PROCEDURES

Procedures may be performed for diagnostic and therapeutic reasons. Unfortunately, diagnostic nerve blocks can be difficult to interpret as confounders are common. Thus, it is important to have a clear sense of the anatomical directed therapy used (Table 31.6).

TABLE 31.6 Treatment Modalities

Pelvic Organs	Spinal Innervation	Sympathetic and Peripheral Nerves
Fallopian tubes, superior portion of uterine segment, ureters and bladder, appendix, broad ligament, proximal large bowel	T9–T12, L1	Celiac plexus, hypogastric plexus
Abdominal wall	T12–L1, L1–L2	Ilioinguinal, genitofemoral
Inferior portion of uterine segment, ureters and bladder, superior vagina, distal colon, rectum, uterosacral ligaments	S2–S4	Inferior hypogastric plexus, inguinal, genitofemoral
Lower vagina, vulva, perineum	S2–S4	Ganglion of impar, pudendal, genitofemoral, inguinal

Temporary but consistent responses to nerve blocks may lead to more permanent procedures such as pulsed radiofrequency neuromodulation or neurolytic nerve blocks if pain lasts. Usually, these more permanent procedures are indicated more towards cancer pain. A simplified version that can be used for directed interventional therapy is seen in the algorithm below ordered by level of invasiveness (Fig. 31.1).

As with any intervention, it is essential that appropriate attention is given to safety and sterility and that a skilled support staff and appropriate monitoring and resuscitation equipment are available. The use of block needles, nerve location devices, and imaging (i.e., X-ray image intensifier, ultrasound, or computerized tomography) appropriate for the procedure is essential.[42]

Trigger Point Injections

Myofacial pelvic pain (MFPP) is common and may contribute 14%–78% of the incidence of CPP.[21,80,81] Trigger point injections show promise as effective techniques for myofascial pain: local anesthetics, saline, botulinum toxin A (botox), and even dry needling have been employed.[82] Some applications include levator ani trigger point injections in CPP with positive results.[83] Trigger point injections have also been tried in chronic prostatitis with promising results; however, the literature lacks power.[84] Trigger point injections pose several challenges including success rates dependent on clinical experience, notoriously difficult referred pain patterns making physical diagnosis challenging, and MFPP being commonly overlooked by first-line health care providers.[21] Additionally, trigger point interventions have also been associated with causing pain and voiding symptoms and a nidus for neurogenic bladder inflammation for patients with interstitial cystitis and urethral syndromes.[85,86]

One particularly active area of researching utilizing trigger points is investigating botulinum toxin A. The role of Botox in health care is publicly known for its use

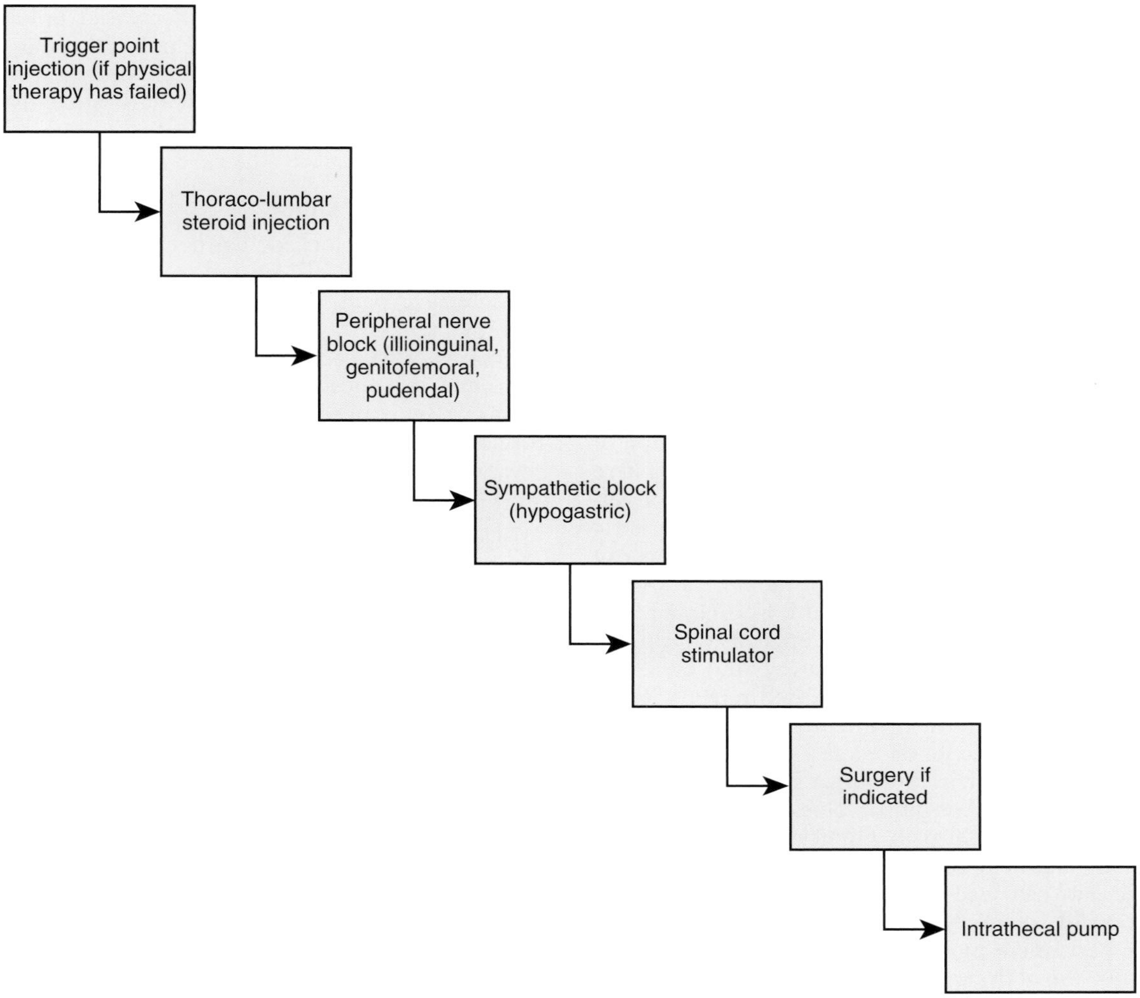

FIG. 31.1 Interventional pain algorithm.

in cosmetic medicine; however, Botox is also useful as an effective chronic pain medicine. For example, a pilot study demonstrated that Botox effectively treats CPP and associated spasm of pelvic floor muscles in women.[87] Several meta-analyses have investigated its efficacy with some showing positive results, while the majority of meta-analyses report limited data and too much heterogeneity for formal recommendations.[88–91] In a study comparing Botox and bupivacaine trigger point injections for myofascial pain treatment, both treatments had similar rates of success compared to placebo; however, it should be noted that bupivacaine remains a more cost-effective treatment. Currently, Botox remains an off-label use for the treatment of CPP; however, this indication is currently being assessed for US Food and Drug Administration (FDA) approval.[92]

Epidural Steriod and Facet Joint Injections

Epidural steroid injections (ESI) and facet joint injections are targeted therapy procedures used as dermatomal-directed therapy, especially in radiculopathy. Caudal epidural interventions are particularly relevant in CPP. Similar to MFPP, radiculopathatic pain is often overlooked and confused with entities such as interstitial cystitis and urinary dysfunction.[86] Evidence for the use of this modality lacks large-scale randomized controlled trials (RCTs); however, case studies and small RCTs do report its success.[86,93,94] Larger studies are needed to increase the power of these conclusions, and similar injections with local anesthetic serve as powerful diagnostic tools if radiculopathic CPP is suspected.

Peripheral Nerve Blocks

As with epidural blocks and facet arthropathy, local anesthetic injections into peripheral nerves serve as a diagnostic tool for CPP by identifying the specific innervation. Nerve blocks are well described in the acute pain setting; however, their role in chronic pain is an active field of research that has only recently yielded positive results in major systematic reviews, and even so, most data on specific nerve blocks exists in smaller trials or case reports.[95,96] Specific nerve blocks are listed below with evidence for suggested uses.

Ilioinguinal/iliohypogastric/genitofemoral blocks: May be useful in the management of CPP and have been described in the literature with respect to persistent postoperative pain, and perineal neuralgia.[95–99]

Pudendal nerve blocks and infiltration: May be useful in the management of endometriosis, pelvic adhesions, pudendal neuralgia, and chronic prostatitis. There is a new generation of RCTs showing efficacy for this particular indication.[100–106]

Caudal/sacral nerve: Caudal blocks have been known to be efficacious in interstitial cystitis.[107] On the whole, local anesthetic injections into the caudal space have not been tested for CPP, and there is a lack of evidence for this indication to make formal recommendations.

Sympathetic Blocks and Neuroablation

Neuroablation of sympathetic nerves can be performed by using different techniques, including thermocoagulation (radiofrequency ablation), cryoablation, or injection of chemical agents (alcohol, hypertonic saline, phenol). There are several anatomical sympathetic sites with clinical relevance to CPP, namely, lumbar sympathetic, hypogastric plexus, and ganglion impar blocks. Hypogastric plexus can be subdivided into superior and inferior plexus. The superior plexus is located retroperitoneally at L3–S1 close to the sacrum and iliac vein bifurcation. The inferior hypogastric plexus is located in the presacral tissues ventral to S2–S4 vertebrae.[108] The ganglion impar is located retroperitoneally where the lumbrosacral sympathetic chains end (slightly below the sacro-coccygeal junction) and supplies the distal-most structures of the pelvis.[108] Lumbar sympathetic, hypogastric plexus, and ganglion impar blocks performed by a well-trained interventional pain physician may aid in the diagnosis and treatment of CPP. However, complications are possible and can lead to further painful dysfunction, including possible neuroma formation, neuritis, deafferentation pain, permanent motor and sensory losses, hypotension, diarrhea, sexual dysfunction, and incontinence.[109]

Lumbar sympathetic blocks: May be helpful in the management of chronic cancer pain and possibly a range of pelvic pain conditions with afferents that pass via the L2–L4 levels; however, there is almost no literature regarding outcomes in CPP.[110,111]

Superior Hypogastric Plexus Block

In 1990, Plancarte et al. showed that superior hypogastric plexus block (SHPB) provided a 70% decrease of pelvic pain in patients with cervical, prostate, or testicular cancer without complications.[112] More recently, additional support for the technique was demonstrated in patients with cancer-related pelvic pain using a long-lasting neurolytic blockade that provided relief of pain in 69% of patients.[113,114] Endometriosis and refractory penile pain have been evaluated, and percutaneous catheters have also been successful.[108,115–117] SHPBs should be considered as an adjunctive therapy and not first line.[108,118–120]

Inferior Hypogastric Plexus Block

Inferior hypogastric plexus block (IHPB) may offer analgesic overlap to areas not effectively covered by SHPBs. The inferior hypogastric plexus innervates the lower pelvic organs and has been shown to decrease CPP.[114,121] Sahar et al. demonstrated markedly decreased opioid requirements and pain scores in cancer patients using a neuroablative block.[122] This is a newer technique first described in 2007, and the community is just starting to investigate its efficacy in CPP.

Ganglion Impar Block

Ganglion impar blockade has been tested for several indications including CPP related to tenesmus, perineal pain, pelvic cancer pain, coccygodynia, and proctitis.[123–125] For example, several case reports show successful use in treating coccygodynia and pelvic cancer.[126–129] One RCT demonstrated its efficacy in chronic perineal pain; however, larger trials are needed.[125] The large majority of the literature are case reports, and to our knowledge, no systematic reviews have been performed.

NEUROMODULATION AND SPINAL CORD STIMULATION

Spinal cord stimulators (SCS) were approved in 1989 for their use in chronic pain. SCS are known to decrease average visual analogue scale (VAS) scores, disability indices, and opioid use. Efficacy has been validated by systematic reviews including use in CPP.[130] Indications such as chronic regional pain syndrome (CRPS), radiculopathy, testicular pain, urge incontinence, urinary retention, interstitial cystitis, and cancer pain have been explored.[131–135] This modality involves the placement of leads into the epidural space with electrical stimulation. Trial is on an outpatient basis with no surgery involved; thus, it is reversible. Those for whom trial stimulation is effective can consider more permanent implantation. While this is a minimally invasive procedure far down the pain algorithm, relatively high complication rates are reported (30%–40%), and while these are mostly minor complications, revisions and explanations can greatly affect cost and patient perception.[135]

The best location for SCS lead placement underscores a recently debated topic. There have been several reports that high lead placement for CPP (as high as T6) may be more efficacious.[136–139] A potential explanation for this effect may be that visceral pain fibers do not follow a dermatomal pattern and that higher placements may inhibit a greater proportion of these fibers. Specifically, sacral fibers entering the dorsal columns are medial relative to nerves entering rostrally. Since sacral fibers are the most medial nerves at any point of the dorsal column system, it follows that they can be stimulated at any point along their progression. Theoretically, the higher placement of electrodes would permit sacral stimulation as well as any missed fibers contributing to CPP above this level.[137]

Neuromodulation

Neuromodulation for pain disorders and functional disease of the urinary tract have become a well-accepted concept. Pudendal nerve modulation is a technique that can be attempted when sacral nerve modulation fails; however, it is only practiced at a few institutions around the world, and only recently has standardization been published.[4] There is a lack of large-scale trials evaluating the efficacy of sacral root modulation; however, several smaller studies exist. Most of these trials show significant and long-lasting effects from this treatment; however, larger clinical trials are needed.

TRANSCUTANEOUS ELECTRICAL NERVE STIMULATION

The transcutaneous electrical nerve stimulation (TENS) unit is a pulse generator with an amplifier and electrodes used to deliver continuous or varying duration of electrical nerve stimulation to relieve pain. The stimulation causes myelinated afferents to activate segmental inhibitory circuits with a cumulative effect.[42] Induction time can be cumulative and typical recommendations include 30 minutes to 2 hours twice a day depending on the severity of the pain. Usually, the patient controls a modulated frequency between 0 and 100 Hz for pain control.[140] A Cochrane review from 2008 looking at the effect of the TENS unit on chronic pain found no evidence for or against their use, which is a finding dually noted on several other meta-analyses.[141,142] Additionally, it underlined that most of the studies are fraught with underpowered results and lack methodologic rigor; with almost none specifically looking at CPP.[143] However, since that time, several RCTs investigating CPP have been published, which show dramatic improvement in pain scores and quality of life measures.[13,144,145] The next major systematic review will likely shed more light on this topic.

INTRATHECAL PUMP

Intrathecal pumps are last-line intervention after both medical and surgical interventions have failed.[146] There are few studies available regarding CPP even though its use is widespread, and it is not a solution for the nonpalliative patient.[147,148] Only three agents have been approved for this indication including morphine, baclofen, and ziconotide. Long-term use is associated with complications, namely infection (2.4%–7%) and granuloma formation.[149,150]

SURGICAL TECHNIQUES

Typically, patients elect to have surgery when there is a failure of medical treatment, contraindications to medical treatment, need for definitive diagnosis, exclusion of malignancy, and treatment of infertility with respect to CPP.

DIAGNOSTIC LAPAROSCOPY AND HYSTERECTOMY

Diagnostic laparoscopy is useful in identifying pathology associated with endometriosis, pelvic adhesions, and PCS. Several studies have confirmed the efficacy of diagnostic laparoscopy in endometriosis with improved pain scores and fertility, especially in patients with severe disease.[151–153] One study showed that diagnostic laparoscopy identified pathology in 58% of women with normal pervaginal findings and may be useful for detecting endometriosis, adhesions, and pelvic congestion.[154,155] Approximately 67% of women treated laparoscopically for pain with documented endometriosis note an improvement in pelvic pain that lasted for 1 year.[156] However, surgical interventions frequently fail to diagnose, for example, patients who undergo laparoscopy. Clinical diagnosis findings include endometriosis and adhesions in two-thirds of the cases, and no pathology is noted in the remaining third.[22] More invasive surgery such as a hysterectomy may be warranted in patients who have failed conservative regimens and have extensive endometrial implants. Recurrence can still occur, and up to 25% of women may have no response; however, pain outcomes have been documented with up to 86%–61% having positive outcomes (pain completely gone or greatly improved) with this technique, especially with deep nodules.[20,157] With respect to adhesions, laparoscopic adhesiolysis has been investigated and several RCTs support its use.[158,159] A Cochrane review from 2000 also shows benefit in patients with extensive disease.[31] Laparoscopic ligation in pelvic congestion is gaining popularity, but evidence remains anecdotal.[31,160]

ROBOTIC SURGERY

Robotic surgery offers a new method to surgically address CPP. One recent systematic review found four articles showing that outcomes with robotic procedures are as effective as conventional laparoscopy; however, three of the studies were case reports. Consequently, more research is required to make conclusions.[161] In addition, newer evidence suggests that robotic surgery may be faster than traditional laparoscopy with less blood loss and lower pain scores.[162]

PRESACRAL NEURECTOMY

Presacral neurectomy is the surgical removal of the presacral nerves lying within the boundaries of the interiliac triangle, and this procedure is performed laparoscopically.[163] Several studies report reduction in analgesic use, pain scores, and improved sexual function, and reduction is largely recognized as a treatment for CPP.[164–168] One RCT using robotic surgery reported a 73% reduction in pain.[169] In patients with endometriosis, laparoscopic removal of lesions alone versus endometrioma removal combined with presecral neurectomy demonstrated a 20% higher success rate in treating chronic pain in the latter group; thus, this intervention may be a powerful adjunct.[170] Potential risks include injury to the vena cavae, iliac arteries, chylous acites, back pain, and urine retention; however, complications remain rare.[156,168]

LAPAROSCOPIC UTERINE NERVE ABLATION

Doyle et al. first described dissection of uterosacral ligaments from the cervix with the intention of treating CPP in 1955.[171] In 1994, Sutton et al. completed a randomized, prospective study in which 62% of patients undergoing laparoscopic uterine nerve ablation (LUNA) therapy had relief of symptoms compared to 23% of nonsurgical controls.[152] These findings have been questioned; at least four major systematic reviews and several RCTs have shown inconclusive evidence for its use.[31,170,172–174] This may be because CPP originates from several nerve plexuses with anatomical and physiologic overlap; thus, LUNA may not address all the innervations associated.[172] Considering surgical complications such as urethral or venous injury, LUNA is likely not an ideal treatment in CPP.

ALTERNATIVE/COMPLEMENTARY PAIN MEDICINE

As with all therapies for pain syndromes, our solutions for CPP must be shaped by a multimodal oriented model. In addition to medicinal and interventional treatment, complementary medicine and supportive care must be included in management. Complementary and alternative therapies are growing in popularity and are used by more than a third of the US population.[162,175] For example, psychological therapy, behavioral relaxation, relaxation training, massage, therapeutic heat, ice, electrical stimulation, vitamins, and herbal medications have been used.

PSYCHOLOGICAL THERAPY

Psychotherapy can be incorporated as a multidisciplinary approach to CPP by helping with coping strategies, increasing perceived control, and decreasing catastrophizing; although in most studies, the effect is minimal.[176,177] Additionally, this modality is often underutilized both by clinicians and patients. A Cochrane Review from 2007 demonstrated that behavioral therapy may have some effect on dysmenorrhea, although the study sizes and quality were marginal.[178] Meditation has also shown promise in patients with CPP.[179] Finally, biofeedback, a mind-body technique that utilizes a monitoring machine to give patient information about bodily function (e.g., muscular reeducation) has been used to treat CPP with success.[180–182]

HERBAL THERAPY AND VITAMINS

Herbal therapies and vitamins have been attempted in CPP with most studies showing no benefit. For example, there is insufficient data to recommend any herbal and dietary therapies for the treatment of primary and secondary dysmenorrhea.[48,183,184] Saw palmetto extracts have not achieved statistically significant relief in three RCTs in CPP.[185–187] Several barriers exist for these types of studies, namely the medications are not manufactured in a consistent manner, and ingredients may vary. There are some interesting caveats; for example, thiamine 100 mg for 90 days in 556 patients resulted in an 87% cure rate up to 2 months post treatment in dysmenorrhea.[188,189]

ACUPUNCTURE

Acupuncture is an adjuvant therapy used by more than 2 million people annually in the United States alone.[190] Acupuncture originated in traditional Chinese medicine using a series of sterile needles in acupoints mapped by meridians and channels.[14] The precise mechanism of analgesia remains unknown; however, it likely involves release of endorphins and monoamines with evidence of sustained depression in spinal cord dorsal horn neurons as well as treating trigger points (akin to dry needling).[14,140,191,192] A prospective study of 32,000 consultations with doctors and physiotherapists in 2001 revealed minimal adverse effects of acupuncture.[193] Acupuncture has shown application for many etiologies of CPP including dysmenorrhea, pelvic pain during pregnancy, chronic prostatitis, and pelvic venous congestion.[140,194–197] At the same time, it has been demonstrated that both patient expectation and practitioner behavior can result in greater placebo analgesia.[175,198–200] In fact, some have postulated that acupuncture may have a "placebo-enhancing effect."[175,199,200] Thus, clear studies have not found acupuncture to have enough strong evidence for clear efficacy, and more remains to be explored in the realm of quality acupuncture analgesic assessment.[175]

OTHER MODALITIES

New alternative modalities are constantly being tested. Topical heat at 38.9°C for 12 hours/day has been shown to be equally as effective as ibuprofen in patients with CPP related to primary dysmenorrhea.[188] Additionally, yoga has been investigated with positive results for dysmenorrhea.[201] Pelvic floor massage in patients with CPP has been found to be effective.[85,202] Interest in the field continues to grow, and it is important that clinicians do not ignore the potential efficacy of many of these treatments.

CONCLUSION: WHY MULTIDISCIPLINARY?

A multidisciplinary team represents both the referral basis and the combined perspective for sources of pain and sources of treatment approaches. Gynecologists, psychologists, physiotherapists, urogynecologists, gastroenterologists, neurologists, physiatrists, social workers, internal medicine physicians, general surgeons, and pain medicine physicians are all involved in caring for these patients. It is a multidisciplinary assessment with multimodal combination therapies including medicinal, procedural, and complementary techniques that can allow further success in analgesia for chronic pain sufferers.[42,203] As there is a wide variety of causes of pelvic pain, the treatments can range from tricyclic antidepressants, anticonvulsants, NSAIDs, and opioids to trigger point injections, nerve blocks, SCS, surgical options, and adjuvant treatments. It is this wide range of approaches and synergistic unions of these approaches that may further help many CPP patients.

KEY POINTS

- CPP is a relatively common problem affecting 2%–25% of women and 3.2% of men. It imposes a significant economic, psychosomatic, and quality of life burden on patients.
- Many etiologies of CPP exist (see Tables 31.1 and 31.2), and the pathophysiology is as varied as the differential diagnosis. There are some general theories, namely, the vascular hypothesis which states that CPP can be caused by states of dysregulation of ovarian hormone cycle, leading to vascular reactivity and pelvic venous congestion. Another hypothesis purports a rewiring of stimuli processing with alterations in signal processing in the spinal cord with visceral afferents that may undergo a change similar to nociceptors in states such as CRPS.

- Diagnosis of CPP can be difficult due to nonspecific symptoms that require a careful history and physical. The practitioner should be well versed in specific maneuvers such as a forced Faber test, and he or she should be careful not to ignore psychosomatic components of the history, as many patients have high rates of sexual abuse and depression (see Tables 31.3 and 31.4).
- Medical therapy should be prioritized according to the interventional pain algorithm (see Figure 31.1). NSAIDs and acetaminophen are generally accepted adjuncts in CPP; however, evidence remains largely anecdotal. Opioids should be reserved for cancer patients and highly selected patients. OCPs, GnRH analogues, and danazol have all been utilized with success especially in patients with cyclic pelvic pain related to ovulation and endometriosis.
- TCAs have been a well-supported treatment in chronic pain; however, their evidence is not specific to CPP. It is reasonable to utilize these agents, as they may offer both help for patients with psychosomatic components of pain and directly interfering with nociceptive transmission. Antiepileptic agents such as gabapentin and pregabalin have sufficient evidence for their use in neuropathic pain, with several studies specific to CPP, but they are second-line agents.
- Interventional techniques for treating CPP are further down the pain algorithm (see Fig. 31.1). Trigger point injections are controversial in CPP, as they have a high rate of complications. Epidural steroid injections and facet joint injections have a paucity of literature regarding their role in CPP, and more RCTs are warranted. Facet joint injections may have a significant role in the diagnosis of radiculopathic pelvic pain.
- Peripheral nerve blocks and stimulators including ilioinguinal, iliohypogastric, genitofemoral, pudendal, caudal, sacral, lumbar sympathetic, hypogastric plexus, and ganglion impar blocks have been tried; however, there remains a lack of literature with more RCTs needed to prove their efficacy.
- Surgical techniques such as diagnostic laparoscopy can help to identify the pathology of CPP and lead to an effective treatment. More aggressive therapy may be warranted in patients who have failed conservative therapy including hysterectomy, robotic surgery, adhesiolysis, and presacral neurectomy, which have all been shown to be effective; however, recurrence of CPP symptoms is not unusual. LUNA has a high complication profile and should be avoided.

REFERENCES

Access the reference list online at ExpertConsult.com.

CHAPTER 32

Painful Peripheral Neuropathies

Sarah A. Endrizzi, MD ◎ James P. Rathmell, MD ◎ Robert W. Hurley, MD, PhD

Neuropathy is a general term used to describe disease of nerve function and structures. Neuropathies arise from many different etiologies (diabetic peripheral neuropathy [DPN], postherpetic neuropathy [PHN], chemotherapy-induced peripheral neuropathy [CIPN], human immunodeficiency virus [HIV] neuropathy, neuropathy of chronic renal failure, idiopathic small fiber neuropathy, and complex regional pain syndrome [CRPS] type II), and can be painful or painless. They can affect the central nervous system (CNS), the peripheral nervous system, or both simultaneously. Neuropathy most often results from systemic disease, but can also arise from physical injury, inherited genetic disorders, infection, or autoimmune disorders. Neuropathies can affect solely a single nerve, termed mononeuropathy, or several separate nerves, termed polyneuropathy. Cranial nerves can also be involved, though less frequently.

Pain is considered a normal, adaptive, or physiologic response when it results from nociceptors (pain receptors) having been activated by tissue disease or damage—termed nociceptive pain. On the contrary, neuropathic pain arises from spontaneous activity within the nervous system, or an aberrant response to "normal" sensory stimulation (e.g., light touch evoking pain). Neuropathic pain is very common in the outpatient setting and second only to musculoskeletal pain.[1]

This chapter presents a brief overview of the evaluation of patients with painful peripheral neuropathy, describes an approach to the differential diagnosis of these disorders, and outlines the therapeutic modalities that may be useful in treating patients with neuropathic pain. The main disease process focused upon will be DPN.

TERMINOLOGY AND CLASSIFICATION

Neuropathy is a disturbance of function or pathological change in a nerve. Mononeuropathy reflects changes in a single nerve. Mononeuropathy multiplex reflects changes in multiple single, discrete nerves. Polyneuropathy reflects changes in sensation in a diffuse, often bilateral, pattern that is not restricted to discrete nerves. Neuritis is a subtype of neuropathy wherein an inflammatory process causes nerve injury. Cases of neurapraxia, including a blow, stretch, or epileptic discharge, are not considered neuropathy. The term *neurogenic* is intended to define "temporary" perturbations in nerve function.

Neuropathic pain, originally defined as pain initiated or caused by a primary lesion or dysfunction in the nervous system, has been revised to now include "pain arising as direct consequence of a lesion or disease affecting the somatosensory system."[2,3] The International Association for the Study of Pain adopted a slightly modified definition: "pain caused by a lesion or disease of the somatosensory nervous system."

As there lacks a clear and specific diagnostic tool to diagnose neuropathic pain and differentiate it from the other major categories of persistent pain, a grading system was also incorporated within the definition. Neuropathic pain can be graded as "possible," "probable," or "definite," based on clinical suspicion. Neuropathic pain can result from multiple causes, and it can be categorized according to the site of initial injury (CNS, peripheral nervous system, or mixed) and the condition causing disease (Table 32.1).[4] Injury to the nervous system that results in persistent pain can occur anywhere from the peripheral nerve terminal to the cerebral cortex. Despite the differing locations and the myriad of underlying causes for injury, patients with neuropathic pain often share similar sensations (Table 32.2).[5]

EPIDEMIOLOGY

Neuropathic pain affects approximately 6.9%–10% of the general population.[6,7] This condition results in substantial physical and social disability. The estimated direct cost associated with the treatment of neuropathic pain in the United States ranged from $1600 to $7000 per patient per year.[8,9] It affects the patient's mood, activities of daily living, quality of life, and work performance. As a result, these conditions result in substantial direct costs to the health care system but also indirect costs resulting from use of the health care system for the associated problems that are a result of the pain. These patients generate health care costs that are three times higher than matched controls.[10]

MECHANISMS OF NEUROPATHIC PAIN

Although several mechanisms are thought to be responsible for the development of neuropathic pain, injury to the afferent pathways appears to be a requirement for the development of neuropathic pain.[11] The mechanism of pain appears to be distinct from the causative disease, and many diseases may cause neuropathic pain by the same mechanism. A patient may also experience pain as a result of more than one mechanism.[12] These mechanisms include changes in ion channel number and density, resulting in central and peripheral sensitization, cortical reorganization and disinhibition of neuronal circuitry, and cellular and molecular changes as a result of the immune response following the initial nerve damage. The sympathetic nervous system is also thought to play a role in maintaining neuropathic pain.[13]

PERIPHERAL

Following trauma to a nerve, sodium channels accumulate in a higher than normal concentration around the area of injury and along the entire axon, resulting in

TABLE 32.1 Common Conditions Causing Neuropathic Pain Syndromes

Etiology	Terminology	Peripheral Versus Central Nervous System Etiology
Physical Injury/Trauma		
	Complex regional pain syndrome (CRPS), type I (reflex sympathetic dystrophy or RSD)	Mixed?
	Complex regional pain syndrome (CRPS), type II (causalgia)	Mixed?
	Radiculopathy	Peripheral > central
	Stroke (cerebrovascular accident)	Central
	Spinal cord injury	Central
Inherited/Genetic		
	Charcot-Marie-Tooth	Mixed
	Fabry's disease	
Infections/Autoimmune		
	Human immunodeficiency virus	Peripheral
	Herpes simplex virus	Peripheral > central
	Acute inflammatory demyelinating polyneuropathy	Mixed
Systemic Disease		
	Diabetes mellitus	Peripheral
	Kidney disorders/renal failure	Peripheral > Central
	Vitamin deficiencies (beriberi, alcoholic pellagra, vitamin B12 deficiency)	Mixed
	Vascular disorders	Peripheral > central
	Chemical toxins (isoniazid, chemotherapy agents [platinum, vinca alkaloids, taxanes], arsenic, thallium)	Mixed
	Hypothyroidism	Peripheral
	Amyloidosis	Mixed
	Multiple myeloma	Mixed

hypersensitivity of the nerve and ectopic foci. This is often the basis for the use of sodium channel blockers and membrane stabilizers in neuropathic pain.[14] It has also been suggested that nerve injury can result in the release of neuropeptides that might further cause peripheral sensitization through neurogenic inflammation.[2] Nerve injury can also result in the sprouting of sympathetic fibers into the dorsal root ganglia of the affected nerve. In partially injured nerves, the uninjured fibers may increase expression of alpha-adrenoreceptors. In both of these circumstances, sympathetically mediated pain may occur. This pain can often be blocked, at least temporarily, by the application of sympathetic blocks or by the administration of systemic alpha-adrenoreceptor antagonists (phentolamine).[2] More

TABLE 32.2 Abnormal Sensations of Neuropathic Pain

Paresthesias: abnormal nonpainful sensations that may be spontaneous or evoked (tingling)

Dysesthesias: abnormal pain that may be spontaneous or evoked (unpleasant tingling)

Hyperpathia: an exaggerated painful response evoked by a noxious or nonnoxious stimulus

Allodynia: a painful response to a normally nonnoxious stimulus (e.g., light touch is perceived as burning pain)

Hyperalgesia: an exaggerated painful response to a normally noxious stimulus

Spontaneous pain: painful sensation with no apparent external stimulation

recently, attention has focused on not only changes in the neuronal pathway following nerve damage, but also the complex interplay of neuronal support cells, including Schwann cells, satellite cells in the dorsal root ganglia, spinal microglia, astrocytes, and components of the peripheral immune system. Processes in this interaction could contribute to the development and presence of neuropathic pain.[15] Another proposed but poorly documented mechanism is that of ephaptic transmission—peripheral nerve injury resulting in "cross-circuiting" of peripheral fibers. In theory, sympathetic efferents would be able to activate nociceptive afferent fibers, explaining spontaneous pain and worsening of pain with activation of the sympathetic nervous system in some patients with neuropathic pain. However, there is little evidence to support this long-standing theory.[16]

CENTRAL

The CNS undergoes changes with peripheral nerve injury. In fact, this mechanism may be a primary one in those conditions where peripheral neuropathy results in reduced input to the CNS (postherpetic neuralgia, diabetic neuropathy). In diabetic neuropathy, there is little evidence that peripheral sensitization (as might be seen with increased sodium channels or with ephaptic transmission) occurs; rather, the evidence points toward reduced neural input to the CNS.[17]

Several potential mechanisms exist for a central contribution to the pain from peripheral neuropathy. Loss of large fiber (Aβ) sensory input could result in a reduction in nonnociceptive sensory input, thereby reducing the effectiveness of the "gate," as proposed by Wall and Melzack.[18] In experimental models of nerve injury, opioid and gamma-aminobutyric acid (GABA) receptors (both involved in inhibition of nociceptive transmission in the CNS) are downregulated, and the amount of GABA in the dorsal horn is reduced. Another mechanism suggests death of dorsal horn interneurons in lamina II (many of which are involved in the inhibition of nociceptive transmission in the dorsal horn) by overexposure to excitatory amino acids (EAA). Cholecystokinin, involved in opioid receptor inhibition, has also been found to be upregulated in the spinal cord following experimental nerve injury.[2] The net effect of these changes in the spinal cord results in "disinhibition" of nociceptive transmission, thereby creating an imbalance of painful over nonpainful impulses. These changes might also explain the relative opioid resistance seen in neuropathic pain.

A central mechanism that may explain the allodynia seen in some peripheral neuropathies involves Aβ fiber sprouting and Aβ fiber "phenotypic switching." Aβ fibers normally synapse in all lamina of the spinal cord except lamina II, where C fiber input predominates. However, following peripheral C fiber nerve injury, Aβ fiber "sprouting" into lamina II occurs, therefore allowing mechanical nonnociceptive input via the peripheral Aβ fibers to trigger second-order pain pathways. Aβ fibers in the dorsal horn also do not normally express substance P (as seen in C fibers), but following peripheral nerve injury, they can (phenotypic switching). When this happens, they thereby allow nonnociceptive input to trigger CNS nociceptive transmission.[2]

These mechanisms are likely far from complete in terms of explaining the changes in the CNS following peripheral nerve injury. It is very likely that significant changes also occur throughout the spinal cord, even in levels not directly involved with the peripheral injury, including the contralateral side, midbrain, and cerebral cortex.[19] The wide variability in how individuals respond to peripheral nerve injury is likely the result of genomic differences. Differences in the ability of Aβ fibers or sympathetic fibers to sprout, the amount of neuropeptide available for release peripherally, and the susceptibility of inhibitory interneurons to EAA in the dorsal horn are all likely to be highly variable between patients. This may explain why patients with the same condition (e.g., diabetic neuropathy) may or may not have pain.[2] Animal models of neuropathic nociception demonstrate notable differences between strains in their reaction to peripheral nerve injury and in their responsiveness to analgesics.[20]

EVALUATION OF THE PATIENT WITH NEUROPATHIC PAIN

When a patient presents with signs and symptoms suggestive of neuropathic pain—most frequently allodynia, hypoalgesia and/or hyperalgesia, and paresthesias—the first useful distinction to be made is the pattern of involvement. Focal lesions of peripheral nerves (mononeuropathies) result frequently from processes that produce localized damage and include nerve entrapment; mechanical injuries; thermal, electrical, or radiation injuries; vascular lesions; and neoplastic or infectious processes. In contrast, polyneuropathies often result in a bilateral and symmetric disturbance in function as a result of agents that act diffusely on the peripheral nervous system: toxic substances, deficiency states, metabolic disorders, and immune reactions. The diagnosis of painful polyneuropathy is most often made by history and standard neurologic examination. In some cases, ancillary studies may be needed to document the disease process.[17]

HISTORY

Pain is often the presenting symptom for polyneuropathy, but it rarely presents in the absence of other sensory abnormalities. In fact, most patients have an incongruous presentation of pain, as well as sensory deficits.[12] Many of the terms used to describe these abnormalities are listed in Table 32.2; paresthesias ("tingling" or "pins and needles" sensations) are particularly common. However, since the characteristics of neuropathic pain are almost always multiple (e.g., varying combinations of burning, stabbing, aching, etc.), they cannot be used as a useful guide to determine the etiology of the neuropathy.[17] The location of the pain and other symptoms is frequently the most important piece of historical information.

NEUROLOGIC EXAMINATION

In the patient suspected of having polyneuropathy, the clinician should focus on sensory evaluation. Strength and deep tendon reflexes are preserved in many patients with polyneuropathy. In addition to testing vibration, proprioception, and light touch, the sensory examination should include several special stimuli including light-touch rubbing, ice, single pinprick, and multiple pinpricks. Lightly stroking the affected area with a finger will assess for allodynia (pain provoked by nonnoxious stimuli), which has been shown to be present in 20% of patients with neuropathic pain (and higher in particular neuropathic pain states, such as postherpetic neuralgia).[21] Ice application will test for both temperature sensation and abnormal sensations such as pain and lingering after-sensations. Single pinprick testing may elicit a sensory deficit or hyperpathia (an exaggerated response to a normally painful stimulus). Repeated pinprick testing may elicit summation (pain growing more intense with subsequent stimuli) or lingering after sensations, both common findings in polyneuropathy.

ELECTRODIAGNOSTIC TESTING

Patients suspected of having polyneuropathy can be considered for electromyography (EMG) and nerve conduction velocity (NCV) studies, which may offer insights into whether the process is a demyelinating (reductions in nerve conduction velocities) or axonal (reductions in the amplitude of evoked responses) neuropathy. However, such differentiation rarely offers any change in therapy when managing neuropathic pain. These tests are best used to demonstrate large fiber involvement, but as many painful peripheral neuropathies involve small fibers, these tests may be completely normal in patients with painful polyneuropathy.[22] Quantitative sensory testing (QST) may be the most useful in the assessment and longitudinal monitoring of painful peripheral neuropathies. While large fibers are assessed through the use of sensory thresholds to vibration, small fibers can be assessed by threshold for detection of heat, painful heat, cold, and painful cold stimuli. Thermography has been found to have little role in the assessment, management, or tracking of painful peripheral neuropathies, despite much published literature on the method. The role of skin biopsies remains controversial[23]; however, it has been used to successfully diagnose loss of small peripheral nerve fibers such as nociceptive afferents.[24]

SCREENING TOOLS

There are several screening tools, including the Neuropathic Pain Questionnaire, the painDETECT Questionnaire, ID Pain and the Leeds Assessment of Neuropathic Symptoms and Signs that evaluate patient's description of their pain to differentiate neuropathic pain from nonneuropathic pain. Diagnostic accuracy appears to be highest when these screening tools are used in conjunction with the physical exam.[25]

DIFFERENTIAL DIAGNOSIS

After assembling the historical information, neurologic examination, and results of electrodiagnostic studies, the underlying etiology will most often be readily apparent. Neuropathic pain is often a result of polyneuropathy.[23]

METABOLIC CAUSES OF PERIPHERAL POLYNEUROPATHY—DIABETES

The reported frequency of neuropathy in patients with diabetes mellitus ranges from 4% to 8% at the time of initial presentation, and rises to 15%–50% after 20–25 years of follow-up.[26] Other studies report an incidence of neuropathy (not necessarily painful) of up to 66%, but clearly the likelihood of neuropathy increases with the duration of the disease.[27] The incidence of painful neuropathy was reported in one study to average about 11.6% in insulin-dependent diabetes mellitus (IDDM) and 32.1% in noninsulin-dependent diabetes mellitus (NIDDM).[28] The cause of diabetic neuropathy has not been determined with certainty.[29] Current hypotheses focus on the possibilities of metabolic and ischemic nerve injury.[30] Hyperglycemia may lead to oxidative stress, which in turn decreases the functioning of proteins in the peripheral nerves and can lead to cell death.[30,31] Pathologic examination of nerves taken from diabetic patients has shown evidence of microvascular disease supporting the ischemic nerve theory. Metabolic abnormalities include (1) accumulation of sorbitol in diabetic nerve as excess glucose is converted to sorbitol by the enzyme aldose-reductase, (2) auto-oxidation of glucose resulting in reactive oxygen molecules, and (3) inappropriate activation of protein kinase C.[32] Other theories suggest that impaired nerve regeneration may contribute to the polyneuropathy in diabetes, as demonstrated in animal models of nerve injury.[33]

Therapeutic strategies aimed at reducing sorbitol accumulation (aldose-reductase inhibitors) have demonstrated only minor improvements in neuropathy. There is strong evidence, however, that good glycemic control can prevent the appearance and worsening of polyneuropathy in patients with both IDDM and NIDDM. A major trial found that the incidence of neuropathy was reduced by 60% over a 5-year period with aggressive glycemic control.[34]

Diabetic neuropathy can be divided by the pattern of distribution of involved nerves (Table 32.3). The most common form of diabetic neuropathy is distal symmetric polyneuropathy. It is predominantly a sensory disturbance. Patients often present with gradual onset of paresthesias and pain in the legs and feet. Symptoms begin in the toes and gradually ascend over months to years to involve more proximal levels. The fingertips and hands become involved later, usually when symptoms in the lower extremities have ascended to the knee level. Allodynia and burning pain are common and are often worse at night. Examination shows graded distal sensory loss predominantly affecting vibration and position sensation. Reflexes may be diminished or absent. Electrophysiologic testing shows a decrease in the amplitude of evoked responses to a greater degree than reduction in nerve conduction velocities as the neuropathy progresses.[2] This reflects primarily axonal damage rather than demyelination. Severe sensory loss may allow repeated trauma to go unnoticed, resulting in the development of foot ulcers and diabetic neuroarthropathy (Charcot's joints). This last condition is critical to identify in the diabetic patient with a unilateral, painful, swollen foot.

TABLE 32.3 Classification of Neuropathies Associated With Diabetes Mellitus

Mononeuropathy	Cranial mononeuropathy
	Compression mononeuropathy
Mononeuropathy multiplex	Proximal motor neuropathy
	Truncal neuropathy
Polyneuropathy	Distal symmetric polyneuropathy
	Painful diabetic neuropathy
	Autonomic polyneuropathy

The syndrome of acute painful diabetic neuropathy may also occur in diabetics.[35] This uncommon disorder is characterized by the rapid onset of severe pain in the distal lower extremities characterized by constant burning in the feet, dysesthesia, allodynia, and lancinating leg pains. Examination shows little or no sensory loss with preserved reflexes. Electrophysiologic testing shows decreased amplitude or absent sensory potentials, but may also be normal. This type of neuropathy often remits within a year after blood sugars are controlled.

Autonomic neuropathy manifestation by abnormalities in tests of autonomic function occurs in 20%–40% of diabetics.[35,36] Symptomatic autonomic neuropathy most often occurs as a component of distal symmetric polyneuropathy. Autonomic nervous system abnormalities include postural hypotension, impaired heart rate control (resting tachycardia and fixed heart rate), esophageal dysmotility, gastroparesis, and erectile dysfunction.

Lower extremity proximal motor neuropathy is an uncommon painful disorder associated with diabetes. It is characterized by acute or subacute onset of moderate to marked weakness and wasting of the pelvifemoral muscles, accompanied by back, hip, and thigh pain, with preserved sensation in the regions of pain. The condition may be painless or accompanied by pain described as a constant, severe, deep ache. Complete recovery occurs in 60% of patients over 12–24 months.

Diabetic lumbosacral radiculoplexus neuropathy (DLRPN) is sometimes referred to as diabetic amyotrophy, proximal diabetic neuropathy, diabetic polyradiculopathy, Bruns–Garland syndrome, or diabetic lumbar plexopathy. It usually affects individuals with diabetes mellitus type II over the age of 50 years, and presents as an asymmetric weakness associated with pain in the legs that appears subacutely and progresses over weeks to months. Although motor function recovery is slow and often incomplete, the pain usually resolves.[36] Both microvascular inflammation and autoimmune mechanisms have been proposed, with no one clear treatment plan being particularly effective.[37]

Diabetic truncal neuropathy involves acute or gradual onset of unilateral pain in the chest or abdomen and may mimic myocardial infarction, intraabdominal pathology, or spinal disorders.[38] Examination shows marked allodynia and hyperpathia in the distribution of pain. Truncal neuropathy occurs most often in long-standing diabetics and those over the age of 50 years. EMG typically demonstrates denervation in the abdominal or intercostal musculature.

Cranial mononeuropathies involving the oculomotor, abducens, trochlear, and facial nerves may occur in diabetic patients.[39] The most common of these is oculomotor neuropathy that is manifested as ophthalmoplegia and ptosis. The eye is deviated laterally and has impaired movement vertically and medially. Pain occurs in 50% of patients and may precede ophthalmoplegia by several days.

Entrapment neuropathies are believed to occur more frequently in patients with diabetes mellitus.[35] Carpal tunnel syndrome is believed to occur more than twice as frequently as in the nondiabetic population. This association must be kept in mind when evaluating the diabetic patient with an isolated peripheral mononeuropathy.

OTHER METABOLIC CAUSES OF PAINFUL PERIPHERAL NEUROPATHY

Metabolic causes other than diabetes mellitus (and excluding postherpetic neuralgia) are uncommon.

Amyloidosis is a disease caused by extracellular deposition of amyloid, a fibrous protein. Amyloidosis can be primary, familial, or associated with other conditions such as multiple myeloma, chronic infectious or inflammatory states, aging, and long-term hemodialysis. The biochemical composition of the amyloid protein varies with the associated disease state. Deep aching and occasional shooting pains, distal sensory loss, and autonomic and motor involvement characterize painful peripheral neuropathy in amyloidosis.[35] As the neuropathy progresses, all modalities are affected, reflexes are lost, and there is motor involvement. Treatment of neuropathy associated with amyloidosis is aimed at the underlying condition when such is identifiable.

Multiple myeloma is due to malignant plasma cell growth. Painful neuropathy can appear in myeloma with or without amyloid deposition. The neuropathy is extremely variable in severity and rate of progression, ranging from a mild, predominantly sensory neuropathy to a complete tetraplegia.[40] Pain in myeloma often declines with successful treatment using chemotherapy, radiation therapy (especially for isolated plasmocytomas), or plasmapheresis.

Patients with untreated hypothyroidism may also develop painful sensorimotor neuropathy.[40] This uncommon disorder may present with long-standing pain in either the hands or the feet, accompanied by weakness in the distal limb musculature. The neuropathy often resolves with successful replacement of thyroid hormone.[40]

NUTRITIONAL CAUSES OF PERIPHERAL POLYNEUROPATHY

Thiamine deficiency is seen in alcoholics, chronic dialysis patients, and people on restrictive diets. Thiamine deficiency appears to lead to beriberi, which consists of heart failure, vasodilatation, and peripheral neuropathy. Hand, foot, and calf pains with allodynia, decreased sensation, and motor involvement characterize the neuropathy. Administration of thiamine may reduce the symptoms of neuropathy, including pain.

The incidence of neuropathy in chronic alcoholism is about 9%.[40] Alcoholic neuropathy is characterized by motor and sensory deficits, often accompanied by pain.[40] The pain consists of aching in the legs or feet with intermittent lancinating pains. The upper limbs are rarely involved. Burning of the soles and allodynia may also occur. Alcoholic neuropathy occurs only after chronic and severe alcohol abuse and is invariably accompanied by severe nutritional deficiency. Pathologically, alcoholic neuropathy cannot be distinguished from beriberi, and both likely result from thiamine deficiency. Treatment consists of abstinence and thiamine supplementation.[40]

Pellagra is caused by niacin deficiency and is rarely seen in developed countries. Signs and symptoms include dermatitis, gastrointestinal (GI) complaints, neurasthenia, and spinal cord dysfunction. Pellagra is associated with a mixed, painful polyneuropathy, similar to that seen with beriberi. A predominant feature of the sensorimotor neuropathy is spontaneous pain in the feet and lower legs, with tenderness of the calf muscles and cutaneous hyperesthesia of the feet. Treatment of pellagra with niacin often results in resolution of all symptoms, except peripheral neuropathy.[40]

TOXIC CAUSES OF PERIPHERAL POLYNEUROPATHY

Isoniazid is a frequently used antitubercular drug. Chronic administration in individuals with slow metabolism of the drug (slow acetylators) is associated with the development of painful neuropathy.[13] Initial symptoms of distal numbness and tingling paresthesias are later accompanied by pain, which may be felt as a deep ache or burning. The calf muscles are painful and tender, and walking often aggravates symptoms. Symptoms may be particularly troublesome at night. Prophylactic coadministration of pyridoxine (vitamin B6) prevents development of neuropathy; however, it is not therapeutic once the neuropathy develops.

The most common neurologic complication of cancer treatment is CIPN. CIPN is a common adverse effect of treatment with platinum-derived, taxane and vinca alkaloid chemotherapeutic compounds.[41] These chemotherapeutic agents exert their cytotoxic effect by binding to DNA and producing interstrand and intrastrand cross-linkage, thus impairing DNA synthesis and transcription. These agents are first-line chemotherapeutic agents in the treatment of solid tumors. Although penetration into the CNS is relatively poor, high levels of this drug are found in dorsal root ganglia and peripheral nerves.[42] The development of CIPN is the most common reason a platinum-based chemotherapy regimen is changed to another agent, administered at a lower dose, or given in fewer or less frequent cycles of therapy.[43] This change in therapy represents a deviation from the optimal life-extending therapy. Symptoms of CIPN, therefore, may directly increase morbidity and indirectly mortality. The earliest manifestations of neuropathy are decreased vibration sense in the toes and loss of ankle jerk reflexes. At larger doses, paresthesias may appear and progress to severe dysesthesias. The neuropathy is reversible, but recovery may take more than a year after discontinuation of the agent.

Other toxic agents that can potentially cause neuropathy include acrylamide, arsenic, dinitrophenol, and pentachlorophenol (pesticides).[12]

GENETIC CAUSES OF PERIPHERAL POLYNEUROPATHY

The most common type of inherited neuropathic disorders is Charcot-Marie-Tooth disease (CMT), a group of disorders that affect peripheral nerves. CMT is subdivided into demyelinating and axonal forms, depending on EMG conduction studies. Common symptoms in CMT include lower extremity motor symptoms (foot deformity, difficulty ambulating), hyporeflexia, and sensory loss.

Other rare genetic neuropathies are included in the hereditary sensory and autonomic neuropathy (HSAN) category that, depending on the subtype, appear in the second to third decades of life and manifest with decreased sensation in the feet and distal legs, leaving patients prone to ulcer formation often leading to cellulitis and osteomyelitis, and distal hereditary motor neuropathies (dHMNS) that typically present with length-dependent weakness and no sensory loss. Except for supportive treatment including orthotics, orthopedic interventions (e.g., for scoliosis, foot deformity) and pain management, there is no specific treatment for dHMNS.[44]

Ion channels are responsible for the detection and transmission of painful stimuli. The voltage-gated sodium channels (Na_v) are essential in determining the excitability of the nociceptors. There are multiple HSAN conditions resulting from variations of voltage-gated sodium channels, four of which ($Na_v1.3$, 1.7, 1.8, and 1.9) are known to be involved in propagating painful signals.[45] Mutations of the genes that code these channels result in variable pain perception ranging from congenital insensitivity (null mutation of $Na_v1.7$ or heterozygous activation of $Na_v1.9$) to persistent burning pain (heterozygous activation of $Na_v1.8$) to paroxysmal extreme pain disorder (heterozygous activation of $Na_v1.7$). Erythromelalgia is an example of a channelopathy that results in severe burning and erythema of the hands and feet, exacerbated by heat, exercise, and prolonged standing. Most cases are isolated and primary, but about 5% of cases are familial, a result of mutation(s) in the gene that encodes the $Na_v1.7$ channel.[46]

INFECTIOUS AND INFLAMMATORY CAUSES OF PERIPHERAL POLYNEUROPATHY

In developing countries, infectious or postinfectious neuropathies are very frequent. Mycobacterium leprae, although quite uncommon in North America and Europe, is among the leading cause. It usually affects the skin and nerves, but there also exists a pure neural leprosy in about 4%–10%[43] of all leprosy cases. Symptoms are found primarily in the form of mononeuritis or mononeuritis multiplex.

Hepatitis C has also been linked to neuropathies, although here the clinical picture is varied, spanning from polyneuropathy to mononeuropathy (involving multiple or single nerves) to cranial neuropathy. Prevalence rates have been found as high as 10.6%. Borrelia burgdorferi has also rarely been associated with a chronic diffuse distal polyneuropathy, more frequent in North America than Europe.[47]

With the development and widespread use of highly active antiretroviral therapy (HAART) and the resulting decrease in opportunistic infections of the CNS, polyneuropathy has become the most prevalent neurological complication associated with HIV infection.[48] Although symptomatic neuropathy occurs in 10%–35% of those seropositive for HIV, pathologic abnormalities exist in almost all of those with end-stage AIDS.[49] There are numerous types of the HIV-associated neuropathy classified by onset, putative etiology, pathology of nerve damage, and motor or sensory involvement. The sensory neuropathies associated with HIV (HIV-SN) include distal sensory polyneuropathy (DSP), due to the viral infection, and antiretroviral toxic neuropathy (ATN), due to the medical treatment of the viral illness. DSP represents the more common of the two disorders. Although these HIV-SNs may represent two distinct entities,[50] the clinical syndrome and pathophysiologic manifestation of the two disorders are practically indistinguishable. The time course of the illness and temporal relation to the commencement of antiretroviral therapy represents the primary differentiating characteristic. The onset of DSP can occur in either the subacute or chronic phases, or following the development of an AIDS-defining illness. The clinical manifestation of ATN can appear within the first week to 6 months of the initiation of antiretroviral therapy and may subside after its cessation. The painful peripheral neuropathy results from both direct neuronal inflammatory injury to the nerve itself (DSP) and the treatment using HAART, particularly nucleoside analogue reverse transcriptase inhibitors (NRTIs), leading to mitochondrial dysfunction. The clinical features of HIV-SN are dominated by painful dysesthesia, allodynia, and hyperalgesia. Onset is often gradual and most commonly beginning with bilateral lower extremity involvement. The neuropathy progresses in a length-dependent fashion, with a worsening gradient of disease from distal structures to those more proximal. The dysesthesias commonly first involve the soles of the feet and progress proximally; when the symptoms encompass the dermatomes of the knee, the patient will often report finger involvement. The first symptoms noted are often numbness or burning sensation, following a diurnal cycle with the pain worse at night. Shortly thereafter, patients will report allodynia and hyperalgesia of the involved structures. As a result, wearing shoes and walking become painful, and the patient's gait becomes antalgic. There is minimal subjective or objective motor involvement, and this is generally limited to the intrinsic muscles of the foot. Physical examination shows a diminution or loss of ankle reflexes in addition to the sensory findings.

Reactivation of a latent infection of varicella zoster virus (human herpes virus-3) in the trigeminal ganglia or the dorsal root ganglia can result in facial or peripheral pain in the dermatomal distribution of the affected nerves. The resulting condition, herpes zoster or "shingles," can be excruciatingly painful and can result in a chronic pain condition called PHN. There are approximately 500,000 new cases per year of herpes zoster in the United States, and 9%–35% of these people develop PHN.[51] Advanced age, greater severity of the rash, and presence and severity of a painful prodrome preceding the rash are well-established risk factors for the development of PHN. The clinical presentation is most common in the thoracolumbar region, following a single or multiple dermatomes with a prodromal period, followed by the eruption of a maculopapular vesicular rash. The pain is most often described as burning, stabbing, and/or throbbing, and is commonly associated with cutaneous allodynia of the region. Primary prevention of herpes zoster and PHN was achieved in 51% and 66% of people who received the varicella vaccine.[52] Prevention of PHN in patients who had a herpes zoster reactivation was successful in those who received acyclovir. Patients who received amitriptyline within 90 days of rash onset had a reduced incidence of PHN from 35% to 16%.[53]

Acute inflammatory demyelinating polyradiculoneuropathy (AIDP) caused by Guillain-Barré syndrome is characterized by areflexic and ascending motor paralysis with sensory paresthesias. It is often preceded by an infection—generally an upper respiratory tract infection or gastroenteritis. Most frequently, if an agent is identified, EBV, CMV, *Mycoplasma pneumoniae*, and *Campylobacter jejuni* are found, although vaccines and other viruses have been also associated with GBS.[54] Other rare etiologies include tumors and certain toxins.[55] The onset of symptoms develops over several days—more frequently weeks. Pain is a common early symptom; weakness, usually in the legs, may progress to respiratory failure requiring mechanical ventilation. Sensory symptoms include paresthesias, often in the presence of decreased sensation in a glove-stocking distribution. Autonomic dysfunction is also commonly evidenced by tachycardia and orthostatic hypotension. Pain may occur in up to 80% of patients. The pain is principally an ache, strain, or deep burning sensation in the thigh or buttocks, and can be quite severe. While pain in AIDP may be severe, it is usually transient. Pain is usually worse at night. Nerve conduction studies and lumbar puncture aid the diagnosis. General therapy for AIDP is supportive along with plasmapheresis and IVIG. Glucocorticoids and other immunosuppressants have not been clearly shown to be helpful.

IDIOPATHIC SMALL-FIBER NEUROPATHY

This condition usually presents with painful feet in patients over the age of 60 years. Although most often classified as idiopathic, autoimmune mechanisms are largely suspected in those cases. While diabetes and the metabolic/genetic causes listed previously can cause small-fiber neuropathy, it can also be present in the absence of those conditions, and this state has been the subject of thorough review.[56] It can be defined as the presence of paresthesias (usually painful) with the absence of significant large-fiber dysfunction (atrophy, loss of vibratory sense, or loss of reflexes). Diagnosis is often confirmed through tests of autonomic function, QST, or skin biopsy.

TREATMENT OF NEUROPATHIC PAIN

There has been substantial research and development of treatment options over the past decades for patients suffering from neuropathic pain (Table 32.4). A variety of medications are currently available to the clinician, and there has been a continued increase in randomized, double-blind, and placebo-controlled trials evaluating them. Nonetheless, the effectiveness of even the best of these medications is often highly variable; side effects are common, analgesic effects are delayed, and dosing is complicated. Treatment recommendations are continuously evolving to keep pace with the newest therapy options.[57] Additionally, although evidence for the efficacy of various agents as compared with placebo is increasing, there is a lack of studies comparing various agents against one another and assessing utility of combination therapy. Furthermore, given the inconsistency and variability of most neuropathic conditions and the highly variable genomic contribution between patients, the conclusions from a study of one group of patients with neuropathy will likely not apply to another. Not only treating but also diagnosing and assessing neuropathic pain can often be challenging. Given that it often coexists with other types of pain related to its etiology (e.g., musculoskeletal dysfunction, orthopedic deformities), and that it can produce psychological and psychiatric sequelae ranging from sleep disturbances, to anxiety, to major depression and suicidal ideation, a multifactorial and often even multispecialty approach might be warranted. Clearly, some of the medications used to treat neuropathic pain might also bring symptomatic relief by alleviating cofactors (e.g., a tricyclic antidepressant for a patient suffering from neuropathic pain and depression).

The Special Interest Group on Neuropathic Pain (NeuPSIG) of the International Association for the Study of Pain recently published a meta-analysis of 229 randomized, double-blind studies, including nonpublished trials, of oral and topical medications used for neuropathic pain. They used the number needed to treat (NNT) to obtain 50% or greater pain relief as the primary outcome. The quality of each study was rated using Grading of Recommendations Assessment, Development, and Evaluation (GRADE). Results of the analysis were used to formulate new pharmacologic treatment recommendations. First-line medication recommendations included gabapentin, pregabalin, SNRIs, and TCAs. Second-line recommendations included capsaicin 8% patches, lidocaine patches, and tramadol. Third-line medications were botulinum toxin A (Botox) and opioids.[58] A more in-depth review of each of these categories of medications is discussed as follows.

One of the most thoroughly studied group of medications employed for the treatment of peripheral neuropathic pain are the antidepressants.[59] In this group, there are three major subgroups that have been studied: tricyclic antidepressants (TCAs), selective serotonin norepinephrine reuptake inhibitors (SNRIs), and selective serotonin reuptake inhibitors (SSRIs). There are no head-to-head studies to date concerning efficacy in peripheral neuropathy and neuropathic pain, but TCAs (amitriptyline, nortriptyline, desipramine,

TABLE 32.4 Medications Used to Treat Neuropathic Pain Conditions

Drug	Start Dose	Maximum Dose	Documented Effect	Side Effects
Gabapentin	100–300 mg/day	3600 mg/day	PHN, PDN, HIV, mixed neuropathic pain	Sedation, dizziness, edema
Pregabalin	50–150 mg/day	300 mg/day (600 mg/day fibromyalgia)	PHN, PDN, mixed neuropathic pain, fibromyalgia, central pain	Sedation, dizziness, edema
Tricyclic Antidepressants	10–25 mg/day	50–150 mg/day	PHN, PDN, central pain, mixed neuropathic pain	Cardiac, anticholinergic, sedation, mood changes
Nortriptyline Desipramine Doxepin				
Specific Serotonergic and Noradrenergic Reuptake Inhibitors				
Venlafaxine Duloxetine	37.5 mg/day 20 mg/day	225 mg/day 60 mg/day	PHN, PDN, fibromyalgia	Sedation/fatigue, nausea, sweating, sexual dysfunction, mood changes
Carbamazepine	200 mg/day	1200–1800 mg (1/3 higher dose for oxcarbazepine)	Trigeminal neuralgia	Sedation, dizziness, ataxia, blood dyscrasias
Tramadol	50–150 mg/day	400 mg/day	PHN, PDN	Sedation, dizziness, seizure
Lamotrigine	25 mg/day	400–600 mg/day	Trigeminal neuralgia, poststroke central pain, HIV	Sedation, tremor, rash
Opioids	5–10 mg/day; titrate and substitute with long-acting opioids	Variable, 100–200 mg (OME)/day	PHN, PDN, postamputation pain	Sedation, dizziness, constipation, tolerance, addiction, respiratory depression
Lidocaine patch	5%	3 patches/day	PHN, traumatic nerve injury	Allergic reaction
Capsaicin	0.025 and 0.075% (cream) or 8% (patch)		PHN, PDN, HIV	Allergic reaction
NMDA Inhibitors			CRPS	Sedation, confusion, hallucinations, GI upset, addiction
Ketamine Dextromethorphan Low-dose naltrexone	0.25 mg/kg PO or 10% topical 30 mg/day 1.5 mg/day	Titrate to effect by 0.25 mg/kg 90 mg/day 4.5 mg/day	CRPS, fibromyalgia	Vivid dreams
Botulinum toxin A	50–200 units q3 months		PHN, TN	Weakness, rash

CRPS, *Complex regional pain syndrome;* GI, *gastrointestinal;* HIV, *human immunodeficiency virus;* NMDA, *N-methyl-D-aspartate;* OME, *oral morphine equivalents;* PDN, *peripheral diabetic neuropathy;* PHN, *postherpetic neuralgia;* TN, *trigeminal neuralgia.*

imipramine) are the best studied and the most efficacious, followed by SNRIs (duloxetine, venlafaxine). SSRIs (citalopram, paroxetine) show a limited effect on neuropathic pain.[60,61] The side-effect profile of TCAs, primarily the anticholinergic effects, limits the widespread application of TCAs, especially in patients with autonomic neuropathy, glaucoma, cardiac arrhythmias, and urinary hesitation.

Anticonvulsants are also used very frequently and relatively successfully. Among these are gabapentin and pregabalin, structural analogs to GABA and agonists at the alpha-2-delta subunit of voltage-gated calcium channels. These, along with TCAs and SNRIs, are considered first-line agents, and are used in the treatment of a multitude of neuropathic pain syndromes, including radiculopathy, CRPS type II, diabetic neuropathy, postherpetic neuralgia, and mixed neuropathic pain conditions. Sedation, dizziness, GI complaints, and lower extremity edema are among the more frequently noted side effects. There is no evidence that shows that either gabapentin or pregabalin are more efficacious, and gabapentin is less costly.[60,62] Other antiepileptics such as topiramate, lamotrigine, lacosamide, and valproic acid have been shown to bring symptomatic relief, such as in HIV neuropathy (lamotrigine), painful diabetic neuropathy (lacosamide, topiramate), and postherpetic neuralgia (valproic acid), but these results were inconsistent and could not always be reproduced in subsequent studies. Levetiracetam, another anticonvulsant, has not been effective in the treatment of neuropathic pain.[63]

Topical agents that have shown improvement in neuropathic pain include lidocaine patches (postherpetic neuralgia, posttraumatic neuralgia) and high-concentration (8%) capsaicin creams (HIV neuropathy, postherpetic neuralgia).[64] Historically, neuropathic pain has been considered "opioid resistant."[65] But over the past years, this notion has been challenged as more evidence emerges, showing that opioids are potent treatment modalities for neuropathic pain. A 2013 Cochrane review of 31 trials that studied 10 different opioids for neuropathic pain showed improved pain scores by at least 33% in 57% of patients receiving opioids versus 34% receiving a placebo for a duration of less than 12 weeks. It was noted that most of the studies used methods associated with significant bias. There was a paucity of data regarding chronic, long-term use of opioids. In addition, there was a lack of evidence of any significant functional improvement in patients treated with opioids versus placebo.[66] Perhaps they would even be considered first-line agents if their usefulness were not limited by the many concerns that are associated with their application. The risk for accidental overdose, addictive properties, the development of tolerance, misuse and abuse, and significant side effects (including constipation and nausea) appropriately decrease the routine use of these medications for neuropathic pain. Additionally, there have been concerns that with long-term management for neuropathic patients, these patients could develop hypogonadism, paradoxical hyperalgesia, cardiac ischemia, osteopenia, and impairment of the immune system.[66]

Botulinum toxin A (Botox) has been suggested for the treatment of various neuropathic pain conditions, including trigeminal neuralgia, postherpetic neuralgia, and painful peripheral neuropathy. The NeuPSIG review looked at six RCTs evaluating the efficacy of Botox injected subcutaneously at the site of pain, with mixed results. Several small studies were positive, but one large study was negative. Therefore the group gave botulinum toxin a weak recommendation.[58]

NMDA antagonists have shown mixed results, with some evidence suggesting improvement in neuropathic pain, particularly phantom limb pain and postherpetic neuralgia with ketamine and polyneuropathy with dextromethorphan. Memantine has not been shown to be better than placebo in treating polyneuropathy, PHN, HIV neuropathy, or postamputation pain.[67]

At low doses (about 1/10 the dose used to treat opioid addiction), naltrexone may exert a paradoxical analgesic effect via its antiinflammatory effects. In addition to being a mu- and delta-opioid receptor antagonist, naltrexone is also an antagonist of TLR4 receptors found on microglia. In chronic pain states, such as fibromyalgia and CRPS, the microglia may be chronically activated, leading to an abundance of proinflammatory factors that may be neurotoxic. It is through blockade of the inflammatory cascade that low-dose naltrexone (LDN) is thought to exert its effects.[68]

Several studies have looked at different delivery systems of cannabis for treating neuropathic pain. Seven of the nine reviewed studies of nabiximols, a cannabinoid-based oral/mucosal spray, were negative for the primary outcome of 50% pain reduction in the NeuPSIG study. Cannabinoids were given a weak recommendation against use.[58] Another meta-analysis reviewed five RCTs that looked at inhaled cannabis for treatment of chronic neuropathic pain and showed an NNT for short-term reduction in neuropathic pain was similar to that of TCAs, SNRIs, and gabapentin (as described in other studies). However, the population size of these studies was small and the follow-up was very short (days to weeks).[69] As of December 2015, the prescription and consumption of medical marijuana was legal in 23 states and the District of Columbia, although federally illegal.[70]

Sympatholytic agents have been proposed for both the diagnosis and treatment of peripheral neuropathic pain, based on the concept of expression of alpha-adrenoreceptors in damaged peripheral nerves. Analgesic response to intravenous phentolamine infusion may be predictive of the response to regional sympathetic ganglion blockade[71]; however, this has fallen out of common practice due to high false positive rates and placebo response. The alpha-2-adrenergic agonist clonidine has been reported as a useful analgesic in treating neuropathic pain.[16]

Corticosteroids both systemically and by peripheral application have been used based on empirical response. When injected perineurally (but not systemically), corticosteroids reduce the spontaneous ectopic discharge rate seen in nerve injuries and neuromas, possibly by a membrane stabilizing effect. They also have been found to have a short-lasting suppressive effect on transmission in normal C fibers, but more recent studies on peripheral nerve injury models in the rat confirm that local application of steroid on the area of injured nerve may produce an analgesic effect by suppression of peripheral ectopic sites.[72]

Because there are currently no clinical markers to indicate which medication a particular patient may respond to best, a stepwise, combination approach is frequently used. One RCT found that the combination of nortriptyline and gabapentin was found to produce greater analgesia than either alone.[73] Importantly, these positive results were observed in patients receiving substantially lower doses of each medication than what is commonly used when they are administered as monotherapy. Patients receiving combination therapy received very good analgesia, while experiencing dramatically fewer side effects than those in monotherapy groups. Although, as the authors report, they did not have the appropriate design to establish drug-drug synergism, the results are highly supportive of a synergistic analgesic response. Other trials have shown that a combination of gabapentin or pregabalin and extended-release morphine and pregabalin and topical lidocaine is more efficacious than a single agent alone.[60,74]

Even with broad usage of the previously mentioned medications and treatment choices, there still remains a substantial number of patients—often cited to be greater than 50%—without significant relief of their neuropathic pain. In these circumstances, various alternative options exist, including sympathetic nerve blocks, neurolytic sympathetic blocks, spinal cord stimulation (SCS), deep brain stimulation (DBS), transcutaneous electrical nerve stimulation (TENS), and repetitive transcranial magnetic stimulation (rTMS). Because TENS and rTMS are noninvasive therapy options, the 2006 Task Force of the European Federation of Neurological Societies deemed them suitable as preliminary or add-on therapies.[75] Although more invasive options such as DBS does show benefit, given the extent of intervention needed, this method still requires more research prior to being adopted on a larger scale.[76] The use of SCS is well established in neuropathic pain conditions, including postlaminectomy syndrome, CRPS type I, and DPN.[77–80]

KEY POINTS

- Neuropathic pain arises from disorders of the peripheral nervous system. Although there are many etiologies of peripheral neuropathy, not all of which produce pain, the most prominent and common is diabetic neuropathy.

- Many mechanisms have been proposed for the pain that occurs in peripheral neuropathic states. They can be categorized into peripheral and central. Peripheral mechanisms proposed include formation of ectopic foci, formation of ephapses (unlikely), release of neuropeptides with neurogenic inflammation, and increased expression of alpha adrenoreceptors.
- Central mechanisms of neuropathic pain proposed include loss of large-fiber pain inhibition, downregulation of opioid and GABA receptors, reduction of GABA release, death of inhibitory interneurons, Aβ fiber sprouting, Aβ fiber phenotypic switching, and cholecystokinin upregulation.
- History and physical examination remains the mainstay in evaluating and following peripheral neuropathic pain. EMG provides evidence of large-fiber changes but rarely will alter therapeutic decisions, while QST may aid in diagnosing subtle aspects of peripheral neuropathy and allow monitoring for scientific study. Skin biopsy can be a useful diagnostic tool.
- Pain in diabetic neuropathy may have a strong central component, given that evidence supports a reduced sensory input in those patients suffering from pain. There are specific syndromes within the class of painful diabetic neuropathy that have profound components, which include rapid onset of symptoms and significant motor components. It is important in painful diabetic neuropathy not to overlook the development of Charcot's joints, which can also be painful and progress to significant deformity if not addressed.
- The treatment of neuropathic pain typically involves the use of antidepressants, anticonvulsants, topical agents, and opioids, often in combination. TCAs, SNRIs, gabapentin, and pregabalin are considered first-line agents and used in a multitude of neuropathic pain conditions. Opioids have been shown to be effective in a short time period (12 weeks or less), but efficacy with chronic use has not been demonstrated. Considering their side effect profile and potential for abuse and dependence, opioids should be used cautiously.
- SCS has been shown to be beneficial for patients with a variety of neuropathic pain syndromes. Sympathetic nerve blockade may also be useful in selected cases.

REFERENCES

Access the reference list online at ExpertConsult.com.

CHAPTER 33

ENTRAPMENT NEUROPATHIES

Sophy C. Zheng, MD ◎ Thomas H. Brannagan III, MD

Nerve entrapments can be a common cause of chronic pain, causing debilitating symptoms and loss of function. We discuss six of the most common entrapment neuropathies in detail: carpal tunnel syndrome (CTS), ulnar neuropathy at the elbow, thoracic outlet syndrome (TOC), meralgia paresthetica (MP), tarsal tunnel syndrome (TTS), and Morton's neuroma. Other entrapment neuropathies, such as peroneal palsy at the fibular head, may result in weakness or paresthesia but not pain. These and other neuropathies are summarized in Table 33.1.

Entrapment neuropathies frequently involve a specific nerve distribution, thus, a thorough understanding of anatomic location and function of the nerve is important for diagnosis. A careful history and physical examination will reveal specific sensory and motor deficits that help localize the site of entrapment. Further, electrodiagnostic (EDX) testing can be helpful to confirm diagnosis as well as characterize its severity and chronicity, lending insight to its prognosis. An EDX study has two components: a nerve conduction study (NCS) and electromyography (EMG). NCS is performed by stimulating a sensory or motor nerve and recording conduction velocity and evoked response amplitude as well as, for motor nerves, the distal motor latency. The degree of deficit also helps to gauge severity of the disease. EMG assesses the integrity of the muscle unit by evaluating its firing pattern with and without activation to further confirm neurologic deficit. The usefulness of EDX is variable depending on the specific entrapment discussed. In recent years, imaging has played an increasing role in diagnosis as well. Ultrasound, magnetic resonance imaging (MRI), as well as x-ray and computed tomography (CT) can help to visualize the lesion and identify external causes of entrapment.

Despite advances in diagnosis and increasing recognition of entrapment neuropathies, treatments have largely remained either conservative care or surgery. Conservative care includes a combination of activity modification, physical therapy, and oral analgesics, whereas surgical options are often resorted to in severe or refractory cases. Recently, localized steroid injection at the site of entrapment is now often tried before proceeding with surgery, providing increasing evidence to its efficacy. Our discussion here highlights some of the most common diagnoses and treatments for each of the six entrapment neuropathies. However, there is large variability in presentation and response to treatment. Both diagnosis and treatment must be individualized to achieve optimal results.

CARPAL TUNNEL SYNDROME

Carpal tunnel syndrome (CTS) is the most common and the most studied entrapment neuropathy. It may occur in as many as 1 in 10 people at some point in their lives and even more frequently in high-risk groups.[1]

PATHOLOGY

The syndrome refers to compression of the median nerve as it passes through a fibrous canal, called the carpal tunnel, located at the base of the hand. The tunnel is composed of the carpal or wrist bones at its base, the flexor retinaculum at the roof, the transverse carpal ligament, median nerve, and nine flexor tendons (Fig. 33.1).[2] Because of this crowded arrangement, any tenosynovial proliferation, fluid collection, or arthritic deformity can lead to median nerve compression. In controlled external compression of healthy volunteers, critical compression between 30 mm Hg and 60 mm Hg acutely affected nerve viability. This pressure may double with passive wrist flexion and triple with passive wrist extension of 90 degrees, especially in the proximal aspect of the wrist.[3] Functional experiments have suggested that ischemic injury also play a significant role by impeding blood flow and causing epineural ischemia.[4] At lower pressures, venous return may be reduced, resulting in venous stasis and intraneural edema.

RISK FACTORS

Occupations involving both increased impact and repetitive motion—such as food processing, carpentry, and roofing—pose the largest risks, with odds ratios greater than 4.[5] The risk from typing and computer work is also seen with a long exposure, or at least 12–20 hours a week of intensive work.[6,7] Similarly, patients with osteoarthritis or rheumatoid arthritis are about twice as likely to get CTS than those without.[8] However, there is an association between physiologic states such as pregnancy, menopause, and CTS, which can sometimes be acute, suggesting that hormonal components may play a role in altering the degree of edema in the tunnel.[9] Similarly, abnormal hormonal states such as hypothyroidism, diabetes mellitus, and obesity also pose a risk (up to 1.5–2 times greater) of developing CTS, correlating positively with the severity of disease.[2] The shape of the wrist can also be a risk factor for CTS. Square wrists—that is, those whose dorsal-volar distance is close to the mediolateral distance with a ratio greater than 0.7—are at increased risk for developing CTS. Perhaps this is why CTS is often present in both hands. It may also be the reason why many patients have a positive family history of CTS.

SYMPTOMS

Classically, patients report numbness or pain on the palmar surface of the thumb and on the index, middle, and half of the ring finger along distribution of the median nerve. However, in practice, reports of numbness often

TABLE 33.1 Major Nerves, Possible Sites of Entrapment, and Resulting Entrapment Syndromes With Eponyms

Nerve	Site of Entrapment	Syndrome
Upper Extremity		
Brachial plexus	Anterior and medial scalene muscle	Anterior scalene syndrome
	Subclavius muscle	Costoclavicular syndrome
	Pectoralis minor and coracoid process	Hyperabduction syndrome
	Cervical rib or band, medial antebrachial cutaneous nerve	Thoracic outlet syndrome
Long thoracic		"Rucksack" palsy
Suprascapular	Transverse scapular ligament, scapular notch or foramen	
	Spinoglenoid ligament or notch	
Musculocutaneous	Coracobrachialis muscle	
	Brachial fascia, lateral antebrachial cutaneous nerve	
Axillary	Quadrangular foramen or lateral axillary hiatus (long head of triceps, teres major and minor)	Quadrilateral space syndrome
Radial	Lateral intermuscular septum	"Saturday night" palsy, "honeymooners'" palsy
	Arcade of Frohse (supinator), leash of Henry (brachioradialis, extensor carpi radialis brevis), Monteggia lesion	Supinator syndrome, posterior interosseous syndrome, radial tunnel syndrome, tardy radial palsy, "tennis elbow," "Frisbee flinging"
	Superficial branch	Cheiralgia paresthetica, Wartenberg's disease, "handcuff" or "wristwatch" neuropathy
Median	Ligament of Struthers (supracondylar process: medial epicondyle)	
	Pronator teres muscle, sublimis bridge (flexor digitorum sublimis), lacertus fibrosis	Pronator syndrome, flexor digitorum sublimis syndrome
	Gantzer's muscle (flexor pollicis longus)	Anterior interosseous syndrome, Kiloh-Nevin syndrome
	Transverse carpal ligament	Carpal tunnel syndrome
	Transverse metacarpal ligament	Intermetacarpal tunnel syndrome, "bowlers' thumb"
Ulnar	Arcade of Struthers (internal brachial ligament, medial head of triceps, medial intermuscular septum)	
	Epicondylo-olecranon ligament, cubital tunnel retinaculum, arcuate ligament of Osborne	Cubital tunnel syndrome
	Humeroulnar aponeurosis (flexor carpi ulnaris)	"Tardy" ulnar palsy
	Deep flexor-pronator aponeurosis	—
	Guyon's canal (piso-hamate ligament, volar and transverse carpal ligament)	Ulnar tunnel syndrome, "cyclists'" palsy (*Radfahrerlahung)*
	Deep branch	Piso-hamate hiatus syndrome
	Transverse and oblique heads of adductor pollicis	
Lower Extremity		
T2–6 posterior rami		Notalgia paresthetica
L5 spinal	Iliolumbar ligament (fifth lumbar: wing of the ilium)	Lumbosacral tunnel syndrome
Ilioinguinal	Transverse abdominis muscle	
Genitofemoral	Inguinal canal	
Lateral femoral cutaneous	Inguinal ligament at anterior superior iliac spine	Meralgia paresthetica, Roth's meralgia, Bernhardt's syndrome
Femoral	Iliopectineal arch	Iliacus tunnel syndrome
	Hunter's canal (vastus medialis, adductor longus, sartorius), subsartorial canal	
	Infrapatellar branch of saphenous nerve	Gonyalgia paresthetica, "housemaid's knee"
Obturator	Obturator canal	Howship-Romberg syndrome
Sciatic	Pyriformis muscle	Pyriformis syndrome
	Greater and lesser sciatic foramens, sciatic notch, Gibraltar of the gluteus	
Common peroneal	Fibular neck, peroneus longus muscle	"Cross leg" palsy
	Crural fascia, superficial branch	
	Inferior external retinaculum (ligamentum cruciforme)	(Anterior) tarsal tunnel syndrome
Posterior tibial	Canal calcaneen de Richet (ligamentum laciniatum)	(Posterior) tarsal tunnel syndrome
	Medial plantar nerve	"Jogger's foot," abductor hallucis tunnel syndrome
	Medial plantar proper digital nerve	Joplin's neuroma
	Transverse metatarsal ligament	Morton's neuroma (metatarsalgia)

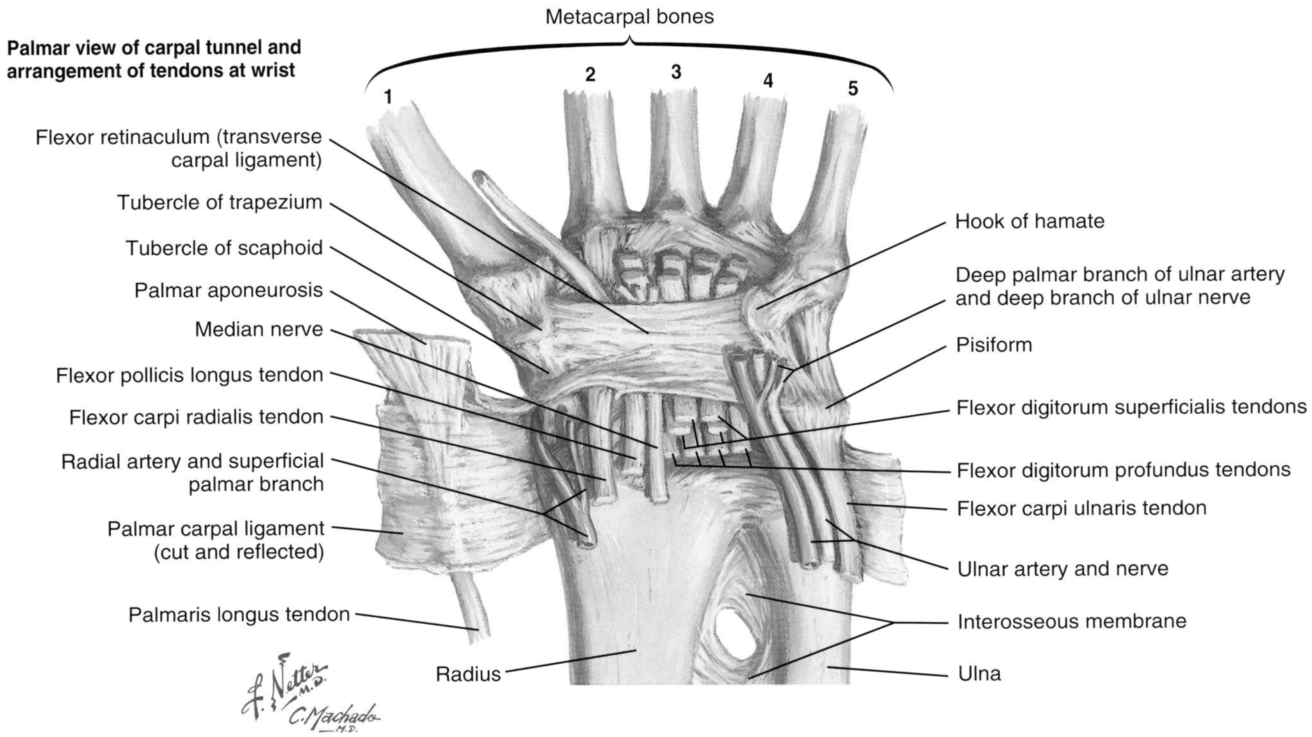

FIG. 33.1 Structures coursing through the carpal tunnel. (Netter medical illustration used with permission of Elsevier. All rights reserved.)

involve only a portion of the median distribution, especially the middle or index finger. The patient may initially report numbness of the entire hand, but when specifically asked to observe which fingers are involved, will observe that the fifth finger is spared. Pain can occur both distal and proximal to the site of compression, including the hand, wrist, elbow, and even shoulder. Symptoms initially present as paresthesia mostly at night or with activities that involve frequent flexion or extension of the hand, as while driving. As the syndrome progresses, patients can have increasing symptoms during the daytime and later weakness expressed by dropping items and difficulty in closing buttons or opening jar lids.

PHYSICAL FINDINGS

The median nerve supplies sensation to the palmar surface of the thumb and index, middle, and half of the ring finger. It also supplies the dorsal tips of these same fingers. However, sensation covered by the palmar branch of the median nerve, including proximal portion of the palm and thenar eminence, is preserved in CTS since it does not go through the carpal tunnel. Two-point discrimination and pinprick testing will often elicit sensory deficits in parts of the median sensory territory. Often, these deficits are noted only when direct comparisons are made with the unaffected hand.

Motor function affected by the median nerve includes five intrinsic hand muscles, as well as the abductor pollicis brevis, one of the easiest to test. To test the strength of the abductor pollicis brevis, the patient should place the thumb perpendicular to the plane of the hand and then resist as the examiner attempts to push the thumb into the plane of the hand. In most patients, weakness will be appreciated only when the result is compared with the unaffected hand or to the flexor pollicis longus muscle of the affected side.

Several provocative tests can further confirm CTS. Two of the most common of these are Phalen's and Tinel's tests. Phalen's test is carried out by placing the patient's wrist in hyperflexion or extension to elicit paresthesia or pain within 60 seconds. This test has sensitivity of 42%–85% and specificity of 55%–98% in various studies.[10] Tinel's test is done with the examiner's middle and index fingers or a reflex hammer gently percussing over the flexor retinaculum 6 times to elicit symptoms. This test has a sensitivity of 38%–100% and a specificity of 55%–100%. However, in one controlled comparison with healthy volunteers, Phalen's test was shown to have sensitivity and specificity of 88% and 89%, respectively, as opposed to 67% and 68% for Tinel's test.[10] The carpal compression test can further confirm CTS. With the patient's affected arm supinated, force is applied over the flexor retinaculum to elicit symptoms within 30 seconds. The tourniquet test can easily be done by applying a pneumatic compression cuff around the arm and inflating it to the patient's systolic blood pressure to elicit symptoms within 60 seconds. Lastly, the hand elevation test can easily compare symptoms on the affected versus unaffected hand by elevating both arms above the head to look for symptoms within 60 seconds. In one comparison study of the five maneuvers discussed, the combination of tourniquet test, carpal compression, and Phalen's test has the highest predictive value, whereas hand elevation provides the best means to rule out CTS.[11]

DIAGNOSTIC STUDIES

Electrodiagnostic (EDX) testing is very sensitive for confirming the diagnosis of CTS. Nerve conductions are especially helpful, having sensitivity and specificity reaching 80%–90% and 95%, respectively.[12] The hallmark of NCS includes decreased conduction velocity especially in digital nerves and across the wrist, with sensory fibers disproportionately affected more than motor fibers. EMG is more useful for excluding concurrent causes of pain, such as cervical radiculopathy or proximal median neuropathies, than in confirming the diagnosis of CTS.[12]

With advances in imaging technology, ultrasonography has grown in popularity as an additional aid in the diagnosis of CTS. Using a high-frequency probe, ultrasound can identify sites of compression with high accuracy. In a recent meta-analysis, ultrasonography was found to have a sensitivity of 78% and specificity of 87% for the diagnosis of CTS compared with clinical presentation.[13] It may be a helpful screening tool that may complement but not replace EDX studies.[14]

TREATMENT

The first line of treatment for CTS is splinting to maintain the wrist in a neutral position along with lifestyle modifications. Splints should be worn both day and night. Oral antiinflammatory treatments may provide relief for select patients. Steroid injection, especially done with ultrasound guidance, has been shown to be more effective than placebo, as well as antiinflammatory medications for reducing symptom severity and rate of surgery at 1 year. However, the majority of patients eventually proceed to surgery.[2] In refractory cases, surgical release is the next step. Surgical procedures can be done via traditional open techniques or endoscopically with no significant difference in outcome between the two methods.[15]

ULNAR NEUROPATHY AT THE ELBOW

Ulnar nerve entrapment at the elbow is the second most common neuropathy in the upper extremity. Entrapment can occur either at several locations within the elbow, with the classic compression occurring at the cubital tunnel.

PATHOLOGY

Ulnar nerve compression may be a result of intrinsic or extrinsic factors. Intrinsic factors contributing to compression include inherent anatomic structural abnormalities, pathologic lesions such as perineuroma, and congenital anomalies such as hamartoma of the nerve itself. External compression by muscle hypertrophy, hematoma or vascular lesions, or tendon proliferation often seen in inflammatory fibrosis are just some examples of extrinsic factors.[16] The ulnar nerve is particularly vulnerable to compression or stretch at the elbow owing to its complex course around multiple aponeuroses, at five common locations (Fig. 33.2). The nerve separates from the axillary artery in the distal arm to emerge on top of the medial head of the triceps. In 70% of the population, a thickened fascia called the arcade of Struthers lies over the nerve and is one source of compression.[16] The nerve then pierces the medial intermuscular septum, another source of compression, to course in the condylar groove between the medial epicondyle and olecranon. When the elbow is in the flexed position, the groove shallows, exposing the more superficial ulnar nerve to injury and creating the "the funny bone" sensation. Nonunion from previous lateral condylar fracture may result in cubitus varus or inward deviation of the forearm, causing "tardy ulnar palsy" or delayed ulnar compression.[17] The nerve then enters the cubital tunnel, a space surrounded medially by the medial epicondyle, laterally by the olecranon, and roofed by the arcuate (Osborne's) ligament, which extends distally to connect the ulnar and humeral heads of the flexor carpi ulnaris. Flexion commonly causes increased pressure in the tunnel, resulting in compression. Deficit in the hand occurs before deficit in the forearm muscle because, topographically, they are in the outer circumference of the nerve bundle.[18] As the nerve leaves the elbow, it pierces through the deep flexor pronator aponeurosis, the fifth potential point of compression.[19]

RISK FACTORS

Ulnar neuropathy at the elbow is aggravated by flexion of the elbow, which can result in both compression and traction of the nerve, leading to injury. This may occur with flexion of the elbow at night while sleeping, prolonged surgical procedures with poor positioning, bed-bound patients with limited mobility, or long flights during which a flexed elbow is pushed against the armrest for extended periods.[20] Certain activities—such as intense gripping while driving, frequent throwing motions by athletes, or work involving repetitive motion—may predispose to ulnar neuropathy either by direct compression or via joint or ligamentous inflammation.[20] Some patients are predisposed to injury. In one study, approximately 37% of the healthy volunteers exhibited hypermobility of the nerve within the condylar groove, increasing the risk of ulnar nerve irritation.[21] Acute elbow fracture or dislocation can also cause acute or delayed ulnar neuropathy.

SYMPTOMS

Symptoms of ulnar nerve entrapment typically start with numbness, tingling, and weakness in the hand in the distribution of the nerve covering the entire fifth digit and ulnar half of the fourth digit. Pain frequently occurs at night, when the elbow is flexed with or without pain radiating to the medial aspect of the elbow. Cramping of the hypothenar eminence may also be felt. In more severe cases, hand weakness, as loss of dexterity or general difficulty with good grip, may be reported. However, weakness without any paresthesia or pain should require further workup to rule out concurrent cervical radiculitis with myelopathy or signs of upper motor neuron disease.[20] Nerve compression can occur at a number of other locations, including the brachial plexus and the ulnar nerve at the wrist, to produce similar symptoms, the exact location can be differentiated based on the position that elicits symptoms. Entrapment at the elbow causes symptoms with elbow flexion, whereas

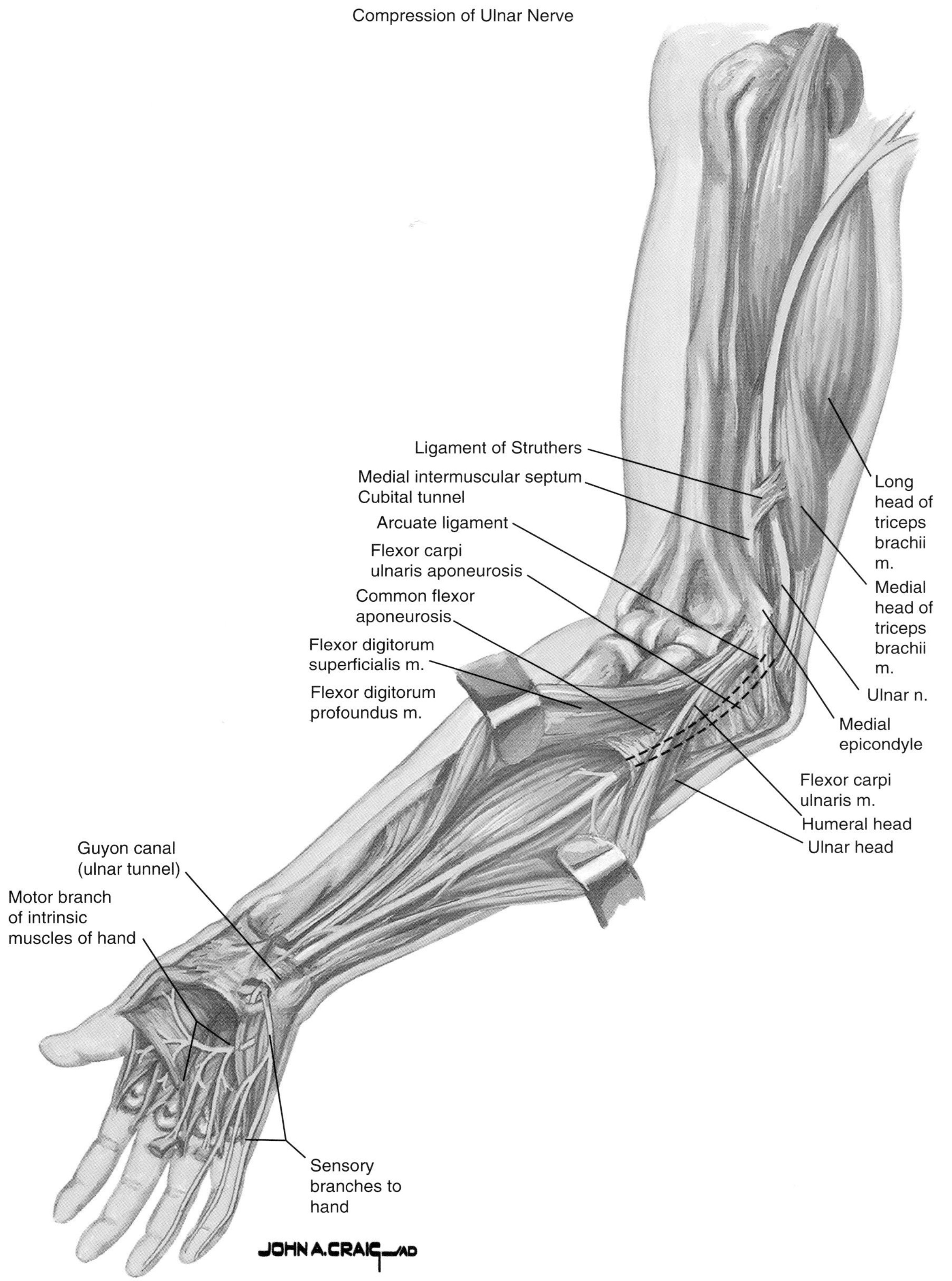

FIG. 33.2 Source of compression of the ulnar nerve. (Netter medical illustration used with permission of Elsevier. All rights reserved.)

entrapment at Guyon's canal results in symptoms with wrist flexion. Compression more proximally at the thoracic outlet results in symptoms with arm elevation.[16] Thus a careful history can be helpful in distinguishing the source of compression.

PHYSICAL FINDINGS

On inspection, atrophy of the hypothenar eminence and first dorsal interosseous muscle may be seen in severe cases.[20] The ulnar nerve supplies sensory fibers to the fifth finger, both palmar and dorsal surfaces, and usually half of

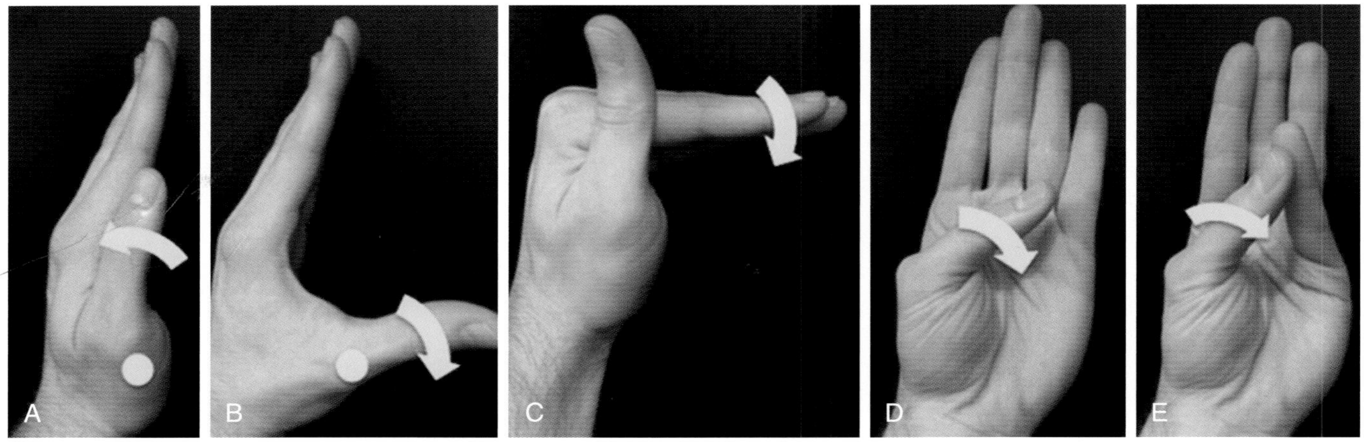

FIG. 33.3 The motor action of (A) the adductor pollicis, (B) the abductor pollicis brevis, (C) the lumbricals, (D) the flexor pollicis brevis, (E) the opponens pollicis. *(Copyright Global Spine J. 2014;4(1):1-6.)*

the ring finger. Sensory deficits that split the ring finger are classic for an ulnar nerve injury. Abnormal sensation limited only to the palmar surface may suggest a more distal compression of the nerve at Guyon's canal at the wrist, since the dorsal sensory branch typically separates 5–6 cm proximal to the ulnar styloid.[22] However, in some individuals the ulnar nerve may supply the whole ring finger and even part of the long finger, making it difficult to distinguish from a C8–T1 radiculopathy. Extension of sensory deficit to medial edge of the forearm, above the wrist, indicates a lesion proximal to the elbow, such as a cervical radiculopathy or brachial plexopathy, since the ulnar sensory distribution ends at the base of the hand whereas the medial edge of the forearm is innervated by the medial antebrachial cutaneous (MABC) nerve, which is supplied by C8–T1 via an independent branch of the medial cord of the brachial plexus.

The ulnar nerve is primarily responsible for all intrinsic motor function of the hand. Entrapment can be seen when pinching with the index finger and thumb or adducting the thumb (Fig. 33.3A). There are five muscles of the hand, however, that are innervated by the median nerve: abductor pollicis brevis, flexor pollicis brevis, opponens pollicis, and the lateral two lumbricals (Fig. 33.3B –D).[22] A positive Jeanne's sign is seen when a flexed interphalangeal joint of the thumb is accompanied by hyperextended metacarpophalangeal joint. It can also be tested by having the patient pinch a paper against resistance with a fully adducted straight thumb and first metacarpophalangeal joint. A positive Froment's test occurs when the patient cannot hold on to the paper and compensate by bending the distal interphalangeal joint of the thumb. The patient may also present with Wartenberg's sign or spontaneous abduction of the little finger in attempting to extend all five fingers.[16] More severe compressions may show "claw hand" or "hand of benediction," for which the fourth and fifth digits are extended in the metacarpophalangeal joints and flexed at the interphalangeal joints while the patient is trying to extend all five fingers. Note that the same sign may be seen in median nerve compression, but with the patient attempting to form a fist rather than to extend the hand.

DIAGNOSTIC STUDIES

EDX testing may be helpful in confirming the diagnosis of ulnar compression, location of compression, and chronicity of disease. Compression neuropathy may present early as dynamic ischemia for which temporary ischemia has been restored. EDX studies are likely normal initially. For more severe compression, demyelination may occur, demonstrating slowing of fastest conducting fibers and associated with recovery 3–4 months after decompression surgery. In long-standing or severe cases of compression, axonal loss is present and nerve conduction studies will show a decrease in amplitude of the compound motor action potential, reflective of an overall decrease in the number of functioning nerves. EMG also demonstrates fibrillations and positive sharp waves at rest as well as long-duration motor unit action potentials and reduced recruitment with maximal effort.[20] Although there are case reports of ultrasound successfully identifying the source of ulnar compression, it remains difficult to visualize the difference between abnormal and normal nerve on imaging.[23] At least one study showed no significant difference in the ultrasound imaging of the nerve as compared with imaging from asymptomatic healthy volunteers.[24] Thus clinical history and EDX testing remain the main sources for diagnosis.

TREATMENT

Mild to moderate cases of ulnar nerve entrapment—as indicated by intermittent symptoms, motor conduction greater than 40 m/s, and no evidence of atrophy—can be successfully managed with nonsurgical options.[16,20] This includes reducing elbow flexion, especially at night, with soft towel or padding; extensive postural education; activity modification; and steroid injection. Improvements are usually seen within 3–6 months and, in one study, 50% of the patients reported improved symptoms with conservative care.[25] For those who fail conservative treatment or in severe cases as indicated by decreased amplitudes on nerve conduction, surgery is the next step. One of three major surgical methods is commonly used for surgical correction: decompression, epicondylectomy, or transposition.

Decompression involves a simple incision and quick postoperative mobilization but poses the risk of incomplete decompression and ulnar subluxation. Epicondylectomy, or resection of the medial epicondyle, involves less dissection than transposition, poses a low risk for ulnar injury, but leads to greater postoperative pain and the potential for elbow instability. Transposition, most commonly an anterior approach, moves the ulnar nerve anterior to the axis of the elbow and thus releases all potential sources for compression and reduces the risk of nerve injury, but it does require extensive dissection and prolonged postoperative immobilization; it is also a technically more demanding procedure.[16] Although there are many studies comparing the results of each approach, the procedure chosen must be tailored to the patient, mechanism of entrapment, and severity of the compression.

THORACIC OUTLET SYNDROME

Thoracic outlet syndrome (TOS) comprises a group of disorders that result from the compression of one or more of the neurovascular structures as they exit the thoracic outlet. There are three major types of TOS: neurogenic, arterial, and venous. Neurogenic TOS (nTOS) is the most common type, accounting for greater than 90% of cases, and is the primary focus of our discussion.[26] Venous and arterial TOSs are much rarer, accounting for 3% and less than 1%, respectively.[27] Neurologic TOS is further categorized as true nTOS, which accounts for only 1% of all cases, which is about 1 per million persons, and the disputed type, which accounts for 99% of the cases.[28] Although true neurologic TOS is relatively rare, there are extensive publications on the topic, ranking it second to CTS in nerve entrapment syndromes.[26] There is growing interest in TOS as well as controversy on its pathophysiology and management approach.

PATHOLOGY

The thoracic outlet is a large space, extending from the base of the neck to the axilla, that can be divided into three portions as it travels superomedial to inferolateral: the interscalene triangle, the costoclavicular space, and the subcoracoid space. Compression of the neurovascular structures—namely the brachial plexus, subclavian or axillary artery, and their veins—is the primary cause of symptoms. The interscalene triangle, bounded by the anterior and middle scalene muscle and the first rib, contains the exiting brachial plexus and subclavian artery. Hyperextension injuries may cause local hematoma, inflammation, and subsequent fibrosis of the scalene muscles.

The brachial plexus, subclavian artery, and vein exit the costoclavicular space, which comprises the middle third of the clavicle anteriorly, the first rib posteriorly, and the upper border of the scapula at its posterolateral edge. The space can be narrowed by prolonged shoulder abduction or extension such as seen in archery or in poor posture. In one case-controlled study, patients with TOS were more likely to have a low shoulder girdle (complex of clavicle, coracoid, and scapula), as measured by radiography, than those in the control group. This suggests that inherent anatomic differences play a role as well.[29]

The subclavian vessels are renamed the axillary vessels as they cross the lateral border of the first rib. They then enter the subcoracoid space, which is surrounded by the coracoid process superiorly; the pectoralis minor muscle (PMM) overlies the space. Shortening of the PMM in contractures causes abduction of the scapula and shoulder girdle protraction, narrowing the space.[30] Similarly, hypertrophy of the PMM with repeated use in overhead sports may create hypertrophy, swelling, and fibrosis, causing nTOS.

RISK FACTORS

Like many other entrapment neuropathies, the risk factors for TOS include anatomic predisposition, repeated activities, and various anatomic anomalies. TOS is more frequently seen in women, especially in the third and fourth decades.[31] An anatomically lower shoulder girdle position, which results in compression of neurovascular structures by the clavicle, has been hypothesized to be a cause.[30] The presence of a cervical rib, which is quite common in the general population, accounts for 20% of nTOS, although not all patients with a cervical rib have nTOS.[30] Abnormal position of the first rib or a supernumerary scalene muscle may increase risk by decreasing the size of the interscalene triangle.[30] Repeated activities that involve unnatural shoulder postures, as sometimes seen in computer users or players of string instruments, can further aggravate symptoms. Acquired conditions such as local trauma, tumor, infection, or inflammatory procedure can further predispose individuals to the development of TOS.

SYMPTOMS

Symptoms of TOS depend, in part, on whether the impingement affects the brachial plexus, the artery, or the vein. True nTOS presents with predominantly motor deficits, including loss of dexterity, weakness, and atrophy.[26] Upon further inquiry, some patients may also have sensory symptoms, such as pain or paresthesia.[30] In contrast, the disputed type of nTOS presents with predominantly sensory deficits, including pain and myalgia of the neck, shoulder, medial arm, or forearm with paresthesia of the hand usually in a C8–T1 distribution.[26] This is because compression typically affects the lower trunk of the brachial plexus. In both cases, symptoms are often exacerbated with arm elevation. Also, anterior flexion of the shoulder or frequent abduction and supination of the arm can further trigger symptoms. Unlike the other forms of TOS, disputed nTOS is frequently bilateral.[32]

Similarly, arterial TOS may also present with pain in the neck, shoulder, or arm triggered by increasing activity, but hand or arm ischemia is also seen if arterial embolization occurs. A subset of patients will also present with symptoms of neurologic TOS from simultaneous compression of the brachial plexus. Venous TOS, sometimes referred to as Paget-Schroetter syndrome, was shown in a large series to present with visible collateral circulation (99% of cases) in the shoulder and arm, upper extremity edema (96%),

TABLE 33.2 Common Provocative Maneuvers for Testing Thoracic Outlet Syndrome

Maneuver	Provocation	Positive Test	Affected Region	Caveats
Adson maneuver (Scalene's test)	Head rotated to affected side, neck hyperextended, check the radial pulse while patient takes a deep inspiration.	Reproduces symptoms and loss of radial pulse.	Causes anterior scalene compression.	
Wright maneuver	Externally rotated the affect arm and abduct 180 degrees. Palpate for radial pulse.	Reproduces symptoms and loss of radial pulse.	Narrows the subcoracoid space.	Keep elbow extended to avoid cubital tunnel syndrome, keep wrist neutral to avoid also testing for carpal tunnel syndrome
Roos test/EAST	Abduct the arm of affected side 90 degrees, flexed at elbow, externally rotated, repeatedly open and close hands in "I surrender" motion every 2 seconds for 1–3 minutes	Reproduces symptoms and diminution of radial pulse or inability to maintain position for 3 minutes	Narrows the costoclavicular space.	High rate of false positives with carpal tunnel syndrome
Halsted test (military brace maneuver)	Patient in military stance: shoulder depressed and retracted	Reproduces symptoms and diminution of radial pulse or inability to maintain position	Narrows the costoclavicular space.	

EAST, *Elevated arm stress test.*

and bluish discoloration of the distal extremity (94%). Relatively fewer patients present with pain, which usually occurs with exercise (33%).[33]

PHYSICAL FINDINGS

General inspection and palpation is the best initial exam for identifying TOS, especially when compared with the unaffected limb. Palpation for presence of a cervical rib, asymmetry, or mass may indicate the cause of compression. In true nTOS, inspection often leads to motor findings such as atrophy of the thenar eminence muscles with or without patchy sensory deficit in the forearm and medial arm, while disputed nTOS has a relatively unremarkable neurologic exam. Tenderness to palpation of the anterior chest wall and the scalene, pectoralis, and trapezius muscles may be seen in both subtypes of nTOS.[30] Vascular compression can be evident from a discrepancy in blood pressure between the affected and unaffected upper extremity as well as evidence of bruit or digital ischemia more distally.[27] A palpable mass in the location of the thoracic outlet would suggest a vascular type of TOS. Several provocative tests can further confirm pathology, although most have limited sensitivity and specificity. The specific maneuvers are listed in Table 33.2.

DIAGNOSTIC EVALUATION

EDX studies are reproducible for true nTOS but are equivocal for disputed nTOS. In addition to confirming the diagnosis of true nTOS, they may be beneficial for evaluating the differential diagnosis, such as cervical radiculopathy, cubital tunnel syndrome, and CTS. One of the first EDX abnormalities seen in true nTOS is a reduction in the amplitude of the MABC sensory response. Later ulnar sensory responses in the hand will be diminished. The amplitude of the median compound motor action potential is reduced more than the ulnar and radial responses. Late responses, such as F waves, will become prolonged as the plexopathy progresses. Needle examination may elicit denervation in the median nerve to a greater degree than ulnar innervated hand muscles in advanced cases.[34]

Additional imaging is very helpful for identifying the source of compression. Plain radiographs of the cervical spine and chest may reveal bony abnormalities such as a cervical rib or clavicular fracture. MRI, especially when comparing the provocative and neutral positions, is especially helpful in revealing anatomic changes at the site of compression. Demirbag et al. have shown that MRI showed no significant difference in neutral position between TOS and healthy controls; however, with provocative maneuvers, the angle between the first rib and the horizontal axis and the minimum costoclavicular distance was significantly decreased.[35] MRI also has the advantage of providing excellent detail about the brachial plexus and eliminating radiation exposure.[36] If vascular TOS is suspected, duplex ultrasound looking for any aneurysm, thrombosis, or abnormal flow is an excellent initial approach, while CT angiography can further delineate the flow pattern and identify the source of compression. For both MRI and CT, imaging is most effective if done in both the neutral position and in the position that elicits symptoms, such as arm elevation. The gold standard of imaging remains catheter-based arteriography or venography for vascular TOS, but it is largely limited to intraoperative use due to its invasiveness and limited visualization of surrounding structures.[27]

TREATMENT

True nTOS is managed aggressively and often requires surgical intervention to prevent further nerve damage. There are multiple surgical approaches depending on the source of compression. Disputed nTOS warrants a trial of symptom control with medications, physical therapy, and posture modifications. However, it is important to note that strengthening and resistance exercises as well as neck traction may worsen symptoms.[37] Some authors propose that patients who are not responsive to 3 months of conservative treatment may warrant surgical evaluation. A review compared two surgical approaches and determined that transaxillary first rib resection had superior results compared with supraclavicular neuroplasty of the brachial plexus, but they have provided no randomized evidence that either approach was better than no treatment.[38] Poor predictors for surgery include chronic pain syndrome, opioid use, and tobacco use. Because of poor outcomes after surgery, some guidelines require EDX evidence of brachial plexus involvement before surgery can be implemented, including (1) an absent or reduced amplitude ulnar sensory response or an absent or reduced MABC response with a normal contralateral MABC response; (2) an absent or reduced median compound muscle action potential (CMAP) amplitude or an absent or prolonged F-wave response with normal F-wave responses on the contralateral side, or needle EMG showing active denervation of at least two muscles innervated by the lower trunk of the brachial plexus with normal EMG of cervical paraspinal muscles and normal EMG of at least one muscle supplied by the middle or upper trunk of the brachial plexus and to exclude the presence of other focal neuropathies or polyneuropathy to explain the abnormalities; (3) a normal median sensory amplitude; and (4) normal conduction velocity of the ulnar nerve across the elbow.[39]

Increasingly, injection serves as the next step before surgery. Jordan and Machleder demonstrated that diagnostic injection of the anterior scalene muscle was helpful in predicting response to surgery.[40] About 90% of those with a clinical diagnosis of TOS had positive responses to block, and 94% of those with a positive block responded to surgical decompression compared with only a 50% response to surgery among those who did not improve with the block.[40] Botulinum toxin (Botox), a neurotoxin that inhibits acetylcholine release from presynaptic endings at the neuromuscular junction, has been shown to have both muscle-relaxing and pain-relieving properties both centrally and peripherally.[41] Several case studies have suggested that Botox injection at the site of compression provides significant relief ranging from 30 to 88 days.[31,42–45] This may offer a new alternative to surgery or provide relief while awaiting surgery.

MERALGIA PARESTHETICA

MP is the entrapment of the lateral femoral cutaneous nerve (LFCN) of the thigh, resulting in pain and discomfort down the lateral and anterolateral thigh. It has also been known as Bernhardt-Roth syndrome or lateral femoral cutaneous neuralgia. The word *meralgia* comes from the Greek *meros*, meaning "thigh" and *algo*, meaning "pain," and this condition has been well described for over 100 years.

PATHOLOGY

The LFCN of the thigh arises from the L2 to L3 roots of the lumbar spine and courses with the lumbar plexus through the pelvis at the lateral border of the psoas muscle, crossing the iliacus muscle anteriorly to just medial to the anterior superior iliac spine (ASIS). It then courses under the inguinal ligament and over the sartorius muscle as it enters the thigh, where it splits into anterior and posterior branches to provide sensation to the anterolateral thigh. There are five variations on how this nerve travels through the inguinal ligament, named types A–E, with certain variation being at higher risk for compression (Fig. 33.4). Specifically, type B is the most common and, based on a cadaveric study of 52 individuals, types A–C are the most susceptible to compression.[46] The most common cause is an external compression at the pelvis as the nerve courses past the inguinal ligament, although internal compression via increased intraabdominal pressure in weight gain and pregnancy or iatrogenic injury relative to surgery may also occur.[47] Since the LFCN is a purely sensory nerve, no motor loss should be seen, which also often limits functional deficits.

RISK FACTORS

Risk factors for spontaneous compression include the following: anatomic variability, as discussed earlier; obesity (body mass index [BMI] ≥30); pregnancy; and tight-fitting clothing (jeans, corsets, and accessories such as armor or belts), although other anatomic abnormalities such as leg-length discrepancy or a pelvic mass may also be risk factors.[48–51] Metabolic factors that affect neuronal function—such as diabetes, alcoholism, and lead poisoning—have also been implicated.[48] Affected patients are typically in their 30s and 40s, with a higher incidence in men than in women.[52] Iatrogenic causes of nerve compression are also commonly seen in hip surgeries, including the anterior approach to total hip arthroplasty (67%) and hip resurfacing (91%), although the majority of those affected had no significant functional deficits.[53] Other surgeries at risk for MP include lumbar spine surgery, with an incidence of 12%–20%.[54] This is postulated to be related to patient positioning and equipment factors.[55] Pelvic osteotomies are associated with about a 30% incidence of postoperative MP.[56] Other lower abdominal or pelvic surgeries may also place the patient at risk.

SYMPTOMS

Patients complain of burning pain, numbness, tingling, or dysesthesia in the thigh with a predominance of symptoms in the lateral thigh 73% of the time and the anterolateral thigh 26% of the time.[57] Dysesthesias such as allodynia and tingling are more common than pain. Pain is often exacerbated with prolonged standing or walking due to tension in the inguinal ligament or movement of the nerve that improves with sitting.[58]

PHYSICAL FINDINGS

The LFCN is a purely sensory nerve that supplies the lateral thigh only. Therefore physical findings are completely sensory. Some patients may also have pain to percussion of the lateral inguinal ligament, known as Tinel's sign; its sensitivity and specificity have not been validated. Inguinal compression of the LFCN can be relieved by the pelvic compression test, done by having the patient lie laterally with the symptomatic side up and compress for 45 seconds

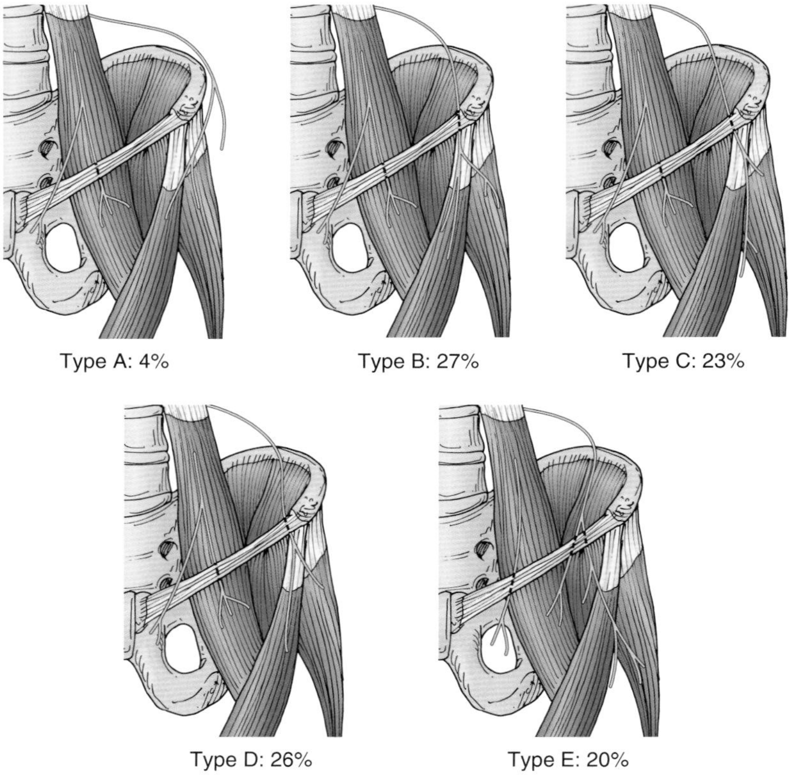

FIG. 33.4 Five variations on the course of the lateral femoral cutaneous nerve through the inguinal canal. *(Images reproduced from Aszmann OC, Dellon ES, Dellon AL: Anatomical course of the lateral femoral cutaneous nerve and its susceptibility to compression and injury.* Plast Reconstr Surg. *1997;100:600-604. Lippincott Williams & Wilkins.)*

to elicit resolution of symptoms as a positive indicator of MP. In a small study of 20 patients, this was shown to have 95% sensitivity and 93% specificity as compared with neurophysiologic testing (gold standard). However, no large studies have confirmed this technique.[59]

DIAGNOSTIC STUDIES

MP can be further confirmed by EDX testing. Somatosensory evoked potentials have 81% sensitivity and nerve conduction studies have 65% sensitivity.[60,61] The exam itself can be technically difficult even in normal individuals and especially in patients with large habitus.[57] Electrodiagnosis is better suited to ruling out other possible diagnoses such as lumbar radiculopathy. Imaging may be considered to identify the source of compression. Magnetic resonance neurography (MRN), a modified MRI with higher resolution for the nerve, can be utilized to follow the course of the LFCN. One isolated small study of 11 patients and 28 controls demonstrates positive and negative predictive value of up to 71% and 94%, respectively, with up to 90% diagnostic accuracy using MRN.[62] The full utility of MRN, however, remains to be determined.

TREATMENT

The majority of patients (85%) improve, over 4–6 months, with conservative treatment such as activity modification, physical therapy, medications, and nerve blocks.[63] Activity modifications such as avoidance of compression activities or wearing loose clothing may help reduce compression. Physical therapy has not been fully studied but is generally recommended. A number of neuropathic medications have been used to treat the syndrome including tricyclic antidepressants, antiarrhythmics, and anticonvulsants, as well as capsaicin and topical lidocaine ointment with good effect. Nerve blocks have been shown to be a very effective treatment. This is done at the exit of the nerve from inguinal ligament 1 cm medial and inferior to the ASIS or at point of maximal tenderness under ultrasound guidance. Block is done initially for diagnostic confirmation but can be followed by therapeutic injection with steroids. Taglifiaco reported 100% resolution of symptoms after 2 months in a small study of 16 patients, 80% of whom responded to the first injection.[64] Pulse radiofrequency may be attempted to achieve longer relief by modulating nerve firing. In nonresponsive cases, surgical intervention either by neurolysis or by resection is the remaining option. Neurolysis is less invasive but has a slightly higher risk of recurrence whereas nerve resection causes permanent loss of sensation in the area with virtually no risk of recurrence. There is no consensus on the best surgical approach.

TARSAL TUNNEL SYNDROME

The term TTS is typically used to describe entrapment of the posterior tibial nerve or its branches at the fibro-osseous tunnel in the medial ankle. It is a rare but often underdiagnosed condition.

PATHOLOGY

The tarsal tunnel is located just posterior and inferior to the medial malleolus, wrapped by the flexor retinaculum at its superior, inferior, and roof segments. The tunnel contains, from medial to lateral, the tibialis posterior tendon, flexor digitorum longus, posterior tibial artery and vein, posterior tibial nerve, and flexor hallucis longus tendon. The tibial nerve divides into a calcaneal branch, which continues to innervate the heel, as well as medial and lateral plantar nerves, which exit the tunnel to innervate the sole of the foot. The medial plantar nerve pierces the flexor retinaculum to innervate the posterior and medial aspects of the heel as well as passing deep to the abductor hallucis muscle to terminate as the medial three pairs of digital nerves. The lateral plantar nerve pierces the abductor hallucis muscle belly and terminates as the lateral digital nerves, primarily supplying the fourth and fifth digit of the toes. Although symptoms often involve both the medial and lateral plantar nerve distribution, the medial branch can divide and split before reaching the retinaculum in 5% of individuals and course external to the tarsal tunnel, thus sparing it from compression.[65]

RISK FACTORS

Compression of the tibial nerve at the tarsal tunnel may be due to intrinsic causes such as hypertrophic retinaculum, tendinopathy, or hemorrhage and later fibrosis or extrinsic causes such as constrictive footwear, significant lower extremity edema (seen in pregnancy or venous congestion), and hind foot and varus or valgus deformity.[66] Inflammatory arthropathies (including rheumatoid arthritis), obesity, and hypothyroidism inherently increase the risk of all neuropathies, including TTS. Athletes or individuals with prolonged weight bearing are also at increased risk.[67]

SYMPTOMS

Patients often report paresthesia, dysesthesia, and pain just posterior to the medial malleolus, heel, sole, and toes or any combination of these depending on which of the three branches of the posterior tibial nerve are affected. Pain may also radiate upward into the calf with percussion of the tarsal tunnel in a condition known as the Valleix phenomenon.[68] Symptoms are usually worse toward the end of the day and peak at night. Weakness of the abductor and flexor muscles of the foot or loss of movement of the big toe in any direction may be seen in chronic compression.

The differential diagnosis for TTS is quite broad; thus subtle differences in history may help rule in the diagnosis. Plantar fasciitis, an overuse injury caused by tension on the fascia, often mimics TTS but lacks the dysesthesia and paresthesia seen in TTS and other nerve compressions. Morton's neuroma may also present with involvement of the distal sole of the foot but produces lancinating pain instead of burning dysesthesia. Although spinal stenosis and peripheral neuropathy often present with intermittent symptoms, they tend to involve both feet, whereas TTS is most often unilateral.

PHYSICAL FINDINGS

On inspection, evidence of foot edema or external injury may be seen. Provocative maneuvers such as the Hoffmann-Tinel sign can be elicited by percussion over the tarsal tunnel, causing paresthesia or pain at the site of compression or radiation into the foot; it is positive in 50% of patients.[69,70] Pain can also be reproduced by the dorsiflexion-eversion test, in which the foot (including the toes) is passively dorsiflexed and everted at the ankle, creating significant tension of the posterior tibial nerve and lateral plantar nerve. This maneuver aggravates symptoms in 82% of affected patients and has no effect in healthy controls.[71] The Trepman test can further confirm TTS by applying the plantarflexion-inversion maneuver to reduce the overall width of the tarsal tunnel and also compress the lateral plantar nerve.[72] When results of these three provocative maneuvers are done within 30 seconds, they have a 86% sensitivity and 100% specificity.[73]

DIAGNOSTIC STUDIES

EDX studies have traditionally been used to assist with diagnosis. Abnormalities include prolonged distal motor latencies, stimulating the tibial nerve above the tarsal tunnel; compound muscle action potential less than 4 mV for the abductor hallucis muscle (correlates to medial plantar nerve), less than 3 mV for the abductor digiti quinti (correlates to lateral plantar nerve); or difference in amplitude decrease greater than 50% compared with the unaffected foot. Absent or reduced amplitude sensory responses of the medial and lateral plantar nerves compared with the unaffected foot are seen. Denervation on needle EMG may be seen in the foot muscles supplied by the tibial nerve, though this must be interpreted with caution, since this is a frequent finding in normal subjects without symptoms.[74] A fair amount of false-negative as well as false-positive results are seen with EDX studies alone; thus results may be helpful adjunctively but are not the sole source of diagnosis.

Imaging is useful for diagnosis as well as assessing extent of compression for TTS. Ultrasound imaging is able to provide direct visual evidence of nerve injury as seen by focal enlargement and change in echogenicity of the nerve, especially compared with the unaffected side.[75,76] MRI further aids in diagnosis by offering measurable detail of the thickness of flexor retinaculum, location of the three branches of the posterior tibial nerve as well as the depth, boundary, and source of compression. One study showed that MRI was positive in 88% of symptomatic patients.[77] Imaging not only confirms compression but also outlines its depth and extent.[78] Plain weight-bearing radiographs or CT of the foot may be indicated in cases where structural abnormalities of the foot are thought to be the cause.

TREATMENT

The majority of TTS is initially treated conservatively by strapping the affected foot in neutral or slight inverted position, custom orthotics to support the arches, as well as stretching and strengthening of the gastrocnemius muscle. Analgesic medications, including antiinflammatory and neuropathic pain medications, have also been used.[79] Patients may benefit from aspiration of a ganglion cyst for temporary relief or corticosteroid injection to the tarsal tunnel to reduce neural edema. In severe or refractory cases for which clear source of entrapment can be identified, surgical decompression is the next step in treatment. The exact approach depends on location and cause of compression and success rates vary widely from 44% to 96%.[72,80] One of the most positive predictors of success is the presence of Tinel's sign, since its absence may indicate that the nerve is too damaged to achieve full recovery.[66]

MORTON'S NEUROMA

Morton's neuroma, also known as interdigital neuroma or Morton's metatarsalgia, is a common painful condition of the foot. Pain is typically due to neural inflammation in the third web space at the plantar surface of the foot. It is 10 times more likely to affect women than men and typically presents at age 50. The condition was first described by Civinini in 1835 then later published by Durlacher, Queen Victoria's chiropodist, but receives its eponymous name from Thomas Morton, an American orthopedic surgeon, who described a case series of patients with the condition in 1876.[81] This may be the earliest entrapment neuropathy to have been described.

PATHOLOGY

Pain from Morton's neuroma can be visualized as an enlarged nerve bundle on the plantar surface of the foot. It most frequently occurs in the third web space, although it may also occur in the second web space and rarely the first web space. The plantar nerves terminate as digital nerves of the foot just superficial to the deep transverse intermetatarsal ligament. The medial plantar nerve innervates the medial three digits, and the lateral plantar nerve supplies the lateral two digits. The third digital nerve, located between third and fourth toes, is unique in that in addition to medial plantar nerve branches it receives a communicating branch from the lateral plantar nerve, forming a larger nerve bundle that makes it more susceptible to injury or compression. Although called a "neuroma," nerve bundle enlargement is not due to an intrinsic neuronal tumor but rather proliferative fibrosis of perineural tissue.[81] Four theories on the cause of Morton's neuroma have been proposed by Hassouna and Singh.[82] Chronic trauma theory proposes that recurrent trauma from heavy weight bearing or metatarsophalangeal joint abnormalities may result in recurrent injury. Intermetatarsal bursitis theory suggests inflammation of the bursae just above the nerve may cause adherence, swelling, and compression or irritation of the nerve itself. The entrapment theory suggests that there is repeated compression of the nerve during walking, which causes irritation and subsequent inflammation and fibrosis.[82] Lastly the ischemia theory proposes poor blood flow as the primary reason for pain, although later studies have disproven this idea, pointing out that similar arterial damage has been seen in patients with no symptoms.

RISK FACTORS

Activities that increase trauma to the foot can increase one's risk for interdigital neuropathy. Ill-fitting shoes, especially high heels, which causes hyperextension and stretching of the nerve, or a narrow toe box, are all risk factors from stretching of the nerve.[82]

SYMPTOMS

The primary symptom of Morton's neuroma is intermittent lancinating pain in the forefoot radiating into the toes with occasional paresthesia or a burning sensation in the toes. Pain is aggravated with weight bearing and relieved by massage of the forefoot or toes. Occasionally, paresthesia alone or pain in the entire forefoot may be the only presenting symptom. Note that synovitis may present similarly, although pain is typically distal to the metatarsophalangeal joint.[82]

PHYSICAL FINDINGS

In addition to basic inspection of the foot and footwear for deformity, several provocative maneuvers can be done to confirm the diagnosis. The best-known test is Mulder's sign, where the examiner compresses all toes together looking for a click or pain signal. This had 95% sensitivity and 100% specificity in a small case series.[83] The digital nerve stretch test can also be done by passively fully extending the lateral two toes with the ankle dorsiflexed, looking for pain or discomfort in the web space. In a case series of 22 patients, this was found to have a 95% positive predictive value.[83] Lastly, percussion of the affected web space analogous to Tinel's test to reproduce pain or paresthesia indicates a positive result. Tinel's test for Morton's neuroma, however, has the lowest sensitivity of the three maneuvers. Having more than one positive provocative maneuver significantly increases the likelihood of the diagnosis.

DIAGNOSTIC STUDIES

EDX studies of the interdigital nerves are difficult and often unreliable. Both orthodromic and antidromic sensory or mixed nerve studies using both surface electrodes and near-needle electrodes have been described, but none are routinely performed. However, electrodiagnosis is very useful for excluding other neural pathologies that also manifest with foot pain and numbness such as TTS, lumbosacral radiculopathy, and generalized peripheral neuropathy.

Imaging is an important tool for diagnosis. Ultrasound is a convenient and inexpensive way to reach diagnosis by looking for a hypoechoic mass parallel to the metatarsal joint. However, ultrasound cannot distinguish between neuroma and mucoid degeneration in adjacent connective tissue; moreover, quality and interpretation of results are operator-dependent.[81] MRI provides significant quality and soft tissue detail and is a viable alternative or addition to ultrasound (US). Both imaging techniques, however, are less sensitive than the clinical exam and thus should not be relied on as the only source for diagnosis.

TREATMENT

Conservative measures—including physical therapy, orthotics, and avoiding offending footwear—are generally successful in some 41% of patients, although they provide a lower level of satisfaction than steroid injection.[84,85] Interdigital

TABLE 33.3 Common Entrapment Neuropathies, the Primary Nerves Involved, Exam Findings, and the Utility of Diagnostic Studies

Entrapment	Nerve (s) Involved	Provocative Maneuvers	Electrodiagnostic Studies	Imaging
Carpal tunnel syndrome	Median	Tinel's test Phalen's maneuver Tourniquet test Hand elevation test	Diagnostic	US may be helpful for confirmation and injection
Ulnar entrapment at the elbow	Ulnar	Jeanne's sign Froment's test Wartenberg's sign Claw hand	Helpful for confirming diagnosis	Equivocal
Thoracic outlet syndrome	Brachial plexus (in neurogenic types)	Adson maneuver Wright maneuver Roos test Halsted test	Helpful especially for true neurogenic TOS	CT or MRI with provocative maneuvers may help identify source of compression
Meralgia paresthetica	Lateral femoral cutaneous	Tinel's test Pelvic compression test	Helpful for confirming diagnosis	May be helpful in confirming diagnosis
Tarsal tunnel syndrome	Posterior tibial or its branch(es)	Tinel's test Trepman's test Plantar flexion-inversion maneuver	Helpful for supporting diagnosis	May be helpful in supporting diagnosis
Morton's neuroma	Digital nerve	Mulder's sign Digital nerve stretch test Tinel's test	Equivocal	Very helpful for diagnosis

TOS, *Thoracic outlet syndrome;* US, *Ultrasound.*

anesthetic nerve blocks, often with corticosteroids, have been effective in some patients. Those who have temporary relief may undergo thermal radiofrequency ablation (RFA), which has a reported success rate of 18%–83%. A pulsed RFA or cryotherapy can also be tried. In those who fail conservative therapy, surgery remains the final treatment option. A variety of surgical interventions have been used, all with some success. Morton himself, in the late 19th century, advocated removal of the metatarsal head, which had a surprisingly good success rate; however, neurolysis of the interdigital nerve or removal of the neuroma (neurectomy) are the most common surgical options today. The larger the neuroma, especially if it is greater than 5 mm in diameter, the more likely neurectomy is to be successful. Surgical risks include permanent loss of sensation and recurrent neuroma.

SUMMARY

An entrapment neuropathy usually involves a specific nerve distribution; therefore a thorough understanding of anatomy and function of the nerve greatly helps in the diagnosis and treatment of the symptoms. The most common neuropathies are CTS, ulnar neuropathy at the elbow, TOS, MP, TTS, and Morton's neuroma. The symptoms, physical examination findings, and diagnostic studies for each of the syndromes are summarized in Table 33.3. Treatment often begins with conservative management, including splints, physical therapy, injections or nerve blocks. RFA, thermal or pulsed, can be tried. In recalcitrant cases or when the relief from conservative measures is temporary, surgery can be instituted.

KEY POINTS

- Pressure in the carpal tunnel increases with flexion and extension of the wrist, often provoking symptoms.
- The ulnar nerve is most vulnerable to impingement at the elbow as well as at the wrist.
- The thoracic outlet is the site of several syndromes—vascular, neurologic, and positional—that are not mutually exclusive.
- Mapping the sensory deficit to the territory of the LFCN is diagnostic of MP.
- TTS may be distinguished from plantar fasciitis in the presence of paresthesia.
- Morton's neuroma commonly causes unilateral lancinating pain between the third and fourth digit of the toes.
- EDX studies are very useful for CTS, ulnar neuropathy, true neurogenic TOS, and MP. It is not especially reliable for Morton's neuroma.
- Imaging is helpful for most entrapment neuropathies but especially important for TOS.

ACKNOWLEDGMENTS

Drs. Michael M. Minieka, Takashi Nishida, and Hubert A. Benzon wrote the previous version.

REFERENCES

Access the reference list online at ExpertConsult.com.

SECTION V

CANCER PAIN AND PAIN IN SPECIAL SITUATIONS

SECTION OUTLINE HEAD

CHAPTER 34

Approach to the Management of Cancer Pain

Britni L. Lookabaugh, MD ◎ **Charles F. Von Gunten, MD, PhD**

Pain is one of the most prevalent and distressing symptoms reported by patients with cancer.[1] It is also underreported by patients, underrecognized by health care providers and consequently undertreated. In its report *Ensuring Quality Cancer Care*, the Institute of Medicine identified management of cancer-related pain as a fundamental element of quality cancer care.[2]

ASSESSMENT OF CANCER PAIN

Effective pain management must begin with comprehensive pain assessment. Since pain perception is inherently subjective, the gold standard for assessing pain is the patient's self-report.[3] Patients with chronic cancer pain may fail to display any signs of adrenergic stimulation, such as tachycardia and hypertension, even though the patient reports severe pain. Thorough assessment includes report of location, type, temporal profile, and severity of each significant pain.

TYPE

Cancer pain can be classified as nociceptive, neuropathic, or a combination of the two.[4] Each type typically presents with a number of relatively distinct qualities.

Nociceptive pain results when pain-sensing neuronal pathways are stimulated and function normally. Specialized receptors at the distal end of neuronal axons, termed nociceptors, detect noxious mechanical, chemical, and thermal stimuli, and generate neuronal electrical activity. These signals are transmitted normally along neuronal pathways to the brain.

Nociceptive pain can originate from somatic or visceral sources, or both. Somatic pain originates from skin, muscle, bone, and fascia. It is mediated by the somatic nervous system. As innervation is highly specific, localization of the pain is precise. Somatic pain is often described as sharp, aching, or throbbing. An oncology example would be the well-localized pain experienced from a spinal compression fracture due to bone metastasis. Visceral pain originates from internal structures. It is mediated by the autonomic nervous system. As there is a lack of specificity of innervation, and considerable neuronal crossover, visceral pain is typically difficult for the patient to localize or describe, and may encompass an area that is much larger than might be expected for a single organ. Visceral pain is often characterized as diffuse and intermittent. Examples can include the abdominal pain experienced with malignant bowel obstruction or from liver metastasis.

Neuropathic pain has been defined as a primary lesion or dysfunction of the pain-sensing nervous system.[5] The lesion can be either peripheral in the somatic or visceral nervous system, or central. The nerves themselves may be subject to damage from compression, infiltration, ischemia, metabolic injury, or transection.[6] The myelin sheath that insulates one nerve from another may also be damaged. Alternatively, neuropathic pain may also be caused by dysfunction of the nervous system, as in central facilitation or "wind-up,"[7] where an event that is normally not painful, such as the pressure from a bed sheet or clothing on the chest of a patient with recurrent breast cancer, causes pain.[8] Neuropathic pain is often described as burning, shooting, stabbing, or electriclike, and may be associated with numbness, tingling, and/or sensory deficits. An example can be the peripheral neuropathy experienced with certain chemotherapy agents.

TEMPORAL PROFILE

The temporal profile of a pain will provide further clues to its etiology.[3] The patient should be asked about the duration of the pain. When did it first start? How long has it been present? Did it come on slowly, or suddenly? One can ask what the baseline or background pain is like. Does it vary over time (e.g., worse at night)? Is the patient ever pain-free? Are there times when the pain gets much worse? What factors exacerbate or relieve the pain (e.g., activity, touch, clothing, cold/heat, or procedures)? As an example, spontaneous pain of short duration could be the paroxysmal firing of a neuroma. Back pain that occurs only with weight bearing could indicate a spinal bony metastasis. Most cancer pain is continuous over time, with some variation in intensity, particularly at night. Without intervention, it rarely disappears completely. Cancer pain is also frequently associated with intermittent paroxysms of pain that occur with activity (e.g., movement, chewing, swallowing, breathing, defecating, urinating, dressing, touch, etc.), or during a procedure.

SEVERITY

Sequential measurement of severity using a validated severity assessment scale will provide an indication of the changing intensity of the pain experienced by a given patient over time. It will also guide analgesic management. In a given patient, the same tool should be used for each assessment.

A numerical analogue scale is the simplest. The patient is asked to indicate the severity of the pain on a 10-point scale, where 0 represents "no pain" and 10 represents the "worst possible pain."

Alternatively, a visual analogue scale can provide more visual cues and be more reliable. The patient is asked to indicate the severity of the pain by marking a 100-mm line at a point that indicates the intensity of her/his pain (delimited by the descriptors "no pain" at one end [usually the left] and "worst possible pain" at the other end). A few patients will find it easier to understand a vertical line where "no pain" is at the bottom and "worst possible pain" is at the top. For children and adults who do not understand numerical or visual analogue scales, the Wong–Baker or other faces scales are similarly reliable assessment tools.

To understand how the pain varies over time, one can ask about the intensity of the continuous pain now, the worst it has been in the last 24 hours, the best it has been in the last 24 hours, and the intensity of intermittent pain at its peak.

TOTAL PAIN

Together with a careful physical examination and select laboratory and imaging studies, it is usually possible to identify the relevant pathophysiology leading to a pain state. However, a particular pain syndrome is part of a whole person's experience. The concept of "total pain" emphasizes that multiple nonphysical factors can also contribute to pain—that is, psychologic factors (e.g., anxiety, depression), social factors (e.g., familial estrangement), and spiritual or existential factors (e.g., loss of meaning in life, fear of death). It may not be possible to control pain successfully without also addressing each of these other sources of suffering.[9]

TREATMENT OF CANCER PAIN

WORLD HEALTH ORGANIZATION THREE-STEP LADDER

In 1988 the World Health Organization (WHO) first promoted the Canadian three-step ladder for cancer pain management (Fig. 34.1).[10] Recent pain guidelines from the Royal College of Physicians and the European Association for Palliative Care both use the WHO guidelines as a basis.[11,12] Today it is the cornerstone for the WHO's public health initiative to treat cancer pain worldwide.

The ladder provides a clinically useful strategy for classifying the available analgesics, and guiding initial analgesic selection based on the severity of the patient's pain. If the pain is mild (1/10 to 3/10), an analgesic can be chosen from step one. If it is moderate (4/10 to 6/10), one can start with an analgesic from step two. If it is severe (7/10 to 10/10), one can start with an opioid from step three. At any step, adjuvant analgesics can be added to optimize pain control.[13]

STEP ONE: Acetaminophen and the nonsteroidal antiinflammatory drugs (NSAIDs) including acetylsalicylic acid (ASA) are the mainstay of step one of the WHO analgesic ladder for the management of mild pain. They obey first-order kinetics and may be dosed up to recommended maximums (Table 34.1). Many are available without prescription. Sustained-release preparations or NSAIDs with longer half-lives (e.g., piroxicam) that require less frequent dosing may encourage adherence. When pain is more than mild, step-one analgesics can be combined with opioids at steps two and three.

STEP TWO: Several opioid analgesics are conventionally available in combination with acetaminophen, ibuprofen, or ASA, and are commonly used to manage moderate

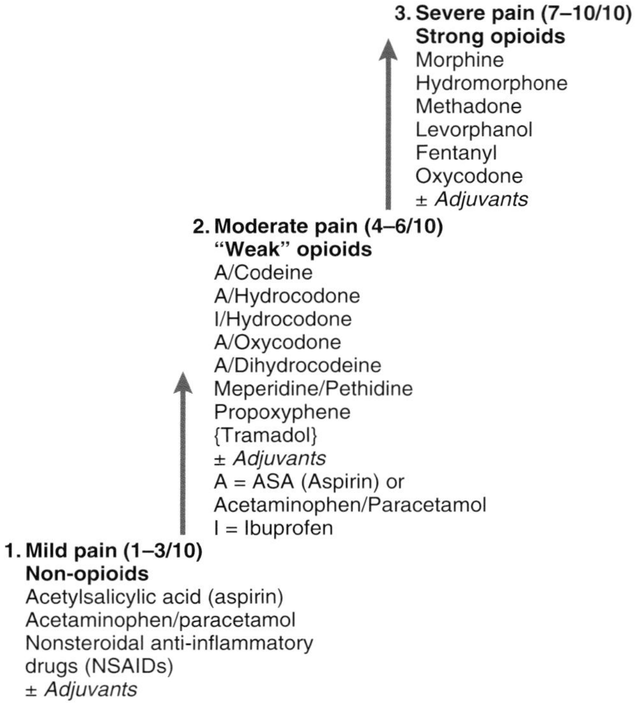

FIG. 34.1 World Health Organization three-step ladder.

TABLE 34.1 Selected Step-One Analgesics

Drug	Suggested Maximum Dose
Acetaminophen (APAP, Tylenol)	650 mg PO q4h
Acetylsalicylic acid (ASA, aspirin)	650 mg PO q4h
Ibuprofen (Motrin)	800 mg PO qid
Choline magnesium trisalicylate	1500 mg PO bid (Trilisate)
Celecoxib (Celebrex)	100 mg PO bid
Diclofenac (Cataflam)	50 mg PO qid
Diclofenac: extended release (Voltaren)	75 mg PO bid
Diflunisal (Dolobid)	500 mg PO tid
Etodolac (Lodine)	400 mg PO bid
Indomethacin (Indocin)	50 mg PO qid
Ketoprofen (Orudis)	75 mg PO qid
Nabumetone (Relafen)	1 g PO bid
Naproxen (Naprosyn)	500 mg PO tid
Oxaprozin (Daypro)	1800 mg PO qd
Sulindac (Clinoril)	200 mg PO bid
Salsalate (Disalcid)	1500 mg PO bid
Ketorolac (Toradol)	60 mg IM/IV then 30 mg IV/IM q6h; 10 mg PO qid; not to exceed 5 days

TABLE 34.2 Selected Step-Two Analgesics

Drug	Suggested Maximum Dose
Codeine	60 mg PO q4h
Codeine 30/mg/300 mg APAP (Tylenol #3); codeine 30 mg/324 mg ASA	2 PO q4h
Hydrocodone 5 mg/325 mg APAP (Vicodin)	2 PO q6h
Hydrocodone 10 mg/650 mg APAP (Lortab)	1 PO q6h
Hydrocodone 7.5 mg/200 mg ibuprofen (Vicoprofen)	1 PO q4h
Oxycodone 5 mg/325 mg APAP (Percocet); oxycodone 5 mg/325 mg ASA (Percodan)	2 PO q4h
Tramadol 50 mg (Ultram)	2 PO q6h

ASA, *Acetylsalicylic acid.*

pain. They are listed in Fig. 34.1 under step two of the WHO analgesic ladder. With the exceptions of propoxyphene (that truly has weak analgesic activity), tramadol (that has a unique combination of weak opioid activity with other analgesic properties), meperidine, and codeine (methylmorphine, which has one-tenth the potency of morphine), the opioids in this class are close in potency to morphine (mg for mg).[14] However, they have been called "weak" opioids because, in combination, they have a ceiling to their analgesic potential due to the maximum amounts of acetaminophen or ASA that can be administered per 24 hours (e.g., 4 g acetaminophen per 24 hours).[15]

The combination medications of step two all obey first-order kinetics and may be dosed up to recommended maximums (Table 34.2). The potential adverse effects are those of the component drugs.[16,17]

Frequently, patients are simultaneously given prescriptions for several step-two drugs, even though pain is poorly controlled. This usually occurs when physicians are reluctant to prescribe a step-three opioid. Aside from propoxyphene, there is no evidence that maximal dosing of any "step-two" medication is better than another, and trials of several step-two medications are likely to prolong the patient's pain. In addition, when a step-two drug inadequately relieves pain, patients may combine two or more medications, or take more than the prescribed amount in an attempt to obtain pain relief. In doing so, they may unknowingly put themselves at increased risk for significant toxicity from either the acetaminophen or ASA component of the medication. If pain persists, or increases, despite a maximum dose of a step-two drug, a step-three drug should be prescribed instead.

STEP THREE: The pure agonist opioid analgesics comprise step three of the WHO analgesic ladder. Morphine is the prototypical drug because of its ease of administration and wide availability. Other widely prescribed opioids are listed in step three of Fig. 34.1. Many patients with chronic pain are best managed with an appropriately titrated strong opioid that is combined with one or more coanalgesics. In contrast with the step-one and step-two analgesics, there is no ceiling effect or upper limit to the dose of opioids when titrating to relieve pain.

"STEP FOUR": Several studies of the WHO three-step ladder have demonstrated that its application results in the adequate control of up to 90% of patients with cancer pain.[3] Several authors have informally invoked "step four" to indicate approaches that should be reserved for patients whose pain is not controlled by competent use of the analgesic approaches outlined in the first three steps. In general, "step four" involves invasive approaches for pain relief that can be summarized as follows.

Subcutaneous (SC) or intravenous (IV) administration of opioid analgesics and coanalgesics may be required for patients where oral (PO), buccal mucosal, rectal (PR), or transcutaneous approaches are not possible or practical, or where doses of oral opioids lead to undesirable adverse effects. Adverse effects may be minimized as a result of the uniform delivery of the drug parenterally, the change in route of administration, or the reduction in first-pass metabolite production.

Intraspinal administration of opioid analgesics either epidurally or intrathecally may be required in selected patients.

Intraventricular application of opioid analgesics and other drugs has been investigated for selected central pain syndromes.

Neuroablative techniques such as peripheral neurolytic blockade, ganglionic blockade, cordotomy, and cingulotomy may be appropriate in highly selected patients. An example includes celiac plexus block for pain management due to pancreatic cancer.

Alternative therapies such as acupuncture, massage, meditation, and others may also add additional nonpharmacologic benefit at any step of the WHO ladder.

COMMON ANALGESICS

ACETAMINOPHEN

Despite its wide use, the precise mechanism of action remains unclear. Although it is analgesic and antipyretic, it is not antiinflammatory, at least systemically. Its analgesic activity is additive to other analgesic agents, including the NSAIDs and opioids.

Acetaminophen is associated with significant liver toxicity. It is generally recommended that the total dose not exceed 4 g per 24 hours for routine dosing of patients with normal liver function.

NONSTEROIDAL ANTIINFLAMMATORY DRUGS (INCLUDING ACETYLSALICYLIC ACID)

Normally the enzyme cyclooxygenase (COX) catalyzes the conversion of arachidonic acid to prostaglandins and thromboxanes. These inflammatory mediators sensitize nerve endings to painful stimuli and stimulate a group of silent nociceptors that only fire in an inflammatory milieu. In the spinal cord, COX plays a role in setting up the dysfunctional signaling pattern involved in neuropathic pain.

NSAIDs are potent antiinflammatory medications that inhibit the activity of COX and decrease the levels of these inflammatory mediators. As a result, there is less sensitization of nerve endings, less recruitment of silent nociceptors, and less risk of central "wind-up." While primary analgesia may be achieved at low doses, for their antiinflammatory effects, maximum doses should be used. As they act through an alternate mechanism to opioids and other adjuvant analgesics, NSAIDs may be combined with other analgesics to achieve better pain relief than is possible with a single medication.

The morbidity and mortality associated with NSAIDs, including ASA, are significantly higher than for any of the other analgesics. The adverse effects of NSAIDs are related to their mechanism of action. Inhibition of COX leads to inhibition of platelet aggregation and microarteriolar constriction/decreased perfusion, particularly in the stomach and kidneys. In the stomach, the relative ischemia compromises the production of gastric mucus by the chief cells, and significantly increases the risk of gastric erosions and bleeding. In the kidneys, the relative ischemia increases the risk of renal papillary necrosis and renal failure.

COX exists in two forms: a constitutive form, COX-1, and a form that is inducible under conditions of inflammation, COX-2. There are both COX-2-selective and nonselective NSAIDs that target both forms of COX. Whereas renal insufficiency is a risk of both nonselective and COX-2-selective NSAIDs, the risk of gastropathy and platelet inhibition is significantly decreased with COX-2-selective NSAIDs.

Patients (particularly the elderly) who are dehydrated, malnourished, cachectic, or have a history of nausea, gastritis, or gastric ulceration with NSAIDs are at increased risk for adverse effects from NSAIDs. However, the dyspepsia and abdominal pain that limit the use of NSAIDs in some patients do not correlate with significant gastric erosions and gastrointestinal bleeding.

To minimize the risk of ischemia, the patient should be well hydrated. The use of an H_2 blocking antacid (e.g., cimetidine or ranitidine) to treat NSAID dyspepsia and abdominal pain does not prevent gastric erosions and gastrointestinal bleeding. Only misoprostol, a prostaglandin-E analogue that reverses the effect of NSAIDs on the microarteriolar circulation of the stomach, and the proton pump inhibitors (such as omeprazole, pantoprazole) have been shown to heal gastric erosions and reduce the risk of significant gastric bleeding.

The nonacetylated salicylates (choline magnesium trisalicylate and salsalate), nabumetone, and the COX-2 inhibitors do not significantly affect platelet aggregation. They may be useful in patients who are thrombocytopenic and for whom other NSAIDs are contraindicated. Sulindac is thought to be least likely to induce renal failure because of its minimal effect on prostaglandin synthesis at the level of the proximal renal tubule.

In contrast to the opioids, NSAIDs and acetaminophen have a ceiling effect to their analgesic potential, do not produce pharmacological tolerance, and are not associated with physical or psychological dependence.

OPIOIDS

Opioid analgesics act by binding to opioid receptors of three subtypes (mu, kappa, and delta), both peripherally and centrally. The central receptors in the spinal cord and brain are most important for mediating analgesia. The opioid analgesics in common usage may be divided into those that are full agonists, partial agonists, and mixed agonist–antagonists. The pure agonist drugs are the most useful in chronic cancer pain.

OPIOIDS TO AVOID

The mixed agonist–antagonist opioids (such as pentazocine, butorphanol, and nalbuphine) and the partial agonist opioids (such as buprenorphine) are poor choices for patients with severe pain. They have no advantages over the pure agonist opioids. Besides having a ceiling effect to the analgesia they produce, they have the significant disadvantage that, if combined with a pure opioid agonist, may precipitate acute pain and opioid withdrawal symptoms.

ROUTES OF ADMINISTRATION

The oral route of administration is preferred for the management of cancer pain. It provides the simplest, least expensive way to manage most cancer pain. When it is not available, analgesics can be administered buccally and rectally before resorting to more invasive and expensive routes of delivery. In a small number of patients (<5%), subcutaneous, IV, or intraspinal administration may be required. The time to peak serum concentration (C_{max}) correlates with time to peak effect, and this occurs in 1 hour for an oral or rectal dose of a short-acting opioid. Subcutaneous doses reach peak effect in 30 minutes, and IV doses reach peak effect in 8 minutes.

ACHIEVING INITIAL PAIN RELIEF

In a patient with severe pain, opioids should be dosed frequently until the patient achieves pain relief or undesirable side effects. This is accomplished by administering a single dose and reassessing after the dose has reached peak effect (time to C_{max}: 1 hour for an oral dose, 30 minutes for a subcutaneous dose, and 8 minutes for an IV dose). If the patient remains in severe pain, the dose should be doubled and the patient observed again until peak effect. This should be repeated with careful observation until the pain is no longer severe or the patient experiences side effects. For example, if a patient continues to have severe pain and no unacceptable side effects 8 minutes after a single 4-mg IV dose of morphine, they should receive an additional 8 mg of morphine intravenously. If they remain in severe pain 8 minutes later, they should be given a 16 mg dose.

ROUTINE DOSING FOR CONSTANT PAIN

One should distinguish between constant and intermittent pain. For constant, ongoing cancer pain, analgesics should be prescribed on a regular schedule at doses sufficient to keep the pain controlled. For patients with constant pain, dosing solely on an "as needed" or "prn" basis guarantees that the patient will frequently return to pain and may increase both the patient's anxiety and the total dose required to control the pain.

Most of the short-acting drugs used for analgesia, particularly acetaminophen, the NSAIDs including ASA, and the opioids, follow first-order kinetics. When prescribing them on a routine schedule, they should be administered once every half-life in order to achieve steady state and maintain constant serum levels—that is, q4h for oral morphine or oxycodone dosing. Methadone, with its longer half-life, is administered every 8–12 hours.[18–20]

TITRATION

When initiating, titrating, or changing analgesic therapy, drugs that follow first-order kinetics take five half-lives to reach pharmacological steady state. Changes in dosages should only be made once the serum level has reached steady state—for example, once every 20–24 hours when morphine is given PO, or even SC. Waiting longer will not improve pain control or safety. Increasing scheduled dosages before steady state is reached may lead to unnecessarily high serum levels and undesired adverse effects.

SUSTAINED-RELEASE PRODUCTS

Sustained-release medications should not be used alone to adjust or titrate a patient's uncontrolled pain. Using them for titration unduly prolongs the process to bring the pain under control, because they can be titrated only once every five half-lives (~60 hours). However, once the pain is controlled, changing to a sustained-release product may enhance the patient's quality of life and improve compliance and adherence due to the decreased frequency of dosing (e.g., q8h, q12h, q24h, etc.).

Sustained-release preparations of morphine and oxycodone are available for PO administration and should be administered in accordance with the instructions of the manufacturer.

Transdermal fentanyl patches are convenient when patients are receiving stable opioid dosing, but should not be used to titrate unrelieved pain. Approximately 12–18 hours are needed for significant serum levels of fentanyl to accumulate, so appropriate doses of opioids need to be maintained during this window of time. Fentanyl patches may be changed every 72 hours, although a small number of patients may need to have their patch(es) changed every 48 hours. Titration may be done every other day. Caution should be exercised in the setting of cancer cachexia, as there may be variable levels of absorption.[21,22]

ABUSE-DETERRENT FORMULATIONS

With the increase in prescription of opioids for pain relief has come an increase in prescription opioid abuse.[23–25] Abuse-deterrent formulations are intended to prevent, impede, or discourage physical and chemical tampering (e.g., crushing, chewing, extraction, smoking, snorting, injecting), while still being able to provide safe and accurate delivery of the opioid for therapeutic benefit. The sustained-release formulations have seen the most use of these (e.g., crush-resistant coatings, nonextractable gels, sequestered naloxone released only with crushing). Technologies for the immediate-release formulations have lagged. Widespread adoption is limited by cost.

BREAKTHROUGH OR RESCUE DOSING FOR INTERMITTENT PAIN

Changes in pain severity may occur spontaneously because of activity (e.g., movement) or a procedure (e.g., venipuncture, wound dressing change). If the duration and severity of the change are sufficient, extra short-acting doses of the same or similar medication (breakthrough or rescue doses) on an "as needed" or "prn" basis may be appropriate. If a patient regularly requires more than 2–4 breakthrough doses per 24 hours, then the routine scheduled dose should be increased. For intermittent pain of short duration (seconds to a few minutes), breakthrough dosing, particularly of the opioids, may lead to undesired adverse effects without increased analgesia.

Breakthrough doses of an analgesic can be given safely with a frequency equivalent to the time required to reach C_{max}. Again, this is 1 hour for an oral dose, 30 minutes for a subcutaneous dose, and 8 minutes for an IV dose. Making the patient wait any longer when the pain is not controlled simply prolongs the time required to establish optimal pain control.

The size of the breakthrough dose should be related to the routine dose. For the strong opioids such as morphine, hydromorphone, and oxycodone, a simple rule of thumb is for the oral route: Administer 10% of the total 24-hour dose per breakthrough dose every 1 hour as needed. For the IV route, administer 50%–100% of the hourly infusion rate every 5–10 minutes as needed. The dose is then adjusted as the routine dose changes or as the intensity of the intermittent pain requires.

Oral transmucosal fentanyl is available in several preparations, including a candy matrix lozenge on an applicator stick that is twirled against the buccal mucosa, as an orally dissolving tablet that is absorbed transmucosally, or as an adherent film. Additionally, other preparations will likely be commercially available soon, including nasal sprays, inhalers, and active transdermal patches. Relatively quick onset and offset make these preparations useful to treat short-lived breakthrough pain. Dosing of fentanyl preparations must be individualized; it cannot be calculated as an equianalgesic dose.[26,27]

EQUIANALGESIC DOSING

The relative abilities of opioid analgesics to relieve pain have been correlated (Table 34.3). These relationships are not scientifically precise, as there is significant interpatient variability. Further, the data from which these equivalencies are derived are often obtained in clinical settings other than chronic cancer pain. Nevertheless, the equianalgesic tables are useful to approximate the dose of a new analgesic when changes are contemplated. The dose should then be adjusted based on patient response.[28]

When changing between opioids, there is incomplete cross-tolerance. To correct for this when pain is controlled, some advocate reducing the dose of the new medication by 25%–50% after calculating the equianalgesic dose.[29]

Methadone, an opioid with a half-life that ranges from 15 to 40 hours or more, is an important exception.[30] Its apparent equianalgesic efficacy varies with the dose of opioid. In acute dosing, or at low doses, it appears to

TABLE 34.3 Equianalgesic Dosing

Oral Dose (mg)	Analgesic	IV/SC/IM (mg)
100	Codeine	60
15	Hydrocodone	—
15	Morphine	5
10	Oxycodone	—
4	Hydromorphone	1.5
—	Fentanyl	0.050

TABLE 34.4 Adverse Effects of Opioid Analgesics

Common	Uncommon
Constipation	Dysphoria/delirium
Nausea/vomiting	Bad dreams/hallucinations
Drowsiness	Pruritus/urticaria
Dry mouth	Urinary retention
Sweats	Myoclonic jerks/seizures Respiratory depression

be a 1:1 ratio of methadone to morphine. For doses of morphine less than 500 mg/day, the relative potency of methadone to morphine is about 5:1. For patients taking between 500 and 1000 mg of morphine per day, the relative potency of methadone becomes 10:1. For patients taking greater than 1000 mg of morphine per day, the relative potency could be from 15:1 to 20:1. Because of its long and variable half-life, care must be taken when switching from one opioid to methadone, and while titrating to an effective dose. Because of its long half-life, adverse effects may appear several days after doses are adjusted. Without continuous review these may be serious; methadone is the opioid most associated with respiratory depression when dosed on a regular basis.[31,32]

Attempts have been made to correlate the relative analgesia provided by acetaminophen, the NSAIDs, and the opioids. Ketorolac 10 mg orally seems to be roughly equivalent to the combination tablet 60 mg codeine/650 mg acetaminophen PO or 6–9 mg morphine PO in cancer pain. Transdermal fentanyl 25 μg/hour is approximately 50 mg morphine PO q24h.

When changing routes of administration, differences in opioid metabolism (e.g., less first-pass catabolism IV/IM/SC compared with PO) necessitate adjustments to the opioid dose, as indicated in Table 34.3. For example, an equivalent dose of morphine IV/IM/SC will be one-half to one-third that given by mouth.

CLEARANCE/BUILDUP

Most opioids are conjugated in the liver and greater than 90% of the metabolites excreted renally. While most of the opioid metabolites are inactive, some (such as morphine 6-glucuronide) have analgesic activity, and several (such as morphine 3-glucuronide) may be responsible for observed adverse effects (e.g., central nervous system excitation).[33] Mild elevation in transaminases should not have a significant impact on opioid dosing. Patients with severe liver failure should have their opioid doses decreased and/or dosing intervals increased.

Impaired renal excretion will reduce opioid clearance,[34] leading to buildup of metabolites, prolonged analgesia, and increased risk of adverse effects. To reduce these risks, patients receiving morphine should be well hydrated and maintain adequate urine output. If renal function is impaired, morphine doses should be decreased and dosing intervals increased. The patient with anuria may require very little or no extra morphine to maintain analgesia. Routine dosing should be discontinued.

Methadone and fentanyl are not renally excreted, and fentanyl does not have active metabolites.

OPIOID ADVERSE EFFECTS

The common and uncommon adverse effects of opioid analgesics are listed in Table 34.4.

Common adverse effects of the opioid analgesics are easily managed.[35] In the majority of patients, pharmacological tolerance develops to all of the common adverse effects, except constipation, within 1–2 weeks. Consequently, nausea and vomiting may be treated expectantly with antiemetics for the short period that these symptoms are problematic. If nausea and/or vomiting persist, changing the opioid or the route of administration may resolve the problem.

Similarly, patients should be counseled that the drowsiness they experience when initiating an opioid will usually dissipate after the first week or so. Patients can often tolerate a little drowsiness if they are assured that it will not persist for the entire time they are taking opioid analgesics. In fact, once a stable dose of an opioid has been reached, drowsiness will likely settle completely, and function will normalize. Most patients on a stable dose of opioid who have no adverse effects may safely drive a car.[36] Persistent somnolence may be managed by ensuring adequate hydration and renal clearance, changing to a sustained-release product to minimize peak effects, changing the opioid, changing the route of administration, or adding a psychostimulant (such as methylphenidate).

As patients given opioid analgesics will not develop tolerance to constipation, they should be treated with stimulant laxatives (e.g., senna or bisacodyl), osmotic laxatives (e.g., magnesium salts or lactulose), or prokinetic agents (e.g., metoclopramide) on a routine basis. Constipation refractory to usual laxatives can be treated with methylnaltrexone, a peripherally acting mu-opioid antagonist. Simple stool softeners (e.g., sodium docusate) are usually ineffective. Fiber-containing products can worsen opioid-induced constipation in patients with poor oral intake.

Persistent adverse effects from opioids seem to be somewhat idiosyncratic to the drug and individual. Simply changing to an alternative opioid at an equianalgesic dose will often resolve the problem.

The uncommon adverse effects of the opioids are also manageable. The dysphoria and confusion that occasionally occur may be managed by ensuring adequate hydration and renal clearance (thereby minimizing metabolite buildup), lowering the opioid dose, changing the opioid analgesic, or by adding low doses of a neuroleptic drug such as haloperidol, chlorpromazine, or risperidone.

The pruritus and urticaria that occur with opioids are not immune mediated, but a nonspecific release of histamine from mast cells in the skin. This may be managed with long-acting antihistamines, doxepin 10–30 mg PO qhs, or by changing to an alternative opioid analgesic. True allergy presenting as bronchospasm leading to anaphylaxis is extremely rare. Most patients who report allergies have had poorly managed adverse effects (usually nausea/vomiting and/or constipation) or too much medication too fast (leading to drowsiness and/or confusion).

The risk of respiratory depression from opioid analgesics in patients with pain is frequently misunderstood. This side effect occurs at relatively higher doses than those that produce other forms of toxicity, such as sedation. Patients develop pharmacological tolerance to the respiratory depressant effects of opioids over the same time course as other adverse effects. Too frequently, opioids have been withheld or underdosed because of unsubstantiated fear of respiratory depression or the mismanagement of adverse effects. In the patient with uncontrolled pain, opioid analgesics can be judiciously but expeditiously and safely titrated until adequate relief is obtained or intolerable adverse effects are encountered.

OPIOID EXCESS/OVERDOSE

In the setting of pain management, opioid excess presents first as mild drowsiness, proceeds to persistent somnolence, then to a poorly arousable state, and finally to respiratory depression. These changes may be associated with increasing restlessness, agitation, confusion, dreams, hallucinations, myoclonic jerks, or even sudden onset of seizures.

When assessing a patient for respiratory depression, it should be remembered that a respiratory rate of 8–12 per minute is frequently normal, particularly at nighttime. One should first check for arousability: The patient may be sleeping. If early or even moderate excess is present without major compromise, the opioid can be held, and normal metabolism will clear the excess opioid, particularly if the patient is adequately hydrated. Naloxone reversal is not normally necessary.

If the patient is not arousable, has a respiratory rate less than 6–8 per minute, or there is significant hypoxemia or hypotension present, opioid reversal with naloxone may be warranted. A 0.4 or 1.0 mg ampule of naloxone can be diluted with 10 mL of saline and 0.1–0.2 mg IV boluses administered every 1–2 minutes. SC or PO administration is not appropriate. As naloxone has a high affinity for opioid receptors, titration any faster, or with larger boluses, may precipitate opioid withdrawal that presents as an acute pain crisis, psychosis, or severe abdominal pain, and precipitates pulmonary edema or even myocardial infarction. Only if several 0.1–0.2-mg boluses are ineffective should the bolus size be increased.

Naloxone has a high affinity for lipids and will redistribute itself into adipose tissue within 10–15 minutes of administration. Any improvement frequently disappears within this time frame and signs of toxicity return. Repeated naloxone dosing may be necessary to sustain the reversal until the patient has cleared a sufficient amount of the opioid to be out of danger. If the overdose is severe and considerable opioid reversal is required, a continuous infusion of naloxone may be required until the crisis is over.

If a patient who has been well managed on a stable dose of opioid for some time suddenly develops signs of overdose, the opioid should be stopped, and sepsis, renal failure, or other causes should be ruled out. It is unlikely that the opioid alone will be the cause of the "effective overdose."

ADDICTION VERSUS TOLERANCE

Addiction, the psychological dependence on the drug, is a vastly overrated and misunderstood consequence of using opioid analgesics.[3] In patients with chronic cancer pain, the incidence of addiction is less than 1:1000 and is usually related to preexisting dependency.

Physical dependence alone, meaning the development of a withdrawal syndrome upon abrupt discontinuation of the drug, is not evidence of addiction. Physical dependence occurs over the same time course as tolerance develops to the adverse effects of the opioid analgesics, and is the result of changes in the numbers and function of opioid neuroreceptors in the presence of exogenous opioid.

If opioid analgesics are tapered instead of abruptly withdrawn, withdrawal symptoms do not occur. Usually the opioid dose can be reduced by 50%–75% every 2–3 days without ill effect. Occasionally a small dose of a benzodiazepine (e.g., 0.5–1.0 mg of lorazepam) or of methadone (with its longer half-life) may be necessary to settle the feeling of slight uneasiness or restlessness that accompanies a rapid tapering process. If restlessness or agitation is anything more than very mild, the rate of tapering should be slowed.

ADJUVANT PAIN MEDICINES

Adjuvant analgesics are used to enhance the analgesic efficacy of opioids, treat concurrent symptoms that exacerbate pain, and/or provide independent analgesia for specific types of pain. They may be used at all stages of the analgesic ladder. Some of the adjuvants, such as acetaminophen, the NSAIDs, the tricyclic antidepressants, and perhaps the antiepileptics, have primary analgesic activity themselves and may be used alone or as coanalgesics. Two cancer pain syndromes bear particular mention in this regard.

Bone pain from bone metastases is thought to be, in part, prostaglandin mediated. Consequently, the NSAIDs and/or corticosteroids may be particularly helpful in combination with opioids. Bone metastasis pain can also be amenable to radiation therapy. Pain and side effects from sustained-release opioids should be monitored during radiation therapy, due to the possible need for downtitration of regularly scheduled opioids. Spinal cord compression should always be considered if back pain is severe, increasing quickly, or associated with motor, bowel, or bladder dysfunction. In the setting of spinal cord compression, emergent radiation is indicated to preserve function, as well as to have a role in pain relief.

Neuropathic pain is rarely controlled with opioids alone. Chemotherapy-induced neuropathic pain is of increasing clinical importance and prevalence, particularly due to the increased use of platinum-derived agents, taxanes, vinca alkaloids, and proteasome inhibitors for the treatment of solid tumors.[37,38] The noradrenergic tricyclic antidepressants and selective noradrenergic serotoninergic antidepressants, antiepileptics, and corticosteroids are often required in combination with the opioids to achieve adequate relief. Commonly used agents are listed as follows, with a few comments about their use.

NSAIDs and/or acetaminophen may be added to the opioids for adjuvant analgesia, particularly when inflammatory or peripheral mechanisms are thought to be responsible for the painful stimulus.

Corticosteroids provide a range of effects, including antiinflammatory activity, mood elevation, antiemetic activity, and appetite stimulation. They reduce pain both by their antiinflammatory effect of reducing arachidonic acid release to form prostaglandins and by decreasing swelling and pressure on nerve endings. Undesirable effects such as hyperglycemia, weight gain, myopathy, infection, and dysphoria or psychosis may complicate therapy.[39–41]

Anticonvulsants (such as gabapentin, pregabalin, levetiracetam, carbamazepine, valproate, and lamotrigine) are used either alone or in addition to opioids or other coanalgesics to manage neuropathic pain. They have been particularly advocated for neuropathic pain with a shooting or lancinating quality (such as trigeminal neuralgia or nerve root compression).[42–46]

Tricyclic antidepressants (such as amitriptyline, desipramine, imipramine, and nortriptyline) are useful in pain management in general, and neuropathic pain in particular. They have innate analgesic properties and are effective through mechanisms that include enhanced inhibitory modulation of nociceptive impulses at the level of the dorsal horn. If the anticholinergic adverse effects of tertiary amine tricyclics (amitriptyline, imipramine) are undesirable or troublesome, the secondary amine tricyclics (nortriptyline, desipramine) may be effective analgesics and produce fewer adverse effects. The selective serotonin reuptake inhibitor class of antidepressants has not been shown to be useful in similar ways to the tricyclic antidepressants. Selective norepinephrine and serotonin reuptake inhibitor antidepressants (such as duloxetine and venlafaxine) may have a role in the management of cancer pain, but have not been well studied.[47,48]

Bisphosphonates (such as pamidronate and zoledronic acid) and calcitonin have been used as adjuvant analgesics in the management of bone pain from bone metastases.[49] In cancer, bone pain is caused in large part by osteoclast-induced bone resorption, rather than the direct effects of the tumor on periosteal or medullary nerve endings. Both the bisphosphonates and calcitonin inhibit osteoclast activity on bone and have been reported to reduce pain significantly in at least some patients. Bisphosphonates should be used with caution in patients with impaired renal function, as they are excreted intact primarily by the kidney. For the treatment of lytic bone metastases, the recommended doses of pamidronate (90 mg in 250 mL saline or D5W infused slowly over 2 hours) and zoledronic acid (4 mg in 100 mL as an IV infusion over 15 minutes or longer) may be repeated every 3–4 weeks. Calcitonin can be administered either subcutaneously (200 IU SC, testing first for hypersensitivity) or as an intranasal spray (200 IU, one spray q day, increasing to 400-IU sprays if ineffective).

Neuroleptic medications (such as haloperidol 1 mg orally q1h, 1 mg IV q15min, chlorpromazine 50 mg orally q1h, or risperidone 1 mg twice daily) and anxiolytics (such as lorazepam 1 mg orally q1h or q15min IV) are used for the management of specific psychiatric disorders that complicate pain management such as delirium, psychosis, or anxiety disorders. With the exception of methotrimeprazine and clonazepam, none have been shown to have intrinsic analgesic activity.

NMDA (N-methyl-D-aspartate) receptor antagonists, such as dextromethorphan, ketamine, and methadone, may affect the spinal neural circuitry that leads to a neuropathic pain state resistant to high-dose opioids.[50] Clinical studies with dextromethorphan and ketamine have shown some mild pain effects but have been significantly limited by dose-related adverse effects, particularly drowsiness. Methadone, however, is inexpensive and well tolerated. It exists as a racemic mix of levo and dextro isomers. The levo form binds at opioid receptors, while both forms can block the NMDA receptor. It is hypothesized that its NMDA receptor antagonist activity explains the variable potency observed when changing from other opioids to methadone. Recent studies have shown QT prolongation as a potential side effect of methadone, and electrocardiogram (ECG) monitoring is recommended in patients treated long term.

Local anesthetics, such as systemic lidocaine, that are nonselective inhibitors of sodium channels have also been utilized to treat neuropathic pain.[51,52] Oral anesthetics such as mexiletine have also been used in neuropathic pain, but clinical trials to date have not been definitive. Topical lidocaine patches have been approved for use in postherpetic neuralgia. Research has identified many subtypes of Na channels. In the future it may be possible to block a specific subset involved in mediating pain transmission.

Alpha-2-adrenergic agonists such as clonidine can also be effective adjuvant analgesics for both nociceptive and neuropathic pain.[53] They act at the level of the spinal cord in two ways. First they act in a mechanistically similar way to the opioids. They act on the same neurons in the cord and lead to the same intracellular events but act through a different receptor. Thus it is likely that they can enhance the nociceptive effects of opioids. Second, researchers believe alpha-2-adrenergic agonists also decrease sympathetic outflow, which is involved with neuropathic pain. Clonidine can be given systemically or delivered intraspinally. Systemic delivery may be limited by the adverse effects of lethargy, dry mouth, and hypotension.

ADDITIONAL CONSIDERATIONS

While this chapter reviews the pharmacological management of cancer pain, medications are not the only important component of comprehensive cancer pain management. In an attempt to simplify the subject of cancer pain management, pathophysiological processes have been separated from psychological, social, and spiritual factors. This has led to the unfortunate labeling of the former as "real" pain and the latter as "not real" pain. It has also led to the inappropriate extrapolation of research on acute pain, particularly in laboratory animals, to the management of chronic pain, and to the general avoidance of emotional, psychological, social, and spiritual issues by physicians trained in the scientific method. Optimal pain control may not be possible unless suffering in these other dimensions is addressed. Appropriate referral to allied health providers, such as counselors, social workers, chaplains, or hospices may be required.

CONCLUSION

Although cancer pain is a prevalent and severe problem, there are a multitude of effective tools to treat nociceptive, neuropathic, and mixed pain syndromes. The opioids remain the first-line therapy for moderate to severe pain. However, when unsuccessful or limited by adverse effects multiple classes of adjuvant analgesics are available to help optimize pain control. If one class alone is insufficient to control pain or is limited by adverse effects, it is rational to try combining classes. This combination may result in synergistic treatment of pain and may allow individual doses to be decreased, thus lowering the risk of adverse effects. Using these guidelines and keeping in mind the concept of total pain, most cancer pain can be controlled with oral drugs.

KEY POINTS

- Successful treatment of cancer pain is possible most of the time.
- The cancer pain syndrome should be determined: nociceptive, neuropathic, or mixed.
- Cancer pain should be assessed and managed within the dimensions of suffering that a patient and his or her family experience: physical, psychological, social, and spiritual.
- Daily evaluation includes an assessment of the location, type, temporal profile, and severity of each significant pain.
- The WHO's three-step approach to cancer pain management using systemic analgesics has been demonstrated to be effective at managing 90% of the pain experienced by patients worldwide.
- Opioids are essential for the management of moderate to severe cancer pain. Familiarity with each opioid's pharmacokinetics, equianalgesic dosing, adverse effects, and cost are necessary for their safe, effective, and cost-efficient use.
- Adjuvant analgesics combined with opioids will improve cancer pain control, especially in neuropathic and mixed pain syndromes.

REFERENCES

Access the reference list online at ExpertConsult.com.

CHAPTER 35

Management of Pain at End of Life

Judith A. Paice, PhD, RN

Pain is a serious problem for people with life-threatening illnesses. In studies exploring symptoms experienced near the end of life, pain, dyspnea, anxiety, and depression are common.[1–4] Cancer pain has been well characterized, representing a wide array of syndromes. These range from acute episodes related to procedures, such as bone marrow aspiration, to chronic syndromes emanating from direct tumor involvement or cancer therapies. Although it may be common during advanced disease, cancer pain can be relieved in 80% to 90% of patients. Less is known about pain occurring in persons with other life threatening illnesses ordinarily seen in palliative care or hospice, such as congestive heart failure, end-stage renal disease, or neuromuscular disorders. An awareness of the most common syndromes in these populations, specific assessment techniques, as well as therapies used to treat these conditions is essential to providing relief.

Until recently, experimental models that elucidated the neurobiology of pain due to cancer or other life-threatening illnesses did not exist, limiting our understanding of the unique mechanisms of these phenomena. The development of rodent models of bone pain, chemotherapy-induced peripheral neuropathies, and other syndromes provides insights into the neurobiology of cancer pain.[5–7] These discoveries are leading to the new, targeted, mechanism-based therapies.[8] Furthermore, greater understanding of cancer pain biology may enhance knowledge related to other symptoms common in end of life care. For example, initial evidence surrounding the role of inflammatory cytokines suggests a common biological mechanism between pain, fatigue, depression, and other symptoms.[9] These investigations are critical to complete our understanding of symptom management for those in palliative care or hospice.

PALLIATIVE CARE AND HOSPICE

All health care professionals, regardless of their specialty area, are responsible for care of the dying; therefore, they must gain the necessary knowledge and skills to care appropriately for those patients.[10] Pain and symptom management, along with advance care planning, are key elements of primary palliative care.[11] Resources, such as palliative care services and hospices, are available to assist clinicians as these teams provide specialized care to patients with life-limiting diagnoses and their families.

Palliative care is the "active total care of patients whose disease is not responsive to curative treatment. Control of pain, of other symptoms, and of psychological, social, and spiritual problems is paramount. Palliative care affirms life and regards dying as a normal process."[12] Palliative care is best integrated into the patient's care early in the course of the disease, rather than being segregated to the last days or weeks of a person's life.[13] Palliative care is often provided through consultation services, inpatient units, outpatient clinics, home care, day programs, and other creative models. Studies reveal that palliative care can lead to improved quality of life, enhanced mood, longer survival, and cost savings when compared with those individuals receiving standard care.[14,15] Palliative care services are expanding rapidly in the United States, with almost universal access in large hospitals and academic medical centers.[16]

Hospice care in the United States is a philosophy of care with similar tenets to palliative care. Goals include attention to alleviation of physical and emotional suffering, along with focus on the patient and family as the unit of care. Most hospice care in the United States is provided within the home, although a few free-standing units exist for patients unable to be cared for in the home. Hospice is reimbursed through the Medicare hospice benefit. Qualified patients must be certified as having a life expectancy of 6 months if the disease takes its natural course. Recent studies reported that families of patients dying of cancer were more satisfied with end-of-life care when treatment is focused on comfort in a hospice rather than aggressive treatment in a hospital's intensive care unit.[17]

PAINFUL SYNDROMES IN CANCER AND OTHER LIFE-THREATENING ILLNESSES

Awareness of the painful syndromes seen in those with cancer and other life-threatening illnesses promotes accurate diagnosis and management. Other chapters in this book describe a variety of pain syndromes that, although primarily seen in the general population, also may occur in people with life-threatening illnesses. However, several syndromes occur uniquely in those with cancer or other advanced diseases.

CANCER

Cancer pain syndromes can be grouped in a variety of categories: acute versus chronic, somatic versus neuropathic, and disease versus treatment related.[18,19] Acute pain is generally due to invasive procedures, such as diagnostic or surgical interventions, and is not unlike the experience of patients with nonmalignant disease.[20] Examples of treatment-related acute pain unique to individuals with cancer are noted in Table 35.1. Chronic pain syndromes often include involvement of bone, soft tissue, the viscera, and the nervous system. Bone

TABLE 35.1 Acute Cancer Pain Syndromes

Chemotherapy
Arthralgia and myalgia induced by paclitaxel
Cold allodynia induced by oxaliplatin
Headache due to methotrexate or L-asparaginase
Mucositis commonly due to pretransplant chemotherapy regimen
Pain due to infusion of chemotherapy into peritoneum or bladder
Growth Factors
Myalgia, bone pain, fever, headache
Hormonal therapy
Flare syndrome (myalgia, arthralgia, and headache) in prostate or breast cancer
Immunotherapy
Myalgia, arthralgia, and headache due to interferon
Radiation
Bone pain flare (due to radionuclides)
Enteritis and proctitis
Mucositis
Myelitis when spinal cord is irradiated

Adapted from Koh M, Portenoy RK: Cancer pain syndromes. In Bruera E, Portenoy RK, editors: Cancer Pain: Assessment and Management, *ed 2, Cambridge: Cambridge University Press, 2010, pp 53-85.*

TABLE 35.2 Chronic Neuropathic Pain Syndromes Seen at End of Life

Cancer-Related
Brachial, cervical, or sacral plexopathies
Chemotherapy-induced neuropathy
Bortezomib
Cisplatin
Oxaliplatin
Paclitaxel
Vincristine
Vinblastine
Cranial neuropathies
Postherpetic neuropathy
Postradiation plexopathies
Surgical neuropathies
Phantom pain
Postmastectomy syndrome
Postthoracotomy syndrome
Noncancer Causes of Neuropathies
Alcohol-induced neuropathy
Brachial plexus avulsion (trauma)
Carpal tunnel syndrome
Complex regional pain syndrome
Diabetic neuropathy
Fabry's disease
Failed back syndrome
Guillain-Barré syndrome
HIV-associated neuropathy
Viral involvement
Antiretrovirals
Poststroke pain
Trigeminal neuralgia
Vitamin deficiencies

HIV, *Human immunodeficiency virus.*
Source: Koh M, Portenoy RK. Cancer pain syndromes. In Bruera E, Portenoy RK, editors: Cancer Pain: Assessment and Management, *ed 2, Cambridge: Cambridge University Press, 2010, pp 53-85.*

metastases are common sources of pain, particularly in patients with breast, lung, or prostate cancers. Lymphedema, occurring in approximately 20% of women who undergo axillary node dissection, is an example of soft tissue pain associated with significant physical and psychological morbidity. Visceral pain may arise from involvement of tumor within the liver, intestine, kidney, peritoneum, bladder, or other organs. In addition, neuropathic pains can evolve from numerous causes, may be difficult for patients to describe, and are often complex to treat (Table 35.2). Finally, many people with cancer experience syndromes unrelated to the cancer or its treatment, such as osteoarthritis.

OTHER LIFE-THREATENING ILLNESSES

The prevalence and types of pain experienced by patients with specific nonmalignant diseases at the end of life have not been fully characterized. Examples include neuropathic pain associated with multiple sclerosis, chest pain due to end-stage cardiac disease, and pain due to pressure ulcers or immobility in those who are debilitated (Table 35.3).

ASSESSMENT OF PAIN AT THE END OF LIFE

The assessment techniques described in other chapters should be applied to patients with cancer or other life-threatening illnesses. Intensity, location (or often, multiple locations), quality, temporal nature of the pain, and factors that alter the pain are critical to ascertain. As with all other pain syndromes, a thorough history is followed by a comprehensive physical examination, with particular emphasis on the neurologic evaluation. Radiographic, laboratory, and other diagnostic techniques may be indicated, although in caring for those at the end of life, treatment decisions may be made empirically to avoid uncomfortable scans or invasive procedures.

When patients are unable to verbalize or describe their pain, clinicians can use the furrowed brow as a proxy measure of pain. If there is no response to adequate doses of opioids or other analgesics, additional sources of distress (e.g., distended bladder or fecal impaction) should be explored.[21]

While the general assessment of pain is universal, several additional dimensions are critical at end of life. A psychosocial assessment is indicated and directed towards the meaning of the pain as well as the effect of pain on the patient and their caregiver. The findings of this assessment may suggest the need for education, to mediate fears of addiction, for example. The results of this questioning may also prompt referral to social workers, chaplains, or others who are trained to address the existential distress or suffering experienced by the patient or their family.

Pain does not exist in isolation and symptom clusters are common, particularly at end of life. Several instruments have been designed to measure clinically multiple symptoms, including the Edmonton Symptom Assessment Scale (ESAS), the M.D. Anderson Symptom Inventory (MDASI), and the Memorial Symptom Assessment Scale (MSAS).[22–26] Another tool, the Distress "Thermometer," is a vertical

TABLE 35.3 Pain Syndromes Seen in People With Noncancer Diagnoses at End of Life

Disorder	Pain Syndromes
Cardiovascular disease Cardiomyopathy Congestive heart disease Peripheral vascular disease	Chest pain Ischemia
Cirrhosis	Abdominal pain due to portal hypertension, esophageal varices
Debility	Myalgias due to immobility Painful pressure ulcers Abdominal pain due to constipation, impaction Suprapubic pain due to distended bladder
End-stage renal disease	Painful pruritus
HIV	Abdominal pain due to infectious gastrointestinal disorders Chest pain from pneumocystis pneumonia Headaches Herpetic neuropathy Myalgia Neuropathies due to antiretrovirals and the virus
Neuromuscular disorders ALS Multiple sclerosis (MS) Spinal cord injury	Painful spasticity Lower extremity dysesthesias Periorbital pain and trigeminal neuralgia (MS)
Pulmonary disease Embolism Infection Pneumothorax	Chest pain Dyspnea

ALS, *Amyotrophic lateral sclerosis;* HIV, *human immunodeficiency virus.*

TABLE 35.4 Pain and Other Symptom Assessment Tools Used in Palliative Care

Assessment Tools	Description
Edmonton Symptom Assessment Scale (ESAS)	Consists of nine symptoms; can add one to individualize Measures severity using a 0–10 visual analog or numeric scales Sum of nine symptoms = distress Valid and reliable (See www.palliative.org for instructions)
M.D. Anderson Symptom Inventory (MDASI)	Consists of 13 items; ranked from 0 "not present" to 10 "as bad as you can imagine" Includes 6 interference items; ranked from 0 "did not interfere" to 10 "interfered completely" Valid and reliable (See www.mdanderson.org/departments/prg)
Memorial Symptom Assessment Scale (MSAS)	Measures 32 physical and psychological symptoms using Likert scales Evaluates prevalence, severity, and distress Total score is average of all 32 symptoms Valid and reliable pediatric versions available (See www.promotingexcellence.org)
Distress thermometer	Measures distress using a vertical visual analog designed to look like a thermometer Zero (0) indicates "no distress" and 10 (at the top of the thermometer) indicates "extreme distress" Includes a checklist of physical, psychological, practical, family support, and spiritual/religious concerns (See www.nccn.org)

visual analog scale designed to look like a thermometer, with 0 meaning "no distress" and 10 (at the top of the thermometer) indicating "extreme distress." Accompanying the distress scale is a checklist of various physical, psychological, practical, family support, and spiritual/religious concerns.[27] These are brief, clinically useful tools that quantify the intensity of a variety of symptoms common at end of life (Table 35.4). The specific needs of people enrolled in hospice are addressed in the Brief Hospice Inventory (BHI).[28] The BHI assesses outcomes of hospice patients, including physical and psychological symptoms, patient's perceptions of hospice care, as well as ratings of their quality of life. Each statement is measured using an 11-point scale.

Benefits of these instruments include the systematic assessment of pain and other symptoms. These data inform the clinician as a treatment plan is developed, including challenges in delivering analgesic therapy and particularly when managing complex pain syndromes that occur at the end of life.

MEDICATION ADMINISTRATION AT END OF LIFE

Alternate routes of medication administration are often necessary at end of life.[29] Transmucosal (sublingual, buccal, or nasal), transdermal, enteral, rectal, and parenteral (intravenous or subcutaneous) delivery can be employed, as can epidural or intrathecal approaches.[30] Considerations must be given to caregiver burden, resource availability, safety, and cost. The risks and benefits of each of these routes are discussed in other chapters.

Adverse effects of opioids must be considered and prevented when feasible. Constipation often worsens as disease progresses, opioid intake increases, activity decreases, and oral ingestion changes. Opioids decrease peristalsis, and this effect is compounded by weakness and fatigue at end of life, making it difficult for the patient to generate the strength to evacuate the colon. Other causes of constipation should be considered and managed when possible, including medications (e.g., ondansetron, iron), metabolic alterations (e.g., hypercalcemia), spinal cord compression, and other comorbidities. Laxatives, including senna, bisacodyl, magnesium hydroxide, or magnesium citrate, administered on a routine basis can be effective. When aggressive use of these agents is ineffective, peripherally acting opioid antagonists, such as methylnaltrexone and naloxegol, can produce a bowel movement if the primary cause of constipation is related to opioids.[31,32] These agents should not be used if bowel obstruction is suspected.

TABLE 35.5 Management of Complex Pain Syndromes at End of Life

Malignant Bone Pain
Dexamethasone 8–20 mg PO, IV, SQ every morning (not to be used in conjunction with NSAIDs)
Opioids
Bisphosphonates such as pamidronate or zoledronic acid
Radiation therapy (may be given as single fraction in some cases)
Radionuclides such as strontium-89 or radium-223
Orthotics for braces or slings
Physical or occupational therapy for assistive devices
Intractable Neuropathic Pain
Dexamethasone 8–20 mg PO, IV, SQ every morning (not to be used in conjunction with NSAIDs)
Opioids can be effective but higher doses are indicated (methadone may provide additional benefit over other opioids)
Anticonvulsants
Antidepressants, including novel or atypical agents such as venlafaxine
Local anesthetics (e.g., lidocaine patch, intraspinal infusions in combinations with opioids or parenteral infusions)
Malignant Intestinal Obstruction
Dexamethasone 8–20 mg PO, IV, SQ every morning to reduce inflammation and nausea (not to be used in conjunction with NSAIDs)
Opioids
Octreotide 20 μg/hour IV or SQ to decrease intestinal secretions; increase dose as needed
Scopolamine transdermal patches (1.5 mg, up to 2 patches) may reduce secretions
Nasogastric tube or venting gastrostomy if consistent with patient goals

IV, *Intravenous;* NSAIDs, *nonsteroidal antiinflammatory drugs;* PO, *oral;* SQ, *subcutaneous.*

COMPLEX PAIN SYNDROMES AT END OF LIFE

The management of pain in palliative care and hospice incorporates the same analgesics, routes, and principles described in the chapter on cancer pain and in monographs.[19,30,33] The majority of patients will obtain relief from these therapies or with the addition of interventional techniques. Unfortunately, a small percentage of patients will experience complex syndromes that do not respond to traditional approaches, such as bone pain, intractable neuropathic pain, or malignant bowel obstruction, or will develop severe opioid-induced toxicity.

MALIGNANT BONE PAIN

Bone pain is often difficult to treat in that patients may obtain good relief of movement-associated pain from higher-dose opioid therapy, yet they may be extremely sedated when they stop moving or place pressure on the bone.[34,35] Patients at risk include those with cancers that frequently metastasize to bone, including breast, lung, prostate, or multiple myeloma. Table 35.5 lists treatment options.

INTRACTABLE NEUROPATHIC PAIN

Neuropathies can be difficult to treat.[36] Standard therapies include opioids and adjuvant analgesics, including corticosteroids (see Table 35.5). Additionally, nerve blocks and other interventional techniques can be useful. In more refractory cases intravenous, lidocaine infusions are used to treat intractable pain.[37] Using techniques and protocols originating from pain clinics, intravenous lidocaine 1 to 2 mg/kg is given over 15 to 30 minutes. If effective, a continuous infusion of 1 to 2 mg/kg per hour is started. The analgesic effects can be as prolonged as weeks of relief. Perioral numbness is an early warning sign of potential toxicity. Hepatic dysfunction and significant cardiac conduction abnormalities are relative contraindications to the treatment, viewed in balance with the patient's goals of care and prognosis.

MALIGNANT INTESTINAL OBSTRUCTION

Bowel obstruction is common in progressive gynecologic and colorectal malignancies. The majority of patients with bowel obstruction will die within 6 months. Palliation can include surgery in selected cases, or, more commonly, intravenous or subcutaneous octreotide, nasogastric tube suction, and venting gastrostomy, in addition to analgesics and antiemetics. Table 35.5 lists specific treatment options.

OPIOID NEUROTOXICITY

The neuroexcitatory effects of opioids include myoclonus, hyperalgesia, delirium, and grand mal seizures. These toxicities have been reported in association with morphine, hydromorphone, hydrocodone, fentanyl, methadone, and oxycodone.[38] The 3-glucuronide metabolites are implicated as contributing to these neuroexcitatory effects. Both morphine-3-glucuronide (M3G) and hydromorphone-3-glucuronide (H3G) are believed to produce myoclonus and seizures.[39] Renal failure appears to be a significant, but not absolute, risk factor, as patients are unable to clear the metabolite. Case reports suggest that H3G plasma levels are greatly increased in the presence of renal failure, with the ratio of H3G to the parent compound four times higher than the ratio seen in patients with normal renal function.

The treatment of mild myoclonus generally includes switching to another opioid, lowering the dose of the opioid, and adding a benzodiazepine. Clonazepam 0.5 mg orally twice daily with upward titration may be effective. If the patient is unable to swallow, midazolam or lorazepam may be used. Hyperalgesia frequently is misdiagnosed and the first response by well-meaning clinicians often is to increase the opioid dose.[40] This generally results in greater pain, with potential progression to delirium and possibly seizures.

When these more severe neurotoxicities occur, the opioid dose should be reduced by at least 50%. Some advocate stopping the opioid altogether, since the half-life of these metabolites is long and the patient is unlikely to experience the abstinence syndrome. Naloxone appears to be ineffective in reversing this toxicity. In select cases, spinal delivery of analgesics can be effective in relieving pain and reducing systemic opioid exposure. Should seizures occur, first- and second-line therapies include phenytoin and benzodiazepines, such as diazepam or lorazepam. In some cases, the seizures will progress in frequency and intensity, advancing to status epilepticus. Refractory status epilepticus treatment may require midazolam, barbiturates, and propofol.

- Midazolam is particularly useful in palliative care due to its rapid onset and short duration, as well as its ability to be given subcutaneously, intravenously, orally, buccally, sublingually, or rectally. Furthermore, its only known drug incompatibility is with corticosteroids, particularly betamethasone, dexamethasone, and methylprednisolone.
- The standard dose of phenobarbital in the management of seizures is 20 mg/kg intravenous infusion with a maximum rate of 50 to 100 mg/min.
- The recommended dose of propofol to treat refractory status epilepticus is 1 to 2 mg/kg via intravenous injection over 5 minutes and repeated if necessary. A maintenance intravenous infusion of 2 to 10 mg/kg per hour is then started, using the lowest dose needed to suppress seizure activity.

OTHER SYMPTOMS COMMON AT END OF LIFE

Dyspnea, anxiety, depression, constipation, and other symptoms are common in the face of advanced illness.[41,42] Palliation of these symptoms, which are frequently linked with pain, can result in improved pain control and enhanced quality of life.[42,43]

DYSPNEA

Dyspnea, or air hunger, can occur as a result of a variety of illnesses, including cancer, congestive heart failure, or pulmonary diseases. Opioids are the first drug of choice, often in small doses that do not typically cause sedation.[42,43] Short-acting anxiolytics are indicated in the face of severe anxiety. Simple measures such as bedside fans can provide additional comfort.

ANXIETY

Anxiety is highly correlated with unrelieved pain. Additionally, many medications commonly used in palliative care, such as corticosteroids, neuroleptics (including metoclopramide), bronchodilators, antihistamines, digitalis, and occasionally benzodiazepines (which can cause a paradoxical reaction in elderly patients), can result in motor restlessness and agitation. Abrupt withdrawal from alcohol, opioids, benzodiazepines, and nicotine also produces agitation. Hypoxia, pulmonary embolus, sepsis, hypoglycemia, thyroid abnormalities, and heart failure are associated with anxiety, as are certain tumors, including pheochromocytomas, and some pancreatic cancers.[42,43] Primary or metastatic lung cancers and chronic cardiopulmonary conditions can lead to dyspnea, which can also produce anxiety.

Pharmacologic treatment of anxiety usually consists of benzodiazepines, particularly lorazepam, as it has a short duration of action and produces fewer adverse effects. A typical initial dosage is 0.5 to 2 mg orally 3 or 4 times daily. Lorazepam can be placed sublingually, which is useful when patients have difficulty swallowing, or given parenterally as a bolus or infusion. Haloperidol is frequently used for short-term management of severe anxiety and as an antipsychotic, with initial dosage starting at 0.5 to 1 mg orally twice daily. Frank discussion of patients' fears in a supportive environment, along with the use of relaxation strategies, such as audiotapes, breathing exercises, and guided imagery, may alleviate anxiety.

DEPRESSION

Depression is often poorly recognized in people at end of life. Diagnosis may be difficult in advanced disease, as the usual physical symptoms of depression (fatigue, anorexia, and sleep disturbance) can result from the disease itself or its treatment.[44] Psychological symptoms suggestive of depression in the patient with life-threatening illness include loss of self-worth, unremitting sadness and hopelessness, and suicidal ideation. There is evidence that a simple screening question "Are you depressed?" or "Are you sad?" is the most valid measure of a patient's depression. Supportive psychotherapy may be of benefit, including dignity therapy, although limited life span may be a barrier.[45] Antidepressant medications, such as serotonin-specific reuptake inhibitors (SSRIs), such as citalopram, fluoxetine, paroxetine, and sertraline, are usually well tolerated. However, the 2 to 4 weeks required for the drug to take effect is often too long for patients with an advanced disease and a very short life span. Newer, "atypical antidepressants" (e.g., bupropion, mirtazepine,) have a relatively rapid onset of action and few reported side effects. However, for patients with a very limited life span, stimulants such as methylphenidate provide rapid relief, usually within hours to days. Ketamine is also under study to address significant depression and anxiety at the end of life.[46]

CONCLUSION

Pain, dyspnea, anxiety, and depression are serious symptoms experienced by people with life-threatening illnesses. All health care professionals are responsible for care of the dying; therefore, they must be aware of the most common syndromes occurring in this population, able to conduct specific assessment techniques, and knowledgeable about the therapies used to treat these symptoms. Resources, such as palliative care services and hospices, can assist physicians as they provide care to these patients and their families.

KEY POINTS

- All physicians, regardless of specialty, are responsible for care of patients with life-threatening illnesses.
- Assessment of pain and other symptoms at end of life requires knowledge of common syndromes, as well as skill to conduct a thorough history and physical examination, with particular attention to the neurologic evaluation.
- Complex pain syndromes require novel drug therapies, in addition to standard nonopioid, opioid, and adjuvant analgesics.
- Adequate pain control in those with life-threatening illness requires attention to related symptoms such as dyspnea, anxiety, and depression.

REFERENCES

Access the reference list online at ExpertConsult.com.

CHAPTER 36

Pain Management in the Emergency Department

James Mathews, MD ✪ Arthur Moore, MD

The complaint of pain is the most common symptom presenting to the Emergency Department (ED).[1,2] Over the past 15 years, the Joint Commission has emphasized the recognition of pain, and it now considers pain the fifth vital sign.[3,4] The causes of pain encompass the entire range of human diseases, including psychological illness. The assessment of the severity of pain is subjective, and what appears to be the same problem or injury can affect each individual very differently. Several systems have been developed to quantify the degree of pain, but all rely on the patient's perception of their pain.[5,6] Practitioners must use all their clinical acumen to make an appropriate decision regarding the need for and class of analgesic to use in a given circumstance.

Pain can be divided into two major categories, acute and chronic. Acute pain serves a physiologic function in that it is a warning to the patient that something is wrong and results in the patient seeking help or prevents the patient from doing further harm by limiting activity. The bulk of this chapter is devoted to the discussion of the management of acute pain in the ED. The transition point from acute to chronic pain has been variably defined, ranging from as little as 4 to 6 weeks up to 6 months of pain.

CHRONIC PAIN

Chronic pain serves no useful function to the patient. Patients with chronic pain can be divided into four general groups. These groups are patients with chronic pain secondary to underlying diseases, such as cancer, sickle cell disease, and AIDS; patients with known pain syndromes, such as tic douloureux and migraine headache; chronic pain patients without an identifiable cause; and finally, the group of patients that uses the complaint of chronic pain to obtain drugs or for other personal gains.

Each of these groups of patients requires a different management approach. Cancer patients with new pain or with acute worsening of their previous pain should be evaluated for a new complication, and their pain should be aggressively managed with opiates.[7] For these patients, palliative screening can be initiated in the ED and can be very helpful for their long-term management.[8] Patients with known pain syndromes and without objective cause for their pain require an aggressive team approach, and if they are patients within your institution, prearranged therapeutic plans should be in place for when they appear in the ED. This is particularly helpful for those patients with sickle cell disease and frequent pain crises. The final group is a subset of pain patients that tests the patience and professionalism of emergency physicians and nurses. The majority of these patients are seeking narcotics. The diagnosis of malingering must be a diagnosis of exclusion and cannot be made on the first visit by a patient to the ED. An appropriate workup for the patient's complaint should be done and often needs to be repeated 2 or 3 times before the diagnosis of malingering is made. If malingering is suspected, the patient should be referred to the outpatient pain and psychiatric services for further evaluation and treatment. Each time these patients appear in the ED, the emergency physician should perform at least a basic history and physical examination, but you can refuse to give further narcotics. Nonsteroidal antiinflammatory drugs (NSAIDs) may be offered, but these patients will often refuse them or state that they cannot take them. There are no hard and fast rules as to how to handle this type of patient. All you can do is maintain your professional ethics and practice and do the best you can by performing an adequate assessment and then refer the patient to the appropriate outpatient services.

ACUTE PAIN

Pain is a combination of physical, chemical, and psychological factors. There is no current method to directly measure the degree of pain that a given patient is experiencing from a given injury. However, if a patient presents to the ED with a complaint of pain, an attempt should be made to quantify the patient's perception of the degree of pain. A patient's verbal report is the only way to reliably obtain a patient's evaluation of their pain. Several tools have been developed to grade a given patient's pain and the response to treatment (Table 36.1). Pain scales should be incorporated as part of the triage process and should be located on the record where the vitals are recorded. The severity of pain index should be recorded during the initial assessment process, and early and effective management of pain should be ensured.[9] After treatment, the assessment should be repeated as needed. However, all too often, this does not occur.[10]

There are several difficult to control barriers to the successful management of acute pain in the ED.[11] These include overcrowding, age, ethnicity, and overall attitude of the caregivers. In addition, the emergency physician must focus on diagnosis of the cause of pain which may distract from the management of the pain itself. Numerous studies have documented inadequate use of analgesic agents in the ED.[12,13] This is particularly true in the pediatric population.[14] Many patients do not receive any pain medications while in the ED, even though their primary presenting complaint was pain.[12,15] In addition to no analgesia, there are a number of therapeutic errors that may result in the inadequate use of analgesics in the ED. These include prescribing the wrong agent, inappropriate dosage and dosing intervals, route of administration, improper use of adjunct agents, and concern for medically induced addiction to narcotics.

TABLE 36.1 Pain Assessment Tools

Clinical Tool	Grading Pain	When Used
Verbal quantitative scale	0–10 (None to worst possible)	Routine evaluation
Visual analog device	[____________]. None to worst. Patient places a mark on the line.	Routine evaluation
Global satisfaction question	Are you satisfied with your pain relief? Yes/No	Useful for confusing patients
Pediatric pain scales		
Observer generated	Facial expressions, crying	Neonate to age 3 and some 3–6
Draw a picture of your pain	Est. location, intensity, and character	Over age 6 and some 3–6
Faces		Over age 6 and some 3–6
Pain thermometer	Like visual scale for adults	Over age 6 and some 3–6

Failure to give analgesics is an issue that must be addressed by education of nursing staff and physicians.[16] The goal should be adequate pain relief for all patients. Emphasis of the importance of pain control to the patient is key in this process of changing practice habits. Patient satisfaction may be directly related to adequate pain control.[17,18] In addition, the early control of acute pain appears to reduce the incidence of chronic pain syndromes and may improve the patient's outcome.[19] Finally, health care providers have taken an oath to reduce or prevent pain and suffering.

Correction of the inappropriate usage of analgesics also requires a great deal of physician reeducation, and frequently, major changes in practice habits must be instituted. Severe pain generally requires the use of parenteral opioids. In the acute situation, an intravenous (IV) line should be established, and the dosage titrated for the individual patient. The amount required of a given opiate for adequate pain relief can vary widely from patient to patient. For example, the effective level for morphine has been reported to be as much as 8 times greater from one patient to another. The intramuscular (IM) route should be avoided, as it is painful and the onset of action is variable. If an IV cannot be obtained, the subcutaneous route offers an excellent alternative. In addition, there are newer agents that can be given by the sublingual or nasal route. Fentanyl is available in sucker form, which has great applicability in the pediatric population. Sufentanil and butorphanol, both potent opioids, are effective when given via the nasal mucosa. Once the route and dosage is determined, it should be given at frequent enough intervals to prevent the return of pain.

There is little role for adjunct agents in the management of acute pain in the ED. The exception is the clinical circumstance of persistent nausea and vomiting following the use of opioids or in patients with pain who also have nausea and vomiting. The practice of using an adjunct to reduce the opioid dose simply is not valid and exposes the patient to another set of side effects. This practice should be abandoned.

The risk of addiction to the opioids with medical use must be a concern for physicians, especially when treating patients with chronic pain.[20,21] However, in the acute patient, there seems to be little evidence for undue concern. Of 11,892 inpatients who received opioids while in the hospital, only 4 became addicted without a prior history of substance abuse.[22]

SPECIFIC PROBLEMS

ABDOMINAL PAIN

For years, the conventional teaching was to avoid the use of opioids for abdominal pain until a definitive decision had been made regarding surgery. This was sound and necessary practice prior to the development of modern diagnostic tools, such as computed tomography (CT) scanning. Simply put, this practice is outdated. From the published literature on this subject, there has not been a significant increase in management errors demonstrated nor is there evidence for major morbidity or mortality associated with the early use of opiates in the treatment of abdominal pain.[23–26] The goal in patients with abdominal pain is not to achieve pain free status, but rather to substantially reduce the severity of the pain. Opioids given by the IV route allow for careful titration of these agents. The patient should be kept responsive enough to allow for subsequent examinations. Close observation of the patient's course is mandatory, especially in patients with ulcerative colitis because of the added risk of toxic megacolon. NSAIDs can be effective therapy when treating biliary or renal colic.

HEADACHE

The complaint of headache is commonly seen in the ED.[27] Many of these patients have a known history of a specific type of headache such as migraine or vascular headaches. There are many causes of headache, and a minority of these patients may require extensive workups, including CT scanning, MRI, and lumbar puncture (LP), to exclude a life-threatening cause of headache. By far the majority of patients presenting to the ED with the complaint of headache will need only pain relief and follow-up. A useful reference to assist the emergency physician to sort through this complaint is the *Classification and Diagnostic Criteria for Headache Disorders, Second edition*, published by The International Headache Society in 2004.[28] This handbook provides an organized approach to the diagnosis and management of the various types of headache and facial pain.

Migraine

In the United States, over 1 million patients per year present to EDs with the complaint of migraine. If the patient does not have a clear and reproducible history of migraines, this diagnosis should be made with caution, and a headache workup needs to be done. If the prodromal symptoms, pattern of pain, and associated symptoms are similar to past attacks, the workup may be limited to a history and physical exam unless there is coexisting illness. Most of these patients have had failure of their usual medications to control pain prior to arrival to the ED. Therapy to relieve the pain is indicated. In mild to moderate migraine, acetaminophen or nonsteroidal agents are often effective. In more severe and persistent migraine, such agents as sumatriptan given subcutaneously or by nasal spray, prochlorperazine, and metoclopromide by the IV route may be required to both relieve the pain and to counteract nausea and vomiting. Sumatriptan works best if used early in the onset of a migraine. This agent is contraindicated in patients with known coronary artery disease, hypertension, pregnancy, and peripheral vascular disease. The other two agents may be associated with hypotension, sedation, and dystonic reactions, and an anticholinergic drug should be added if these agents are given in high doses. Patients receiving metoclopromide or similar agents should receive a 500 cc bolus of saline prior to the drug being given to help avoid hypotension. When added to standard acute migraine therapy, 10 mg of dexamethasone given IM or IV appears to reduce the incidence of recurrent migraine over the next 24–72 hours.[29] Opioids should only be given for patients who do not get relief by other means or in those who are unable to receive other agents.[30] Dihydroergotamine is contraindicated in vascular disease, in the elderly, and in patients on monoamine oxidase (MAO) inhibitors or if sumatriptan has already been used. This agent is especially useful for those patients with a refractory attack of migraine, and if used, the patient should first receive an antiemetic.

Cluster Headache

Cluster headaches are seen much less commonly in the ED, and emergency physicians are often less comfortable with management of this clinical problem. If the patient is having a typical pattern of headache, there is little indication for extensive workup, and treatment should be initiated to control the pain. In many cases, sumatriptan will abort the attack. Frequently the patient with this problem has already used this medication, and needs pain control. High flow oxygen will often end the attack. If these attempts fail, dihydroergotamine given by the IV route is effective. Numerous other agents have been used, but if the above fails, neurological consultation should be considered to assist in managing this problem.

Subarachnoid Hemorrhage

Subarachnoid hemorrhage (SAH) remains a difficult diagnosis for the emergency physician, and SAH has a high morbidity and mortality rate, exceeding 50%. Many of these patients will expire before they can get to medical care or arrive at the ED comatose. Patients with SAH often deteriorate rapidly, and early diagnosis is mandatory to maximize the chances for a good outcome.

The speed of onset of the headache is a major diagnostic clue. If the headache has come on over more than a few minutes, it is highly unlikely that the headache is due to an SAH.[31] In many cases, the patient describes the headache as if their head is exploding or that the top of their head felt as if it was going to come off. These patients will frequently state that this is or was the worst headache of their life, but this complaint is not exclusive to SAH. Even if the patient has none of the other features of an SAH, such as meningismus and neurological findings, these complaints should not be ignored.

A patient giving this type of history should be seriously considered for the work-up of SAH. The approach for many years has been to obtain a rapid CT of the brain to look for blood, and if this is negative, an LP should be used. CT cannot be relied on alone, as up to 10% of acute SAH does not show blood on CT. This percentage is based on results from the earlier generations of CT scanners, and it is probably much less today.[32–34] If a cranial CT is performed closer to the time of onset of the headache associated with SAH, then the cranial CT is more reliable. By 1 week after an SAH, the percentage of false negatives on a brain CT may exceed 50%.[35] A diagnostic alternative to an LP is a CT angiogram that is widely available today and is almost as reliable as LP to detect bleeding and diagnose for aneurysms.

Pain relief can be given. Nonsteroidals are contraindicated in the treatment of patients with suspected SAH because of their anticoagulation properties. Treatment similar to that for migraines as described above is often effective and should be tried first. If the headache is rapidly relieved by these agents, it is unlikely that the patient has SAH. Opioids are safe and effective, but it should be titrated to prevent excessive sedation.

Tension Headache

This is the most common cause of headache in the ED and is frequently associated with other medical and psychological problems. Tension headaches are also the most general and difficult to categorize. To a great extent, this is a diagnosis of exclusion and should only be given if the practitioner is satisfied that a more serious problem is not causing the headache. This may require imaging studies. Tension headaches often have a general pattern in that the patient complains of a bandlike pressure around the head and associated neck stiffness. Other symptoms are usually absent, and, if present, they are mild. Pain relief can usually be achieved with acetaminophen or nonsteroidals. If there is associated anxiety, mild tranquilizers may help to prevent recurrence.

Other Causes of Headache

There are numerous other disease processes that either are the direct cause of or are associated with the complaint of headache. An in-depth discussion of these is beyond the scope of this chapter. In many of these conditions, associated neurological symptoms will make the complaint of headache secondary. If the headache is related to a space-occupying lesion in the brain, opioids in careful doses are very useful to relieve the patient's suffering. The patient requires rapid consultation with the appropriate specialty. For headaches associated with underlying medical diseases, such as hypertension, the treatment of the underlying problem will often relieve the headache with minimum need for analgesia. Suffice it to say, the emergency physician must use judgment when prescribing pain medications for the headache patient. Underlying causes for the headache should not be masked by the aggressive use of analgesics. However, the patient should not be denied some relief of their discomfort. Careful selection of the agent used, appropriate titration of the dosage of the agent, and proper delivery route of the drug can go a long way towards achieving these therapeutic goals without overly confusing the clinical picture.

CHEST PAIN

Chest pain is a frequent complaint in the ED. The causes of chest pain are myriad, and the emergency physician must make rapid clinical decisions if the pain is secondary to a life-threatening disease.[36] The three most common serious diseases presenting with chest pain are myocardial ischemia and infarction, pulmonary embolism, and dissection of the thoracic aorta. Clinical pathways, particularly for myocardial ischemia, are well established. Part of these pathways is the use of morphine for the reduction of pain and anxiety. A major role of this agent is in those patients whose pain is not fully relieved by nitrates and beta-blockers. Doses should be given IV and titrated to achieve pain relief without respiratory depression. The clinician must carefully monitor the patient to avoid hypotension. Aortic dissection commonly requires an opioid to relieve the severe pain experienced by patients with this condition. Pulmonary embolism seldom requires heavy analgesia, and good pain relief can usually be obtained with NSAIDs. If required, opioids are safe and effective.

Most of the remaining causes of chest pain are either inflammatory, such as pericarditis, or due to musculoskeletal problems. The majority of these patients will respond well to NSAIDs or to acetaminophen. Adjunct therapy of heat or cold, massage therapy, and physical therapy may be indicated in follow up. A commonly occurring condition where NSAIDs should be avoided is in those patients with gastroesophageal reflux disorder (GERD). Acetaminophen may be used, but primary treatment with antacids and histamine blockers should be initiated.

MUSCULOSKELETAL PAIN

All people experience a variety of aches and pains secondary to contusions, minor arthritis, and soft tissue sprains and strains. By far, the majority of these individuals treat themselves at home with a host of over-the-counter medications of varying degrees of efficacy and other adjunctive measures. The two over-the-counter drugs most frequently used today are ibuprofen and acetaminophen. If these patients present to the ED, a history of what agents and the amount taken needs to be obtained by the emergency physician to give appropriate treatment and to avoid overdosing the patient. Icing sprains and contusions and appropriate splinting and immobilization of the injured extremity is mandated in the acute period, but these adjunct therapies are often overlooked during long waits in the waiting room. This group of patients comprises the largest single source of complaints regarding failure of staff to control pain.

Although there has been little research to support the use of muscle relaxants, they appear to have a role in acute musculoskeletal injury when there is associated severe muscle spasm. Commonly used agents are orphenadrine citrate, methocarbamol, and the benzodiazepines. These agents cannot be a substitute for adequate analgesia. Oral opioids may be required in the management of severe musculoskeletal pain, especially when these patients are discharged. Acetaminophen with codeine has been used for years, but in reality, codeine is a poor analgesic and has not been demonstrated to be more effective than NSAIDs or acetaminophen alone. Other oral opioids are effective in the management of severe pain, but physicians are often reluctant to prescribe them on an outpatient basis because of the fear of causing addiction. Included in this group are hydrocodone, oxycodone, and oral meperidine. These agents should be used if the pain is severe and are generally safe to prescribe for short-term use. All of these agents do have a relatively high potential for abuse, and they should be prescribed with discretion and in limited amounts.

Patients with obvious fractures should be seen as soon as possible, and early immobilization be obtained. This prevents further soft tissue injury and will reduce the pain. Opioids often are required to control the pain, and the safest and most effective method is titration of these agents by the IV route. Patients given IV opioids need to be monitored for respiratory depression, hypotension, and excessive euphoria. If patients require extended "road trips" to radiology for multiple X-rays or CT scanning, they should be accompanied by medical personnel to both monitor their vitals and give additional analgesia if required.

PAIN MANAGEMENT IN PEDIATRICS

It has been well demonstrated that the pediatric population is often overlooked for adequate analgesia.[14] Children over the age of 5 can usually tell you where it hurts and how much. Pediatric scales have been developed and are a useful adjunct for pain assessment (see Table 36.1). Pediatric patients are often overlooked in a busy department because the bulk of their complaints are not life or limb threatening, and they do not openly complain. Their parents may attribute their child's fussiness to being tired and hungry or to being frightened from being in the ED. The same attention and assessment for pain is mandated in the pediatric population, and appropriate doses of analgesics should be given. The same agents that are effective in adults are effective in children when used in proper dosage and if administered by the appropriate route.

ANALGESIA DURING PROCEDURES

The use of "OK, OK" anesthesia has little role in the modern practice of emergency medicine. This is a time-honored but brutal practice that has been used for everything from reduction of small joints to using force to restrain children for repair of small lacerations. Although it is impossible to do any procedure without some pain and discomfort, every attempt should be made to keep these to a minimum.[37] Adequate sedation prior to performing the procedure helps to reduce the anxiety and fear associated with procedures and reduces the memory of the event. Also, it produces muscle relaxation, an important effect for major joint reduction. Numerous regimens have been developed to provide sedation, amnesia, muscle relaxation, and analgesia. The emergency physician needs to have an excellent knowledge of one or two of these regimes and to know what side effects to expect. Patients must be monitored carefully, and specific procedures to ensure that this occurs need to be in place. The American College of Emergency Physicians has published guidelines to assist in developing the approach to safely use procedural sedation and analgesia (PSA), also known as conscious sedation (Box 36.1).[38] The American Society of Anesthesiologists also recommends a period of fasting of 6 hours for solids and 2 hours for liquids prior to PSA.[39] To date, there has been no evidence that PSA as performed in the ED requires prolonged fasting, and prior ingestion of food is not a contraindication. If ingestion of food or liquids has occurred recently, the degree of sedation should be minimized by careful titration of the agent(s) used to obtain PSA.

SPECIFIC AGENTS

FENTANYL AND MIDAZOLAM

This combination is widely used for PSA in both adults and children. Fentanyl is a short-acting opioid with high potency and minimal cardiovascular effects. This agent has a rapid onset of action, usually within 2 minutes, and the duration of action is 30–40 minutes. Serum half-life is approximately 90 minutes. This combination of rapid onset, high potency, and short half-life makes fentanyl an excellent agent for most ED procedures. The usual required dose is between 2 and 3 μg/kg by slow IV push given in increments of 0.5–1 μg/kg every 2 minutes to a maximum of 5 μg/kg for both adults and children. The total amount of the agent required is dependent on the individual's response. Because of its high potency, safety, and relatively short half-life, fentanyl is very easy to titrate by using multiple small doses to achieve the desired effect. Fentanyl can induce severe respiratory depression, especially when used with other agents such as midazolam. This side effect is dose related, and usually appears within 5 minutes of administration of the agent. The doses used for PSA in the ED have not been reported to cause muscular and glottic rigidity or "board chest," which has been well documented when the agent is used in general anesthetic doses of over 50 μg/kg. This reaction can be reversed by either naloxone or succinylcholine. Seizures have not been documented when using fentanyl for ED PSA. General pruritus is usually not present with the use of fentanyl as occurs with many opioids as it does not cause histamine release, and nausea is usually minimal when compared to other opioid analgesics. Fentanyl can also be administered orally in the form of a lollipop, making it useful in children if the IV route is not possible or required. The dose is usually 10–15 μg/kg, and onset of action is between 12 and 30 minutes. It is not feasible to fully titrate the dosage administered when fentanyl is given by the oral route. Nausea and vomiting are more common, but major side effects of seizures and "board chest" have not been reported.

Midazolam is so frequently used in combination with fentanyl that these two agents should be considered together. The usual dose is 0.02–0.1 mg/kg for adults and 0.05–0.15 mg/kg for children. Midazolam also has a rapid onset of action of 1–3 minutes and a relatively short half-life of 30–60 minutes. When given IV, the drug is easily titrated to achieve the desired response. Midazolam provides excellent sedation, a beneficial hypnotic effect, muscle relaxation, amnesia, and antiseizure activity. The major side effect is respiratory depression, which is dose related and is more pronounced in the presence of other central nervous system depressants such as alcohol. The elderly and patients with chronic lung, liver, or renal disease are more sensitive to this agent. In general, cardiovascular side effects are not seen at sedative dosages. If other agents, such as fentanyl, are used in combination with midazolam, hypotension may occur. This will usually respond to a bolus of saline solution. Occasionally children will have paradoxical agitation when midazolam is used. If the IV route is not available, midazolam may be administered by rectal suppository, orally, and by nasal insufflation. This alternative can be useful to sedate children before simple therapeutic or diagnostic procedures. A specific regimen for the use of the combination of fentanyl and midazolam has been developed and appears to be safe and effective. This recommendation is midazolam 0.02 mg/kg IV and fentanyl 0.5 μg/kg IV. Repeat one or both agents as needed every 2 minutes.

BOX 36.1 Recommendations of the Clinical Policies Committee of American College of Emergency Physicians

1. Personnel involved in the administration of agents to and monitoring of PSA patients must understand the drugs given, have the ability to properly monitor the patient, and have the necessary skills to intervene to manage the potential complications. An excellent approach is to have one support person present in addition to the provider.
2. The patient should receive a history of past or present illnesses and allergies, and limited physical aimed at vitals, airway, and cardiovascular status. Recent ingestion of food is not a contraindication.
3. Initial consent to treatment is adequate, but separate consent may be obtained.
4. Advanced life support equipment and oxygen should be available. In addition, antagonists (naloxone for opiates, flumazenil for benzodiazepines) need to be present. An IV line should be obtained.
5. Patient monitoring must include frequent vital signs. Constantly monitoring pulse oximetry and cardiac monitoring are excellent options, but they may not be mandatory in every circumstance. The patient's appearance and response to verbal stimuli should be watched during and after the procedure.
6. Drugs should be administered slowly and titrated to desired effect.
7. The patient should be monitored carefully during the postprocedure period. Discharge occurs when the patient responds appropriately, the vitals are stable and back to normal for the patient, respiratory function is normal, pain has been addressed, minimal nausea, and new symptoms are handled. Patients should be back to baseline before discharge or discharged to a responsible third party.

IV, Intravenous.

KETAMINE

Ketamine has had extensive use in PSA and is especially useful and safe in the pediatric population.[40] It is a derivative of phencyclidine, a notorious street drug. When ketamine is used, dissociation of the limbic and thalamocortical systems occurs, and the patient is essentially unable to perceive pain and other external stimuli while maintaining spontaneous respiration and airway protection. It does not produce muscle relaxation, and if this is required for the procedure, another agent such as midazolam must be added. Hypertension may occur with the use of ketamine, especially in adults. The presence of cardiovascular disease, active pulmonary disease, central nervous system masses or abnormalities, hydrocephalus, eye injury, glaucoma, and hyperthyroidism are relative contraindications for this agent. In the past, emergence phenomena such as hallucinations and nightmares have been reported to be as high as 50% in the adult population, but newer literature suggest an incidence between 0% and 30%.[40,41] Fortunately, most of these reactions are usually mild. The drug should be avoided in patients with a history of personality disorders and schizophrenia. Both of these complications are much less common in the pediatric population. Laryngospasm is a serious complication in children, especially in those less than 3 months old, and it should not be used in this age group. Laryngospasm rarely occurs in children older than 3 months and studies have shown that there is no increased risk in most ED procedures when the posterior pharynx is not overly stimulated. Ketamine can be given by all routes of administration, including IM, although IV remains the preferred option for adults as IV access may be required to treat emergence reactions. The IV route is the most common, and the typical IV loading dose required is 1 mg/kg in adults and 1.5–2.0 mg/kg in children. When ketamine is administered through the IV route, it should be given over 30–60 seconds to minimize the risk of transient respiratory depression. Repeat IV doses of 0.5–1.0 mg/kg can be administered as needed to maintain sedation every 5–15 minutes. Onset of action is within 1 minute of IV infusion, and the duration of action is only 15 minutes. The typical IM loading dose is 4–5 mg/kg for both adult and pediatric populations with a repeat dose of 2–4 mg/kg 10 minutes as needed. Unlike sedative-hypnotics, once ketamine's dosing threshold is reached, additional ketamine administration does not result in deeper sedation, but it may prolong the time of sedation. Ketamine is an excellent first-line agent in the pediatric population and is a good alternative to opioids for adults allergic to opioids and for patients at risk of hypotension and respiratory problems.[38,40]

KETAMINE AND PROPOFOL

The combination of ketamine and propofol is frequently used for PSA. When the agents are combined, they are each given in smaller doses than when used alone. Most dosing regimens use 0.5–0.75 mg/kg of each agent administered intravenously. There are many theoretical and synergistic benefits to combining the two agents. Ketamine induces higher levels of norepinephrine that can reduce the hypotension seen with propofol sedation. Propofol's anxiolytic and antiemetic properties may ameliorate the nausea and emergence phenomenon associated with the use of ketamine alone. This combination can be used safely in both pediatric and adult populations.

Propofol is a unique ultrashort-acting anesthetic agent unrelated to any other anesthetic class.[42] It is administered by slow injection of an initial loading dose 0.5–1 mg/kg IV followed by 0.5 mg/kg IV every 3–5 minutes as needed. Anesthesia occurs within 40 seconds and lasts 6 minutes. Propofol is not recommended for children less than 3 years old. Absolute contraindications include hypersensitivity to egg lecithin and soybean oil. Propofol can induce transient hypotension; consequently, it should be used with caution in patients with hypovolemia, hypotension, or poor cardiac function. Similar to etomidate, propofol injection may be painful and can be prevented by similar techniques, as mentioned above. Propofol provides no analgesia. It is considered first-line for PSA in young healthy patients.

OTHER AGENTS

Numerous agents have been used to provide PSA. These include nitrous oxide and methohexital. These agents appear to be safe and effective, but all have side effects and appear to offer no advantage over the agents previously discussed. In the past, chloral hydrate was used extensively in children, but this agent has little indication today because of its delayed onset of action and prolonged duration. The use of the combination of meperidine, promethazine, and chlorpromazine, known as DPT, should be dropped because of the numerous side effects that are seen with this mixture.

LOCAL ANESTHETICS

These remain a mainstay of anesthesia in the ED. They are used for local and regional anesthesia. The so-called "caine" drugs are divided into two classes, the esters and the amides, and the various agents have different times of onset and duration (Table 36.2). The most commonly used in the ED are lidocaine, bupivacaine, and mepivacaine, all of which are amides. If a patient has a history of allergy to these agents, the allergy is almost always to the ester class. Allergic reactions to the amides are exceedingly rare;

TABLE 36.2 Common Local Anesthetics Used in the Emergency Room

Agent (Trade Names)	Type of Agent	Use, Onset, and Duration
Lidocaine (Xylocaine, Dilocaine, Ultracaine)	Amide	Blocks, infiltration: Onset is rapid. Duration 90–200 min.
Tetracaine (Pontocaine)	Ester	Spinal, topical, eye. Onset slow. Duration 180–600 min.
Mepivacaine (Carbocaine)	Amide	Epidurals, blocks, infiltration. Onset very rapid. Duration 120–240 min.
Bupivacaine (Marcaine)	Amide	Blocks. Onset intermediate. Duration 180–600 min.
Procaine (Novocaine, Neocaine)	Ester	Blocks, infiltrations. Onset slow. Duration 60–90 min.

consequently, they can usually be safely used. Pain during administration is the norm. Efforts should be made to reduce this discomfort. These include using as small a needle as possible, warming the solution to be injected, slow injection of the agent, injecting through the wound edges rather than through skin, and use of topical anesthetics prior to administration. Buffering the injected solution with sodium bicarbonate has been advocated. The amount of bicarbonate solution suggested for lidocaine is 1 cc of bicarbonate per 10 cc of lidocaine solution. All of these agents may produce central nervous system and cardiovascular toxicity if blood concentrations are too high. The potential toxic effects of these agents include seizures and ventricular fibrillation. These tragedies can be avoided by calculating total doses before use and by careful administration of the agent.

Topical anesthesia has been used for years, especially in otolaryngology and dental practice. Cocaine is an excellent topical agent for such things as nosebleed because of its additional vasoconstrictor effect. A 50/50 mixture of topical tetracaine and adrenaline solutions will produce similar results. The major application for topical anesthetics is in treating lacerations in small children. The two agents used most frequently are the combination of lidocaine, epinephrine, and tetracaine (LET) in solution, and EMLA, a eutetic mixture of local anesthetic agents. This compound comes in cream form, and the active ingredients are lidocaine and prilocaine present in equal amounts. The cream is applied directly to the laceration under an occlusive dressing without pain to the child. Within 30–60 minutes, complete anesthesia can be obtained, which lasts up to 5 hours. Depth of penetration is limited, and for deep wounds, additional injection may be required. There are theoretical concerns regarding the effect of this combination on wound healing, but these concerns have largely been refuted. This agent has been a real boon to the management of lacerations in the pediatric population, and has markedly reduced the need to tie them down as was done in the past.

KEY POINTS

- Pain is the most common complaint seen in the ED. The emergency physician must ensure that patients in pain are treated with appropriate analgesics as soon as is feasible.
- With modern diagnostic modalities, such as CT scanning, there is no reason to withhold pain medications for patients with abdominal pain. The goal is to reduce the pain for the patient while they are undergoing diagnostic evaluation. Oversedation should be avoided to enable reliable physical examinations by consultants.
- PSA, also known as conscious sedation, is an integral part of the practice of emergency medicine. The emergency physician must know several of the various regimens well and anticipate each of these regimens' potential side effects and complications. Protocols for the appropriate monitoring of these patients need to be in place.
- Drug seeking is a problem in every ED. However, a patient's complaint should not be attributed to this without adequate diagnostic evaluation. Drug seeking is a diagnosis of exclusion.

REFERENCES

Access the reference list online at ExpertConsult.com.

CHAPTER 37

Chronic Pain Management in Children and Adolescents

Ravi D. Shah, MD ◎ **Santhanam Suresh, MD, FAAP**

Chronic pain is a significant yet underreported problem in the pediatric population that carries psychological, emotional, and social repercussions for both the child and family.[1,2] The potential for such consequences to negatively impact a child's quality of life has fostered the development of a multidisciplinary approach to treat pediatric pain.[3,4] A variety of behavioral, pharmacological, and physical therapies are used in pediatric chronic pain treatment regimens. Interventional procedures may be introduced after patients fail other treatment approaches.[5]

Chronic pain in childhood and adolescence is more common than is reported and prevalence rates vary substantially between data from different studies.[6] Children experiencing persistent or recurrent chronic pain may miss school or withdraw from social activities and are at risk of developing internalizing symptoms in response to their pain. Given these consequences, researchers and clinicians are working to develop effective interdisciplinary strategies to manage chronic pain in children and adolescents.

ASSESSMENT OF CHRONIC PAIN IN CHILDREN

Assessment of children with chronic pain requires a biopsychosocial perspective that accounts for the biologic, developmental, temperamental, cognitive-behavioral, affective, social, and situational factors that shape the child's pain experience.[7,8] Each domain may become a target of assessment and intervention. Several developmentally sensitive validated instruments are now available to measure the varied aspects of a child's pain (Table 37.1).

The Children's Comprehensive Pain Questionnaire (CCPQ)[9] and the Varni-Thompson Pediatric Pain Questionnaire (VTPPQ)[10] are age-specific standardized interviews for school-age and adolescent children and their parents that provide comprehensive evaluations of a child's chronic pain. Both interviews separately assess the child's and parents' experience with a pain-related problem by utilizing open-ended questions, checklists, and quantitative pain-rating scales. Some studies suggest potential limitations to these self-report measures because of cultural or cognitive differences among families.[11] The Pain Behavior Observation Method is a 10-minute observational pain behavior measure that can be used in children who may have difficulty with self-report measures because of age-related or cognitive limitations.[12] Electronic diary assessment of pain and disability has gained popularity in recent years, and studies have supported their use in children with chronic pain, demonstrating increased compliance and accuracy in diary recording when compared to traditional paper diaries.[13]

The ability to function in tasks of daily living is a critical outcome measure to assess when treating children and adolescents with chronic pain. In some cases, pain cannot be completely relieved and the child must learn to cope with and adapt to the pain to participate in normal developmental activities and tasks, such as attending school, participating in extracurricular activities, and maintaining social relationships. Various measures have been developed to assess the child's functional ability.[14–16] The Functional Disability Inventory (FDI) was developed to assess illness-related disability in children and adolescents. It is particularly useful for children with pain disorders that are associated with psychological factors and pain-associated disability. The Child Health Questionnaire may be used to assess general quality of life in children with chronic pain and has the advantage that the scores obtained can be compared with standardized samples of scores obtained by children with other medical illnesses. The Child Activity Limitations Interview (CALI) measures the impact of recurrent pain on the child's daily activities to identify appropriate targets for treatment.[17]

Other instruments used to evaluate psychological factors that are contributing to a child's behavioral adaptation to chronic pain include the Children's Somatization Inventory (CSI),[18] which measures a child's propensity towards somatization, and the Harter Scales of Perceived Competence,[19] which assesses a child's judgment about his or her capabilities in functional domains such as school performance, peer relationships, and athletic abilities. The Patient Reported Outcomes Measurement Information System (PROMIS) is a relatively new tool that is gaining popularity for tracking physical, mental, and social well-being in children with chronic pain.[20]

INTERDISCIPLINARY APPROACH TO PEDIATRIC CHRONIC PAIN MANAGEMENT

The introduction of interdisciplinary chronic pain management programs has allowed children to be evaluated and treated by a number of consultants during a single office visit. Many pediatric pain clinics are composed of an anesthesiologist specialized in pain management, a child psychologist with a special interest in pain, physical therapists, and complementary medicine specialists who incorporate massage therapy, acupuncture therapy, as well as biofeedback. This comprehensive approach enables patients to receive better care with minimal disruption to their lives.

Psychological pain management methods aim to improve the child and family's understanding of the child's pain and its treatment by focusing on factors that may reduce or exacerbate symptoms. The child's cognitive and behavioral coping skills are fostered in an effort to reduce pain-related discomfort and disability. Eccleston and colleagues performed a meta-analysis to evaluate the efficacy of behavioral interventions for treating pediatric

TABLE 37.1 Methods for Assessment of Chronic Pain in Children and Adolescents

Pain Measures	Disability or Quality of Life Assessment Tools	Other Behavioral Measures
Varni-Thompson Pediatric Pain Questionnaire (Ages 5–18 years)	Functional Disability Inventory (Ages 8–17 years)	Children's Somatization Inventory (Ages 8–18 years)
Children's Comprehensive Pain Questionnaire (Ages 5–19 years)	Child Health Questionnaire (Ages 5+)	Harter Scales of Perceived Competence for Children (Ages 4–12)
Pain Behavior Observation Method (Ages 6–17)	Children's Activity Limitations Scale (Ages 8–16 years)	–
Pain Diary (Ages 8+)	–	–

chronic pain.[21] They concluded that strong evidence exists to support psychological treatments, specifically relaxation and cognitive behavioral therapy, as effective methods to reduce the severity and frequency of chronic pain in children and adolescents. Other studies have suggested that interdisciplinary pediatric pain rehabilitation may facilitate increased willingness to self-manage pain, which is associated with improvements in function and psychological well-being.[22]

Physical therapy is geared toward reestablishing adequate functional ability of the child. In children, physical therapy is especially useful in cases of myofascial pain and can be implemented at a rehabilitation facility, home, or school. In younger children, these exercises can take the form of play that is geared toward improving musculoskeletal function, fine and gross motor function, posture, endurance, and circulation. Restoring the patient's physical ability can help the child participate in activities of daily living and improve overall function.

Complementary and alternative medicine (CAM) is defined by the National Center for CAM as "a group of diverse medical and health care systems, practices, and products that are not generally considered to be part of conventional medicine."[23] Biofeedback, hypnosis, guided-imagery, mindfulness, massage, and acupuncture have been used as adjunctive treatments for chronic, acute, and recurrent pain in both pediatric and adult populations.[24–27] Gut-directed hypnotherapy for functional abdominal pain (FAP) and irritable bowel syndrome appears to be superior to traditional medical management of such conditions. Although limited data are available to support the efficacy of CAM in pediatric patients, such treatments offer the potential for pain relief with a relatively low incidence of side effects.[28]

Many tertiary pain centers in the United States have adopted a multidisciplinary approach to pain management that incorporates use of at least a subset of CAM modalities. In a 2005 survey of 43 pediatric anesthesiology fellowship programs, 38 reported that their clinical services to patients included at least one CAM modality, including biofeedback (65%), guided imagery (49%), relaxation therapy (33%), massage (35%), hypnosis (44%), acupuncture (33%), art therapy (21%), and meditation (21%).[29] Tsao et al. have suggested that the longer a child experiences pain, the more likely he or she is to express an interest in trying CAM treatment approaches.[30]

Interventional procedures can serve as useful adjuncts to managing chronic pain conditions in children, especially in cases that are refractory to noninvasive treatments.[31] This differs from the adult cohort for which such procedures are more commonly used as a diagnostic or therapeutic modality. The majority of literature on this topic consists of case reports and retrospective studies. Due to lack of scientific evidence, significant controversy surrounds the utility of invasive techniques for managing pediatric pain states.

FUNCTIONAL IMAGING OF PEDIATRIC CHRONIC PAIN STATES

The introduction of noninvasive neuroimaging techniques has significantly advanced our understanding of how chronic pain affects the structure and function of cortical, subcortical, and brainstem networks.[32] Brain imaging studies of chronic pain in pediatric populations offer unique opportunities to understand changes in the young brain from both developmental and neuroplastic perspectives. In the pediatric population, the brain undergoes rapid changes and may be more likely to recover after an injury.[33] Very few studies have addressed the effects of pain on brain maturation and plasticity processes. The use of noninvasive imaging approaches to evaluate brain changes in pediatric patients may lead to novel treatment approaches, potentially limiting the development of long-term consequences.

Imaging techniques are being utilized in pain research to depict functional, biochemical, and anatomical changes within the brain (Fig. 37.1). Below we provide a brief overview of these techniques and their relevance to the study of pediatric chronic pain states.

FUNCTIONAL IMAGING TECHNIQUES

Functional magnetic resonance imaging (fMRI) determines cortical activation by measuring changes in the local concentration of paramagnetic deoxyhemoglobin. This technique, also referred to as *blood oxygen level-dependent* (BOLD) imaging, assesses regional neuronal activation by measuring changes in blood flow and blood volume, depicting dynamic changes with relatively high spatial resolution. Due to its noninvasive nature, fMRI can potentially be used repeatedly in children, allowing longitudinal studies on neural network development, disease process evolution, and treatment responses.[34]

Lebel and colleagues have utilized fMRI to study cerebral activation patterns in pediatric patients with complex regional pain syndrome (CRPS).[35] Children 9 to

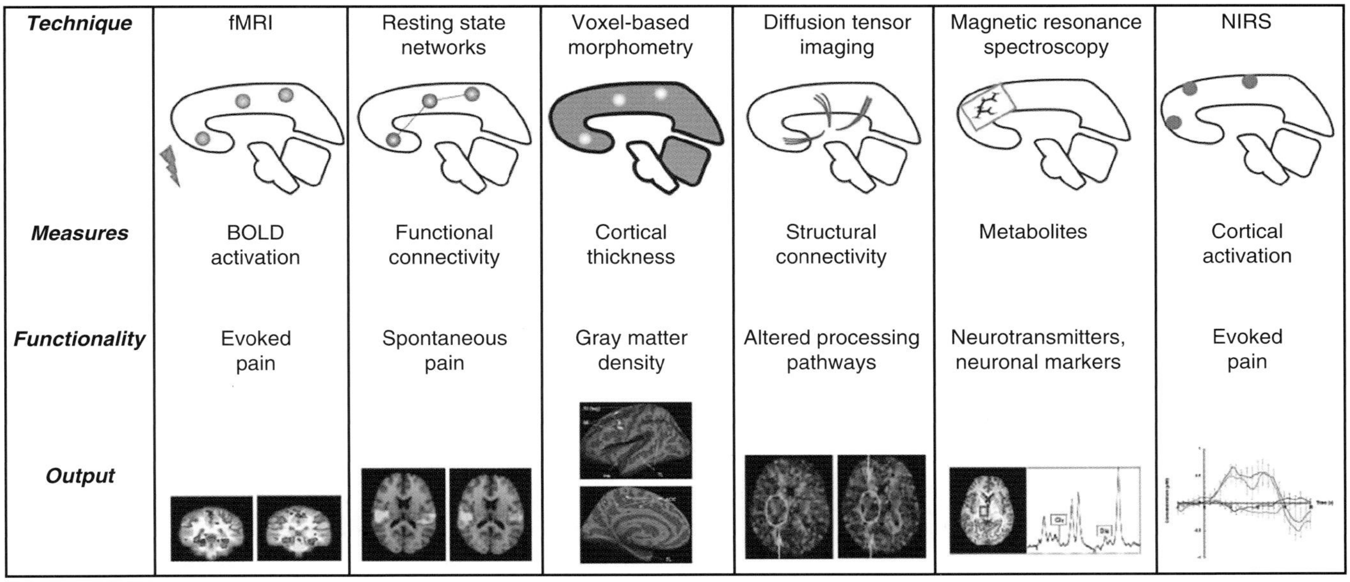

FIG. 37.1 Imaging methods used in pain research. *BOLD*, Blood oxygen level-dependent, *fMRI*, functional magnetic resonance imaging; *NIRS*, cerebral near-infrared spectroscopy. *(From Sava S, Lebel AA, Leslie DS, et al. Challenges of functional imaging research of pain in children.* Mol Pain. *5:30, 2009.)*

18 years of age with lower extremity CRPS-I underwent two scanning sessions; the initial scan was performed during an active period of pain, and a follow-up scan was done after symptomatic recovery. Patients with active symptoms (including mechanical and thermal allodynia) demonstrated BOLD activation patterns that were similar to data reported in adults.[36] Specifically, activation changes were noted in regions involved in pain processing (primary sensory-motor cotices, insula) as well as in areas that presumably contribute to the affective symptoms of pain (parietal, frontal, and temporal cortices).[37] Brain activation patterns continued to differ between symptomatic patients and those who had recovered, suggesting that functional changes in central nervous system processing may outlast the signs and symptoms of CRPS.

Simons and colleagues applied fMRI to evaluate resting state functional connectivity of the amygdala with cortical and subcortical regions in a group of pediatric CRPS patients with age-sex matched control subjects before and after treatment. The investigators observed rapid changes in amygdala connectivity after patients underwent an aggressive physical-biobehavioral pain treatment program, serving as a potential indicator of treatment response.[38] In addition, functional connectivity to several regions key to fear circuitry correlated with higher pain-related fear scores (Fig. 37.2).

Cerebral near-infrared spectroscopy (NIRS), which detects subtle changes in the concentration of natural chromophores such as oxygenated and deoxygenated hemoglobin, has been successfully utilized in newborns, children, and adults to measure the hemodynamic and oxygenation changes related to cortical processing of specific stimuli. NIRS studies in neonates have noted that painful and tactile stimuli elicit specific hemodynamic responses in the somatosensory cortex, implying conscious sensory perception in preterm neonates.[39]

Magnetic resonance spectroscopy (MRS) can be utilized to study alterations in neurotransmitters and neuronal markers. Several in vivo MRS techniques have been developed to provide unique information about brain chemistry. MRS has been used to gain insight into several conditions, including migraine, back pain, and spinal cord injury and has potential to provide biomarkers of disease that precede structural changes within the brain.[40–42] No pediatric pain studies to date have utilized this imaging approach.

Diffusion Tensor Imaging (DTI) has been used to study a number of pain disorders, including migraine and post-stroke centralized pain.[43,44] This approach measures microstructural changes in water diffusion to determine changes in white matter tracts and when combined with fMRI studies, this approach may improve our understanding of functional anatomical mapping of brain activity.[45]

Functional imaging of the brain changes that occur in pediatric chronic pain patients is an emerging field with great potential. Such techniques can serve as powerful noninvasive tools that may be used to perform longitudinal studies in children so we may better characterize the mechanisms of pain and ultimately improve therapeutic strategies.

PEDIATRIC CHRONIC PAIN SYNDROMES

The following section discusses the diagnosis and management of some common pediatric chronic pain syndromes, including CRPS type I, headache, abdominal pain, and cancer pain.

COMPLEX REGIONAL PAIN SYNDROME

CRPS type I (CRPS-I) involves a group of symptoms involving extremity pain with neuropathic features, including allodynia and hyperalgesia, neurovascular degeneration, sudomotor dysfunction, trophic changes, and loss of

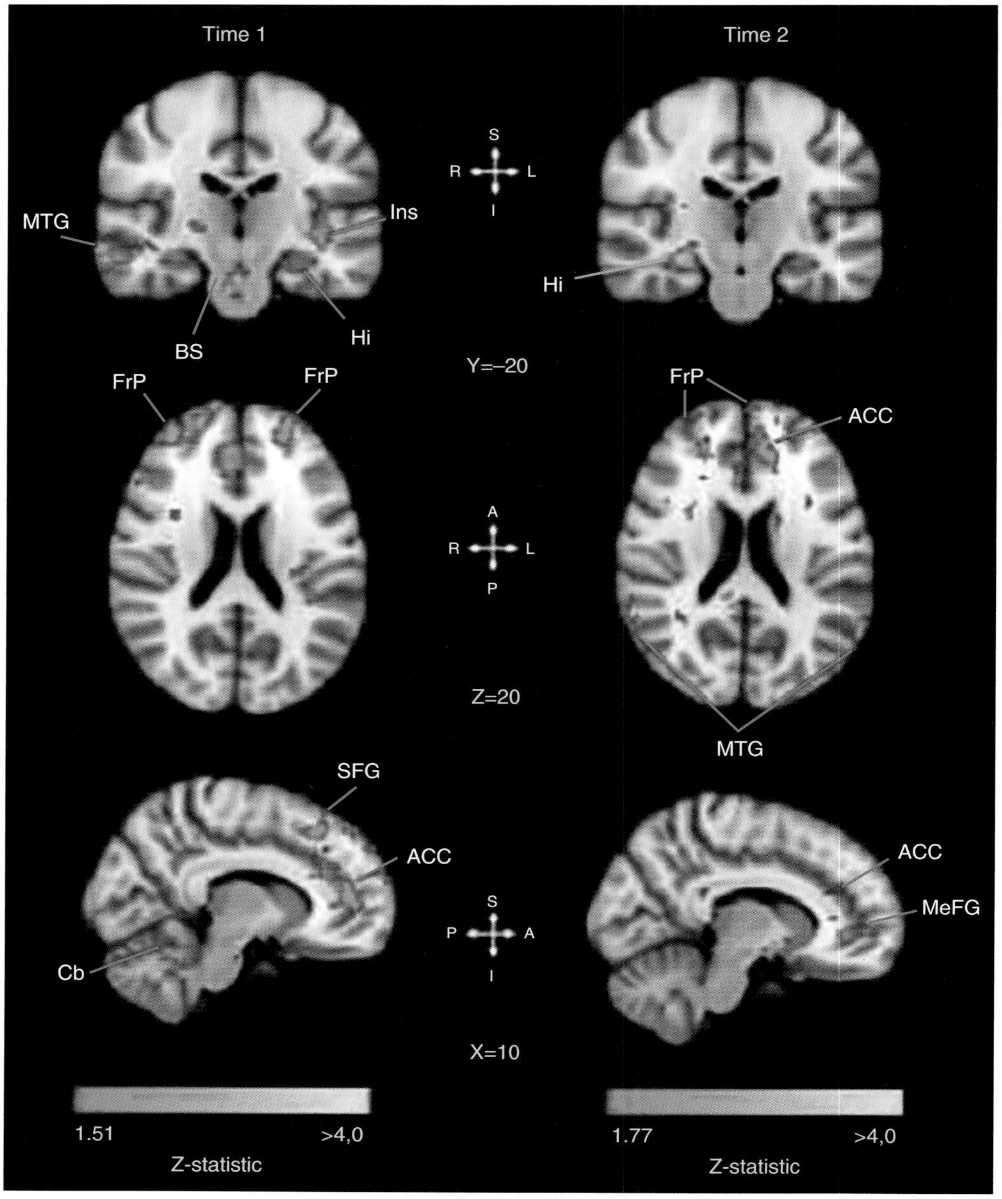

FIG. 37.2 Connectivity strength by levels of pain-related fear in patients (left amygdala). Across time, areas associated with fear circuitry were consistently associated with higher pain-related fear scores. Key: *ACC*, Anterior cingulate cortex; *BS*, brain stem; *Cb*, cerebellum; *FrP*, frontal pole; *Hi*, hippocampus; *Ins*, insula; *MTG*, middle temporal gyrus; *MeFG*, medial frontal gyrus; *SFG*, superior frontal gyrus. *(From Simons LE, Pielech M, Erpelding N, et al: The responsive amygdala: treatment-induced alterations in functional connectivity in pediatric complex regional pain syndrome.* Pain. *155:9, 2014.)*

motor function. Pediatric cases of CRPS-I typically begin in adolescence, and the lower extremity is more commonly affected than the upper extremity (ratio of approximately 5:1).[46,47] Significant trauma is a much less frequent precipitating event than in adults.[48] The majority of children involved appear to be Caucasian females.[49] Studies in adult patients suggest that psychological factors are frequently involved in the CRPS-I pain experience.[50] Contrary to this hypothesis, children with CRPS-I report no greater anxiety or depressive symptoms than children with other pain conditions.[51] Pediatric CRPS-I patients do, however, demonstrate greater enmeshment with their parents and many exhibit a degree of overachievement.[52]

Early recognition and management are the major factors in improving outcome and preventing symptom recurrence. Management should include an interdisciplinary approach. Although medication and procedure-based treatments may be performed in children, rehabilitative treatments thus far show the best evidence of yielding positive outcomes. Outcome reports from pediatric pain rehabilitation programs remain scarce in the literature and have primarily involved inpatient rehabilitative treatments, including hospitalization. Logan and colleagues recently reported disability reduction and improved physical and emotional functioning in pediatric CRPS-I patients who underwent an interdisciplinary day-hospital rehabilitation program.[53]

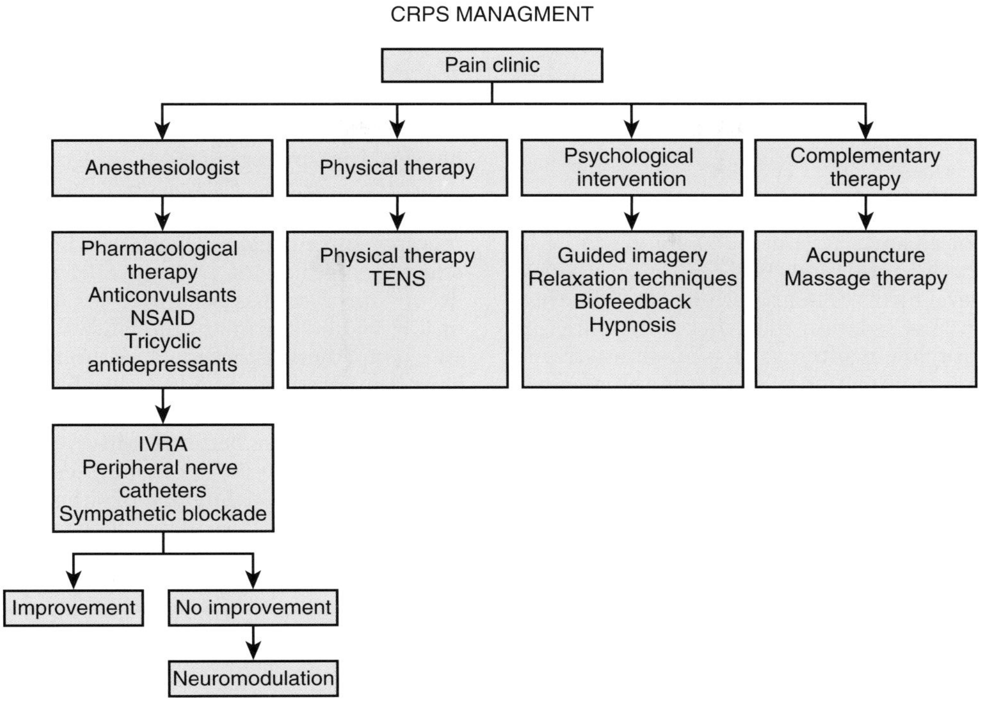

FIG. 37.3 Algorithm for management of pediatric complex regional pain syndrome (CRPS) I. *IVRA*, Intravenous regional anesthesia; *NSAID*, nonsteroidal antiinflammatory drug; *TENS*, transcutaneous electrical nerve stimulation.

EVALUATION

A detailed history of the nature of the injury that includes the type and duration of pain, relieving and aggravating factors, and dependence on medications should be performed prior to physical examination. A thorough and systematic neurologic examination should be performed with evaluation of motor, sensory, cerebellar, cranial nerve, reflex, cognitive, and emotional functioning. A concerted effort should be made to rule out a rare, but possible, malignancy or central degenerative disorder. *Allodynia* is a common finding and *hyperalgesia* to cold is seen more frequently than sensitivity to heat.[54] In children, the distribution is not generally restricted to particular dermatomes and commonly occurs along a glove-and-stocking distribution. *Nerve conduction studies* may provide insight into the nature of a nerve injury; however, the use of invasive electromyography may not be acceptable to children.[55] *Quantitative sensory testing* (QST) in the affected limbs can be compared with data from normal healthy children. Although this involves cumbersome equipment, bedside QST may play a role in the diagnosis of CRPS-I in children and adolescents.[56] *Bone scans* may be helpful in the diagnosis of CRPS-I. Although insufficient data exist to support their diagnostic accuracy in children, they can nevertheless be performed in children and adolescents with suspected CRPS-I.[57]

TREATMENT

Management of CRPS-I can be frustrating for both the caregiver and the patient as no single therapy can uniformly provide relief of symptoms. Children, compared with adults, are thought to have a better response to noninvasive treatments.[58] Therefore, treatments that have been reported effective in adults may not apply to pediatric patients. Despite this, most CRPS-I management techniques that are used in children have been extrapolated from the adult literature (Fig. 37.3).[59]

It is imperative to return the child to a functional state, including attendance at school. Behavioral measures are extremely useful in the management of CRPS-I in children and adolescents. For example, group therapy often helps family members cope with the situation.[60] We generally advocate consultation with a medical psychologist during the initial visit to the pain clinic. Several techniques, including biofeedback, visual guided imagery, and structured counseling, have been shown to assist in the development of adequate coping skills.[61] Participation in a day program for acute psychological intervention has been valuable for some of our patients, specifically those with significant psychiatric coillness.

Physical therapy is geared toward restoring adequate functional ability of the child. Transcutaneous electrical nerve stimulation (TENS) is widely used, and its efficacy has been studied in adults as well as children; therapeutic benefits with TENS in children with CRPS-I have been reported by Kesler and colleagues.[62] We use TENS extensively in our practice, along with physical therapy, which consists of both active and passive physical modalities. The physical therapy program is geared toward individual patients, and the goal is to allow the child to participate in as many activities as possible. Other commonly used modalities include graded motor imagery, desensitization, warm and cold baths, massage therapy, and heat therapy. Such modalities, when used in conjunction with active physical modalities, can help ameliorate pain symptoms.[63]

The following section focuses on therapeutic adjuncts used to treat pediatric CRPS-I, including pharmacotherapy, regional anesthesia, and sympathetic blockade. Most treatment approaches are extrapolated from efficacy data in adults.

TRICYCLIC ANTIDEPRESSANTS

Despite the lack of adequately controlled studies in pediatric patients, tricyclic antidepressants (TCAs) are widely prescribed for several forms of neuropathic pain.[64] Because amitriptyline may cause sedation and other anticholinergic side effects, nortriptyline is often used as an alternative in children. Thorough examination of the cardiovascular system is necessary before instituting TCA treatment because of the associated tachydysrhythmia and other conduction abnormalities of the heart, particularly prolonged QT syndrome.[65,66]

ANTICONVULSANTS

Anticonvulsant medications are commonly used to manage neuropathic pain in pediatric patients, especially since the introduction of gabapentin and pregabalin. Despite the lack of controlled trials in children to demonstrate the efficacy of either drug, both of these medications have been used in our practice with promising results.[67] More controlled trials should be conducted to better determine the dosing and efficacy of this class of drugs in children with CRPS-I. An important side effect that we have noted in our clinic setting is the potential for increased somnolence, as well as the potential for weight gain in children taking pregabalin. This is important to consider, especially when treating adolescent girls who happen to be the majority of this cohort.

SELECTIVE SEROTONIN REUPTAKE INHIBITORS AND SEROTONIN-NOREPINEPHRINE REUPTAKE INHIBITORS

Despite the lack of proven efficacy of the use of selective serotonin reuptake inhibitors in the management of pain in children and adolescents, they are occasionally used to treat psychological comorbidity, including pain-associated depression.[68] More recently, serotonin-norepinephrine reuptake inhibitors (e.g., duloxetine) have been introduced and used successfully to treat neuropathic pain, especially in patients with psychological comorbidity.[69]

SYSTEMIC VASODILATORS

Several patients with CRPS-I have benefited from the use of vasodilators such as prazosin, nifedipine, and phenoxybenzamine. However, overwhelming adverse effects of orthostatic hypotension often offset the efficacy of this therapy.

REGIONAL ANESTHESIA AND SYMPATHETIC BLOCKS

A common treatment of these syndromes is to interrupt the apparent pathologic reflexes by performing sympathetic blocks. Regional anesthesia, which is often utilized in adults for the diagnosis and management of CRPS-I, is generally introduced in children after pharmacological and cognitive-behavioral management have been exhausted. In severe cases, regional anesthesia is used to introduce a physical therapy regimen.

Central neuraxial blockade may be performed in children with severe pain to facilitate the introduction of physical therapy. Intrathecal analgesia has been reported to be an effective method for treating refractory CRPS-I in children.[70] *Bier block* has been used for mild to moderate cases of CRPS-I as a primary modality for providing analgesia and sympathetic blockade.[71] Although various substances have been used to provide a Bier block, a local anesthetic in combination with either an α2-agonist or an NSAID appears to produce better results.[72]

Peripheral nerve blocks can be used to facilitate physical therapy while providing a sympathectomy. Serial peripheral nerve blocks are often performed, after which the patient's pain relief may outlast the duration of conduction blockade. *Continuous peripheral nerve blocks* (CPNBs) have been reported to be effective in both controlling pain and facilitating physical therapy in children with CRPS (Fig. 37.4).[73] Despite such reports, limited data exist regarding the feasibility, safety, and efficacy of CPNBs for the treatment of CRPS-I in children.[74]

Sympathetic blockade is used in children after exhausting the aforementioned techniques. A crossover trial of fluoroscopically guided lumbar sympathetic blocks demonstrated a decrease in allodynia and pain intensity when compared with intravenous injection of lidocaine in adolescents with CRPS.[75] *Neuromodulation*, though commonly performed in adults for refractory cases of CRPS, is very rarely used

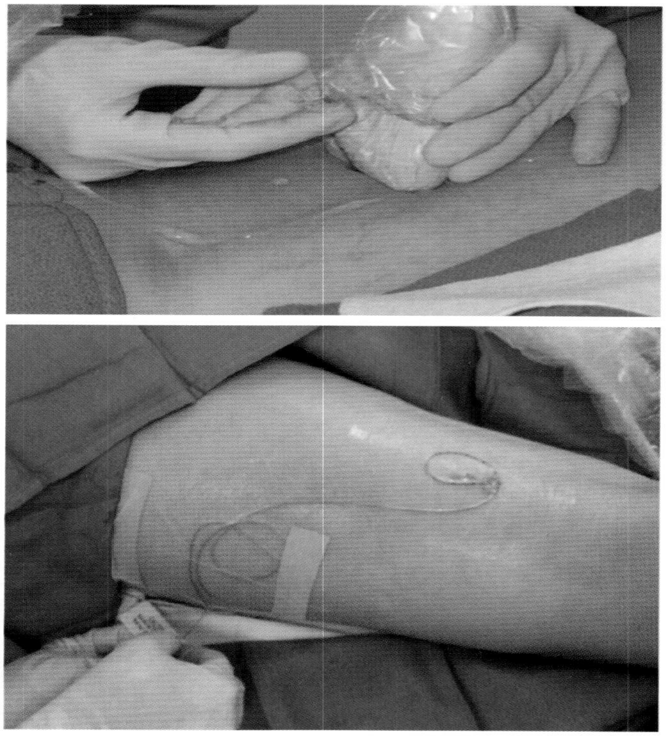

FIG. 37.4 Ultrasound-guided sciatic nerve catheter placement to facilitate physical therapy in a child with complex regional pain syndrome-I.

in the pediatric setting.[76,77] Spinal cord stimulation has, however, been reported to achieve favorable outcomes in adolescents with therapy-resistant CRPS.[78]

Ashwal and associates concluded that the prognosis of childhood CRPS-I is more favorable than that of adult CRPS-I.[79] Neuropathic pain can be puzzling and frustrating, and treatment approaches require a strong alliance with the family and the patient. A multidisciplinary algorithmic management approach can be helpful. The use of physical therapy and psychological management must be stressed while managing these patients.

HEADACHES IN CHILDREN

Headache is a common neurological symptom reported in childhood and adolescence and is associated with several comorbid conditions, particularly with respect to the neurological, psychiatric, and cardiovascular systems. Symptoms in children can cause significant impairment, leading to school absences and withdrawal from daily activities.

Bille et al. reported migraine headaches to occur in 3.9% of children younger than 12 years and noted a 6.8% incidence of nonmigrainous headaches daily.[80] Childhood headaches are commonly associated with psychiatric and neurological comorbidity, in particular depression and anxiety, epilepsy, sleep disorders, and ADHD.[81] Association with cardiovascular disease, especially ischemic stroke and patent foramen ovale (PFO), has also been reported in the pediatric population.[82]

EVALUATION AND MANAGEMENT OF HEADACHE

A thorough history and physical examination should be performed to determine the nature of the headache. Neurologic symptoms such as ataxia, lethargy, seizures, or visual impairment should be noted and other medical conditions such as hypertension, sinusitis, and emotional disturbances must be evaluated. Physical examination should include a thorough neurologic examination and blood pressure measurement. Neuroimaging may be required and a lumbar puncture might be advised in some cases. Benign intracranial hypertension or idiopathic intracranial hypertension is a constellation of symptoms that includes headaches, diplopia, tinnitus, and eye pain in the presence of normal imaging results.[83]

Childhood headaches are associated with comorbid symptoms. Sleep deprivation is a common finding, and delayed sleep is a frequent disorder seen in children with headaches. Many children with headache also report dizziness, which can be associated with postural hypotension and tachycardia (postural orthostatic tachycardia syndrome).[84] A history of a new-onset severe headache, pain that awakens a child from sleep, headaches associated with straining, or the presence of a headache accompanied by nausea or vomiting suggests a more pathologic origin of the headache and must be carefully evaluated.

After careful evaluation and classification of the type of headache, treatment is initiated in stepwise fashion. We use the algorithm shown in Fig. 37.5 for the management of headaches. *Tension-type headache* is perhaps the most common type of headache that is witnessed in our pain clinic. These patients commonly complain of debilitating frontotemporal or frontoparietal headaches, often due to contraction of the temporalis muscle and tension on the scalp muscles.[85] Management of tension-type headaches includes the use of relaxation techniques, as well as biofeedback. These patients frequently benefit from the routine use of nonsteroidal agents.[86] In addition, caffeine has been described as an effective adjuvant to nonsteroidal drugs in treating childhood headaches.[87]

Children occasionally suffer from *persistent neuropathic headaches.* This commonly occurs in those who have undergone ventriculo-peritoneal shunt revision or surgical decompression for a Chiari malformation. After first utilizing cognitive-behavioral therapy and pharmacotherapy,

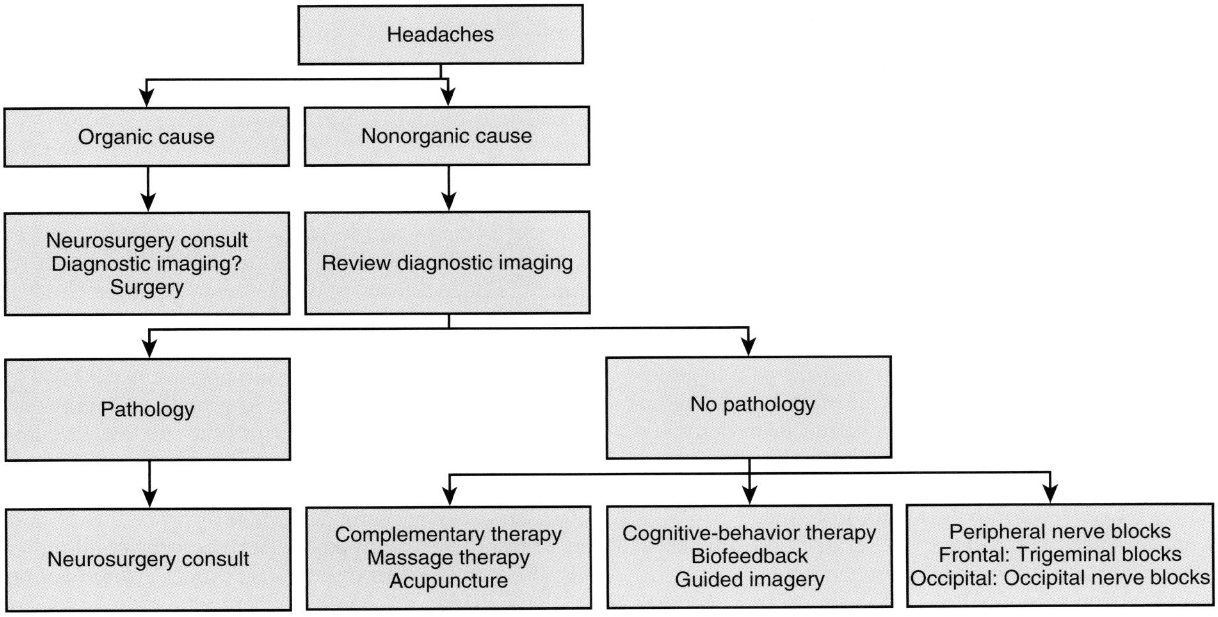

FIG. 37.5 Algorithm for management of headache in children.

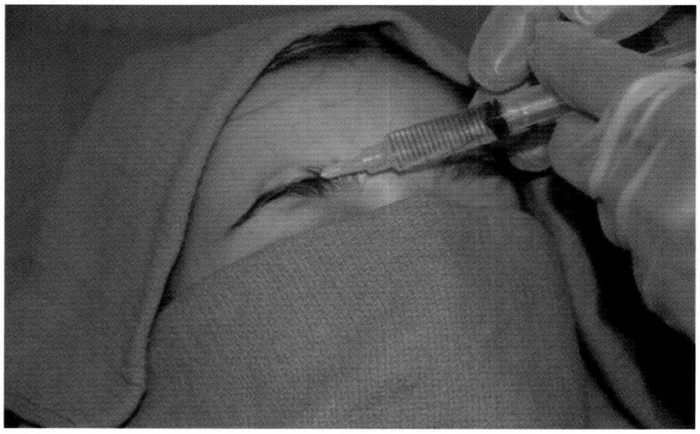

FIG. 37.6 Supraorbital nerve block for management of headache in a child.

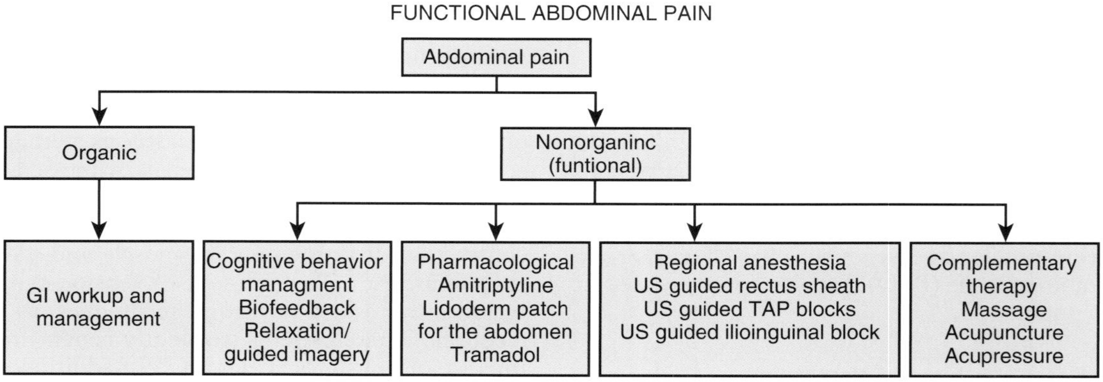

FIG. 37.7 Abdominal pain management. *GI*, Gastrointestinal; *TAP*, transverse abdominis plane; *US*, ultrasound.

we have attempted to use serial peripheral nerve blocks in these patients. This includes trigeminal nerve blocks for frontal headaches and occipital nerve blocks for occipital headaches (Fig. 37.6). An ultrasound-guided approach to the occipital nerve allows easy access to the C2 nerve root, thereby providing a more robust blockade than can be achieved with a peripheral subcutaneous injection.[88]

ABDOMINAL PAIN IN CHILDREN

Abdominal pain is commonly encountered in the pediatric population. FAP is considered to be pain unrelated to an identifiable organic gastrointestinal disorder.[89] Once a diagnosis of FAP is established, cognitive-behavioral therapy combined with family-centered therapy may be initiated.[90] Several authors have described an affective component to FAP.[91] Walker and associates suggested that children with FAP are at increased risk for the development of chronic pain in adulthood.[92] This is potentially due to mechanisms linked to heightened central sensitization.[93] Amitriptyline has been described as an effective treatment of FAP in children, although a prospective randomized controlled trial demonstrated no significant difference between control and amitriptyline.[94]

We demonstrated the efficacy of serial nerve blocks in children with chronic abdominal pain, particularly those in whom neuropathic pain develops after abdominal surgery. Specifically, ultrasound-guided rectus sheath blocks or transversus abdominis plane blocks resulted in decreased pain scores in our cohort (Fig. 37.7).[95] Ilioinguinal neuralgia following hernia repair is an underreported cause of abdominal pain in older children and adolescents.[96] Persistent pain likely results from major dissection during surgery. TENS may be helpful and peripheral nerve blocks can be used to manage pain. Serial ultrasound-guided ilioinguinal nerve blocks have been effectively utilized as a treatment modality in this setting (Fig. 37.8).[97]

PEDIATRIC CANCER PAIN

Cancer is diagnosed in more than 12,000 children annually, and approximately 2200 children die each year of this disease.[98] The incidence of cancer-related pain in children at the time of diagnosis is estimated to be 75%, with ongoing pain affecting 50% of patients.[99,100] During the terminal phase of disease, the incidence of pain approaches 90%.[101] Cancer pain in children can be related to several etiologies: (1) tumor-related pain (e.g., solid tumor or bony metastatic tumors), (2) pain caused by treatment (e.g., mucositis or surgical pain), and (3) neuropathic pain secondary to tumor invasion or surgery. Pain caused by either a treatment or procedure is cited as the most frequent type of pain experienced by children with cancer.[102] Management of pediatric cancer-related pain must be individualized, and caregivers must be empathetic to family needs and concerns. Although most pain complaints can be

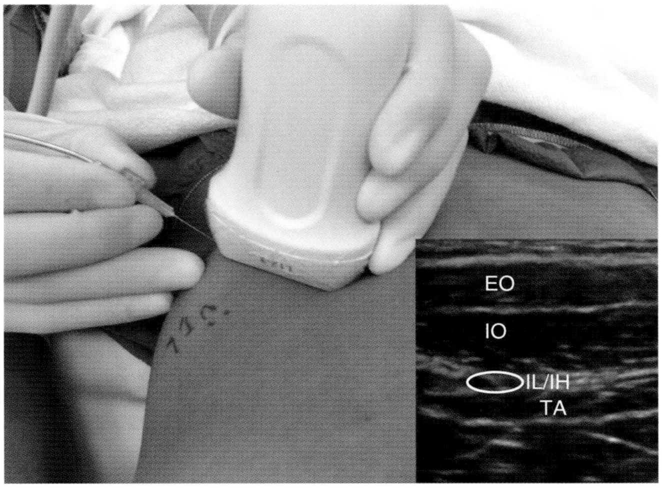

FIG. 37.8 Ultrasound-guided ilioinguinal nerve block performed on a child with inguinal neuralgia.

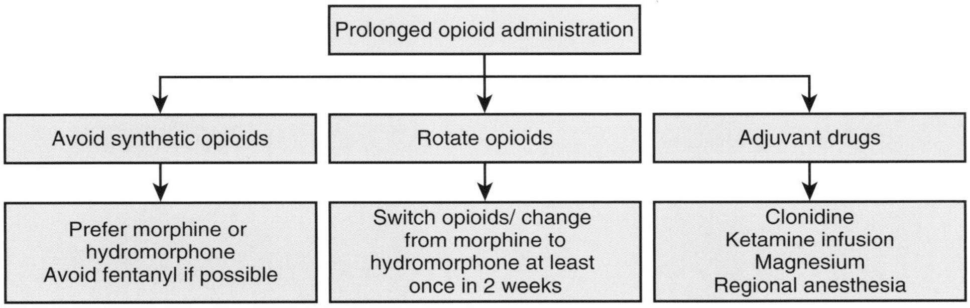

FIG. 37.9 Opioid tolerance management.

managed by implementation of the World Health Organization (WHO) cancer pain ladder paradigm, a significant number of children may require additional therapies or techniques for pain management because of escalating or intractable pain.

Opioid tolerance is a major problem in children and infants who have been exposed to long-duration analgesia with opioids. As treatment possibilities for tumors increase, the number of children with opioid tolerance has been increasing, and proactive steps to decrease tolerance must be set in place from the time of initiation of opioids. Fig. 37.9 illustrates an algorithm that we have developed to manage pediatric opioid tolerance.

Although systemic analgesic therapies are the mainstay of pain treatment in pediatric palliative care, there are cases where they fail to adequately relieve symptoms or produce side effects that undermine effectiveness. Regional anesthesia or other procedural interventions may be considered as a potential therapy for these patients.[103] The use of such techniques in children is supported only by case reports, case series, and very few randomized controlled studies.

CONCLUSION

Chronic pain in children remains an underrecognized entity. Early diagnosis and intervention are helpful in achieving adequate recovery. A multidisciplinary approach is emphasized when treating the child with chronic pain. Future research in the paradigms for managing chronic pain in children needs to be conducted to shape treatment strategies and develop novel approaches to caring for this challenging group of patients.

KEY POINTS

- Assessment of children with chronic pain requires a biopsychosocial perspective that accounts for the various factors influencing a child's pain experience. Multidimensional models elucidate the biologic, developmental, temperamental, cognitive-behavioral, affective, social, and situational factors that shape the child's pain experience.
- The management of pediatric CRPS-I includes physical therapy, regional blocks, pharmacological management, and psychological interventions.
- Several characteristics of headache can suggest a pathological or more serious etiology.
- The management of pediatric headache includes pharmacological management, nerve blocks, psychological techniques, and complementary therapy.
- FAP in children is most commonly treated with cognitive-behavioral measures, antidepressants, and serial rectus sheath or TAP blocks.
- The management of cancer pain is individualized and based on family needs

REFERENCES

Access the reference list online at ExpertConsult.com.

CHAPTER 38 SICKLE CELL DISEASE

Dawn Belvis, MD ◎ Kimberly J. Henderson, MD, JD ◎ Hubert A. Benzon, MD, MPH, FAAP

Sickle cell disease (SCD) is an inherited disorder of hemoglobin that affects approximately 100,000 Americans.[1] The sickle cell gene is found in many ethnic groups, but the majority of those affected are of African or African-Caribbean origins. The average lifespan of those with SCD is about two to three decades less than for Americans without SCD, due in part to acute complications of the disease.[2] Manifestations of the disease occur in every organ system; however, the most common complication is the vaso-occlusive painful episode.[3] These episodes are marked by excruciating corporeal pain and are the most common cause for Emergency Department (ED) visits and hospitalizations in this population.[4] There are approximately 230,000 ED visits related to SCD in the United States each year, and acute care expenditures for SCD are estimated at $1.5 billion annually.[5] For the emergency provider, management of acute sickle cell pain is challenging. Undertreatment can occur due to concerns regarding the etiology of vaso-occlusion as well as the concern for opioid addiction. This chapter provides an overview of pain in SCD and strategies for successful management in the ED and during the hospital stay.

PATHOPHYSIOLOGY

SCD is a family of genetic disorders caused by mutations (resulting in altered protein structure or altered production) at the beta-globin gene on chromosome 11. While several abnormal hemoglobins have been described, the most important is the valine-glutamine substitution at codon 6, which results in the formation of hemoglobin S. Individuals who are homozygous for this mutation have hemoglobin SS, the most severe form of SCD (often referred to as sickle cell anemia). Heterozygotes who have a different mutation on their other beta-globin gene are also classified as SCD. The most common heterozygous forms of SCD include hemoglobin SC and hemoglobin Sβ thalassemia. Patients with HbSS or HbSB-thalassemia typically experience more vaso-occlusive crises (VOCs).[2]

Individuals who carry one normal beta-globin gene and one hemoglobin S mutation are defined as having sickle cell trait. In the United States, approximately 2 million people carry the sickle cell trait.[6] The sickle cell trait is found in 8% of African Americans and is also prevalent in persons of Mediterranean, Middle Eastern, Indian, Caribbean, and Central and South American descent. People with this disease do not have vaso-occlusive pain.[7] Pain in an individual with sickle cell trait should prompt the same evaluation as would be performed on a normal individual. These patients have been found to suffer from certain medical problems during times of increased physical stress. Complications include traumatic hyphema, hyposthenuria, and hematuria, especially during strenuous exercise, doubling the number of urinary tract infections during pregnancy.[8] Acute hyphema is the only manifestation of sickle cell trait that can result in vaso-occlusion. Vaso-occlusion can occur in the anterior chamber of the eye; thus all individuals with hyphemae should be admitted for serial intraocular pressure measurements. Patients carrying the sickle cell trait are also at increased incidence for splenic infarction.

The pathophysiology underlying SCD is characterized by a complex state of ongoing hemolysis, inflammation, altered blood rheology, and endothelial dysfunction.[9–12] Manifestations occur in every organ system; however, the most common manifestation is the vaso-occlusive painful episode or VOCs, typically in the bones and bone marrow. The pathophysiology of vaso-occlusive pain is not completely understood. However, it is presumed that local microvascular occlusion propagates further ischemia, hemoglobin deoxygenation, hemolysis, and tissue damage, which ultimately tips the delicate steady state toward diffuse vaso-occlusion (i.e., the pain is both ischemic and inflammatory in nature). It is thought that recurrent bouts of acute pain can eventually lead to chronic pain, particularly if they are not appropriately treated.

Triggers for such events include stress, dehydration, fever/infection, and trauma, but very often there is no clear precipitating cause. These episodes can be unpredictable, with varying degrees of intensity and frequency.

CLINICAL MANIFESTATIONS

VOC pain usually presents with sudden onset, but may occur gradually in some people. The first episode may occur as early as 6 months of age. Pain may occur at any site, but the most common locations for pain are the lower back and the legs.[13] Patients may describe the pain as sharp, throbbing, stabbing, dull, or aching. The pain may be localized or move to different places in the body. In children, painful episodes may be associated with physical findings such as the swelling of digits in dactylitis. With the loss of active bone marrow in small bones, these manifestations wane. In adults, there are no objective physical findings associated with VOC. Vital signs are of no utility in determining if a patient is having a VOC, as blood pressure and heart rate are usually normal.[14] A common misconception is that hemoglobin drops during vaso-occlusion. In fact, hemoglobin is typically at or above baseline during painful episodes. Furthermore, SCD patients with higher steady state hemoglobin are more likely to have painful manifestations of SCD.[15]

Other clinical manifestations of SCD relevant to a discussion of pain include acute chest syndrome, fever, neurological complications, organ infarction, hepatobiliary complications, acute anemia, splenic sequestration, and venous thromboembolism. Acute chest syndrome is the second most common cause for hospitalization and the most common cause of death. The syndrome is clinically identical to lobar pneumonia, presenting with chest pain, fever, and pulmonary opacities. Therapy includes correcting dehydration, if present, pain control, respiratory support, antibiotics, and transfusion therapy.[16] Individuals with SCD are functionally asplenic and thus susceptible to infection with encapsulated bacteria. Additionally, high prevalence of bone disease (osteoporosis and avascular necrosis) further predisposes individuals to infections of the bone. Neurological complications of SCD include ischemic and hemorrhagic stroke, and there is also evidence that individuals with SCD have elevated rates of venous thromboembolic disease.[17–22] These manifestations are important in the consideration of pain, because an appropriate differential diagnosis must always be formed before the provider assumes the etiology of pain is simply vaso-occlusion.

DIFFERENTIAL DIAGNOSIS AND EVALUATION

For individuals with chest pain, always consider acute chest syndrome, pulmonary embolism, and other life-threatening causes. Abdominal pain should prompt consideration of biliary etiologies, splenic or renal infarction, in addition to other standard non-SCD related causes of abdominal pain (appendicitis, diverticulitis, ovarian torsion, renal stones, etc.). Limb pain should prompt consideration of osteomyelitis and necrotizing fasciitis. There are no laboratory tests or imaging studies that can validate pain. Listening to the patient is key, as they often know what their "typical crisis" feels like and if what they are experiencing is different. Patients have often attempted to control their pain at home, and upon arrival in the ED have already experienced a few days of pain already.[23] It is important to note that a majority of painful episodes are treated at home.

History should focus on triggers for pain, location, intensity, and how it compares with prior episodes. Physical examination should focus on areas of pain and assessment for infection. Laboratory evaluation should include a complete blood count, electrolyte panel, and bilirubin. Reticulocyte count, a commonly ordered test in SCD, is useful in differentiating etiologies of an acute drop in hemoglobin. For simple vaso-occlusion, reticulocyte counts are not necessary. Once alternative etiologies have been ruled out, the emergency provider can proceed with management of acute vaso-occlusive sickle cell pain.

MANAGEMENT OF ACUTE SICKLE CELL PAIN

In 2014 the National Heart, Lung, and Blood Institute (NHLBI) released evidence-based guidelines for the management of SCD.[2] Because of a lack of scientific evidence, most recommendations were based on published guidelines by professional organizations and expert consensus. Recommendations included in this publication reflect those of the NHLBI guidelines, and whenever possible are evidence based. The following discussion assumes a diagnosis of simple vaso-occlusive pain and that more serious etiologies of pain have been ruled out.

KEYS TO SUCCESSFUL MANAGEMENT OF ACUTE SICKLE CELL DISEASE PAIN IN THE EMERGENCY DEPARTMENT

1. Rapid triage and administration of analgesics is encouraged.
   Upon presentation to the ED, the patient should be rapidly triaged and examined to rule out other pain causing pathologies. Proper management of acute SCD pain inevitably involves administration of appropriate doses of parenteral opioids. For a variety of reasons, patients will often fail to tolerate doses of opioid that they have tolerated in the past. All SCD patients with acute pain should be managed in a monitored setting, with continuous pulse oximetry at a minimum. More conservative measures such as cardiac monitoring and (if available) end-tidal CO_2 monitoring should be considered. Taking these precautions will enable the emergency provider to safely administer the necessary doses of analgesic medication required for vaso-occlusive pain.
2. Choose starting opioid dose based on an individualized pain plan or prior opioid consumption.
   For the individual with acute sickle cell pain, intravenous (IV) opioids are first-line therapy.[8] It is considered best practice to administer analgesia within 30 minutes of presentation, although there is no empirical data showing this results in better outcomes. The majority of adults with SCD suffer from chronic pain,[24–26] and chronic opioid use and tolerance are common in the adult SCD population. Thus individuals with SCD often require extraordinarily high opioid doses to achieve adequate pain reduction. Appropriate initial doses will allow patients to receive less opioid overall, which reduces resource demands on nursing and shortens the time to adequate pain relief. There are three methods to determine opioid doses in the ED: patient-specific, consumption-based, and weight-based. Patient-specific opioid dosing involves administering a dose of opioid that has worked successfully for the patient in the past. Patients are often aware of their prior treatment and know what was successful. Patients should be part of the discussion of their treatment plan. Whenever possible, providers of long-term care should work to develop patient-specific ED pain management plans, as this is the preferred method for ED pain management. These pain management plans should be readily accessible to ED personnel upon presentation of the sickle cell patient to the ED. Consumption-based opioid dosing involves calculating the total dose of opioid taken by the patient over the last 24 hours and administering 20% of this total as a first IV dose in the ED. Opioid conversion calculators available online are helpful with this process (http://www.globalrph.com/narcoticonv.htm).

For the patient who does not have an individual pain plan and is unable to give a reliable medication history for the provider to calculate a consumption-based dose, weight-based dosing is appropriate. IV hydromorphone is recommended because it is a synthetic opioid with less histaminergic effects, and its time to peak onset is faster than morphine, which allows for safer redosing. The proper weight-based dose of hydromorphone is 10–20 mcg/kg. Morphine can be used as an alternative at a dose of 0.1–0.2 mg/kg. Some patients will give a history of intolerance to both these medications, or have coexisting renal dysfunction. In these cases, fentanyl 1–2 mcg/kg can be used. Meperidine should be avoided, as it is a poor analgesic and its renally cleared metabolite, normeperidine, is neurotoxic.

Medication	Dosage
Hydromorphone	10–20 mcg/kg
Morphine	0.1–0.2 mg/kg
Fentanyl	1–2 mcg/kg

3. When IV access is difficult or delayed, use oral or subcutaneous opioids; avoid intramuscular.
For patients with difficult access or milder symptoms of vaso-occlusion, oral or subcutaneous opioids are an appropriate alternative. Intramuscular administration is not recommended because it is more painful without pharmacologic advantage.
4. Titrate to pain reduction.
The cornerstone of successful ED pain management in SCD is redosing of opioid analgesics every 15–30 minutes. If the previous dose did not substantially improve the patient's pain (i.e., <2-point improvement on a 0–10 numerical pain scale), the next dose should be escalated by 25%–50%. The interval between doses is essential. Administration every 15–30 minutes allows for stacking of doses in order to achieve sufficient analgesia. It is common practice among emergency physicians to admit all patients who require more than three doses of opioids. There is very limited data on this topic, and the decision to admit should be made on an individual basis. Hospital admission exposes individuals with SCD to increased risk of venous thromboembolism, infection, and acute chest syndrome (a leading cause of death), and should be avoided whenever possible. Experience from SCD day hospitals suggest that patients can successfully be discharged after more than three doses of opioid without increased complications.[27]
5. Achieve pain reduction before starting patient controlled analgesia (PCA).
PCA is recommended for individuals admitted to the hospital for painful episodes.[28] PCAs are also an attractive alternative to bolus-dosed opioids for patients in the ED, because they alleviate some nursing demands and may result in faster pain relief.[28] It has been shown that PCA can lead to less opioid consumption compared with clinician-administered analgesia. When using PCA (either inpatient or in the ED), it is very important to achieve at least moderate pain reduction before starting the PCA. PCAs deliver small doses of opioid over short intervals (typically every 6–8 minutes). Achieving pain reduction through high-dose opioid boluses prior to PCA initiation is critical for two reasons. First, it helps the provider calculate the proper PCA settings (i.e., a patient who requires 12 mg of hydromorphone before initiation of PCA will require different settings than the patient who requires 6 mg of hydromorphone). Second, it also helps the patient because analgesia will not be delayed.
6. Choose proper PCA settings.
Individuals with SCD often require complex, nonstandard PCA dosing strategies. Basal rates are often appropriate, especially during early phases of VOCs. For opioid tolerant individuals with SCD, consultation with a pain specialist is recommended to ensure that PCA settings adequately mirror the opioid doses required to achieve adequate analgesia. If pain consultation services are unavailable, and the emergency provider is not comfortable starting nonstandard PCA settings, then it is preferable not to use PCA. In this setting, nurse administered bolus opioids in conjunction with oral long-acting medication may be preferred.
7. Continue long-acting home oral meds.
A large percentage of patients take daily long-acting opioids. If the patient is taking long-acting opioids at home, the decision to continue these medications should be made on an individual basis. It may be advisable to continue long-acting opioids, including methadone, to ensure adequate pain relief and avoid withdrawal symptoms. However, long-acting oral opioids may need to be withheld or reduced to prevent oversedation. During the course of admission, as IV medications are tapered down, the patient can return to a dose of long-acting opioid that is appropriate.
8. Do not overhydrate; use appropriate volumes of hypotonic fluids.
Dehydration can precipitate vaso-occlusive pain episodes; therefore, one would think that aggressive rehydration would be therapeutic. However, overhydration—especially with isotonic crystalloid—does not cure crisis and may have detrimental effects.[29] One undesirable effect of normal saline is that large amounts can cause hyperchloremic metabolic acidosis, and lowering the serum pH promotes sickling. Excessive IV fluids have been anecdotally associated with the development of atelectasis. A prospective observational cohort of 3751 patients with SCD identified atelectasis as a risk factor for the development of acute chest syndrome.[30] Therefore isotonic fluids should be avoided unless the patient is overtly hypovolemic. No studies have established which type or quantity of IV fluid is ideal for the patient with VOC.[31] However, hypotonic fluids are associated with reduced sickling in vivo and in vitro.[32] At our institution, we use 5% dextrose in half normal

saline at an infusion rate not exceeding maintenance to avoid overhydration.

9. Adjuvant acetaminophen.
   There are no clinical trial data to support the use of acetaminophen during vaso-occlusive pain; however, anecdotal experience suggests it may have opioid sparing effects. As acetaminophen is safe and well tolerated, we recommend oral acetaminophen as a first-line therapy in conjunction with IV opioids in the treatment of acute sickle cell pain. IV acetaminophen is attractive because it crosses the blood-brain barrier rapidly and does not undergo first-pass liver metabolism (which limits the potential for hepatotoxicity). Because of the costs of IV acetaminophen, we cannot broadly recommend its use without additional data. At our institution, we use IV acetaminophen for patients with poorly uncontrolled pain who cannot receive additional opioids because of concern for side effects (typically respiratory depression) and in whom nonsteroidal antiinflammatory drugs (NSAIDs) are contraindicated.
10. NSAID use for acute pain.
   NSAIDs should be used cautiously in the treatment of acute SCD pain. For acute episodes, NSAIDs may have the ability to improve analgesia when used in conjunction with IV opioids. Four small studies compared NSAIDs with placebo as adjunctive treatment for SCD pain, and only one found reductions in opioid requirements.[33-36] The potential for NSAIDs to cause or worsen renal damage is particularly concerning for individuals with SCD.[37,38] Individuals with SCD have hyposthenuria, which leads to increased clearance of creatinine, despite declining glomerular filtration rates. The clinical implication is that creatinine is an unreliable marker of renal function in SCD. As all individuals with SCD have some degree of renal injury due to chronic medullary infarcts, NSAIDs should be used sparingly, even when creatinine levels are normal. However, the current recommendation is to continue NSAIDs if there is no contraindication.
11. Minimize supplemental oxygen.
   Monitor oxygen saturation with pulse oximetry. Common practice in the many EDs is to administer supplemental oxygen to all individuals with vaso-occlusive pain. There is evidence, however, that excess administration of oxygen may be harmful because of the potential to reduce endogenous erythropoietin levels.[39,40] Chronic hypoxemia, associated with pulmonary hypertension and sleep-disordered breathing, is common in SCD and supplemental oxygen is recommended in the ED to keep hemoglobin oxygen saturations above 95%. For individuals who are not hypoxic, supplemental oxygen is not indicated.[4]
12. Nonpharmacologic measures: warm blankets, limit blood pressure measurements.
   Nonpharmacologic measures can improve SCD pain management in the ED and during admission. For adults, use manual blood pressure cuffs when possible, and limit unnecessary measurements. Warm blankets or heating pads are helpful, especially when the surrounding environment is cold. For children, distraction from pain by the provider, parent, or child-life specialist is recommended.
13. Address drug seeking behavior, tolerance, dependence, addiction, and diversion.

Keys to successful management of acute SCD pain in the emergency department

1. Rapid triage and administration of analgesics is encouraged.
2. Choose starting opioid dose based on an individualized pain plan or prior opioid consumption.
3. When IV access is difficult or delayed, use oral or subcutaneous opioids; avoid intramuscular injections.
4. Titrate to pain reduction.
5. Achieve pain reduction before starting PCA.
6. Choose proper PCA settings.
7. Continue long-acting home oral meds.
8. Do not overhydrate; use appropriate amounts of hypotonic fluids.
9. Adjuvant acetaminophen.
10. NSAID use for acute pain.
11. Minimize supplemental oxygen.
12. Nonpharmacologic measures: warm blankets, limit blood pressure measurements.
13. Address drug seeking behavior, tolerance, dependence, addiction, and diversion.

IV, Intravenous; *NSAID*, nonsteroidal antiinflammatory drugs; *PCA*, patient controlled analgesia; *SCD*, sickle cell disease.

Reports from the literature indicate varying perceptions among health care providers about rates of addiction and other self-destructive opioid related behaviors.[41-52] A large percentage of individuals with SCD are highly opioid tolerant, because they require daily or frequent chronic opioids; however, rates of true addiction in SCD are similar to the general population.[41] Acute pain management of opioid tolerant individuals is challenging, and it is important for long-term care providers to minimize chronic opioid use and aggressively address problematic opioid-related behaviors. Emergency providers can assist in the effort to minimize chronic opioid use by strongly encouraging patients to maintain follow-up with a comprehensive SCD clinic when available within 1 week. For patients who have an active relationship with a hematologist or comprehensive SCD clinic, emergency providers should limit opioid prescriptions to short courses, or preferably have all prescriptions written by a central provider in the SCD clinic. While it is appropriate to limit outpatient prescriptions and strongly encourage outpatient follow-up, it is not appropriate to withhold IV opioids during visits for acute pain, even when addiction or secondary gain is a concern. For individuals with concerning opioid related behaviors or inappropriate ED utilization patterns, we recommend multidisciplinary meetings between ED, hematology, and pain management specialists to devise a specific plan for each individual.

The following are the recommendations from NHLBI for management of patients with SCD and VOCs.[2]

RECOMMENDATIONS

The recommendations labeled "consensus" in this section were based on those developed by the American Pain Society or on panel expertise. The remaining recommendations are based on the evidence review conducted by the methodology team. These recommendations are intended to be for all settings where patients present with VOC.

1. In adults and children with SCD and pain,
   - When indicated, initiate diagnostic evaluation of causes of pain other than a VOC while beginning to treat pain.

   (Consensus-adapted)
2. In adults and children with SCD and a VOC,
   - Determine characteristics, associated symptoms, location, and intensity of pain based on patient self-report and observation. If the VOC pain is atypical, investigate other possible etiologies of pain.

   (Consensus-adapted)
   - Rapidly assess the patient's recent analgesic use (opioid and nonopioid).

   (Consensus-adapted)
   - Rapidly initiate analgesic therapy within 30 minutes of triage or within 60 minutes of registration.

   (Consensus-panel expertise)
   - Base analgesic selection on pain assessment, associated symptoms, outpatient analgesic use, patient knowledge of effective agents and doses, and past experience with side effects.

   (Consensus-adapted)
3. In adults and children with SCD and a VOC,
   - Use an individualized prescribing and monitoring protocol (written by the patient's SCD provider) or an SCD-specific protocol whenever possible to promote rapid, effective, and safe analgesic management and resolution of the VOC.

   (Consensus-panel expertise)
4. In adults and children with SCD and a VOC associated with mild to moderate pain who report relief with NSAIDs.
   (Moderate recommendation, low-quality evidence)
5. In adults and children with SCD and a VOC associated with severe pain, rapidly initiate treatment with parenteral opioids.
   (Strong recommendation, high-quality evidence)
6. In adults and children with SCD and a VOC associated with severe pain,
   - Calculate the parenteral (IV or subcutaneous) opioid dose based on total daily short-acting opioid dose currently being taken at home to manage the VOC.

   (Consensus-panel expertise)
   - Administer parenteral opioids using the subcutaneous route when intravenous access is difficult.

   (Consensus-panel expertise)
   - Reassess pain and readminister opioids if necessary for continued severe pain every 15–30 minutes until pain is under control per patient report.

   (Consensus-adapted)
   - Maintain or consider escalation of the dose by 25% until pain is controlled.

   (Consensus-panel expertise)
   - Reassess after each dose for pain relief and side effects.

   (Consensus-panel expertise)
   - Initiate around-the-clock opioid administration by patient-controlled analgesia (PCA) or frequently scheduled doses versus "as requested" (PRN) administration.
7. If ordering around-the-clock, continuous infusion of opioids via the PCA, carefully consider whether there is a need to withhold long-acting oral opioids to prevent oversedation.
   (Consensus-panel expertise)
   - If demand dosing only is ordered via the PCA, continue use of long-acting opioids.

   (Consensus-panel expertise)
   - At discharge, evaluate inpatient analgesic requirements, wean parenteral opioids prior to conversion to oral opioids, and adjust home dose of long- and short-acting opioid prescriptions to prevent opioid withdrawal after discharge.

   (Consensus-panel expertise)
8. In adults and children with SCD and a VOC, do not use meperidine, unless it is the only effective opioid for an individual patient.
   (Consensus-adapted)
9. In adults and children with a VOC, administer oral NSAIDs as an adjuvant analgesic in the absence of contraindications.
   (Consensus-adapted)
10. In adults and children with a VOC who require antihistamines for itching secondary to opioid administration, prescribe agents orally and do not readminister with each dose of opioid in the acute VOC management phase. Readminister every 4–6 hours if needed.
    (Consensus-panel expertise)
11. To reduce the risk of acute chest syndrome in adults and children hospitalized for a VOC,
    - Encourage use of incentive spirometry while awake.
      (Strong recommendation, moderate-quality evidence)
    - Encourage ambulation and activity as soon as possible.

    (Consensus-panel expertise)
12. In adults and children with VOC, use adjunctive nonpharmacologic approaches to treat pain such as local heat application and distraction.
    (Consensus-adapted)
13. In euvolemic adults and children with SCD and a VOC who are unable to drink fluids, provide intravenous hydration at no more than maintenance rate to avoid overhydration.
    (Consensus-adapted)
14. In adults and children with SCD and a VOC being treated with opioids, monitor for excessive sedation by measuring sedation with an objective measurement sedation scale and oxygenation levels.
    (Consensus-panel expertise)
15. Gradually titrate down parenteral opioids as VOC resolves.
    (Consensus-panel expertise)
16. In adults and children with SCD and a VOC, do not administer a blood transfusion unless there are other indications for transfusion.
    (Moderate recommendation, low-quality evidence)
17. In adults and children with SCD and a VOC with an oxygen saturation <95% on room air, administer oxygen.
    (Consensus-Panel Expertise)

IV, Intravenous; *NSAID,* nonsteroidal antiinflammatory drugs; *SCD,* sickle cell disease; *VOC,* vaso-occlusive crises.
From Buchanan GR, Yawn BP: *Evidence-based Management of Sickle Cell Disease.* Bethesda, MD: US Department of Health and Human Services, National Institutes of Health, National Heart, Lung, and Blood Institute, 2014; Chapter 3. Available from: https://www.nhlbi.nih.gov/sites/www.nhlbi.nih.gov/files/sickle-cell-disease-report.pdf (with permission).

14. Chronic pain and SCD.
    Patients with SCD can have chronic pain in addition to acute pain episodes. Chronic pain is typically defined as pain lasting longer than 3 months. It appears to be more common in adults compared with children. Neuropathic pain is often a component of chronic pain. Its etiology stems from nerve damage from occlusion of blood vessels supplying the nerves, or it is the result of persistent pain. The mainstay of managing chronic pain in SCD is to restore function, thereby improving quality of life. Medications useful in treating chronic pain in SCD include NSAIDs, opioids, antidepressants, and anticonvulsants. In addition, nonpharmacologic therapies should be used, such as cognitive-behavioral therapies, occupational and physical therapy, acupuncture, and physical activity.

There is limited data on the treatment of chronic pain in SCD. The following recommendations by NHLBI are formulated from research in other chronic pain settings.[53,54]

RECOMMENDATIONS

1. Determine the cause and type of SCD-related chronic pain. This includes chronic pain with objective signs such as avascular necrosis (AVN) and leg ulcers, and chronic pain without objective signs due to neuroplasticity of the peripheral or central nervous system.
(Consensus-adapted)
2. Use a combination of the patient's response to treatment—including pain relief, side effects, and functional outcomes—to guide the long-term use of opioids.
(Consensus-adapted)
3. Encourage people to use deep tissue/deep pressure massage therapy, muscle relaxation therapy, and self-hypnosis as indicated.
(Weak recommendation, low-quality evidence)
4. Use long- and short-acting opioids to manage chronic pain that is not relieved by nonopioids.
(Consensus-adapted)
5. Assess all people with SCD for chronic pain annually or more often as needed. This assessment should include descriptors of the pain; its severity on a numerical scale; its location; factors that precipitate or relieve it, including biopsychosocial factors; and its effect on the patient's mood, activity, employment, quality of life, and vital signs.
(Consensus-adapted)
6. Use a partnership agreement leading to a written, individualized treatment plan (to include risks, benefits, and side effects) with the patient if long-term opioids are indicated. The partnership agreement should list the patient's rights and responsibilities, and the treatment plan should list the type, amount, and route of administration of the opioid in question, including random drug urine testing.
(Consensus-adapted)
7. Appoint one physician or other clinician to write the biweekly to monthly prescriptions for long-term opioids. Refills without seeing the patient should be kept to a minimum, and people on chronic opioid therapy must be evaluated in person every 2–3 months.
(Consensus-adapted)
8. Document all encounters with a patient, including medical history, physical exam, diagnosis, plan of management, type and amount of opioids prescribed and their side effects, if any, and lab data as needed.
(Consensus-adapted)
9. Encourage people receiving opioids to increase their fluid intake, maintain dietary fiber intake per the current dietary fiber recommendations, and use stool softeners and bowel stimulant laxatives such as senna and/or docusate as needed.
(Consensus-adapted)
10. Believe the patient's report of pain and optimize therapeutic outcomes to achieve adequate pain relief and improve the patient's quality of life.
(Consensus-adapted)
11. Refer patients for evaluation by a mental health professional such as a psychiatrist, social worker, or addiction specialist as needed.
(Consensus-adapted)
12. Assess all people for other types of non-SCD-related chronic pain, including postoperative pain due to trauma, pain due to therapy, iatrogenic pain, and pain due to comorbid conditions.
(Consensus-adapted)

SCD, Sickle cell disease.

From Buchanan GR, Yawn BP: *Evidence-based Management of Sickle Cell Disease.* Bethesda, MD: US Department of Health and Human Services, National Institutes of Health, National Heart, Lung, and Blood Institute, 2014; Chapter 3. Available from: https://www.nhlbi.nih.gov/sites/www.nhlbi.nih.gov/files/sickle-cell-disease-report.pdf (with permission).

SUMMARY

Despite the challenges associated with managing acute sickle cell pain in the ED, the structured approach presented is likely to improve patient and provider satisfaction. The cornerstones of proper pain management are early treatment with IV opioids with frequent reassessments and redosing until adequate analgesia is achieved. Close follow-up with a physician is necessary to minimize ED utilization and improve compliance and follow-up. The adjuvant measures discussed will improve safety and patient satisfaction, and minimize opioid consumption when possible.

KEY POINTS

- Patients with sickle cell trait do not have vaso-occlusive disease.
- VOCs usually present with sudden onset of pain, usually in the lower back and legs. In children, there may be swelling of the digits. Vital signs and laboratory tests are of little use during these episodes.
- The management of acute sickle cell pain includes the use of analgesics, judicious use of hypotonic fluid solutions, appropriate use of supplemental oxygen, and use of pharmacologic measures, including warm blankets.
- The use of opioids during acute sickle cell crisis should be individualized and titrated to reduction of the acute pain. Pain should be reduced before an IV PCA is started. Acetaminophen may be used as an adjuvant, NSAIDs should be used cautiously; and meperidine should be avoided.
- Chronic sickle cell pain not relieved by nonopioids can be managed with long- and short-acting opioids.
- Patients with SCD pain should be assessed annually.
- The recommendations of NHLBI on the management of patients with SCD and VOCs should be followed.

REFERENCES

Access the reference list online at ExpertConsult.com.

CHAPTER 39

PAIN MANAGEMENT DURING PREGNANCY AND LACTATION

Jeanette Bauchat, MD, MS ◌ Cynthia A. Wong, MD

Complaints of pain occur commonly in pregnant and lactating women. Nonpharmacologic methods to treat pain during pregnancy and lactation should be considered before turning to pharmacologic agents, because almost all drugs administered to the mother cross the placenta to the fetus or are secreted in breast milk.[1]

The mechanisms of drug transport are similar to the transport of drugs across any membrane.[2,3] Diffusion is primarily passive and the drug concentration in the umbilical vein or breast milk depends on the concentration gradient, drug lipid solubility, degree of ionization and protein binding, and the diffusion capacity of the membrane (this may change as pregnancy progresses).[4] The effects on the fetus or nursing child will depend on the gestational or postconceptual age, as well as the amount and duration of drug exposure, and the specific drug.

In the United States, nonopioid and opioid analgesics are commonly ingested during pregnancy.[5,6] The benefit of analgesic medications should justify the risk (e.g., the untreated illness may pose a greater risk to the fetus than the medications used to treat the illness)[3] and the minimum effective dose should be used. Consideration should be given to using nonpharmacologic methods of pain control, or using nonsystemic methods of drug administration.

DRUGS DURING PREGNANCY

PHARMACOKINETIC CHANGES DURING PREGNANCY

The myriad physiologic changes of pregnancy influence drug absorption, distribution, and elimination.[7] Changes in gastrointestinal function can alter oral drug absorption. Renal elimination is generally increased because of an increase in glomerular filtration rate. Hepatic metabolism may be increased, unchanged, or decreased, and the increase in total body water may alter drug distribution and peak concentrations. Protein binding is usually decreased; however, the free drug concentration may be unchanged because of increased drug clearance.

TRANSFER OF DRUGS ACROSS THE PLACENTA

The amount of drug that crosses the placenta depends on maternal cardiac output, fetal cardiac output, placental binding, and placental metabolism, as well as factors that influence passive diffusion across the placenta.[8] Maternal plasma levels of a drug depend on the site of administration (e.g., oral, intravascular, or epidural space), the total dose, the dosing interval, and other drugs that may be coadministered (e.g., epinephrine). The amount of drug to which the fetus is exposed also depends on fetal metabolism (fetal blood carrying drugs away from the placenta passes first through the fetal liver), fetal protein binding (about half of maternal protein binding), and the distribution of fetal cardiac output (fetal distress results in redistribution of blood flow to the vital organs).[9]

In general, good studies of human placental drug transfer and fetal exposure are limited. Interspecies differences in placental anatomy and function make animal model comparisons with humans risky. Ethical concerns have limited studies in pregnant women. Most studies of the placental transfer of anesthetic agents administered to the mother intrapartum report single measurements of drug concentration in the maternal and umbilical vein serum at the time of delivery (the fetal:maternal or F/M ratio). The measured fetal concentration does not reflect the effects of drug passage through the fetal liver, or the possibility of altered pharmacokinetics and pharmacodynamics in the fetus compared with the mother.

TERATOGENICITY

Possible adverse effects on the fetus of in utero drug exposure include structural malformations, intrauterine fetal death, altered fetal growth, neurobehavioral teratogenicity, acute neonatal intoxication, or neonatal abstinence syndromes.[2] A major determinant of the effect of a drug on the fetus is the gestational age of the fetus. Traditionally, teratogenic effects of drugs have been defined as structural malformations. However, functional and behavioral effects are also likely to occur, and are much harder to identify because the effects of fetal drug exposure may be delayed and only apparent later in life.[2] The mechanisms by which drugs cause teratogenicity are poorly understood, and may be direct or indirect (direct effect on the mother indirectly effects the fetus). There is interspecies variation in the ability of a drug to cause a specific congenital defect (e.g., thalidomide is not teratogenic in nonprimates).

The period of classic teratogenesis corresponds with the critical period of organogenesis and begins approximately 31 days after the first day of the last menstrual period until about 71 days after the last period.[10] Exposure to teratogens before 31 days results in an all-or-none effect (survival without a defect or loss of pregnancy). Fetal development, particularly the central nervous system, continues into the second and third trimesters, and indeed after birth. Therefore fetal drug exposure at this time is not risk free.

Information on the teratogenic potential of many drugs comes from large-survey studies. These studies are often flawed because of reporting bias. They often do not control for other variables, including environmental exposures, exposure to multiple drugs (including alcohol, tobacco, nonprescription and illicit drugs), and the influence of the disease itself. Case reports of an association between in utero drug exposure and fetal anomalies are more likely to be published than if no anomaly occurred.[11]

FOOD AND DRUG ADMINISTRATION RISK CLASSIFICATION

The US Food and Drug Administration (FDA) previously required labeling of drugs using the Pregnancy Category System (Table 39.1). The FDA recognized that this system was often not helpful to the prescribing physician and pregnant patient. Starting in 2015, the FDA mandated a new drug labeling system (Pregnancy and Lactation Labeling Rule, or "Final Rule"), which requires three new subsections in the pregnancy and lactation sections of the package insert: risk summary, clinical considerations, and data sections (Table 39.2).[12]

SPECIFIC DRUGS

Aspirin use during pregnancy may be associated with an increased risk of gastroschisis. Pregnant women should not use aspirin (>150 mg/day) regularly.[13] Ibuprofen and naproxen during the first trimester do not appear to be teratogenic.[13] Prostaglandin inhibitors have been associated with narrowing of the ductus arteriosus in utero. This effect increases with gestational age, although it appears reversible when the medication is stopped.[2,13] Aspirin and other prostaglandin inhibitors may decrease amniotic fluid volume secondary to decreased fetal urine output, and they may prolong pregnancy and labor. An increased incidence of neonatal intracranial hemorrhage has been found in premature infants whose mothers ingested aspirin near birth. For these reasons, full-dose aspirin and nonsteroidal anti-inflammatory drug (NSAID) therapy should be avoided in the third trimester.[2,13] If a mild analgesic is indicated during pregnancy, acetaminophen is the drug of choice.

Fourteen percent of pregnant women fill an opioid prescription during their pregnancy.[5] Chronic in utero exposure to opioids can lead to neonatal abstinence syndrome, and maternal opioid use should be minimized if possible.[14] Neonatal abstinence syndrome presents at 24–72 hours of life.[14] Infants have variable features and presentations, including central nervous system hyperirritability (i.e., excessive crying, tremors, increased muscle tone); autonomic nervous system dysfunction (i.e., nasal stuffiness, yawning, sweating); and gastrointestinal disturbances.[14] There is no evidence that opioid agonist or agonist–antagonist exposure during pregnancy is teratogenic.[2] Opioid analgesics should be reserved for patients with moderate to severe pain who have failed nonpharmacologic interventions and nonopioid multimodal analgesic medications.

Bupivacaine and lidocaine were not associated with risk of teratogenicity in the Collaborative Perinatal Project.[2,9] The incidence of fetal anomalies was increased twofold in women who were exposed to mepivacaine; however, this group included a very small number of women, and so it is difficult to draw any conclusions from the data.

Several surveillance studies have found an association between maternal steroid use and orofacial clefts, while others have not.[2] A limited trial of epidural steroid therapy is probably associated with minimal fetal risk after the first trimester of pregnancy.

Antidepressant medications are frequently used in the treatment of chronic pain. There is no evidence that tricyclic antidepressant drugs are teratogenic.[2] First trimester exposure to most selective serotonin reuptake inhibitors (SSRIs) appears to have similar rates of congenital malformations than the general population.[15,16] Paroxetine is the

TABLE 39.1 US Food and Drug Administration Pregnancy Category System

Category	Drugs
A	None
B	Acetaminophen; butorphanol, nalbuphine; caffeine; oxycodone IR,[a] Ibuprofen, naproxen, indomethacin; prednisone, prednisolone
C	Amitriptyline; aspirin, ketorolac; betamethasone, cortisone; codeine,[a] fentanyl,[a] hydrocodone,[a] hydromorphone,[a] methadone,[a] meperidine,[a] morphine,[a] oxycodone ER,[a] oxymorphone,[a] tramadol[a]; gabapentin, pregabalin; lidocaine; propranolol; sumatriptan; sertraline, fluoxetine; bupropion
D	Imipramine; carbamazepine; diazepam; paroxetine; phenobarbital; phenytoin, valproic acid
X	Ergotamine

[a]*Opioid agonists and agonist–antagonists are considered risk category D when used at high doses near term.*

TABLE 39.2 US Food and Drug New Pregnancy and Lactation Classification System

Category	Risk Summary	Clinical Considerations	Data
Pregnancy	Risk of adverse developmental outcomes	• Disease-associated maternal and/or embryo/fetal risk • Dose adjustments during pregnancy and postpartum • Maternal adverse reactions • Fetal/neonatal adverse reaction • Labor and delivery	Human or animal data providing the scientific basis for the risk summary and clinical considerations
Lactation	Summarizes information on drug and/or active metabolite(s): • Presence in human milk • Effects on the breastfed child • Effects on milk production	Information for prescribing and risk/benefit analysis to limited exposure and monitor child for adverse reactions	Human or animal data providing the scientific basis for the risk summary and clinical considerations

only SSRI that is associated with increased risk of major congenital heart anomalies.[15] There is limited data, but studies with duloxetine suggest it may increase rates of spontaneous abortion in the first trimester.[16] Exposure to SSRIs in the third trimester before delivery may lead to a neonatal withdrawal syndrome[15] and transient QT interval prolongation.[17] The long-term clinical consequences of these changes are not known. The noradrenergic and specific serotonergic antidepressant, venlafaxine and the serotonin-noradrenalin reuptake inhibitors, mirtazapine, appear to confer no risk of malformation or neonatal withdrawal syndrome, but these are newer drugs with fewer studies.[15] Data on the teratogenicity of bupropion in pregnant women are limited, but suggest an increased risk of cardiac malformations.[18,19]

Anticonvulsants have been implicated in fetal growth restriction and congenital malformation. The Medical Birth Registry of Norway compared 2600 children exposed to antiepileptics with 771,412 unexposed children.[20] Carbamazepine, lamotrigine, oxcarbazepine, gabapentin, and pregabalin had low malformation rates, similar to the general population.[20,21] Topiramate increased fetal growth restriction and microcephaly, and valproic acid increased risk for hypospadias and septal heart defects.[20] Children of women with epilepsy who take anticonvulsants carry a higher risk of developmental delay and cognitive impairment than those who do not require therapy during pregnancy. Human studies demonstrate that phenytoin and valproic acid confer the highest potential for neurodevelopmental disorders, whereas lamotrigine and carbamazepine are least likely to lead to these adverse outcomes.[22]

Ergotamine is contraindicated in pregnancy, as it may be teratogenic, and it also causes uterine contractions.[23] There is no evidence that beta-blockers are teratogenic; however, they may be associated with intrauterine growth retardation.[24,25]

DRUGS DURING LACTATION

The amount of drug to which an infant is exposed during lactation depends on a number of maternal and infant factors. Maternal factors include maternal dose and dosing interval, the elimination half-life of the drug, the infant nursing pattern (volume and timing), and the amount of drug that actually crosses into breast milk.[2,3] The milk to plasma (M:P) ratio is an index of the amount of drug that is excreted into breast milk. Breast milk is slightly more acidic than plasma, and therefore passive diffusion favors drugs that are weak bases, lipid soluble, and have low protein binding.[3] The amount of drug to which the infant is actually exposed depends on infant pharmacokinetics, which may differ from maternal pharmacokinetics. The average infant dose is generally 1%–2% of the maternal dose.[3] Even when the M:P ratio approaches one, the infant plasma concentration rarely attains therapeutic levels.

Because the volume of colostrum is small, nursing neonates are exposed to minimal amounts of the drugs administered to the mother in the postpartum period.[3] Most milk is made during and immediately following nursing. Administration of drugs shortly after nursing, and avoiding long-acting drugs, may help minimize infant exposure. For mothers taking chronic medications, the in utero exposure is greater than the exposure during lactation. In general, the lowest effective dose should be used, and older drugs with a history of widespread use should be chosen.[3] It is best to use drugs that do not have an active metabolite.

AMERICAN ACADEMY OF PEDIATRICS

The American Academy of Pediatrics believes the benefit of breast-feeding usually outweighs the risk of drug exposure in breast milk. The Committee on Drugs previously listed drugs that could be used safely during lactation and their effects on the infant and/or on lactation. This committee now refers practitioners to a more comprehensive and current database at LactMed (http://toxnet.nlm.nih.gov). A summary of analgesics that should be avoided in breast-feeding mothers is presented in Table 39.3.

The following should be considered when prescribing drugs to lactating women[3]:

- Is drug therapy really necessary?
- The safest drug and lowest therapeutic dose should be chosen—for example, acetaminophen rather than aspirin for mild analgesia.
- Preterm infants or neonates may be more vulnerable to adverse events because of immature organ function or medical conditions.
- If there is a possibility of risk to the infant, one should consider monitoring infant serum levels of the drug.

SPECIFIC DRUGS

Acetaminophen is considered the safest analgesic for nursing mothers. The infant of a mother taking acetaminophen 4 g/day was exposed to less than 5% the therapeutic infant dose.[26] There is controversy as to the use of aspirin in nursing mothers. Intermittent use should not pose a risk, but infants of mothers receiving chronic aspirin therapy should be observed for adverse side effects.[26] NSAIDs are considered compatible with nursing.[13,27]

Opioid agonist and agonist–antagonists cross freely into breast milk. The American Academy of Pediatrics considers opioids compatible with breast-feeding, because most undergo significant first-pass metabolism in the infant. However, oxycodone, pentazocine, meperidine, and codeine are not recommended in the lactating mother, because clinically therapeutic levels are achieved and produce adverse effects in breastfeeding infants.[27] The infants of nursing mothers ingesting opioids should be monitored for adverse effects.

TABLE 39.3 Drugs Achieving Greater Than 10% Therapeutic Maternal Dose in Breastmilk

Class	Drugs
Nonopioid analgesic	Aspirin, ergotamine
Opioids	Oxycodone, pentazocine, meperidine, codeine
SSRIs, SNRIs	Bupropion, citalopram, fluoxetine, venlafaxine
Anticonvulsants	Lamotrigine nonsteroidal antiinflammatory drugs, opioid agonists, opioid agonists–antagonists, steroids, sumatriptan

SNRIs, *Serotonin-norepinephrine reuptake inhibitors;* SSRIs, *selective serotonin reuptake inhibitors.*

Less than 1% of the maternal dose of prednisone or prednisolone is recovered in breast milk.[2] Even at high maternal doses, this is unlikely to be enough to suppress infant adrenal function.[11]

Current guidelines suggest that the choice of a specific antidepressant or anticonvulsant be based on maternal clinical factors, particularly previous efficacious therapies. The American Academy of Pediatrics warns that infant plasma concentrations that exceed 10% of therapeutic maternal plasma concentrations have been reported in several of these drugs, and should be avoided in nursing mothers if possible (bupropion, fluoxetine, citalopram, venlafaxine, and lamotrigine).[27] The anticonvulsants carbamazepine, phenytoin, and valproic acid may be used safely during lactation. Low and undetectable serum concentrations of many antidepressants are detected in the serum of nursing infants, but long-term studies are lacking.[28] Sertraline, duloxetine, and paroxetine are preferred in lactating women who require antidepressant drugs for the first time.[15,16,28]

Maternal administration of beta-blockers results in subtherapeutic levels in nursing infants.[26] Serum concentrations of propranolol in the nursing infant are less than 1% of the therapeutic dose.[26] There are no data regarding the use of gabapentin or pregabalin during lactation.[29] Ergotamine has been associated with neonatal convulsions and gastrointestinal disturbances and should not be used in nursing mothers.[2,26] Sumatriptan is the most studied tryptan during lactation.[26] It is present in low concentrations in breast milk and has poor oral bioavailability, so the American Academy of Pediatrics considers sumatriptan compatible with breast-feeding.[26,27]

IMAGING DURING PREGNANCY

The two factors that determine the possible effects of radiation exposure on the developing fetus are the gestational age and fetal dose of absorbed radiation. Risks of fetal radiation exposure include abortion, genetic mutation, and carcinogenesis.[30] At doses of less than 50 mGy, the risk of abnormalities is thought to be negligible; significant risk of malformation is increased only at doses greater than 150 mGy.[31] Although radiation exposure from imaging studies generally falls below 50 mGy, exposure should be avoided if possible until after the 15th week of gestation, since radiation can be lethal to the fetus or cause severe defects with doses as low as 50 mGy.[30]

Although there is theoretical risk to using magnetic resonance imaging (MRI), no detrimental effects to the fetus have been documented. MRI is indicated during pregnancy when other nonionizing imaging methods (e.g., ultrasonography) are unsatisfactory, and the information obtained would otherwise require exposure to ionizing radiation.[30] Normal fluoroscopy can deliver 10–50 mGy/min of exposure time and thus should be avoided in pregnancy, if possible.[31]

PAIN SYNDROMES DURING PREGNANCY AND LACTATION

PELVIC GIRDLE PAIN AND LOW BACK PAIN

Although definitions differ, the term *pelvic girdle pain* is used to describe pain in the regions of one or both sacroiliac (SI) joints and the gluteal region sometimes involving the symphysis pubis, whereas *pregnancy-related low back pain* refers to pain in the lumbar region.[32–34] The incidence of these syndromes during pregnancy is about 45% and around 25% in the postpartum period.[33] Risk factors include strenuous work, previous low back pain, or pain syndromes in a previous pregnancy.[32] The etiology of pelvic girdle pain and low back pain (LBP) are likely related to mechanical, traumatic, hormonal, metabolic, or degenerative changes during pregnancy. Pain usually begins in the second trimester and resolves for most women within several weeks to months of delivery.[32] About 10% of women continue to have chronic pain.[33]

Pelvic girdle pain is usually located between the posterior iliac crests near the SI joints. It may occur in conjunction with symphysis pubis pain and may radiate into the posterior thighs.[32,34] Few treatments have undergone rigorous scientific scrutiny. Patient education, pelvic belts, physiotherapy, and acupuncture may be of benefit to some patients.[32,35] Pregnancy-related LBP is described as pain in the lumbar region, above the sacrum, and it may radiate into the leg. The pain is often dull and exacerbated by forward flexion.[33] It is important to distinguish low back pain from posterior pelvic joint pain using specific provocation tests to optimize physical therapy and exercise recommendations.[32,33]

If pharmacologic agents are required, acetaminophen and cyclobenzaprine are the drugs of choice for minor pelvic and back pain. The short-term use of NSAIDs may be appropriate during the first and second trimesters. Severe back pain may require opioid therapy. Epidural steroid injection(s) may be indicated for acute radicular pain, consistent with lumbar nerve root compression.

NEUROPATHIC PAIN: CARPAL TUNNEL SYNDROME

The incidence of carpal tunnel syndrome ranges from 7% to 62% and is attributed to the hormonal changes and tissue edema that occur during pregnancy.[36] Conservative management with nighttime splinting, physical therapy or local injections with local anesthetic and steroid medications are effective in most cases. Surgery is reserved for severe cases with neurologic injury.[37]

HEADACHE

Migraine headaches are unusual during pregnancy.[26] The initial presentation of a migrainelike headache in pregnancy should prompt a search for another serious cause.[38]

KEY POINTS

- Pain is frequent during pregnancy and lactation. Many women suffer from pelvic girdle pain and back pain.
- Physiologic changes during pregnancy may alter drug pharmacokinetics and pharmacodynamics.
- Most drugs cross the placenta and cross into breast milk.
- Drug effects on the fetus may be direct or indirect (effect on the mother).
- Efforts should be made to minimize maternal exposure to drugs during pregnancy and lactation.

- Possible adverse effects of in utero drug exposure include structural malformations, intrauterine fetal death, altered fetal growth, neurobehavioral teratogenicity, acute neonatal intoxication, and neonatal abstinence syndromes.
- The effects of drugs on the fetus or nursing infant depend on the gestational or postconceptual age, the type/amount of drug and duration of exposure.
- Drug pharmacokinetics and pharmacodynamics are altered in the fetus and neonates compared with the older child and adult.
- Information about fetal and neonatal effects of drugs administered to mothers is frequently incomplete, but new FDA labeling requirements may aid in clinical decision making.
- The decision to use drugs to treat pain during pregnancy and lactation should involve a risk: benefit analysis.

REFERENCES

Access the reference list online at ExpertConsult.com.

CHAPTER

40 Pain Control in the Critically Ill Patient

Abbas Al-Qamari, MD ◎ Michael Lynn Ault, MD, FCCP, FCCM

Management of pain, agitation, and delirium is vital in the critical care setting. Within the intensive care unit (ICU), the concepts of analgesia, hypnosis, and cognition are inexorably intertwined. Adequate treatment of pain and anxiety has been shown to decrease the stress response and psychological illness, improving outcomes in critical care patients.[1] Importantly, critically ill patients are at great risk of developing delirium, negatively affecting the trajectory of care. Critically ill patients experience both pain and anxiety from a multitude of factors. Along with obvious etiologies of pain such as preexisting diseases and trauma, patients in critical care settings often experience pain from prolonged immobility, routine nursing care (airway suctioning, dressing changes, and patient mobility), monitoring and therapeutic devices (catheters, drains, and endotracheal tubes), and air hunger. Understandably, critical care patients also experience a significant degree of anxiety. Anxiety may stem from pain, being in an unfamiliar environment, and lack of control or even a fear of impending death. Significant anxiety may lead to agitation and eventually delirium, complicating diagnosis and interfering with treatment, leading to increased morbidity and mortality. Certainly, anxiolysis is difficult to achieve in a patient experiencing significant pain or delirium. Furthermore, many of the medications used to treat pain have hypnotic effects. Thus it is easy to understand how the concepts of hypnosis and analgesia have become interdependent goals of critical care therapy. Complicating matters is the possibility of delirium altering the ability to assess and attain these goals. However, the close relationship between these distinct goals should not confuse the clinician as to the specific aim of each therapeutic agent. By understanding the tools for appropriate patient assessment and management, one can better choose the appropriate pharmaceutical agents for analgesia, hypnosis, and delirium management, providing an integrated, patient-centered therapeutic regimen to the critically ill.[2]

ASSESSMENT

ANALGESIA

Analgesia assessment tools are difficult to implement in the critical care setting. An ideal assessment tool should provide simple, reliable data that guide therapy in a critical care setting. The most reliable and valid indicator of pain is a patient's self-report. Unidirectional tools such as the numeric rating scale and visual analog scale rely on a patient's perception of their pain (Fig. 40.1). The numeric rating scale requires patients to rate their pain from 0 to 10, with 0 representing no pain and 10 representing the worst pain possible. The visual analog scale consists of a 10-cm horizontal line with descriptive phrases at either end, from no pain to worst pain ever. Variations of the visual analog scale include simplistic facial images rather than descriptive phrases. Despite the simplicity and reliability of these unidirectional pain assessment tools, they often are not useful in the critical care setting, because patients may be unable to communicate. Behavioral-physiologic scales use pain-related behaviors such as posturing and facial expressions, along with physiologic indicators such as heart rate, blood pressure, and respiratory rate to assess pain intensity in patients who are unable to participate in unidirectional pain assessment scales. However, physiologic markers are not specific for pain and may be misinterpreted in a critical care setting. The Behavioral Pain Scale (BPS; Fig. 40.2) and the Critical-Care Pain Observation Tool (CPOT) are the most reliable in critically ill patients who are unable to self-report their pain. The BPS allows for pain assessment in mechanically ventilated patients by assigning a score of 1–4 for three different behaviors.[3] The CPOT allows for evaluation of both intubated and extubated patients by scoring four different behaviors on a scale of 0–2.[4] Both these tools allow for standardized assessment of pain based on patient behaviors. Anxiety and delirium often cloud the behavioral-physiological pain picture, resulting in overestimation of a patient's pain.[5] Although both unidirectional and behavioral scales provide reliable assessment in a majority of patients, pain assessment in patients requiring critical care therapy remains challenging to assess.

HYPNOSIS

Titrating therapy to sedation levels allows for better outcomes as sole assessment of pain is complicated in critically ill patients. Both oversedation and undersedation can result in clinically significant adverse events. Undersedation may result in ventilator dyssynchrony, increased oxygen requirements, self-removal of devices, and possibly posttraumatic stress disorder from a stay in the critical care unit. Alternatively, oversedation may result in prolonged tracheal intubation and mechanical ventilation, increasing the chance of pneumonia and respiratory deconditioning. To this end, several sedation monitoring scales (Table 40.1) have been developed to aid in appropriate monitoring and titration of sedation levels. With sedation assessment scales, sedation levels can be maintained by different care providers, and therapeutic agents may be titrated to achieve desired levels of sedation. The Richmond Agitation Sedation Scale (RASS) and Riker Sedation-Agitation Scale (SAS) are the most valid and reliable sedation assessment tools. The RASS is a user-friendly and therefore commonly used sedation scale, with scores ranging from +4 (a violent dangerous patient) to −5 (an unarousable patient).[6] A sedation score of 0 is most often therapeutically targeted, as it correlates with

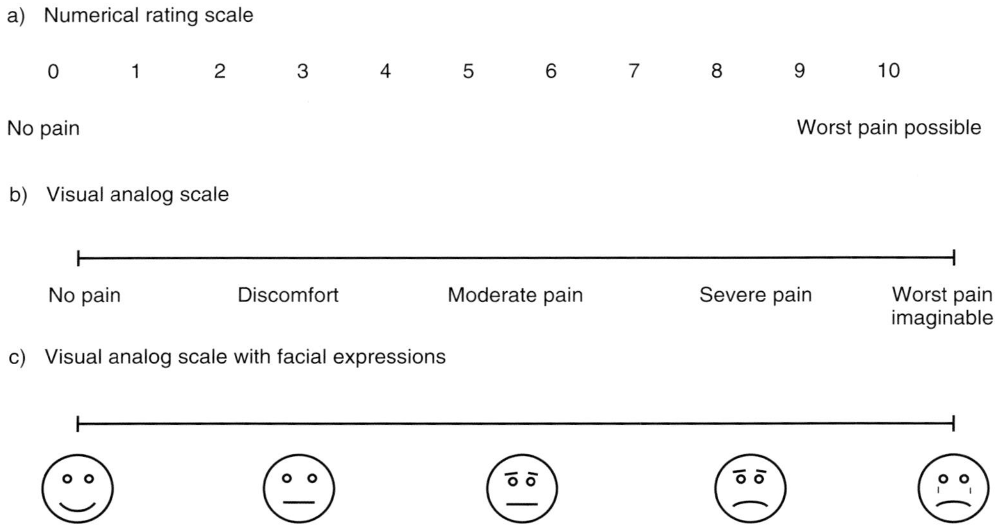

FIG. 40.1 Unidirectional Pain Assessment Scales.

Item	Description	Score
Facial expression	Relaxed Partially tightened (e.g., brow lowering) Fully tightened (e.g., eyelid closing) Grimacing	1 2 3 4
Upper limbs	No movement Partially bent Fully bent with finger flexion Permanently retracted	1 2 3 4
Compliance with mechanical ventilation	Tolerating movement Coughing but tolerating ventilation most of the time Fighting ventilator Unable to control ventilation	1 2 3 4

FIG. 40.2 Behavioral Pain Scale. *(Payen JF, Bru O, Bosson JL, et al.: Assessing pain in critically ill sedated patients by using a behavioral pain scale.* Crit Care Med. *29:2258-2263, 2001.)*

TABLE 40.1 Sedation Assessment Scales

(a) Richmond Agitation Sedation Scale

Score	Term	Description
+4	Combative	Overtly combative or violent; immediate danger to staff
+3	Very agitated	Pulls on tubes or has aggressive behavior toward staff
+2	Agitated	Frequent nonpurposeful movement or ventilator dyssynchrony
+1	Restless	Anxious but movements not aggressive or vigorous
0	Alert and calm	
−1	Drowsy	Not fully alert but sustained (>10 seconds) awakening
−2	Light sedation	Briefly (<10 seconds) awakens with eye contact
−3	Moderate sedation	Any movement (but no eye contact) to voice
−4	Deep sedation	No response to voice, but any movement to physical stimulation
−5	Unarousable	No response to voice or physical stimulation

TABLE 40.1 Sedation Assessment Scales—cont'd

(b) Ramsay Sedation Scale

Score	Arousal	Description
1	Awake	Patient anxious, agitated, or restless
2	Awake	Cooperative, orientated, and tranquil
3	Asleep	Patient responds to commands only
4	Asleep	Brisk response to loud auditory stimulus or glabellar tap
5	Asleep	Sluggish response to loud auditory stimulus or glabellar tap
6	Asleep	No response to loud auditory stimulus or glabellar tap

(c) Riker Sedation Agitation Scale

Score	Term	Description
7	Dangerous agitation	Pulling at catheters, climbing out of bed, striking staff, thrashing
6	Very agitated	Does not calm despite verbal reminders; requires restraints
5	Agitated	Anxious, attempting to sit, calms down with verbal instruction
4	Calm and cooperative	Calm, awakens easily, follows commands
3	Sedated	Difficult to arouse, awakens to verbal stimuli but drifts off again
2	Very sedated	Arouses to physical stimuli but does not follow commands
1	Unarousable	Minimal or no response to noxious stimuli

(d) Motor Activity Assessment Scale

Score	Term	Description
6	Dangerously agitated	Patient is pulling tubes, striking staff
5	Agitated	Spontaneously moving and not following commands
4	Restless and cooperative	Follows but spontaneous uncomfortable activity
3	Calm and cooperative	Spontaneous movement and patient with calm activity
2	Response to name/touch	Opens eyes, turns head, moves limb with name or touch
1	Response to noxious stimuli	Moves in response to noxious stimuli
0	Unresponsive	Does not move with noxious stimuli

an alert and calm patient. The Ramsay Sedation Scale is the most simplistic and allows for a numeric score from 1 to 6, based on responsiveness of the patient. However, it is more subjective and lacks clear descriptors between different levels. The SAS scores a patient's level of sedation from 1 to 7 and is especially adapted to warn the clinician of extremes of sedation and agitation, which is not provided by the simplistic Ramsay Sedation Scale.[7] The Motor Activity Assessment Scale has been derived from SAS and categorizes a patient's sedation level based on behavioral response to stimulation.[8] Other complex sedation scoring systems have also been constructed, but it is most important to become familiar with one system and standardize its use in an ICU. Scoring should be consistent and reliable by different care providers to ensure patients are not oversedated or undersedated. Once sedation goals are met for a particular patient, they should be regularly reevaluated to ensure therapy is being properly guided. Importantly, requirements for sedation are dynamic, generally declining as illness improves, and thus must be reassessed frequently.

Few objective measures are available to assess sedation. Vital signs such as heart rate, blood pressure, and respiratory rate are not specific or sensitive to sedation in the critically ill. Heart rate variability and lower esophageal sphincter tone are beginning to be used to objectively measure sedation. The bispectral index (BIS) aims to provide an objective measure of a patient's sedation by assigning a numerical value to a patient's electroencephalogram activity. The BIS has been shown to correlate with hypnotic drug effect in healthy elective surgery patients, but the BIS has not been as useful in the critical care setting.[9] BIS scores may vary between individuals with the same subjective level of sedation, resulting in marked variability. Furthermore, the BIS may not correlate with sedation in patients with muscle activity or impairments of the brain. However, there may be a role for the BIS in patients receiving neuromuscular blocking agents (NMBAs), as other assessment tools for hypnosis are useless. Currently, subjective scoring of sedation is the standard for assessing sedation in the critical care setting, until more reliable objective tools are available.

DELIRIUM

Patients requiring intensive care therapy often become delirious, complicating the assessment of pain and

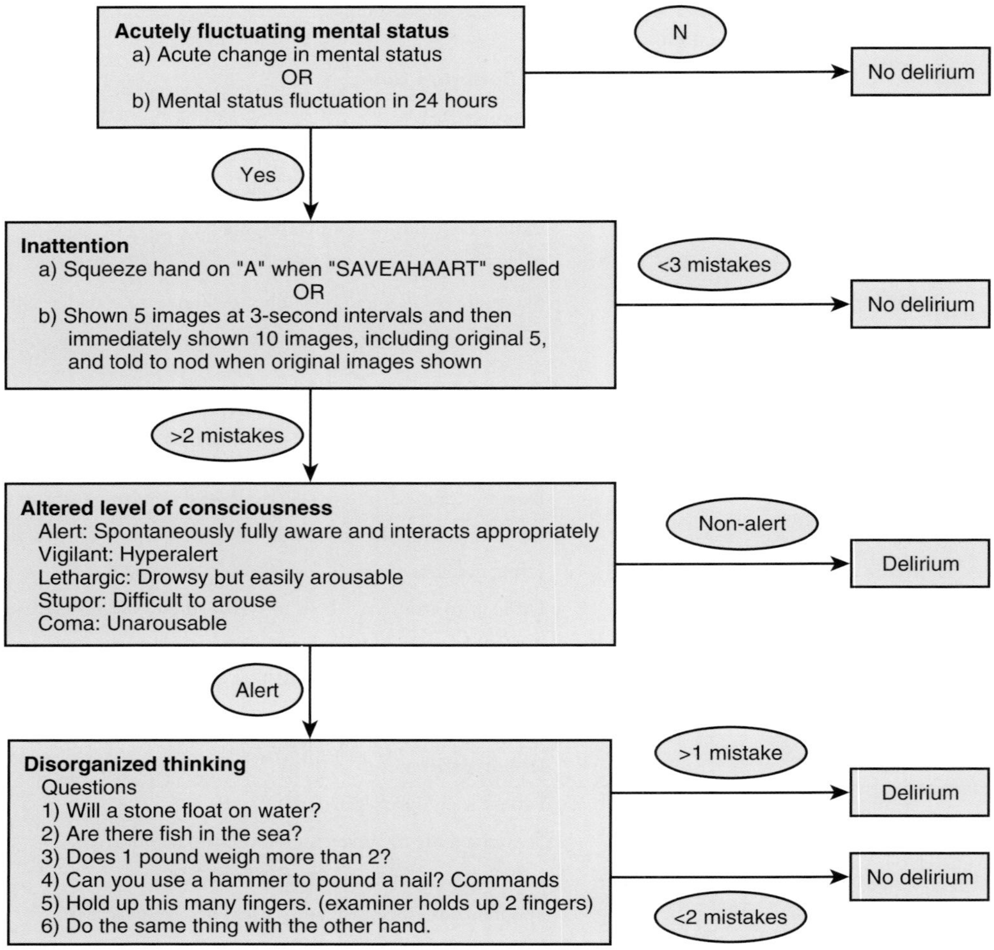

FIG. 40.3 The Confusion Assessment Method for the intensive care unit.

anxiety. Delirium is often confused with dementia. Dementia is a progressive disease with a decline in memory and cognitive skills and rarely presents acutely. Conversely, delirium is an acute reversible change in mental status. It is characterized by fluctuating levels of arousal associated with sleep–wake cycle disruption brought on by the reversal of day–night cycles and is associated with worse outcomes and increased long-term mortality. Patients suffering from delirium can be hypoactive, hyperactive, or even have mixed levels of activity. Hyperactive delirium is easily recognized, as patients are agitated and combative interfering with therapeutic measures; however, hypoactive delirium, which is characterized by calm appearance, decreased mobility, and inattention, is actually associated with a worse prognosis. Ideally, delirium should be assessed using the DSM-IV criteria by a psychiatric expert. The DSM-IV assessment, however, is involved and often impossible in an acutely ill patient. The Confusion Assessment Method for the ICU (CAM-ICU; Fig. 40.3) and the Intensive Care Delirium Screening Checklist (ICDSC; Fig. 40.4) rapidly and accurately assesses delirium in critically ill patients. The CAM-ICU assessment is a flow-diagram assessment, while the ICDSC is a scoring assessment in determining the presence of delirium.[10] In a critically ill patient with an acute change or fluctuating mental status, the CAM-ICU aims to evaluate inattention, altered level of consciousness, and disorganized thinking. In order to be diagnosed with delirium, a patient must not be heavily sedated and demonstrate inattention, along with either altered level of consciousness or disorganized thinking. The ICDSC, on the other hand, does not evaluate disorganized thinking but incorporates alterations in sleep-wake cycle, orientation, psychomotor function, appropriateness, and delusions.[11] The development of delirium assessment has improved the ability to provide appropriate therapy, and more importantly enlightened caregivers, on the occurrence of this complicated disease.

THERAPEUTIC AGENTS

Patient comfort in the critical care setting is obtained with the use of both hypnotic and analgesic agents. Focusing first on providing analgesia and then on hypnosis may provide more effective sedation. The lack of appropriate analgesia may lead to hyperesthesia and paradoxical agitation in the face of disinhibition from sedative drug administration. Once adequate analgesia has been established, the remainder of the sedation regimen should be targeted at maintaining patient comfort, behavioral control, and an appropriate degree of amnesia with hypnotic agents. The value of a standardized approach to sedation with treatment using analgesic and sedation agents has been demonstrated to reduce oxygen

1. Altered level of consciousness, choose one from A to E		
A. Exaggerated response to normal stimulation	SAS = 5, 6, 7 or RASS = +1 to +4	(1 point)
B. Normal wakefulness	SAS = 4 or RASS = 0	(0 points)
C. Response to mild or moderate stimulation (follows commands)	SAS = 3 or RASS = −1 to −3	(1 point)
D. Response only to intense and repeated stimulation (e.g., loud voice and pain)	SAS = 2 or RASS = −4	Stop assessment*
E. No response	SAS = 1 or RASS = −5	Stop assessment*
2. Inattention (1 point if any present)		
A. Difficulty in following commands or		
B. Easily distracted by external stimuli or		
C. Difficulty in shifting focus		
Does the patient follow you with their eyes?		
3. Disorientation (1 point for any abnormality)		
A. Mistake in either time, place, or person		
Does the patient recognize ICU caregivers who have cared for him/her and not recognize those who have not? What kind of place are you in? (list examples)		
4. Hallucinations or delusions (1 point for either)		
A. Equivocal evidence of hallucinations or a behavior due to hallucinations (hallucination = perception of something that is not there with no stimulus) or		
B. Delusions or gross impairment of reality testing (delusion = false belief that is fixed/unchanging)		
Any hallucinations now or over past 24 hr? Are you afraid of the people or things around you? (fear that is inappropriate to the clinical situation)		
5. Psychomotor agitation or retardation (1 point for either)		
A. Hyperactivity requiring the use of additional sedative drugs or restraints in order to control potential danger (e.g., pulling IV catheters out or hitting staff) or		
B. Hypoactive or clinically noticeable psychomotor slowing or retardation		
based on documentation and observation over shift by primary caregiver		
6. Inappropriate speech or mood (1 point for either)		
A. Inappropriate, disorganized, or incoherent speech or		
B. Inappropriate mood related to events or situation		
Is the patient apathetic to current clinical situation (i.e., lack of emotion)?		
Any gross abnormalities in speech or mood? Is patient inappropriately demanding?		
7. Sleep/wake cycle disturbance (1 point for any abnormality)		
A. Sleeping <4 hr at night or		
B. Waking frequently at night (do not include wakefulness initiated by medical staff or loud environment) or		
C. Sleep ≥4 hr during day		
Based on primary caregiver assessment		
8. Symptom fluctuation (1 point for any)		
Fluctuation of any of the above items (i.e., 1–7) over 24 hr (e.g., from one shift to another)		
Based on primary caregiver assessment		
Total intensive care delirium screening checklist score (add 1–8) ____________		

FIG. 40.4 Intensive Care Delirium Screening Checklist. *ICU*, Intensive care unit; *RASS*, Richmond Agitation Sedation Scale; *SAS*, Riker Sedation-Agitation Scale. *(Bergeron N, Dubois MJ, Dumont M, et al.: Intensive care delirium screening checklist: evaluation of a new screening tool.* Intensive Care Med. *27:859-864, 2001.)*

consumption and autonomic hyperactivity, and improve outcomes. Ideally, therapeutic agents should possess a rapid onset and offset of action, with easy titration to therapeutic goals without the development of consequential side effects.

ANALGESIA

Appropriate attention to analgesia is an important step in all sedation protocols, because most critically ill patients experience some degree of pain. Critical care staff should aim to minimize the production of pain by minimizing irritating stimulation, such as endotracheal tube traction on the carina and prolonged immobility. Despite aims to minimize pain production, supplemental analgesic therapy is often necessary for adequate pain control. Both opioid and nonopioid pharmacologic agents should be used to help control pain. With proper treatment of pain, better outcomes with quicker and more positive return to health can be expected.

TABLE 40.2 Comparison of Commonly Used Opioid Agents

Property	Morphine	Fentanyl	Sufentanil	Alfentanil	Remifentanil	Hydromorphone
Volume of distribution	334	335	123	27	30	91.5
Protein binding (%)	35	84	93	92	93	7.7
Metabolism	**Hepatic**	**Hepatic**	**Hepatic**	**Hepatic**	**Hepatic**	**Hepatic**
Active metabolites	+	–	–	–	–	–
Rapid onset	–	+	+	++	++	–
Short duration	–	±	+	+	++	–
Accumulation with long-term infusion		++	+	–	–	–
Inexpensive	++	+	–	–	– –	+

Nonopioids

Acetaminophen and nonsteroidal antiinflammatory drugs (NSAIDs) are recommended first-line therapy for the treatment of pain. Despite this recommendation, their use in the ICU is a frequently forgotten adjunct to pain control. NSAIDs nonselectively inhibit cyclooxygenase, blocking the production of inflammatory mediators. Ketorolac, an NSAID, has been shown to have an efficacy comparable to moderate doses of commonly used opioids at doses of 30 mg intravenously (IV) every 6 hours. However, clinical concerns of renal insufficiency and bleeding from platelet dysfunction and gastrointestinal tract mucosa limit the use of NSAIDs in the ICU. Renal insufficiency results from the decreased of production of prostacyclins that increase renal blood flow. Normally, inhibition of prostacyclin production does not result in a decrease in renal function; however, in patients with hypoperfusion, hypovolemia, or baseline renal impairment, or in older age, ketorolac may increase the incidence of NSAID-induced renal injury.[12] Additionally, use of ketorolac for greater than 5 days has been associated with an increased risk of renal dysfunction and both gastrointestinal and operative site bleeding. Acetaminophen is commonly used to treat mild to moderate pain, and as an antipyretic. The addition of acetaminophen, at doses of 1 g every 6 hours, to opioid therapy has been shown to produce greater pain relief than opioids alone. With the availability of intravenous acetaminophen, use of this medication has shown benefits in conjunction with opioids immediately postoperatively.[13] Care should be taken to ensure that toxic doses of acetaminophen are avoided, given that oral pain medications are routinely given as a combination of opioid and acetaminophen. Particularly, patients with liver dysfunction or a history of alcohol abuse are at risk for hepatoxicity from acetaminophen.

Patients suffering from neuropathic pain may prove difficult to manage with opioid medication alone. Enterally administered gabapentin and carbamazepine are often helpful in the treatment of neuropathic pain.[14] Gabapentin can be administered in doses of 100–1200 mg 3 times a day with precautions in patients with renal dysfunction as the drug is excreted unchanged. Carbamazepine is dependent upon hepatic metabolism, and dosing starts at 50 mg twice a day uptitrated to a maximum of 1200 mg per day. Although opioids remain the mainstay of analgesic therapy in the ICU, nonopioids should be considered as possible supplemental agents.

Analgesic Agents: Opioids

A careful understanding of the properties of individual opioids (Table 40.2) is essential to the appropriate use of these agents in the ICU.[15] Intravenous opioids are first-line agents for the treatment of nonneuropathic pain in the critically ill, with all being equally effective when titrated to patient needs. Lipid solubility, protein binding, and metabolism account for the pharmacokinetic differences between these agents. Opioids produce analgesia, mainly by stimulating μ, δ, and κ-receptors located both centrally and peripherally; however, interaction with other opioid receptors may lead to adverse effects. Unwanted effects of opioids include nausea, constipation, urinary retention, pruritus, and excessive sedation with possible respiratory depression. Severe constipation leading to ileus has been treated with some success using intravenous and parenteral opioid antagonists. Respiratory depression occurs because the ventilatory response to hypercapnia is decreased, while the response to hypoxia is obliterated. These respiratory depressive qualities, however, are often helpful in treating ventilator-patient dyssynchrony. Hypotension is occasionally seen in hypovolemic patients, as a decrease in sympathetic tone occurs after treatment of pain with opioid administration. The full opioid agonists, hydromorphone and fentanyl, are the most frequently used analgesics in critically ill patients. Opioids combined with hypnotic agents result in a synergistic effect that may permit dose reduction, thereby reducing the occurrence of undesirable side effects of both opioids and hypnotics.

Fentanyl is an opioid that has a rapid onset and short duration of action, often necessitating continuous infusion therapy of 1–2 $\mu g.kg^{-1}.h^{-1}$, with 1–2 μg/kg initial loading doses to provide adequate pain control. Prolonged effects, however, can be seen with protracted continuous administration necessitating frequent monitoring to avoid detrimental narcosis. Sufentanil and alfentanil are close chemical relatives of fentanyl, with shorter onset and duration of action times. Sufentanil is a potent lipophilic narcotic with greater protein binding and smaller volume of distribution than fentanyl, resulting in a shorter duration of action. However, similar to fentanyl, accumulation of sufentanil may occur with prolonged infusion, resulting in difficulty in predicting the duration of action. Alfentanil possesses a small volume of distribution secondary to protein binding and low lipid solubility, allowing for predictable duration of action. Despite the shorter duration of action of sufentanil and alfentanil when compared with fentanyl, the cost and unfamiliarity with use of both alfentanil and sufentanil limit the routine use of these agents in the critical care setting. Hydromorphone has a longer onset of action than fentanyl, but also a longer duration of action, allowing for intermittent dosing at ranges of 10–20 μg/kg per 1–2 hours. Metabolism of hydromorphone may be influenced by the presence of underlying liver disease, renal disease, or alterations in protein binding. Thus hydromorphone is reluctantly used in long-term infusions, because accumulation of metabolites can lead to much difficulty in appropriate dosing. Morphine has a pharmacokinetic profile similar to hydromorphone, but has a potent active metabolite that depends on renal excretion, limiting its use in the critical care setting. Morphine may also rarely lead to significant hypotension mediated by vasodilatation from histamine release. Although popular in the past, meperidine is generally avoided for prolonged therapy due to accumulation of its neuroexcitatory metabolite, normeperidine, which can cause seizures. Meperidine also has vagolytic and histamine releasing side effects, both of which may result in tachycardia. Remifentanil is an ultra-short-acting opioid, as it is metabolized by nonspecific plasma esterases, providing the most predictability of duration of action of all the opioid agents.[16] Remifentanil-based sedation regimens, at doses of 0.01–0.2 μg.kg^{-1}.min^{-1}, have shown to produce better sedation and decrease the length of ICU stays when compared with hypnotic-based regimens.[17] However, the cost of prolonged continuous infusions of remifentanil is prohibitive for its routine use in the critical care setting. Because critically ill patients often have altered peripheral blood flow, the use of intravenous dosing over intramuscular, subcutaneous, or transdermal delivery systems is often preferred. Thoracic epidural anesthesia is beneficial for patients undergoing abdominal aortic surgery or suffering from rib fractures.[18] Interestingly, however, this same benefit is not supported by the literature with thoracic epidurals for nonvascular thoracoabdominal surgery. More importantly, no analgesic benefit is seen with lumbar epidurals compared with parenteral opioid pain management after major abdominal surgery in high-risk patients.[19] Demand-based patient-controlled analgesia (PCA) is often useful in allowing appropriate opioid dosing for pain control without oversedation and respiratory depression.[20] Because of their underlying critical illness, many patients in the ICU do not possess the level of cognitive interaction required for appropriate PCA opioid dosing. Thus the use of continuous opioid infusions has become quite popular, but warrants concern about potential oversedation. More importantly, dosing of opioids must be carefully undertaken in critically ill patients. Understandably, a debilitated elderly patient may have drastically lower opioid requirements than a young, healthy trauma patient. It is best to diligently titrate medication to ensure adequate pain control without the development of harmful narcosis.

HYPNOSIS

Hypnosis plays an important role in providing comfort to critically ill patients. Multiple studies have demonstrated the consequences of prolonged deep sedation, compared with the benefits of maintaining a lighter sedation level. Deep levels are associated with longer duration of mechanical ventilation and longer ICU stays. After adequate treatment of pain, hypnotic agents should be appropriately titrated to provide anxiolysis, sedation, and amnesia, often decreasing analgesic requirements. Benzodiazepines, propofol, and dexmedetomidine are the most commonly used hypnotic agents in the critical care setting, with current trends favoring nonbenzodiazepine agents.

Hypnotic Agents: Benzodiazepines

Within the ICU, benzodiazepines are commonly used hypnotic agents. They possess anxiolytic, amnestic, sedating, and anticonvulsant properties, but no analgesic activity. Benzodiazepines interact with the γ-amino-butyric acid (GABA) receptor, creating an increase in intracellular chloride concentration and subsequent hyperpolarization of the cellular membrane. This hyperpolarization of neuronal membranes explains the utility of the benzodiazepines, as sedatives in addition to their frequent use as anticonvulsants. These agents block encoding of new information, resulting in anterograde amnesia and possibly decreasing the incidence of posttraumatic stress disorder from unpleasant intensive care therapy. Midazolam and lorazepam are the most commonly used benzodiazepines in the critical care setting, and vary in their onset, duration of action, and metabolism (Table 40.3). Furthermore, individual patient characteristics, such as age and metabolism induction or inhibition, alter the pharmacokinetics and pharmacodynamics, requiring individualized titration of these agents. Often, loading doses are needed to achieve a therapeutic level, but then smaller as-needed doses are often adequate to maintain a desired sedation level. If frequent doses are required to maintain desired sedation goal, continuous intravenous infusions should be cautiously considered, because patient awakening times after continued prolonged use are quite unpredictable. The use of flumazenil, a benzodiazepine antagonist, may cause withdrawal symptoms, resulting in increased oxygen consumption, and is therefore avoided in the critical care setting.

Diazepam may possess the most enduring track record for use as a sedative. Its original formulation in propylene glycol made its use difficult, secondary to the frequent venous irritation and thrombophlebitis, but this has been overcome by the use of a fat emulsion. Additionally, it is important to note that although diazepam has a relatively rapid onset of action and rapid awakening after small doses, lengthy therapy results in a prolonged sedative effect, as the hepatic metabolism of diazepam results in the production of an active metabolite known as desmethyldiazepam, forcing diazepam to be considered a long-acting agent. Interestingly the primary metabolic pathway of diazepam, the CYP2C19 hepatic enzyme subfamily, demonstrates significant genetic polymorphism, resulting in marked metabolic variation. Many medications inhibit or stimulate the CYP2C19 enzymes, complicating diazepam dosage

TABLE 40.3 Comparison of Commonly Used Hypnotic Agents

Property	Lorazepam	Midazolam	Propofol	Dexmedetomidine
Rapid onset	–	+	++	+
Short duration	–	±	+	–
Cardiovascular depression	–	±	+	+
Respiratory depression	–	±	+	–
Inactive metabolites	+	–	+	+
Hepatic metabolism	+	+	+	+
Hepatic conversion to inactive products	++	–	+	+
Renal elimination of active metabolite	–	+	–	–
Inexpensive	+	±	–	– –

requirements. As diazepam relies on hepatic metabolism, patients with hepatic dysfunction may experience a significant increase in the duration of action of this agent. The titration of diazepam to achieve appropriate levels of sedation in the critically ill patient is often challenging, given the active metabolic byproduct and dynamic pathophysiologic nature of critically ill patients, altering hepatic metabolism.

Lorazepam is used frequently in the ICU, at doses of 1–2 mg every 1–2 hours. Lorazepam is the least lipophilic benzodiazepine and thus has a slower onset of action than other benzodiazepines. This drug has a favorable metabolic profile, as it relies on hepatic glucuronidation, producing an inactive metabolite that makes elimination more predictable. Regardless, it is essential for the clinician to note that this intermediate acting benzodiazepine will require consistent vigilance in its use, to prevent oversedation. Large doses of prolonged intravenous lorazepam should be avoided, as they have been associated with acute tubular necrosis, lactic acidosis, and hyperosmolar states. These are secondary to pathology from the carrying solvents, propylene glycol, and polyethylene glycol.[21] Therefore as-needed bolus doses of lorazepam are often preferred over continuous intravenous infusions.

Midazolam is frequently used in the preoperative and intraoperative areas at doses of 1–5 mg secondary to its water-soluble characteristics that allow the drug to become highly lipid soluble at physiologic pH, allowing for a rapid onset. Midazolam relies on hepatic metabolism, and significant accumulation of midazolam may occur in patients with hepatic dysfunction during prolonged therapy because of its high lipophilicity and large volume of distribution. Additionally, it possesses an active metabolite, alpha-hydroxymidazolam, which relies on renal excretion, prolonging its duration of action in patients with renal disease. Although the rapid onset of this agent is ideal for acute therapy, the possible prolonged sedative effect of midazolam makes its use in the critical care setting objectionable.

Hypnotic Agents Propofol

Like benzodiazepines, propofol is also a GABA receptor agonist, but also binds to glycine, nicotinic, and muscuranic receptors in the central nervous system. Propofol is commonly used to induce general anesthesia but can be used at lower doses as a hypnotic agent, producing a degree of amnesia less than benzodiazepines. Propofol is highly lipophilic, easily crossing the blood-brain barrier for quick onset of action. Hypnosis from propofol rapidly resolves even in patients with hepatic and renal impairment, because redistribution of the medication away from the central compartment results in arousal. Propofol also acts as a vasodilator and a cardiac depressant, resulting in a dose-dependent decrease in blood pressure and possibly heart rate, respectively. Additionally, higher doses of propofol result in depression of respiratory drive. Despite the cardiovascular and pulmonary depression, the rapid onset and resolution of hypnosis make propofol a commonly used agent in the ICU at doses between 10 and 50 $\mu g.kg^{-1}.min^{-1}$.[22] Furthermore, propofol therapy may also have antioxidant or antiinflammatory properties secondary to the preservatives ethylenediaminetetraacetic acid (EDTA) or metabisulfite, respectively.[23]

Long-term continuous infusions of propofol, however, should be used cautiously. Propofol is prepared with a lipid emulsion carrier that may support bacterial growth. It is recommended that propofol be discarded 6 hours after initiation of use, and that tubing carrying propofol be changed every 12 hours to avoid contamination. The phospholipid emulsion of propofol should be counted as a calorie source and may result in triglyceridemia and eventually pancreatitis.[24] A rare but morbid complication of prolonged high-dose propofol therapy above 50 $\mu g.kg^{-1}.min^{-1}$, propofol infusion syndrome, results in mitochondrial injury, lactic acidosis, dysrhythmias, hyperkalemia, and rhabdomyolysis. Propofol provides superb short-term hypnosis, as arousal is rapid. For longer-term sedation, surveillance of propofol complications is warranted.

Hypnotic Agents Dexmedetomidine

Dexmedetomidine is an α_2-agonist with an affinity for the α_2-receptor seven times greater than clonidine. Activation of the postsynaptic α_{2A}-receptor results in hypnosis, mild amnesia, and significant analgesia that reduce the need for supplemental opioids. A hypnotic effect is produced by dexmedetomidine that resembles induction of normal sleep at doses between 0.2 and 1.0 $\mu g.kg^{-1}.min^{-1}$. The hypnotic effect of dexmedetomidine is unique, in that patients, when left undisturbed, will sleep, but when aroused with gentle stimulation, patients will be cooperative and follow commands. This effect is mediated by activation of the α_{2A}-receptor in the locus ceruleus. Attention to environmental control becomes essential, as disturbances easily awaken patients. Dexmedetomidine also provides for mild anterograde amnesia; however, benzodiazepines should be considered to ensure amnesia. The major advantages of dexmedetomidine are that it produces virtually no respiratory depression, while providing sedation and reducing analgesic opioid requirements.[25] It has been shown to facilitate extubation in patients who have previously failed extubation attempts due to severe agitation.[26] Dexmedetomidine may have a superior antiinflammatory profile with improved immune function, compared with other hypnotic agents that could be particularly beneficial in patients suffering from sepsis.[27]

Some adverse effects of α_2-agonists include enhancement of vagal effects by creating a pharmacologic sympathectomy, resulting in hypotension and bradycardia. However, if therapy is initiated rapidly at a high dose, a transient hypertension and tachycardia may occur. This is then followed by hypotension and bradycardia, mediated by the α_{2A}-receptor inhibiting sympathetic tone in the peripheral vascular system. However, the hemodynamic effects of α_2-agonists are relatively similar to those induced by other drugs used commonly in sedation regimens. Interestingly, dexmedetomidine has been recently associated with a lower incidence of delirium compared with other hypnotic agents.[28] The cost of dexmedetomidine is cited as prohibitive for routine use, but both favorable clinical and economic outcomes have been reported.[29]

Hypnotic Agents: Ketamine

Ketamine provides sedation by acting as both a functional and electrophysiological dissociative agent in the brain. Ketamine is highly lipophilic and results in a rapid onset of sedation and analgesia through stimulation of NMDA and opioid receptors. Importantly, ketamine decreases cathecholamine reuptake and preserves respiratory drive and reflexes. Despite not being widely used as a sedative in the critical care settings, the sympathomimetic effects of ketamine make it a viable alternative for patients with cardiovascular or pulmonary instability.[30] Furthermore, ketamine is thought to decrease opioid requirements. Ketamine, however, is associated with pronounced salivation and an emergence phenomenon notable for severe confusion and hallucinations. In patients with concern of cardiac function, ketamine may worsen myocardial ischemia, as it may cause tachycardia and hypertension. Ketamine may also increase intracranial pressure, limiting its use in patients with intracranial pathology. Experience with ketamine is limited, but it may be a reasonable supplemental agent in patients receiving exceptionally high doses of traditional agents or patients suffering from hemodynamic compromise.[31]

DELIRIUM

If after adequate analgesia and hypnotic therapy, delirium is suspected, therapy geared toward delirium should be initiated. Sleep is essential for recovery from illness. Critically ill patients are often rendered unconscious by sedative agents, but hypnotic-induced coma is not equivalent to natural sleep. Cognitive, cardiopulmonary, and immune functions suffer with sleep deprivation.[32] In particular, disruption of the sleep cycle is associated with the development of delirium. Modifying the critical care environment to promote the normal day–night sleep–wake cycle can promote sleep. In particular, controlling noise, lighting, and minimizing therapies during nighttime will allow for better sleep. Relaxation, massage, and music therapy have also been used to promote sleep in the critically ill. Additionally, zolpidem, a potentiator of GABA receptors, at 5–10 mg may provide benefit as a sleep aid in the critically ill. More importantly, ramelteon, a melatonin agonist, has been demonstrated to decrease the incidence of delirium in critically ill patients with insomnia.[33] In addition to sleep and normalizing the day–night cycle, reorientation, informing patients of their ongoing clinical situations, and allowing patients to have some control of their care are thought to improve delirium. Early mobilization in critical illness is important, as it has been shown to improve both delirium and outcomes.[34] Control of pain and anxiety is essential to avoid delirium. Undermedication with hypnotics and analgesics may drive a patient to agitation, leading to delirium. On the other hand, overmedication with sedatives and analgesics may lead a patient to be more confused, leading to a paradoxical increase in agitation and delirium. Current guidelines do not support or refute the use of medication to treat delirium. However, routinely after appropriate sedation and analgesic therapy, haloperidol 0.5–5 mg every 5 minutes until agitation is controlled is often used as an adjunct in patients who have a component of hyperactive delirium. Haloperidol antagonizes dopamine-mediated neurotransmission, stabilizing cerebral function. Unstructured thought patterns are thought to be inhibited, producing a flat sedative affect. Intravenous loading dose injection of haloperidol with repeat loading doses is routinely used to treat delirium acutely. Once delirium is controlled, haloperidol therapy should be regularly scheduled over a few days, followed by tapering doses over several days. Monitoring for extrapyramidal symptoms, neuroleptic malignant syndrome, hypotension, and QT prolongation is recommended specifically, as QT prolongation can lead to torsades de pointes. Fortunately, such idiosyncratic effects are rarely seen, and haloperidol remains helpful in treating delirium in many critically ill patients.[35] Olanzapine, a newer agent for the treatment of delirium, has similar efficacy to haloperidol, but with fewer extrapyramidal side effects at doses of 2.5–5 mg daily.[36] Quetiapine, an atypical antipsychotic with a very low incidence of extrapyramidal side effects, has some support for its use in the treatment of hyperactive delirium. Hypoactive delirium, on the other hand, may actually be exacerbated by sedative medications. Interestingly, lorazepam has been found to be an independent risk factor for the development of delirium in ICU patients.[37] A newer atypical antipsychotic, ariprazole, has some stimulating properties, and may show some benefit in patients suffering from hypoactive delirium.[38] Delirium is a common occurrence in critical care patients. Surveillance for this morbid complication of critical care, along with appropriate pharmaceutical and environmental therapy, is essential for improved critical patient care.

NEUROMUSCULAR BLOCKING AGENTS

A discussion of NMBAs may seem inappropriate when considering patient comfort in the ICU. However, the frequent use of NMBAs and confusion about their mechanism of action warrants some discourse. With the aggressive use of sedation regimens and recognition of prolonged weakness from NMBAs, neuromuscular blockade use has declined significantly in the critical care unit. However, on rare occasion, paralysis with neuromuscular blockade is desired for the critically ill patient.[39] One of the most common reasons to utilize NMBAs in the intensive care is patient–ventilator dyssynchrony. Such dyssynchrony can result in increased airway pressures, which may predispose the patient to ventilator induced lung injury. Additionally, adequate oxygenation and ventilation can become extremely difficult in many patients with dyssynchrony. In the past, the most frequent form of treatment for this problem was administration of neuromuscular blockade. However, it is essential to realize that these drugs do not provide analgesia. They merely provide paralysis. Thus not only does it become difficult to assess pain, agitation, and mental status, these agents can actually worsen patient anxiety by preventing patient movement in the presence of inadequate sedation. As one can imagine, many patients would find such a situation emotionally distressing. Thus frequently the best approach to treatment of these patients consists of increasing opioid delivery to the patient. Because opioids provide respiratory depression, patient–ventilator dyssynchrony can be ameliorated by the use of an agent, which will depress the patient's ventilatory drive without risking the side effects of prolonged paralysis from an NMBA.

In addition to treating dyssynchrony, NMBAs are also used to decrease oxygen consumption in patients with tenuous oxygen supply versus demand. Such individuals may benefit from neuromuscular paralysis by decreasing metabolic oxygen consumption needs to the minimal. Individuals with evidence of anaerobic metabolism, despite maximal maneuvers to increase tissue oxygen delivery, may be able to return to a state of aerobic metabolism. Such treatment with an NMBA must not be viewed as definitive, but rather a temporary means of controlling an oxygen supply versus demand imbalance.

In addition to the risk of prolonged weakness due to neuromuscular blockade, the decision to use NMBAs in patients with a history of frequent tonic-clonic seizures or status epilepticus must occur only after careful consideration. It is important to realize that intact neuromuscular function provides the clinician with a constant monitor of potentially life-threatening seizure activity. However, in the patient who has received an NMBA, this monitor is now unavailable. Thus a risk exists that the patient may develop cerebral seizure activity without the awareness of health care providers. Such unrecognized, untreated, prolonged cerebral seizure activity can then lead to irreversible neurologic injury and even brain death.

The greatest concern to neuromuscular blockade use is prolonged paralysis, particularly in patients receiving steroid therapy. The most commonly used NMBA in the critical care unit is cisatracurium at infusion rates of 1 to 5 $\mu g.kg^{-1}.min^{-1}$ as it undergoes Hoffman degradation. Only temperature and pH alter the pharmacokinetics; therefore patients with renal and hepatic dysfunction can be treated with cisatracurium with minimal concern for prolongation of action. Ideally, before neuromuscular blockade use is initiated, plans should be made to discontinue use of the agent with conversion to another therapy. Often this entails increasing the sedation regimen, but may also entail improving oxygen delivery or treatment for seizure activity.

CONCLUSION

Maintaining sedation is an extremely important goal in the care of critically ill patients, but this aspect of their care frequently becomes lost in the myriad of physiologic derangements encountered in the critically ill patient. All sedation regimens have potentially adverse side effects that can endanger the patient's well-being and can prolong the clinical course. Sedation regimens have been implicated in the development of depression and posttraumatic stress disorder after ICU stays.[40] Furthermore, daily interruption of sedative treatment has been shown to reduce the length of a patient's ICU stay. Even patients with coronary artery disease have been shown to have reduced lengths of critical care unit stays, despite the surge of catecholamines and resultant cardiac stress associated with daily sedation interruptions.[41] The current clinical trend is to provide a lighter level of sedation using shorter-acting agents. However, discontinuation of sedative and analgesic medications must be undertaken carefully. Patients with continued use of medication for greater than a week are at risk for neuroadaptation and physiologic dependence, and may develop withdrawal symptoms with discontinuation of therapy.[42] Additionally, chronic pain syndromes are increasingly recognized in survivors of critical illness.[43] In order to design a proper sedation regimen, multiple critical endpoints and factors must be considered. These include duration of desired sedation, drug side effects, potential complications of the sedation regimen, and costs; such costs include not only the drugs alone, but also the aforementioned side effects and complications. Thus it is essential that all members of the critical care team be aware of the sedation and analgesia plan, adhere to it, and be aware of the potential shortcomings of the plan so that appropriate adjustments can be made as the patient's condition changes or adverse effects emerge. Only with a systematized and consistent approach to sedation can efficacious and cost-effective care to tenuous critically ill patients be provided.

KEY POINTS

- Patient assessment for analgesia, hypnosis, and delirium needs with targeted therapeutic plans for each one of these components is essential to ICU patient management. There is significant interplay between each of these three concepts; for example, both inadequate analgesia from an opioid and oversedation with a hypnotic may cause delirium.
- When critically ill patients cannot communicate their pain perception to others, the use of behavioral and physiological indicators of the patient's pain are essential to managing analgesia in critically ill patients.

- Nonopioid analgesics should be used as first-line patient therapy to decrease the reliance on opioid medications in the ICU, thereby decreasing the incidence of nausea, pruritus, respiratory depression, and ileus in critically ill patients.
- Neuropathic pain in ICU patients may be treated with gabapentin and carbamazepine. Chronic pain syndromes are increasingly recognized in patients after ICU stays.
- Benzodiazepines have much different effects when administered as intermittent bolus doses versus infusions. Of diazepam, lorazepam, and midazolam, only lorazepam is noted to lack active metabolites and therefore the most dependable pharmacokinetics.
- Propofol and dexmedetomidine are both short-acting intravenous hypnotics often used in the ICU. Vigilance is necessary to prevent propofol infusion syndrome and dexmedetomidine-associated bradycardia and hypotension.
- Ketamine can be a valuable adjunct to sedation and analgesia in the ICU via its action on both the NMDA and opioid receptor. Unfortunately, its side effects of emergence delirium and sympathetic stimulation may limit its use in the ICU, particularly in patients with coronary artery disease and intracranial pathology.
- Sleep deprivation in the ICU is a significant contributor to ICU delirium. Hypoactive delirium is often underrecognized. Haloperidol and the atypical antipsychotics (olanzapine and quetiapine) are useful in managing delirium, and ariprazole may be particularly useful in managing hypoactive delirium.
- NMBA use in the ICU should be a rare event secondary to the risk of both unrecognized convulsive seizures, particularly in the neurologically injured patient, and prolonged weakness after ICU discharge. However, when necessary, cisatracurium provides the most dependable pharmacokinetic profile.

REFERENCES

Access the reference list online at ExpertConsult.com.

CHAPTER 41

GERIATRIC PAIN

Gwendolyn A. Sowa, MD, PhD ◎ Debra K. Weiner, MD ◎ Alejandra Camacho-Soto, MD

It is estimated that the number of individuals aged 65 and older will grow to 1.5 billion by 2050, with 83.7 million older adults in the United States.[1] Given the rapidly changing demographics, the aging population will require the care of physicians from all disciplines; therefore they should be familiar with the unique medical aspects related to the older adult. Advances in health care and improvements in prevention strategies have allowed individuals to live longer with chronic illnesses and functional and cognitive impairments. In older adults, additional factors such as reduced physiologic reserve, polypharmacy, and decreased activity further contribute to this functional and cognitive decline. Understanding how pain presents in the older adult and implementing treatment strategies to reduce pain is critical, but more important is the need to maintain functional independence.

PRESENTATION OF DISEASE/COMORBIDITY

Chronic pain can be considered a geriatric syndrome, a multifactorial health condition that occurs when the accumulated effects of impairments in multiple systems render the older adult vulnerable to situational challenges.[2] The quest for a unifying diagnosis to explain the presenting signs and symptoms in the older adult with chronic pain often fails, as more often than not there are multiple contributing factors. These include altered biomechanics, sleep and mood disturbances, cognitive deficits, and other chronic comorbidities. For example, the treatment targets in the older adult with fibromyalgia may be weight management through activity and diet, the optimization of sleep and mood rather than direct treatment of the area of pain. Another example is that of the older adult with chronic low back pain (CLBP). A recent series titled "Deconstructing Chronic Low Back Pain in the Older Adult" examined other diagnostic contributors to CLBP that may require a unique treatment approach.[3]

AGING-ASSOCIATED PHYSIOLOGY AND PATHOLOGY

Many physiologic changes occur with aging. Medical conditions such as dementia, peripheral neuropathy, osteoporosis, osteoarthritis, and cancer are found more commonly in older adults. The evaluation of older adults with chronic pain requires a working knowledge of how these diagnoses affect evaluation and management decisions. Based on this understanding, the goal of the pain practitioner should be to optimize function when possible and minimize adverse effects when deciding on appropriate treatment plans.

NERVOUS SYSTEM

Decreases in short-term memory and cognitive processing speed are known to occur with aging, although cognitive decline widely differs among older adults, with varying degrees of neuronal loss, neurotransmitter changes, and alterations in synapses within the nervous system.[4] The prevalence of dementia increases, with Alzheimer's disease being the most common form. Current figures suggest that 25% to 30% of people 85 years of age and older have dementia.[1] These individuals may be unable to communicate their source of pain or may fixate on pain itself when the underlying process may be anxiety or fear.

Aging is associated with a decline in the number of myelinated and unmyelinated fibers, an increase in the number of damaged nerve fibers, and slowed nerve conduction velocity, resulting in alterations in proprioception, postural instability, and balance deficits. Peripheral neuropathy is more common in older adults due to comorbidities such as diabetes, chronic kidney disease, and chemotherapy and/or radiation treatments for cancer. In an older adult with cognitive, visual, or hearing deficits, superimposed impairments in proprioception can affect balance adversely, leading to falls in an individual who is already vulnerable.[5] An estimated 30% of adults older than 65 and 50% of adults older than 85 are estimated to have had at least one fall,[6,7] with more recent evidence suggesting that pain increases this risk.[8] Thus assessment of balance should be a routine part of assessing the older adult with pain.

MUSCULOSKELETAL

Sarcopenia is common with advancing age; it is defined as progressive loss of muscle mass associated with muscle cell atrophy and increased fat content. The latter may result in increased retention of fat-soluble medications, which may increase the risk of adverse side effects. There is also a decreased number of motor units. It is estimated that by age 70, there are reductions in the cross-sectional area of skeletal muscle (25%–30%) and muscle strength (30%–40%), which may affect mobility.[9,10] Decreased muscle strength, decreased range of motion, and common conditions such as degenerative arthritis and osteopenia/osteoporosis may place the older adult at increased risk for falls and resulting fractures. It also should be highlighted that older adults frequently have radiographic evidence of degenerative disease, whether

TABLE 41.1 Physiologic Changes Associated With Aging and Frailty That Can Affect the Pharmacokinetics and Pharmacodynamics of Drugs

Pharmacokinetics			
Absorption	**Distribution**	**Metabolism**	**Elimination**
Remains unchanged	↓ Plasma albumin[a,b]	↓ Liver volume[a,b,c]	Measurable and predictable decline in renal function with age[a,b]
↑ Gastric pH[a] ↓ Secretory capacity[a] ↓ GI blood flow[a]	↓ Protein affinity ↑ α_1-acid glycoprotein[a] ↓ Total body water[a,b] ↑ Expression and activity of P-glycoprotein in liver[a]	↓ Hepatic blood flow[a,b,c] ↑ Interindividual variability with age[a,b] ↓ First-pass metabolism[b] ↓ Phase I metabolism[a,c]	↓ Glomerular filtration rate[a] ↓ Renal plasma flow[a]
		↔ Phase II metabolism[a,c] ↓ Phase II metabolism in frail patients	

Pharmacodynamics	
Body Composition	**Central Nervous System**
↑ Body fat[a] ↓ Lean and total body mass[a,b] Cardiovascular Function ↓ Resting heart rate, stroke volume, and cardiac output[a]	↓ Blood supply to brain[a] ↓ Baroreceptor activity[a] Renin-Angiotensin-Aldosterone System ↓ Plasma renin[a] ↓ Urine aldosterone[a]

GI, *Gastrointestinal.*
[a]*Human/clinical studies.*
[b]*Pharmacokinetic and/or pharmacodynamic change is accentuated in the frail.*
[c]*Animal studies.*
Source: Mitchell SJ, Hilmer SN, McLachlan AJ: Clinical pharmacology of analgesics in old age and frailty. Rev Clin Gerontol. *19:103-118, 2009.*

or not they have pain. For example, degenerative disc disease is nearly ubiquitous in older adults[11,12]; thus history and physical examination should be the main tools used to identify potential pain generators in those with chronic musculoskeletal pain.[3] Imaging alone should rarely guide management and treatment in the older adult with chronic pain. Older adults often have multiple degenerative musculoskeletal conditions influencing the kinetic chain and leading to additional pathology. For example, older adults with pain associated with knee and hip osteoarthritis may alter their gait and posture, subsequently leading to back pain from altered spine mechanics.[13,14]

VISION AND HEARING

Aging-associated sensory deficits can exacerbate and contribute to pain-related disability. Common eye diseases (e.g., cataract, glaucoma, macular degeneration, and diabetic retinopathy) associated with aging may result in moderate to severe vision loss. Reduced visual acuity, particularly at night, and presbyopia, may predispose the older adult to falls. Poor eyesight may affect how medication is administered or how therapy is performed; for example, use of visual aids such as mirrors or pictures of correct performance of exercises may not be effective. Presbycusis, defined as the loss of hearing with age, is estimated to affect one third of patients over the age of 65 and half over the age of 85. Resulting communication errors may be wide-ranging and include, for example, misunderstanding of pain education delivered by the provider or errors in treatment implementation. Assistive technologies such as hearing aids and a frequency modulation (FM) device for those patients with speech recognition difficulty may be helpful when practitioners evaluate these patients, as they afford the opportunity to engage in more meaningful conversation and improved care.[15,16]

DRUG METABOLISM[17]

A number of physiologic changes associated with aging, summarized in Table 41.1, may lead to alterations in pharmacokinetics and pharmacodynamics. The pain practitioner must be cognizant of these changes to optimize analgesia while also minimizing adverse effects.

ANALGESICS AFFECTED BY ALTERED PHARMACOKINETICS

Medications that have a high hepatic extraction ratio may undergo decreased clearance and experience a longer half-life in older adults because of diminished liver size and blood flow. Meperidine (contraindicated in older adults because of its renally cleared active metabolite that can cause seizures) and morphine are high-extraction-ratio analgesics whose first-pass effect and clearance is reduced with age. The following nonsteroidal antiinflammatory drugs (NSAIDs) with long half lives are hepatically metabolized and their clearance may be reduced in older adults: celecoxib, diflunisal, naproxen, oxaprozin, piroxican, salsalate, and sulindac. The opioids levorphanol and methadone may be similarly affected.

Analgesics that are affected by aging-associated decline in renal function include codeine, duloxetine, gabapentin, meperidine, pregabalin, propoxyphene, salicylate, tramadol, and the opioids morphine, oxycodone, hydromorphone, fentanyl, and methadone. The dosing schedule for gabapentin by renal function is shown in Table 41.5.[18]

Geriatricians widely use the Cockcroft-Gault equation, shown below, to estimate creatinine clearance (CLcr); it helps to guide the dose adjustment of renally cleared medications:

$$\text{CLcr} = \frac{[(140 - \text{age}) \times \text{Weight}]}{[\text{SCr} \times 72]}$$

Multiply the value by 0.85 for females.
CLcr (mL/min) = creatinine clearance, SCr (mg/dL) = serum creatinine
Age (years), weight (kg)

ANALGESICS AFFECTED BY ALTERED PHARMACODYNAMICS

Pharmacodynamics refers to tissue sensitivity and how a drug interacts with its end organ. The body's response to medications may be therapeutic or adverse. The effectiveness of a medication may be influenced by age-related changes in receptors and signal processing—that is, the target organ's sensitivity. Opioid sensitivity increases with the associated decline in mu opioid receptor density and increase in opioid affinity. Thus older adults may respond to opioid doses that are significantly smaller than those used in younger individuals.

COMPREHENSIVE PAIN ASSESSMENT

Chronic pain assessment in older adults requires comprehensive identification of the multiple contributing biologic, mechanical/physical, social, and psychologic factors. The assessment and monitoring of patient-identified goals should be implemented in all patient encounters. To identify the efficacy of prescribed interventions, it also is critical to identify the meaningful outcomes to be tracked in the course of treatment. Tables 41.2 and 41.3 suggest approaches for assessing pain and offer outcome measures to be followed during pain treatment.

Assessment of pain alone is not sufficient; providers should inquire about changes in cognition or memory, appetite, sleep, mood disturbances, a loss or decrease in mobility, falls, and diminished activity level with changes in performance related to activities of daily living. Assessment of the type of pain—whether nociceptive and/or neuropathic, pain intensity, and how this directly affects daily activity, discomfort, or change in health status—is critical. Nociceptive pain may be associated with fractures, arthritic/musculoskeletal disorders, or myofascial dysfunction. Neuropathic pain can include conditions such as postherpetic neuralgia, trigeminal neuralgia, and painful diabetic or compression neuropathies. The assessment of pain intensity in older adults should include an in-depth assessment of changes in functional status. Older adults may underreport pain as a result of several preconceived notions regarding pain, such as the belief that pain is a normal part of aging or fear that no treatments are available. By obtaining collateral information from a spouse, family members, caregivers, or friends of the patient, the physician may gather additional information that would otherwise have been missed during the evaluation.

TABLE 41.2 Brief Pain Impact Assessment for Verbal Patients

How strong is your pain (right now, worst/average over past week)?
How many days over the past week have you been unable to do what you would like to do because of your pain?
Over the past week, how often has pain interfered with your ability to take care of yourself, for example, with bathing, eating, dressing, and going to the toilet?
Over the past week, how often has pain interfered with your ability to take care of your home-related chores such as going grocery shopping, preparing meals, paying bills, and driving?
How often do you participate in pleasurable activities such as hobbies, socializing with friends, travel? Over the past week, how often has pain interfered with these activities?
How often do you do some type of exercise? Over the past week, how often has pain interfered with your ability to exercise?
Does pain interfere with your ability to think clearly?
Does pain interfere with your appetite?
Does pain interfere with your sleep? How often over the past week?
Has pain interfered with your energy, mood, personality, or relationships with other people?
Over the past week, how often have you taken pain medications?
How would you rate your health at the present time?

Source: Weiner DK, Herr K, Rudy TE: Persistent Pain in Older Adults: An Interdisciplinary Guide for Treatment. *New York: Springer, 2002.*

KEY ASSESSMENT TOOLS FOR THE OLDER ADULT WITH PAIN

Unlike acute pain events where abnormalities in blood pressure, heart rate, or respiratory rate are common, there are no objective clinical measurements to assess chronic pain. Providers often rely on self-reported measurements, functional and cognitive assessments, and collateral sources. For cognitively intact older adults, pain rating tools such as the numeric rating scale (NRS) and verbal descriptor scales (VDS) are commonly used and sensitive to changes in pain. These self-reported instruments can be used reliably in patients with mild to moderate dementia.[19]

In patients with advanced dementia who have difficulty using self-report instruments, caregivers rely on behavioral cues such as facial grimacing, guarding, bracing, rubbing, and sighing to determine the presence and severity of pain (Table 41.4). Several behavioral instruments are available to detect pain in those with advanced dementia. These include the Pain Assessment in Advanced Dementia (PAINAD), the Doloplus-2, and the Pain Assessment Checklist for Seniors with Limited Ability to Communicate (PACSLAC).[20]

As described previously, screening for mobility impairments should be done routinely in patients with chronic pain, since changes in function may be an early sign of pain. Although there are no gold-standard tests to assess

TABLE 41.3 Assessing Functional Response to the Treatment of Persistent Pain in Older Adults: Suggested Outcome Measures

Domain Functional	Parameters	Comments
I. Physical	Basic and instrumental activities of daily living (ADL, IADL) Mobility/activity level Sleep Appetite Pain intensity	Look at the degree of assistance needed. Decreased activity, such as the diminished participation in advanced activities of daily living (AADL) in the community dweller, or decreased ability to participate in AM care in the nursing home resident may indicate pain. Ask about pain awakening from sleep, difficulty falling asleep because of pain, time spent in bed during the day. Many persistent pain patients experience appetite suppression from pain. Follow caloric intake and weight. In nursing home residents, use pain thermometer, behavioral indicators of pain, and rate of prn analgesic ingestion. In community dwellers, use numeric or verbal scales.
II. Psychosocial	Mood Interpersonal interactions/behavior	Anxiety and depression may coexist and worsen in patients with pain. Reclusiveness and/or irritability/agitation may occur. In nursing home residents, tone of interactions with staff, family, and other residents may be helpful.
III. Cognitive	Mental status Beliefs and attributions	Consider pain as causative in the patients who experience decline in mental status or delirium. The Mini Mental State Examination may not be sensitive enough to detect subtle changes. Note if the patient has changed orientation from a "fix-me" mentality to a "teach-me" mentality.

Source: Weiner DK, Herr K, Rudy TE: Persistent Pain in Older Adults: An Interdisciplinary Guide for Treatment. *New York: Springer, 2002.*

TABLE 41.4 Common Pain Behaviors in Cognitively Impaired Elderly Persons

Facial Expressions
Frown; sad, frightened face Grimace, wrinkled forehead, tightened eyes
Verbalizations, Vocalizations
Sighing, moaning, groaning, grunting Calling out, asking for help Noisy breathing; verbally abusive
Body Movements
Rigid, tense body posture; guarding, fidgeting Pacing, rocking; restricted movement Gait or mobility changes
Changes in Interpersonal Interactions
Aggressive, combative, resisting care Decreased social interactions, withdrawn Socially inappropriate, disruptive
Changes in Activity Patterns or Routines
Refuses food, appetite change Sleep, rest pattern changes Sudden cessation of common routines
Mental Status Changes
Crying, tears Increased confusion Irritability or distress

From AGS Panel on Persistent Pain in Older Persons: The management of persistent pain in older persons. J Am Geriatr Soc. *50:S205-S224, 2002.*

an older adults' functional capacity, gait speed has been described as a good predictor of disability[21] and may be a useful measure to incorporate into clinical practice.

In patients with suspected cognitive deficits, the Quick Mild Cognitive Impairment (Qmci) screen is a 3- to 5-minute screening tool that assesses for mild cognitive impairment.[22] In more advanced cases of cognitive impairment, the Montreal Cognitive Assessment (MoCA),[23] a 10-minute screening tool, or the Mini-Cog,[24,25] a brief delayed-recall and clock-drawing test, can be used. In the case of abnormal scores, the provider should refer the patient for neuropsychologic testing or to a physician who specializes in cognitive impairments.

RED FLAGS

For all patients presenting with pain, consideration of possible serious conditions (i.e., red-flag symptoms) that require immediate attention is of paramount importance. Examples of red-flag symptoms in the older adult include but are not limited to pain following a fall or other trauma, fever, sudden unexplained weight loss, acute onset of severe pain, new-onset weakness or sensory loss, loss of bowel or bladder function, jaw claudication, new headaches, bone pain in a patient with a history of malignancy or that awakens the patient from sleep, and sudden pain in an extremity that is associated with pallor, pulselessness, and paresthesias. Further workup—including bloodwork or imaging—is needed to exclude these serious conditions when red flags are present.

TREATMENT

For the older adult with chronic pain, treatment should be approached from both a nonpharmacologic and pharmacologic standpoint, often in the context of an interdisciplinary team. Given the risk of polypharmacy and potential drug-drug and drug-disease interactions as well as medication nonadherence, treatment should ideally start with nonpharmacologic approaches.

NONPHARMACOLOGIC TREATMENT

There is evidence that nonpharmacologic interventions may be helpful in older adults with chronic pain.[26] Common nonpharmacologic approaches that may be helpful include weight management, exercise, physical and occupational therapies, activity modification, prescription of assistive devices,[27] and cognitive-behavioral therapy.[28,29]

Additionally, there is evidence for reducing pain in older adults with acupuncture, mindfulness meditation (MM),[30,31] and massage.[32] A critical review of behavioral mind-body interventions for chronic pain in older adults—specifically biofeedback, progressive muscle relaxation, meditation, guided imagery, hypnosis, tai chi, qi gong, and yoga—suggested that such interventions may improve not only pain but also pain-related comorbidities such as depression, anxiety, and disability.[33]

A randomized controlled trial of 282 community-dwelling older adults with CLBP randomized to an 8-month MM program (8 weekly followed by monthly booster sessions for 6 months) versus a health education control demonstrated significantly improved function as measured by the Roland Morris questionnaire at 8 weeks and reduced long-term current and average pain.[34]

Lumbar percutaneous electrical nerve stimulation (PENS) has been studied in older adults with CLBP demonstrating both reduction in pain and improvement in function.[35,36] Periosteal stimulation therapy facilitated by acupuncture needles was shown to reduce pain in older adults with advanced knee osteoarthritis in a randomized controlled trial.[37] However, there are no clear guidelines on the intensity, duration, or frequency of these interventions. These treatments should be individualized to the patient in order to optimize function and reduce pain to a tolerable level, thus allowing the highest level of function.

Physical modalities, such as thermotherapy (cold or heat) or manual therapy, may be helpful adjuncts for treating nociceptive and myofascial pain. Spinal manipulative therapy may be effective in reducing disability in older individuals with CLBP.[38] Patients with altered sensation and/or cognitive deficits should not undergo heat/cold treatment without direct supervision and a structured guideline including frequency and intensity. Based on a systematic review, the Ottawa panel recommended aerobic activity with a walking program, stretching, strengthening exercises, and education as a method to help improve pain and function in cognitively intact patients with mild to moderate osteoarthritis.[39] A combination of aerobic activity, endurance, resistance, balance, and flexibility exercises may be effective in reducing pain, improving mood, and augmenting functional capacity. Aquatic therapy may be considered in patients with balance impairments or a history of falls. Individualized exercise programs should be created based on the patient's medical comorbidities and current functional status.

Therapies such as occupational and physical therapy can be effective in managing pain and optimizing function in the older adult. It is important to distinguish between these two disciplines. Occupational therapists work on maximizing one's ability to perform activities of daily living and instrumental activities of daily living independently. They can also assist with the proper prescription of activity modification, pacing, or an assistive device that may be used to optimize activities of daily living, including but not limited to cooking, eating, grooming, self-care, and dressing. Physical therapists can help the older adult with pain conditions affecting mobility, which includes transfers, balance, and ambulation. Providers should identify therapists who are both knowledgeable and comfortable managing the older adult with pain. Medical comorbidities, such as cognitive impairment, osteoarthritis, and cardiovascular and pulmonary diseases, are common in the older adult and may impact the therapist's assessment and therapy plan.

PHARMACOLOGIC TREATMENT

Pharmacologic treatment may be delivered topically, by the oral route, or by injection (i.e., intraarticular, epidural, intramuscular).

TOPICAL THERAPIES

Topical agents may be preferred to oral agents because they have less systemic effects and drug-drug interactions; they are also easier to apply, particularly for older adults with dysphagia. Topical lidocaine 5% is approved by the US Food and Drug Administration (FDA) for postherpetic neuralgia, which is more common in older adults; it may be considered for localized neuropathic pain in individuals who are unable to tolerate oral medications.[40] Capsaicin cream, an agent that depletes substance P, is FDA-approved for use in both neuropathic pain and musculoskeletal pain. Several NSAIDs can be applied topically and may be a safer alternative to oral NSAID use. Topical diclofenac is FDA-approved for use in osteoarthritis. Gastrointestinal (GI) side effects may be less frequent than with oral NSAIDs.[41] Compounded topical preparations are available and may be helpful for some patients who have failed other treatment options; however, rigorous investigation of their efficacy is lacking.[42] Typical side effects associated with topical medications include local irritation, rash, and/or a burning sensation, the latter occurring most commonly with capsaicin cream.

ORAL ANALGESICS

The practitioner who determines that oral analgesics are needed must begin with a careful medication history that includes all prescription and over-the-counter medications, herbal and dietary supplements, vitamin preparations, illicit drugs, and alcohol. Table 41.5 provides a list of oral analgesics to consider for the treatment of nociceptive and/or neuropathic pain in older adults. Consideration should be given to discontinuing any medication included among the Beers criteria, last updated in 2015.[43] These medications are considered potentially inappropriate and best avoided in older adults because of their high risk of adverse effects. Table 41.6A and B lists an abbreviated version of pain and pain-related medications included in Beers criteria.

Acetaminophen continues to be recommended as first-line treatment in patients with nociceptive pain, specifically low back pain and osteoarthritis.[32] The most common side effects associated with the use of acetaminophen include adverse hepatic effects, which often occurs with simultaneous use of over-the-counter medications, prescription opioid-acetaminophen combinations, and premorbid hepatic injury. Use of analgesics, 30 to 60 minutes prior

TABLE 41.5 Oral Analgesics

Medication Class	Medication	Recommended Dosing	Pharmacokinetics	Key Drug-Drug Interactions	Key Drug-Disease Interactions	Important Adverse Effects
Oral Analgesics for Nociceptive Pain						
Other analgesic	Acetaminophen	325–1000 mg q4–6 hours Maximum daily dose 4000 mg	Metabolized via glucuronidation Clearance may be reduced in frail older adults	Hepatic injury can occur with modest doses when concomitant use of hepatic enzyme-inducing medications (e.g., rifampin, carbamazepine, phenytoin, phenobarbital).	None	Hepatic necrosis with acute 10 g ingestion or chronic use of >4 g/day. Increased toxicity from chronic use occurs with heavy alcohol use, malnourishment, preexisting liver disease; decrease maximum daily dose to 2 g. Nephrotoxicity (dose-dependent)
Nonacetylated salicylates	Salsalate	500–750 mg bid Maximum dose 3000 mg/day	Metabolized by hydrolysis to salicylate; also metabolized via glucuronidation.	No significant drug-drug interactions.	See other NSAIDs below.	Does not interfere with platelet function; GI bleeding rare.
Other NSAIDs	Ibuprofen Naproxen	400 mg tid-qid 250–500 mg bid	CYP2C9/19 CYP2C9 and CYP1A2; clearance significantly reduced with advanced age.	Concomitant use of NSAIDs with diuretics and antihypertensives may decrease their effectiveness. Use with corticosteroids and/or warfarin increases the risk of peptic ulcer disease. Increases concentration of lithium and methotrexate.	Use NSAIDs with caution in patients with chronic renal failure, heart failure, hypertension, and peptic ulcer disease history.	Risk of GI bleeding increased in persons ≥60 years. Cognitive impairment possible with higher doses. These NSAIDs should be reserved for short-term use in the older adult. Because of relatively long half-life, naproxen should not be the first choice for older adults.
COX-2 inhibitors	Celecoxib	100 mg bid	CYP2C9/19	Same as NSAIDs above.	Same as NSAIDs above.	COX-2 inhibitor has less GI toxicity but similar renal toxicity to other NSAIDS. Given long half-life and perhaps greater cardiac toxicity, it is not a preferred agent for older adults.
Weak opioids	Codeine Hydrocodone	15–30 mg q4–6 hours 5–10 mg q4–6 hours (alone or in combination with acetaminophen)	Prodrug metabolized by CYP2D6 CYP2D6; not studied in older adults.	Few clinically significant drug-drug interactions. Quinidine can inhibit the analgesic effect of codeine.	For all opioids, increased risk of falls in patients with dysmobility. May worsen or precipitate urinary retention when BPH present. Increased risk of delirium in those with dementia. Codeine has active renal metabolites that can accumulate with advancing age and renal insufficiency.	Because of increased sensitivity to opioids older adults at greater risk for sedation, nausea, vomiting, constipation, urinary retention, respiratory depression, and cognitive impairment.
Opiate receptor agonist/SNRI	Tramadol	Initiate at 25 mg qd. Increase by 25–50 mg daily in divided doses every 3–7 days as tolerated to max dose of 100 mg qid. Renal dosing 100 mg bid.	Prodrug metabolized by CYP2D4, 2B6, and 2D6.	Sedative medications and other opioids. Risk of serotonin syndrome in combination with SSRI and triptans. Seizure risk with MAOIs. Rare reports of interaction with warfarin and digoxin. Quinidine can inhibit the analgesic effect.	Seizure disorder (avoid if history of seizures). Adjust dose with renal insufficiency; maximum dose 100 mg bid.	Seizures and orthostatic hypotension. Other side effects similar to traditional opioids, including sedation, confusion, respiratory depression.

Strong opioids	Oxycodone (short- and long-acting)	Start with 5 mg (short-acting) q4–6 hours; after 7 days, determine dose requirements, then convert to long-acting.	CYP2D6	As above.	As above. Oxycodone and morphine have active renal metabolites that can accumulate with advancing age and renal insufficiency.	As above. Strong opioids to be avoided in older adults: pentazocine, meperidine.
	Morphine (short- and long-acting)	Start with 2.5 mg q+4 hours and titrate by 2.5-mg increments q7 days. Convert to long acting after dosing requirements determined.	Large first-pass effect and high hepatic extraction ratio results in higher serum levels and decreased clearance; glucuronidation to active renally cleared metabolites.			Constipation is very common with all opioids but not universal; a stimulant laxative (e.g., senna) should be prescribed if needed.
	Hydromorphone	Start with 2 mg q4 hours. Increase after 7 days if needed.	Glucuronidation; not studied in older adults			Dose of opioid required (for weak, strong, and tramadol) can be reduced by combining with a nonopioid agent such as acetaminophen.
	Fentanyl transdermal	Start with 12-μg patch q72 hours. If ineffective after 1 week, increase to 25 μg. 48-hour dosing interval may be required.	CYP3A4			Fentanyl patch, methadone and other sustained-release opioids should be avoided in those who are opioid-naïve.
	Methadone	Start with 1 mg q12–24 hours (po, buccal, sc). Titrate ≥ q7 days.	CYP3A4; not studied in older adults.	Phentyoin can increase clearance.		ECG should be obtained and monitored in those on methadone, as it may be associated with prolonged QT interval.
Oral Analgesics for Neuropathic Pain						
Anticonvulsants	Gabapentin	Initiate at 100 mg nightly. Increase by 100 mg weekly. Renal dosing: CLcr 30–59 mg/min, titrate to 600 mg bid. CLcr 15–29 mg/min, titrate to 300 mg bid. CLcr < 15 mg/min, titrate to 300 mg qd. Supplemental dosing after dialysis.	Renal elimination. Nonlinear pharmacokinetics. Plasma concentration increases disproportionately to dose.	Other CNS/sedative medications	Dementia, ataxia	Confusion, dizziness, somnolence, peripheral edema, weight gain. Withdrawal syndrome with abrupt discontinuation.

Continued

TABLE 41.5 Oral Analgesics—cont'd

Medication Class	Medication	Recommended Dosing	Pharmacokinetics	Key Drug-Drug Interactions	Key Drug-Disease Interactions	Important Adverse Effects
	Pregabalin	Initiate at 25–50 mg nightly. Increase by 25–50 mg weekly up to 100 mg bid. Max dose 300 mg qd. Renal dosing: CLcr 30–60 mg/min adjust dose to 150–300 mg qd. CLcr 15–30 mg/min adjust dose to 75–150 mg qd. CLcr < 15 mg/min adjust dose to 25–50 qd. Supplement dose after dialysis.	Renal elimination. Linear pharmacokinetics (plasma concentration is dose proportionate).	Other CNS/sedative medications	Dementia, ataxia	Confusion, dizziness, somnolence, peripheral edema, weight gain.
	Carbamazepine	Initiate at 50 mg nightly. Increase by 50 mg every week up to 100 mg bid. Target dose 200–600 mg qd. Max dose 1200 mg qd. Adjust dose for serum levels (4–12 mg/L). Patients on multiple CNS medications may have toxicity at lower serum levels.	Metabolized by CYP4503A4; induces CYP450.	CYP3A4 inhibitors increase serum CBZ levels. CYP3A4 inducers decrease serum CBZ levels. CBZ induces hepatic activity and can lower concentration of numerous drugs.		Slurred speech, gait instability, poor coordination; SIADH; rare severe reactions: Stevens–Johnson syndrome, aplastic anemia, hepatotoxicity, drug-induced lupus. Monitor LFTs, CBC, and serum sodium after initiation and during treatment.
Tricyclic antidepressants	Nortriptyline Desipramine	10 mg at night. Increase by 10 mg weekly. Max dose 50 mg at night.	Metabolized by CYP2D6.	CYP2D6 inhibitors increase serum levels. CYP2D6 inducers decrease serum levels. Other CNS/sedative medications	Myocardial infarction and bundle branch block; seizures, narrow-angle glaucoma, prostatic hypertrophy; dementia, falls	Arrhythmia, prolongation of QT interval and conduction block. Severe cases may lead to torsades de pointes. ECG prior to use in older adults. Orthostatic hypotension, sedation, confusion, constipation, urinary retention, SIADH.
Dual reuptake inhibitors (SNRIs)	Venlafaxine	Initiate at 37.5 mg daily. Increase by 37.5 mg weekly up to 150 mg daily. Max dose 225 mg daily.	Metabolized by CYP2D6	Contraindicated within 14 days of MAOI use. May precipitate serotonin syndrome when combined with triptans, tramadol, and other antidepressants.	HTN and uncontrolled narrow-angle glaucoma. Precipitation of mania in bipolar disorder.	Sedation/falls, insomnia, nausea, xerostomia, and constipation. Abrupt discontinuation may result in withdrawal syndrome.
	Duloxetine	Initiate at 20–30 mg daily. Increase to 60 mg after 1 week. Max dose 60 mg. Not recommended in ESRD or with CLcr < 30 mL/min.	Metabolized by CYP1A2 and CYP2D6.	CYP2D6 inhibitors; contraindicated within 14 days of MAOI use. May precipitate serotonin syndrome when combined with triptans, tramadol, and other antidepressants.	HTN, uncontrolled narrow-angle glaucoma, and seizure disorder. Precipitation of mania in patients with bipolar disorder.	Nausea, dry mouth, sedation/falls, urinary retention, and constipation. Abrupt discontinuation may result in withdrawal syndrome; low risk of hepatotoxicity, but contraindicated with hepatic disease and heavy alcohol use.

Topical agents	Lidocaine patch 5%	1–3 patches topically 12 hours on, 12 hours off. Only 3±2% of lidocaine patch absorbed. 95% lidocaine remains in patch form.	Hepatically metabolized. Unknown if lidocaine is metabolized in the skin. Negligible serum metabolite levels after topical application, that is, minimal systemic absorption.	Use with caution in patients taking class I antiarrhythmics (tocainamide and mexiletine).	Severe hepatic disease and nonintact skin.	Site reactions. Symptoms of lidocaine toxicity rare; they include nausea, nervousness, tinnitus, metallic taste, confusion, and tremor. Toxicity seen with serum lidocaine levels of >5 μg/mL. Serum levels with lidocaine patch typically 0.13 μg/mL.
	Capsaicin	Apply thin layer to affected area qid.	Cutaneous action. Maximum effect noted after 4–6 weeks of use.	None known.	Irritation on nonintact skin.	Skin reactions and burning. Avoid contact with eyes and sensitive skin areas. Respiratory irritation/cough if inhaled.
Muscle relaxants	Baclofen	Initiate at 5 mg nightly. Increase by 5 mg every week as tolerated. Max dose 10 mg tid. Dose adjustment with renal insufficiency.	Minimal metabolism; 85% excreted unchanged in liver and feces.	CNS depressants	Ataxia, renal disease, dementia, and seizures.	Confusion, nausea, sedation. Abrupt withdrawal syndrome with hallucinations, seizures, muscle rigidity, high fever. If severe may lead to rhabdomyolysis, multiorgan system failure, and death.
Opioid analgesics	See above under "Oral Analgesics for Nociceptive Pain."					

BPH, *Benign prostatic hyperplasia;* CBC, *complete blood count;* CBZ, *carbamazepine;* CLcr, *creatinine clearance;* CNS, *central nervous system;* CYP, *cytochrome P450;* ECG, *electrocardiogram;* ESRD, *end-stage renal disease;* GI, *gastrointestinal;* HTN, *hypertension;* LFTs, *liver function tests;* MAOI, *monoamine oxidase inhibitor;* NSAIDs, *nonsteroidal antiinflammatory drugs;* SIADH, *syndrome of inappropriate antidiuretic hormone secretion;* SNRI, *serotonin-norepinephrine reuptake inhibitor ;* SSRI, *selective serotonin reuptake inhibitor.*

Based in part on: Weiner DK, Karp JF, Bernstein C, et al.: Pain medicine in older adults: how should it differ? In: Deer T, Ray A, Gordin V, et al., editors: Comprehensive Treatment of Chronic Pain by Medical, Interventional and Behavioral Approaches: The American Academy of Pain Medicine Textbook on Patient Management. *New York: Springer, 2013. Reproduced with permission of the American Academy of Pain Medicine.*

TABLE 41.6A Beers List: Pain and Pain-Related Medications

Organ System, Therapeutic Category, Drugs	Rationale	Recommendation	Quality of Evidence	Strength of Recommendation
Central nervous system Antidepressants, alone or in combination Amitriptyline Desipramine Nortriptyline	Highly anticholinergic, sedating, and cause orthostatic hypotension.	Avoid	High	Strong
Pain medications				
Meperidine	Not effective oral analgesic in dosages commonly used; may have higher risk of neurotoxicity, including delirium, than other opioids; safer alternatives available.	Avoid, especially in individuals with chronic kidney disease.	Moderate	Strong
Noncyclooxygenase–selective NSAIDs: oral Aspirin > 325 mg/day Diclofenac Diflunisal Etodolac Fenoprofen Ibuprofen Ketoprofen Meclofenamate Mefenamic acid Meloxicam Nabumetone Naproxen Oxaprozin Piroxicam Sulindac Tolmetin	Increased risk of gastrointestinal bleeding or peptic ulcer disease in high-risk groups, including those aged >75 or taking oral or parenteral corticosteroids, anticoagulants, or antiplatelet agents; use of proton-pump inhibitor or misoprostol; reduces but does not eliminate risk. Upper gastrointestinal ulcers, gross bleeding, or perforation cause by NSAIDs occur in approximately 1% of patients treated for 3–6 months and in ~2%–4% of patients treated for 1 year; these trends continue with longer duration of use.	Avoid chronic use unless other alternatives are not effective and patient can take gastroprotective agent (proton-pump inhibitor or misoprostol).	Moderate	Strong
Indomethacin	Indomethacin is more likely than other NSAIDs to have adverse CNS effects. Of all the NSAIDs, indomethacin has the most adverse effects.	Avoid.	Moderate	Strong
Ketorolac, includes parenteral	Increased risk of gastrointestinal bleeding, peptic ulcer disease, and acute kidney injury in older adults.	Avoid.	Moderate	Strong
Pentazocine	Opioid analgesic that causes CNS adverse effects, including confusion and hallucinations, more commonly that other opioid analgesic drugs; is also a mixed agonist and antagonist; safer alternatives available.	Avoid.	Low	Strong

CNS, *Central nervous system;* NSAIDs, *nonsteroidal antiinflammatory drugs.*
American Geriatrics Society 2015 Beers Criteria Update Expert Panel. American Geriatrics Society 2015 updated Beers criteria for potentially inappropriate medication use in older adults. J Am Geriatr Soc *6:432-442, 2015. [Advance online publication].*

TABLE 41.6B Abbreviated Version of 2015 American Geriatrics Society Beers Criteria

Disease or Syndrome	Drug (s)	Rationale	Recommendation	Quality of Evidence	Strength of Recommendation
Heart failure	NSAIDs and COX-2 inhibitors	Potential to promote fluid retention and exacerbate heart failure	Avoid	NSAIDs: moderate	Strong
Syncope	Tertiary TCAs	Increases risk of orthostatic hypotension or bradycardia	Avoid	TCAs: moderate	TCAs: strong
Chronic seizures or epilepsy	Tramadol	Lowers seizure threshold; may be acceptable in individuals with well-controlled seizures in whom alternative agents have not been effective	Avoid	Low	Strong
Delirium	Corticosteroids Meperidine	Avoid in older adults with or at high risk of delirium because of the potential of inducing or worsening delirium.	Avoid	Moderate	Strong

TABLE 41.6B Abbreviated Version of 2015 American Geriatrics Society Beers Criteria—cont'd

Disease or Syndrome	Drug (s)	Rationale	Recommendation	Quality of Evidence	Strength of Recommendation
History of falls or fractures	Anticonvulsants TCAs Opioids	May cause ataxia, impaired psychomotor function, syncope, additional falls. If one of the drugs must be used, consider reducing use of other CNS-active medications that increase risk of falls and fractures and implement other strategies to reduce fall risk.	Avoid unless safer alternatives are not available; avoid anticonvulsants except for seizure and mood disorders. Opioids: avoid, excludes pain management due to recent fractures or joint replacement.	High Opioids: moderate	Strong Opioids: strong
History of gastric or duodenal ulcers	Aspirin (>325 mg/day) Non–COX-2-selective NSAIDs	May exacerbate existing ulcers or cause new or additional ulcers.	Avoid unless other alternatives are not effective and patient can take gastroprotective agent (i.e., proton pump inhibitor or misoprostol)	Moderate	Strong
Chronic kidney disease Stages IV or less (creatinine clearance < 30 mL/min)	NSAIDs (non-COX and COX-selective, oral and parenteral)	May increase risk of acute kidney injury and further decline of renal function.	Avoid	Moderate	Strong

CNS, *Central nervous system;* NSAID, *nonsteroidal antiinflammatory drug;* TCA, *tricyclic antidepressant.*
American Geriatrics Society 2015 Beers Criteria Update Expert Panel. American Geriatrics Society 2015 updated Beers criteria for potentially inappropriate medication use in older adults. J Am Geriatr Soc. *63(11):2227-2246, 2015. [Advance online publication].*

to exercise, or therapy sessions may prove synergistic and optimize the treatment program.

Oral NSAIDs, used at the lowest effective dose, may be indicated for short-term use in the patient with inflammatory pain or in cases where acetaminophen efficacy is suboptimal. Nonacetylated salicylates may be considered for pain control, given their safer side-effect profile compared with traditional NSAIDs. Chronic use of NSAIDs should be avoided, given the risks of congestive heart failure, exacerbation of hypertension, renal insufficiency, and GI bleeding. Coprescription of a proton pump inhibitor (PPI) with an NSAID should be considered in older adults, as this will reduce but not eliminate GI side effects. However, the use of a PPI does not appear to reduce the risk of lower GI adverse effects (e.g., colitis, acute diverticulitis). Both the frequency and severity of upper and lower GI side effects were found to be lower with use of a COX-2–selective NSAID, specifically celecoxib.[44]

In carefully selected older adults with moderate to severe pain from inflammatory disorders, cancer-related pain, or severe neuropathic pain who have failed nonpharmacologic and nonopioid pharmacologic treatments or those with advanced osteoarthritis who are not candidates for surgery, opioids may be an effective option. These individuals require close monitoring and regular follow-up given their broad side-effect profile that includes constipation, glucose intolerance, sleep-disordered breathing, hypertension, psychosis, and osteoporosis. In older adults, potential side effects such as delirium, urinary retention, falls, and fractures should be considered in the risk-benefit analysis.

Before starting an opioid in an older adult, several precautions should be taken. Educating the patient about potential side effects is critical. In addition to the side effects listed above, this education should include issues of tolerance and dependence and the potential for abuse. Screening tools such as the Opioid Risk Tool, a concise office-based instrument for detecting potential for abuse or deviant behavior (Table 41.7), and/or the Screener and Opioid Assessment for Patients with Pain Revised (SOAPP-R), a method for assessing the potential for misuse with long-term opioid treatment,[45,46] can be used. The Current Opioid Misuse Measure is recommended for assessing ongoing misuse.[47] When the older adult is opioid naive, a short-acting preparation at the lowest effective dose should be initiated, with frequent evaluation of pain control and consideration of a long-acting agent at a later stage. Constipation should be monitored closely; many providers routinely prescribe a stimulant laxative and/or a stool softener at the same time that an opioid is initiated. Opioids should be avoided in older adults with a history of falls or fractures if at all possible, with the exception of short-term use related to posttraumatic or postoperative pain.[43] If opioid prescription cannot be avoided in the older adult with impaired balance and mobility, an assistive device should first be prescribed and the patient referred to a physical therapist for guidance

TABLE 41.7 Predicting Aberrant Behaviors in Opioid-Treated Patients: Preliminary Validation of the Opioid Risk Tool

Item	Mark Each Box That Applies	Item Score If Female	Item Score If Male
1. Family history of substance abuse			
Alcohol	[]	1	3
Illegal drugs	[]	2	3
Prescription drugs	[]	4	4
2. Personal history of substance abuse			
Alcohol	[]	1	3
Illegal drugs	[]	2	3
Prescription drugs	[]	4	4
3. Age (mark box if 16–45)		1	1
4. History of preadolescent sexual abuse	[]	3	0
5. Psychologic disease			
Attention deficit disorder, obsessive-compulsive disorder, bipolar, schizophrenia	[]	2	2
Depression	[]	1	1
Total		—	—
Total score risk category			
Low risk: 0–3			
Moderate risk: 4–7			
High risk: ≥8			

Source: Webster LR, Webster RM: Predicting aberrant behaviors in opioid-treated patients: preliminary validation of the Opioid Risk Tool. Pain Med. *6:432-442, 2005.*

on using the device correctly in addition to working on minimizing fall risk.

There is strong evidence for the use of antidepressants and antiepileptic medications such as tricyclic antidepressants (TCA), serotonin-noradrenaline reuptake inhibitors (SNRIs), pregabalin and gabapentin and weak evidence for use of lidocaine patches, capsaicin patches, tramadol, and strong opioids for treatment of neuropathic pain in adults.[48] However, in adults older than 65 years of age, TCAs are not recommended, given their anticholinergic side effects (sedation, delirium, urinary retention, constipation, exacerbation of glaucoma), risk of falls, and cardiac toxicity in higher doses.[43] The SNRI duloxetine and anticonvulsant pregabalin are effective drugs for the treatment of painful diabetic neuropathy. Both gabapentin and pregabalin are used to treat pain associated with postherpetic neuralgia, a condition more commonly found in older adults. In adults with trigeminal neuralgia, carbamazepine or oxcarbazepine is recommended as first-line treatment. Oxcarbazepine is associated with fewer side effects and potential drug-drug interactions and may be preferred in older adults.[49]

Oral corticosteroids are often prescribed for short-term use in the older adult with inflammatory disorders (i.e., giant cell arteritis, polymyalgia rheumatica, rheumatoid arthritis) and cancer-related pain. Long-term use of steroids should be limited unless absolutely necessary due to common side effects including glucose intolerance, decreased bone density, hypertension, increased cardiovascular risk, GI ulcers and bleeding, mental status changes, glaucoma, and cataracts.

INJECTION THERAPIES

Injection therapies may be an effective treatment option in patients who are unable to tolerate oral or topical agents and where pain is significantly limiting adherence with rehabilitation interventions. Injection therapies can target the spine, peripheral joints (e.g., knee, hip, shoulder), muscles, and tendons with medications that include corticosteroids, analgesics, and prolotherapy.

CORTICOSTEROID INJECTIONS

Epidural steroid injections (ESIs) are commonly performed for pain associated with discogenic disease with radiculopathy and lumbar spinal stenosis. A recent randomized trial of ESIs in older adults with spinal stenosis did not show any benefit compared with the use of lidocaine alone. In this study, some of the most common side effects reported included fevers, infection, and headaches.[50]

Intraarticular corticosteroid injections may be beneficial in reducing pain in patients with knee osteoarthritis[51,52] and hip osteoarthritis.[53] Based on a retrospective review[54] and a small prospective study,[55] joint injections may still be safe to perform on patients taking warfarin for anticoagulation if the international normalized ratio (INR) is therapeutic. Patients with diabetes should be counseled on the possible risk of hyperglycemia following steroid injections and the need for close monitoring.

TRIGGER-POINT INJECTIONS

Trigger-point injections using local anesthetics such as lidocaine may be effective adjunctive treatment for reducing pain associated with myofascial pain syndrome.[56,57] Dry needling also can be effective. Side effects can include pain or swelling at the site, skin infection, and excessive bleeding, which may be more common among patients on anticoagulation. There are few adverse side effects associated with trigger-point injections with no severe life-threatening issues reported in randomized controlled trials.[56,58]

PROLOTHERAPY

Prolotherapy is defined as an injection of "growth factors or growth factor stimulants" that can be categorized as irritants, osmotics, or chemotactics.[59] Although there are studies investigating the use of prolotherapy for musculoskeletal conditions such as knee osteoarthritis, the evidence is inconclusive and not specific to older adults.[60,61]

FIBROMYALGIA: INTERDISCIPLINARY TREATMENT APPROACH EXAMPLE

Fibromyalgia is one of the more common chronic nonmalignant and widespread pain problems in older adults, with symptoms occurring for longer than 3 months varying from morning stiffness, fatigue, and nonrestorative sleep to headaches, myofascial pain, and pelvic pain.

Fibromyalgia, like many chronic pain conditions, often requires an interdisciplinary treatment approach. Effective treatments for fibromyalgia include 30 minutes of low- to moderate-intensity aerobic exercise with supervision and/or cognitive-behavioral therapy. The FDA-approved medications for fibromyalgia include SNRIs such as duloxetine, venlafaxine, pregabalin, and milnacipran.[62] Complementary and alternative modalities have also been studied as viable treatment options in patients with fibromyalgia. There is some evidence to support the benefits of acupuncture, homeopathy, hydrotherapy, and massage.[63] However, more studies are needed regarding the efficacy and safety of these interventions for older adults.

CONCLUSION

We continue to reinforce the importance of an interdisciplinary approach in caring for the older adult. All health care providers will be exposed to the older adult with chronic pain and should have familiarity with this patient population. The most important goal of treatment should be to promote functional independence, prevent functional decline if possible, and/or manage disability. In the practice of pain medicine, it is important to consider geriatricians, geriatric psychiatrists and psychologists, physiatrists, rheumatologists, neurologists, sports and spine specialists, endocrinologists, social workers, physical and occupational therapists, and complementary medicine practitioners as important potential collaborators in the care of frail older adults with complex conditions.

KEY POINTS

- Sarcopenia is common with advancing age and is defined as progressive loss of muscle mass associated with muscle cell atrophy and increased fat content. This may result in increased retention of fat-soluble medications; there is also a decrease in the number of motor units.
- Medications such as morphine that have a high hepatic extraction ratio may undergo decreased clearance and experience a longer half-life in older adults because of diminished liver size and blood flow.
- The following long half-life NSAIDs are hepatically metabolized and their clearance may be reduced in older adults: celecoxib, diflunisal, naproxen, oxaprozin, piroxican, salsalate, and sulindac.
- Analgesics that are affected by aging-associated decline in renal function include codeine, duloxetine, gabapentin, meperidine, pregabalin, propoxyphene, salicylate, tramadol, and the opioids morphine, oxycodone, hydromorphone, fentanyl, and methadone.
- Chronic pain assessment in older adults requires comprehensive identification of the multiple contributing biologic, mechanical/physical, social, and psychologic factors. Providers should also inquire about changes in cognition or memory, appetite, sleep, mood disturbances, a loss or decrease in mobility, falls, and diminished activity level with changes in performance related to activities of daily living.
- In patients with advanced dementia who have difficulty using self-report instruments, caregivers rely on behavioral cues such as facial grimacing, guarding, bracing, rubbing, and sighing to determine the presence and severity of pain. There are assessment tools that can help the practitioner detect pain in this patient population.
- Red-flag symptoms that require immediate attention include pain following a fall or other trauma, fever, sudden unexplained weight loss, acute onset of severe pain, new onset of weakness or sensory loss, loss of bowel or bladder function, jaw claudication, new headaches, bone pain in a patient with a history of malignancy, and sudden pain in an extremity that is associated with pallor, pulselessness, and paresthesias.
- Acetaminophen continues to be recommended as first-line treatment in patients with nociceptive pain, specifically in patients with low back pain and osteoarthritis.
- For opioids, several tools are available to detect abuse and aberrant behavior. Constipation should be monitored closely; opioids should be avoided in patients with history of falls.
- There is strong evidence for use of antidepressants and antiepileptic medications such as TCAs, SNRIs, pregabalin, and gabapentin and weak evidence for use of lidocaine patches, capsaicin patches, tramadol, and strong opioids for treatment of neuropathic pain in adults. TCAs are not recommended in adults older than 65 years of age because of their anticholinergic side effects.

REFERENCES

Access the reference list online at ExpertConsult.com.

SECTION VI

PHARMACOLOGY AND PHARMACOLOGIC MODALITIES

SECTION OUTLINE HEAD

CHAPTER 42

MAJOR OPIOIDS IN PAIN MANAGEMENT

Samir Sheth, MD ◎ Mark Holtsman, PharmD ◎ Gagan Mahajan, MD

Opioids remain an important option for the treatment of substantial pain despite the recognition of heightened risks and growing analgesic options from other drug groups. Over the past several decades, opioid prescribing for chronic nonmalignant pain (CNMP) has become more widespread, resulting in opioids being the most frequently prescribed class of drugs in the United States.[1–4] Looking at the top 25 most dispensed prescriptions in the United States, hydrocodone, tramadol, and oxycodone ranked as number 1, 21, and 22, respectively.[4] In 2012, some 259 million opioid prescriptions were written by health care providers, and there was a parallel increase in the rate of overdose deaths associated with opioid analgesics.[5] From 1999 to 2014, there were approximately 165,000 overdose deaths due to opioid pain relievers.[5,6] In 2014, 61% of drug overdose deaths involved opioids (including heroin).[7] Equally important are the nonfatal opioid overdoses, which have increased sixfold over the past 15 years.[7] The Drug Abuse Warning Network (DAWN) reported that of the greater than 1.2 million Emergency Department visits in 2011 involving nonmedical use of prescription medicines, over-the-counter drugs, or other types of pharmaceuticals, opioids accounted for 29%; and nonmedical use of opioids accounted for an increase of 183% in medical emergencies from 2004 to 2011.[8] Dart et al., in analyzing the Researched Abuse, Diversion and Addiction-Related Surveillance (RADARS) System data from 2002 to 2013 for opioid-related adverse events, found a parallel relationship between the legitimate dispensing of opioids and opioid diversion and abuse.[1] In addition to this is the parallel increase in the rate of opioid addiction, affecting 2.5 million adults in 2014.[7] Emerging data, however, suggest that prescription opioid abuse may be decreasing.[1] Although the legitimate use of opioids in select and monitored patients with CNMP has been supported by consensus statements developed by national organizations, such as the American Pain Society (APS) and American Academy of Pain Medicine (AAPM), prescribing remains increasingly controversial, with polarized arguments on both sides of the debate over the risk and effectiveness of opioids in treating CNMP.[9–16]

RATIONALE

Opioids produce reliable analgesia, and their adverse effects (e.g., constipation, nausea and vomiting, sedation, and respiratory suppression) often can be preempted, treated, or reversed. Opioid therapy can be an integral part of a multidisciplinary approach to acute and chronic pain management. An attempt to optimize a patient's pain management may include concurrently combining opioids with nonopioid adjuvant analgesics (nonsteroidal antiinflammatory drugs [NSAIDs], acetaminophen, antidepressants, anticonvulsants, etc.), physical therapy, psychological therapy, and/or injection therapies. Much of the debate concerning the role of chronic opioid therapy (COT) for the management of CNMP, however, has centered on whether opioids should be used as a first-line treatment or whether they should be used at all on a chronic basis. The Centers for Disease Control (CDC) recently produced guidelines that suggest use of nonpharmacologic as well as nonopioid pharmacologic therapy prior to opioid therapy.[5,6] Health care professionals should not utilize opioid therapy as a first-line treatment for CNMP for the following reasons: (1) nonpharmacological and nonopioid medications, such as NSAIDs and anticonvulsants or tricyclic antidepressants (TCAs), can be efficacious as first-line treatments for CNMP secondary to arthritic pain[17] and neuropathic pain,[18] respectively; (2) injection therapies may be effective and obviate the need for opioids; and (3) opioid treatment carries substantial side effects as well as liability profiles (see further on), and the risk-benefit ratio often demands that alternative treatments be implemented before instituting COT. An opioid trial may be considered when alternative analgesics, injection therapies, physical therapy, and psychological therapy have been inadequate, contraindicated, or otherwise exhausted. Although nonopioid drugs may appear to be better and/or safer choices for patients with CNMP, long-term use of such agents also may have deleterious or life-threatening effects.[5,19]

GUIDELINES

Since opioids are controlled substances with potential for abuse, they are regulated by federal and state agencies. In addition to unintentional overdose, major concerns for opioid prescribers include the potential of diversion through fraud, theft, forged prescriptions, or illegal activities of unprincipled health care professionals. In 1998 the House of Delegates of the Federation of State Medical Boards (FSMB) of the United States established and adopted the Model Guidelines for the Use of Controlled Substances for the Treatment of Pain, which offered prescribing expectations for state medical boards. These guidelines have been updated multiple times, most recently in 2013, and have been converted to a model policy.[20,21] The policy includes definitions of addiction, pseudoaddiction, tolerance, physical dependence, and substance abuse (Box 42.1).[20] It emphasizes the importance of an evaluation, physical examination, and follow-up to monitor and evaluate for therapeutic efficacy, which includes the patient's functional status. The model policy also recommends the use of specialty consultations and additional referrals when patients present with complex histories, troubling adverse effects, lack of progress toward analgesia or improved function, or any issues outside the purview of the prescriber's expertise. Other organizations have published guidelines for the use of chronic opioids in patients with CNMP. The APS and

BOX 42.1 Definitions Related to Opioid Use

SECTION III: DEFINITIONS

For the purposes of these guidelines, the following terms are defined here:

Addiction—Addiction is a primary, chronic, neurobiologic disease, with genetic, psychosocial, and environmental factors influencing its development and manifestations. It is characterized by behaviors that include the following: impaired control over drug use, craving, compulsive use, and continued use despite harm. Physical dependence and tolerance are normal physiological consequences of extended opioid therapy for pain and are not the same as addiction. According to the 2013 Federation of State Medical Board's Model Policy, there are updated definitions that have been adopted by the American Society of Addiction Medicine that state addiction is "a primary, chronic disease of brain reward, motivation, memory and related circuitry" and that "without treatment or engagement in recovery activities, addiction is progressive and can result in disability or premature death."

Physical Dependence—Physical dependence is a state of adaptation that is manifested by drug class–specific signs and symptoms that can be produced by abrupt cessation, rapid dose reduction, decreasing blood level of the drug, and/or administration of an antagonist. Physical dependence, by itself, does not equate with addiction.

Pseudoaddiction—The iatrogenic syndrome resulting from the misinterpretation of relief-seeking behaviors as though they are drug-seeking behaviors that are commonly seen with addiction. The relief-seeking behaviors resolve upon institution of effective analgesic therapy.

Substance Abuse—Substance abuse is the use of any substance(s) for nontherapeutic purposes or use of medication for purposes other than those for which it is prescribed.

Tolerance—Tolerance is a physiologic state resulting from regular use of a drug in which an increased dosage is needed to produce a specific effect, or a reduced effect is observed with a constant dose over time. Tolerance may or may not be evident during opioid treatment and does not equate with addiction.

The terms "pain," "acute pain," and "chronic pain" are defined in Chapter 3, Taxonomy.

TABLE 42.1 Risk-Assessment and Monitoring Tools and Websites

Risk assessment tool	Screener and Opioid Assessment for Patients with Pain (SOAPP) Version 1.0-14Q Opioid Risk Tool (ORT) DIRE (Diagnosis, Intractability, Risk, Efficacy) Score: Patient Selection for Chronic Opioid Analgesia
Monitoring tools	Pain Assessment and Documentation Tool (PADT) Current Opioid Misuse Measure (COMM)

From Chou R, Ganciullo GJ, Fine PG, et al.: Clinical guidelines for the use of chronic opioid therapy in chronic noncancer pain. J Pain. *10:113-130, 2009.*

AAPM have published consensus guidelines for rational approaches to prescribing opioids and avoiding potential adverse effects. In these guidelines, information regarding risk assessment tools is included (Table 42.1).[9] Finally, as stated earlier, the CDC also published comprehensive guidelines in 2016 with regards to opioid prescribing in patients with CNMP (Table 42.2).[5,6]

Although federal and state law enforcement agencies are the principal regulators of prescription drug abuse, public and congressional outcry over opioid misuse, addiction, and diversion prompted the US Food and Drug Administration (FDA) to get involved. By authority of the FDA Amendments Act (FDAAA) of 2007, the FDA can require drug manufacturers to implement Risk Evaluation and Mitigation Strategies (REMS) to ensure that the benefits of the drug outweigh the risk. Although REMS can include any drug, in 2009 the FDA notified manufacturers of sustained-release opioids (SROs) and long-acting opioids (LAOs) that a "class-wide" opioid-specific REMS would be required to include proposed communication and education materials, a medication guide, elements to ensure safe use, a patient package insert, enrollment forms, and prescriber and patient agreements. Because of the significant abuse potential of transmucosal immediate release fentanyl (TIRF) products, in December 2011 the FDA also required "class-wide" opioid REMS for this class of medications in addition to the SRO and LAO medications.[22] The TIRF REMS Access Program applies to all rapid-onset fentanyl preparations, which currently applies to the Abstral (fentanyl) sublingual tablet, Actiq (fentanyl citrate) oral transmucosal lozenge and its generic equivalents, Fentora (fentanyl citrate) buccal tablet, Lazanda (fentanyl) nasal spray, and Onsolis (fentanyl) buccal.[23] Pharmaceutical companies are required to implement an opioid REMS program, but participation for clinicians is voluntary. Whether this might change in the future remains to be seen.

To date, REMS programs for SROs and LAOs have increased knowledge with regard to opioid prescribing and a significant number of clinicians are reported to be implementing changes as a result of REMS programs.[24] However, the full impact of REMS on opioid prescribing remains to be seen. Listed below are important websites detailing the REMS blueprint as well as access to the current list of opioids that require REMS:

- http://www.fda.gov/forindustry/userfees/prescriptiondruguserfee/ucm361870.htm#Training, accessed June 1, 2017.
- http://www.accessdata.fda.gov/scripts/cder/rems/index.cfm?event=RemsDetails.page&REMS=17, accessed May 24, 2016
- http://www.accessdata.fda.gov/scripts/cder/rems/index.cfm?event=RemsDetails.page&REMS=60, accessed May 24, 2016

INITIATION OF CHRONIC OPIOID THERAPY

In the absence of comorbid risk factors (e.g., hepatic or renal impairment, age, etc.), there is no direct evidence to support the use of one opioid over the other.[9] Due to recent evidence comparing LAOs/SROs with SAOs,[5] the CDC guidelines recommend that clinicians should initiate an opioid trial with an SAO instead of an LAO/SRO and that the lowest effective dose should be prescribed for patients.[5,6] A patient with moderate to severe acute and/or chronic pain who has not improved with nonopioid therapies is a potential candidate for opioid analgesics. Although opioids lack an absolute upper limit to dosing necessary to control a patient's pain, dose escalation should be carried out in a judicious manner, as opioids do not have any known benefits for CNMP but the risks of opioids are well documented and dose-dependent.[5,6,25]

The severity and frequency of the patient's pain should determine whether "as needed" (PRN, *pro re nata*) versus "around-the-clock" dosing is necessary. For example, in

TABLE 42.2 Centers for Disease Control Guideline for Prescribing Opioids for Chronic Pain

- Nonpharmacologic therapy and nonopioid pharmacologic therapy are preferred for chronic pain. Clinicians should consider opioid therapy only if expected benefits for both pain and function are expected to outweigh risks to the patient. If opioids are used, they should be combined with nonpharmacologic therapy and nonopioid pharmacologic therapy, as appropriate.
- Before starting opioid therapy for chronic pain, clinicians should establish treatment goals with all patients, including realistic goals for pain and function, and should consider how opioid therapy will be discontinued if benefits do not outweigh risks. Clinicians should continue opioid therapy only if there is clinically meaningful improvement in pain and function that outweighs risks to patient safety.
- Before starting and periodically during opioid therapy, clinicians should discuss with patients known risks and realistic benefits of opioid therapy and patient and clinician responsibilities for managing therapy.
- When starting opioid therapy for chronic pain, clinicians should prescribe immediate-release opioids instead of extended-release/long-acting opioids.
- When opioids are started, clinicians should prescribe the lowest effective dosage. Clinicians should use caution when prescribing opioids at any dosage, should carefully reassess evidence of individual benefits and risks when considering increasing dosage to ≥50 morphine milligram equivalents (MME) per day, and should avoid increasing dosage to ≥90 MME/day or carefully justify a decision to titrate dosage to ≥90 MME/day.
- Long-term opioid use often begins with the treatment of acute pain. When opioids are used for acute pain, clinicians should prescribe the lowest effective dose of immediate-release opioids and should prescribe no greater quantity than needed for the expected duration of pain severe enough to require opioids. Three days or less often will be sufficient; more than 7 days will rarely be needed.
- Clinicians should evaluate benefits and harms with patients within 1–4 weeks of starting opioid therapy for chronic pain or of dose escalation. Clinicians should evaluate benefits and harms of continued therapy with patients every 3 months or more frequently. If benefits do not outweigh harms of continued opioid therapy, clinicians should optimize other therapies and work with patients to taper opioids to lower dosages or to taper and discontinue opioids.
- Before starting and periodically during continuation of opioid therapy, clinicians should evaluate risk factors for opioid-related harms. Clinicians should incorporate into the management plan strategies to mitigate risk, including considering offering naloxone when factors that increase risk for opioid overdose, such as history of overdose, history of substance use disorder, higher opioid dosages (≥50 MME/day), or concurrent benzodiazepine use, are present.
- Clinicians should review the patient's history of controlled substance prescriptions using state prescription drug monitoring program (PDMP) data to determine whether the patient is receiving opioid dosages or dangerous combinations that put him or her at high risk for overdose. Clinicians should review PDMP data when starting opioid therapy for chronic pain and periodically during opioid therapy for chronic pain, ranging from every prescription to every 3 months.
- When prescribing opioids for chronic pain, clinicians should use urine drug testing before starting opioid therapy and consider urine drug testing at least annually to assess for prescribed medications as well as other controlled prescription drugs and illicit drugs.
- Clinicians should avoid prescribing opioid pain medication and benzodiazepines concurrently whenever possible.
- Clinicians should offer or arrange evidence-based treatment (usually medication assisted treatment with buprenorphine or methadone in combination with behavioral therapies) for patients with opioid use disorder.

From Dowell D, Haegerich TM, Chou R: CDC guideline for prescribing opioids for chronic pain—United States, 2016. MMWR Recomm Rep. *65:1-49, 2016; Dowell D, Haegerich TM, Chou R: CDC guideline for prescribing opioids for chronic pain—United States, 2016.* JAMA. *315(15):1624-1645, 2016.*

those with acute pain secondary to an injury or surgery, PRN dosing with an SAO may be sufficient if the anticipated healing process is rapid and short. In those with either a slow and prolonged recovery process or persistent chronic pain, an SAO used on a PRN basis can produce a "rollercoaster" effect, whereby patients have pain, take analgesics, and experience brief periods of relief followed by repetition of this cycle when the pain returns. Typically COT aims to avoid perpetuation of this phenomenon by producing stable analgesia that is targeted less at total abolition of pain and more toward augmentation of the patient's function at a tolerable level of pain. Recent guidelines suggest starting with an SAO as an initial trial even if use of an LAO is anticipated.[1,14] Since the usual goal of opioid administration for the treatment of chronic pain is to achieve sustained analgesia over regular intervals,[26] SAOs may be given at fixed dosing intervals, just as with an LAO or SRO. Such a strategy permits consistent delivery for reaching steady-state levels and may avoid the peak-and-trough effect associated with on-demand dosing.

If a patient responds to an SAO and tolerates its side effects, COT may be best delivered by converting to an equianalgesic LAO or SRO if dosing permits. Ideally, an LAO or SRO should not be combined with an SAO.[5,6] Benefits of using an LAO or SRO include achievement of safe, effective steady-state levels with regard to fixed dosing intervals[27] and lack of a compounded nonopioid analgesic which may impose a ceiling dose. Although fixed dosing with an SRO or an LAO has been presumed to provide more sustained levels of analgesia, improved compliance, less reward-associated reinforcement of potentially dysfunctional cycles where pain and pain medication become a conditioned part of the patient's life, and poses less risk of addiction or abuse, these beliefs have becoming increasingly challenged. Published studies have failed to conclusively prove these proposed benefits of SROs and LAOs over SAOs or fixed dosing over PRN dosing.[9] Nonetheless, the use of fixed dosing may prevent the delays in delivery that can occur with PRN dosing. Still, consensus in this area of pharmacotherapy remains elusive at present.

ADMINISTRATION

The convenience of orally administered opioids has made this the preferred route of delivery. Many patients with cancer or acute postoperative pain, however, are unable to tolerate oral ingestion or temporarily are not permitted oral ingestion. Therefore having multiple means of administering opioids is advantageous.[28] An intravenous (IV) or subcutaneous (SQ) infusion is commonly used in terminally ill patients in pain, often with fixed dosing for constant effect. Both routes avoid the first-pass effect and can be supplemented by PRN doses for breakthrough pain. The SQ route has several advantages, including faster onset of analgesia compared with most oral preparations (although slower than IV administration), uncomplicated access in patients with poor venous access, and safer administration compared with the intramuscular (IM) route in patients with bleeding disorders or reduced muscle mass.

A common system for delivering IV opioids is patient-controlled analgesia (PCA), most commonly using morphine, hydromorphone, or fentanyl. Widely used for treating postoperative pain, PCA is rapidly finding broader use in treating cancer pain. PCA immediately delivers a preprogrammed IV or SQ dosage of an opioid when the patient activates a handheld button, thereby permitting rapid analgesia without needing a nurse to deliver an IV PRN dose. By placing a maximum limit on the dose and frequency of opioid administered, the physician helps the patient titrate his or her opioid requirement. Because the PCA machine records the patient's individual dosing and frequency parameters, useful information can be obtained about the patient's analgesic requirements, which also simplifies subsequent conversion to a non-PCA opioid regimen.

Alternatives for patients unable to use IV or oral preparations include rectal (suppositories are available containing morphine, hydromorphone, and oxymorphone), sublingual, buccal, intranasal, transdermal, epidural, or intrathecal routes of administration. Epidural and intrathecal opioids—commonly used in the perioperative, postoperative, obstetric, and cancer populations—make opioids directly available to the opiate receptor–rich neuraxis. These two forms of selective analgesia have the advantage of requiring relatively small quantities of opioids, thereby reducing the risk of central and autonomic complications. Patient-controlled epidural analgesia (PCEA), a newer variant of patient-controlled drug delivery systems, administers epidural dosages of opioid, and potentially other drugs, via a similar mechanism such as IV PCA.

TREATMENT ENDPOINTS AND OPIOID SELECTION

Since pain is an untestable hypothesis that can neither be proved nor disproved, using pain relief as the endpoint of opioid therapy is also untestable and subjective. One of the most feared adverse effects from COT is drug addiction, which manifests as the compulsive use of a drug that causes dysfunction and its continued use despite the harm related to that dysfunction. In 2013, the estimated rate of opioid misuse and abuse affected nearly 2 million people.[5] Thus clinicians are advised to focus on functional improvement as an objective endpoint of analgesia, since this also offers evidence of opioid efficacy in contrast to addiction. The challenge, however, is to develop outcome measures for COT beyond a lower pain score that distinguish function from dysfunction and that emphasize therapy expectations, goal setting, goal monitoring, and collaboration with the patient's entire treatment team. Two critical issues related to treatment endpoints in COT include (1) defining what outcomes should be expected and followed to demonstrate an effective and safe trial of opioids and (2) determining when and how opioid therapy should be discontinued (or tapered) if the treatment is either effective or ineffective. Clinical studies in this area are limited.

Markers of opioid benefit in patients treated for CNMP include subjective pain reduction and evidence of improved functional status and quality of life. Determining functional improvement can be accomplished with standardized instruments (Short Form [36] Health Survey and Oswestry Disability Index, among others) or through a simple process of ascertaining limitations in function and quality of life prior to treatment and following these endpoints through the course of opioid therapy. The ideal functional assessment model should be simple, brief, individualized, and comprehensive—something that most formalized scales fail to accomplish. There are many examples of functional goals, including daily exercise, returning to work, and sleeping in a bed as opposed to a lounge chair. Supporting evidence of these functional goals is important for validation and documentation purposes.[21]

Psychological and social factors as well as coexistent diseases that may influence pain perception and suffering can affect the overall assessment of pain.[29–31] Initiation of opioid therapy is unlikely to offer concomitant and proportional improvement in all of these areas. If the psychological amplifiers of pain perception have not been adequately addressed, opioid-induced analgesia may not be maximally effective. Likewise, analgesia and functional improvement resulting from opioid therapy may be discordant with improvements due to psychological treatment. Many possible variations in efficacy and functional gain may dictate flexibility in ascertaining treatment endpoints.

Because pain reduction is subjective, it can serve as only a single aspect of adequate COT. Consider, for example, the patient who has constant pain rated "6 out of 10" ("0" being no pain and "10" being severe pain) with significantly associated disability. Although opioid therapy may only decrease the patient's pain from a 6 to a 5, a successful outcome has been achieved if the patient demonstrates improvements in activities of daily living (ADL), ability to participate in physical rehabilitation, and/or ability to return to work. Conversely, an opioid trial can be considered counterproductive if the patient reports increased pain relief without observable functional gains and possibly even signs of functional loss (daytime sedation, impaired cognition, voluntary unemployment, dysfunctional interpersonal or family relationships, diminished physical activity, or legal difficulties).

Although the effectiveness of opioid therapy is a primary concern, an equally important part of opioid management relates to deciding when to discontinue treatment if it is deemed to be unsatisfactory. Determination of a treatment failure requires consideration of multiple contributing factors, including (1) underdosing; (2) inappropriate dosing schedule; (3) improper drug delivery route; (4) potentially diminished opioid responsiveness relating to the nature of the pain generator (e.g., neuropathic pain); (5) involvement of unresolved contributors to pain, such as physical, psychological, and social disability; and (9) development of side effects that limit dose escalation. Apparent opioid ineffectiveness from a single opioid may not predict the same ineffectiveness from other opioids.[32]

The duration of opioid therapy remains a question with no clear consensus among practitioners and minimal science to guide the debate. Pharmacologic tolerance to opioids can develop during treatment and may require either escalating the dose to maintain the same level of analgesia or switching to a different opioid. Deciding to raise the dose requires reassessment of the risks and benefits and medical decision making that would warrant accepting these increased risks. The need to rotate to another opioid is expected to arise in less than 2% to 3% of cases.[33] Although some clinical studies have suggested stabilizing the opioid dose requirement following an initial dose increase, it is possible that periodic increases may be warranted during COT. For opioid-tolerant patients, changing from one opioid to another requires knowledge of equianalgesic dosages. Since cross-tolerance between opioids may be incomplete, a patient who has become tolerant to one opioid can respond with effective analgesia to another opioid of less than equianalgesic dose. Management of pain in tolerant patients can be a challenge because typical dosages for the opioid-naive patient do not apply. In such cases, opioids are slowly and incrementally increased until analgesia with tolerable side effects is reached. However, it is important to note that the risks of opioid therapy are dose-dependent and that CDC guidelines now suggest specific dose ranges for opioid prescribing.[5,6,25] Analgesia occurring only in conjunction with intolerable side effects indicates that the particular opioid is suboptimal and that there may be a need to change to a different opioid or that the pain is not opioid-sensitive. Analgesia occurring only in combination with sedation after an individual trial of most or all opioids suggests opioid-insensitive pain. Additionally, analgesia may also be related to effects associated with sedation rather than direct antinociceptive properties of the drug. As one would expect, side effects without analgesia indicate failure of that particular opioid. In such cases, another opioid may be worth trying, as it may not share the same profile. Clearly, determining the duration of effective opioid therapy must be individualized based on treatment efficacy balanced with side effects and progression or regression of the underlying disease process. Ultimately it may be impossible to know how much pain would be present without opioid therapy unless the medication is tapered.

SELECTED OPIOIDS

MEPERIDINE

Although meperidine (Demerol) is a common analgesic, particularly by the IM route, its primary use in the pain management setting has steadily declined due to its potential for neurotoxicity. Meperidine was developed in Nazi Germany as a synthetic opioid with relatively weak μ-opioid receptor agonist properties. Compared to morphine, it is one-tenth as potent and has a slightly more rapid onset and shorter duration of action.[34] At equianalgesic doses, meperidine produces less sedation and pruritus and may be more effective in treating neuropathic pain.[34] However, it possesses significant cardiac (orthostatic hypotension and direct myocardial depression),[34] anticholinergic, and local anesthetic properties, which decrease its therapeutic window.[35] Epidural or spinal administration of meperidine, unlike other opioids, can produce sensory, motor, and sympathetic blockade.[34] Meperidine has been used in the operative setting for the treatment of postanesthesia shivering.

Meperidine has a relatively short half-life of 3 hours and prolonged administration (>3 days) is problematic due to the potential for accumulation of normeperidine, its neurotoxic metabolite. Meperidine is demethylated in the liver to normeperidine, which has a half-life of 12 to 16 hours and is well documented to produce central nervous system (CNS) hyperactivity and ultimately seizures.[36] Since normeperidine is excreted by the kidneys, its adverse effects are most commonly although not exclusively seen in patients with renal impairment. Normeperidine toxicity initially manifests as subtle mood alteration and may progress to potentially naloxone-irreversible tremors, myoclonus, and seizures. Because the hyperexcitability due to normeperidine can also occur in patients with normal renal function, chronic administration of meperidine is not recommended. Finally, for patients on monoamine oxidase inhibitors, coadministration of meperidine can have potentially fatal outcomes. Caution may be prudent in coadministering meperidine and any other serotonergic drugs such as selective serotonin reuptake inhibitors (SSRIs), tramadol, or methadone.

MORPHINE

Morphine is the prototypical mu-opioid receptor agonist against which all other opioids are compared for equianalgesic potency. It can be given via oral, IV, epidural, or intrathecal routes for perioperative and postoperative pain management. As an SAO, it is available in instant-release (IR) formulations (morphine, MSIR, and Roxanol). As an SRO (MS-Contin, Oramorph-SR, Kadian, and Embeda), its dosing frequency ranges from every 8 to every 24 hours. Unique among currently available SROs, Embeda contains both morphine (an opioid agonist) and naltrexone (an opioid receptor antagonist). It was the first "abuse-deterrent" opioid formulation on the market. When taken as directed, naltrexone remains inert. However, if the medication is crushed for IV injection, naltrexone will antagonize the effects of morphine.

With repeated dosing, morphine's oral bioavailability ranges from 24% to 40%.[37,38] Morphine's low bioavailability and relative hydrophilicity make it less than ideal as an analgesic. Because of the delay in transport across the blood-brain barrier, morphine has a slower onset of action than other opioids. Conversely, morphine has a relatively longer analgesic effect of 4 to 5 hours relative to its plasma half-life (2–3.5 hours), thereby minimizing its accumulation and contributing to its safety.[36] The disproportionate duration of analgesia versus plasma half-life is due in part to its low solubility and slower elimination from the brain compartment relative to the plasma concentration.[35] Although morphine's pharmacologic activity is primarily due to the parent compound, morphine's efficacious and toxic effects can also be mitigated or perpetuated by two of its major metabolites: morphine 3-glucuronide (M3G) and morphine 6-glucuronide (M6G). M3G lacks any μ- and δ-opioid receptor activity and accounts for approximately 50% of morphine's metabolites. It has been shown in animals to cause generalized hyperalgesia, CNS irritability, seizure, myoclonus, and development of tolerance.[39] Whether this explains why neuroexcitatory side effects occur in humans exposed to chronic dosing of morphine has yet to be conclusively proven. Although M3G is devoid of opioid receptor activity, its true mechanism of action remains unknown. Conversely, M6G is a μ- and δ-opioid receptor agonist and accounts for approximately 5% to 15% of morphine's metabolites. M6G has intrinsic opioid agonism and sustains analgesia in addition to side effects. The route of morphine administration may account for variations in concentration of both glucuronide metabolites. Because the IV and rectal routes of administration avoid hepatic biotransformation, their glucuronide concentrations are less than with oral administration.[40,41] Chronic use of oral morphine ultimately results in higher circulating concentrations of the glucuronides (mean ratios of M3G:M6G range from 10:1 to 5:1) than the parent compound.[35] Patients experiencing side effects attributable to M3G and/or M6G may be candidates for rotation to an alternative opioid.

Since morphine's elimination is dependent on hepatic mechanisms, it should be used with caution in cirrhotic patients. However, enterohepatic cycling and extrahepatic metabolism of morphine have also been reported to occur in the gastric and intestinal epithelia.[35] The glucuronides can also undergo deconjugation back to morphine by colonic flora and subsequently be reabsorbed.[35] Because morphine metabolites are excreted through the kidneys, the dose should be adjusted in those with renal impairment in order to minimize the risk of adverse side effects associated with the accumulation of glucuronide metabolites. Smith reported that although respiratory depression, sedation, and vomiting due to relatively high concentrations of M6G can be reversed by naloxone, the most concerning adverse effect in patients with compromised renal function is encephalopathy and myoclonus.[39] Studies have found that the ratio of M6G and M3G to morphine correlated with increased blood urea nitrogen or creatinine levels.[40,42] Ultimately, morphine's analgesic effects and side effects are likely related to complex interactions between the parent compound and its glucuronide metabolites. Exactly how specific diseases, polypharmacy, and patient age influence ratios of the individual glucuronide metabolites to morphine remains unclear.[35]

OXYCODONE

Oxycodone is a semisynthetic congener of morphine that has been used as an analgesic for over 80 years.[43] As an SAO, it is available in IR preparations as a single agent (oxycodone, OxyIR, or Roxicodone) or compounded with acetaminophen (Percocet, Endocet, or Roxicet) or aspirin (Percodan or Endodan). IR oxycodone has been shown to deliver equivalent analgesia as the sustained-release (SR) version (OxyContin).[44] In April 2010, the FDA approved a ("tamper-resistant") formulation of OxyContin that is more difficult to break, crush, chew, or dissolve for snorting or IV injection. In July 2014, the FDA approved an "abuse-deterrent" version of SR oxycodone-naloxone named Targiniq Extended-Release (ER): The naloxone blunts the euphoric effects of oxycodone if the user crushes and snorts or injects the drug. Postmarketing studies are still needed to determine its efficacy in reducing misuse and abuse.

SR oxycodone possesses many of the characteristics of an ideal opioid, including no ceiling dose, minimal side effects, minimal active metabolite, easy titration, rapid onset of action, short half-life, long duration of action, and predictable pharmacokinetics.[45] In comparison to SR morphine, it has a prolonged pharmacokinetic profile, which theoretically allows it to be administered solely on an every-12-hour dosing schedule. This, however, reflects a characteristic of the drug delivery system rather than a property of the drug itself. The oral bioavailability of oxycodone (55%–64%)[46] relative to morphine (24%–40%) can account for variations in dose conversion ratios between the two drugs. Milligram-to-milligram, oral oxycodone is more potent than morphine and has a shorter onset of analgesia with less plasma variation. Accordingly, oxycodone is associated with fewer side effects (hallucinations, dizziness, and pruritus) than morphine.

Although it possesses some intrinsic analgesic properties via activation of the κ-opioid receptors, oxycodone appears to have lower affinity than morphine for the mu-opioid receptor in rat studies. It undergoes hepatic metabolism via the cytochrome P450 2D6 enzyme, where it is converted into oxymorphone, an active metabolite with high affinity for the μ-opioid receptor, and via CYP3A4 to noroxycodone, an inactive metabolite. In the approximately 10% of the population with genetically low levels of the cytochrome P450 2D6 enzyme, lower concentrations of oxymorphone may account for the fact that higher than usual doses of oxycodone may be necessary to obtain pain relief. Analgesic efficacy may also be decreased in those concurrently taking medications that competitively inhibit the P450 2D6 enzyme. Analgesic efficacy may be increased in those patients concurrently taking medications that inhibit the P450 3A4 enzyme. Whether the relationship between impaired hepatic metabolism and decreased analgesia has anything to do with lower levels of oxymorphone remains uncertain. Therefore careful dose titration must be ensured for those concurrently taking medications with potential drug interactions such as SSRIs, TCAs, azoles, mycins, or neuroleptics. Finally, because the kidneys excrete oxycodone and its metabolites, the dose should be adjusted in cases of renal dysfunction.[47]

OXYMORPHONE

Oxymorphone is a semisynthetic opioid that has been available as an IV preparation (Numorphan) since 1959 and subsequently as a rectal suppository (Numorphan). It was not until 2006 that an oral formulation (Opana IR and ER) was released.[48] Oxymorphone is primarily a μ-opioid receptor agonist that has more affinity for the μ-opioid receptor than morphine and is 10 times as potent as morphine when given intravenously.[48–54] Oxymorphone's affinity for the δ-opioid receptor is greater than that of morphine, with agonism decreasing tolerance as well as potentiating μ-opioid receptor–mediated analgesia. In general oxymorphone has little or no affinity for the κ–opioid receptor, has less histamine release from mast cells than morphine, and is more fat-soluble than morphine and oxycodone.[48,49,52,54] However, oxymorphone does not redistribute into fat stores but rather dissociates slowly from receptors in the CNS.[51] The increase in lipophilicity leads to maximum plasma concentrations in 30 minutes, compared with 1.2 hours for immediate-release morphine.[48]

Although well absorbed in the gastrointestinal (GI) tract, oxymorphone's bioavailability is only 10% due to extensive first-pass hepatic metabolism. Even though the bioavailability of oxymorphone is lower than that of morphine (24%–40%) or oxycodone (55%–64%), oxymorphone's greater lipid solubility facilitates its ability to cross the blood-brain barrier and may account for its rapid onset of analgesia: The time to maximum plasma concentration is shorter for oxymorphone IR (30 minutes) compared with morphine IR (1.2 hours) and oxycodone IR (1.5 hours).[48–50,53,54] The onset of analgesia for the IR formulation occurs in 30 to 60 minutes and follows linear pharmacokinetics, allowing for predictable dosing.[48–51,53,54] For the ER formulation, steady-state occurs in 3 days with every-12-hour dosing.[53]

Oxymorphone is hepatically metabolized and renally excreted. It requires dosing adjustment for hepatic and renal impairment.[50,54] For those with moderate to severe hepatic impairment, oxymorphone is contraindicated.[48] Because moderate to severe renal impairment can result in bioavailability as high as 57% to 65%, clinicians should proceed with caution and reduce dose accordingly.[48] The main metabolite of oxymorphone, oxymorphone-3-glucorinide, has unknown activity and is produced in the liver via uridine diphosphate glucuronosyl transferase enzymes after reduction or conjugation with glucuronic acid.[48–51,53,54] A secondary metabolite, 6-OH-oxymorphone, is formed by reduction by an unknown enzyme and possesses analgesic activity.[48,53] There appears to be minimal interaction with the cytochrome P450 enzyme systems such that oxymorphone is not metabolized by the CYP2D6 enzyme and does not interact with the CYP2C9 or CYP3A4 enzymes.[53] Compared with other strong opioids, oxymorphone has similar efficacy in the treatment of acute, chronic, and cancer pain and a similar side-effect profile.[53,54] Since taking this medication with food can greatly increase the maximum plasma concentration, it is advisable to avoid eating at least 1 hour prior to or 2 hours after taking this medication.[48–51,54] Alcohol should be avoided, as it can produce an almost 300% increase in the plasma concentration.[49,51]

HYDROMORPHONE

Hydromorphone is a hydrogenated ketone analogue of morphine that can be formed by the N-demethylation of hydrocodone. It can be given via oral, IV, epidural, or intrathecal routes for perioperative and postoperative pain management. As an oral medication, it is available in an IR formulation (hydromorphone or Dilaudid) and an SR formulation (Exalgo), with the latter affording once-daily dosing for chronic pain management.

Like morphine, hydromorphone is hydrophilic, possesses strong μ-opioid receptor agonist activity, and has a similar duration of analgesic effect (3 to 4 hours). However, side effects of pruritus, sedation, and nausea and vomiting occur less frequently with hydromorphone than with morphine.[33] Depending on whether it is administered orally or intravenously, hydromorphone's milligram-to-milligram potency is estimated to be 5 to 7 times that of morphine, respectively. Hydromorphone bioavailability ranges from 20% to 80% when administered by the oral route. Onset of analgesic effect occurs within 30 minutes when administered orally and 5 minutes when administered intravenously. The peak analgesic effect of IV hydromorphone occurs within 8 to 20 minutes, most likely because its hydrophilicity impairs its ability to cross the blood-brain barrier.[55]

Although it is hydrophilic, it is 10 times as lipid-soluble as morphine. This feature, plus its greater milligram-to-milligram potency compared with morphine, allows equianalgesic doses to be infused subcutaneously but in smaller volumes (10 or 20 mg/mL). Possessing 78% of the bioavailability of IV hydromorphone,[33] subcutaneously administered hydromorphone offers a safe alternative for hospice patients with impaired GI function and requires less maintenance than would be required with an IV site.

Hydromorphone undergoes hepatic biotransformation into hydromorphone-3-glucuronide (H3G), its primary metabolite, with both the parent compound and metabolite being renally excreted. Like morphine's M3G metabolite, H3G is an active metabolite that lacks analgesic efficacy but possesses potent neuroexcitatory properties that are 10 times stronger than those of the parent compound and that have been shown to produce neuroexcitation (allodynia, myoclonus, and seizures) when administered directly into the lateral ventricle of rat brains.[35] Because H3G is produced in such small quantities, its effects are negligible except in cases of renal insufficiency, where it may accumulate. Nonetheless, because H3G is produced in such small amounts, hydromorphone is preferable to morphine in patients with renal insufficiency. Concentrations of H3G are dose-dependent and clear with time once hydromorphone is discontinued.

METHADONE

According to the *American Heritage Dictionary*, the name *methadone* is a derivative merging of the words that describe its chemical structure, 6-dimethylamino-4,4-diphenyl-3-heptanone.[56] When one hears the word *methadone*, many images come to mind. Although clinicians trained in the use of methadone to treat pain may envision the drug as a potential source of analgesia, patients and other health care providers may have difficulty separating the idea of methadone from heroin addiction and drug rehabilitation programs. In 2008, a total of 268,071 patients in the United States were using methadone in opioid treatment programs and nearly 720,000 patients were using methadone to treat chronic pain.[57,58] The wide use of methadone is likely due to its many attractive features as an analgesic medication: low cost (wholesale price is approximately 5% to 7% that of the more expensive proprietary SROs), high bioavailability with absorption and activity within 30 minutes, multiple receptor affinities, and lack of known metabolites that produce neurotoxicity. Methadone is well absorbed and has an oral bioavailability (approximately 80%; range 40% to 99%) that is approximately threefold that of morphine.[59,60] Its sublingual bioavailability ranges from 34% to 75%, with higher absorption favored by a higher pH of 8.5 in the sublingual space.[61,62] Unfortunately methadone's pharmacokinetics and pharmacodynamics, exemplified by unpredictable bioavailability and high interindividual variability in steady-state serum levels, can make it a challenge to initiate and titrate, thereby increasing the potential for delayed methadone-related side effects. As methadone use as an analgesic has risen, it has gained attention because of a significant increase in unintentional overdoses and has led the FDA in 2006 to issue a manufacturer's black box warning for QT prolongation and serious arrhythmia. Although methadone accounts for only 2% of the prescribed opioids, it is responsible for 30% of the deaths due to prescription opioid medications.[63] Indeed, initial dosing or escalation of methadone requires more frequent follow-up than other LAOs/SROs.[5,6]

Methadone, which is structurally unrelated to other opium-derived alkaloids, is available as a hydrochloride powder that can be reconstituted for oral, rectal, or IV administration. It is lipophilic, basic (pK_a, 9.2), and usually exists as a racemic mixture of its two isomers, d-methadone (S-met) and 1-methadone (R-Met), both of which have separate modes of action. The d-isomer antagonizes the NMDA receptor, blocks the hERG (human ether-a-gogo related gene) voltage-gated potassium channel, and inhibits serotonin and norepinephrine reuptake, while the l-isomer (R-met) possesses the opioid receptor agonist properties.[64] Among opioid receptor subtypes, methadone demonstrates variable affinity. Animal models demonstrate that it has a lower affinity than morphine for the μ-opioid receptor, which may explain why methadone may have fewer μ-opioid receptor–related side effects.[65] Conversely, methadone has a greater affinity than morphine for the δ-opioid receptor.[66] Although δ-opioid receptor activity is felt to be crucial to the development of morphine-induced tolerance and dependence, methadone's δ-opioid receptor agonism leads to its desensitization. This feature may partially account for methadone's ability to counteract opioid-induced tolerance and dependence.[67] Aside from acting as an opioid receptor agonist, methadone also acts as an NMDA receptor antagonist.[68–71] Numerous studies have demonstrated the involvement of the NMDA receptor mechanisms in the development of opioid tolerance and neuropathic pain.[70,71] In theory, methadone's ability to mitigate opioid-induced tolerance and treat neuropathic pain remains an intriguing but unproven concept.

Methadone's lipophilicity most likely accounts for its extensive tissue distribution (mean volume of distribution, 6.7 mL/kg) and slow elimination (mean half-life, 26.8 hours; range, 15 to 55 hours).[60,72] Its delayed clearance (mean 3.1 mL/min per kilogram) provides the basis for once-daily dosing for methadone maintenance therapy, thereby preventing the onset of opioid withdrawal syndrome for 24 hours or more.[72] Unfortunately the same does not hold true for analgesia. Furthermore, there is extensive interindividual variation in the relationship between changes in plasma methadone concentration and analgesia.[73] The ability to use methadone for either opioid detoxification or analgesia can be explained by methadone's biphasic elimination phase. The α-elimination phase (distribution phase), which lasts 8 to 12 hours, equates to the period of analgesia that typically does not exceed 6 to 8 hours. Consequently initial dosing for analgesia may need to be frequent, because steady-state kinetics is required for reaching the biphasic profile. The β-elimination phase (clearance), which ranges from 30 to 60 hours, may be sufficient for preventing opioid withdrawal symptoms but is insufficient for providing analgesia. This provides the rationale for prescribing methadone every 24 hours for opioid maintenance therapy versus every 6 to 12 hours for analgesia.

Unlike other opioids whose breakdown products contribute to potential neurotoxicity, methadone has no known active metabolites. It undergoes hepatic metabolism, primarily N-demethylation, by the cytochrome P450 (CYP) family of enzymes. As a result, methadone has multiple potential drug interactions that can result from induction, inhibition, or substrate competition at several of the CYP enzymes, including CYP3A4, CYP2D6, and CYP2B6.[74] In the absence of other drugs, CYP3A4 is an autoinducible enzyme, which means that methadone can bring about its own metabolism and increase its clearance over time.[65] However, one study found that methadone and its metabolite (2-ethyl-1,5-dimethyl-3,3-diphenylpyrrolidine) did not change significantly over a 9-month period, indicating that autoinduction by methadone may not occur.[75] Patients who have the CYP2B6 *6/*6 genotype, approximately 6% of Caucasians, are poor metabolizers of racemic methadone and are at increased risk of prolonged QTc interval due to high plasma concentrations of (S)-methadone (d-methadone).[64,76] In addition to the possibility of drug interactions, gastric pH can affect methadone's degree of absorption. For example, patients who are also taking omeprazole will absorb more methadone.

For most patients, renal excretion of unchanged methadone is insignificant. However, decreases in urinary pH can significantly increase methadone excretion. For example, in patients with acidic urine who are taking high doses of ascorbic acid, about 34% of an administered dose could be excreted in the urine as unchanged methadone.[77,78] Although changes in urinary pH can also influence the renal excretion of methadone, it does not accumulate in renal failure and does not appreciably filter during hemodialysis.[79] Thus the possibility of methadone toxicity is increased in the setting of polypharmacy and/or changes in either gastric or urinary pH. Finally, variability in protein binding, excretion, and equianalgesic potency can further contribute to methadone's potential instability by provoking either overdose or withdrawal symptoms. Although signs of toxicity are often clear, signs of decreased analgesia or withdrawal symptoms due to involuntary decreases in free circulating methadone may not be as apparent. Such patients may be erroneously characterized as drug-seeking because they display signs and symptoms of pseudoaddiction, requiring higher doses of methadone.

Methadone has an inherently longer duration of effect than other nonmodified opioids or SROs. Unlike the SROs, methadone tablets can be broken in half or chewed. Methadone is also available in an elixir formulation (1 mg/mL or 10 mg/mL), which is advantageous for those with a gastrostomy feeding tube, thus minimizing the risk of clogging the tube by not having to crush a tablet. In addition, the low-concentration elixir theoretically allows for a relatively more careful and precise titration of methadone, which can potentially minimize the risk of delayed-onset toxicity. Ultimately, methadone's pharmacodynamic property as an LAO makes it beneficial for those with impaired GI absorption secondary to "short-gut syndrome" or "dumping syndrome." It can also be used for patients with renal impairment, since it does not accumulate in renal failure and is insignificantly removed during dialysis.

The many attractive features of methadone relate to its pharmacologic complexity. This, however, can increase the risk of side effects, especially in patients with cardiac issues, those with concomitant illness, or those on multiple medications. As awareness of the proarrhythmic potential—prolongation of QTc interval resulting in torsades de pointes—of methadone has increased, experts have developed consensus guidelines to help clinicians safely prescribe methadone and minimize the risk of cardiotoxicity.[5,6,80] The guidelines suggest that clinicians inform patients of methadone's risk of proarrhythmia, look for a history of cardiac disease, obtain a baseline electrocardiogram followed by periodic monitoring of the QTc interval, and be aware of other factors or medications that might contribute to a QTc prolongation (Table 42.3).[80] Furthermore, uncertainty remains regarding methadone's equianalgesic dosing conversion. A recent review of opioid conversion ratios used with methadone found a relatively strong positive correlation between the previous morphine dose and the final methadone dose and dose ratio, but ratios varied widely.[81] Contrary to logic as it relates to tolerance, methadone appears to have greater potency (milligram-per-milligram) in patients rotating from high dosages of other opioids. Its antagonism of the NMDA receptor may help explain why methadone appears to have increasing potency as a patient's daily morphine-equivalent dose increases when converting from another opioid to methadone.[65] In the opioid-tolerant patient, the exact equianalgesic dose for methadone as a conversion from morphine-equivalents is uncertain. Older equianalgesic tables are usually based on studies that included normal controls or opioid-naive patients; therefore they do not take into account chronic opioid exposure. This tends to lead to excessive dosages. A panel comprising experts from the American Academy of Pain Medicine and American Pain Society recommended that a safe starting dose in most opioid-naive adults is 2.5 mg orally every 8 hours with subsequent dose increases no more often than weekly.[9] This same panel could not recommend a particular method for converting patients from other opioids to methadone but did suggest that opioid-tolerant patients generally should start at doses no higher than 30 to 40 mg/day, even those previously on high doses of other opioids. Converting from methadone to another opioid is even less clear due to the small number of studies available to offer uniform guidelines. A recent study attempted to quantify the conversion ratio when transitioning from methadone to morphine and determined that it is approximately 1:5.[82] Therefore methadone presents the inexperienced clinician with the challenge of predicting effects, not only in the face of unreliable and confusing equianalgesic dosing ratios but also because of its potential for drug interactions, metabolic instability related to altered hepatic metabolism or renal clearance, and protein-binding changes. In making a conversion to or from methadone, use extreme caution and reference the methadone package insert for the most updated information.

TABLE 42.3 Consensus Guidelines for Prescribing Methadone

- The panel suggests that for patients with risk factors for QTc interval prolongation, any prior electrocardiogram (ECG) demonstrating a QTc > 450 ms, or a history of syncope, clinicians perform follow-up ECG 2–4 weeks after initiation of methadone therapy and following significant dose increases.
- The panel suggests that for all patients, clinicians perform follow-up ECG when the methadone dose reaches 30–40 mg/day in patients started at lower doses, and again at 100 mg/day.
- The panel suggests that clinicians perform follow-up ECG for all patients prescribed methadone with new risk factors for QTc interval prolongation or signs or symptoms suggesting arrhythmia.
- The panel recommends that clinicians switch methadone-treated adults with QTc interval ≥500 ms to an alternate opioid or immediately reduce the methadone dose; in all such cases, the panel recommends that clinicians evaluate and correct reversible causes of QTc interval prolongation, and repeat the ECG after the methadone dose has been decreased.
- The panel recommends that clinicians consider switching methadone-treated adults with QTc interval ≥450 ms but <500 ms to an alternative opioid or reducing the methadone dose. In patients in whom there are barriers to switching to alternative opioids, or who experience decreased treatment effectiveness with methadone dose reductions, the panel recommends that clinicians discuss with patients the potential risks of continued methadone. In all cases, the panel recommends that clinicians evaluate and correct reversible causes of QTc interval prolongation, and repeat the ECG after the methadone dose has been decreased.

From Chou R, Cruciani RA, Fiellin DA, et al.: A clinical practice guideline from the American Pain Society and College on Problems of Drug Dependence, in collaboration with the Heart Rhythm Society. J Pain. *15(4):321-337, 2014.*

BUPRENORPHINE

Buprenorphine is a highly lipophilic Schedule III semisynthetic opioid that is a derivative of the thebaine, the morphine alkaloid that was developed in the late 1960s. Used primarily as an alternative to methadone maintenance therapy, it is regaining popularity as an analgesic for treating chronic pain.[83–86] Buprenorphine is available in sublingual, buccal, transdermal, and IV formulations. Several of the sublingual and buccal formulations (Suboxone, Bunavail, Zubsolv) also contains the μ-opioid receptor antagonist naloxone. The ratio of buprenorphine to naloxone is generally 4:1.[85] Although buprenorphine has low abuse potential, the addition of naloxone will block opioid effects in opioid-naive patients and potentially produce withdrawal in opioid-sensitive patients who try to inject this formulation.[83,85,87] For maintenance dosing in addicted patients, dosing ranges from once daily to as infrequently as three times a week.[83,88]

Buprenorphine has complex pharmacologic activity at the μ-opioid receptor that may be misunderstood because of extrapolation of results from early animal studies and poor description of endpoints used to define its activity. A simple but accurate way to describe buprenorphine activity separates its effects on respiratory depression from analgesia.

Buprenorphine is a full agonist at the at μ-opioid receptor when measuring analgesia as the endpoint. Buprenorphine is a partial agonist at the μ-opioid receptor when measuring respiratory depression as the endpoint.[89,90] Buprenorphine has antagonist activity at κ- and δ-opioid receptors. Its unique properties as a full μ-opioid receptor agonist for analgesia, partial μ-opioid receptor agonist for respiratory depression, and κ-opioid receptor antagonist make this drug appealing as an analgesic, especially with regard to its adverse effects. Compared with other opioids, buprenorphine alone has a ceiling effect for respiratory depression but no ceiling for analgesia; however, when it is combined with other medications that suppress respiratory drive, such as benzodiazepines, buprenorphine can have respiratory depressant effects.[91] Buprenorphine appears to cause less euphoria and stimulate less craving due to antagonism at the κ-opioid receptor.[83,85,86] Studies also suggest that there may be less tolerance with buprenorphine.[84,88] Limited spinal analgesia, dysphoria, and psychotomimetic effects are due to its antagonist effects at the κ-receptor.[85] Buprenorphine also acts on opioid receptor like-1 (ORL-1) receptors, which may contribute to antihyperalgesia, but it may counteract its antinociceptive effects. One proposed explanation for these opposing effects suggests that binding to ORL-1 receptors in different parts of the body has diverse clinical effects.[84,92]

Pharmacodynamically, sublingual buprenorphine has a slow onset of action (approximately 90 minutes) and a relatively long half-life (4 to 5 hours).[93] Its slow dissociation from the μ-opioid receptor may help to explain its prolonged duration of action, leading to once-daily dosing in opioid treatment programs.[83,85,86,88,94,95] The slow dissociation from the mu-opioid receptor may also be the reason why cessation of buprenorphine induces only mild withdrawal symptoms.[86,96] Buprenorphine exhibits high affinity for the μ-opioid receptor and is thought to be 30 to 40 times more potent than morphine, which allows for the attainment of effective analgesia at low receptor occupancy rates. Because its high affinity for the μ-opioid receptor blocks other opioids from binding, this may necessitate the use of a higher dose of a full μ-opioid receptor agonist if added to a patient's existing buprenorphine regimen.[85] Conversely, introduction of buprenorphine to a patient already taking an alternate opioid may precipitate opioid withdrawal symptoms. In a small retrospective study, single-step conversions appeared safe as long as the clinician carefully calculated the optimal buprenorphine dose and provided adequate doses of conventional opioids for breakthrough pain when starting buprenorphine in an opioid-tolerant patient.[97] However, more research is needed in this regard. Finally, buprenorphine's high affinity for the receptor means that usual doses of naloxone may not readily reverse any buprenorphine-induced respiratory depression. Although most opioid overdoses resulting in respiratory depression respond to doses of naloxone given in a range of 0.4 to 1 mg, buprenorphine-induced respiratory depression may require bolus doses of 2 to 3 mg of naloxone followed by a continuous infusion running at 4 mg/h.[98] The respiratory stimulant doxapram may be more appropriate in this setting.[34,99]

The bioavailability of oral buprenorphine, owing to its first-pass hepatic metabolism, is approximately 10% to 15%. However, when tablets are taken sublingually, the absolute bioavailability increases to 21% (range 12% to 33%).[100] Buprenorphine buccal films have even greater absolute bioavailability of approximately 46% to 65%.[101] Buprenorphine is hepatically metabolized primarily via the cytochrome P450 3A4 enzyme into nonactive and active metabolites. The nonactive metabolites (80% to 90%) are the result of glucoronidation, and the active metabolite (norbuprenorphine) results from N-dealkylation.[102,103] Because norbuprenorphine is more potent with regard to respiratory depression, use of buprenorphine must be closely monitored in patients with moderate to severe liver dysfunction or those who are on concomitant medications that may induce the CYP 3A4 enzyme.[85] However, buprenorphine appears to be safe in patients with renal disease, including those on dialysis.[85,86,88,94] Overall, the addition of buprenorphine as an alternative opioid offers a distinctive medication with a favorable safety profile as compared with other strong opioid medications.

FENTANYL

Originally formulated as part of a balanced anesthetic for use during surgical procedures, fentanyl continues to be used via the IV, epidural, and intrathecal routes for perioperative and postoperative pain management. Because fentanyl is highly lipophilic, it can present advantages or disadvantages, depending on the desired effect, due to its limited spread along the neuraxis when administered in the epidural or intrathecal space. Fentanyl possesses predominantly μ-opioid receptor agonist properties and little affinity for the κ- and δ-opioid receptors.[104] Compared with morphine, it has an inherently faster onset of action and is 75 to 125 times as potent.[34,36] It is hepatically metabolized by CYP3A4 into the inactive metabolite norfentanyl. When given intravenously, it has a high first-pass effect and 30- to 60-minute duration of analgesia.[104] Its greater degree of potency compared with other opioids allows for the delivery of smaller quantities of the drug measured in micrograms per hour. Although considered short acting, its lipophilicity allows for transdermal application for the management of chronic pain and transmucosal and buccal applications for the management of breakthrough cancer pain. Based on several studies reporting a 20% incidence of hypoventilation when it was used in acute postoperative pain management, transdermal fentanyl (Duragesic patch and other generic fentanyl patches) is recommended for use only in opioid-tolerant patients with chronic or cancer pain.[105]

In addition to a peel strip that protects the adhesive, the Duragesic patch consists of four layers: (1) the polyester backing layer, which is impermeable to drug loss or moisture penetration; (2) the drug reservoir, which contains fentanyl gelled with hydroxyethyl cellulose and ethanol, thus enhancing the transdermal absorption of fentanyl; (3) the rate-controlling membrane, which helps to control the rate of drug absorption (whereby 50% of the absorption rate is controlled by the membrane and 50% by the inherent resistance of the skin); and (4) the silicone adhesive layer, which keeps the patch in place when affixed to the skin.[106] Several newer generic patches use matrix technology that allows for cutting the patch without undermining drug delivery. The patch should be placed on the upper body on a hairless (clipped, not shaved), flat surface of skin that is free of defects. Once applied to the skin, sustained levels of analgesia can be achieved via fentanyl's continuous transdermal absorption.

Transdermal fentanyl permits 3-day dosing with avoidance of the first-pass effect of the liver, where fentanyl is metabolized primarily by the cytochrome P450 family of enzymes. Because transdermal fentanyl does not pass through the GI tract, it theoretically causes less constipation than oral opioids. Furthermore, not having to depend on the GI tract provides the rationale for prescribing it for those who are unable to tolerate oral medications secondary to chronic nausea and vomiting, in those with impaired GI absorption secondary to "short-gut syndrome" or "dumping syndrome," and in those with trouble adhering to oral medication regimens.

Unlike the titration of oral LAOs, dose titration of the patch can sometimes be difficult due to individual variations in the rate of transdermal absorption, faulty adherence of the patch to the skin due to perspiration (~10%), and other factors such as skin temperature, fat stores, and muscle bulk.[106] Because of the slow and variable rate of absorption after initial patch application or increase in patch dose, it can take 1 to 30 hours (mean value of 13 hours) before therapeutic serum levels are achieved.[107] Therefore, during the first 12 hours, patients may require an SAO or IV PCA to address breakthrough pain and to minimize withdrawal symptoms if rotation is from another opioid, especially since it takes approximately 3 days before steady-state is achieved.[108] The amount of SAO required after steady state is achieved may also determine if the patch dose needs to be changed, although caution is recommended in making rapid dose adjustments. Conversely, because it takes at least 16 hours before serum fentanyl concentrations drop by 50% after the patch is removed, one would also expect a delay in effects on analgesia or side effects on removing the patch. Patients should be advised to avoid submerging the patch in hot water, placing a heating pad over the patch, or placing the patch over broken skin, as all of these can influence the rate of drug absorption and attendant side effects. The most common side effects of the transdermal delivery system (<1%) are related to reactions with the patch adhesive, including erythema, itching, and occasional pustule formation.[62]

Breakthrough pain typically peaks in 3 to 5 minutes, lasts an average of 30 minutes, and usually occurs about 1 to 4 times per day.[109–111] Because onset of analgesia after administration of oral SAOs for breakthrough pain often lags behind the painful episode (30–45 minutes to reach peak effect) owing to variable GI absorption and/or first-pass hepatic metabolism, an alternative formulation of opioids was developed: rapid-onset opioids (ROOs), which are defined by an onset of analgesia of 15 minutes or less.[112–115] The currently available ROOs are fentanyl preparations (oral transmucosal fentanyl citrate [OTFC, brand name Actiq]; fentanyl buccal tablet [FBT, brand name Fentora]; fentanyl buccal soluble film [FBSF, brand name Onsolis]; sublingual fentanyl orally disintegrating tablet [sublingual fentanyl ODT, brand name Abstral]; fentanyl nasal spray [brand name Lazanda], and fentanyl sublingual spray [brand name Subsys]). All are approved only for breakthrough cancer pain and have the benefit of bypassing first-pass hepatic metabolism. All of these products require the prescribers to participate in an FDA-approved REMS training program.

OTFC was the first submucosal ROO to come to market. Unlike transdermal fentanyl, OTFC has a rapid onset of analgesia (15 minutes), short duration of action, and serum half-life of 193 to 386 minutes.[108] Compared with the IV route, it has 47% bioavailability.[104] Rapid absorption occurs via the buccal mucosa combined with slower absorption via the GI tract for the amount swallowed. OTFC yields peak serum concentrations within 20 to 40 minutes of starting a 15-minute application.[116] In a study comparing OTFC to IV morphine in acute postoperative pain, both demonstrated a similar onset of analgesia.[117] Absorption depends on the patient's application technique and is thus dependent on patient effort. Because OTFC contains sugar and has been associated with dental caries, attention to dental hygiene is recommended.[118]

The FBT was the second submucosal ROO approved for the treatment of breakthrough cancer pain. When placed in the buccal cavity, the FBT undergoes an effervescent reaction, theoretically to enhance buccal absorption, and dissolves in an effort-independent manner within 30 minutes.[115,119,120] Advantages of the FBT over OTFC include faster median time to maximum peak serum concentration (47 minutes vs. 91 minutes), greater proportion of transmucosal dose (48% vs. 22%), greater early systemic exposure of fentanyl, and lack of sugar.[115,119]

The FBSF (brand name Onsolis) was initially approved but subsequently removed from the market owing to issues related to its physical appearance. The FDA recently reapproved this medication after these issues were rectified.[121] This bilayer delivery technology uses a dual-layer polymer film consisting of a mucoadhesive layer containing the active drug and an inactive layer that facilitates unidirectional flow to prevent diffusion of drug into the oral cavity.[120] As with the FBT, application of the FBSF is effort-independent, produces greater early systemic exposure to fentanyl, and lacks sugar. It requires minimal saliva to dissolve upon immediately adhering to a moist mucosal membrane, completely dissolves within 15 to 30 minutes, and has an absolute bioavailability of 71%.[109,120]

The sublingual fentanyl ODT (brand name Abstral) is a sublingual fentanyl preparation combining a rapidly disintegrating tablet with soluble carriers coated with mucoadhesive agents which enables the quick dissolution of fentanyl, thus taking advantage of the highly permeable sublingual mucosa.[110,111] In one study, first detectable fentanyl plasma levels and peak serum concentrations were noted as early as 8 to 11 minutes and 40 to 57 minutes, respectively.[122] Like the FBT and FBSF, application of the sublingual ODT is effort-independent.

The fentanyl pectin nasal spray (FPNS, brand name Lazanda) was approved by the FDA in 2011. The FPNS uses the addition of pectin to help bind to cations of calcium ions in the nasal mucosa. This binding helps to prolong the duration of action of fentanyl compared with fentanyl nasal sprays without pectin.[123] Time taken to achieve maximal plasma concentration is between 15 and

21 minutes, depending on dose.[123] The fentanyl sublingual spray (FSS, brand name Onsys) is the latest ROO to be approved. The sublingual formulation allows a very rapid onset of the fentanyl medication. According to Parikh et al. in 2013, "after 10 minutes, plasma concentration of fentanyl reached 53.7% of C_{max} with FSS compared with 6.1% of C_{max} with OTFC."[116] The bioavailability of the FSS was reported to be 76%.[124]

Since dosing based on the total daily amount of a fixed opioid regimen is unpredictable, patients taking ROOs should be advised to start at the lowest dose and gradually titrate to effect.[119,125,126] This same dosing strategy is recommended even in converting from one rapid-onset fentanyl preparation to another, since variations in absorption and bioavailability among the three preparations makes them unequal on a microgram-to-microgram basis. Rapid absorption and short duration of effect make all four of the rapid-onset fentanyl preparations ideal analgesics for breakthrough cancer pain, especially in patients with impaired swallowing or an impaired GI tract.

SUFENTANIL

Used primarily in the operative setting as an IV or neuraxial analgesic, sufentanil (Sufenta) is a thiamyl analogue of fentanyl. Like fentanyl, sufentanil is lipophilic, predominantly hepatically metabolized by the CYP3A4 isoenzyme, and has a rapid onset with short duration of effect. Although the pharmacokinetics and pharmacodynamics of sufentanil and fentanyl are similar, sufentanil has a smaller volume of distribution, greater analgesic potency (IV, 5 to 7 times; epidural or intrathecal, 2 to 5 times), shorter half-life (2.7 hours vs. 3.1 to 7.9 hours), and more rapid onset of analgesia (IV, 1 to 3 minutes; epidural or intrathecal, 4 to 10 minutes) with a shorter duration of effect (IV, 20 to 45 minutes; epidural or intrathecal, 2 to 4 hours).[34,35] Sufentanil may also produce dose-related skeletal muscle rigidity.

ALFENTANIL

Also used primarily in the operative setting as an IV or neuraxial analgesic, alfentanil (Alfenta) is less lipophilic than fentanyl and sufentanil. Its lower lipid solubility means that it has a smaller volume of distribution (~25% of that of fentanyl and sufentanil). This, coupled with its short elimination half-life (70 to 111 minutes) and rapid onset of analgesia (IV, 1 to 2 minutes; epidural, 5 to 15 minutes) with a short duration of effect (IV, 10 to 15 minutes; epidural 4 to 8 hours), makes it ideal in an operative setting due to the lower probability of accumulation with repeated dosing or continuous infusion and its ease of rapid titration.[34,35] Like fentanyl and sufentanil, alfentanil is extensively metabolized in the liver by the CYP3A4 isoenzyme.

REMIFENTANIL

The most potent μ-opioid receptor agonist of the opioids discussed here, remifentanil (Ultiva), is administered intravenously for the induction and maintenance of anesthesia.[35] More lipophilic than fentanyl, sufentanil, and alfentanil, remifentanil also has a larger volume of distribution, a more rapid distribution and metabolism, a shorter elimination half-life (3 to 10 minutes), and a more rapid analgesic onset (1 minute), with a shorter duration of effect (5 to 10 minutes).[35] Unlike fentanyl, sufentanil, and alfentanil, remifentanil is not metabolized to any appreciable degree by the liver. Instead, its ester side-chain linkage subjects it to rapid degradation by tissue and plasma esterases into an inactive carboxylic acid metabolite that is renally excreted.[35] This confers unique pharmacokinetic and pharmacodynamic parameters that make remifentanil's actions brief and unaffected by renal or hepatic insufficiency. Brisk clearance and lack of accumulation with repeated dosing are advantageous features in an operative setting, but discontinuation of the infusion results in a rapid loss of analgesia.

KEY POINTS

- With an informed and cautious approach, opioids may be safe and effective for treating moderate to severe pain of both malignant and nonmalignant origin.
- Clinicians who choose to offer chronic opioid therapies must formulate rational and individualized regimens according to strategies such as those described by the CDC, FSMB Model Policy, and the APS/AAPM consensus guidelines.
- Safe opioid therapy requires a program for continuous and close observation of analgesia and possible adverse effects.
- Subjective reports of pain relief should be corroborated by documentation of objective signs of success, such as improvement in function.
- Experience dictates that improvements in functionality are more frequently encountered when a multidisciplinary treatment plan is employed.

REFERENCES

Access the reference list online at ExpertConsult.com.

CHAPTER 43 OPIOIDS USED FOR MILD TO MODERATE PAIN

Mark Holtsman, PharmD ◌ Charity Hale, PharmD

With 97 million prescriptions written in 2015 in the United States, the most commonly prescribed opioids are formulations combining the opioid (hydrocodone) with a nonopioid (acetaminophen).[1] When opioids are administered with aspirin, acetaminophen, or ibuprofen, these medications are referred to as "weak opioids." This is a misnomer referring to the limit to which they can be prescribed due to the restrictive dosing of the nonopioid component. For example, when a patient takes 12 hydrocodone/acetaminophen 10/325-mg tablets per day, they are receiving an impressive amount of opioid equivalent to approximately 180 mg oral morphine per day.[2] These products may not provide the optimum opioid sparing effects that are desired by patients when compared to patients utilizing these medications in separate formulations. These commonly prescribed combination formulations create a potential problem by mixing an opioid that has no dose ceiling effect with acetaminophen or a nonsteroidal antiinflammatory drug (NSAID), which may cause toxicity beyond a certain dose. Patients are often unaware of the potential renal or hepatic toxicity from the nonopioid component and may take over-the-counter (OTC) acetaminophen along with their prescribed combination formulation containing an opioid with acetaminophen.

Acetaminophen-related adverse events are a significant public health burden with an average of 112,000 poison center calls, 59,000 emergency department visits, and 38,000 hospitalizations annually in the United States.[3] Approximately half of all acetaminophen-related hepatotoxicity is caused by unintentional overdose, and 63% of these cases involve opioid combination products.[4,5] The National Poison Data System annual report from 2012 listed acetaminophen combination products as the sixth highest cause of fatalities related to substance poisoning.[6]

In 2009, a Food and Drug Administration (FDA) advisory committee voted in favor of eliminating prescription acetaminophen/opioid combination products, but the FDA has not followed this recommendation.[7] In 2011, the FDA announced that manufacturers of prescription acetaminophen-combination products would be required to limit the amount of acetaminophen in products to 325 mg per tablet, capsule, or other dosage with a January 2014 deadline for implementation.[3] By January 2014, over half of the pharmaceutical manufacturers had complied with this recommendation.[4] The FDA said that it would begin proceedings to withdraw approval of prescription combination drug products that contain more than 325 mg acetaminophen per dosage unit that remained on the market; it completed those proceedings in March 2014.[8]

There are few studies investigating the usual period of time that patients require opioid analgesics after surgery. As a result, clinicians are often unsure about the best quantity of opioids to prescribe for postoperative pain. A retrospective review of hydrocodone 5 mg and acetaminophen 500 mg (10 tablets 1 refill) prescriptions after orthopedic surgery (arthroscopies, anterior cruciate ligament, etc.) found 61% of patients did not refill their prescriptions and 89% required less than or equal to 20 tablets.[9] In another study, 250 patients given 30 tablets of oxycodone, hydrocodone, or propoxyphene were interviewed about medication usage after outpatient upper extremity surgery. Overall, each patient reported about 19 unused tablets, leaving approximately 4700 unused tablets for the entire study population.[10] Other investigators have shown that many patients use only 50% to 60% of their prescribed opioids after cesarean section, thoracic surgery, and urologic procedures.[11,12] Further research is needed to determine the optimal number of opioid tablets to prescribe to patients with different sources of pain because unused tablets are often ingested by people other than the patient, thereby contributing to the current opioid overdose epidemic in the United States.

This chapter reviews the use of short-acting opioids, and provides the reader with a practical approach to using these medications in clinical practice. It also reviews significant pharmacokinetic and pharmacogenetic variables that can influence analgesic efficacy, toxicity, and clearance, as well as potential drug interactions.

SPECIFIC SHORT-ACTING OPIOIDS

OXYCODONE

Oxycodone is found in the following branded combination products: Percocet, Roxicet Solution, Xartemis XR, Combunox, and Percodan. Oxycodone is a semisynthetic opioid processed from thebaine, an organic chemical found in opium. Oxycodone is available as an immediate-release tablet combined with acetaminophen, aspirin, or ibuprofen. It is also available as an immediate release (IR) solution and controlled-release tablet combined with acetaminophen. With so many formulations available, it is one of the most popular opioids in the United States. The popularity of oxycodone is, in some part, due to its suitability for oral administration due to high bioavailability (60%); oral oxycodone is 1.5 times more potent than oral morphine. Unfortunately, this property may also contribute to its abuse. Even though oxycodone in combination products has been placed in the more restricted Schedule II controlled substance category in the United States, its abuse has been a recurrent problem with law enforcement authorities. Clinicians also need to be aware that oxycodone is converted by P450 CYP2D6 hepatic enzymes to oxymorphone and P450 CYP3A4 to noroxycodone.

Patients that are poor metabolizers at CYP2D6 are at risk for accumulation of oxycodone if they take a drug such as fluconazole, a moderate CYP3A4 inhibitor. Similarly, patients taking a strong CYP2D6 inhibitor (paroxetine) and strong CYP3A4 inhibitor (itraconazole) are at risk for the accumulation of oxycodone.[13,14] It is less clear whether CYP2D6 phenotypes correlate with analgesia or risk of toxicity because physiologic effects correlate best with exposure to the parent compound, oxycodone.[15]

HYDROCODONE

Hydrocodone, an opium derivative, found in both combination products and single entity extended-release (ER) formulations was rescheduled from Schedule III to Schedule II on October 6, 2014 by the Drug Enforcement Administration. Hydrocodone is slightly less potent than oxycodone and is found in the following combination products: Norco, Hycet oral solution (hydrocodone and acetaminophen), and Vicoprofen (hydrocodone and ibuprofen). Clinicians need to be aware that hydrocodone is converted by P450 hepatic enzymes CYP2D6 to hydromorphone and CYP3A4 to norhydrocodone. Patients who are poor metabolizers at CYP2D6 are at risk for the accumulation of hydrocodone when given a potent CYP 3A4 inhibitor. A case report describing a fatal hydrocodone overdose provides evidence for the seriousness of drug interactions in patients that are poor metabolizers at CYP2D6. In this case, a young girl was given hydrocodone 3 times per day for cold symptoms, and clarithromycin for an ear infection. The patient used approximately 30 mg of hydrocodone over 24 hours along with clarithromycin, a potent CYP3A4 inhibitor. Postmortem hydrocodone blood concentration was 0.14 μg/mL, a concentration associated with fatality while the hydromorphone concentration was below the limit of detection 0.008 μg/mL (a finding expected in a poor metabolizer at CYP2D6). Postmortem analysis showed the patient had a CYP2D6 * 2A/*41 genotype, which is associated with poor metabolizer status.[16,17] As pharmacogenetic testing becomes more widely available, pharmacists with access to this patient data will be able to anticipate significant pharmacogenetic–drug interactions and help clinicians manage them.

CODEINE

Codeine has a very similar chemical structure to morphine, but has approximately 200 times less affinity for the mu-opioid receptor than morphine.[18] Approximately 5% to 10% of codeine is metabolized via the hepatic microsomal enzyme cytochrome P450 2D6 to morphine. In patients with poor metabolizer phenotype at CYP 2D6 (~5% to 10% of patients), there is greatly reduced morphine formation after codeine administration, leading to insufficient pain relief. In patients with ultrarapid metabolizer phenotype (~1% to 2% of patients), there is greatly increased morphine formation after codeine administration, leading to a higher risk of toxicity. The FDA issued a Boxed Warning that codeine is contraindicated in children undergoing tonsillectomy and/or adenoidectomy because deaths have occurred postoperatively in children with obstructive sleep apnea who received codeine for pain relief following a tonsillectomy and/or adenoidectomy. These children had evidence of being ultrarapid metabolizers of codeine.[19] When codeine (≤90 mg per dosage unit) is administered in combination with acetaminophen as an analgesic, it is placed in the Schedule III controlled substance category. This allows clinicians to prescribe codeine combination products with less regulatory restrictions than combination products containing oxycodone or hydrocodone. Many physicians view codeine as a safer analgesic than morphine as evidenced by the 13.2 million patients in the United States that received codeine-containing products in 2014.[20] On December 10, 2015, an FDA advisory committee recommended codeine be contraindicated for pain and cough management in children and adolescents younger than 18 years of age due to concerns about respiratory depression and death.[21]

TRAMADOL

Tramadol (Ultram) is a Schedule IV controlled substance and has a dual mechanism of action. Tramadol is a weak mu agonist and inhibits norepinephrine and serotonin reuptake. Tramadol is metabolized via CYP2D6 to the active metabolite *O*-desmethyl tramadol (M1).[22] The parent compound is primarily responsible for norepinephrine and serotonin reuptake inhibition, whereas M1 is primarily responsible for mu agonistic properties. Tramadol has approximately 6000 times less affinity for mu receptors than morphine. M1 has approximately 300 times greater affinity for mu receptors than the parent drug.[23] In contrast to tramadol and M1, tapentandol, which is discussed below, is a relatively strong opioid agonist and norepinephrine reuptake inhibitor. Patients who are poor CYP2D6 metabolizers form less M1 after tramadol administration, leading to inadequate pain relief. Patients who are ultrarapid CYP2D6 metabolizers produce an increased amount of M1 after tramadol administration, leading to higher risk of toxicities, such as respiratory depression and over-sedation. On September 21, 2015, the FDA issued a safety alert stating that the use of tramadol is under investigation when used in children 17 years and younger, due to increased risk for respiratory depression.[24] This alert was in response to the case report of a 5-year-old who experienced difficulty breathing after one dose of tramadol. It was later discovered the child was an ultrarapid metabolizer of CYP2D6 and had high levels of M1.[24] This risk may be increased in children following a tonsillectomy and/or adenoidectomy, or potentially after any other use in children. The risk of inadequate pain relief and toxicities can be reduced with preemptive genetic testing. Tramadol is mostly renally excreted (30% as unchanged drug and 60% as metabolites). In normal renal function, the maximum total daily dose is 400 mg.[22] In severe renal dysfunction (CrCl less than 30 mL/min), the IR formulation should not exceed 200 mg/day, and the dosing interval should be increased to 12 hours. The ER formulation of tramadol should be avoided in patients with severe renal dysfunction.[22–26]

TAPENTADOL

Tapentadol (Nucynta), a Schedule II controlled substance, is an opioid agonist and a norepinephrine reuptake inhibitor that works at both the ascending (excitatory) and descending (inhibitory) pathways.[27,28] Tapentadol appears to be 2 to 3 times less potent than morphine, even though its binding affinity for opioid receptors is 50 times lower.[29] Data suggest that 3.3 mg of oral tapentandol is equivalent to 1 mg of oral morphine equivalence in both opioid naïve and tolerant patients.[27]

Currently tapentadol is available in both IR (50, 75, and 100 mg) and ER (50, 100, 150, 200, and 250 mg) formulations. It is more expensive compared to other generically available opioids. Tapentadol has been shown equal to and noninferior to equianalgesic doses of oxycodone and morphine with a lower incidence of gastrointestinal side effects, including vomiting and constipation.[27,31–37] Tapentadol is generally well tolerated, but it may cause nausea, vomiting, dizziness, and drowsiness.[30] Although tapentadol does not directly increase serotonin levels, data suggest norepinephrine reuptake inhibition may indirectly elevate serotonin. This is demonstrated by case reports of serotonin syndrome, implying that additional serotonergic drugs should be avoided when prescribing tapentadol.[28] The IR formulation of tapentadol is FDA approved for moderate to severe acute pain, and has further shown efficacy for acute lower back pain and associated radicular leg pain, osteoarthritis pain, and postoperative pain secondary to dental and orthopedic surgeries.[31–33,38–40] The ER formulation is FDA approved for diabetic peripheral neuropathy severe enough to require daily, long-term, around-the-clock opioid use, and when alternative treatments are inadequate. The ER formulation has shown efficacy for chronic lower back pain, osteoarthritis knee pain, and moderate to severe chronic malignant tumor pain.[34–37,41,42] For acute moderate to severe pain, the IR formulation dose is 50 mg to 100 mg by mouth every 4 to 6 hours as needed. On the first day of therapy, a second dose may be administered one or more hours after the initial dose (maximum total daily dose is equal to 700 mg). Subsequential maximum total daily doses are 600 mg daily.[29–31,43]

Clinicians should be aware of how to transition a patient from a long-acting opioid to ER tapentadol. A general approach is to discontinue all other long-acting opioids, and then initiate ER tapentadol at 50% of the patient's current 24-hour oral morphine equivalence. Titration should be limited to 50 mg twice daily every 3 days until the most effective dose is achieved. During the titration process, an IR opioid may be used for breakthrough pain.[43,44]

Renal dose adjustments are not required for creatinine clearances greater than or equal to 30 mL/min; however, tapentadol should be avoided if creatinine clearance is less than 30 mL/min.[28,43]

Tapentadol is mostly metabolized to tapentadol-*O*-glucuronide via glucuronidation and, to a lesser degree, through oxidation via CYP2C9, CYP2C19, and CYP2D6 pathways. All metabolites are inactive. Hepatic dose adjustments are not required for mild dysfunction (Child–Pugh score 5 to 6). For moderate dysfunction (Child-Pugh score 7 to 9), the initial IR tapentadol dose should not exceed 50 mg by mouth every 8 hours, and the initial ER tapentadol dose should be limited to 50 mg by mouth once daily with a maximum ER dose of 100 mg daily. Tapentadol is not recommended for severe hepatic dysfunction (Child–Pugh score 10 to 15).[28,30,44]

CONCLUSION

Caution should precede the use of any opioid including "minor opioids" that are wrongly viewed as less potent or less dangerous than other opioids. Codeine and tramadol should not routinely be used for treatment of mild to moderate pain, since significant numbers of patients have unpredictable responses resulting in toxicity or inadequate analgesia. An FDA advisory committee has recommended against the use of codeine in children younger than 18 years of age. The same logic that went into that decision could be used to recommend against its use in adults as well. As IR hydrocodone is only available as a combination formulation with acetaminophen or an NSAID, it is difficult to utilize in a multimodal regimen with the goal of minimizing opioid consumption. Utilizing a multimodal approach, patients would be better served by around-the-clock acetaminophen and/or an NSAID as a single agent, plus the addition of a potent opioid analgesic, such as morphine, hydromorphone, or oxycodone, rather than a combination product containing codeine, tramadol, hydrocodone, or oxycodone. These combination products are not optimal components of a multimodal analgesic regimen, and they expose patients to an increased risk of toxicity. The pediatric population with acute and postoperative pain can benefit from oral solution formulations of opioid analgesics that make them more palatable in this age group (Table 43.1). Acetaminophen with codeine is included in this table for completeness, but it is not recommended for routine use in children or adults. Patients taking oxycodone or hydrocodone, who are poor metabolizers at CYP2D6, are at risk for significant drug interactions that can result in overdose and death.

Randomized trials have shown that multimodal analgesia involving simultaneous use of several medications acting at different receptors is associated with superior pain relief and decreased opioid consumption compared with the use of a single medication.[45–47]

When utilizing multimodal analgesia, the basis for using nonopioid analgesics is to reduce opioid consumption and lessen opioid-related adverse effects. There are several scenarios in which opioids may be preferable. As NSAIDs cause platelet dysfunction, their use in a patient with a low platelet count or a high risk for bleeding is relatively contraindicated. Likewise, the patient with a low threshold for bronchospasm may do better perioperatively with an opioid. Women may want to avoid NSAIDs during pregnancy as these medications may increase the risk of miscarriage. NSAIDs as a group tend to exacerbate reflux esophagitis and peptic ulceration. Individuals prone to these conditions may have less risk exposure with brief opioid therapy. Also at risk are patients with congestive heart failure, intrinsic renal disease, liver failure with ascites, and those receiving diuretics. Acetaminophen overdose toxicity is a growing concern and patients with hepatic impairment may have heightened risk from acetaminophen exposure.[48] Although opioid analgesics might appear to be advantageous in these scenarios, they must be used with caution because most are excreted by the kidneys and metabolized by the liver, and they carry many other risks.

TABLE 43.1 Opioid Oral Solutions

Generic Name	Brand Name	Formulation	Dose in Children Weighing <50 kg
Codeine	Tylenol with Codeine #3	Solution (120 mg acetaminophen/12 mg codeine per 5 mL)	Start at 0.5–1.0 mg/kg every 4 h as needed based on codeine
Hydrocodone	Hycet (hydrocodone with acetaminophen)	Solution (108 mg acetaminophen/2.5 mg hydrocodone per 5 mL)	Start at 0.1–0.2 mg/kg every 4 h as needed based on hydrocodone
Oxycodone	Roxicet (oxycodone with acetaminophen)	Solution (325 mg acetaminophen/5 mg oxycodone per 5 mL)	Start at 0.1–0.2 mg/kg/dose every 4 h based on oxycodone
Morphine	Roxanol	Morphine oral solution (100 mg/5 mL)	Start at 0.2–0.5 mg/kg/dose every 3–4 h as needed
Oxycodone	Roxicodone	Oxycodone oral concentrate (20 mg/mL)	Start at 0.1–0.2 mg/kg/dose every 4–6 h as needed
Hydromorphone	Dilaudid	Hydromorphone oral liquid (1 mg/mL)	Start at 0.03–0.08 mg/kg/dose every 3–4 h as needed

KEY POINTS

- The most commonly prescribed opioids in the United States—formulations combining hydrocodone and acetaminophen—are responsible for a significant number of acetaminophen-related adverse events due to unintentional overdose.
- Clinicians electing to utilize opioid analgesics combined with acetaminophen, ibuprofen, or aspirin should educate their patients to avoid taking OTC acetaminophen, ibuprofen, or aspirin to avoid unintentional overdose.
- Clinicians need to carefully consider the usual period of time patients require opioid analgesics after surgery, because several investigators have shown that many patients only utilize 50% of their prescribed opioids after surgery. These unused opioids may be ingested by people other than the patient, and further contribute to the opioid overdose epidemic in the United States.
- Patients with a CYP2D6 genotype associated with a poor metabolizer phenotype will not experience significant analgesia after taking codeine or tramadol.
- Patients with a CYP2D6 genotype associated with an ultrarapid metabolizer phenotype are more likely to experience toxicity after taking codeine or tramadol.
- Codeine and tramadol should not routinely be used for the treatment of mild to moderate pain because significant numbers of patients have inadequate analgesia or toxicity.
- Patients with a CYP2D6 genotype associated with a poor metabolizer phenotype, who are taking oxycodone or hydrocodone are at higher risk for significant drug interactions with medications that are CYP3A4 inhibitors. CYP3A4 inhibition in these patients can result in the accumulation of oxycodone or hydrocodone, which can lead to sedation and respiratory depression.
- Tapentadol is a unique analgesic with a dual mechanism of action making it useful for the treatment of neuropathic pain. It may have a lower incidence of gastrointestinal side effects when compared with equianalgesic doses of morphine or oxycodone.

REFERENCES

Access the reference list online at ExpertConsult.com.

CHAPTER 44

The Prescription Drug Abuse Epidemic and Emerging Prescribing Guidelines

Lynn R. Webster, MD

Around 100 million people in the United States struggle with some level of chronic pain,[1] and the prevalence is expected to worsen as the population ages.[2] Chronic pain isolates the sufferer and affects all aspects of social, family, and occupational life. Frequently, those who suffer speak of the irrevocable change pain wreaks upon their lives. Extended-release/long-acting (ER/LA) opioids are powerful analgesics that are indicated for pain that is severe enough to require daily, around-the-clock, long-term opioid treatment, and for which alternative treatment options are inadequate.[3] A careful risk-benefit analysis is essential to prescribing ER/LA opioids to prevent significant risk of associated harm from misuse, addiction, and overdose mortality. The same caution and clinical vigilance is necessary with opioids and any other central nervous system (CNS) depressants that may form part of a pain management regimen. Assessment of the potential benefits of opioid prescribing should include recognizing that long-term benefits are not proven by science, while risks are well established. Laws and regulations surrounding the use of opioids vary by state and are evolving at the federal level; however, consensus-based guidelines are available to assist health care providers. A common thread in guidelines is the need for careful risk assessment and management, including candidate selection, screening, and frequent clinical follow-up in patients treated with controlled substances for pain.

EMERGING PRESCRIBING GUIDELINES

Prescribers of opioids need awareness of multiple federal and state laws, regulations, and guidelines surrounding the use of controlled substances to treat pain. Some of these parameters have evolved rapidly in recent years, as policymakers move to reduce overdose mortality, the spread of nonmedical use, and the illicit diversion of pharmaceuticals. State strategies include the increasing use of prescription drug monitoring programs (PDMPs), leveraging state-run health plans to address inappropriate prescribing, widening access to naloxone to reverse opioid overdose, more access to substance-abuse treatment, and the promotion of state-published opioid prescribing guidelines.[4]

In addition, medical boards regulate practice within states to assure professional standards are met. Practice requirements are frequently listed on the website of each state's medical board or professional licensing agency. Many states have adopted—in whole or in part—the criteria set by the Federation of State Medical Boards (FSMB) for the use of opioids to treat chronic pain (Table 44.1).[5] In 2016, the Centers for Disease Control and Prevention (CDC) released a "Guideline for Prescribing Opioids for Chronic Pain," discouraging the use of opioids in treating chronic pain, excluding cancer and end of life (Table 44.2).[6] Unfortunately, insurance benefits are lacking for interdisciplinary pain treatments and alternatives to opioids, and dose limits fail to acknowledge individual analgesic response; these are matters the CDC does not adequately address in its guideline.[7] It should be noted that strong recommendations are backed by low-quality evidence, a feature common to many opioid-prescribing guidelines.

Common elements are found in practice guidelines developed by professional medical societies, states, or federal agencies. The CDC, in partnership with other federal agencies, reviewed eight guidelines developed before 2013. These guidelines, which were intended for general practitioners, failed to address specific conditions or subpopulations and excluded guidelines intended for specialists.[8–16] In addition, a systematic review of 13 opioid-prescribing guidelines[17] gave high marks to the joint guideline of the American Pain Society (APS) and American Academy of Pain Medicine (AAPM)[9] and

TABLE 44.1 Federation of State Medical Boards Model Policy for the Use of Opioid Analgesics in the Treatment of Chronic Pain

1. Thorough evaluation and risk stratification with an indication for prescribed opioids supported by history, physical, and appropriate tests before prescribing
2. Written treatment plan with stated objectives and consideration of pharmacologic and nonpharmacologic treatment modalities as appropriate
3. Informed consent on risks/benefits and an agreement for treatment outlining physician/patient responsibilities
4. Opioid trial following consideration of safer alternatives at lowest possible dose, titrated to effect
5. Regular review of the course of treatment to evaluate progress toward treatment objectives and to monitor adherence with medical direction, adjusting treatment when necessary, using "5A's": analgesia, activity, adverse effects, aberrant substance-related behaviors, and affect.
6. Periodic drug testing to ensure patient adherence (e.g., urine testing, pill counts, prescription database checks)
7. Referrals for additional and specialist evaluation and treatment if necessary
8. Continually weigh benefits versus risk of opioid therapy and institute opioid discontinuation plan if necessary (e.g., resolution of pain, intolerable side effects, inadequate analgesia, significant aberrant use, deteriorating function)
9. Accurate and complete records that include documentation of all of the above and all prescription orders
10. Familiarity and compliance with all state and federal laws and regulations regarding controlled substances

TABLE 44.2 Centers for Disease Control and Prevention Recommendations for Prescribing Opioids for Chronic Pain Outside of Active Cancer, Palliative, and End-of-Life Care

1. Nonpharmacologic therapy and nonopioid pharmacologic therapy are preferred for chronic pain. Clinicians should consider opioid therapy only if expected benefits for both pain and function are anticipated to outweigh risks to the patient. If opioids are used, they should be combined with nonpharmacologic therapy and nonopioid pharmacologic therapy, as appropriate
2. Before starting opioid therapy for chronic pain, clinicians should establish treatment goals with all patients, including realistic goals for pain and function, and should consider how opioid therapy will be discontinued if benefits do not outweigh risks. Clinicians should continue opioid therapy only if there is clinically meaningful improvement in pain and function that outweighs risks to patient safety
3. Before starting, and periodically during opioid therapy, clinicians should discuss with patients known risks and realistic benefits of opioid therapy and patient and clinician responsibilities for managing therapy
4. When starting opioid therapy for chronic pain, clinicians should prescribe immediate-release opioids instead of ER/LA opioids
5. When opioids are started, clinicians should prescribe the lowest effective dosage. Clinicians should use caution when prescribing opioids at any dosage, should carefully reassess evidence of individual benefits and risks when considering increasing dosage to ≥50 MME/day, and should avoid increasing dosage to ≥90 MME/day or carefully justify a decision to titrate dosage to ≥90 MME/day
6. Long-term opioid use often begins with treatment of acute pain. When opioids are used for acute pain, clinicians should prescribe the lowest effective dose of immediate-release opioids and should prescribe no greater quantity than needed for the expected duration of pain severe enough to require opioids. Three days or less will often be sufficient; more than 7 days will rarely be needed
7. Clinicians should evaluate benefits and harms with patients within 1–4 weeks of starting opioid therapy for chronic pain or of dose escalation. Clinicians should evaluate benefits and harms of continued therapy with patients every 3 months, or more frequently. If benefits do not outweigh harms of continued opioid therapy, clinicians should optimize other therapies and work with patients to taper opioids to lower dosages or to taper and discontinue opioids
8. Before starting, and periodically during continuation of opioid therapy, clinicians should evaluate risk factors for opioid-related harms. Clinicians should incorporate into the management plan strategies to mitigate risk, including considering offering naloxone when factors that increase risk for opioid overdose, such as history of overdose, history of substance use disorder, higher opioid dosages (≥50 MME/day), or concurrent benzodiazepine use, are present
9. Clinicians should review the patient's history of controlled substance prescriptions using state PDMP data to determine whether the patient is receiving opioid dosages or dangerous combinations that put him or her at high risk for overdose. Clinicians should review PDMP data when starting opioid therapy for chronic pain, and periodically during opioid therapy for chronic pain, ranging from every prescription to every 3 months
10. When prescribing opioids for chronic pain, clinicians should use UDT before starting opioid therapy and consider UDT at least annually to assess for prescribed medications as well as other controlled prescription drugs and illicit drugs
11. Clinicians should avoid prescribing opioid pain medication and benzodiazepines concurrently whenever possible
12. Clinicians should offer or arrange evidence-based treatment (usually medication-assisted treatment with buprenorphine or methadone in combination with behavioral therapies) for patients with opioid use disorder

ER/LA, *Extended-release/long-acting;* MME, *morphine milligram equivalents;* PDMP, *prescription drug monitoring programs;* UDT, *urine drug testing.*

the guideline from the Canadian National Opioid Use Guideline Group[13]; the same review rated 7 other guidelines to be of intermediate quality and determined that 4 additional guidelines could not be recommended. Taken together, the two reviews found commonly endorsed recommendations in the guidelines that include the following[8,17]:

- Conducting and documenting a physical exam, pain history, past medical history, and family and social history
- Assessing for abuse and addiction, perhaps using an opioid-specific tool
- Conducting urine drug testing (UDT), when appropriate
- Checking the state prescription drug monitoring database where available for past or present patterns of unauthorized prescriptions
- Considering all treatment options, weighing the benefits and risks of opioid therapy, and using opioids when alternative treatments are ineffective
- Initiating opioids with the lowest effective dose
- Implementing pain treatment agreements to set parameters and expectations of therapy
- Monitoring pain and treatment progress with documentation
- Using greater vigilance at high doses and/or greater abuse risk
- Possessing special knowledge to prescribe methadone
- Recognizing risks of fentanyl patches
- Considering opioid rotation with adverse effects or ineffective analgesia
- Reducing doses by ≥25% to 50% when rotating to a different opioid
- Treating high-risk patients with more frequent and stringent monitoring and comanagement with mental health and addiction specialists
- Considering reasons for repeated escalations in opioid dose
- Discontinuing opioid therapy when repeated aberrant drug-related behaviors are observed
- Using safe and effective methods for discontinuing opioids, such as tapering and making appropriate referrals to medication-assisted treatment or substance-abuse specialists

Newer or updated guidelines, particularly those developed to assist recovery from occupational injuries, emphasize dose-dependent risks of opioids, functional improvement of the patient, opioid-sparing techniques, and exhaustion of nonopioid pain modalities.[18,19]

In addition to numerous practice guidelines, a number of initiatives to reduce harm and regulate prescribing have been enacted at the federal level. The US Food and Drug Administration (FDA) has made changes to labeling for ER/LA opioids to clarify indication and to add warnings regarding misuse and addiction, life-threatening respiratory depression, accidental ingestion, consumption during pregnancy, and coingestion with alcohol.[3] Furthermore, the FDA has issued a risk evaluation and mitigation strategy (REMS), including patient medication guides and a blueprint for provider education programs, to help ensure that the benefits of opioids outweigh the risks.[20] The US Substance Abuse and Mental Health Services

Administration (SAMHSA) has published a toolkit to help communities and local governments prevent opioid overdose with information for patients, prescribers, first responders, community members, and family members.[21]

A synthesis of these sources underscores that the administration of opioids for pain requires significant risk management in key domains through careful assessment of benefits to risks, candidate selection, stratifying by risk category, monitoring for adherence to the regimen, periodic reassessment of progress toward treatment goals, and thorough documentation in the patient record. These fundamentals of practice are discussed along with some additional, often underappreciated, risks of opioid therapy.

PATIENT EVALUATION AND RISK STRATIFICATION

Most guides specify a new patient evaluation beginning with a physical exam to include health and pain-specific information, a review of medical history, and a personal history to collect psychiatric, social, and substance-use data.[5,9,11,13,14,16] Who has been caring for the patient in the past, plus the medications that have been prescribed and for what indications, should be determined; and the patient's substance history, including their use of alcohol, prescription and over-the-counter medications, and illicit drugs should be assessed.[21]

Problematic opioid use by the patient is behavior that threatens the integrity of pain management. Definitions related to problematic opioid use include the following[22]:

- Misuse: Use of a medication for a medical purpose other than that directed or indicated, regardless of the patient's intention
- Abuse: The intentional self-administration of a medication for a nonmedical purpose
- Diversion: The act of removing a prescription medication from its intended and lawful use
- Addiction: A disease state with genetic, psychosocial, environmental factors, and behavioral characteristics that include impaired control over drug use, compulsive use, continued use despite harm, and/or craving

The motive underlying problematic opioid use is not always clinically apparent and may have various causes, including addiction, uncontrolled pain, fear of withdrawal symptoms, recreational use, or an untreated mental disorder. This is why a thorough evaluation of risk for substance abuse and of psychiatric history should take place before opioids are initiated or continued.[20]

Clinicians need knowledge of factors that may contribute to an opioid-use disorder in a patient with pain. These include, but are not limited to, family and personal history of substance abuse, a history of legal problems, a craving for prescription medication, mood swings, nicotine dependence, and a younger age.[23] Patient risk factors for overdose death include middle age, high opioid dose, history of substance abuse, comorbid mental disorders, methadone use, benzodiazepine coprescribing, unemployment, polysubstance abuse, and sleep apnea.[24,25,21]

Tools to assess risk for problematic opioid use may be predictive or diagnostic, but should be brief enough to include in regular clinical practice. Validated opioid-specific tools include the Opioid Risk Tool,[26] the revised 24-item Screener and Opioid Assessment for Patients with Pain,[27] and the Diagnosis, Intractability, Risk, Efficacy inventory.[28] A baseline UDT[10–14,16] and initial check of the state PDMP[5,10,13,15,16] are common recommendations. The state PDMP can help a clinician determine whether a patient is filling prescriptions appropriately, and whether the patient is obtaining unauthorized prescriptions from other providers. Within limits, UDT may confirm the presence or absence of a specific drug or its metabolites. Many initial assessment strategies will also form part of the ongoing monitoring process.

DEVELOPMENT OF A TREATMENT PLAN AND GOALS

To develop a treatment plan, discuss the goals for analgesia and function with the patient and document in the record.[21,29] Patients should understand that the removal of all pain may not be possible, and that pain management is usually most successful using a variety of modalities based on the biopsychosocial model of interdisciplinary care.[30,31] The treatment plan is to be revisited throughout the course of therapy.

INFORMED CONSENT AND TREATMENT AGREEMENT

Patient education begins with a discussion of the expected benefits and risks of opioid therapy. An informed consent document detailing the risks should be signed by the patient and retained in the medical record.[5] The patient should understand that physical dependence and tolerance are likely; that risks exist for oversedation, drug interactions, misuse, addiction, and overdose; and that numerous side effects may develop, including constipation and cognitive impairment.[5]

Treatment agreements set forth the parameters of treatment and usually require adherence to medical direction, require a full patient report on other medications or substances that could affect the course of therapy, limit the patient to one provider for controlled substances prescriptions, and outline policies on early refills, medication refills, and the circumstances under which opioid therapy may be discontinued.[5,21] Although most regulators and some insurance payers expect treatment agreements, evidence of the benefit of preventing opioid-related harm is sparse.

INITIATING AN OPIOID TRIAL

If nonopioid pain modalities have failed, would not be effective, or are not available due to insurance coverage restrictions, and no other contraindications are present, opioid therapy may be trialed at the lowest possible effective dose, and titrated to effectiveness as part of an individualized pain management plan.[5] To select an appropriate opioid, consider the patient's severity of symptoms, their reliability in taking medication, and the dependence-producing potential of the opioid.[21] Genetic individual variability may also affect the choice of an opioid.[29] Consider also prescribing naloxone along with the patient's initial opioid prescription.[21] The patient is closely monitored for the 5A's of analgesia therapy: analgesia, adverse effects, activities of daily living, aberrant

TABLE 44.3 Monitoring Measures by Risk Category for Problematic Opioid Use[a]

Low Risk (Routine)	Moderate Risk	High Risk
• Pain assessment • Substance misuse/abuse assessment via validated tool • Informed consent • Signed treatment agreement • Regular follow-up visits, prescriptions based on clinical need and behaviors • Initial prescription database check and every 6–12 months • Review previous medical records and as directed by behaviors and state regulations • Specialist consult as clinically determined • Medication choices as clinically determined • Document 5A's • Document clinical interactions	• More visits when appropriate • More frequent prescription intervals when appropriate • Regular prescription database check every 6 months or more often, depending on state regulations • Verification via patient's family members/friends • Random UDT with any aberrant behavior or every 3–6 months • Evaluate for comorbid mental health disease • Consider psych/pain specialist evaluation • Consider pill counts • Consider limiting RO analgesics	• Avoid opioids if possible • Use alternative therapies if possible • Weekly visits or more often as necessary • Weekly prescriptions (on attendance) or more often where possible • Quarterly prescription database check or more frequent depending on state regulations • Friend/family member controls medication • UDT every visit • Consider blood screens • Psych/addiction specialist evaluation • Consider pain specialist evaluation • Limit RO analgesics • Consider limiting SAO

[a]*All recommendations from lower risk columns continue to apply as risk increases.*
5A's, *Analgesia, activities of daily living, adverse effects, aberrant drug-related behaviors, affect;* RO, *rapid onset;* SAO, *short-acting opioids;* UDT, *urine drug test.*

drug-related behaviors, and affect.[5] The courses of action after the trial period may include: to continue opioids, to change doses or rotate to a different opioid, to add adjuvant medications, or to discontinue opioid therapy.[22]

ONGOING MONITORING AND ADAPTING THE TREATMENT PLAN

Clinicians should monitor patients according to risk levels, intensifying monitoring measures for patients who are at higher risk or who exhibit signs of problematic opioid behaviors during treatment (Table 44.3).[29,32,33] Unfortunately, research shows that close oversight of opioid-treated patients is uncommon in primary care, even for patients at highest risk for misuse.[34] The following triage scheme for patient management was developed by Gourlay et al.[32] and stratifies patients into three treatment groups:

- *Low:* No personal or family history of substance abuse, no major or untreated psychological disorder, and may be managed in primary care; if aberrant behaviors are observed, consider increasing the risk category
- *Medium:* No active addiction, but a history of treated substance abuse, significant family history of substance abuse, and/or past or comorbid psychological disorder; to be comanaged with the help of addiction and/or pain specialists
- *High:* Active substance abuse or addiction and/or major untreated psychological disorder; primary care should consider referring the management to specialists

Remember that patients may change risk categories over time, particularly if the stress in the patient's environment changes.[28] The patient is continually reassessed for analgesia, adverse effects, activities of daily living, aberrant drug-related behaviors, and affect.[5] Regular review provides for adjustments to the course of treatment, the evaluation of progress toward treatment goals, and the monitoring of adherence to medical direction.

Family members or friends of the patient may be helpful in checking for the following signs of opioid overmedication[21]:

- Unusual sleepiness or drowsiness; snoring
- Mental confusion, slurred speech, intoxicated behavior
- Slow, shallow breathing
- Pinpoint pupils
- Slow heartbeat, low blood pressure
- Difficulty waking the person from sleep

Family members should understand the use of naloxone to reverse overdose and know how to respond in an emergency. See the toolkit to prevent overdose published by SAMHSA for more information.[21]

PERIODIC DRUG TESTING

Follow-up UDT is based on patient risk level (see Table 44.3) or manifestations of clinical signs of abuse with the understanding that all patients are assumed to be at some risk.[29,32,33] In clinical usage, UDT checks for the presence of prescribed medications and for unauthorized prescription and illegal drugs. Testing usually requires two parts: immunoassay drug panels, which usually are not able to identify specific drugs within a class and, if necessary, based on the initial result, follow-up testing using specific techniques, such as gas chromatography/mass spectrometry (GC/MS) to confirm specific drugs or their metabolites.[5] The clinician must also appreciate the potential for false positives or false negatives with UDT, caused by variables, such as individual patient and drug metabolism, and test unreliability.[5,33] For this reason, UDT is only one part of a comprehensive monitoring program, not a sole determinant of discharge from care.

Periodic pill counts may also be helpful as well as periodic checks of the state PDMP. Checks of the state prescribing database are now required in many states.[35] Discuss any unexpected results from UDT, pill counts, or prescribing database checks with the patient, and document the rationale for the decision to continue or discontinue treatment in the medical record.

MENTAL HEALTH CONSULTATION AND REFERRAL

Consultation and referral are often necessary when the patients' needs are beyond the prescriber's expertise.

People with mental health disorders are frequent consumers of therapeutic opioids and are at risk for adverse outcomes, which include abuse, overdose, and drug-drug interactions.[36]

When indicated, referrals may be made to experts in mental health or substance-abuse treatment fields, who may comanage the patient or take over treatment.[37] Consider also referral for pain management when the prescriber has reached the limit of comfort with opioid prescribing, the disease has progressed, or uncontrolled pain remains. It is recognized that the ability to refer is affected by the availability or lack of insurance coverage for the consultation.[30]

Signs that opioids may not be appropriate for a patient include the following manifestations[38]:

- Impulsivity
- Catastrophizing
- Chemical coping
- Failure to accept limits
- Personality disorders
- Demoralization, existential distress
- Sensation seeking
- Escapism

DISCONTINUING OPIOID THERAPY

The decision of whether and when to end opioid therapy may be based on the resolution of pain, insufficient analgesia, significant side effects, or ongoing or egregious aberrant drug-related behaviors, among other causes.[29,31] Tolerance dictates that tapering should be gradual: expert guidelines set a reduction of 10% per week as the most conservative taper[10,12,13,16]; slower or faster tapering may accommodate individual need, but should be monitored to prevent withdrawal symptoms. Appropriate referrals for addiction treatment or nonopioid pain management are indicated. Opioids are only one tool for pain management, and interdisciplinary care is optimal.[30,31] If illegal diversion has occurred, immediate discharge from the clinic practice is advised.[29]

DOCUMENTATION IN MEDICAL RECORDS

Thorough documentation in the medical record is necessary for medicolegal reasons and to assist optimal clinical decision making. Details to document include the indication for prescribing the opioid, past pain history and treatments tried, types and dosages of current medications, and enough detail to reflect the rationale for all clinical decisions.[5] Clinical monitoring tools that facilitate good documentation practices include the Pain Assessment & Documentation Tool[39] and the Current Opioid Misuse Measure.[40]

COMPLIANCE WITH CONTROLLED SUBSTANCE LAWS AND REGULATIONS

To comply with federal law, health care providers must ensure that the prescribing of controlled substances, including opioids, occurs for a legitimate medical purpose in the usual course of professional practice.[41] In addition, the Drug Enforcement Administration requires reasonable measures on the part of the practitioner to prevent abuse and diversion, and warns against ignoring signs that abuse is taking place.[42] These requirements leave room for broad interpretation by investigators. Furthermore, whenever federal and state law overlap, the more stringent law applies and, in some cases, it is the state law that is the more restrictive.[5]

ADDITIONAL PRACTICES FOR SAFER PRESCRIBING

Building on the basic principles of practice described above, some additional factors may adversely affect opioid therapy if not addressed.

Conventional conversion tables can cause harm and should be used cautiously when rotating from one opioid to another.[37] Equianalgesic tables provide insufficient guidance to determine the equivalent doses of different opioids, and individual consideration is necessary for every patient. To switch between opioids, slowly decrease one opioid while slowly titrating the new opioid to effect.[7,37]

Coprescribing benzodiazepines with opioids should be avoided, especially during sleep hours.[12,15,16,37,43] Consider an alternative treatment for anxiety disorders, and when a sleep aid is indicated, consider an anticonvulsant or low-dose trazodone. For patients with neuropathic pain, low-dose trazodone at bedtime may be dually beneficial.

Methadone for pain carries heightened risks relative to most other prescribed opioids. If deemed necessary, methadone must be started at a very low dose (e.g., ≤15 mg/day in divided doses) and slowly titrated (e.g., by no more than 25% to 50%, no more frequently than weekly), regardless of a patient's opioid tolerance.[37] Practitioners without experience and knowledge of methadone should seek expert consultation before prescribing.

Sleep apnea is a risk with high daily doses of methadone (>50 mg) or other opioids (>150 mg/day of morphine equivalent dose), and in patients with a predisposition.[37] It is advisable to refer these high-risk patients for a sleep study and possible inpatient evaluation of opioid therapy safety.

Upper respiratory compromise from flu, pneumonia, upper respiratory infections, cigarette use, chronic obstructive pulmonary disease, asthmatic episodes, or other causes should trigger patient counseling to reduce opioid dose.[37]

Avoid ER/LA opioid formulations for acute, postoperative, or trauma-related pain.[3,36]

ACKNOWLEDGMENT

Beth Dove of Dove Medical Communications, LLC, Salt Lake City, Utah, provided medical writing for this manuscript.

KEY POINTS

- Relief of pain is an important goal for health care providers
- Concerns about misuse, abuse, addiction, and overdose raise significant barriers to the use of opioids for treating pain
- Clinicians need an understanding of the risk factors for problematic opioid use or overdose in patients

- Risk assessment leading to stratification can help match appropriate monitoring to the risk of problematic opioid use
- Ongoing monitoring of the patient's therapeutic goals and adherence with the elements of pain therapy is necessary
- Patients who may need to discontinue opioid therapy include those who fail to achieve sufficient analgesia, whose pain resolves, or who display repeated or egregious aberrant drug-related behaviors

REFERENCES

Access the reference list online at ExpertConsult.com.

CHAPTER 45

Legal and Regulatory Issues in Pain Management

Aaron M. Gilson, MS, MSSW, PhD ◎ Ben A. Rich, JD, PhD

The legal and regulatory landscape of pain management has, perhaps unsurprisingly, continued to be shaped (critics might say distorted) by what can plausibly be characterized as "the politics of pain."[1–3] Over the last decade there has been the convergence of two "perfect storms" in the domain of pain management. According to an Institute of Medicine report, there continue to be many patients in the health care system who do not receive adequate pain relief.[4] Yet there is also compelling evidence that there has been a substantial increase in recent years in deaths from prescription drug overdose.[5] Physicians who care for patients with pain have vociferously expressed their concerns that, in attempting to fulfill their professional responsibility to patients, these laws and litigation (civil, criminal, and administrative) place them between the proverbial "rock and a hard place" or "damned if they do and damned if they don't." A gulf between practice standards (established by laws, clinical practice guidelines, and legal determinations) and actual clinical practice continues to persist, perhaps due, in part, to the fact that most pain management is provided by primary care physicians rather than pain medicine specialists who are primarily involved in formulating such standards. In this chapter, we provide an overview of the policy and legal environment that informs pain care.

LAWS AND POLICIES AFFECTING PAIN MANAGEMENT

Legislative bodies typically create laws (i.e., statutes) that are broad and general, and depend on the relevant regulatory agency to interpret and implement the laws. For medicine, the legislature grants authority to the state medical board to operationalize and uphold its laws through regulation. Such professional boards generally have updated their pain management policies in reaction to changing professional standards. Alternatively, pain-related statutes do not as consistently keep pace with advances in medical and scientific understanding.[6]

The purpose of this section is to review relevant legislative and regulatory policies governing the treatment of pain, including opioid analgesics. Of course, a variety of therapeutic modalities (both pharmacological and nonpharmacological) are required for a comprehensive approach to pain management for cancer, HIV/AIDS, or other more chronic conditions, including interventional techniques, nerve blocks, acupuncture, psychological interventions, and nonopioid analgesics. Many of these treatments are discussed throughout this textbook. However, practitioners generally do not receive training in legal and regulatory issues related to opioid prescribing, and are not familiar with the federal and state laws that govern their practice. Nevertheless, they are increasingly being called on to have knowledge of the policies under which they practice.[7,8]

FEDERAL CONTROLLED SUBSTANCES LAWS

Controlled substances laws govern the distribution of prescription medications that have an abuse liability (i.e., that fulfill the potential to produce psychological or physical dependence), and which the Food and Drug Administration (FDA) have approved for medical use. The federal Controlled Substances Act (CSA)[9] is the principal drug control law in the United States, and establishes a closed distribution system to minimize the substances' trafficking, abuse, and diversion.

The CSA is designed to prohibit the nonmedical use of controlled substances and establishes criminal penalties for their illicit possession, manufacture, and distribution, while at the same time recognizing that they have a useful and legitimate medical purpose, and that they are necessary for public health.[10] "Controlled substances" status of any medication is not meant to diminish its medical usefulness or create the perception that practitioners should avoid its use when it is clinically justified. The legislative history, as well as the language contained in the CSA itself (which is implemented through its related regulations called the Code of Federal Regulations [CFR]), makes it clear that efforts to prevent drug abuse and diversion should not interfere with legitimate medical practice and appropriate patient care.[11] This position conforms to a long-standing medico-legal principle, referred to as "Balance," which was established by the *Single Convention on Narcotic Drugs of 1961*.[12]

The CSA specifies five classification schedules for controlled substances, each carrying different penalties for unlawful uses. Both a drug's medical usefulness and abuse liability form the basis for the decision to assign it to a particular schedule.[13] Schedule I controlled substances (e.g., heroin, LSD, and ecstasy) have no currently accepted medical use, no accepted safety for use under medical supervision, and a high potential for abuse, and are available only for scientific research. Controlled substances that have an FDA-approved medical use are placed in Schedules II through V according to the potential for abuse (Box 45.1). For example, on October 6, 2014, hydrocodone-combination products were reclassified from Schedule III to Schedule II of the CSA.[14] As a result, Schedule II now contains single-entity hydrocodone products as well as those of hydrocodone combined with acetaminophen, aspirin, or ibuprofen. Under federal law, the Drug Enforcement Administration (DEA) is the primary federal agency responsible for enforcing the CSA and, thus, has regulatory authority over controlled substances in every schedule.

Licensed practitioners must be registered with the DEA to prescribe, dispense, and administer controlled substances.[15] To minimize harm to patients and to protect the

BOX 45.1 Controlled Substances Schedules for Opioid Analgesics

- Schedule II medications have the highest potential for abuse, and include opioids such as codeine, fentanyl, hydrocodone, hydromorphone, meperidine, methadone, morphine, and oxycodone.
- Schedule III medications have a lower abuse potential than Schedule II drugs, and include opioids such as dihydrocodeine combinations with aspirin and paracetamol, and codeine combinations with aspirin or acetaminophen.
- Schedule IV medications have a lower abuse potential relative to drugs in Schedule III, and include opioids such as dextropropoxyphene, pentazocine, and tramadol.
- Schedule V medications have a lower abuse potential compared to drugs in Schedule IV and include compounds or preparations containing limited quantities of opioids such as codeine or opium, which may be used for over-the-counter preparations to treat cough or diarrhea, respectively.

public health, conditions of registration involve, among other things, adhering to statutes and regulations that limit medication availability to legitimate medical uses and patients[16,17]; incorporating into practice safeguards against diversion[18]; and reporting to the DEA the medication amounts that are lost or stolen.[19] Prescriptions for controlled substances must be issued only for legitimate medical purposes and in the usual course of professional practice.[16] Prescriptions for Schedule II medications may not be refilled,[20] while five refills are permitted for medications in Schedules III and IV.[21] Federal law allows oral authorization of prescriptions for Schedule II controlled substances in medical emergencies if certain requirements are met.[22] It is also possible under federal law to partially dispense or fax prescriptions under specific circumstances.[23] Importantly, in 2010 the DEA issued an interim final rule, including a request for comment, to revise the CFR to provide practitioners with the option of electronically writing prescriptions for controlled substances.[24] The regulation became effective on June 1, 2010. According to the DEA, the new regulations:

> "*...will reduce paperwork for DEA registrants who dispense controlled substances and have the potential to reduce prescription forgery. The regulations will also have the potential to reduce the number of prescription errors caused by illegible handwriting and misunderstood oral prescriptions. Moreover, they will help both pharmacies and hospitals to integrate prescription records into other medical records more directly, which may increase efficiency, and potentially reduce the amount of time patients spend waiting to have their prescriptions filled.*" (*p. 16236*)[24]

Federal law was also recently developed in recognition of the need for more controlled substance disposal options, as a means to reduce the volume of unused medications and, ultimately, curtail opportunities for diversion. The CFR was changed, effective October 9, 2014, to permit certain DEA-registrants to become "collectors" of controlled substances for the purpose of destruction using a number of specified methods.[25] Under the new regulations, manufacturers, distributors, reverse distributors, opioid treatment programs (OTPs), hospitals/clinics with on-site pharmacies, and retail pharmacies can volunteer to be registered as a collector.[26] In addition, a registered hospital/clinic with an on-site pharmacy or a retail pharmacy can be a collector to maintain a medication drop box at long-term care facilities (LTCFs), to dispose of medications from residents of those LTCFs.[27] The regulation also permits law enforcement to voluntarily conduct collection activities for controlled substances through a variety of methods (e.g., take-back events and mail-back programs).[28] Importantly, however, practitioners cannot be designated as a collector and, therefore, have no more disposal opportunities than previously (e.g., medication transfer to a reverse distributor or delivery to a DEA agent).[29] It would be beneficial for practitioners to at least have access to a current list of volunteer collectors so that they could inform their patients about a greater array of disposal options, to reduce the volume of unused medications possibly entering into the illicit market.

In addition to these policy developments, other provisions demonstrate that federal drug control laws are not intended to interfere with medical practice or limit the availability of controlled medications for patient care.

Assuring Medication Availability

The CSA authorizes the DEA to establish production quotas for a number of opioids and other controlled substances as a means to curtail diversion resulting from excessive unused supplies.[30] Such quotas, however, are meant to maintain sufficient supplies for accommodating all medical and scientific needs.[31] Although a recent US Government Accountability Office (GAO) report has identified a notable increase in shortages of controlled medications in recent years, officials from the DEA and the FDA are now working to update a shared memorandum of understanding to prevent future shortages.[32]

Medical Practice Is Not Regulated

The authorization to regulate medical practice belongs to the states and underlies the medical practice acts that are designed to protect the public health and safety.[33] Thus, the CSA provides no authority for the DEA to define or regulate medical practice.[9] The DEA's enforcement authority is intended to relate to clinicians involved in unlawful distribution of controlled substances that is outside legitimate health care practice (i.e., behaviors that are clearly criminal).

Treating Addiction Versus Treating Pain

Under federal law, it is unlawful for a practitioner to administer or dispense (but not prescribe) methadone or administer or dispense (including prescribe) buprenorphine to treat addiction unless separately registered by the federal government as an OTP for the purpose of maintenance or detoxification of opioid addiction, and is in compliance with regulations governing such treatment.[34,35] However, methadone, a Schedule II medication approved for the purpose of addiction treatment, can be prescribed as an analgesic according to the same laws for prescribing any other Schedule II opioid. In addition, the CSA[36] and the CFR[37] place no prohibitions on the use of opioids to treat pain in a patient who has a history of substance use or a current addictive disease, although such practices may be addressed in state law. Critically, determining the legitimacy of a particular prescribing practice must be based on the purpose of the prescribing and not solely the type of patient being treated.

Prescription Amount and Duration

Federal laws do not set limits on the amount or duration of medication that a practitioner can prescribe, administer, or dispense at one time.[38] Importantly, the DEA clarified that this standard did not change when the CFR was amended to allow practitioners to issue multiple prescriptions of a Schedule II controlled substance, each issued on the same date and filled sequentially (called a "prescription series").[39] With the CFR amendment, the DEA's stated intent was to permit health care professionals to better manage chronic pain in stable patients while exercising improved control over potential medication abuse and diversion, which is consistent with the principle of balance.[40]

STATE CONTROLLED SUBSTANCES AND HEALTH CARE LAWS

Both federal and state laws govern the prescribing, dispensing, and administering of controlled substances. However, only states have the authority to regulate health care practice, including medical, pharmacy, and nursing practice, and such regulatory policies can be used to address concerns that professionals hold about investigation or sanction for prescribing pain medications. Unlike federal law, state laws generally do not recognize that controlled medications are important to public health.[10] Some state laws also consign more frequent restrictions than do federal laws regarding the prescribing and dispensing of opioids, which ultimately can hinder medical decision making that should be based both on the expertise of the practitioner and the individual patient needs. The messages and requirements contained in state policies that govern health care practice, including opioid prescribing, has been shown to influence clinical care decisions.[41–43,43a] As a result, state policy content must be considered a necessary part of a multifaceted plan to improve pain and symptom management, while at the same time stemming prescription medication abuse and diversion.[44]

Evaluating the Quality of State Pain Policy

Since the early 2000s, a criteria-based policy research methodology has existed to evaluate and promote more balanced state drug control and health care regulatory policies related to pain management, including for palliative care and end-of-life care. As indicated earlier, balanced state policies maintain drug controls and avoid undue restrictions to appropriate health care practice and patient care, and will support pain treatment, including the use of controlled substances when warranted, as an essential part of quality medical practice. Although separate efforts are necessary to assess the presence and effectiveness of current state-level drug control frameworks to minimize abuse and diversion, the purpose of this evaluation has been to characterize pain-related issues covered in state policies.

The evaluation uses 16 criteria from two categories: (1) positive provisions—policy language that can *enhance* pain relief; and (2) negative provisions—language that can *impede* pain relief. Periodic reports have been developed containing a complete description of the criteria, the evaluation methodology, and the identified policy language from all states (including the District of Columbia) that satisfies each criterion. State policy evaluations have been conducted periodically since 2000. The findings presented in Table 45.1 represent policies in effect by the end of 2015, which is the most recent year to date for which policies were evaluated.

TABLE 45.1 Frequency of Criteria Fulfilled During Evaluation of State[a] Pain Policies in Effect in 2015

Positive Provisions: Criteria That Identify Policy Language With the Potential to Enhance Pain Management	
1.	Controlled substances are recognized as necessary for the public health (in 4 states)
2.	Pain management is recognized as part of general medical practice (in 45 states)
3.	Medical use of opioids is recognized as legitimate professional practice (in 51[a] states)
4.	Pain management is encouraged (in 40 states)
5.	Practitioners' concerns about regulatory scrutiny are addressed (in 39 states)
6.	Prescription amount alone is recognized as insufficient to determine the legitimacy of prescribing (in 32 states)
7.	Physical dependence or analgesic tolerance are *not* confused with "addiction" (in 38 states)
8.	Other provisions that may enhance pain management Category A: Issues related to health care professionals (in 47 states) Category B: Issues related to patients (in 44 states) Category C: Regulatory or policy issues (in 50 states)
Negative Provisions: Criteria That Identify Policy Language With the Potential to Impede Pain Management	
9.	Opioids are relegated as only a treatment of last resort (in 0 states)
10.	Medical use of opioids is implied to be outside legitimate professional practice (in 6 states)
11.	Physical dependence or analgesic tolerance are confused with "addiction" (in 12 states)
12.	Medical decisions are restricted Category A: Restrictions based on patient characteristics (in 5 states) Category B: Mandated consultation (in 7 states) Category C: Restrictions regarding quantity prescribed or dispensed (in 1 state) Category D: Undue prescription limitations (in 2 states)
13.	Length of prescription validity is restricted (in 2 states)
14.	Practitioners are subject to additional prescription requirements (in 6 states)
15.	Other provisions that may impede pain management (in 0 states)
16.	Provisions that are ambiguous Category A: Arbitrary standards for legitimate prescribing (in 14 states) Category B: Unclear intent leading to possible misinterpretation (in 14 states) Category C: Conflicting (or inconsistent) policies or provisions (in 5 states)

[a]*Includes the District of Columbia.*

Overall, policy language that promotes the concept of appropriate pain management and that maintains patient access to pain care opportunities is common in policies from state regulatory agencies, rather than from legislative drug control statutes.[6] A state's drug control laws often focus on the abuse potential of controlled medications to the exclusion of recognizing their public health and medical benefit when used as directed for legitimate purposes, unlike more positive provisions contained in federal law (see, e.g., Refs. 10 and 45). It has been, and continues to be, possible to adopt state policies designed to prevent drug abuse and the transfer of medications to an illicit distribution system without creating additional requirements that unduly restrict health care decision making, that conform to and do not conflict with current standards of professional practice, and that eschew imposing excessive burdens on patients. Indeed, many of the policy actions identified in these reports reinforce state governments' willingness to work collaboratively to avoid unduly restricting access to controlled medications for the people who need them while taking precautions against activities that could contribute to patient or public harm. Such an approach corresponds to the continued call from international and national authoritative bodies (representing legal, regulatory, and health care communities) to reduce the misuse, abuse, and diversion of prescription medications, while at the same time addressing inadequate treatment for debilitating pain (see, e.g., Refs. 46–49).

Grading the Quality of State Pain Policy

Findings from each criteria-based evaluation of state pain policy also has served as the basis for a methodology to quantify a state's policy based on its quality, creating a single metric that can then be used to compare all states and track policy change over time. In the last report, grades (ranging from A to F) were calculated for the state policies in effect in 2015. A higher grade means a state's policies has many positives and few negatives and is, therefore, more balanced in relation to appropriate pain management. An "A" is achieved only if a state has a high number of positive provisions and no instances of unduly restrictive or ambiguous language. A lower grade is associated with the presence of provisions that contradict current medical knowledge, are inconsistent with policy guidance recommendations from authoritative sources, or fail to communicate the appropriate messages about pain management to professionals, patients, and the public. An "F" results when a state has abundant negative provisions and no positive language.

The grades, and the methodology used to calculate them, are contained in a recent report that is available at www.acscan.org/painreportcard.[50] In the aggregate, the last decade was a time of notable improvement in the quality of many states' drug control and professional practice policies. This policy change seems to represent continued progress in response to evolving national and state acknowledgment that adopting positive policies governing health care practice and patient care is part of improving pain treatment for patients with cancer, HIV/AIDS, and other diseases or conditions. By and large, states avoided adopting new policies that could impede pain management and the medical use of controlled substances when clinically justified. Members of government and regulatory agencies, as well as health care professionals, are in a position to continue seeking policy approaches that eschew undue restrictions on medical decision making or unintentional consequences on pain treatment.

Much of the improvement in the quality of state pain policies results from individual health care regulatory boards taking advantage of the Federation of State Medical Boards' (the Federation's) policy templates to promote consistency in state medical board policy.[51–53] Throughout the templates, the importance of documenting various aspects of treatment is mentioned. These templates also encourage safe and effective pain relief, perpetuate the message that pain management and the appropriate use of controlled substances is an accepted part of professional practice, and reassure clinicians that they have nothing to fear from their licensing agency if reasonable professional practices are followed when using controlled substances for patient care. In addition, the policies promote the assessment of both potential benefits and risks when considering opioid treatment, especially for patients with more chronic conditions. Patient risk assessment, as well as the periodic monitoring for adverse events and the manifestation of abuse-, addiction-, and diversion-related behaviors, have been an explicit component of the Federation's templates since their inception[54,55]; in fact, the clinical need for risk stratification strategies was emphasized even more in the most recent policy issued in 2013.[53] Importantly, health care regulatory boards (e.g., medical, osteopathic, pharmacy, and nursing) in many states have worked together to adopt joint guidelines for pain management, palliative care, or end-of-life care.[56] Such policies tend to emphasize the value of an integrative and multidisciplinary approach to treating pain; they recognize that the goal of pain treatment should include improvements in patient functioning and quality of life; and they assure that a broader variety of health care practitioners should not fear disciplinary action from their licensing board for practice that generally conforms to the included treatment standards.

Given this notable regulatory progress, most states now can focus on maintaining policy improvement and consider efforts to remove long-outdated restrictive or ambiguous language from law, some of which has been present for almost 40 years. This is especially the case with drug control laws that contain outdated definitions of "drug-dependent person" (or "narcotic-dependent person," "addict," "active addiction," "narcotic addict," or "habitué") that are based on the concept of physical dependence and developing a withdrawal syndrome. Such definitions should be abrogated because they can legally classify any patient who is taking an opioid to treat pain as an addict.[57] Repeal from law of archaic restrictive language has received less attention compared to the work of professional licensing boards to adopt positive policy.[56] Although states must be allowed to vary in their approaches to public policy, the creation of undue restrictions is not obligatory in laws designed to control drug diversion or regulate professional practice. Avoiding such language ensures that patient care decisions requiring medical judgment are not overly limited by governmental laws.

THE IMPORTANCE OF PRACTITIONERS IN IMPROVING STATE POLICY

Inadequately treated pain is a multifactorial phenomenon and, as such, focusing solely on changing state policy is likely insufficient to guarantee better patient access to appropriate pain relief and symptom control.[58] Addressing this single factor, however, often remains a necessary activity to attain a supportive professional practice and a regulatory environment for the appropriate treatment of pain. Adoption of state policies also requires broad dissemination and communication to relevant practitioners to help enhance compliance to the policy recommendations or requirements,[59] since an evaluation of practice generally involves a determination regarding adherence to applicable policy.[8]

Improving state policies covering pain-related issues requires a strategic approach, often beginning simply by determining the types of policies in need of improvement. For example, revising statutory law requires legislative activity, whereas changing regulatory policy involves engaging with the relevant health care administrative agency, such as the medical, pharmacy, or nursing board. Health care practitioners increasingly have assumed a leadership role in collaborating with legislators or members of administrative agencies to help construct state policy that avoids undue restrictions, recognizes the professional obligation to treat pain, and promotes effective patient pain care.[59] This activity has been accomplished when practitioners have acted alone, in conjunction with a state pain initiative or other organization, or as a member of a legislatively created advisory committee.[44]

OTHER IMPORTANT POLICIES TO CONSIDER

Although the aforementioned policy evaluation reports synthesize the content of numerous state-level statutes and regulatory policies governing drug control and medical and pharmacy practice, as well as nursing practice for certain years, various other policy types fall outside the scope of the research but may nevertheless affect pain care. Such unevaluated policies include physician assistants practice, controlled substances scheduling, advance directives or living wills, workers' compensation, institutional (including chain pharmacies) policies, and program grants to state agencies. Especially important also are the multitude of federal and state laws establishing standards for reimbursement of therapeutic interventions, covering such areas as prior authorization, drug formularies, medication synchronization, and abuse-deterrent formulations for opioid medications. Efforts to understand the positive and negative aspects of these policies, as well as the impact of such policy content on professional practice and patient care, are warranted. In addition, it is often important to be aware of the content of statutes being proposed in the state legislature but which have not yet become laws (i.e., bills). Some recent bills have been designed with the objective of improving public health and safety by reducing prescription medication abuse and diversion, but may inadvertently establish barriers to the availability of medications needed by people who use them therapeutically for pain relief and to maintain quality of life (see http://sppan.aapainmanage.org/legislation). Coordinated responses to introduced legislative bills, and to proposed regulatory policies whenever possible, provide opportunities to make policy makers aware of potential unintended consequences. Engagement with legislators and regulators during policy development can effectively reduce the prospect of future policy impediments.

One of the most prevalent policies recently promoted to reduce opioid-related overdoses and other harmful consequences is dosing thresholds based on daily cumulative morphine milligram equivalence (MME) amounts. At this time, most of the thresholds are limited to the treatment of patients with chronic noncancer pain. These thresholds have been described as "a precautionary signal to get the prescriber to press pause before moving forward with dose escalation."[60] When the dosage threshold is met or exceeded, prescribers are then recommended to obtain an expert consultation (see, e.g., Ref. 61). Beginning in 2007 in Washington, with a recommended 120 MME threshold established in clinical practice guidelines,[62] some states (including Washington) eventually established such amounts in law (see, e.g., Ref.63). Now that these dosage amounts are imposed by laws, there is a legal liability established for failing to comply with the requirements. This concern is especially relevant in a state like Maine, which, in 2016, adopted a 100 MME amount for treating chronic pain that, for all intents and purposes, cannot be exceeded.[64]

In addition to the dosing equivalence threshold itself, the American Academy of Pain Management[65] (now the Academy of Integrative Pain Management) has identified a number of provisions from the Washington policy, and therefore contained in similar policies adopted subsequently by other states, which could create ambiguity for practitioners attempting to follow the rules. Such provisions include (1) the use of a written prescriber/patient agreement for those judged to be at a high risk of substance abuse, have a history of substance abuse, or have psychiatric comorbidities; (2) the requirement of certain prescribers to obtain a consultation with a "pain management specialist" under certain circumstances, including exceeding the dosing threshold; and (3) the establishment of qualifications for prescribers who can serve as adequately prepared specialist consultants. It is possible, though, that practitioner confusion may relate more to an inaccurate understanding of the legal requirements, rather than to the requirements themselves.[65] Indeed, policy can become a barrier to practice due equally to misunderstandings about policy requirements as from perceptions of legal liability based on actual policy content.

A recent commentary by Ziegler,[60] however, has identified substantive concerns related to policies establishing dosage thresholds, such as the emphasis on potential harms only at higher dosage levels, the neglect of other factors contributing to harms, the errors in morphine equivalent conversions, and the lack of pain management specialists required for consultation. Given these considerations, there is a clear need to thoroughly assess the various reasons for practitioners' concerns to determine appropriate next steps. This is especially feasible now since some of these policies have been in effect for a few years. Ultimately, the question remains: Will identified practitioner concerns be better addressed through changes (by any extent) to the laws or other regulatory policies, enhanced resources to aid implementation, or improving practitioners' knowledge about the policy standards and promoting their clinical utility, or by a combination of approaches?

THE IMPORTANCE OF CONSIDERING DIVERSION

Along with policy efforts to enhance benefits and minimize harms for pain treatments, drug control measures must be in place to reduce the potential for transferring prescription medications into illicit channels. Despite the preponderance of legislative and regulatory requirements governing the closed distribution of controlled medications, it remains possible for opioid analgesics to be diverted from all levels of the distribution system.[66] Once diverted, they can become illegally available for sale and nonmedical use, which may result in harmful consequences, such as overdose and death. Indeed, using controlled medications without a valid prescription issued by a properly licensed practitioner for a legitimate medical purpose, or in ways that are contraindicated, compounds the risk of harmful effects.

To this end, health care professionals who prescribe opioid medications have a responsibility to protect public safety by avoiding unintentionally contributing to abuse and diversion. Some practitioners may prescribe or dispense more dosage units than medically necessary, which often remain unused and become susceptible to theft or perhaps accidental use by others.[67] When such prescribing reaches a level or pattern considered "excessive," it can further be designated as "unprofessional conduct" and make the practitioner vulnerable to license revocation or other civil penalties under law (see, e.g., Ref. 68).

Patients receiving prescription-only controlled medications also share responsibilities under law, which has yet received little attention up to this time.[69] Prescription labeling includes a warning for patients that it is a violation of law to transfer the medications prescribed for them to any other person.[70] More generally, it is illegal under federal and state laws for any person to possess controlled substances, including opioid analgesics, without a valid prescription, as well as to acquire these medications by theft, fraud, or misrepresentation. Even when opioids are prescribed legitimately, but then are not stored securely in the patient's home, they become susceptible to diversion through loss or theft. As a result, when attempting to mitigate diversion, learning that a person acquired an opioid from peers or family, for example, remains insufficient. Further investigation is necessary to determine the *circumstances* through which the opioid became available for nonmedical uses (e.g., through a dispensed prescription, through a forged prescription, or when medication is lost or stolen).

Since opioid medications are diverted from throughout the entire medication distribution system, including before they are prescribed, there are many potential sources feeding their use for illicit purposes. Examples of such activities include:

- Criminal diversions of large quantities are reported by manufacturers, distributors, and pharmacies
  - Often involving armed robberies and night break-ins
- Criminal activities by organizations and individuals, including some patients, to obtain opioid analgesics unlawfully
  - Thefts, including employee pilferage, occur from pharmacy supplies in nursing homes and hospitals
  - Fraud and misrepresentation, such as "doctor shopping" or prescription form theft, forgery, or alteration
  - "Script doctors" and "Pill Mills," which are illegal activities by rogue physicians who still have the necessary authority to prescribe, or to purchase and dispense, controlled substances
  - Misuse of Medicare and Medicaid drug coverage.

It is essential, therefore, that efforts to reduce nonmedical drug use and diversion should include, but must be more comprehensive than, focusing on prescribing and dispensing practices and patient access.

As of today, little empirical evidence exists about the degree to which these numerous possible diversion sources play a role in prescription medication-related abuse, addiction, overdose, and death. However, an appreciation for the multiple determinants of diversion substantiates the benefit of a broad, multifaceted, approach to effectively address the nonmedical use of opioid analgesics. Such an approach is exemplified at a federal level by the Office of National Drug Control Policy's (ONDCP) *Prescription Drug Abuse Prevention Plan*, which was published in April 2011 and has been updated annually. The ONDCP's Plan is a multiagency collaboration of federal, state, and local enforcement activities to enhance practitioner and public awareness about the risks and benefits of prescription medications; investigate the production of analgesics with less or no abuse liability; reduce pill mills, doctor-shopping or pharmacy-hopping; and reduce the volume of unused medications.[71] The ONDCP's collaborative and systematic strategy is auspicious, because it seeks to more comprehensively address the multiple means by which prescription medications can become available for illicit use, including through the practitioner/patient relationship. Such an approach, as well as broad policy initiatives now underway in some states, appropriately focuses on the intricate nature of the national public health problem of nonmedical drug use.[72,73]

LITIGATION INVOLVING PAIN MANAGEMENT

The provision of pain management by health care professionals has been the subject of litigation in all four domains of the law: administrative proceedings, civil litigation, criminal litigation, and constitutional challenges. Cases have arisen in both state and federal tribunals. We will consider the general nature and trends of proceedings in each of these domains, with brief mention of particular cases. Readers are encouraged to directly access the referenced cases for more details on those of particular interest.

ADMINISTRATIVE PROCEEDINGS

The most influential and frequently discussed proceedings are those of state medical licensing boards. Until very recently, medical boards generally were viewed by physicians as hostile to the prescribing of opioid analgesics except for patients in an advanced stage of terminal illness.[74] The phenomenon of opiophobia and the pervasive myths and misinformation concerning opioid analgesics were as prevalent among members of medical boards as in the medical profession generally as well as the general public.[75] Prior to 1999, there was no record of a state medical board initiating any disciplinary proceeding against a physician for failure to provide adequate pain relief to a patient, yet proceedings for excessive or otherwise inappropriate prescribing of opioids was common. The recognition of excessive prescribing and disproportionate use of opioids in the United States relative to all other countries suggests that undertreatment of pain is not supportable, and that inadequate treatment may involve both to too little and too much treatment.

A case that demonstrates the traditional negative attitudes of state medical boards toward opioid prescribing, particularly regarding chronic noncancer pain, was *Hoover v. Agency for Health Care Administration*, a disciplinary action by the Florida medical licensing board. Dr. Katherine Hoover was a board-certified internist who cared for a number of patients with serious chronic pain problems that were effectively manageable only with opioids. The board singled out seven of her patients as the basis of disciplinary proceedings. The hearing officer in the case ruled in favor of Dr. Hoover, finding that the board's "experts" (two physicians who did not treat chronic pain patients and who had only reviewed pharmacy computer printouts) failed to establish that her prescribing for these patients was excessive. Nevertheless, the board imposed sanctions against Dr. Hoover, which she appealed. The Court of Appeals reversed the board's disciplinary action stating: "[T]he board has once again engaged in the uniformly rejected practice of overzealously supplanting a hearing officer's valid findings of fact regarding a doctor's prescription practices with its own opinion in a case founded on a woefully inadequate quantum of evidence."[76]

What changed gradually during the 1990s was a growing public and professional recognition that "opiophobia" and "pseudo-addiction" were demonstrable phenomena with the potential to negatively influence a patient's access to pain medication.[77] In 1999, the Oregon Board of Medical Examiners became the first state board to successfully discipline a physician for inadequate management of pain. Dr. Paul Bilder, a pulmonary specialist, was found to have failed to properly manage the pain or severe symptom distress of six seriously ill or dying patients over a period of 5 years.[78] Despite a formal reprimand, a requirement to complete the board's Physician Education Renewal Program, and a 10-year probation, Dr. Bilder was the subject of board discipline 2 years later for further instances of undertreating pain.[79]

Largely through the efforts of the Federation's Model Guidelines[51] and Model Policies[52,53] on opioid prescribing, a majority of state medical boards are now on record emphasizing the need for physicians to incorporate sound pain management practices into their patient care.[80] In other words, both manifest overprescribing and underprescribing of opioids may constitute substandard or unprofessional practice giving rise to disciplinary proceedings. Nevertheless, the gulf between policy and practice persists at both ends of the prescribing continuum.

CIVIL LITIGATION

As with administrative proceedings regarding pain management practices, the civil litigation climate has changed markedly in the last 2 decades. Before 1990, there were no civil actions solely or primarily grounded on an alleged failure of a health care institution or professional to provide effective pain relief. In the next decade, several cases revealed that, in fact, undertreated pain could be shown to be substandard patient care. The first such case was successfully litigated in North Carolina in 1991, when a skilled nursing facility (SNF) was subjected to a multimillion-dollar-damage jury verdict because one of its nurses had deliberately deprived an elderly patient dying of metastatic prostate cancer of the strong pain relievers previously prescribed by a community physician. This conduct was deemed to be so egregious that millions of dollars of punitive damages were assessed in addition to compensatory damages.[81]

Ten years later, a California jury determined that a physician had perpetrated elder abuse when he failed to adequately manage the pain of a hospitalized patient who was within weeks of death from lung cancer. Again, damages in excess of a million dollars were awarded to the deceased patient's family, and the jury came within one vote of also assessing punitive damages.[82] The case was particularly significant for several reasons. First, as an elder abuse claim, the plaintiff's burden of proof was the much more challenging "clear and convincing evidence" standard rather than the "preponderance of the evidence" standard generally applicable in medical malpractice claims. Second, the jury found liability not for a mere departure from the standard of acceptable care, but rather for a gross departure or reckless disregard for the patient's well-being. They did so despite testimony by defense experts that the defendant's treatment was consistent with the usual custom and practice among physicians. What may have enabled the jury to find the custom and practice itself to be deficient was the admission into evidence of the Agency for Health Care Policy and Research Clinical Practice Guidelines for the Management of Cancer Pain.[83] The therapy recommended in these guidelines was in stark contrast to that provided by the defendant physician. It should be noted that the family initiated the litigation only after their complaint against the physician that was filed with the Medical Board of California failed to result in any disciplinary action against the physician, even though the Board's own expert reported that the pain management provided was inadequate.

The third case also involved an elderly cancer patient, but this one was suffering from mesothelioma. The allegations in the suit brought by his widow and daughter were that, at both a local community hospital and the SNF to which he was subsequently transferred, his pain management was woefully inadequate, resulting in weeks of unnecessary suffering before he died.[84] Because this case was in California, as was the previous one just noted, all defendants elected to settle with the plaintiffs prior to trial. Also, state regulatory agencies took disciplinary action against the SNF and the physician responsible for the patient's care.[85]

The reaction of the medical profession generally to these trends toward holding health care professionals and institutions responsible for the effective management of pain has been quite mixed. Proponents of the proposition that good pain management is an essential element of quality patient care argue that such changes in approach are long overdue. Critics argue that they place clinicians between a rock and hard place, still very much vulnerable to punitive measures for "overprescribing," yet now also at risk for administrative sanction and civil liability for undertreating pain.

With the increase in the nonmedical use of prescription medications in the last decade, it should come as no surprise that some patients with such addiction disorders file suit against the prescribing physician alleging that the addiction was caused by the physician's negligent practice. Such a case recently came before the West Virginia Supreme Court for consideration of certain legal questions submitted by a trial court. The case involved eight separate civil actions brought by 29 individual respondents against a clinic, four physicians practicing at the clinic, and three pharmacies where the medications prescribed by the physicians were filled.[86] The case is remarkable for several reasons. First, many of the plaintiffs admit that they abused controlled substances before they were treated by the defendant physicians. Second, all of the plaintiffs admitted that they had engaged in some or all of the following illegal activities associated with the prescribing and dispensing of controlled substances: criminal possession of pain medications; criminal distribution, purchase, and receipt of pain medications ("off the street"); criminal acquisition of narcotics through misrepresentation, fraud, and forgery; misuse or abuse of pain medications by taking more than the amount prescribed or snorting or injecting the medications to enhance their effects. These problematic behaviors led to the certification of two questions for the state's supreme court: (1) May a person maintain an action if, in order to establish the cause of action, the person must rely, in whole or in part, on an illegal or immoral act or transaction to which the person is a party? (2) May the doctrine of *in pari delicto* (in equal fault) be employed as a bar to tort claims under state law?

The West Virginia Supreme Court majority opinion holds that wrongful or illegal conduct of plaintiffs will not, in this jurisdiction, act as an absolute bar to a claim of negligence. The better approach, according to the majority, is the application of the doctrine of comparative negligence, according to which, as interpreted and applied in West Virginia, a plaintiff may recover damages for negligence unless his/her negligence equals or exceeds that of the defendant. There were vigorous dissenting opinions noting that the wrongful conduct rule has been adopted in 13 states and the rule has been used to deny similar liability claims for drug addiction. According to these dissenting opinions, West Virginia is an outlier in its approach to a lawsuit by a patient against a prescribing physician when the patient's wrongful, perhaps even criminal conduct, caused or contributed to the addiction that is the source of the patient's injury. Whether such claims will be viable in other jurisdictions will be a matter of interpretation of state law.

Interestingly, one of the physician defendants in the West Virginia case, described above, is Dr. Katherine Hoover, who successfully challenged disciplinary proceedings in Florida. She was the number one prescriber of opioids in West Virginia at the time authorities raided the Mountain Medical Care clinic where she practiced, and alleged numerous instances of illegal prescribing. Ultimately, Dr. Hoover did not face criminal charges and reportedly no longer resides in the United States.

As will be noted hereafter in more detail, the concept of "illegal prescribing" that would justify criminal prosecution of a physician is somewhat ambiguous. In general, it involves the prescribing of a controlled substance without any legitimate medical purpose, hence warranting the claim that it was done outside the scope of any legitimate practice of medicine. The West Virginia Mountain Medical Care case is perhaps distinguishable from the numerous cases (often criminal prosecutions) against so-called "pill mills." This term lacks a well-recognized and consistently applied definition. The writing or dispensing of prescription medications without a legitimate medical purpose and, hence, outside the bounds of the legitimate practice of medicine or pharmacy is the *sine qua non* of a pill mill. As a practical matter, health care professionals involved in practices to which the term "pill mill" would legitimately apply are not simply treating a high volume of patients with serious pain problems, but rather are intentionally engaged in the criminal enterprise of selling controlled substances for profit in violation of state and federal law. A PowerPoint presentation on the DEA website provides a detailed description of such activities, where they have been found to be most extensive, and efforts are underway to curtail and punish them.[87]

Given the extent of harms associated with the nonmedical use of prescription opioids, numerous lawsuits have been filed against Purdue Pharma LP over its marketing of OxyContin. In addition to claims by individuals, suits are pending by the State of Kentucky, the city of Chicago, Illinois, as well as Santa Clara and Orange counties in California.[88] The common thread in these complaints is that the company's marketing strategy for OxyContin intentionally and deceptively sought to downplay the risks of abuse and addiction to which those who were prescribed the drug would be subjected. Thus far, the company has managed to win dismissals of over 400 personal injury lawsuits related to the drug, as well as defeating over 10 attempts to pursue class actions. It was reported in late 2014 that Purdue Pharma LP had never gone to trial in a case alleging OxyContin abuse.[89] The Kentucky case was originally filed in 2007 and has been working its way through both state and federal courts ever since.

CRIMINAL LITIGATION

Criminal prosecutions of physicians at either the state or federal level are relatively rare, and generally reserved for egregious departures from acceptable care.[90] Those concerning pain management usually involve allegations that excessive prescribing of opioids either lead to a patient's untimely death and therefore constitute homicide, or that the prescriptions had no legitimate medical purpose and therefore violated provisions of the federal CSA. These cases vary significantly based on their underlying facts, but the following are illustrative of the two general types.

In 1994, the attorney general of Kansas filed a two-count indictment against small-town Kansas physician,

L. Stanley Naramore, relating to his care of two terminally ill patients. One of these patients, Ruth Leach, was dying of advanced breast cancer metastatic to bones, lungs, and brain. Dr. Naramore was charged and convicted of her attempted murder based on the doses of Versed and fentanyl that he prescribed to control her pain when she was in the hospital, and his plan to subsequently administer morphine. Shortly after explaining the need to ensure her comfort, he was told by the patient's son that he would be held accountable for the patient's death, whereupon he withdrew as her physician. Mrs. Leach was subsequently transferred to another hospital where she died several days later of her cancer. At the criminal trial, the state's expert witnesses testified that the types and doses of pain medications prescribed by Dr. Naramore were excessive and would have shortly thereafter resulted in respiratory failure. Dr. Naramore's expert witnesses testified that his plan for controlling Ruth Leach's pain was well within the standard of acceptable care given her pain and distress, and her impending death from cancer.

Perhaps the most significant aspect of the Naramore prosecution was the disposition of the conviction on appeal.[91] The Kansas Court of Appeals noted that the transcript of this trial looked very much like the typical "battle of the expert witnesses" that characterizes medical malpractice cases. While in such civil actions a jury has substantial discretion as to what evidence it finds persuasive, in a criminal prosecution the jury must find beyond a reasonable doubt that all elements of the offense charged have been proven. The court concluded that on the record before it, no reasonable jury could have found that beyond a reasonable doubt Dr. Naramore intended to kill Ruth Leach rather than to control her pain and symptom distress as she was dying of her underlying disease. The case should stand not only as reassurance to physicians caring for dying patients, but also as a cautionary tale for prosecutors that if the defendant can provide competent, credible expert testimony in support of the appropriateness of the care provided, the state's burden of proof cannot be met, and in the reasonable exercise of prosecutorial discretion no charges should be filed.

Federal prosecutions for violations of the CSA have often involved physicians caring for large numbers of patients with chronic noncancer pain. A typical, and closely followed, case was *United States v. Hurwitz*. Dr. William Hurwitz operated a pain medicine practice in McLean, Virginia; patients from 39 states came to his practice seeking opioids to manage their chronic pain conditions. He was indicted in 2004 by a federal grand jury on 62 counts, including drug trafficking resulting in death and serious bodily injury, and health care fraud, among others. The prosecution claimed that Dr. Hurwitz knew, or in the exercise of sound clinical judgment should have known, that many of the persons to whom he prescribed opioids either were addicts or sought drugs for misuse or diversion. He was subsequently convicted of 50 counts. On appeal, the 4th Circuit Court of Appeals reversed the convictions and remanded the case for a new trial on the grounds that he had not been allowed to argue to the jury that his prescribing had been a good faith exercise of clinical judgment.[92] When retried, Dr. Hurwitz was convicted of 16 counts and sentenced to 57 months in prison.

There is a legitimately concerning element that is common to many of these prosecutions. The government and its expert witnesses have been able to persuade juries that there are only two types of situations and that a clear line of demarcation separates them. The first constitutes adherence to the standard of care for prescribing opioids. The second is a material departure from the standard of care that takes the physician's action outside the bounds of medical practice and renders the prescribing physician nothing more than a drug dealer with a medical degree. In fact, whether one is prescribing opioids for chronic pain or practicing any other form of medicine, there are many levels of care, only one of which can be properly characterized as "outside the bounds of medicine." At the pinnacle of the hierarchy of practice would be "best practices," such as consistently following nationally recognized clinical practice guidelines. Below that would be the usual custom and practice or acceptable care, which may or may not track the guidelines. Further down would come isolated instances in which a practitioner's care falls below the standard of care and may give rise to a malpractice claim or minor action by a state medical board. Below this would be serious or repeated departures from acceptable practice, which might not only lead to multiple adverse medical malpractice verdicts but also lead to suspension or revocation of medical licensure. The final category would be practices so far removed from the standard of care as to be characterized as "outside the bounds of medicine." Unless and until drug regulators, prosecutors, and juries come to recognize these distinctions, there will continue to be a profound chilling effect on prescribing practices from high-profile and successful prosecutions like that of William Hurwitz.

Three recent cases against individual physicians also are of particular significance. A southern California physician, Dr. Hsiu-Ying "Lisa" Tseng, was convicted of second-degree murder when three of her patients died from drug overdoses. Her attorney argued that at worst these should constitute the basis for professional liability claims, not criminal homicide. She also stated that the jury verdict would be appealed.[93] One month earlier, a Florida jury acquitted a pain clinic physician of murder and other charges of drug trafficking, but did convict him of a single count reported to involve a benzodiazepine medication. It is of unclear significance that the patient was reported to have been prescribed this drug at the time he was employed as a chef for Donald Trump, the 2016 republican candidate for the US presidency.[94]

It is often challenging to explain different outcomes in what appear to be similar cases. While cases at the trial court level have no precedential value, that fact may be lost on both lay people and health care professionals. The case that follows offers a good illustration of the kind of professional practice that will minimize the likelihood that criminal charges will be filed in the first place and, in the unlikely event that they are, that will maximize the likelihood of a favorable outcome.

Finally, a federal jury acquitted a board-certified physical medicine and rehabilitation physician in Fort Meyers, FL, who was criminally charged with 10 counts of prescribing controlled substances outside the bounds of acceptable medical practice, thereby causing her patients to become addicted. The charges stemmed from "Operation Pill Mill

Nation 2." Her defense team attributed the outcome to the defendant's meticulous record-keeping on each of her patients, clearly documenting the medical basis for prescribing the medications. Her attorneys said the federal prosecutors unsuccessfully sought to persuade the jury that a high opioid dosage was *per se* criminal and necessarily led to addiction.[95]

CONSTITUTIONAL CASES

The cases involving pain management that involve constitutional interpretation have, for the most part, concerned the phenomenon of prohibitions on or attempts to regulate the practice of providing a lethal prescription at the request of a terminally ill patient. In 1997, the US Supreme Court ruled unanimously that there is neither a constitutional right to nor a constitutional prohibition of what was then characterized as "physician-assisted suicide." Thus, the matter was left to "the laboratory of the states" as one of the justices phrased it.[96] In the early years of President George W. Bush's administration, Attorney General John Ashcroft sought to nullify the Oregon Death with Dignity Act, which legalized and regulated the provision of lethal prescriptions for terminally ill patients. He insisted that such prescriptions violated the CSA since there was no legitimate medical purpose to support them. The case took many years to litigate and, by the time it reached the Supreme Court, Ashcroft had been succeeded by Alberto Gonzales. In 2006, the Supreme Court ruled (by a 6 to 3 vote) that the Attorney General had exceeded his authority when he issued an interpretive ruling that such prescriptions violated the CSA and could therefore be the basis of physician sanction.[97] The reasoning of the majority was that regulation of the medical profession has been traditionally a matter of state law, and nothing in the language or history of the CSA supported the Attorney General's position.

CONCLUSION

The prudent practice of pain management requires more than up-to-date knowledge and skills in the assessment and management of pain. It also requires a basic familiarity with the legal and regulatory landscape described in this chapter. For the most part, health care professionals who encounter significant legal problems associated with their pain management practices remain a distinct and insular minority. Often, but not always, their prescribing practices are aberrational in the extreme. Providing appropriate pain management, now more than ever, requires a familiarity with and adherence to a wide assortment of state and federal laws, regulations, and judicial decisions. As with any other form of professional practice, continually updating one's knowledge and skills through regular reference to leading professional journals, continuing professional education conferences in one's primary areas of practice, and familiarity with applicable laws and policies are important components in a risk minimization strategy. If there is a single technique likely to serve the adequately informed and skilled prescribing professional well, it is scrupulous documentation of all patient encounters in a level of detail that transparently illuminates medical decisions and supports the appropriateness of the care provided.

KEY POINTS

- Appropriate health care practice is a function of clinicians' understanding of and conforming to both federal and state statutes and regulations governing medication prescribing.
- Many states' laws contain addiction-related definitions (i.e., "drug dependent person," "narcotic-dependent person," "addict," "active addiction," "narcotic addict," or "habitué") that could legally apply to patients being treated for pain with prescription opioid medications.
- The University of Wisconsin Pain & Policy Studies Group has developed resources to inform clinicians about the content of federal and state policies related to pain management.
- The Federation of State Medical Boards has a history of encouraging responsible opioid medication prescribing for pain management.
- Attempts to reduce prescription opioid-related harms requires addressing diversion activities in addition to clinician prescribing.
- Litigation involving pain management may involve all four domains of law: administrative, civil, criminal, and constitutional.
- Allegations of inappropriate pain management may arise from either excessive or insufficient utilization of opioid analgesics.
- Prescribing practitioners can be held legally accountable for failure to practice pain management consistently with federal and state statutes and regulations, as well as the prevailing standards of their profession.
- As with all other aspects of professional practice, careful, thorough, and timely documentation of each patient encounter can be critical, not only to sound clinical practice but also in successfully defending against allegations that may arise in subsequent legal proceedings.

REFERENCES

Access the reference list online at ExpertConsult.com.

CHAPTER

46 URINE DRUG TESTING IN PAIN MEDICINE

Gagan Mahajan, MD

The recent Institute of Medicine report declared that greater than 100 million Americans have chronic pain with an associated cost of up to $635 billion each year due to medical treatment and lost productivity.[1,2] The explosion in opioid prescribing since the 1990s has resulted in opioids being the most frequently prescribed medication in the United States.[3–5] Manchikanti et al.'s study revealed a 149% increase in retail opioid sales and a 402% increase in average sales of opioids per person in the United States from 1997 to 2007.[6] Looking at 1999–2012, the National Center for Health Statistics found that among patients aged 20 or older prescription opioid use increased from 5% to 6.9% until 2006 and then stayed at 6.9% until 2012.[7] However, the percentage of patients using an opioid stronger than morphine dramatically increased from 17% to 37% over the same time period.[7] Among the top 25 dispensed prescriptions in the United States, hydrocodone, tramadol, and oxycodone accounted for the number 1, 21, and 22 dispensed prescriptions, respectively.[5] Opioids represent one of many therapeutic options to treat chronic nonmalignant pain (CNMP), but their widespread use has resulted in a concomitant increase in misuse, abuse, addiction, overdose, and diversion. While there is evidence of short-term benefit of opioids for treating pain based on randomized trials lasting less than 3 months, there are few studies reporting outcomes at 12 months or longer.[8,9]

While few studies have demonstrated the long-term benefits of chronic opioid therapy (COT), mounting evidence has demonstrated the potential adverse risks (opioid use disorder, overdose, and motor vehicle injury) associated with COT.[2,10] Death due to opioid overdose has occurred in 165,000 individuals from 1999 to 2014,[11] and while most patients who are on COT will not develop an opioid-use disorder, the likelihood is greater than in the general population. One study demonstrated that an opioid-use disorder occurred in 3.8% of those on COT versus 0.9% of the general population, and other studies suggest abuse rates can be as high as 18% to 41%.[12,13] Among patients with chronic pain who were either taking or not taking a controlled substance, illicit substance abuse was noted in 14% to 16% and 34%, respectively.[2] In 2014, approximately 27.0 million Americans aged 12 or older were current (past month) illicit drug users.[14] While marijuana was by far the most commonly used illicit drug (22.2 million Americans), use of pain relievers (opioid and nonopioid) for nonmedical purposes was second (4.3 million Americans).[14] Of the people aged 12 or older who had a prescription pain reliever use disorder (1.9 million people, or 0.7% of the people aged 12 or older), the percentage was largely the same as it was from 2005 to 2013.[14] Based on an analysis of 2.1 million patient urine drug testing reports, the most recent annual Quest Diagnostics Health Trends *Prescription Drug Monitoring Report 2015* revealed consistent results in 47% and inconsistent results in 53%; and of the inconsistent results, 44% had no drug, 35% had additional drugs, and 21% had different drugs (Fig. 46.1).[15] While the inconsistent results are high, it represents a decline from 63% in 2011, likely due to a multitude of factors: implementation and use of the prescription drug monitoring program in the prescriber's state, federal and state legislation on opioid prescribing guidelines, practitioner education, public awareness campaigns, and utilization of law enforcement.[15]

For those patients in whom opioids might be beneficial, many clinicians express reluctance to prescribe them for various reasons, such as lack of education and training in opioid prescribing; concerns about misuse, abuse, addiction, tolerance, side effects; fear of regulatory investigation; and lack of evidence proving COT is efficacious for managing CNMP.[2,16] Such concerns present barriers to the use of COT for CNMP. Numerous screening instruments have been developed to risk-stratify patients on COT for substance misuse and addiction, but it is up to the clinician to decide which one(s) to use since no one instrument has been shown to be superior to all others. Use of risk-assessment tools (e.g., Screener and Opioid Assessment for Patients with Pain [SOAPP] and Opioid Risk Tool [ORT], and Drug Abuse Screening Test [DAST]) and obtaining a

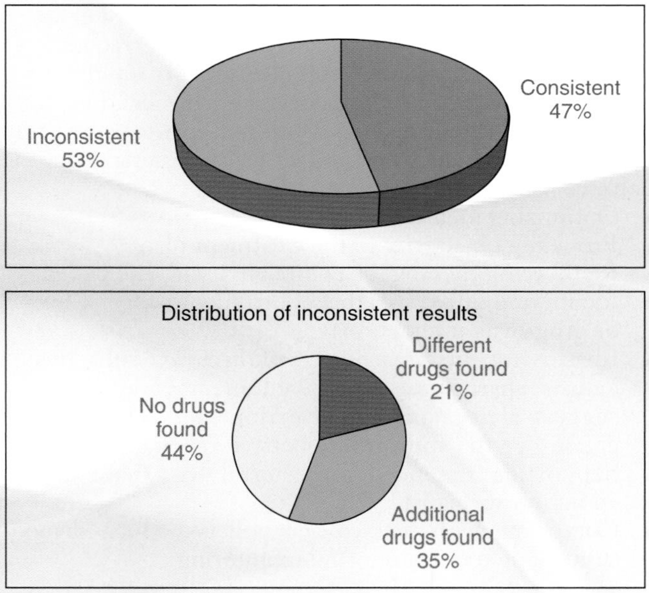

FIG. 46.1 Distribution of urine drug testing reports for Quest Diagnostics (January 2014 to December 2014). *(From Blatt A, Chen Z, McClure L, Niles J, Kaufman M: Prescription drug misuse in America: diagnostic insights in the continuing drug epidemic battle. Quest Diagnostics Health Trends Prescription Drug Monitoring Report 2015, 16.)*

careful history and physical exam can assist the clinician in determining the level of risk associated with prescribing opioids for a patient and the associated level of monitoring needed.[17]

In a retrospective analysis of urine drug testing results in 470 patients, one study found that noncompliance with COT occurred in 45%.[18] Not taking a medication as a reason for noncompliance can be due to the following: patient personality and beliefs, sociodemographic and environmental issues, patient-clinician communication, severity and chronicity of health problems, comorbid illnesses, complexity of the treatment plan, side effect profile, and drug-drug interactions.[19,20] Taking a medication not as prescribed as a reason for lack of compliance can be due to difficulty seeing a clinician, self-escalation, abuse, addiction, and diversion. All of these problems have significant medical and/or societal consequences.[21] For patients on COT, urine drug testing represents one of many ways to objectively monitor for compliance with a designated treatment plan, identify substance misuse or abuse, and support medical decisions for continuing or discontinuing COT.[21] Numerous studies have shown that patient self-reports are notoriously inaccurate, with patients underreporting or denying noncompliance or illicit drug abuse.[12,13,17,22] Patients may fail to report or underreport a past or current history of addiction or drug misuse for fear of not having their pain treated.[23] Furthermore, profiling based on a patient's race, socioeconomic status, and gender is poor at determining who will have an abnormal urine drug testing result.[12,17,18,22]

The rationale for performing urine drug testing, which is to support patient care, should be explained to the patient. Consent for urine drug testing should be included in an opioid treatment agreement and prior to initiating COT, thereby reducing a patient's confusion or surprise when a specimen is requested. Urine drug testing should be included as part of a comprehensive monitoring program that includes accessing the prescription drug monitoring program (PDMP); behavior monitoring (self-escalation, reports of lost or stolen prescriptions, frequent phone calls to the clinic, requesting a same-day appointment for a refill, allegations of multiple drug intolerances or allergies); and documenting relief, functional improvement, and side effects. With appropriate patient education, a thoughtfully structured urine drug testing policy can enhance patient care by[23–25]:

- Optimizing medication therapy
- Providing objectivity to the treatment plan
- Reinforcing therapeutic compliance with the patient
- Identifying substances that contribute to adverse events or drug-drug interactions
- Identifying the presence of undisclosed substance(s) and/or absence of prescribed medication(s), which suggest abuse, misuse, diversion, and addiction, to encourage the appropriate behavioral changes
- Supporting the need for referral to a pain and/or addiction specialist
- Complying with medicolegal policies, which demonstrate patient evaluation and monitoring

HISTORY OF URINE DRUG TESTING

To assure a drug-free workplace, the *Mandatory Guidelines for Federal Workplace Drug Testing Programs* came about as a result of the Federal Drug Free Workplace Act established in the 1980s.[26] The five drugs tested for in a federal urine drug test (UDT) include opiates, marijuana, cocaine, phenylcyclohexyl piperidine (PCP), and amphetamine/methamphetamine. Eventually, urine drug testing as a means of deterring and detecting illicit drug use expanded to nonfederal workplaces, sports organizations, schools, forensics, and the health care arena.[17] Unfortunately, the type of urine drug testing performed and method of testing employed by federal testing is suboptimal for the health care setting. With federal testing, thresholds for the detection of opioids and illicit substances are higher as determined by statutes, the testing panel is limited with a fewer number of opioids tested, specimen collection may be witnessed, there is a strict chain of custody, and there is no therapeutic relationship between the individual and testing entity.[27]

BODILY SPECIMENS THAT CAN BE TESTED

Why test urine as opposed to other bodily specimens, such as blood, hair, sweat, or saliva? Unless a patient has a neurogenic bladder requiring intermittent catheterization, **urine** is an easily obtainable noninvasive specimen, is cheap to analyze, can be analyzed with in-office point-of-care (POC) tests, is detectable for days, has higher concentrations of the parent drug and/or metabolites than serum, and has the most extensively published information and evidence for adherence testing.[2,28] The disadvantages of urine specimens include ease of adulteration or substitution, a short to intermediate window of detection, and difficulty of same patients to spontaneously provide a specimen.[28] Other bodily specimens possess apparent advantages, but limitations currently override widespread use as part of an adherence-monitoring program.

Measuring a drug's **serum** concentrations is useful in the setting of the anuric patient or for detecting recent substance use, such as in the intoxicated patient seen in an Emergency Department setting. There are established testing methods for serum.[28] The disadvantages of serum specimens are the cost, the narrow window of detectability (hours), and invasiveness.[17,28,29] Because drawing blood requires a trained professional, use of this specimen in the workplace setting is not practical or economically feasible.[17]

Saliva concentrations reflect serum concentrations since the salivary gland is highly perfused.[30] In addition to being noninvasive, testing saliva offers more potential advantages compared to testing urine: ease of specimen collection, ability to witness collection in a less embarrassing manner than a urine specimen, low likelihood of adulteration, ability to target the parent drug instead of the metabolite, and availability as a POC test.[28,31,32] Saliva testing, however, has limitations: salivary concentration is influenced by salivary pH, with basic drugs being found in a higher concentration; low concentrations of a drug may be difficult to detect if the salivary volume is low; elution solvent must adequately remove the drugs adsorbed to the collection device; drug-interference patterns, cross-reactivity, and impact of potential adulterants are not as well studied; and because it reflects serum concentrations, the window of detectability is only hours.[17,28,29,33]

Hair testing presents a number of advantages: minimally invasive; specimen is easy to store and transport; collection can be observed with minimal embarrassment or risk of substitution; and, depending on the length of the hair sample, the window of detectability expands from days to months.[28] Clinical application of hair testing is challenged by a number of factors: unclear relationship to timing and dosing of the drug versus hair length; difficulty detecting low-level use and low drug concentrations; difficulty obtaining a sufficient hair sample from those who shave or who otherwise have minimal body hair; hair can be adulterated by using dyes or other stylistic treatments; a drug is more readily identified in naturally occurring dark-colored hair versus lighter colored or white hair, thereby inherently biasing test results; and costly and time-consuming sample preparation.[28,29,33] Ultimately, hair analysis is really useful from a forensics standpoint as it is most reliable for detecting chronic drug use as opposed to recent and infrequent drug use.[28,29]

Sweat testing presents a number of advantages as it is minimally invasive, difficult to adulterate, and has a window of detectability that allows detection of drug that has been used within 24 hours (using a sweat wipe) or up to weeks (using a sweat patch worn for 1 to 2 weeks), which is ideal for monitoring in a chemical dependency or probation program.[28,29] Sweat patch testing requires two visits for application and removal of the patch.[28] Drug detection depends on the drug's diffusion from the vasculature to the sweat gland, molecular mass, pKa, protein binding, lipophilicity, where the patch is applied, patch adherence to the skin, and impact of potential adulterants.[17] Development of more successful technical and scientific guidelines is needed for these alternate specimens before they can be used as a substitute for a urine specimen.

URINE DRUG TESTING

Comprehensive urine drug testing is a two-step process (Table 46.1). The first step is an enzyme-mediated immunoassay screen (IAS), which is strictly a qualitative test used to screen for the presence or absence of drug classes.[21,23] IASs included in the federal workplace test for five classes mandated by the Substance Abuse and Mental Health Services Administration (SAMHSA): amphetamine, cocaine, marijuana, PCP, and opiates (limited to codeine, morphine, and 6-monoacetyl-morphine to test for heroin use). Most IASs performed in the clinical setting test for the same "SAMHSA-5," but maintaining such a limited panel is not recommended.[34] Other drugs or classes, such as benzodiazepines, barbiturates, methamphetamine, semisynthetic opioids, methadone, and buprenorphine should also be included. Since it is neither cost efficient nor practical to test for all drugs and illicit substances, clinicians may need to customize their IAS and UDT panels to identify the most commonly used drugs and illicit substances. Furthermore, because it is impossible to identify all drugs present in a specimen, let alone all drugs within the same class, astute clinicians must recognize that an IAS is not definitive. Therefore, an IAS is only helpful for making preliminary treatment decisions.

IASs typically work by measuring an antigen-antibody reaction. Antigens—the free drug and/or free drug metabolite and the same labeled drug and/or labeled drug metabolite—compete for antibodies to elicit an enzymatic reaction.[20,34] When the free drug and metabolite are absent, the labeled drug and metabolite bind the antibody to prevent enzymatic activity.[20,34] However, when the free drug or metabolite is present, it displaces the labeled drug or metabolite to create an enzymatic reaction that is measurable and proportional to the concentration of the free drug or metabolite.[20,34] Regarding an IAS's antigen-antibody specificity, this can account for why an immunoassay can be specific for particular drugs (e.g., it principally detects the cocaine metabolite, benzoylecgonine, which has a longer half-life than cocaine itself and, if used as a legitimate topical anesthetic, does not cross-react with any other local anesthetic); it can be so specific for a particular drug that it excludes similar drugs (e.g., it detects morphine and codeine, but not methadone); or it can be so nonspecific that it has difficulty differentiating drugs in the same class (e.g., it cannot distinguish morphine from codeine, and it has low sensitivity for detecting semisynthetic opioids); or it cross-reacts with unrelated drugs which are structurally similar enough to trigger a false positive for a particular drug class (Table 46.2).[23]

TABLE 46.1 Comprehensive Urine Drug Testing

	Step 1: Immunoassay Screen	Step 2: Urine Drug Test (GC/MS or LC/MS)
WHERE	In-office or laboratory	Laboratory
TURNAROUND TIME	Minutes	Hours-days
ASSESSMENT	Drug classes Some medications Some illicit substances	Measures concentrations of parent compound and metabolite(s)
PLAN	Preliminary treatment decisions	Mostly definitive
CROSS-REACTIVITY	Common: more false positives	Less common: fewer false positives
THRESHOLD OF DETECTABILITY	Higher: more false negatives	Lower: fewer false negatives

From Webster LR: The Role of Urine Drug Testing in Chronic Pain Management: 2013 Update. New York: McMahon Publishing; 6:2013.

In addition to identifying illicit drugs, advantages of an IAS are that it is cheap, yields results within minutes, and is convenient (either performed with an in-office POC test or sent to a laboratory for testing).[17] Originally developed to monitor workers for illicit substance use, a POC IAS offers the advantage of a faster turnaround time (minutes to hours) while the patient could still be in the clinic than a laboratory-based IAS.[12,28,35] However, performance of a POC IAS depends on having clinic personnel who are trained in precisely following the manufacturer's specific instructions (e.g., amount of sample to use, sample application, and timing of reaction) and understanding how to interpret the result given the test's inherent limitations.[12,17,21,28] Since a POC IAS is a noninstrumented test, in most cases, the person handling

TABLE 46.2 Drugs That May Cause False Positive Results on an Immunoassay Screen[77]

Opiates	Dextromethorphan, diphenhydramine, fluoroquinolones, poppy seeds, quinine, rifampin, verapamil
Amphetamines	Amantadine, bupropion, chlorpromazine, desipramine, fluoxetine, L-methamphetamine (nasal decongestant), labetalol, phentermine, phenylephrine, promethazine, pseudoephedrine, ranitidine, thioridazine, trazodone
Benzodiazepines	Oxaprozin, sertraline
PCP	Dextromethorphan, diphenhydramine, ibuprofen, imipramine, ketamine, venlafaxine, meperidine, thioridazine, tramadol, venlafaxine
Cocaine	Topical anesthetics that contain cocaine
Tetrahydrocannabinol	Dronabinol, nonsteroidal antiinflammatory drugs, proton pump inhibitors

PCP, *Phenylcyclohexyl piperidine.*
From Standridge JB, Adams SM, Zotos AP: Urine drug screening: a valuable office procedure. Am Fam Phys. *81:635-640, 2010.*

the "device" (dipstick, cup, card, or cassette) must visually interpret its appearance and manually enter the data into the electronic medical record.[17] Because interpretation of some devices depends on a color change after application of a specimen, any delay in when the change is interpreted, even as little as 10 minutes, can result in an inaccurate analysis since the color can continue to change over time.[26] Some POC IASs, however, can be read by a meter, which then transfers the result electronically to the electronic health record.[17] A POC IAS should also include a "control" to be certain that the device is working as expected.[26]

Because manufacturers of POC IASs may differ in terms of threshold of detectability, specificity for identifying the target drugs of interest, reproducibility, and complexity of performing the test, the IAS results can differ between brand manufacturers. But not only can there be variation between brand manufacturers, there can also be variations between manufactured lots/batches that can lead to differing outcomes.[26,34] Studies have also demonstrated inconsistencies in product performance versus the manufacturer's claims and deviations in threshold reporting (identifying drugs or metabolites below the threshold or not identifying drugs or metabolites above the threshold).[36] Crouch et al. compared the utility and accuracy of five POC IAS brand manufacturers (800 specimens) and found that each brand had a false-negative rate of less than 1% for all drug classes and false-positive rates of less than 0.25% (marijuana, cocaine, and opiates), less than 1.5% (PCP), and less than 1.75% (amphetamine).[37] While studies comparing the accuracy of POC IASs and laboratory-based IASs suggest both provide similar results, limitations of the studies were due to the fact that laboratory-trained personnel performed the POC IASs, and challenges in interpreting the results were greatest when at the lower end of threshold of detectability.[17]

For clinicians who opt to use a POC IAS, it must be certified by the Clinical Laboratory Improvement Amendments of 1988 (CLIA) depending on the Food and Drug Administration's (FDA) categorization of test complexity (e.g., waived, moderate, or high).[34] Medicare reimbursement also requires this certification. A CLIA Certificate of Waiver can be obtained for those POC IASs that the FDA approves for use in nonlaboratory settings (e.g., home and office) provided the POC IAS is easy to use and interpret and the clinic follows the manufacturer's explicit testing instructions.[36] To minimize testing errors and maximize quality assurance, the Centers for Disease Control and Prevention's Division of Laboratory Systems created "Good Laboratory Practices for Waived Testing Sites."[38] In addition, the manufacturers of POC IASs include specific instructions on specimen collection, handling, storage and testing, reference values, and recording of test results. It is up to the clinician to review the device manufacturer's instructions on whether confirmatory testing is or is not needed. Violating the manufacturer's instructions may otherwise invalidate the device's CLIA-waived status.[26] It is up to the clinician to determine which POC IAS is covered by any given insurance company and to compare the cost and expediency of performing a POC versus laboratory-based IAS. If one requires an immediate result to assist with making a clinical decision while the patient is still in the clinic, a POC IAS would be most prudent. If an immediate result is not needed, then the clinician may consider sending the specimen to the laboratory. From an insurance standpoint, Medicare will not reimburse for both a POC IAS and laboratory-based IAS at the same clinical encounter.[25]

In a laboratory setting, the IAS is performed by licensed personnel using automated analyzers. The advantage of using an automated analyzer is that results can be automatically exported to the patient's electronic health record. Similar to a POC IAS, a laboratory IAS is also subject to variability among testing products. Because of its complex regulatory status (ensuring both quality control of the test product and analyzer and proficiency of the personnel doing the testing) and overhead (equipment and trained personnel), the cost and reimbursement is higher than with a POC IAS.[26]

The second step in comprehensive urine drug testing is a confirmatory UDT, which requires laboratory-based testing using gas chromatography-mass spectrometry (GC/MS) or liquid chromatography-mass spectrometry (LC/MS). A UDT is a quantitative test that adds a much higher level of sensitivity and specificity than an IAS and identifies, where applicable, the specific drug within a class as well as drug metabolite and drug concentration. Unlike an IAS, most UDTs can identify codeine, fentanyl, hydrocodone, hydromorphone, methadone, morphine, oxycodone, and oxymorphone. This is especially important for those chronic pain patients who are on more than one type of opioid. With some opioids, metabolism of the parent opioid can lead to a metabolite of an alternate opioid (e.g., codeine is metabolized to morphine and oxycodone is metabolized to oxymorphone). If both a prescribed drug and its metabolite or only the metabolite is identified on an IAS, it is unclear if the patient is compliant versus abusing nonprescribed opioids and highlights why one might see conflicting results with an IAS versus UDT.[17] Because an IAS is only a qualitative screening test, quantitative confirmatory testing with a UDT should also be performed as part of the adherence-monitoring program.

From a simple technical standpoint, chromatography is a separation method that involves both a stationary phase (contained with the analytical column) and a mobile phase (gas or liquid).[26] A drug that does not interact with the stationary phase exits at the same flow rate as the mobile phase, whereas a drug that interacts with the stationary phase gets retained in a column and exits at a slower rate. There are two different types of chromatography: gas chromatography (GC) and liquid chromatography (LC). And there are two different types of LC: ultra-performance liquid chromatography (UPLC) and high-performance liquid chromatography (HPLC). While GC is the most popular method, UPLC is increasingly a method of choice because of its many advantages over GC: greater sensitivity, requirement for a smaller sample size, faster analysis time, and less laborious sample preparation time.[20]

While chromatography separates the analytes in a specimen, mass spectroscopy (MS) can be combined with both GC and LC to identify the specific molecular structure of individual drugs and/or metabolites based on their mass-to-charge ratio along with their concentrations.[17] Because GC/MS and LC/MS allow for a qualitative and quantitative analysis of the specimen, ambiguous immunoassay results can be resolved by analyzing the concentration of both the parent compound and its metabolite. This improvement in sensitivity and specificity allows for a reduction in false positives and false negatives. The secondary benefit to testing for drug metabolites is greater assurance that the drug has been consumed and processed by the body, whereas the presence of only the parent drug does not rule out the possibility that the urine specimen was adulterated by directly adding the parent drug.[26]

THRESHOLD OF DETECTABILITY

The accuracy of both an IAS and UDT in identifying a drug or illicit substance depends on a number of factors: the IAS's antigen-antibody specificity, the drug concentration in the sample, and the threshold of detectability.[17] Where a laboratory chooses to set its threshold of detectability may depend on whether it is being run for nonclinical (e.g., workplace or forensic) purposes versus clinical purposes. Unlike nonclinical testing standards, the threshold concentrations in a pain management setting are not standardized.[26]

The threshold of detectability intentionally may be set higher in nonclinical testing to yield the fewest false negatives and false positives. For example, morphine's threshold of detection is set at 2000 ng/mL for a workplace IAS compared with 300 ng/mL for a clinical IAS or 50 ng/mL for a clinical UDT.[2] When the drug is absent or the concentration falls below the threshold of detectability, the result is reported as negative, and where the concentration rises above the threshold of detectability, it is reported as positive.[39] For clinical purposes, one should ask the lab to set the lowest threshold of detectability to yield the most true positives and fewest false negatives. However, the by-product of setting a low threshold is that higher sensitivity may also detect impurities or contaminants associated with manufacturing process; for example, two different opioids manufactured on the same equipment may result in low levels of a nonprescribed opioid being detected on an IAS despite the patient using only one prescribed opioid. While a laboratory could conceivably eliminate its threshold, there is a certain concentration below which a laboratory cannot reliably report the result with a high level of confidence, thereby yielding inaccurate results.[17]

WHY PERFORM AN IMMUNOASSAY SCREEN AND URINE DRUG TEST

Even though a diabetic patient may self-report good glycemic control, clinicians still periodically obtain laboratory tests to objectively confirm the retrospective level of diabetes control without accusing the patient of lying.[27] This thought process should be no different with respect to performing an IAS and UDT in the patient on COT. This includes not only monitoring for the prescribed opioid(s), but also for nonprescribed opioid(s) or illicit substances that identify a treatable substance use disorder. For some patients, knowing they are being monitored may reinforce healthy lifestyle changes; and for those who engage in or relapse into problematic drug use, an unexpected test result may provide a safe harbor for the patient and/or clinician to explore treatment options for a substance use disorder.[27] A testing policy also signals to patients, law enforcement authorities, and regulatory authorities that one's vigilance demonstrates a commitment to patient and community safety.[27] Used in this manner, testing is one tool that can be used in supporting the clinician's decision to continue versus discontinue COT.

Caution should be exercised when interpreting test results because of limitations related to thresholds of detection, variables that affect drug concentration (pharmacokinetics, pharmacodynamics, and pharmacogenetics), and variables related to the specimen itself (collection, handling, and analysis).[40] These limitations and variables also, in part, explain why there is no scientifically validated relationship between the urine drug concentration and the amount of drug taken, the timing of when the drug was last taken, or the source of the drug.[24]

WHO SHOULD GET AN IMMUNOASSAY SCREEN AND URINE DRUG TEST

While every patient is entitled to pain management, COT may not be the safest option for every patient. When a risk-benefit analysis suggests benefits outweigh risks, testing should be performed in patients in whom a trial of COT is being considered, patients already on COT who are transferring care, patients in whom an opioid rotation is being considered, patients being referred to a pain specialist, as part of a random process to monitor for adherence, or when behavioral signs suggest concern (lost or stolen medications, requests for early refills, unannounced clinic visits, doctor shopping, frequent Emergency Department visits, request for certain opioid(s), or allergies to multiple opioids).[23,24,41] Those who are candidates for COT and consent to their use must also accept responsibility for using the medication as prescribed and under the conditions stipulated by the opioid agreement the patient signs with the clinician.[27] One of the conditions of prescribing

TABLE 46.3 Suggested Frequency of Urine Drug Testing[25,42,43]

Risk Category Based on Opioid Risk Tool	Baseline	Random	Number of Times	Frequency
Low risk	Yes	Yes	1–2	Every 12 months
Moderate risk	Yes	Yes	1–2	Every 6 months
High risk or opioid dose >120 mg morphine equivalents per day	Yes	Yes	1–3	Every 3 months
Aberrant behavior (lost prescriptions, multiple requests for early refills, opioid prescriptions from >1 provider, self-escalation, intoxication)	—	—	—	At time of visit

COT should include the patient consenting to random testing. While the patient is within his/her rights to object to random testing, the clinician is not obligated to initiate or continue the COT since opioid analgesics are not a required therapy. For the patient who states he/she cannot submit a specimen (e.g., because he/she already urinated, is late for work, or has another appointment to attend), options include holding the prescription until the patient can urinate later that day vs. giving a limited supply (e.g., one-day supply) and making further refills contingent upon submitting a specimen within a specified period of time (e.g., 24 hours).[27] A uniform practice policy is helpful in avoiding bias in determining who gets tested and reducing the stigma associated with submitting an IAS and UDT.[23]

WHEN TO GET AN IMMUNOASSAY SCREEN AND URINE DRUG TEST

Katz et al. showed that urine drug testing only those who have a history of addiction or exhibit aberrant behavior missed a significant number of patients who had unexpected test results.[22] To confirm the veracity of a patient's responses to questions about his/her controlled substance use or illicit substance use, the clinician should consider obtaining an IAS and UDT prior to the initiation of COT, upon inheriting a patient who is already on COT that was initiated by another provider, prior to dose escalation or opioid rotation, in those instances when a patient exhibits behaviors or makes statements that may arouse suspicion, and randomly during maintenance therapy as part of an ongoing monitoring program.[23] Combining urine drug testing with other monitoring techniques makes the most sense.[21] Using this formulaic approach helps the clinician avoid profiling and stigmatizing patients based on race, ethnicity, socioeconomic status, or gender.

HOW OFTEN TO GET AN IMMUNOASSAY SCREEN AND URINE DRUG TEST

Because there is no evidence-based guideline that pinpoints which patients with chronic pain should be tested, definitive criteria for frequency of testing similarly do not exist. The frequency of testing beyond baseline urine drug testing is left to the clinician's discretion based on individual patient needs and documented medical necessity.[25] Table 46.3 shows one suggestion on monitoring frequency.[25,42,43] However, some state guidelines may suggest or require certain frequencies.

WHAT IS THE EVIDENCE FOR GETTING AN IMMUNOASSAY SCREEN AND URINE DRUG TEST?

Numerous consensus guidelines authored by national and state pain societies and federal and regulatory agencies have commented on the usefulness of urine drug testing as one strategy for adherence monitoring to increase patient safety (by identifying nonprescribed opioid or illicit drugs) and to decrease diversion (by identifying absence of prescribed opioid), but recommendations on who should get tested and frequency of testing vary.[44–55] In 2009, Chou et al. reported on the quality of evidence and recommendations for monitoring patients on COT (Table 46.4).[44] While the quality of evidence was low for how to monitor patients on COT, the authors strongly recommended that clinicians should at least assess patients periodically and as determined by circumstances (changes in the pain condition, comorbid illness, or psychosocial status) by documenting pain scores, functional improvement, presence of side effects, and adherence to the prescribed therapy to ascertain whether the treatment plan needs to be modified. For those patients determined to be high risk for COT, the quality of evidence was "*low*" for periodic testing, but the authors' recommendation for testing was "*strong.*" The likelihood of picking up abnormal test results is greater in high-risk patients.[44] For those patients determined to be low risk for COT, the quality of evidence was similarly "*low,*" but for this group, the authors' recommendation for periodic testing was "*weak.*" While there remains insufficient evidence that testing leads to improved clinical outcomes or deters against substance use, some studies suggest testing may enhance compliance when patients know that random tests may be performed.[17,44,56] Furthermore, cross-sectional studies and case series show that it can be a useful tool to monitor for adherence beyond patient self-report and behavioral monitoring.[56]

HOW TO INTERPRET AN IMMUNOASSAY SCREEN AND URINE DRUG TEST

Given the controversies surrounding COT for CNMP, as well as the many guidelines that recommend IAS and UDT as an expected part of COT, one would assume that random testing should be routine. However, while testing in addiction management is routine, it is not so in chronic

TABLE 46.4 Monitoring Recommendations[44]

	Strength of Recommendation	Quality of Evidence
Reassess patients on COT periodically and as warranted by changing circumstances. Monitoring should include documentation of pain intensity and level of functioning, assessments of progress toward achieving therapeutic goals, presence of adverse events, and adherences to prescribed therapies.	Strong	Low-quality
Periodic urine drug testing should be done to confirm adherence to the COT plan of care in patients who are HIGH-risk or who have engaged in aberrant drug-related behaviors.	Strong	Low-quality
Periodic urine drug testing should be done to confirm adherence to the COT plan of care in patients who are LOW-risk and who have engaged in aberrant drug-related behaviors.	Weak	Low-quality

COT, *Chronic opioid therapy.*

pain management.[2] Studies show that in the primary care setting, few clinicians actually perform urine drug testing or are knowledgeable in interpreting the results.[57] In a retrospective review of 209 patients being taken care of by 74 PCPs, Adams et al. showed only 8% of PCPs performed urine drug testing.[58] Based on a written survery completed by 248 PCPs, Bhamb et al. showed only 7% of PCPs performed urine drug testing before initiating COT, and only 15% did so on existing patients.[16] Reasons for not urine drug testing included discomfort with discussing the premise of testing with patients, lack of access to tests, difficulty interpreting and responding to test results, and believing that testing is not needed because the patient is not at risk for opioid misuse.[23,57,59]

Similar to results from any other laboratory, imaging, or electrodiagnostic study, IAS and UDT results only should be used as one tool to assist with clinical decision-making. (Other tools include carefully taking a history, performing a relevant physical and mental status examination, assessing for risk, monitoring behavior, accessing one's state prescription drug monitoring program, and reviewing past medical records.) Results should be carefully interpreted, documented, and reviewed with the patient. Interindividual variability in drug metabolism can result in drug concentrations that are higher or lower than expected, both potentially leading to inaccurate conclusions.[12] Because an IAS and UDT can result in potentially false positive or false negative results, overinterpretation or underinterpretation of the result can lead to erroneous conclusions, thereby leading to problematic recommendations that can unintentionally harm the patient.[2] One must be knowledgeable regarding drug interference patterns/cross-reactivity and drug metabolism to confidently interpret the results. Some results will include this information for the clinician to facilitate interpretation of the results. However, if a detailed explanation is not included with the results, or if one is in doubt as to the meaning of the results, the clinician should communicate with the laboratory. One study showed that clinicians often have difficulty interpreting test results, and another showed only 23% of clinicians stated they would contact the laboratory if the patient had an abnormal or unexpected result.[12,17]

Outcomes from an IAS and UDT can be broken down into the following general categories:

1. Expected results
   a. Presence of prescribed opioid
   b. Absence of nonprescribed opioids
   c. Absence of any opioid
   d. Absence of any illicit drugs
2. Unexpected results
   a. Absence of prescribed opioid
   b. Presence of nonprescribed opioid
   c. Presence of an illicit drug
   d. Adulterated specimen

However, one must keep in mind that the results are not always definitive, as limitations of an IAS or UDT can sometimes lead to false negative and false positive results. It is incumbent upon the clinician to understand these limitations.

A **false negative** result technically means that a drug whose concentration should be present above the threshold of detection is not detected.[39] This type of false negative can be due to laboratory error (e.g., inappropriate storage/handling of the specimen, performing the test incorrectly, or analyzing the wrong patient's specimen), intentional adulteration of the urine specimen, or limitations of a particular test.[12,23,26] For example, limitations of an IAS include that it is designed to detect opiates (codeine and morphine), but it is unreliable for detecting the presence of semisynthetic (buprenorphine, hydrocodone, hydromorphone, oxycodone, and oxymorphone) and synthetic opioids (fentanyl, meperidine, and methadone) due to variable cross-reactivity (see Table 46.5).[34,39] Furthermore, an opioid metabolized by the cytochrome P450 enzyme system may result in only the metabolite being present. An IAS does not detect these metabolites, which is important to understand given the metabolite can be present in the absence of the parent opioid within 6 to 24 hours of ingestion and metabolite prevalence as the sole marker can range from 2.2% to 53.1%.[34] The higher threshold of detectability of an IAS makes it possible that a short-acting opioid taken with low frequency is not detected.[39] For example, if greater than 8 hours has elapsed from when the short-acting opioid is taken and the specimen is submitted, the concentration may fall below the level of

TABLE 46.5 Limitations of an Immunoassay Screen[41]

	Opiates (Natural Alkaloids Derived from Opium)	Semisynthetic Opioids	Synthetic Opioids	Detectable on Immunoassay
Codeine	✔	—	—	**YES**
Morphine	✔	—	—	**YES**
Hydrocodone	—	✔	—	Unreliable
Hydromorphone	—	✔	—	Unreliable
Oxycodone	—	✔	—	Unreliable
Oxymorphone	—	✔	—	Unreliable
Buprenorphine	—	✔	—	Unreliable
Fentanyl	—	—	✔	Unreliable
Meperidine	—	—	✔	Unreliable
Methadone	—	—	✔	Unreliable
Pentazocine	—	—	✔	Unreliable
Tapentadol	—	—	✔	Unreliable
Tramadol	—	—	✔	Unreliable

detectability and lead to the potentially false conclusion of noncompliance or diversion.

A **pseudo-false negative** result means the test correctly fails to identify the presence of a drug even though the patient is truly taking the drug. For example, this can occur in a patient who is genetically predisposed to rapid opioid metabolism, or in a patient who is taking another drug, which inadvertently accelerates opioid metabolism.[26,39]

A **false positive** result technically means that a drug that is truly absent, is inaccurately identified as present.[39] This is due to either laboratory error (performing the test incorrectly or analyzing the wrong patient's specimen) or drug interference/cross-reactivity (see Table 46.2).[26]

A **pseudo-false positive** result means the test correctly identifies the presence of a drug, but it is not due to the patient taking that specific drug.[39] The metabolic conversion of a parent opioid to an alternate opioid might lead a clinician to falsely conclude that the patient is also taking an unprescribed opioid (Fig. 46.2). For example, the presence of morphine could be due to the metabolism of codeine to morphine or the metabolism of heroin to morphine. Even the consumption of foods with poppy seeds can trigger a positive IAS result for opiates.[60] Another example includes marijuana testing. Since marijuana and the synthetic cannabinoid compounds dronabinol (Marinol) and nabiximols (Sativex) contain 11-nor-delta-9-tetrahydrocannabinol-9 (THC), they will all trigger positive results for the THC metabolite 11-nor-delta-9-tetrahydrocannabinol-9-carboxylic acid (THCA).[24] (Since nabilone [Cesamet] does not contain THC, it should not trigger an immunoassay-positive result for THCA.[24]) Inaccurate interpretation of this type of pseudo-false positive result might suggest that the patient has a substance abuse disorder.

A **true negative** result means that the drug is absent.[39] A true negative can be particularly puzzling to interpret if an expected drug is absent. Lack of detection in such a case could be explained by any one of the following plausible scenarios: laboratory error (mislabeled specimen, mishandled specimen, device/equipment error), the patient is not taking the medication (e.g., hoarding, diverting, or not picking up the prescription) or the result is actually a false negative or pseudo-false negative (see above). Of these scenarios, lab error due to device/equipment error is the easiest to rule out by having the lab rerun the specimen. However, one must know their laboratory's policy for retention of a specimen, as it may be discarded after a specified amount of time.

A **true positive** result means that the drug is present above the threshold of detectability.[39] However, there is no correlation with the urine concentration and the amount of drug used, when the drug was taken, or the source of the drug.[17,23] This limitation makes it nearly impossible to discern whether a patient is only taking a portion of the prescribed opioid and diverting the remaining drug because he/she can take just the right amount or take it at just the right time to trigger a positive result. In some instances, unexpected true positive results may have a medical explanation. For example, some otolaryngology procedures may involve the use of cocaine, which could then trigger a positive result for cocaine if the test is done within the window of detectability of the cocaine metabolite, benzoylecgonine. Another explanation is that the drug discovered is an impurity of the manufacturing process; use of morphine reveals codeine, and use of oxycodone reveals hydrocodone.[17] Another explanation is the drug discovered is a metabolite of the parent compound. For example, codeine and heroin both metabolize to morphine. Confirming use of heroin is particularly challenging because it metabolizes to 6-monoacetyl-morphine (6-MAM), an intermediary metabolite, within minutes; and 6-MAM metabolizes to morphine within hours.[17] Other examples of metabolism to an "alternate" opioid include oxycodone to oxymorphone; hydrocodone to hydromorphone; and morphine to hydromorphone. In both of these instances, the "alternate" opioid only appears in low concentration in relation to high concentrations of the primary opioid. Fig. 46.2 summarizes the metabolism of some of the more common opioids.[20]

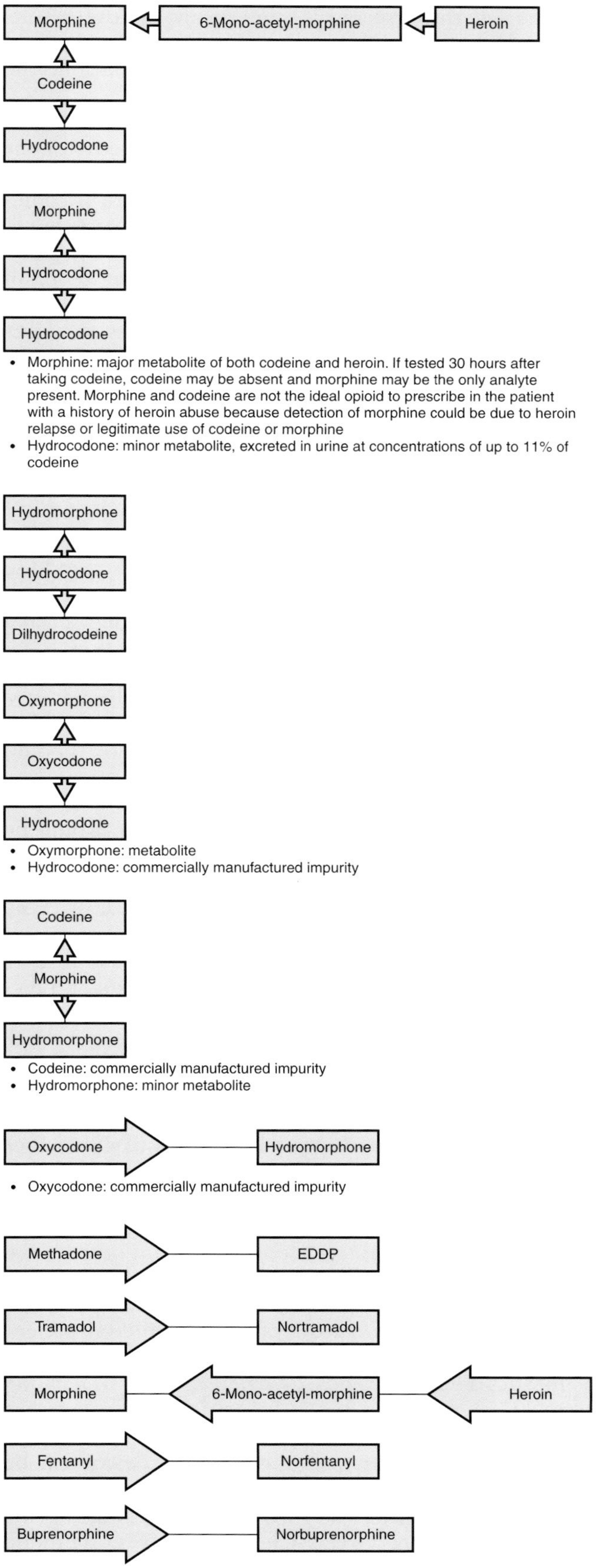

FIG. 46.2 Metabolism of some of the more common opioids with the parent opioid designated in the *arrow*. EDDP, 2-ethylidene-1,5-dimethyl-3, 3-diphenylpyrrolidine. *(From Carlozzi A, Fornari F, Siwicki D, et al: Urine Drug Monitoring: Opioids, New York: McMahon Publishing, 2009, 96.)*

TABLE 46.6 Window of Detection[17,20]

Fentanyl	2–3 days
Codeine, hydrocodone, hydromorphone, meperidine, morphine, oxycodone, oxymorphone, tramadol	2–4 days
Buprenorphine	Up to 11 days
Methadone	Up to 14 days
Cocaine	1–3 days
Heroin	Low dose (3 mg IV): <1/2 day High dose (6–12 mg IV): 1–2 days
Marijuana	1–3 days, casual use Up to 30 days, chronic use —
Amphetamines, methamphetamines	2–4 days
Barbiturates	2–4 days (short-acting) Up to 30 days (long-acting)
PCP	2–7 days, casual use Up to 30 days, chronic use

PCP, *Phenylcyclohexyl piperidine.*

Reference tables identifying drug detection times are often based on single dose administration and can underestimate the detection time when a patient is taking a medication or drug frequently or chronically.[17] For example, marijuana's detection time may be 1 to 3 days for a casual user but, because of its lipophilicity, the detection time may be up to 30 days for a heavy user.[17] With respect to smoked marijuana, a positive result is consistent with the use of marijuana and not due to second-hand inhalation.[24] Benzodiazepines, which are the second most commonly identified drug class in patients with chronic pain, have variable cross-reactivity because the IAS is typically formulated for identifying oxazepam, a metabolite of diazepam, and chlordiazepoxide, which is an older benzodiazepine.[25,34] This, coupled with each benzodiazepine drug having a different elimination half-life (the window of detection can be as little as 3 days if a therapeutic dose is ingested and as long as 4 to 6 weeks after extended use or with abuse quantities), means benzodiazepines, such as clonazepam and lorazepam, are difficult to detect and lead to high potential for false negative results.[23,25,34] To improve the probability of identifying a specific benzodiazepine, confirmatory testing should be done.

The window of detection for a drug and/or its metabolite represents how long after taking a drug the person continues to excrete the drug and/or metabolite above the test's limit of detection (Table 46.6).[23] This window of detection is influenced by the drug's pharmacokinetics (what the body does to the drug—absorption, distribution, metabolism, and elimination), pharmacodynamics (what the drug does to the body—the relationship between drug concentration at the site of action and its resulting biochemical and physiological effect), and pharmacogenetics (how genes that code for drug enzymes, receptors and transporters affect drug response).[17] Both the pharmacokinetics and pharmacodynamics of a drug are influenced by the complex interplay of numerous variables: drug dose; dosing frequency; chronicity of drug use; route and rate of administration; site of administration; route, rate, and volume of distribution; state of hydration; drug-protein binding; drug-drug interaction; genetics; upregulation or downregulation of enzymatic systems; urine pH, volume, and frequency; renal and hepatic function; comorbid illness; diet; age; sex; pregnancy; cardiac output; body weight; and environmental factors.[17]

Variations in first pass metabolism, genetic polymorphisms of both the cytochrome (CYP) P450 and uridine 5′-diphospho-glucuronyltransferase enzyme systems, and genetic polymorphisms of the transporter contribute to the variations in systemic concentration that can even be seen giving a drug with the same dose and route of delivery.[2] For example, CYP2D6 metabolizes the prodrug codeine to morphine and exhibits a wide variability of action.[2,61] Poor metabolizers of CYP2D6 will have higher concentrations of codeine and lower concentrations of morphine, and ultra-rapid metabolizers of CYP2D6 will have lower concentrations of codeine and higher concentrations of morphine. Thus, the genetic variety of CYP2D6 determines a patient's analgesic response to codeine as well as the urine concentration of codeine and morphine.[2,61] It is also important to recognize that opioid metabolism can be affected by the other drugs or foods an individual is consuming or by comorbid illness. Even the route of delivery (oral, transdermal, transmucosal, rectal, intravenous, subcutaneous, or intrathecal) can yield interindividual and intraindividual variability in the time course of a drug's absorption, bioavailability, distribution, metabolism, excretion, efficacy, and side effects.[2] These pharmacokinetic variables are affected by both the chemical properties of a drug and patient-related properties (e.g., hepatic and renal function, genetics, sex, age), and these then determine the drug's onset, duration, and intensity of action.[62]

Inaccurate conclusions based on an incomplete understanding of the test result, which then result in opioid discontinuation, can be harmful for patients and have even resulted in legal implications for the prescriber.[63] To minimize errors in interpretation of the results, the clinician should be knowledgeable about the limitations of (both POC and laboratory) IASs, always order the confirmatory UDT, and gather relevant information from the patient. Below are questions that may be helpful for the clinician to ask the patient to support optimal understanding in advance of ordering drug testing:

- What prescribed and nonprescribed (conventional, over-the-counter, and naturopathic) medications are you taking?
- How often are you taking your opioids?
- When did you last take your opioids?
- Are you taking any medications I am not prescribing?
- Are you using any illicit substances?

As in ordering any other diagnostic study (e.g., labs, imaging, EKG, EMG), urine drug testing should meet the basic standard of medical necessity by documenting at least the following three items.[27]

- Why was the test ordered?
- What was the test result?
- Based on the test result, the review of the results with the patient and the clinical assessment, what was the action plan (even if plan remains to continue the same)?

Unexpected results offer an opportunity for a compassionate discussion with the patient, as opposed to confrontation, and a reassessment of the treatment plan.[27] It is important to have a consistent policy when it comes to addressing unanticipated findings, that is, patients get a "second chance" versus "only one chance." A full discussion of opioid discontinuation is beyond the scope of this chapter. It should be noted that although it may be necessary, the rate of discontinuation requires thoughtful medical judgment and should never be an excuse for patient abandonment. If a patient's IAS and UDT reveal an absence of the prescribed opioid or the presence of nonprescribed opioids or illicit substances, the clinician is faced with the following considerations:

- Should the IAS and UDT be repeated? Yes, if lab error is likely.
- Should the prescribed opioid be continued? Yes, if lab error is likely, the frequency and amount of opioid use falls below the level of detectability, or there is a reasonable medical explanation to account for the unexpected finding (e.g., the patient was administered or prescribed an alternate opioid by his/her dentist). If the result is inconclusive and the clinician decides to continue prescribing, the clinician can consider dispensing a smaller quantity of opioids with more frequent follow-up and drug testing to justify ongoing prescribing.
- Should the prescribed opioid be discontinued? Yes, if the frequency and amount of opioid use would be expected to fall above the level of detectability, if a nonprescribed opioid is present without a reasonable explanation, if an illicit substance is detected, or if the specimen has been adulterated.
- Should the patient be referred to an addictionologist? Yes, in many cases when a nonprescribed opioid is present or if an illicit substance is detected.
- Should the patient be discharged from the practice? No, because one can still offer nonopioid therapeutic options (e.g., nonopioid medications, injection-based therapies, behavioral therapy, and physical therapy) in addition to addressing a possible substance misuse/abuse disorder.

ADULTERATION

Some patients intentionally try to subvert the tests by using simple or sophisticated adulteration techniques, products, and devices. Based on an analysis of 2.1 million patient urine drug testing reports, the most recent annual Quest Diagnostics Health Trends *Prescription Drug Monitoring Report 2015* revealed 33,396 (1.5%) urine specimens were adulterated by various means (Fig. 46.3).[15] Information about adulteration techniques, products, and devices can be readily found on the internet. Products purchased on the internet can be broadly categorized as "cleansing" agents (e.g., XXTra Clean; Green Clean), additives, synthetic urine substitutes, and prosthetic devices.[39,64–67] There are commercially available products that claim to dilute the urine or, alternatively, patients will ingest copious amounts

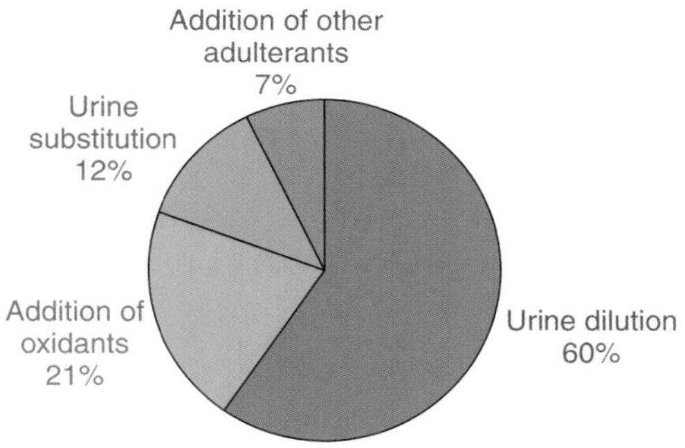

FIG. 46.3 Distribution of adulteration strategies for urine drug testing reports for Quest Diagnostics (January 2014 to December 2014). *(From Blatt A, Chen Z, McClure L, Niles J, Kaufman M: Prescription drug misuse in America: diagnostic insights in the continuing drug epidemic battle. Quest Diagnostics Health Trends Prescription Drug Monitoring Report 2015, 16.)*

of water for the same purpose, thereby decreasing the concentration of substance that could be detected.[17] Because ingestion of large volumes of water can result in pale colored urine, some patients will concurrently consume niacin and/or vitamin B to give the urine a yellow color. Urine specimens can also be directly adulterated by adding water from a sink or toilet bowl, household products (bleach, vinegar, and detergent), over-the-counter medications (eye drops and sodium chloride), and commercially purchased chemicals (glutaraldehyde, sodium or potassium nitrite, pyridinium chlorochromate, or peroxide/peroxidase).[34,68] Glutaraldehyde (e.g., "Clean X") may mask the presence of marijuana, opioids, cocaine, morphine, amphetamine, and PCP.[17,68] Sodium or potassium nitrite (e.g., "Klear" or "Whizzies") may mask the presence of marijuana metabolites and THCA.[17,68] Pyridinium chlorochromate (e.g., "Urine Luck") may mask the presence of THCA and morphine.[17,68] Peroxide/peroxidase (e.g., "Stealth") may mask detection of THCA.[17,68] Some patients will bring a pouch, which may include a heating device to warm the specimen to body temperature and/or appropriately skin tone colored prosthetic penis that can be catheterized, filled with drug-free human, animal, or synthetic urine.[39,69,70] The synthetic urine can be purchased as a dehydrated product for reconstitution (e.g., "Dr John's Concentrated Urine") or as a liquid solution (e.g., "Quick-Fix" and "Sub-Solution").[69,70] Some patients will go even further by emptying their bladder and then, using a catheter, instill unadulterated urine from another individual.

Various strategies can be implemented to reduce the chance that adulteration attempts are successful. Recognizing that no one strategy is 100% foolproof and that simply looking at the appearance of the specimen is insufficient, many of these strategies can be readily employed prior to submission of the specimen or at the point of submission and/or analysis of the urine specimen. Strategies to consider prior to submission include the following[17,41]:

- Have the patient submit his/her specimen in the morning when urine is most concentrated.
- Shut off the water supply to the bathroom sink to prevent using it to dilute the specimen. For hygiene purposes, access to a working sink that is external to the bathroom and in view of clinic personnel is needed.
- Add a colored dye to the toilet's water tank to prevent the patient from taking water from the toilet bowl or tank to dilute the specimen. If the patient does so, the specimen will have a similar hue as the dye.
- Ensure that no bathroom cleaning agents, chemicals, or medications are stored in the bathroom.
- Besides the patient, friends or family members should not be allowed to enter the bathroom with the patient. If the patient needs assistance, a nurse or medical assistant should help the patient.
- Witness the patient giving the specimen and document the chain of custody of the specimen. Specific protocols may be needed when urine specimens are submitted as a part of an employment requirement or addiction management treatment program, and there is a concern for adulteration. This is rarely performed for clinical purposes, as such protocols can prove to be difficult to implement from a resource standpoint and can make patients feel like they are being treated as criminals.

Validity testing ensures the reliability and accuracy of the specimen tested.[23] For laboratory submitted specimens, verify with a technician that the measurements below are included in the analysis.

- **Temperature:** ranges between 90°F and 100°F, provided it is measured within 4 minutes of collecting the specimen.[23] For POC tests that include a temperature strip within the specimen cup, the validity of the reading depends entirely on the person reading the strip within the period of time delineated by the manufacturer.
- **Random urine creatinine concentration:** a reliable indicator of how well hydrated a patient is, it ranges from 20 to 400 mg/dL in individuals greater than 12 years of age.[71] Since creatinine levels are affected mostly by muscle mass renal clearance, individuals who have less muscle mass and/or renal impairment will have lab values that fall at the lower end of spectrum. According to SAMHSA, a random urine concentration ranging from 2 to 19 mg/dL is consistent with dilution (either by ingestion or adulteration), and less than 2 mg/dL is inconsistent with adult urine and, therefore, reflects substitution.[17,72]
- **Specific gravity:** measures the density of urine relative to the density of water, which is 1.000. Since one of the kidney's main jobs is to eliminate waste molecules while minimizing the loss of water and nutrients, the concentration of waste molecules dissolved in the specimen determine the urine's specific gravity, which in adults ranges from 1.003 to 1.030.[73] According to SAMHSA, a specific gravity greater than 1.001 but less than 1.003 is consistent with dilution; and ≤1.001 or ≥1.020 is consistent with substitution.[72] The results, though, must be interpreted with caution since, in isolation, an elevated or depressed specific gravity can have medical explanations. For example, an elevated specific gravity can be due to dehydration, diarrhea, emesis, excessive sweating, bladder infection, glucosuria, renal artery stenosis, hepatorenal syndrome, decreased blood flow to the kidney, and syndrome of inappropriate antidiuretic hormone (SIADH). Conversely, a depressed specific gravity can be due to renal failure, pyelonephritis, diabetes insipidus, acute tubular necrosis, interstitial nephritis, and psychogenic polydipsia. Findings of specific gravity

should instead be correlated with the other measurements listed above.[73]

- **pH:** fluctuates throughout the day but ranges from 4.5 to 8.0, such that adulteration with additives, such as bleach and vinegar, explains a pH less than 3 or greater than 11, respectively.[17,72]
- **Oxidants:** can cause decreased levels of certain drugs by disguising the drug or destroying it. One must ask the lab to include testing for oxidants in general or in specific (bleach, nitrate, chromate, iodate, and peroxidase).[17]

TESTING ALCOHOL

Patients should be discouraged from consuming alcohol of any frequency while on opioid therapy, as alcohol increases the risk of opioid side effects. In the case of some oral extended-release opioids, alcohol can degrade the coating that makes the drug long lasting, thereby causing a potentially fatal burst release of the opioid. Testing for alcohol in serum and urine is impractical in a chronic pain management setting, because it has an extremely narrow window of detection (<12 hours) due to rapid metabolization and does not provide information about long-term use.[17,41] The window of detection is influenced by the amount of alcohol ingested, but not the frequency of consumption.[17] Testing urine for the alcohol biomarkers, ethyl glucuronide (EtG) or ethyl sulfate (EtS), provides a longer window of detectability of up to 24 to 72 hours, but positive results can occur with other alcohol-containing products such as mouthwash, antitussive medicines, nonalcoholic beer, communion wine, and certain foods.[17,41] Due to the high sensitivity of both biomarkers, even incidental exposure to alcohol vapors (cleaning products and hand sanitizers) can trigger a positive result.[41] Regarding threshold levels for detection, there are currently no agreed upon values.[41] For all of the aforementioned reasons, extreme caution is advised when interpretation of a positive UDT for alcohol or one of its biomarkers may result in changing the treatment plan.

CONCLUSION

An estimated 100 million Americans experience chronic pain and 1.9 million aged 12 or older have a pain reliever use disorder.[1,14] The expansion of opioid prescribing for CNMP has led to a concurrent increase in diversion and deaths from overdose.[10,74,75] To preserve legitimate access to these potent but potentially dangerous pain relievers, clinicians must employ tools to guard against diversion, misuse, and abuse. Patient selection is critical to identify individuals who are most likely to benefit from COT. Risk stratification based on a detailed history and physical exam can help determine the level of surveillance that is needed to monitor for compliance or avoid prescribing in the first place. Tools, such as a PDMP and urine drug testing, objectively evaluate adherence with a COT plan and can help support clinical decisions. Given the dire need to reduce risk related to opioid-related adverse events, various medical societies and regulatory agencies have erred on the side of making urine drug testing recommendations now even though the evidence is weak or indirect as opposed to waiting for the outcomes from more rigorous studies.[54] The Federation of State Medical Boards (FSMB) Model Guidelines for the Use of Controlled Substances for the Treatment of Pain, which provides state regulatory authorities with guidelines on how to assess whether a clinician's prescription of opioids is medically appropriate, recommends periodic drug testing for adherence monitoring.[45] Likewise, the recent Centers for Disease Control and Prevention (CDC) guidelines published in 2016 recommend that clinicians obtain an IAS and UDT before initiating COT and at least annually.[10] Clinicians are responsible for knowing and complying with regulatory policies pertaining to opioid prescribing and monitoring as established both by the federal government and individual state government(s) where they practice.

Targeted urine drug testing strictly based on suspicious behavior will miss a reasonable number of patients in need of testing who do not exhibit such behavior. Due to the unreliability of self-reporting and clinician observation, both an IAS and UDT should be incorporated as a part of a consensual adherence-monitoring program.[12,76] Remember that an IAS is only useful as a screening tool and that a laboratory-based confirmatory UDT should always be performed to minimize false positives and false negatives. Although urine drug testing is performed to monitor for compliance with prescribed medications and to confirm the absence of nonprescribed medications and illicit drugs, remember that the test reflects only a single "snapshot" in time. The presence of a prescribed medication only suggests, but does not necessarily confirm adherence. In addition, the absence of illicit substances only means that an illicit substance was not used within the window of detection of the test and not that the patient is not using illicit substances. The inherent uncertainties with drawing conclusions from a single test result explain why urine drug testing should be performed on a random basis. Knowing how to interpret a drug test requires that the clinician understand the limitations of both an IAS and UDT and how opioids are metabolized.[44] When uncertain about the meaning of the results, contacting the laboratory for assistance in interpreting the results is critical to avoid drawing the wrong conclusions, which could then negatively impact a patient's care. Proper interpretation of the results depends on the reliability, accuracy, and completeness of the test, which then impacts important clinical decisions. Remember, the differential diagnosis for an "abnormal" IAS or UDT is broad: appropriate but infrequent opioid use (which may explain absence of the opioid), diversion, self-treatment of pain, psychological problems, drug abuse, or addiction.[44] Therefore, the tests should be used in conjunction with other tools to assist the clinician in developing, continuing, or modifying the treatment plan as needed. For those who have a dual diagnosis of addiction and chronic pain, neither disease can be addressed in isolation, and only treatment of both diseases will successfully treat the other.[23] Urine drug testing should be included as part of a risk evaluation and mitigation plan. Similar to other risk management protocols (e.g., checking blood pressures to monitor for hypertension, performing pap smears to prevent cervical cancer, performing colonoscopies to prevent colon cancer), urine drug testing can be coupled with clinical findings to improve patient care.[27] Finally, having a urine drug testing policy may make one's practice less attractive to individuals targeting physicians for opioids and may suggest to law enforcement and regulators that one has a risk management protocol in place.[27]

REFERENCES

Access the reference list online at ExpertConsult.com.

CHAPTER 47

Substance Use Disorders and Detoxification

J. Gregory Hobelmann, MD, MPH ◌ Michael R. Clark, MD, MPH, MBA

SUBSTANCE USE AND CHRONIC PAIN

The prevalence of substance use disorders in patients with chronic pain is higher than in the general population.[1] Over the past 2 decades, opioid analgesic prescriptions have increased to patients with chronic nonmalignant pain, yet prescriptions for nonopioid analgesics did not significantly change.[2–3] Approximately two-thirds of patients in clinics specializing in pain management are prescribed opioid analgesics, which is about 8 million people in the United States.[4–6] In a study of primary care outpatients with chronic noncancer pain who received at least 6 months of opioid prescriptions during 1 year, behaviors consistent with opioid abuse were recorded in about 25% of patients.[7] Review articles have indicated that addiction in patients with chronic noncancer pain ranges from 0% to 50%, with 20% being the most consistent approximation.[8–10] This compares to an estimated 8.6% in the general population, according to the National Institute on Drug Abuse.[11] Specifically for opioid use disorders, one study showed that the frequency of opioid use disorders was 4 times higher in patients receiving opioid therapy than in the general population (3.8% vs. 61.3%) and even higher in patients who received methadone maintenance therapy for the treatment of opioid dependence (55.3% to 61.3%).[12–13]

Determining the presence of a substance abuse disorder usually involves the problem of how to evaluate the patient with chronic pain who is prescribed controlled substances with abuse potential.[14–15] Individuals with substance use disorders are more often initiated and continued on opioid therapy for noncancer pain than those without substance use disorders and rates of opioid use were 4 times higher for those with substance use disorders than those without substance use disorders. In those with an opioid use disorder specifically, that rate of opioid use was 7 to 8 times higher. In addition, those with substance use disorders were much more likely to receive higher doses, a larger supply, and more potent medications.[16] A recent review of the effectiveness and risks of long-term opioid therapy for the treatment of noncancer pain found that no study of opioid versus nonopioid therapy evaluated long-term outcomes related to pain, function, quality of life, opioid use, or addiction. It also confirmed that there is evidence that opioid therapy is associated with increased risk for abuse and overdose and that this risk is dose dependent.[17]

Comorbid psychiatric disorders also play a role in the complexity of treating patients with chronic pain. Psychiatric disorders are associated with increased physical symptoms, more subjective pain, more aberrant drug behaviors, and are linked to increased opioid use.[18–20] For example, pain arising from chronic medical disorders are rated as more severe in the presence of major depression.[21] A large prospective trial indicated that common psychiatric disorders, such as depression, anxiety, and drug use disorders, predict initiation and ongoing regular use of opioids in patients with chronic pain.[22]

The causes and onset of substance use disorders have been difficult to characterize in relationship to chronic pain. During the first 5 years after the onset of chronic pain, patients are at the highest risk for developing new substance use disorders and additional physical injuries.[23] This risk is highest in patients with a history of a substance use disorder, childhood physical or sexual abuse, and psychiatric comorbidity as opioid misuse occurs for a variety of reasons, including self-medication, use for reward, compulsive use because of addiction, and diversion for profit.[24–25] Chronic pain is associated with long-term substance use after substance abuse treatment and detoxification. Therefore, addressing and treating patients for their chronic pain could improve their long-term outcome.[26] The mechanisms of relapse into substance abuse after treatment in patients with chronic pain are not well understood and probably involve multiple factors; however, a cycle of pain followed by relief after taking medications is a classic example of operant reinforcement of future medication use that eventually becomes abuse. Careful monitoring of patients is essential to prevent this complication in the treatment of chronic pain.[27] Research in patients with substance abuse has demonstrated abnormalities in pain perception and tolerance. An increased sensitivity to pain and the reinforcing effects of relieving pain with substance use suggest a different mechanism for the development of substance abuse in patients with chronic pain. Patients with substance use disorders have increased rates of chronic pain and are at the greatest risk for undertreatment with appropriate medications and subsequent self-medication with illicit drugs.[28] Almost a quarter of patients admitted to an inpatient residential substance abuse program and over a third of patients in a methadone maintenance program reported severe chronic pain, many of whom also had pain-related interference in functioning.[28] It also appears that patients with co-occurring substance abuse and pain are less likely to complete a substance abuse program than those without pain.[29] Ethical principles such as beneficence, quality of life, and autonomy can provide particularly useful guidance for the use of chronic opioid therapy, recognizing that benefits should be optimized in a context of risk management.[30]

RISKS OF PHARMACOLOGICAL TREATMENT FOR CHRONIC PAIN

OPIOIDS

Opioids are effective in the treatment of chronic nonmalignant pain in reducing pain, pain-related disability, depression, insomnia, and physical dysfunction in the short term (months), but evidence is lacking for their long-term (>1 year) effectiveness.[17,31] Nonetheless, opioids are widely considered to be appropriate treatment for various chronic pain conditions. For example, opioids are considered second-line medications for the treatment of neuropathic pain conditions and may be considered first-line treatments in certain circumstances (i.e., acute neuropathic pain, during periods of titration of first-line agents, and exacerbations of neuropathic pain).[32] In the past, it was felt that a constant, rather than intermittent "as needed," dosing should be followed to maintain analgesic effect, but more recent recommendations indicate that long-acting opioids at high doses are recommended only in specific circumstances with severe intractable pain that is not amenable to short-acting or moderate doses of long-acting opioids.[33] Using an intermittent schedule can reduce tolerance and dependence. If continuous scheduling is used, most experts agree that opioids with slow onset of action and longer duration of action are preferred to minimize the initial euphoria and interdose withdrawal symptoms. Extended-release oral medications and transdermal routes of administration decrease these qualities and are generally preferred for long-term use.

Opioid dependence is mediated by the actions and interactions of opioid receptors.[34] Mesolimbic dopaminergic projections to the nucleus accumbens have been implicated in the development of psychological dependence. In contrast, physical dependence on opioids is probably due to adrenergic activity in the locus ceruleus. However, the treatment of nonmalignant chronic pain with opioids remains the subject of considerable debate with fears of regulatory pressure, medication abuse, and the development of tolerance and dependence. This has created a reluctance to prescribe opioids and, possibly, their underutilization. Despite this, the prescribing of long-term opioids is an accepted practice and the number of opioid prescriptions for noncancer pain continues to increase. With this has come a rise in nonmedical use of prescription opioids, which many feel has reached "epidemic" proportions in the United States. In some cases, this nonmedical use progresses to heroin use, often intravenous use, which has devastating consequences.[35] In addition, chronic pain conditions may facilitate the development of tolerance to opioid analgesia.[36] This can lead to escalating doses of opioids, and at some point, the side effects (tolerance, dependence, opioid-induced hyperalgesia, constipation, sedation, delirium, urinary retention, immunosuppression) outweigh the benefits of analgesia.[37] A thorough evaluation, careful patient selection, and close monitoring are all essential for the safe and effective prescribing of opioids for noncancer pain. There are several useful guidelines for responsible opioid prescribing that are readily available to help practitioners.[33,38–39]

Predicting which patients are at risk for developing an addiction to opioids has been studied. Demographic factors have not been consistent. Strong predictors include a personal history of substance use disorder and/or mental health disorders.[40–41] Self-reported craving has also been shown to be a possible risk factor.[42]

BENZODIAZEPINES

Benzodiazepines are commonly prescribed for anxiety and insomnia in patients with chronic pain, but no studies have demonstrated any benefit for these target symptoms.[43–44] Almost 50% of patients with chronic pain report anxiety symptoms, and 30% of chronic pain patients have a diagnosed anxiety or disorder, such as panic disorder.[45–46] In general, however, benzodiazepines are less effective for these conditions than other pharmacotherapies such as antidepressants, anticonvulsants, and mood stabilizers.[47] Only a limited number of chronic pain conditions such as trigeminal neuralgia, tension headache, and temporomandibular disorders were found to improve with benzodiazepines.[48] In addition, patients may take benzodiazepines for reasons other than treating these conditions, and data suggest that the majority of benzodiazepine use is recreational rather than therapeutic.[49] Benzodiazepines have been used for the detoxification of patients with chronic pain from sedative/hypnotic medications and were superior to barbiturates for minimizing symptoms of withdrawal.[50] Higher levels of withdrawal symptoms during detoxification predicted relapse to future use of benzodiazepines.[51]

Benzodiazepines also cause cognitive impairment as demonstrated by abnormalities on neuropsychological testing and electroencephalogram (EEG).[52] In patients with chronic pain, use of benzodiazepines was associated with decreased activity levels, higher rates of health care visits, increased domestic instability, depression, and more disability days.[53] Combining benzodiazepines with opioids may cause additional problems. Patients often notice the enhanced feelings of euphoria when benzodiazepines are used in combination with opioids, especially if the drugs are misused or abused.[49] This combination can also have severe, and sometimes fatal, consequences. From 2000 to 2010, hospital admission rates related to coabuse of benzodiazepines and opioids increased by a staggering 570%, while those related to all other substances declined by approximately 10%.[54] In a study of 278 opioid related deaths in Utah, benzodiazepines played a role in up to 80% of the deaths.[55] In methadone-related mortality, almost 75% of deaths were attributable to a combination of drug effects and benzodiazepines were present in 74% of the deceased.[56–57] Benzodiazepines have also been associated with exacerbation of pain and interference of opioid analgesia, which is mediated by the serotonergic system.[58] Concomitant use was also associated with higher mean doses of opioids, longer periods of being prescribed opioids, greater risk of receiving a psychogenic pain diagnosis, and higher rates of being diagnosed with other substance use disorders.[59–60]

DIAGNOSIS OF SUBSTANCE USE DISORDERS

The fifth edition of the *Diagnostic and Statistical Manual of Mental Disorders* (DSM-V) of the American Psychiatric Association differs considerably from the fourth edition (DSM-IV). The DSM-IV uses the terms *substance abuse* and *substance dependence*, with substance dependence being distinguished from abuse by more than a continuum of severity. It was important to distinguish dependence from abuse, because dependence reliably predicted more severe medical sequelae, poorer treatment outcomes, higher rates of relapse, and worse overall prognosis. The DSM-V utilizes the term "substance use disorder" (i.e., opioid use disorder and sedative, hypnotic, or anxiolytic use disorder). To be diagnosed with a substance use disorder, patients must demonstrate a pattern of substance use leading to impairment or distress, as manifested by at least 2 of 11 criteria, such as taking the substance in larger amounts or over a longer period of time than was intended, continued use despite negative consequences, tolerance, and dependence. The DSM-IV further specifies among severity: mild (presence of two to three symptoms), moderate (presence of four to five symptoms), severe (presence of six or more symptoms).[61] A comparison of patients diagnosed using both the DSM-IV and DSM-V indicated that the majority of patients with a lifetime DSM-IV opioid dependence were now classified as having mild opioid use disorder using the DSM-V.[62]

The core criteria for substance use disorder in patients with chronic pain include the loss of control in the use of medication, excessive preoccupation with the medication despite adequate analgesia, and adverse consequences associated with the use of the medication.[63] Items from the Prescription Drug Use Questionnaire that best predicted the presence of addiction in a sample of patients with problematic medication use were the following: (1) patients believing they were addicted; (2) increasing analgesic dose/frequency; and (3) a preferred route of administration. The diagnosis of addiction in the patient with chronic pain must demonstrate certain drug-taking behaviors that interfere with the successful fulfillment of life activities. Access to opioids may not be a specific problem, because a physician has been prescribing them. If addiction is present, however, the patient may fear that the opioid access will be limited and therefore try to conceal any problematic use of the medication. The presence of maladaptive behaviors is emphasized to diagnose addiction, because physical dependence and tolerance should be recognized as normal physiological phenomena. Increased function and opioid analgesia without side effects, not the avoidance of high dose opioids, are the goals of treatment.[64]

The evaluation of a patient suspected of misusing medications should be thorough and include an assessment of the pain syndrome as well as other medical disorders, patterns of medication use, social and family factors, patient and family history of substance abuse, and a psychiatric history.[65] Reliance on medications that provide pain relief can result in a number of stereotyped patient behaviors that are often mistaken for addiction. Persistent pain can lead to increased focus on opioid medications. Patients may take extraordinary measures to ensure an adequate supply even in the absence of addiction. This may be manifested as frequent requests for higher medication doses and larger quantities of medication or seeking medication from additional sources. Patients may understandably fear the reemergence of pain and withdrawal symptoms if they run out of medication. Drug-seeking behavior may be the result of an anxious patient trying to maintain a previous level of pain control. In this situation, the patient's actions define pseudoaddiction that results from the therapeutic dependence and current or potential undertreatment, but no addiction.[66–68] These behaviors resolve once adequate opioid therapy is prescribed.

In patients with higher risk of addiction, prevention begins with a treatment contract to clarify the conditions under which treatment with opioids will be provided. Elements of a contract emphasize a single physician being responsible for the prescription of the medication, and, in advance, describe for the patient all conditions under which continued use of opioids would be inappropriate. Under optimal circumstances, opioid contracts attempt to improve compliance by distributing all information and utilizing a mutually designed, agreed upon treatment plan that includes consequences for aberrant behaviors and incorporated the primary care physician to form a "trilateral" agreement with patient and pain specialist.[69–71] When there is concern that a patient will have difficulty taking medications as directed, a policy of prescribing small quantities of medications, performing random pill counts, and not refilling lost supplies should be explicitly discussed and then followed. External sources of information such as urine toxicology testing, interviews with partners or family members, data from prescription monitoring programs, and review of medical records can improve detection of substance use disorders.[72–73] Patients who denied using illicit substances that were detected on urine toxicology are more likely to be younger, receiving workers' compensation benefits, and have a previous diagnosis of polysubstance abuse.[72]

The occurrence of any aberrant medication-related behaviors should prompt evaluation for addiction. Even when the diagnosis of a substance use disorder is suspected in patients taking opioids for chronic pain, behaviors such as stealing or forging prescriptions is relatively uncommon.[74] The more serious aberrant behaviors consistent with addiction also include selling medications, losing prescriptions, using oral medications intravenously, concurrent abuse of alcohol or other illicit drugs, repeated noncompliance with the prescribed use of medications, and deterioration in the patient's ability to function in family, social, or occupational roles. Concerns by family or friends about the patient's pattern of medication use, an appearance suggesting intoxication, or the patient having difficulties with functional abilities require in-depth evaluation. Any unwillingness to discuss the possibility of addiction or changes in chronic opioid therapy requires discussion about the patient's worries and the possible aberrant behaviors, including medication misuse.

TREATMENT OF SUBSTANCE USE DISORDERS IN PATIENTS WITH CHRONIC PAIN

In general, an active substance use disorder is a relative contraindication to chronic opioid therapy. However, it can be accomplished successfully if the clinical benefits are deemed to outweigh the risks. The treatment of this extraordinary subset of patients with chronic pain will always require considerably more effort and frustration on the part of the physician. A strict treatment structure with therapeutic goals, landmarks to document progress, and contingencies for noncompliance should be made explicit and agreed upon by the patient and all the providers of health care. The first step for the patient is acknowledging that a problem with medication exists. The first step for the clinician is to stop the patient's behavior of misusing medications. Then, sustaining factors must be assessed and addressed. These interventions include treating other medical diseases and psychiatric disorders, managing personality vulnerabilities, meeting situational challenges and life stressors, and providing support and understanding. Finally, the habit of taking the medication inappropriately must be extinguished.

The patient should be actively participating in an addictions treatment program that will reinforce taking medications as prescribed and examine the possible reasons for any inappropriate use. Relapse is common and patients with addiction require ongoing monitoring even if the prescription of opioids has ceased. Traditional outpatient drug treatment or 12-step programs can provide support for recovery. Relapse prevention should rely on family members or sponsors to assist the patient in getting prompt attention before further deterioration occurs. If relapse is detected, the precipitating incident should be examined, and strategies to avoid another relapse should be implemented. Although the misuse of medications is unacceptable, complete abstinence is not always the most appropriate or optimal treatment of patients with chronic pain. Data suggest that buprenorphine-naloxone may be a safer alternative to provide pain relief for the chronic pain patient with an opioid use disorder.[75] Restoration of function should be the primary treatment goal and may improve with adequate, judicious, and appropriate use of medications.[76]

LONG-TERM OPIOID THERAPY

Long-term opioid therapy remains controversial and may be complicated by many adverse outcomes.[77–78] Published guidelines on the use of opioids for chronic nonmalignant pain have been largely based on expert consensus due to lack of strong evidence.[79] Outcomes from trials have been inconclusive and there have been no long-term studies comparing opioids to placebo. Nonetheless, long-term treatment with opioids is a widely accepted practice and several up-to-date guidelines exist for the use of opioids in chronic nonmalignant pain. A total approach to the patient including a history of substance abuse, psychosocial comorbidities, and aberrant drug-related behaviors must be considered in an evaluation. Only if these potential risks can be minimized or treated should chronic opioid treatment be considered.[33,38–39] Although a risk of addiction exists in all patients, a review and meta-analysis showed that only a small percentage of patients (0.05%) with no previous substance abuse problems developed an addiction when treated with long-term opioids.[80] Close monitoring and random drug screening may serve as a deterrent for substance abuse in this population.[8] Regardless, each patient requires a careful risk-benefit analysis when starting long-term opioid therapy.

WHY IS DETOXIFICATION NECESSARY?

Detoxification does not necessarily imply that a patient has been given the diagnosis of a substance use disorder. It is simply the process of withdrawing a person from a specific psychoactive substance in a safe and effective manner. Conversely, not all patients diagnosed with a substance use disorder will require detoxification. While addiction may necessitate detoxification at the onset of drug rehabilitation treatment, there are many reasons that patients must undergo detoxification. Since long-term treatment will have resulted in physiological dependence, discontinuation or substantial dose reduction requires gradual tapering of medication. In the treatment of chronic nonmalignant pain, the ongoing assessment of a therapeutic trial of medication such as opioids may result in the conclusion that the risk-benefit ratio is no longer acceptable (Table 47.1). A carefully planned and monitored detoxification will avoid withdrawal syndrome in a patient who has become physiologically dependent on medications such as opioids or benzodiazepines.

TABLE 47.1 Indications for Detoxification

Intolerable side effects
Inadequate response or benefit
Aberrant drug-related behaviors
Noncompliance
Loss of control of medication use
Preoccupation with the medication
Continued use despite adverse consequences
Refractory comorbid psychiatric illness
Lack of functional improvement or impairment in role responsibilities

OPIOID DETOXIFICATION

Although physiological opioid dependence can be demonstrated experimentally within days, most patients will not experience withdrawal symptoms unless they have taken opioids regularly for at least several weeks. Withdrawal symptoms vary among individuals, but patients with a history of physiological opioid dependence, opioid withdrawal, or any other drug withdrawal will generally be more likely to experience opioid withdrawal after shorter periods of use.[81] Regardless of total daily dose, once physiological dependence is established, abrupt discontinuation of opioids will precipitate acute withdrawal. Even a reduction in dose can precipitate withdrawal to a lesser degree. Patients taking opioid analgesics on a variable schedule are at higher risk for experiencing intermittent withdrawal if they have become physiologically dependent. Even a long overnight dosing hiatus from a short half-life opioid can cause significant withdrawal symptoms. However, patients on a variable schedule may be at less risk for developing dependence if low and infrequent dosing is maintained. Exacerbations of pain or intermittent withdrawal symptoms relieved by taking medications are highly reinforcing and a common factor in failure of detoxification. Patients with these experiences will require longer tapering schedules and more support to overcome this conditioned habit.

The essential element for successful opioid detoxification is gradual tapering of the dose of medication. Opioid withdrawal is generally not dangerous except in patients at risk from increased sympathetic tone (e.g., increased intracranial pressure or unstable angina).[81] However, opioid withdrawal is very uncomfortable and distressing to patients with symptoms including cravings, nausea, emesis, diarrhea, agitation, anxiety, muscle tension and aches, bone pain, insomnia, increased lacrimation, yawning, and shaking. Patients with pain are often particularly miserable during opioid withdrawal because of the phenomenon of rebound pain. Increases in pain can occur even if the analgesic effects of opioid therapy had not been appreciable. Although it is generally not possible to avoid discomfort completely, the goal of detoxification is to ameliorate withdrawal as much as is clinically practical. Explaining the treatment plan to patients before detoxification begins is critical. In particular, patients should know to expect worsening of pain and should have concrete short-term goals on which to focus, such as improvement in withdrawal symptoms, increasing functional abilities, or an alternative analgesic trial when withdrawal has resolved. The projected length of taper is typically a balance between the expected severity of withdrawal symptoms (increased with faster tapers) and their expected duration (shorter with faster tapers).

SETTING

Although detoxification can be accomplished in either inpatient or outpatient settings, the inpatient setting offers more intensive monitoring, supervision, and other support that generally allows for a faster taper schedule. Indications for inpatient detoxification include the failure of outpatient detoxification attempts, medically unstable patients, comorbid psychiatric illness, unreliable or noncompliant patients, and complicated pharmacological regimens requiring taper of more than one medication or illicit drug.[82] However, usually opioid detoxification can be accomplished in the outpatient setting. Outpatient detoxification should be planned not only for discomfort, but also for temporary emotional lability and reduction in function. Compensatory planning might include warning family and work supervisors, planning for a decrease in workload on the job, and even taking vacation or sick leave days. Extensive support with frequent monitoring substantially increases the likelihood of a successful taper.

Higher success rates have been reported for patients with better therapeutic relationships or formal treatment programs that have included a period of stabilization on long half-life opioids and then proceed with a taper slowly over a period of months. Office visits should occur at least weekly, but daily contact with the patient proves a major advantage of ensuring success. Most contact with the patient does not have to involve the physician and often can be accomplished with a phone call. A nursing visit to check vital signs and assess the severity of withdrawal can provide enormous help to the patient. This should include allowing the patient to express discomfort and frustration but then focus on the treatment plan and patient's progress.[83] Formal checklists of signs and symptoms such as the Subjective Opioid Withdrawal Scale (SOWS) and the Objective Opioid Withdrawal Scale (OOWS) allow for the objective rating of withdrawal and documentation of the patient's condition over time (Table 47.2).[84] Adjustment to the treatment plan is then based on several sources of information and not just the patient's complaints.

AGENTS

The primary principle for detoxification is that medication should not be prescribed by a "cookbook" approach but through ongoing patient evaluation and subsequent dosage titration. The simplest strategy institutes a taper of agents that the patient is currently using. This may be a short half-life agent, but offers the advantages of using an agent already familiar to the patient, simplifies an anxiety-filled process, and avoids the imperfect calculation of dosage equivalence and incomplete cross-tolerance. Short half-life agents possess the disadvantage of pharmacokinetics that may not allow a smooth taper. Serum levels will fluctuate more with increasing dosing intervals. Patients will usually experience mild withdrawal within 4 to 8 hours of dosage reduction. The severity of withdrawal will usually peak with a short half-life agent at 8 to 36 hours; however, it can occur as late as 72 hours. When using these agents, certain procedures can minimize the risks of severe withdrawal symptoms (Table 47.3).

The preferable pharmacological strategy is to choose a long half-life pure agonist such as methadone, sustained-release morphine or oxycodone, and transdermal fentanyl patches (Table 47.4). Methadone is the only medication approved by the US Food and Drug Administration for detoxification in opioid use disorders.[81] This strategy has the primary advantage of more consistent opioid serum

TABLE 47.2 Opioid Withdrawal Rating Scales

The Objective Opiate Withdrawal Scale	
Score one point for each sign that is present during a 10-min observation period	
__	Yawning (≥1 yawn per observation period)
__	Rhinorrhea (≥3 sniffs per observation period)
__	Piloerection (gooseflesh: observe patient's arm)
__	Perspiration
__	Lacrimation
__	Mydriasis
__	Tremors (hands)
__	Hot and cold flashes (shivering or huddling for warmth)
__	Restlessness (frequent shifts of position)
__	Vomiting
__	Muscle twitches
__	Abdominal cramps (holding stomach)
__	Anxiety (from mild fidgeting to severe trembling or panic)
Total score __ (maximum severity = 13)	
The Subjective Opiate Withdrawal Scale	
Patients should rate each symptom statement on a scale of 0–4: 0 = not at all, 1 = a little, 2 = moderately, 3 = quite a bit, 4 = extremely	
__	I feel anxious
__	I feel like yawning
__	I am perspiring
__	My eyes are tearing
__	My nose is running
__	I have goose flesh
__	I am shaking
__	I have hot flashes
__	I have cold flashes
__	My bones and muscles ache
__	I feel restless
__	I feel nauseous
__	I feel like vomiting
__	My muscles twitch
__	I have cramps in my stomach
__	I feel like taking [name of opioid] now
Total score __ (maximum severity = 64)	

TABLE 47.3 Short-Half-Life Opioid Taper

Determine the total daily dosage being used by the patient
Adopt a fixed interval schedule with equal doses every 4–6 h for 48 h
Increase the prescribed dose until the patient has no opioid withdrawal symptoms for 48 h
Taper the amount of each dose without lengthening the interval between doses
Taper the total daily dose approximately 10% every 3–7 days
Slowing the taper may be accomplished by the following:
1. Increasing the number of days at a given total dose
2. Decreasing a single dose amount while keeping the remaining doses the same
3. Increasing the time between doses only if the smallest individual dose has been reached

TABLE 47.4 Long-Half-Life Opioid Taper

Determine the total daily dose of the prescribed agent being taken by the patient
Estimate by conversion the equivalent total daily dose of the long-half-life opioid
Adopt a fixed interval schedule with equal doses every 6–8 h for 48 h
Increase the prescribed dose of long-half-life opioid until the patient has no withdrawal symptoms for 3–5 days
Taper the amount of each dose unless the patient can tolerate an interval schedule of dosing every 8–12 h
Taper the total daily dose approximately 10% every 3–7 days
Increase the number of days at a given total daily dose to slow the taper

TABLE 47.5 Buprenorphine Taper

Test for the precipitation of acute withdrawal symptoms by giving an initial dose of 0.1 mg SQ/IM or 1.0 mg SL
Determine the total daily dose of the prescribed agent being taken by the patient
Estimate the equivalent total daily dose of buprenorphine (0.2 mg SQ/IM = morphine 10 mg PO)
Adopt a fixed interval schedule with equal doses every 8–12 h
Titrate the dosage until the patient has no withdrawal symptoms for 24–72 h
Taper the dose and interval to 0.1 mg SQ/IM or 1.0 mg PO qd
Discontinue the medication when the patient experiences no or tolerable withdrawal symptoms

IM, *Intramuscular;* PO, *oral (per os);* qd, *daily (quaque die);* SL, *sublingual;* SQ, *subcutaneous.*

TABLE 47.6 Adjunctive Agents for Symptoms of Opioid Withdrawal

Symptom	Agent Type	Agent
Diarrhea	Bismuth products	Pepto-Bismol
Rhinorrhea	Antihistamines	Diphenhydramine, loratadine
Muscle aches	Muscle relaxants	methocarbamol
Abdominal cramps	Anticholinergics	Dicyclomine HCl
Insomnia	Antihistamines	Diphenhydramine
	Antidepressants	Trazodone, doxepin

levels with less chance of intermittent withdrawal between doses. With a long half-life agent, the onset of withdrawal symptoms should be expected at 12 to 24 hours, although 24 to 48 hours is the usual reported time course. The severity will usually peak at 36 to 96 hours, but can occur up to 1 week later. Substitution, which is not exact, may require some initial titration to achieve dosing equivalence. An initial test dose of the agent can be given to determine the total dose needed. Switching from short to long half-life opioids in anticipation of detoxification may serendipitously prove an effective analgesic strategy. Side effects, intermittent withdrawal, and rebound pain may serve as a general guideline to estimate equivalent opioid doses. Clinical judgment should be used and individual patient characteristics should be considered when applying any table, since there is variance between equivalence charts.[85]

Another detoxification strategy utilizes the partial agonist/antagonist opioids. The agent most commonly used in this category is buprenorphine or the buprenorphine-naloxone combination (Suboxone) (Table 47.5). The buprenorphine-naloxone combination comes in a 4:1 ratio, respectively, and naloxone is added to prevent intravenous use as it only becomes bioavailable when dissolved and injected.[86–87] The use of partial agonist/antagonists is designed to reduce the severity of withdrawal and cause less reinforcing drug effects. As a result, the taper should be easier and more successful. There is also less risk of respiratory depression, which is an infrequent consequence of overestimating the dosing equivalence with pure agonist substitution. When using partial agonist/antagonists such as buprenorphine, it is important to give a small test dose under the supervision of a provider because of the rare precipitation of withdrawal symptoms secondary to the partial antagonist effects. The patient should not take the agonist/antagonist until withdrawal symptoms have begun because taking it too soon after the last dose of a pure agonist will likely precipitate withdrawal. If the patient tolerates the test dose, then the titration of dose equivalence substitution can proceed. Buprenorphine-naloxone is effective for outpatient or inpatient detoxification, and improved outcomes when compared to clonidine for detoxification.[88–89] Evidence indicates that buprenorphine and methadone are similar with regards to treatment retention and decreasing use of other opioids in patients with nonmalignant pain and an opioid use disorder.[90] Buprenorphine-naloxone has been shown to be safe and well tolerated.[88–90]

ADJUNCTIVE AGENTS

Several nonopioid pharmacological agents are commonly used as adjunctive agents to provide patients additional relief from withdrawal symptoms (Table 47.6). Clonidine, an alpha-2-adrenergic agonist that decreases adrenergic activity, is the most commonly prescribed. Clonidine can help relieve many of the autonomic symptoms of opioid withdrawal, such as nausea, cramps, sweating, tachycardia, and hypertension, which result from the loss of opioid suppression of the locus ceruleus during the withdrawal syndrome.[91–92] Other adjunctive agents include nonsteroidal antiinflammatory drugs for muscle aches, bismuth subsalicylate (Pepto-Bismol) for diarrhea, dicyclomine (Bentyl) for abdominal cramps, and antihistamines for insomnia and restlessness. Gabapentin (Neurontin) has also been shown to decrease the severity of coldness, diarrhea, dysphoria, yawning, and muscle tension during opioid withdrawal.[93]

SCHEDULE

Unless patients are involved with dangerous aberrant drug-taking behaviors, there is generally no urgency to shorten the duration of opioid detoxification. There is only scant literature examining the pace of tapering in opioid-dependent patients, so clinical judgment must be used.[81] The longer the patient has been taking opioids, the more difficulty they are likely to have with withdrawal. The taper will then require more time to be completed. Other factors that tend to increase the difficulty and length of a taper are medical comorbidity and complexity, older age, female gender, and detoxification from multiple agents simultaneously. Detoxification occurs if more difficult in the last stages of the taper, and it should be anticipated that decreases in the dose of opioids would need to be more gradual during this time. If a taper becomes more complicated, the schedule should be extended by decreasing the dosage reductions or lengthening the intervals between reductions. As long as patients are demonstrating ongoing progress, there is generally no reason not to extend an opioid taper over several weeks or even months. Progress can be demonstrated by simple compliance with taper instructions, not using illicit substances, improvement in side effects of opioids, and maintenance of function.

FOLLOW-UP

The process of detoxification does not end with the completion of the opioid taper. Patients can have lingering subacute withdrawal symptoms for weeks. In some circumstances, they can last for months. Insomnia and rebound pain are the most common symptoms, but any of the withdrawal symptoms can reemerge. After the taper, patients who had difficulty with aberrant drug-taking behaviors continue to need increased levels of monitoring and supervision in their treatments because the risk of relapse is high. Patients without a history of addiction and aberrant drug-taking behaviors do not require specialized substance abuse treatment. These patients should be reassured that they do not have an addiction or the diagnosis of substance abuse/dependence. However, any detoxification precipitated by the diagnosis of addiction or medication misuse should have further evaluation and treatment. Referral to an addiction specialist is usually a helpful first step. Furthermore, active ongoing participation in the treatment prescribed for addiction should be a condition of continued pain treatment. For these patients, the prevention of relapse requires a long-term outpatient program of substance abuse rehabilitation.

TABLE 47.7 Signs and Symptoms of Sedative-Hypnotic Withdrawal

Hyperarousal
Agitation Anxiety Hyperactivity Insomnia Fever
Neurological
Ataxia Fasciculation/myoclonic jerks Formication Headache Myalgia
Paresthesias/Dysesthesias
Pruritus Tinnitus Tremor Seizures Delirium
Genitourinary
Incontinence Loss of libido Urinary urgency, frequency
Psychiatric
Depersonalization Depression Hyperventilation Malaise Paranoid delusions Visual hallucinations
Gastrointestinal
Abdominal pain Constipation Diarrhea Nausea Vomiting Anorexia
Cardiovascular
Chest pain Flushing Palpitations Hypertension Orthostatic hypotension Tachycardia Diaphoresis

BENZODIAZEPINE DETOXIFICATION

The technique of a benzodiazepine taper follows the same general principles of an opioid taper.[94–95] If patients have been using benzodiazepines only intermittently, there is generally no need for a taper. However, anyone who has been using benzodiazepines continuously for more than two weeks should be tapered to avoid the unpleasant experience of mild withdrawal and the risk of unexpected major withdrawal symptoms. A higher total daily dose and longer duration of use produces a higher risk of significant and potentially life-threatening withdrawal with abrupt cessation. The general features of benzodiazepine withdrawal are similar to those of opioid withdrawal with hyperarousal and hypersympathetic states. However, in its more specific features, the withdrawal syndrome is more similar to the syndrome observed with alcohol (Table 47.7). Similarly, benzodiazepine withdrawal is much more dangerous than opioid withdrawal and includes the potential for seizures, hallucinations, hyperthermia, and delirium tremens. Similar to alcohol withdrawal, when untreated, severe benzodiazepine withdrawal has a higher rate of morbidity and mortality.

The two main techniques for detoxification include a taper of the agent a patient has been taking and the substitution of an equivalent dose of a long half-life agent such as diazepam or clonazepam. Another strategy for benzodiazepine detoxification utilizes phenobarbital solution, especially in cases of complex detoxification from multiple agents such as opioids, sedative-hypnotics, and alcohol. The phenobarbital dose should be determined by a series of test doses and subsequent observation to determine the level of tolerance. In addition, infrequently, the "second generation" benzodiazepines (clonazepam, alprazolam, oxazepam, triazolam) are not fully cross-tolerant with each other or with the more traditional agents. A patient may require higher doses than expected to avoid significant withdrawal symptoms when taking these medications. Benzodiazepine tapers will generally require more time than opioid tapers with less frequent dose reductions. A taper of 6 weeks or more, especially with long half-life agents, is not unusual, and some have recommended a 6-month taper.[96] Carbamazepine has been shown to have modest benefit in reducing symptoms of benzodiazepine withdrawal, and, more recently, gabapentin has been utilized by some practitioners, but it has not been studied.[95]

CONCLUSION

Patients with chronic pain are at increased risk of substance use disorders. However, it is crucial to appreciate that there are many causes for aberrant medication-related behaviors. Misuse of medication is a clinical problem that can be the result of dependence, but it is often the result of inadequate analgesia. This can be due to undertreatment with opioids and other analgesics, disease progression, or tolerance to medications. Eventually, instead of consulting with their physician, the patient may simply take more medication. Without proper instructions, they will often take it inappropriately. If the patient does have an addiction, they will be preoccupied with the medication, have lost control of its use, and continue taking it regardless of the negative consequences they are now suffering. This patient requires specialized evaluation and treatment in addition to the management of their chronic pain syndrome. If careful planning and common principles are applied, detoxification will facilitate the transition from ineffective or problematic treatments to other potentially more effective treatments for pain. Treatments may include drug rehabilitation, but it should not be prescribed for every inpatient undergoing detoxification. By avoiding unpleasant or dangerous withdrawal syndromes and providing the patient with the reinforcement that all treatments should result in benefits that outweigh their risks, the therapeutic relationship will be strengthened and the chances for successful treatment are optimized.

KEY POINTS

- The prevalence of substance use disorders in patients with chronic pain is higher than in the general population.
- Individuals with substance use disorders are more often initiated and continued on opioid therapy for noncancer pain than those without substance use disorders.
- Comorbid psychiatric disorders are associated with increased physical symptoms, more subjective pain, more aberrant drug behaviors, and are linked to increased opioid use.
- Research in patients with substance abuse has demonstrated abnormalities in pain perception and tolerance.
- Opioids are effective in the treatment of chronic nonmalignant pain in reducing pain, pain-related disability, depression, insomnia, and physical dysfunction in the short term (months), but evidence is lacking for their long-term (>1 year) effectiveness.
- A thorough evaluation, careful patient selection, and close monitoring are all essential for the safe and effective prescribing of opioids for noncancer pain.
- Benzodiazepines have little to no role in treating chronic noncancer pain and are associated with significant risk.
- To be diagnosed with a substance use disorder (DSM-V), patients must demonstrate a pattern of substance use leading to impairment or distress, as manifested by at least 2 of 11 criteria, such as taking the substance in larger amounts or over a longer period than was intended, continued use despite negative consequences, tolerance, and dependence, among others.
- The occurrence of any aberrant medication-related behaviors should prompt evaluation for addiction.
- An active substance use disorder is a strong relative contraindication to chronic opioid therapy.

REFERENCES

Access the reference list online at ExpertConsult.com.

CHAPTER 48

Psychopharmacology for Pain Medicine

Mohammed A. Issa, MD ◌ Zwade Marshall, MD, MBA ◌ Ajay D. Wasan, MD, MSc

Burgeoning evidence suggests that psychiatric factors play a critical role in the experience of pain and the development of chronic pain syndromes. One of the early studies that described this phenomenon was performed by Atkinson et al. at the Veterans Affairs Medical Center Low Back Pain Clinic.[1] They studied 100 consecutive admissions to the clinic and compared lifetime and current rates of depression, alcohol abuse, and anxiety between controls and the chronic back pain cohort. The 6-month and lifetime rates of major depression were 22% and 32%, respectively, versus 6% and 16% for controls.[1] Subsequent to the onset of pain, patients had a relative risk of 9.0 for developing major depression. The lifetime alcohol abuse rate for chronic pain patients was 65%, compared with 39% for controls.[1] Patients with pain and psychiatric comorbidity are commonly referred to pain medicine clinics and frequently present with prescribed psychoactive medications. Many of these medications, such as antidepressants and anticonvulsants, also have analgesic properties and are a mainstay of the drug armamentarium of the pain physician. Consequently it behooves the astute pain practitioner to be familiar with the psychiatric comorbidities of patients with chronic pain and to understand the therapeutic benefits and risks associated with the use of psychoactive medications to treat both pain and/or psychopathology. Psychotherapeutic modalities, such as cognitive behavioral therapy, relaxation training, and biofeedback, play an important role in the treatment of both psychiatric and chronic pain syndromes; in some cases they are the preferred method of treatment. However, this chapter focuses on the use of medications as they pertain to treating patients with pain and psychiatric comorbidity. As with many of the medications used in pain medicine, psychoactive medications with reported analgesic properties do not always have an indication from the US Food and Drug Administration (FDA) for this purpose, but they can legally be prescribed for off-label use.

EPIDEMIOLOGY

Over three decades, studies of US pain clinic populations have shown that by the criteria of the *Diagnostic and Statistical Manual of Mental Disorders* (DSM), 60% to 80% of these patients have psychiatric illnesses.[2–4] Estimates are lower for persons with pain in primary care, institutional, and community settings, but regardless of setting, given the prevalence of persistent pain in adults, which is estimated at 20% to 45%, pain combined with psychiatric comorbidity constitutes an important public health problem.[5,6] Patients with psychiatric illness report greater pain intensity, more pain-related disability, and a larger affective component to their pain.[7–9] The majority of patients with psychiatric comorbidity developed their psychiatric illness after the onset of chronic pain. Major depression alone affects 30% to 50% of all pain clinic patients, followed by anxiety disorders, personality disorders, somatoform disorders, and substance use disorders.[2,10,11] Virtually all psychiatric conditions can be treated with variable improvement and the majority of patients who are provided with appropriate treatment show significant improvement. Of the disorders that most frequently affect patients with chronic pain, major depression and anxiety disorders are the most common and have the best response to medication. Regardless of the specific psychopathology, however, improvement in psychiatric illness results in diminished pain levels, greater acceptance of the chronicity of pain, improved functionality, and improved quality of life. Although this chapter focuses on psychopharmacologic treatment, it is important to note that in general combined pharmacologic and psychotherapeutic treatments are more effective in alleviating depression and anxiety than pharmacologic treatment alone. Psychotherapeutic treatments (e.g., cognitive-behavioral therapies, relaxation and biofeedback, interpersonal therapies, and group therapies) are covered in other chapters of this book.

PSYCHIATRIC NOSOLOGY

Mental health practitioners utilize the fifth edition of the DSM (DSM-5) or the tenth revision of the *International Statistical Classification of Diseases and Related Health Problems* (ICD-10) as an aid in making psychiatric diagnoses.[12] Although these manuals outline the suggested criteria for psychiatric diagnosis elegantly, they are not very good at highlighting which symptoms are more or less important in making a diagnosis. Although the criteria have high reliability—that is, two psychiatrists applying the criteria to the assessment of the same patient will very often come up with the same diagnosis—the criteria do not all have equally high validity. That is, there is no universal agreement that the symptoms listed under diagnostic criteria for a particular condition are the best description of that illness.[13] In this light, and in an attempt to demystify psychiatric diagnosis for the pain physician, the following descriptions of psychopathology emphasize the hallmark features of each illness.

MAJOR DEPRESSION AND SUBTHRESHOLD DEPRESSION

Symptoms: According to the DSM-5, *major depressive disorder* (MDD) requires the presence of depressed mood and loss of interest or pleasure in most activities (anhedonia) for at least 2 weeks. The lifetime risk of MDD is 7% to 12% in men and from 20% to 25% in women.[14] But the risk of major depression in patients with pain is at least twice as high. As the most prevalent of the psychiatric comorbidities, major depression can be distinguished from *situational depression* (also termed *demoralization* or *adjustment disorder with depressed mood*) by the triad of persistently low mood, self-attitude changes, and changes in vital sense, all lasting at least 2 weeks.[13] Low mood manifests itself by emotions of "feeling blue," down, or depressed. *Anhedonia*, or the inability to experience pleasure, is a key reflection of low mood. A *diminished self-attitude* is seen in feelings of guilt or thinking that one is a bad person. *Changes in vital sense* means changes in sleep, appetite, or energy level. Patients with major depression often feel that their thinking is slow or fuzzy, and they have difficulty concentrating. Depressed patients may feel anxious, have panic attacks, or experience symptoms of posttraumatic stress disorder (PTSD), which, if they occur in the presence of significant depression, are consistent with an MDD and not a separate anxiety disorder. Depressive symptoms may present as Beck triad, with patients feeling hopeless, hapless, and helpless. They see the future as bleak; they feel that they cannot help themselves and that no one else can help them.[15] Suicidal thoughts reflect the severity of depressive symptoms. Untreated or undertreated major depression has a lifetime risk of death through completion of suicide of 10% to 15%.[16] Major depression is a serious complication of persistent pain; if not treated adequately, it will reduce the effectiveness of all pain treatment. Even low levels of depression ("subthreshold depression") may worsen the physical impairment associated with chronic pain conditions and should also be treated.[8]

TREATMENT

Antidepressants can take up to 2 to 4 weeks to produce an initial response, but all can take 4 to 8 weeks for full clinical improvement after a typical dose is reached, and remission may take longer. This can be particularly the case for depressed patients who also suffer from comorbid pain. Patients should remain on their medications for 6 to 12 months for the treatment of an initial depressive episode and for 5 years for the treatment of a recurrent depressive episode. Regardless of the medication chosen, approximately 60% of patients will respond (have at least a 50% improvement) to the initial antidepressant prescribed. At least 80% of patients will respond to at least one medication, either with or without an augmentation agent such as lithium, an anticonvulsant, or another antidepressant.[17] There is some evidence that pain patients with major depression have increased treatment resistance, particularly when their pain is not effectively managed.[6] Older adults tend to respond at lower doses of antidepressants, and dose titration should occur more slowly in this group because of their heightened sensitivity to side effects and toxicity.[18] A good rule of thumb in starting antidepressants in any age group is to begin with one quarter to one half of the standard initial treatment dose for a week and then advance gradually over the next 2 to 3 weeks to the treatment dose. This minimizes side effects and increases treatment compliance.

Often, patients with chronic pain are on multiple medications that can potentiate the side effects of antidepressants, such as headache, nausea, constipation, or sedation; therefore "starting low and going slow" is even more important in this population. Typically, in the initial treating period, reevaluations are done every 2 to 4 weeks, with dose adjustments if indicated. Monoamine oxidase inhibitors (MAOIs), such as phenelzine, which are rarely prescribed any longer, should not be prescribed concurrently with other antidepressants. Because of the inherent risks of these medications, they should be used only by experienced psychopharmacologists.[19]

Cognitive-behavioral therapy (CBT) in conjunction with antidepressant therapy is the most efficacious treatment for major depression. CBT examines negative and destructive thoughts that arise in conjunction with low moods, helping patients to see the unrealistic and maladaptive qualities of thoughts and behaviors.[20]

SELECTIVE SEROTONIN REUPTAKE INHIBITORS

Since the introduction of fluoxetine (Prozac) in 1987, many selective serotonin reuptake inhibitors (SSRIs) have been introduced. They have an immediate effect on the blockade of the presynaptic serotonin reuptake pump in the central nervous system (CNS), which has been shown in animals to increase the duration of serotonin in the synaptic cleft, increasing the effects of neurotransmission.[21] The antidepressant efficacy of SSRIs and their low side-effect profiles have made them the most widely prescribed class of antidepressants. However, the SSRIs have few independent pain properties. Pain patients whose depression responds to an SSRI may have diminished pain that is attributable to improvements in the affective components of their pain, but there is little evidence supporting independent analgesic activity of SSRIs. Although a few case reports have shown improvements in diabetic neuropathic pain treated with SSRIs, double-blind, placebo-controlled clinical trials that exclude patients with depression have not consistently demonstrated analgesic benefit.[22–26]

Before prescribing an SSRI, all medications/supplements that the patient is taking must be carefully reviewed along with their general medical condition, since SSRIs are commonly associated with easy bruising/bleeding[27] and osteoporosis.[28,29] SSRIs can cause serotonin syndrome when given with other medications, including serotonin-norepinephrine reuptake inhibitors (SNRIs), tricyclic antidepressants (TCAs), MAOIs, triptans (e.g., sumatriptan), and antiemetics (e.g., ondansetron, metoclopramide). Moreover, serotonin syndrome can be precipitated by a combination of SSRIs and multiple analgesics, including tramadol, meperidine, fentanyl, and pentazocine. The use of SSRIs in combination with tramadol can lower the seizure threshold, and caution is called for if these drugs are combined.[30] No additional laboratory workup is required in starting SSRIs, and dose titration is based on clinical response and side effects. Fluoxetine tends to be more activating and is prescribed in the morning, whereas paroxetine, with its anticholinergic effect of activating muscarinic receptors, is more sedating and has greater anxiolytic properties. It is generally prescribed in the evening. Paroxetine has a relatively shorter half-life than most SSRIs and is often associated with withdrawal symptoms upon

TABLE 48.1 Selective Serotonin Reuptake Inhibitors

Drug	Usual Start Dose	Average Dose	Maximum Dose
Citalopram (Celexa)	10 mg qd	20–40 mg qd	60 mg/day
Fluoxetine (Prozac)	10 mg qd	20–40 mg qd	80 mg/day
Fluvox-amine (Luvox)	25 mg qd	50–100 mg bid	300 mg/day
Paroxetine (Paxil)	5–10 mg qd	20–40 mg qd	60 mg/day
Sertraline (Zoloft)	25 mg qd	50–150 mg qd	200 mg/day

discontinuation. Sertraline and citalopram tend to be less sedating than paroxetine and are generally prescribed in the morning.[19]

Patients should begin on half of the usual dose for a week (Table 48.1) and then go on to the standard dose so as to minimize the side effects of nausea, diarrhea, tremor, and headache. Some patients can experience sedation or overstimulation. Approximately 75% to 80% of patients on SSRIs can experience sexual side effects, such as decreased libido, impotence, ejaculatory disturbances, or anorgasmia. This can be particularly the case in elderly patients who may already have diminished libido owing to possible comorbid pain and depression. Rare side effects include dystonia, akathisia, palpitations, a lowered seizure threshold, serotonin syndrome, or the syndrome of inappropriate antidiuretic hormone (SIADH).[31]

SSRIs are metabolized by hepatic oxidation, and their use may alter the serum levels of other hepatically metabolized drugs. SSRIs induce and/or inhibit various cytochrome P450 (CYP450) enzymes. Most significantly, they can increase levels of TCAs and benzodiazepines (BZDs).[32] They may also affect levels of carbamazepine, lithium, antipsychotics, and commonly used analgesics, such as methadone, oxycodone, and fentanyl.[33] Fluoxetine, paroxetine, and to a lesser extent fluvoxamine are inhibitors of cytochrome 2D6; fluoxetine and fluvoxamine also interfere with cytochrome 3A4.[14] There is also evidence that sertraline at doses greater than 100 mg may inhibit these enzymes[34] and thus may increase the circulating metabolites of certain opioids. Citalopram and escitalopram have less of an effect on CYP450 enzyme activity. If taken in overdose, SSRIs are rarely, if ever, lethal. In discontinuing SSRIs, they should be tapered down slowly to avoid a withdrawal syndrome, which has the same symptoms as initiation of SSRIs (headache, nausea, diarrhea, or myalgias).

TRICYCLIC ANTIDEPRESSANTS

TCAs are one of the oldest classes of antidepressants and they act by inhibiting both serotonergic and noradrenergic reuptake. This lengthens the time serotonin and norepinephrine (NE) remain in the synaptic cleft, enhancing their neurotransmission.[35] The analgesic properties of TCAs are independent of their treatment effects on depression, thus making them a good choice for treating depression in patients with chronic pain, particularly if cost is a factor.

All TCAs are equally effective for the treatment of depression; the choice of a particular one is determined by side effects. The magnitude of anticholinergic and antihistaminic effects is the largest determinant. Amitriptyline and imipramine are more sedating, with more weight gain and orthostatic hypotension. Other anticholinergic side effects include dry mouth, constipation, blurred vision, urinary retention, sexual side effects, excessive sweating, and confusion or delirium. TCAs also decrease the seizure threshold. Desipramine and nortriptyline have fewer anticholinergic side effects, and of all of the TCAs, desipramine has the fewest anticholinergic side effects. Serum plasma levels can be monitored for TCAs, and this is particularly important for desipramine, imipramine, and nortriptyline, which have the best correlation of blood levels to therapeutic antidepressant response.[18] The therapeutic blood level for nortriptyline ranges from 50 to 150 ng/mL; it is 75 to 225 ng/mL for both desipramine and imipramine, as desipramine is simply the desmethyl metabolite of imipramine.[14]

Prior to initiating treatment, patients should have laboratory screening of electrolytes, blood urea nitrogen (BUN), and creatinine as well as liver function tests (LFTs). TCAs also have quinidine-like properties, are potentially proarrythmic, and can prolong the QTC interval. It is recommended that patients with a history of cardiac disease or who are taking other QTC-prolonging medications have a baseline electrocardiogram (EKG), with particular attention to the QTC interval.[36] TCAs are strongly protein-bound (85%–95%) and undergo first-pass hepatic metabolism. Subsequent stages involve demethylation, oxidation, and glucuronide conjugation. Amitriptyline is demethylated to nortriptyline, and imipramine is demethylated to desipramine. Hepatic clearance involves the P450 enzyme system, so drugs such as SSRIs, cimetidine, and methylphenidate can increase TCA plasma levels. SSRIs and TCAs should not be prescribed at the same time unless plasma levels are carefully monitored. Phenobarbital, carbamazepine, and cigarette smoking induce the P450 enzyme system and thus decrease serum TCA levels.[32]

As with SSRIs, to minimize side effects and increase adherence, initiation of TCAs should begin at lower doses (usually 25 mg for a week) than the target doses for antidepressant effect (typically 75 to 150 mg) (Table 48.2). The elderly are more sensitive to their side effects, and many psychiatrists begin at doses of 10 to 20 mg in this age group.[18] With diminished or altered metabolism of TCAs, as well as the multiple medications older patients are frequently taking, they are more prone to develop toxic serum levels, and monitoring should be more frequent. There is a withdrawal syndrome with abrupt discontinuation of TCAs, characterized by fever, sweating, headaches, nausea, dizziness, and/or akathisia. Unlike the SSRIs, overdose can be lethal. TCA overdose is a leading cause of drug-related overdose and death. Three to five times the therapeutic dose is potentially lethal, so this narrow therapeutic range must be respected, and serial blood levels monitored. Toxicity results from

TABLE 48.2 Tricyclic Antidepressants

Drug	Usual Start Dose	Average Dose	Maximum Dose
Amitriptyline (Elavil)	10–25 mg qd	75–150 mg qd	300 mg/day
Amoxapine (Asendin)	25 mg bid	75–200 mg bid	600 mg/day
Clomipramine (Anafranil)	25 mg qd	150–250 mg qd	250 mg/day
Desipramine (Norpramin)	10–25 mg qd	75–150 mg qd	300 mg qd
Doxepin (Sinequan)	10–25 mg qd	75–150 mg qd	300 mg qd
Nortriptyline (Pamelor)	10–25 mg qd	75–150 mg qd	200 mg qd
Protriptyline (Vivactil)	5 mg qd	10 mg tid	60 mg/day

TABLE 48.3 Miscellaneous Antidepressants

Drug	Usual Start Dose	Average Dose	Maximum Dose
Bupropion (Wellbutrin)	75 mg bid	100–150 mg bid	600 mg qd
Duloxetine (Cymbalta)	30 mg qd	60 mg qd	120 mg
Mirtazepine (Remuron)	15 mg qhs	30–45 mg qd	60 mg qd
Nefazodone (Serozone)	100 mg bid	150–300 mg bid	600 mg/day
Trazodone (Desyrel)	50 mg qhs	150–250 mg bid	600 mg/day
Venlafaxine (Effexor)	37.5 mg qd	75–112.5 mg bid	375 mg/day

anticholinergic and proarrythmic effects such as seizures, coma, and QTC widening.[36]

Also, unlike the SSRIs, TCAs have independent analgesic properties. A series of studies by Max and others have illustrated the analgesic properties of TCAs, which are independent of its effects on improving depression.[37,38] TCAs have been shown to be modestly effective for diabetic neuropathy pain, chronic regional pain syndrome, chronic headache, poststroke pain, and radicular pain.[17,37–41] Additionally, TCAs are useful as preemptive analgesics, being opioid-sparing in the postoperative period.[42] Although the initial studies were done with amitriptyline and desipramine, subsequent studies have confirmed that the other TCAs have equivalent analgesic properties. Of note, the typical doses for the analgesic benefit of TCAs (25 to 75 mg) are lower than the typical doses for antidepressant effect (75 to 150 mg). However, many patients are referred to a pain specialist after a failed trial of TCAs at lower doses. And yet there is a dose–response relationship for analgesia. So even if one is using a TCA solely for pain relief, patients may benefit with a dose in the antidepressant range in conjunction with blood level monitoring.

SEROTONIN-NOREPINEPHRINE REUPTAKE INHIBITORS

The nontricyclic SNRIs are a newer group of antidepressants that, like the TCAs, act by inhibiting serotonin and NE reuptake. This appears to be one of the mechanisms accounting both for the higher rates of depression remission and the analgesic efficacy associated with TCAs and SNRIs as compared with SSRIs.[28] Venlafaxine, desvenlafaxine, duloxetine, and milnacipran are the main drugs in this category. They have significantly less alpha-1, cholinergic, and histamine inhibition and thus fewer side effects than the tricyclics, with equivalent antidepressant and potentially equal analgesic benefits. Placebo-controlled studies have demonstrated modest efficacy in neuropathic pain for both venlafaxine[43,44] and duloxetine.[45] A numbers-needed-to-treat analysis suggested superior analgesic properties of TCAs (particularly amitriptiline), which may be due to their properties of *N*-methyl-D-aspartic acid (NMDA) antagonism and sodium channel blockade in addition to their combined SNRI effect.[43]

Venlafaxine is given in two or three divided daily doses (even with extended-release formulations), beginning at 37.5 mg/day for a week and then slowly increased to as high as 375 mg/day (Table 48.3). A typical dose is 150 to 225 mg/day. Generally patients are escalated over a month to 75 mg/day; then, depending on clinical response, the dose is adjusted.

Laboratory studies are not needed prior to starting venlafaxine, but patients with hypertension should be treated with caution. Particularly at doses over 150 mg/day, venlafaxine may increase systolic blood pressure by 10 mm or more. This is likely due to the onset of NE reuptake inhibition, which occurs at the higher doses of venlafaxine[43] that appear to be needed for analgesic efficacy in neuropathic pain, unlike tricyclics, which may be effective at lower than antidepressant doses. Other side effects include nausea, somnolence, dry mouth, dizziness, nervousness, constipation, anorexia, and/or sexual dysfunction. Venlafaxine may affect hepatic metabolism of other medications, but it is a weak inhibitor of the CYP450 system.[34]

Venlafaxine (Effexor) is structurally similar to tramadol; in mice, venlafaxine demonstrates opioid-mediated analgesia that is reversed by naloxone. Both controlled studies and case reports indicate that venlafaxine has analgesic properties independent of its antidepressant effects in a variety of neuropathic conditions.[46–49] Many patients are unable to tolerate the side effects of tricyclics, so venlafaxine and duloxetine are promising agents in patients with major depression and chronic pain. Desvenlafaxine (Pristiq) is the active metabolite of venlafaxine and was recently approved by the FDA for the treatment of MDD. Preliminary studies have shown success in treating neuropathic pain at higher doses.[50] It is classified as a combined serotonin (5-HT) and NE reuptake inhibitor (SNRI) but also inhibits the reuptake of dopamine to a lesser degree. Unlike venlafaxine, the affinity of desvenlafaxine for the 5-HT and NE receptors does not increase with escalating doses of the medication.[50] An initial dose of 50 mg/day is recommended that can be titrated up to 100 mg/day for treatment of depression. However, higher doses up to 400 mg/day have shown some efficacy in treating neuropathic pain. Venlafaxine was shown to be as effective at treating painful polyneuropathy as imipramine in a recent randomized study.[44]

Duloxetine (Cymbalta) is an SNRI approved for use in the United States for diabetic peripheral neuropathy, fibromyalgia, major depression, and generalized anxiety disorder. It is the only major psychotropic drug approved in the United States for both pain and psychiatric conditions; thus it is the treatment of choice for patients with neuropathic pain and psychiatric comorbidity. The typical starting dose is 30 mg at dinnertime for a week, then increasing to 60 mg at dinnertime. Dosing in the evening tends to mitigate the side effects of nausea and tiredness. Other side effects include dry mouth, dizziness, constipation, and sexual dysfunction. Dosing in the elderly should begin lower, at about 20 mg/day, because of increased side effects and less tolerability in these patients.[51] The maximum dose that has been studied is 120 mg/day. Most of the studies show no significant benefit above doses of 60 mg/day, but there is a range of individual responses and some patients will preferentially respond at the higher dose. Duloxetine is a moderate inhibitor of the CYP2D6 liver enzyme and thus may increase TCA and antipsychotic levels.[34] No laboratory tests are needed prior to prescribing duloxetine. It should not be prescribed to patients with renal or liver insufficiency.

Milnacipran (Savella): In the United States, milnacipran is FDA-approved for the treatment of fibromyalgia but not depression. However, in Europe, milnacipran has an established use for both chronic pain and depression. It is an SNRI that has shown some efficacy in treating neuropathic pain and fibromyalgia at a dose of 100 mg to 200 mg/day.[52] A recent Cochrane systematic review indicates that milnacipran provides at least a 30% reduction in pain caused by fibromyalgia for 40% of patients compared with a similar level of pain relief in 30% of patients given placebo.[52] There was insufficient evidence to evaluate a higher threshold of pain relief (50%) and there were no data to support its use in other neuropathic pain conditions.[53,54] The magnitude of the effect is relatively modest but it may be clinically significant, since fibromyalgia has been extremely difficult to treat. Adverse events were more often associated with the dose of 200 mg/day than with that of 100 mg/day, with a number needed to harm of 23 and a number needed to treat of 8.8.[54] Nausea and constipation were the most common events reported with this treatment regimen. The mechanism of action is not fully understood, but it is theorized to be involved in the modulation of endogenous analgesic mechanisms via descending inhibitory pathways. The increase in serotonin and NE with milnacipran augments the inhibition of painful signals, resulting in a reduction of pain intensity.[53]

OTHER ANTIDEPRESSANTS

Bupropion (Wellbutrin) is a noradrenergic and dopaminergic reuptake pump inhibitor, prolonging the time that NE and dopamine remain in the synaptic cleft.[21] Unlike many of the other antidepressants, it has significant psychostimulant properties. It is used in the treatment of depression, attention deficit hyperactivity disorder (ADHD), and smoking cessation at doses up to 600 mg/day (see Table 48.3). Studies have shown that bupropion has independent analgesic effects in a variety of neuropathic conditions.[55] Anecdotal reports have also indicated that bupropion is effective in alleviating the sedative effects of opioids. Consequently bupropion has an important use in pain medicine. Enthusiasm was dampened, however, by a randomized controlled trial (RCT) in 44 patients with chronic low back pain showing no significant improvement.[56]

Treatment with bupropion should start at 75 to 100 mg in the morning to avoid insomnia, which may occur if the drug is started at night. After 5 days, this dose is advanced to the average treatment dose of 100 to 150 mg bid, even for sustained-release preparations. At these doses there is a very slight decrease in seizure threshold. Doses from 450 to 600 mg/day may cause seizures in 4% of patients, so these doses should be avoided.[57] Bupropion should not be prescribed to patients with seizures, eating disorders, or those taking MAOIs. Caution is needed in coprescribing bupropion with tramadol, since lowering of the seizure threshold is most likely additive. Side effects include nervousness, headache, irritability, and insomnia.

Mirtazapine is an antidepressant with antagonism of serotonin and central presynaptic alpha-2 adrenergic receptors, stimulating serotonin and NE release. This serves to potentiate serotonergic and noradrenergic transmission while having no anticholinergic effects.[32] It is thought to preferentially augment serotonergic transmission and have an antihistaminic effect at lower doses of 15 to 30 mg/day. At higher doses, 45 to 60 mg/day, it augments more noradrenergic transmission (see Table 48.3). As a result, at lower doses it is more sedating and has antianxiety effects, with the side effect of weight gain. At higher doses it is more activating and can provoke anxiety symptoms. Agranulocytosis and neurotropenia can rarely occur with this medication at an incidence of 0.3%.[19] One case report and an open-label study indicate that there may be analgesic benefits to mirtazapine, but improvements in depression were not adequately controlled.[58,59]

Trazodone, like nefazodone, is a serotonin-2 antagonist/reuptake inhibitor (SARI) used to treat major depression and insomnia. The sedative qualities of trazodone are so great that few patients are able to get to a dose that is high enough to be in the effective antidepressant range. Trazodone is most often prescribed for insomnia accompanying symptoms of depression, anxiety, or pain and is the preferred treatment of many pain physicians for insomnia.[17] Typical dosing for sleep is 25 to 100 mg at bedtime (see Table 48.3). For depression, dosing for trazodone and nefazodone is 50 to 600 mg/day in two divided doses. A rare but serious side effect of trazodone is priapism, occurring in 1 in 1000 to 1 in 10,000 cases.[60] Side effects common to both medications are sedation, dizziness, dry mouth, orthostatic hypotension, constipation, and headache. Studies have shown that trazodone has few analgesic properties. No such studies have been done with nefazodone, but one would not expect a different result.

ANXIETY DISORDERS

There are many anxiety disorders, including generalized anxiety disorder, panic disorder, and obsessive-compulsive disorder. PTSD had been included in this group, but DSM-5 has reclassified PTSD into its own category. Nevertheless, most psychiatrists still widely regard PTSD as part of the cluster of anxiety disorders, since it shares many common features with others in this group. There is a high prevalence of anxiety disorders in chronic pain clinic populations, with 30% to 60% of patients having anxiety at pathologic levels.[3,5,61] Generalized anxiety disorder is the most frequent anxiety disorder affecting pain patients.

Anxiety is a broad concept with many dimensions. Anxiety can be an enduring personality trait that at times becomes excessive. It can be a symptom among a constellation of symptoms as part of another disorder, such as major depression. Alternatively, it may be an episodic disorder, provoked by stressful and taxing challenges, such as chronic pain. Anxiety also has a biologic component and is responsive to medications.[2] It is difficult to determine when anxiety is pathologic, but one guideline is when anxiety interferes with normal functioning. There is both trait anxiety and situational anxiety. Trait anxiety is excessive worry and concern, often about routine matters. The amount of worry and anxiety is out of proportion to the likelihood of the negative consequences occurring, and the patient has great difficulty controlling worry.

In pain patients, situational anxiety is often anxiety about pain and its negative consequences. Patients may be conditioned to be excessively fearful that some activities will cause uncontrollable pain, causing avoidance of those activities, which in some patients can be extreme, almost phobic. Also, pain may activate thoughts that one is seriously ill.[62] Pain-specific anxiety as well as generalized anxiety amplify pain perception and pain complaints through several biopsychosocial mechanisms, including sympathetic arousal with noradrenergically mediated lowering of nociceptive threshold, increased firing of ectopically active pain neurons, excessive cognitive focus on pain symptoms, and poor coping skills. Patients with pathologic anxiety are often restless, fatigued, and irritable; they also have poor concentration. They may have muscle tension and sleep disturbances. Their mood is often low, but not at the severity of MDD.[17]

TREATMENT

Overall, CBT demonstrates the best treatment outcomes for anxiety disorders. Significant improvements are further obtained with relaxation therapy, meditation, and biofeedback.[63] Antidepressants are effective, but generally at higher doses than what is typically prescribed for depression. Anxiolytics, such as BZDs and buspirone, are most useful in the initial treatment stages to stabilize a disorder. However, the side effects and physiologic dependency associated with BZDs in particular make them a poor choice for long-term treatment.

ANTIDEPRESSANTS

In the treatment of depression, it may take 4 to 8 weeks after a patient is on the target dose to see improvement. To improve compliance, escalation of doses must be done very slowly, because anxious patients are poorly tolerant of side effects. Antidepressants are useful in diminishing the overall level of anxiety and preventing anxiety or panic attacks, but they have no role in treating acute anxiety. Both the SSRIs and SNRIs are effective agents among antidepressants. Paroxetine tends to have greater antianxiety effects, but all of the SSRIs have good anxiolytic properties.[64] Effective doses for SSRIs are higher than those for depression, typically 60 to 80 mg/day.[65]

Of the TCAs, clomipramine is the most effective, with particular usefulness in obsessive-compulsive disorder. Nefazodone has antianxiety effects, as does venlafaxine at higher doses. Mirtazapine has anxiolytic properties at the lower, more sedating doses; higher doses of 45 to 60 mg can worsen anxiety with its activating qualities.[66] Similarly, although there are reports that bupropion is effective in treating depression with anxious features, its stimulating effects make it less attractive as a primary antianxiety agent.

SNRIs, specifically venlafaxine and duloxetine, have also demonstrated efficacy in generalized anxiety, and have an FDA indication for the treatment of generalized anxiety disorder.[67]

BENZODIAZEPINES AND BUSPIRONE

These medications are useful in the treatment of acute anxiety, panic attacks, and the stabilization of generalized anxiety. Occasionally, anxiety cannot be stabilized with antidepressants and patients remain on BZDs in the long term. BZDs bind to the benzodiazepine component of the gamma-aminobutyric acid (GABA) receptor, an inhibitory neurotransmitter. They depress the CNS at the levels of the limbic system, brain-stem reticular formation, and cortex.[21] Although they are widely prescribed by pain practitioners, studies indicate that they have few independent analgesic properties. However, these medications are also used as muscle relaxants and to treat pain associated with muscular spasticity. Issues of tolerance often limit their long-term use for anxiety or muscle pain.

Acute anxiety or panic attacks can be treated with short-acting BZDs, such as lorazepam, which has a rapid onset of action (10 to 15 minutes) and a half-life of 10 to 20 hours.[32] (Table 48.4 lists the features of many BZDs.) Caution should be taken in prescribing short-half-life drugs such as alprazolam. Although alprazolam has a rapid onset of action, it typically lasts only 2 to 3 hours, and many patients have significant rebound anxiety. This results in a roller coaster of peaks and valleys of anxiety during the day.

Buspirone (Buspar), which acts as a serotonin agonist, is also an effective anxiolytic. It is especially useful in treating patients with a history of substance abuse who may abuse BZDs. It has no addictive properties and does not impair psychomotor or cognitive function. It is started at 5 mg tid and can be advanced as high as 10 mg tid.[35] Unlike the short-acting BZDs that deliver anxiolysis with the first dose, buspirone requires 1 to 4 weeks of administration for antianxiety benefits to appear. Patients can experience headache, dizziness, paresthesias, and gastrointestinal upset.

Clonazepam (Klonopin), a long-acting BZD, is often used in conjunction with a short-acting agent or an antidepressant to stabilize persistent anxiety or prevent acute anxiety attacks. Diazepam, which also has psychoactive metabolites lasting several days, and flurazepam are other agents with long half-lives.

TABLE 48.4 Benzodiazepines

Drug	Onset	Half-Life (h)
Alprazolam (Xanax)	Intermediate	6–20
Chlordiazepoxide (Librium)	Intermediate	30–100
Clonazepam (Klonopin)	Intermediate	18–50
Clorazepate (Tranxene)	Rapid	30–100
Diazepam (Valium)	Rapid	30–100
Estazolam (ProSom)	Intermediate	10–24
Flurazepam (Dalmane)	Rapid-intermediate	50–160
Lorazepam (Ativan)	Intermediate	10–20
Midazolam (Versed)	Rapid	2–3
Oxazepam (Serax)	Intermediate-slow	8–12
Temazepam (Restoril)	Intermediate	8–20
Triazolam (Halcion)	Intermediate	1.5–5

The side effects of BZDs limit their use as long-term agents. Acutely, all of the BZDs can cause profound sedation, confusion, or respiratory depression; they can be fatal in overdose. Caution is required in prescribing these medications concurrently with opioids, which can compound the risk of these side effects. Rarely but with more frequency in the elderly, BZDs can be disinhibiting agents and can lead patients to become agitated. All BZDs have physiologic dependence potential depending on the dose and duration of treatment. All of them can cause physical and psychologic dependence and often require long tapering schedules from 1 to 3 months to minimize withdrawal symptoms.[17] Abrupt discontinuation of BZDs can cause insomnia, anxiety, delirium, psychosis, or seizures. Recent evidence indicates that long-term prescription of BZDs adversely affects short- and long-term memory as well as learning ability.[68] Furthermore, given that CBT with coping skills training is one of the most effective treatments for anxiety disorders, treatment with an anxiolytic can undermine this approach because it may reinforce the notion that only a pill can solve a patient's anxiety problems, thus decreasing his or her sense of self-efficacy for anxiety control.

MOOD STABILIZERS

Mood stabilizers are agents that have both antimanic and antidepressant properties. Some of these medications are antiepileptic drugs. In psychiatry, they are most frequently prescribed for bipolar disorder. There is no evidence that bipolar disorder occurs at a higher frequency in patients with chronic pain.[61] This class of medications is often used to treat patients with chronic neuropathic pain, trigeminal neuralgia, and headache. Some of the medications in this class are lithium, valproic acid (Depakote is the longer-acting brand name formulation), carbamazepine, and lamotrigine. Although many of the other anticonvulsants have antimanic properties if prescribed either as sole agents or in combination with other agents, they have little, if any, antidepressant effects of their own and thus are not true mood stabilizers.

LITHIUM

Lithium is the most commonly prescribed mood stabilizer for bipolar disorder and is the only one demonstrating a clear decrease in suicide attempts among those taking it.[69] It is also used as an augmentation agent for MDD, administered in conjunction with antidepressants to which a patient has had a partial response. With mixed results, lithium has been used as prophylaxis for chronic daily headaches and cluster headaches. Lithium has a narrow therapeutic range for both benefit and toxicity; thus it is important to monitor serum levels. Lethal overdoses can involve as little as 4 to 5 times the daily dose. Lithium has effects on the thyroid and kidney, hence their function must be monitored. These difficulties in using lithium and its sparse analgesic benefits make it less useful to the pain practitioner. Typically, patients with chronic pain on lithium are followed by a psychiatrist.

VALPROIC ACID

Depakote is the brand name of long-acting valproic acid, with a duration of action of 8 to 12 hours. It has both antimanic and antidepressant effects, although with less antidepressant effect than lithium. It is also useful as an augmentation agent in depression. Depakote can also be used for the treatment of impulsivity and aggression. Valproic acid has an established use in migraine prophylaxis, and neurologists have extensive experience with it in seizure treatment. The starting dose is 250 mg/day, and a typical dose used in pain medicine is 250 mg tid. Doses used in the treatment of bipolar disorder are higher, 500 to 1000 mg tid.[32] Serum levels are monitored for therapeutic and toxicity ranges. Prior to initiating treatment, complete blood count (CBC) and liver function tests are obtained. Anemia and neurotropenia are rare side effects of valproic acid, but thrombocytopenia is more common. Platelet levels should be checked at least 2 weeks after the start of treatment and 2 weeks after reaching a therapeutic dose. Fortunately, platelet levels quickly rise after discontinuation of valproic acid. Sedation, dizziness, and hepatitis are other side effects. Hepatotoxicity/hepatic failure and pancreatitis are also rare but serious potential side effects. As a result, this medication is contraindicated in patients with hepatic disease. This medication should not be given to pregnant women, since it is associated with neural tube defects.

LAMOTRIGINE (LAMICTAL)

Lamotrigine is an antiepileptic medication commonly prescribed for seizure control by neurologists and for mood stabilization by psychiatrists. It is often prescribed for bipolar patients with prominent depressive symptomatology, and it appears to be more effective in preventing depression than mania.[14] Its mechanism for treating bipolar disorder is not known. Lamictal has been reported to reduce neuropathic pain in case reports,[70] but two RCTs in a variety of neuropathic pain conditions show no effect.[71,72] Lamotrigine does have an established use as a preventive agent in headache management, and a recent systematic review concludes that it is efficacious in reducing the frequency of migraines.[73] Although this drug is generally well tolerated, rash may occur in up to 10% of individuals, and Stevens–Johnson syndrome, also known as toxic epidermal necrolysis, has been reported in 0.08% of individuals.[14] The rash appears to be related, in part, to the starting dose and the rate of increase. As a result, this medication is often started at 25 mg/day for 2 weeks, then 50 mg/day for 2 weeks, then 100 mg/day for 1 week, and finally 200 mg/day for most patients.

CARBAMAZEPINE (TEGRETOL)

Carbamazepine is an anticonvulsant used to treat partial and generalized seizures. Carbamazepine is a well-established mood stabilizer and is also the first-line treatment for trigeminal neuralgia and other neuropathic pain disorders with a lancinating quality.[14] This medication is usually started at doses between 200 and 400 mg/day in divided doses with a therapeutic dose range of 750 to 2500 mg/day in divided doses. Caution must be exercised when using this medication as it can have serious side effects, including rash, agranulocytosis, and aplastic anemia; regular laboratory monitoring is therefore required. Carbamazepine also interacts with other medication through the induction of liver enzymes, including the induction of its own metabolism.

The other anticonvulsants are useful as secondary or tertiary agents in bipolar disorder or as augmentation agents in the treatment of major depression. The anticonvulsants, such as gabapentin and pregabalin, are frequently prescribed in pain medicine and are documented analgesics for a variety of conditions, most often neuropathic pain and headache (Table 48.5).[74–79] Their use is covered in more detail in other chapters of this text.

OTHER ANTIEPILEPTIC DRUGS

TOPIRAMATE (TOPAMAX)

Topiramate is an antiepileptic and prophylactic medication for chronic migraines; it has shown some efficacy in the treatment of neuropathic pain and fibromyalgia. It has several modes of action that are theorized to be beneficial in the treatment of neuropathic pain. Topiramate inhibits activity-dependent, voltage-gated sodium channels, blocks L-type voltage-gated calcium channels, and further enhances the action of GABA-A receptors.[80] All of the aforementioned pathways are implicated in the transmission of neuropathic pain signals. In a randomized double-blind trial, topiramate was shown to be more effective than placebo in reducing pain associated with diabetic neuropathy.[81] The medication was initiated at 25 mg/day and increased by 25 mg/wk to a daily dosage of 100 mg/day or a maximum dose of 400 mg/day (see Table 48.5). At the conclusion of the study, patients taking topiramate had significantly less pain than those on placebo ($P = .039$).[81] Studies have also shown that topiramate has modest efficacy in the treatment of trigeminal neuralgia and intercostal neuralgia. Data are equivocal regarding complex regional pain syndrome.[82] The side effects most commonly associated with topiramate are somnolence, dizziness, nausea, weight loss, and difficulty with concentration.[83] The medication also mildly inhibits enzymatic activity of carbonic anhydrase, which may lead to more serious adverse effects like metabolic acidosis, compensatory hyperventilating respiratory alkalosis, nephrolithiasis, and perioral paresthesias.[80]

TABLE 48.5 Other Antiepileptic Drugs

Drug	Usual Dose	Maximum Dose
Gabapentin (Neurontin)	300–900 mg tid	3600 mg/day
Pregabalin (Lyrica)	150 mg/day	600 mg/day
Topiramate (Topamax)	50–200 mg/day	400 mg/day
Levetiracetam (Keppra)	500 mg bid	3000 mg/day

LEVETIRACETAM (KEPPRA)

Levetiracetam is a unique antiepileptic with wide-ranging anticonvulsant activity and a high safety margin. Its mode of action stems from its effect on the GABA-A receptor, a novel mechanism as compared with other anticonvulsants.[84] The evidence supporting the therapeutic benefit of levetiracetam for chronic pain is scant. There has been a systematic review of six randomized, double-blind trials investigating levetiracetam for the treatment of multiple neuropathic pain conditions (e.g., postherpetic neuralgia, postmastectomy pain, polyneuropathy, central poststroke pain, spinal cord injury, and multiple sclerosis).[85] These studies enrolled a total of 344 patients and compared levetiracetam with placebo. Finnerup et al. reported that 3 of 34 patients treated with levetiracetam and 4 of 32 given placebo experienced a 33% reduction in pain over the treatment period.[86] Vilholm et al. showed that 8 of 25 participants benefited from a 50% pain reduction in both the levetiracetam and placebo groups.[87] The most common adverse events reported were fatigue, dizziness, headache, constipation, and nausea.[85]

NEUROLEPTIC DRUGS

Also termed antipsychotics, neuroleptic drugs have been available for almost 50 years. They are used to treat any psychotic process, the hallmark illness being schizophrenia; psychotic symptoms in depression, mania, and delirium are also indications for their use. Both the typical and newer-generation atypical neuroleptics have independent analgesic properties and are effective in the treatment of nociceptive and neuropathic conditions.[88] Historically, the serious side effects of parkinsonism and tardive dyskinesia have limited their use in pain medicine (particularly for the older generation of antipsychotics, such as haloperidol or fluphenazine). More often, neuroleptics are used in inpatient settings where other analgesic agents have produced delirium.

However, based on a recent review of the literature, there is evidence demonstrating a role for antipsychotics in treating many different types of pain, including cancer pain and chronic noncancer pain, such as fibromyalgia, chronic headache, low back pain, musculoskeletal pain, chronic pain in older patients, chronic facial pain, and diabetic neuropathy.[89] The mechanism of antipsychotic pain relief

TABLE 48.6 Selected Typical Neuroleptics

Drug	Usual Dose	Maximum Dose
Fluphenazine (Prolixin)	5–10 mg bid-tid	40 mg/day
Haloperidol (Haldol)	2–5 mg bid-tid	100 mg/day
Perphenazine (Trilafon)	8–16 mg bid-tid	64 mg/day
Thiothixene (Navane)	5–10 mg tid	60 mg/day
Trifluoperazine (Stelazine)	5–10 mg bid	40 mg/day
Loxapine (Loxitane)	20–50 mg bid-tid	250 mg/day
Chlorpromazine (Thorazine)	10–50 mg bid-qid	2000 mg/day
Thioridazine (Mellaril)	100–200 mg bid-qid	800 mg/day

has not been clearly delineated. It may be that antidopaminergic properties play a role in analgesia, whereas the serotoninergic antagonism may also be important for pain relief.[90] Antipsychotic antagonism of alpha-2 adrenoceptors may also mediate analgesia.[91]

TYPICAL NEUROLEPTIC DRUGS

Typical neuroleptic drugs (Table 48.6) act as antipsychotics through their antagonism of dopamine receptors, particularly the D2 receptors. They also have actions on histaminic, cholinergic, and alpha-1 adrenergic receptors. Haloperidol is the prototypical agent in this class, with a molecular structure similar to that of morphine. All of the typical neuroleptics have varying degrees of anticholinergic side effects: dry mouth, dizziness, sedation, weight gain, constipation, or blurred vision. They are also associated with varying degrees of extrapyramidal effects: tremor, dystonia, akathesia, and, most seriously, tardive dyskinesia, which is permanent once it has occurred. All of these agents very slightly lower the seizure threshold and may elevate serum glucose levels. Cardiovascular effects include hypotension, tachycardia, nonspecific electrocardiographic changes (including torsades de pointes), and, exceedingly rare, sudden cardiac death.[32]

ATYPICAL NEUROLEPTIC DRUGS

The first atypical neuroleptic was clozapine, which is used in treatment-refractory schizophrenia. Subsequently, several other agents have been released in this class: risperidone, olanzapine, quetiapine, aripiprazole, and ziprasidone (Table 48.7). The atypicals have a lesser degree of dopamine D2 receptor antagonism and a greater degree of D4 receptor antagonism than the typical neuroleptics.[57] Additionally, they have some degree of serotonin-2 receptor blocking activity. This mixed receptor profile results in far fewer extrapyramidal, anticholinergic, and cardiac side effects. However, virtually all the side effects of the typical agents can occur with atypicals. Caution should be exercised in prescribing this class for patients with diabetes. Emerging evidence indicates that the atypicals, particularly olanzapine, lower glucose tolerance and can elevate serum glucose levels.[92] Overall, since the atypicals are better tolerated than typical neuroleptics, they are quickly becoming

TABLE 48.7 Atypical Neuroleptics

Drug	Usual Dose	Maximum Dose
Abilify (Aripiprazole)	5 mg qd	30 mg qd
Clozapine (Clozaril)	100–300 mg qd-bid	900 mg/day
Olanzapine (Zyprexa)	5–15 mg qd	20 mg/day
Quetiapine (Seroquel)	50–150 mg bid-tid	800 mg/day
Risperidone (Risperdal)	2–4 mg qd-bid	16 mg/day
Ziprasidone (Geodon)	20–40 mg bid	160 mg/day

the first-line treatment for psychotic symptoms. Both classes are equally as effective for the "positive symptoms" of psychosis: hallucinations and delusions. However, the atypicals are more effective for the "negative symptoms" of flat affect, poor motivation, and social withdrawal. Additionally, these agents are increasingly used as augmentation agents for treatment-resistant depression or anxiety, and may be very useful in helping patients disabled by pain and comorbid agitated depression in controlling their anger.[17,93]

The use of atypical neuroleptics in pain medicine will continue to grow. Case reports and retrospective studies indicate that they may be effective as secondary or tertiary agents for migraine and chronic daily headache prophylaxis.[91] They have been effective as abortive agents for cluster headache.[91] A small study showed analgesic benefit for patients with cancer pain.[94] In mice, studies of risperidone demonstrate an opioid-mediated analgesia to thermal pain.[95] In one animal pain model, the strong antinociceptive effect of risperdone was attributed to its selective opioid antagonism via m1, m2, kappa1 opioids and delta-opioid systems.[90] Zyprexa has been shown to provide pain relief from alpha2-adrenoceptors, opioid, and serotonergic receptor activity.[90] The dosage range for the analgesic benefit of atypicals remains unclear.

Whether an atypical or typical neuroleptic drug is prescribed, patients must initially be warned about the side effects, especially the risks of tardive dyskinesia, which becomes permanent if it occurs. In a nonpsychotic patient, the initial dose of a neuroleptic should be very low with a slow escalation, since these patients are neuroleptic-naive and are very vulnerable to the side effects.

CONCLUSION

Some 60% to 80% of patients with chronic pain attending pain clinics have significant psychiatric pathology. This comorbidity worsens their pain and disability, and this mental distress is an independent source of suffering, further reducing quality of life. The boom in psychotherapeutic medications over the past 25 years, combined with more effective psychotherapies, has resulted in significantly improved treatment. Many of these medications have analgesic benefits independent of their treatment effects on depression, anxiety, or psychosis. The antidepressants, anticonvulsants, and antipsychotics are the most notable for their pain properties. The improved treatment results for psychopathology and the emergence of additional analgesics is a boon to the practice of pain medicine.

KEY POINTS

- Antidepressants can take up to 2 to 4 weeks to produce an initial response, but all can take 4 to 8 weeks for full clinical improvement after a typical dose is reached, and remission may take longer.
- SSRIs have an immediate effect on the blockade of the presynaptic serotonin reuptake pump in the CNS, increasing the duration of serotonin in the synaptic cleft.
- TCAs inhibit both serotonergic and noradrenergic reuptake, lengthening the time serotonin and NE remain in the synaptic cleft and enhancing their neurotransmission. The analgesic properties of TCAs are independent of their treatment effects on depression.
- TCAs also have quinidine-like properties, are potentially proarythmic, and can prolong the QTC interval. Patients with history of cardiac disease or taking other QTC-prolonging medications should have a baseline electrocardiogram.
- Amitriptyline is demethylated to nortriptyline, and imipramine is demethylated to desipramine.
- SNRIs, like the TCAs, act by inhibiting serotonin and NE reuptake. This accounts for the higher rates of depression remission and the analgesic efficacy associated with TCAs and SNRIs as compared with SSRIs.
- Duloxetine is the only major psychotropic drug approved in the United States for both pain and psychiatric conditions; thus it is the treatment of choice for patients with neuropathic pain and psychiatric comorbidity.
- Milnacipran is FDA-approved for the treatment of fibromyalgia but not depression. The increase in serotonin and NE with milnacipran augments the inhibition of painful signals, resulting in a reduction in the intensity of pain.
- Bupropion is a noradrenergic and dopaminergic reuptake pump inhibitor, prolonging the time that NE and dopamine remain in the synaptic cleft. It has significant psychostimulant properties.

REFERENCES

Access the reference list online at ExpertConsult.com.

CHAPTER 49

Membrane Stabilizers

Stacy Peterson, MD ◌ Honorio T. Benzon, MD ◌ Robert W. Hurley, MD, PhD

INTRODUCTION

The treatment of neuropathic pain presents a distinct challenge to health care practitioners. A wide range of conditions resulting in chronic neuropathic pain include, but are not limited to, diabetic polyneuropathy, postherpetic neuralgia, central neuropathic pain, traumatic/surgical nerve injury, incomplete spinal cord injury, trigeminal neuralgia, multiple sclerosis, radiculopathy, complex regional pain syndrome (CRPS), and human immunodeficiency virus (HIV)-associated peripheral neuropathy. Defined as pain initiated or caused by a primary lesion or dysfunction in the nervous system, neuropathic pain is often described as burning, lancinating, or tingling in nature.

Neuropathic pain is the unfortunate consequence of detrimental changes that occur after tissue injury.[1] Pathologic changes after injury result in plasticity or alterations in the way peripheral nerve fibers respond to and deliver input to the central nervous system. The source of neuropathic pain may be related to damage of a peripheral nerve, with or without associated autonomic changes or central nervous system dysfunction. Examples of these changes include prolonged central sensitization, damage to neuronal inhibitory functions, and alterations in the effects of pain on the sympathetic nervous system. When abnormal neural activity persists beyond the expected duration of healing, the pain sensation becomes chronic in nature and continues without ongoing disease.

Following tissue injury, the threshold of activation of A delta and C fibers decreases and an augmented response to a given stimulus occurs. In addition, alterations in ion channels located at the site of injury take place. Sodium and calcium channels play a fundamental role in the propagation of hyperexcitability in central and peripheral neurons.[2] After nerve injury, the number of ion channels accumulates in excess, leading to ectopic, spontaneous firing of sensory nerves and dorsal root ganglion cell bodies. The result of neuronal membrane hyperexcitability is the chronic perception of pain.

Research into the physiologic source and pharmacologic management of neuropathic pain has led to the study of sodium and calcium channel blockade.[3,4] The pathology leading to epilepsy was extrapolated and studied as a possible source of the development of neuropathic pain. Membrane stabilizers include agents typically used for the treatment of epileptic foci in the brain. As a result of this inferential leap, these agents have been used in patients with neuropathic pain. There are multiple classes of medications that fall under the membrane stabilizer classification, including sodium channel blocking agents (antiepileptics, anticonvulsants, local anesthetics, tricyclic antidepressants, and antiarrhythmics) and calcium channel blocking agents (Table 49.1).

When evaluating the effectiveness of medications for neuropathic pain, outcome measures most commonly include changes in the average daily pain score by a 10-cm (100-mm) visual analog scale (VAS) and on an 11-point Likert scale (0, no pain; 10, worst possible pain), or a numeric rating scale (NRS); patient reported pain relief of 30% or greater (moderate benefit); patient reported pain relief of 50% or greater (substantial benefit). "Numbers needed to treat" (NNT) is used to allow a comparison between different drugs and diseases to better judge the efficacy of an agent more precisely.[5,6] The NNT is the number of patients treated with a particular drug to obtain one patient with a defined degree of relief. Usually, the parameter of NNT greater than 50% pain relief is used because it is easily understood and seems to be related to relevant clinical effect.[5] The "numbers needed to harm" (NNH) is the number needed to treat with a certain drug before a patient can experience a significant side effect. The NNH of several drugs for pain management is not yet known. The drugs with a low NNT/NNH ratio are superior to the drugs with high NNT/NNH ratio.

SODIUM CHANNEL BLOCKERS

These agents include the antiepileptics/anticonvulsants, local anesthetics, tricyclic antidepressants, and antiarrhythmics. As a group, they inhibit the development and propagation of ectopic discharges. The primary agents used for neuropathic pain are antiepileptics/anticonvulsants and local anesthetics. Gabapentin and pregabalin, also anticonvulsants, are discussed separately under calcium channel antagonists, as their mechanism of action differs from other agents that are typically used for epilepsy and convulsions.

Sodium channel blockers are used for primary therapy or adjunctive treatment for processes such as trigeminal neuralgia, CRPS, diabetic neuropathy, radicular extremity pain, chemotherapy-induced peripheral neuropathy, and postherpetic neuralgia. When using these agents, as with all membrane stabilizers, it is crucial to be knowledgeable of the proper dosages, toxicities, and their effects when coadministered with other drugs. As a general rule the dose should be titrated to patient comfort within safety standards.

ANTICONVULSANTS

PHENYTOIN (DILANTIN)

The initial dosage of phenytoin is 100 mg 2 or 3 times daily (Table 49.2). It is primarily used for the treatment of

TABLE 49.1 Commonly Used Membrane Stabilizers: Their Mechanisms of Action and Common Side Effects

Membrane Stabilizer	Mechanism	Side Effects	Clinical Comment
Carbamazepine	Na channel blockade	Sedation, dizziness, gait abnormalities, hematologic changes	Blood count every 2–4 months
Gabapentin/pregabalin	Binds to alpha-2 delta subunit of voltage-gated Ca channel	Dizziness, sedation	Discontinue gradually
Lamotrigine	Stabilizes slow Na channel; suppresses release of glutamate from presynaptic neurons	Rash, dizziness, somnolence	Drug interactions[a]
Levetriacetam	Exact mechanism not determined	Asthenia, somnolence	No significant drug interactions
Lidocaine cream/TD	Na channel blockade	Skin irritation	—
Mexilitine	Na channel blockade	Nausea, blurred vision	Monitor serum level, CBC (for dyscrasias)
Oxcarbazepine	Na channel blockade	Hyponatremia, somnolence, dizziness	—
Phenytoin	Na channel blockade disturbances	Sedation, motor	—
Topiramate	Na channel blockade; potentiates GABA inhibition	Sedation, kidney stones, glaucoma	—
Valproic acid	Na channel blockade; increase GABA	Somnolence, dizziness, gastrointestinal upset	Drug interactions[a]
Zonisamide	Calcium and sodium channel blockade	Ataxia, renal calculi	—

[a]*Amotrigine: Increased efficacy when combined with valproate (reduce dose); decreased efficacy when combined with phenytoin and carbamazepine.*
CBC, *Complete blood count;* GABA, *gamma aminobutyric acid;* TD, *transdermal.*

TABLE 49.2 Dosing Recommendations for Neuropathic Pain

Membrane Stabilizer	Initial Dosage	Titration	Maximum Dosage
Carbamazepine	100–200 mg twice daily	Increase by 200-mg increments gradually	1200 mg/day
Gabapentin[a]	100–300 mg at bedtime or 100–300 mg 3 times daily	Increase by 100–300 mg 3 times daily every 1–7 days, as tolerated	3600 mg (1200 3 times daily)
Lamotrigine	25–50 mg at bedtime	Increase by 50 mg every 1–2 weeks	300–500 mg/day
Levetiracetam	500 mg bid	Increase by 500 mg/week	3000 mg/day
Lidocaine cream	2%, 5%, 10%	—	—
Lidocaine patch	5%	—	12–18 h on and 6–12 h off
Mexilitine	150 mg/day	Increase to 300 mg in 3 days then 600 mg	10 mg/kg per day
Oxcarbazepine	600 mg twice daily	Increase by 300 mg	1200–1800 mg every 3 days
Phenytoin	100 mg 2 to 3 times daily	—	—
Pregabalin[a]	50 mg 3 times daily or 75 mg twice daily	Increase to 300 mg/day after 3–7 days, then by 150 mg/day every 3–7 days as tolerated	600 mg/day (200 mg 3 times daily or 300 mg twice daily)
Topiramate	50 mg daily at bedtime	—	1500 mg twice daily
Valproic acid	250 mg twice daily	Increase by 250 mg/week	500 mg twice daily
Zonisamide	100 mg/day	Increase by 200 mg/week	600 mg/day

[a]*Reduce if impaired renal function.*

diabetic neuropathy; however, due to the mixed results of its efficacy and high side effect and medication interaction profile, it has fallen into disuse. Phenytoin provides pain relief by blocking sodium channels, thereby preventing the release of excitatory glutamate and inhibiting ectopic discharges.

Studies have been performed in trials regarding the efficacy of phenytoin for diabetic neuropathy, with conflicting results.[7] A recent Cochrane review did not find evidence to routinely use phenytoin in the treatment of neuropathic pain as prior studies have failed to demonstrate effective long-term improvement in pain.[8] Therefore this agent should not be considered first-line therapy for neuropathic pain. Some evidence is present to suggest improvement in acute pain. Intravenous phenytoin has been investigated in the pain management setting. Doses of this agent at 15 mg/kg have provided relief of acute pain when administered over a 2-hour period. Side effects include somnolence and slowing of mentation, with nystagmus and ataxia seen in some patients. Among the antiepileptic drugs, a feature unique to phenytoin is the development of facial alterations, including gum hyperplasia and a coarsening of facial features. Fosphenytoin, an intravenously administered prodrug that is converted to phenytoin, is used by some to avoid long dosing intervals or initial burning at the injection site.

Phenytoin activates the cytochrome P450 enzyme system in the liver, and, hence, careful assessment of cotherapy is warranted. For example, phenytoin decreases the efficacy of methadone, fentanyl, tramadol, mexiletine, lamotrigine, and carbamazepine. As a result, dosages of these medications should be adjusted accordingly. Coadministration with antidepressants and valproic acid could lead to increased blood concentrations of phenytoin, lowering the subsequent doses required for effect. Phenytoin in the treatment of neuropathic pain is considered a therapy of last resort.

CARBAMAZEPINE (TEGRETOL)

The initial dosage of carbamazepine is 100 to 200 mg twice daily, titrated to effect, with typical dose ranges of 300 to 1200 mg/day administered in two divided doses. Common maintenance doses are 600 to 800 mg/day. The chemical structure of this compound is similar to that of the tricyclic antidepressants, although the mechanism of action for analgesia is quite different. This agent is thought to inhibit pain via peripheral and central mechanisms. Carbamazepine selectively blocks active fibers, having no effect on normally functioning A delta and C nociceptive fibers. Major uses of the drug include primary therapy for trigeminal neuralgia (tic doloreux), thalamic-mediated poststroke pain, postherpetic neuralgia, and diabetic neuropathy. Drowsiness, dizziness, and nausea and vomiting are common side effects, which can often be limited by slow titration. Carbamazepine is associated with very deleterious side effects, including pancytopenia (necessitating a complete blood count and monitoring while on this therapy), Stevens-Johnson syndrome, and toxic epidermal necrolysis.

Carbamazepine is considered to be the pharmacologic treatment of choice for trigeminal neuralgia, a sharp severe facial pain in one or more of the distributions supplied by the trigeminal nerve.[9] Although the pathology of this process has not fully been determined, the majority of cases are believed to be caused by compression of the trigeminal nerve at the pontine origin of the nerve by an aberrant loop of an artery or vein.

With an NNT of less than 2, carbamazepine is the most studied treatment for trigeminal neuralgia, and many studies have highlighted its usefulness.[9] One study noted the effect of carbamazepine in 70 patients with trigeminal neuralgia and demonstrated a 68% decrease in pain episodes and a 58% decrease in the severity of pain.[10] Research from other studies noted a verbal response by patients of "excellent" or "good" upon initiation of therapy for 2 weeks.[11] Additionally, the positive effect of carbamazepine on trigeminal neuralgias has been tested by crossover, placebo, and controlled double-blind studies[12]; yet despite these positive results, trigeminal neuralgia is a disease process that, in many patients, is difficult to treat adequately, often requiring multiple agents.

Carbamazepine has also been investigated for use in pain states caused by diabetes mellitus. Its application in animals resulted in a decrease in hyperalgesia to various stimuli. This agent has been shown to be more beneficial than placebo in the human diabetic patient population.[7] Carbamazepine therapy, when compared with nortriptyline/fluphenazine in patients with painful diabetic neuropathy, was found to be equally effective and with fewer side effects.

Patients on carbamazepine therapy should have blood tests done every 2 to 4 months, as there is an increased risk of developing agranulocytosis and aplastic anemia with this agent. Studies noted that the NNH for severe adverse effects was 24 and for minor adverse effects, such as sedation, was 3.[9] A recent retrospective review study on the use of carbamazepine for the treatment of trigeminal neuralgias showed a high discontinuation rate secondary to adverse effects. In this study of 100 patients, 27% treated with carbamazepine suffered an adverse effect that led to the discontinuation of therapy. The mean time to adverse effect in this review was 8.6 months.[13]

OXCARBAZEPINE (TRILEPTAL)

Oxcarbazepine, the keto-analogue of carbamazepine, was developed to preserve carbamazepine's membrane-stabilizing effects while minimizing minor adverse effects, such as sedation and serious or life-threatening reactions. A major advantage of oxcarbazepine is that monitoring of drug plasma levels and hematologic profiles is generally not necessary. Similar to carbamazepine, oxcarbazepine blocks sodium channels; it does not affect gamma-aminobutyric acid (GABA) receptors.

Significant hyponatremia (sodium < 125 mmol/L) may develop during treatment with oxcarbazepine. This typically occurs during the first 3 months, with normalization of sodium levels within a few days of discontinuing the drug. Monitoring of sodium levels should be performed when instituting oxcarbazepine therapy. Frequently reported adverse effects of oxcarbazepine include dizziness, somnolence, and nausea and vomiting, which are generally well tolerated.

In a randomized placebo-controlled trial over 16 weeks, oxcarbazepine was evaluated in patients with painful diabetic neuropathy.[14] They were treated with 300 mg/day that was titrated to a maximum of 1800 mg/day. Oxcarbazepine-treated patients reported less pain on VAS, global improvement, and less sleep disturbances due to pain.

The superior side-effect profile of oxcarbazepine compared with carbamazepine has led to its increased use. Although it is better tolerated, there is still a significant incidence of adverse effects. In a retrospective review of 100 patients successfully treated for trigeminal neuralgia with oxycarbazepine, there was an 18% discontinuation rate secondary to adverse effects.[13] In several countries oxcarbazepine is now the drug of choice for trigeminal neuralgia. Although a case series reported its efficacy in the treatment of neuropathic pain,[13] prospective randomized controlled studies are lacking at this time.

VALPROIC ACID (DEPAKOTE)

This drug acts at the GABA-A receptor. There are conflicting reports in the literature as to the efficacy of this agent in treating neuropathic pain, although studies have demonstrated that valproic acid was effective in migraine therapy at dosages of 800 mg/day for a period of 3 months in patients with medication overuse headache and a history of migraines following detoxification.[15] Side effects include gastrointestinal upset, somnolence, and dizziness. The exact role of this agent in the armamentarium of the pain practitioner is yet to be elucidated.[6]

LAMOTRIGINE (LAMICTAL)

The initial dosage is 25 to 50 mg at bedtime, which can be increased to 50 mg twice daily after 2 weeks. Subsequently, it may be increased by 50-mg increments every 1 to 2 weeks as tolerated to a dose of 300 to 500 mg/day in two divided doses. Upon discontinuation, drug administration should be slowly tapered over a 2-week period. Like other agents discussed, lamotrigine is an agent that blocks sodium channels in actively firing nerves. It has no effect on sensation in the native, normally functioning nervous system. Unique to lamotrigine is the fact that, in addition to acting as a sodium channel blocker, it prevents release of the excitatory transmitter glutamate.

A major use for lamotrigine is in the treatment of trigeminal neuralgia. Although carbamazepine has been advocated as the first-line therapy for trigeminal neuralgia, it is not effective in all patients. Lamotrigine has been investigated in this patient model for use as a coadministered drug and as a substitute for carbamazepine.[16] A total of 21 trigeminal neuralgia patients who had received no benefit from carbamazepine therapy were treated with lamotrigine.[7] In a population of 7 men and 14 women, 14 of the patients noted significant to complete relief of their symptoms after the institution of lamotrigine therapy, and the remaining 7 patients had no benefit. The use of lamotrigine may therefore be indicated in carbamazepine-resistant trigeminal neuralgia. This positive result has also been seen in follow-up with a group of 15 patients with trigeminal neuralgia receiving lamotrigine therapy. In this paper,[17] 73% of patients were free of their painful symptoms at the conclusion of the study. Subsequent interval follow-up revealed a continued positive result, with no change in pain scores reported by patients. As a result of these studies, lamotrigine may have a role in the prevention of trigeminal neuralgia in susceptible patients.

Lamotrigine has also been evaluated in the diabetic neuropathy population. Patients suffering from diabetic neuropathy may receive benefit from lamotrigine therapy. In two replicate randomized, double blind, placebo-controlled trials, a total of 360 patients were treated with lamotrigine. In patients receiving 400 mg/day, a reduction in pain-intensity score versus placebo was observed in one of the two studies. Doses of 200 and 300 mg/day did not demonstrate any benefit.[18] A group of 15 patients with peripheral neuropathy induced by diabetes (types I and II combined) were treated in an open study. They were tested with brush and cold stimuli for allodynia and pinprick for hyperalgesia. Upon completion of the study, patients were tested and reported improvement of pain in all settings, and their relief persisted as noted during the subsequent 6-month interval follow-up.

In one randomized controlled trial (RCT), lamotrigine (300 mg/day) was found to significantly reduce pain in distal sensory polyneuropathy (DSP) but not in antiretroviral toxic neuropathy (ATN) associated with HIV disease.[19] HIV-associated neuropathy is believed to be on the rise, concomitant with the increase in the number of patients who become diagnosed with the virus. Patients with distal sensory peripheral neuropathy associated with HIV infection were subjected to a placebo-controlled, randomized double-blind study to identify the benefit of lamotrigine therapy. Although both placebo-treated patients and patients receiving lamotrigine had a decrease in pain, the rate of decrease was more rapid in the lamotrigine group. Patients administered antiretrovirals and lamotrigine, however, were noted to have slower pain relief than those maintained on lamotrigine without the antiretroviral agents. In a subsequent larger trial, lamotrigine was found to be effective for both DSP and ATN HIV-related pain.[20] The effect of lamotrigine as an adjunctive therapy was also studied in 220 patients with a variety of neuropathic pain conditions uncontrolled by monotherapy.[21] This randomized, double-blind, placebo-controlled study evaluated the efficacy and tolerability of lamotrigine in addition to gabapentin, a tricyclic antidepressant, and a nonopioid analgesic. The study patients suffered from diabetic peripheral neuropathy, postherpetic neuralgia, traumatic/surgical nerve injury, incomplete spinal cord injury, trigeminal neuralgia, multiple sclerosis, or HIV-associated peripheral neuropathy. Lamotrigine was generally well tolerated but did not demonstrate effective pain relief as evaluated by pain score or use of rescue medication.

A rash is the most common side effect seen in patients. This can occur in up to 10% of patients. This rash is more likely to develop in pediatric patients, especially when lamotrigine is combined with valproic acid. Stevens-Johnson syndrome has occurred in rare cases. Prescribing physicians should also be aware that when lamotrigine is combined with the CYP450 inhibitor valproate, the initial dose should be reduced to 12.5 mg/day and titration should be done cautiously. Additionally, when combined with anticonvulsants that induce hepatic enzymes, such as phenytoin and carbamazepine, the efficacy of lamotrigine may be diminished and a higher dose required for symptomatic improvement.

TOPIRAMATE (TOPAMAX)

In addition to affecting sodium channels and calcium channels, topiramate enhances the action of the GABA (inhibitory) neurotransmitter and inhibits the α-amino-3-hydroxy-5-methyl-4-isoxazolepropionic acid (AMPA)-type glutamate (excitatory) receptor. The initial dose is 50 mg at bedtime, increasing to an upper limit of 200 mg thrice daily. Studies have demonstrated that pain relief begins to occur at doses of 200 mg/day.

Topiramate has been assessed for use in patients with diabetic neuropathy. A 12-week, double-blinded study showed that topiramate therapy had more efficacy than placebo in relieving the pain sensed by patients with diabetic neuropathy.[22] A review[7] of other double-blinded studies have not corroborated these results, however. In a double-blinded, randomized crossover trial, topiramate 50 to 400 mg was assessed in patients with chronic, lumbar radicular pain; it resulted in an improved global pain relief score but did not reduce leg pain.[23] The study was limited by frequent side effects and a high dropout rate. The exact role of topiramate is yet to be determined; thus it may best be reserved as an adjunct for pain management with other membrane stabilizing agents. Case reports in the literature have also highlighted the use of this agent for additional forms of neuropathic pain, including postherpetic neuralgia, intercostal neuralgia, and CRPS.

The role of topiramate in migraine prevention is well established and is also approved for migraine prevention in the adolescent population. In a 26-week double-blind, placebo-controlled study, 483 patients were randomized to placebo, topiramate 50, 100, or 200 mg/day. Of this group, 463 patients completed postbaseline efficacy reports. Statistically significant reductions in migraine frequency were seen at the doses of 100 and 200 mg/day. In addition to a reduction in migraine frequency, less rescue medication was reduced at these doses.[24]

The primary side effect seen with topiramate is sedation. Other unique consequences of this agent include the potential for development of kidney stones and ocular glaucoma, since topiramate is an inhibitor of carbonic anhydrase.[12] Weight loss associated with topiramate may be a benefit for some and problematic for others.

LEVETIRACETAM (KEPPRA)

Levetiracetam is structurally unrelated to other antiepileptic agents and its mechanism of action has yet to be determined. A starting dose of levetiracetam is 500 mg twice daily, and may be increased to a recommended 3000 mg/day in divided doses. Dosages up to 5000 mg/day have been assessed in the treatment of neuropathic pain.[25] Linear pharmacokinetics allow for predictable effects as the dosage is increased. Levetiracetam is not metabolized by the cytochrome P450 system and thus does not have significant drug interactions.[26]

Levetiracetam was found to be ineffective in the treatment of neuropathic pain secondary to a spinal cord injury[27] and in postmastectomy pain.[28] There is some evidence to support the use of levetiracetam 500 mg/day as prophylaxis therapy for migraine headaches; however studies done to date are small.[29,30] Adverse effects include asthenia, dizziness, somnolence, and headache.

LOCAL ANESTHETICS

Local anesthetics are used in neuropathic pain states to block the aberrant firing of abnormal nerves, although they also block normally conducting (nonnociceptive) nerves. As a group, they are effective in the treatment of postherpetic neuralgia, trigeminal neuralgia, radiculopathies, and peripheral neuropathies.

LIDOCAINE

The typical intravenous infusion dose is 1 to 5 mg kg^{-1} h^{-1} over 30 to 60 minutes. Side effects include dizziness, blurred vision, and seizure, typically presenting at a plasma level of 10 mg/mL.[12] Given that lidocaine is an antiarrhythmic, bradycardia and cardiac depression (present at a plasma concentration of 20 to 25 mg/mL) is a potential risk with this agent; therefore, obtaining electrocardiography studies is indicated for long-term or high-dosage use of lidocaine. A formulation of 5% lidocaine is available in transdermal application, which has proven benefit to patients with various types of neuropathic pain, including postherpetic neuralgia, postthoracotomy pain, intercostal neuralgia, and meralgia paresthetica.[31]

The eutectic mixture of local anesthetics (EMLA)—comprising prilocaine and lidocaine—has also been advocated for use as a topical local anesthetic. This agent is sometimes used as an adjunct for venipuncture in the pediatric population; care must be taken with the amount of EMLA cream used so as to avoid toxicity. Prilocaine is readily metabolized to o-toluidine, which can lead to methemoglobinemia.[32]

There is also promise when examining perioperative use of lidocaine infusions to prevent chronic pain in certain cases. A recent double-blind, placebo-controlled trial of 80 patients undergoing mastectomy showed a significantly decreased risk of developing chronic postoperative surgical pain when a lidocaine infusion was utilized in the perioperative period.[33] There are mixed reports of the efficacy of intraoperative and perioperative lidocaine infusion to decrease postoperative opioid consumption and pain (see also Chapter 12).[34,35]

MEXILETINE

The standard starting dose is 75 to 150 mg/day, with a target of 300 to 450 mg/day. This agent is an antiarrhythmic and, for pain relief, can be considered an oral analogue of lidocaine. Pain physicians may provide intravenous lidocaine for pain management with monitoring of dose and effect. When there is relief from the intravenous infusions, and although supportive studies are lacking, treatment can be maintained by oral mexiletine.[36]

Mexiletine can be used for diabetic neuropathy, thalamic stroke pain, spasticity, and myotonia, although its effects are minimal.[37] Common side effects, including somnolence, irritability, blurred vision, and nausea and vomiting, severely limit the utility of this medication. Patients are also at risk for developing blood dyscrasias and should have blood tests on a regular basis.

CALCIUM CHANNEL BLOCKERS

Recommended first-line treatment agents for neuropathic pain include the calcium channel blockers.[38] Six different types are found in nervous tissue: L, N, P, Q, R, and T. Calcium channel blockers used for the treatment of neuropathic pain bind to the alpha-2 delta subunit of L-type voltage-gated calcium channels and result in the decreased release of glutamate, norepinephrine, and substance P.[39,40] Although structurally derived from the inhibitory neurotransmitter GABA, neither gabapentin nor pregabalin bind to or have activity at the GABA receptor. They also have no effect on the uptake or metabolism of GABA.

GABAPENTIN (NEURONTIN)

The standard initial dose is 100 to 300 mg/day with a gradual increase to a maximum of 3600 mg/day in three divided doses. To minimize adverse effects, the initial dose is often given at bedtime. After 2 to 5 days, the dose is increased to 300 mg twice daily, and after another 2 to 5 days to 300 mg 3 times daily. Subsequently the dose can be increased by 300 to 600 mg every other week as tolerated until an effective dosage is obtained or the maximum daily dose is reached. The main dose-limiting side effects are fatigue, somnolence, and dizziness, which are often attenuated by gradual dose titration. Although gabapentin has few drug interactions, dosage reduction is necessary in patients with renal insufficiency. Introduced in 1994, gabapentin is now available in generic form, which may make it a more cost-effective option. However, starting dosages of gabapentin often do not provide immediate pain relief, and the slow titration requirements may result in adequate therapeutic pain relief taking up to 2 months.

Gabapentin has many uses for patients suffering from multiple pain conditions. Studies have been performed on patients being treated for postherpetic neuralgia, CRPS, painful diabetic neuropathy, and other forms of neuropathic pain.[41,42] Gabapentin has been assessed in postherpetic neuralgia pain through double-blinded studies. Patients with postherpetic neuralgia being maintained on opioids and/or tricyclic antidepressants (TCAs) were identified and divided into two groups: 113 receiving gabapentin and 116 receiving placebo therapy in addition to their current background pain regimen. For a period of 8 weeks, patients were maintained on their respective therapies, with increased titration of the drug to a maximum dose of 3600 mg/day, achieved in 4 weeks.[42] Results indicated that the gabapentin patients had a decrease in their visual analogue score (VAS) for pain of nearly 2 points, compared with a decrease of only 0.5 in the placebo-treated patients. Along with a decrease in pain, patients also reported improvement in their SF-36 (quality of life) scores, noting improved functionality, feeling better, and more restful sleep at night.

The effect of gabapentin on the neuropathic pain of diabetes has also been evaluated.[41] A randomized double-blind placebo-controlled trial pooling patients from multiple centers showed a decrease of 2.5 on the VAS for patients receiving gabapentin up to 3600 mg/day versus a decrease of 1.4 for patients in the control group.[41] As with the postherpetic neuralgia study, patients also had an increase in their SF-36 scores, more restful sleep at night, and an overall improvement in functioning.

Gabapentin has also been studied in patients with lumbar spinal stenosis. In a pilot study, both patient groups received the standard care, including physical therapy, lumbosacral bracing, and nonsteroidal antiinflammatory drugs (NSAIDs).[43] The treatment group also received gabapentin, 900 to 2400 mg divided into three daily doses. After 4 months, patients who received gabapentin reported improvement in pain scores, increased walking distance, and decreased sensory and motor deficits. Given these results, it appears that gabapentin can be indicated as adjunctive therapy for symptomatic spinal stenosis.

In a double blind randomized placebo-controlled 8-week trial, patients with CRPS, postherpetic neuralgia, radiculopathy, postlaminectomy syndrome, poststroke syndrome, phantom limb pain, and other neuropathic pain syndromes were included. Gabapentin was initially started at 900 mg/day for 3 days and then increased to a maximum of 2400 mg/day at the end of week 5. The conclusion of the study showed that gabapentin reduced pain and improved some quality-of-life measures in these patients.[44] Gabapentin has also been found to be effective in reducing the pain associated with multiple sclerosis, specifically paroxysmal pain with a throbbing, pricking, and cramping quality rather than the dull, aching pain experienced by multiple sclerosis patients.[45] Finally, gabapentin appears to improve the analgesic efficacy of opioids in patients with neuropathic cancer pain.[46]

Studies of gabapentin in postamputation pain and phantom limb pain have been less effective than in other neuropathic pain states. Nikolajsen and colleagues[47] administered gabapentin to patients following limb amputation and found no effect on postamputation or phantom limb pain. In a small cohort-control study, gabapentin was found to be effective in the treatment of chemotherapy-induced painful peripheral neuropathy.[48] However, an earlier, larger RCT found no benefit to gabapentin therapy for the same condition.[49]

In patients with either painful diabetic neuropathy or postherpetic neuralgia, the combination of gabapentin and morphine was noted to be more effective than either drug given alone.[46] The mean daily pain scores at the maximum tolerated doses were 5.7 at baseline, 4.5 with placebo, 4.1 with gabapentin, 3.7 with morphine, and 3.06 with the gabapentin-morphine combination. The combination resulted in a higher frequency of dry mouth than with morphine alone and a higher frequency of constipation than with gabapentin alone.

In an extremely important and well-performed trial, combination therapy of gabapentin and the tricyclic antidepressant nortriptyline was found to be highly effective in the treatment of neuropathic pain resulting from diabetes and varicella zoster.[50] Although this study was not designed to show synergism between the two medications, the results are highly suggestive of a synergistic analgesic effect. Patients achieved greater pain relief on a combination of low dosages of gabapentin (600 mg by mouth thrice daily) and nortriptyline (50 mg by mouth at bedtime) than with either medication given alone at high doses. Importantly, patients on combination therapy received good analgesia without the significant side effects suffered by those on monotherapy. This trial, supported by the Canadian Institutes of Health, is a rare study in that the investigators had no influence from pharmaceutical companies and two inexpensive generic medications were studied.

In addition to gabapentin's well-established role in the treatment of neuropathic pain, there is also evidence to support the use of gabapentin as a preventive medication for primary headache syndromes, including chronic daily headaches.[51] There is less evidence to suggest that it is an appropriate primary therapy for migraine-type headaches, but it can be considered an alternative when first-line therapies prove ineffective.

PREGABALIN (LYRICA)

Initial pregabalin dosing is 150 mg/day given in two or three divided doses or 75 mg/day given at bedtime in elderly patients. Upward dose titration can be completed after 3 to 7 days to 300 mg/day; subsequently the dose can be increased to a maximum of 600 mg/day within 2 weeks of initiation. Like that of gabapentin, the dose of pregabalin must be decreased in patients with reduced kidney function. The advantages of pregabalin over gabapentin include a more rapid onset of pain relief; linear pharmacokinetics with low intersubject variability[52]; fewer dose-related side effects, allowing for faster upward titrations; and twice daily versus thrice daily dosing. Additionally, maximum benefit often occurs after 2 weeks of treatment at target doses of 300 to 600 mg/day compared with up to 2 months in gabapentin-treated patients. A retrospective analysis of data from nine controlled trials of pregabalin for painful diabetic neuropathy and postherpetic neuralgia showed the time to onset of neuropathic pain reduction was within a week (usually 2 to 3 days) with pregabalin compared with 2 weeks for gabapentin.[53]

Pregabalin is an alpha-2 delta ligand structurally related to gabapentin. It similarly binds to calcium channels and modulates calcium influx into hyperexcited neurons, leading to its antinociceptive and antiseizure effects.[39] Although it is structurally derived from the inhibitory neurotransmitter GABA, it does not bind to GABA or benzodiazepine receptors. Pregabalin is approved for the treatment of peripheral and central neuropathic pain, including postherpetic neuralgia and painful diabetic neuropathy.

In patients with postherpetic neuralgia, a trial was conducted in 370 patients, evaluating doses of 150, 300, and 600 mg/day versus placebo.[54] The randomized, controlled trial demonstrated reduced mean pain scores and improvement in sleep interference. Patients responded at all dosages, with the greatest response noted at 600 mg/day. Patients responded as early as the first week, and beneficial effects were sustained throughout the 13-week study duration. Adverse effects were generally mild to moderate, and 13% of patients withdrew from the study, most commonly due to dizziness or somnolence.

In a randomized, double blind study, the effects of pregabalin on neuropathic pain due to diabetic neuropathy was evaluated.[55] A total of 395 patients were randomized to receive 150, 300, or 600 mg/day. Of the patients who received 600 mg/day, 46% reported greater than 50% improvement of pain scores from baseline, and the NNT to achieve this response was 6.3. Pregabalin also improved pain-related sleep interference, and overall was well tolerated with an NNH of 10.3 in patients treated with 600 mg/day.

In patients with central neuropathic pain due to spinal cord injury, pregabalin was evaluated in a 12-week multicenter study.[56] A total of 137 patients were randomized to either a flexible-dose regimen of 150 to 600 mg/day or placebo and were allowed to continue an existing stable pain regimen. Pregabalin was found to be significantly more effective in relieving central neuropathic pain than placebo.

Pregabalin has also been studied for use in patients with refractory neuropathic pain.[57] A 15-month open label study was conducted in 81 patients with postherpetic neuralgia and diabetic neuropathy refractory to treatment, including gabapentin, a TCA, and a third medication (e.g., other anticonvulsant, opioid, SSRI, tramadol). Patients took 150 to 600 mg/day for 3-month intervals and then had a 3- to 28-day "drug holiday." As evaluated by the VAS, patients had a clinically meaningful and sustained reduction in pain intensity during the treatment cycle, with return of pain during "drug holidays." In patients with unsatisfactory responses to other medications, pregabalin may be considered as an adjunctive therapy.

Pregabalin has been noted to be effective in the treatment of fibromyalgia. A double-blind study examined 748 patients with fibromyalgia taking placebo versus pregabalin at 300, 450, and 600 mg/day over 13 weeks. The results showed a statistically significant reduction in pain intensity for all doses of pregabalin.[58] There was a 21% dropout rate owing to adverse effects, with the majority of the dropouts being in the 600-mg/day group. There has not been great evidence to suggest benefit of a dose of 600 mg/day versus 450 mg/day.

In addition to its role in treatment of neuropathic pain, there is increasing evidence to support the use of pregabalin in preemptive analgesia in operative cases such as spine surgery, shoulder arthrosocopy, septoplasty, and thoracotomy.[59,60]

The advantage of pregabalin is its early response and favorable side-effect profile. Most common adverse effects include somnolence and dizziness and are noted more frequently with higher doses. When pregabalin is being discontinued, it should be tapered gradually over at least a week to minimize symptoms, including insomnia, nausea, headache, and diarrhea.

ZONISAMIDE (ZONEGRAN)

The initial dose is 100 mg/day for 2 weeks, increasing by 200 mg/week for a target of 600 mg/day. This agent acts by blocking T-type calcium channels and sodium channels; its action also increases GABA release. It has uses in various types of neuropathic pain.

An open-label dose-titration study resulted in minimal change in VAS scores after 8 weeks of therapy.[61] Similar results were seen in a randomized, double blind, placebo-controlled, pilot study in patients with painful peripheral neuropathy.[61] Side effects include ataxia, decreased appetite, rash, and renal calculi (due to the carbonic anhydrase inhibitor effect). In children there is an increased risk of oligohydrosis and susceptibility to hyperthermia. The exact role of zonisamide in the management of patients with neuropathic pain is yet to be elucidated, and further research is needed. It is important to note that zonisamide does have a role in headache prevention. A double-blind study of 80 patients comparing zonisamide titrated up to 200 mg/day was shown to be as effective at decreasing headache frequency as topiramate, and headache severity was reduced with zonisamide more than with topiramate.[62]

ZICONOTIDE (PRIALT)

Ziconotide is a ω-conopeptide (previously known as SNX-111) that is administered intrathecally owing to its peptidic structure. It is derived from the venom of a marine snail (genus *Conus*). Ziconotide blocks calcium influx into N-type calcium channels that are present in the dorsal horn lamina of the spinal cord, thus preventing the afferent conduction of nerve signals.[63] Administration is via an intrathecal infusion pump, and dosing should be started low, at a recommended dose of 2.4 μg/day (0.1 μg/h). Due to a lag time, it should be titrated up slowly, at intervals of no more than 2 to 3 times per week, to a recommended maximum of 19.2 μg/day.[63] Ziconotide does not cause tolerance, dependence, or respiratory depression, and adverse effects—including dizziness, ataxia, confusion, and headache—primarily involve the CNS.

Ziconotide has been evaluated in randomized double-blind placebo-controlled trials for severe, chronic, and treatment-refractory pain in both malignant and nonmalignant conditions.[64] Patients experienced a significant improvement in mean pain score and global pain relief. The response rate was higher in patients receiving a maximum of 21.8 μg/day; however, pain relief was accompanied by a high incidence of adverse effects—including sedation, confusion, aphasia, dizziness, nystagmus, and hallucinations—which resulted in frequent interruptions of the trial. A slow titration schedule with a lower maximum infusion rate was associated with significantly lower dropout rates but also resulted in a more modest treatment effect. At the conclusion of one trial, nearly 90% of patients elected to continue receiving ziconotide. Rare but serious adverse effects include hallucinations; thus, ziconotide is not recommended for use in patients with a history of psychosis. Elevations in creatine kinase (CK) were noted in some studies to be related to ziconotide. The etiology remains unclear, and CK levels should be monitored periodically. In addition, a recent case series suggests that there is possibly a significant dropout rate after the initial titration not seen in previous short-term studies. This study looked at 11 patients over 24 months and had 7 patients discontinue ziconotide due to adverse effects. All of those patients had successful trials.[65]

The role of ziconotide for chronic pain management has yet to be fully elucidated. Currently, ziconotide is approved for the management of severe chronic pain in patients for whom intrathecal therapy is warranted and who are intolerant of or refractory to other treatments, including intrathecal opioids.

NIMODIPINE (NIMOTOP)

Nimodipine has been shown to decrease the dose of morphine for cancer pain in 9 of 14 patients.[66] In a colorectal surgery population, concomitant therapy with a calcium channel blocker did not decrease opioid requirements.[67] Nimodipine taken concurrently with antiretroviral medications demonstrated a trend toward improvement and/or the stabilization of HIV-associated neuropathy as compared with placebo.[68]

MAGNESIUM

Research has recently been performed evaluating the antagonists of the *N*-methyl-D-aspartate (NMDA) receptor, including the effect of magnesium. In a study of seven patients with postherpetic neuralgia, the intravenous infusion of 30 mg/kg of magnesium sulfate over 30 minutes was found to be more effective in relieving the pain than an intravenous infusion of saline.[69]

KEY POINTS

- Neuropathic pain is associated with altered processing and changes in central modulation. This includes pathologic activity in injured nerves (resulting in hyperexcitability as well as spontaneous and evoked pain); loss of C fibers; sprouting of the large fibers in the outer laminae of the dorsal horn, where the nociceptive-specific neurons are located (resulting in allodynia); and increased activity in the sympathetic nervous system.
- Some of the molecular changes in neuropathic pain include the accumulation and novel expression of sodium channels in peripheral nerves, increased activity of glutamate receptor subpopulations (especially the NMDA receptor), reduction of GABA inhibition, and changes in the penetration of calcium into the cells.
- The mechanisms of action of the membrane stabilizers include blockade of the sodium channel, suppression of the release of glutamate or blockade of glutamate activity, increase in GABA content, and binding to the alpha-2 delta subunit of GABA (see Table 49.1).
- The most common side effect of lamotrigine is the development of a rash. This is usually seen in pediatric patients and upon rapid titration of the dose of the drug.
- The most common side effect of oxcarbazepine is hyponatremia.
- Gabapentin is an effective drug in the treatment of neuropathic pain, specifically postherpetic neuralgia and painful diabetic neuropathy. It is well tolerated, and its common side effects include dizziness and sedation.
- The beneficial effects of pregabalin include linear pharmacokinetics, a shorter time to therapeutic effect, and lower effective dosages.

REFERENCES

Access the reference list online at ExpertConsult.com.

CHAPTER 50

Recommendations for Pharmacologic Therapy of Neuropathic Pain

Simon Haroutounian, MScPharm, PhD ◎ Nanna Brix Finnerup, MD, PhD

NEUROPATHIC PAIN—EPIDEMIOLOGY AND ASSESSMENT

Neuropathic pain (NeuP) is defined by the International Association for the Study of Pain (IASP) as "pain caused by a lesion or disease affecting the somatosensory system."[1] From a taxonomy standpoint, it is typically divided into central and peripheral NeuP, depending on whether the anatomic location of the nerve lesion or disease affects the central or the peripheral nervous system, respectively. Classic examples of peripheral NeuP include polyneuropathies such as painful diabetic peripheral neuropathy (DPN), chemotherapy-induced peripheral neuropathy (CIPN), and human immunodeficiency virus (HIV)–induced sensory neuropathy as well as focal neuropathies such as in postherpetic neuralgia (PHN), posttraumatic nerve injury, postamputation pain, and entrapment neuropathies. Central NeuP conditions include, but are not limited to, pain after spinal cord injury (SCI), central poststroke pain (CPSP), and multiple sclerosis (MS) pain.

There are various epidemiologic estimates of the prevalence of NeuP. Some estimates suggest a prevalence of about 3%, others point toward 6%–10% in the general population.[2–4] This substantial discrepancy is derived primarily from NeuP assessment methodology and the criteria used for defining "neuropathic pain" or "pain with neuropathic characteristics."[3] One of the current limitations in performing reliable population-wide surveys is the lack of a "gold standard" for diagnosing NeuP. Recently, the criteria for identifying NeuP and grading its probability have been revised by the Neuropathic Pain Special Interest Group (NeuPSIG) of the IASP and are intended to allow more consistent and accurate assessment of NeuP in large-scale studies and in clinical practice.[5]

Briefly, the probability of NeuP can be determined based on the three following criteria:

1. Patient's history of signs, symptoms, and descriptors suggestive of pain related to a neurologic lesion or disease *and* pain distribution that is consistent with the suspected lesion or disease
2. Presence of sensory disturbances upon examination in the painful area and with a neuroanatomically plausible distribution
3. Diagnostic tests that confirm a lesion or disease of the somatosensory nervous system

Unmet criterion 1 implies unlikely NeuP, whereas the fulfillment of each criterion in this sequence grades NeuP as possible, probable, or definite. Obtaining probable or higher grading of NeuP should be sufficient for initiating treatment per the NeuP guidelines discussed in this chapter.

Interdisciplinary management of chronic pain typically yields higher response rates than individual drug or nondrug approaches; however, pharmacotherapy has been the key approach to NeuP management. Several guidelines and their iterations have been available over the past decade,[6–11] each using a somewhat different approach for creating the evidence base and the recommendations. This chapter focuses on the process and the contents of the 2015 recommendations for the pharmacotherapy of NeuP based on the work carried out by the IASP NeuPSIG treatment guidelines committee.[10]

CONSTRUCTING THE EVIDENCE BASE FOR RECOMMENDATIONS FOR NEUROPATHIC PAIN PHARMACOTHERAPY

The NeuPSIG treatment guidelines were generated by an international committee representing 17 members from 10 countries; they included experts in neurology, anesthesiology, neuroscience, pain medicine, psychology, pharmacy, biostatistics, and epidemiology.

As the first step, a systematic literature search has been performed in PubMed, Medline, and Embase databases and in the Cochrane Central Register of Controlled Trials for identifying all NeuP treatment articles published since 1966. In addition, a web search was performed on the website of the US Food and Drug Administration (FDA), clinical trial registries such as ClinicalTrials.gov, and the pharmaceutical company websites to identify any unpublished research studies with available results. The details of the web search are available in the appendix of the published guidelines.[10]

It is important to mention that exclusion criteria have been applied, and several studies have been excluded from analyses. Only randomized, double-blind, placebo-controlled studies were included. The included interventions were of systemic or local treatments of at least 3 weeks' duration or single-administration treatments with follow-up of at least 3 weeks' duration. Studies of shorter duration were excluded. All conditions meeting the IASP criteria of NeuP were included. Importantly, conditions such as complex regional pain syndrome type 1, low back pain without radicular pain, fibromyalgia, and atypical facial pain were not included because they do not meet the current definition of NeuP.[5]

Studies with enriched-enrollment randomized withdrawal[12] designs were analyzed separately.

The primary outcome of effectiveness was based on NeuP intensity, considering the proportion of responders to active treatment versus responders to placebo. The response of a reduction in pain intensity equal to or greater than 50% (or, if unavailable, ≥30% reduction in pain intensity or at least moderate pain relief) was the primary outcome measure, which was used to calculate the numbers needed to treat (NNT) for each intervention. NNT is the number of patients needed to treat with a drug to achieve a response (i.e., ≥50% reduction in pain intensity) that is not attributable to placebo.

The NNT is the inverse of absolute risk reduction. It was calculated based on the following formula:

$$NNT = 1/\left[P\,(\text{active}) - P\,(\text{placebo})\right]$$

where P is the proportion of responders. For example, if 60 of 100 subjects in the active arm and 27 of the 100 subjects in the placebo arm report a reduction in pain intensity equal to or greater than 50%, the NNT is calculated as follows:

$$NNT = 1/\left[(60/100) - (27/100)\right] = 1/(0.60 - 0.27) = 3$$

Subsequently, of every three patients treated with the drug, one will have an important (≥50%) degree of pain relief not attributable to placebo. In the real clinical scenario, the objective response rate might be somewhat higher, considering that the patients might experience an additional placebo response effect added to the "true" drug effect, although these effects are not necessarily additive.[13]

For determining the balance between the benefit and the potential risks of each intervention, the numbers needed to harm (NNH) were calculated for each drug/drug group. NNH is calculated similarly to NNT (but from the ratios of subjects who withdrew from the study owing to side effects) for active drug versus placebo. Contrary to NNT, a larger NNH implies a safer drug (i.e., a smaller ratio of patients is harmed). It is important to note, though, that although NNH provides a measure of tolerability, it does not, by itself, indicate the seriousness of adverse effects. Rare but serious risks as well as side effects that develop over long periods of treatment are unlikely to be captured by clinical trials of a few weeks' duration.

All identified studies have been assessed for methodologic quality using the five-point Oxford Quality Scale. Two investigators independently extracted the data from each manuscript, and the findings were compared for any inaccuracies to produce a single extraction dataset from each study for data analyses.

The majority of randomized controlled trials (RCTs) have been performed in DPN and PHN with fewer studies in other NeuP conditions, such as painful radiculopathy, phantom pain, and postsurgical NeuP. There is a considerable overlap in symptoms and signs in different NeuP conditions[14] and there was no evidence for effectiveness of particular drugs in specific disorders. Therefore the NeuPSIG recommendations do not divide NeuP conditions based on etiology or pathophysiology but rather present the evidence on the safety and effectiveness of each drug (or drug class) in a variety of NeuP conditions. Although some differences may exist, there is no current evidence to support that a given drug is more effective in a certain peripheral or central NeuP condition. The main exception is trigeminal neuralgia (TGN), which has quite a different presentation of symptoms and signs. Most TGN studies did not meet NeuPSIG inclusion criteria; therefore TGN treatment recommendations offered here are based on a separate body of work that systematically addressed the evidence of safety and effectiveness of drugs in TGN.[6,15]

In general, poorer effectiveness of pharmacotherapy in conditions such as painful radiculopathy, CIPN, and HIV sensory neuropathy have also been suggested; however, there is a limited number of studies and no direct comparison studies to confirm this with certainty. In addition, studies in HIV sensory neuropathy in general tend to have higher placebo response rates and may thus not have sufficient assay sensitivity, while studies in CIPN often include patients with nonpainful symptoms, which are less likely to be responsive to analgesic treatments.

To minimize bias in translating evidence into recommendations, the NeuPSIG treatment guidelines committee used the Grading of Recommendations Assessment, Development, and Evaluation (GRADE), which is a systematic, transparent approach to making judgments about quality of evidence and strength of recommendation.[16,17]

PHARMACOLOGIC THERAPY OF NEUROPATHIC PAIN—SUMMARY OF EVIDENCE

The current NeuP guidelines are based on 229 randomized, placebo-controlled trials of pharmacologic agents in NeuP. Of these, 191 have been published, and 21 have not been published, but results were publicly available.

Table 50.1 presents the results of meta-analyses for drugs that had sufficient data to allow NNT and NNH analysis. Based on these analyses incorporated into GRADE framework, the drugs were categorized to lines of treatment according to the strength of recommendation for or against their use in NeuP.

DRUGS WITH STRONG GRADE RECOMMENDATION FOR USE AND RECOMMENDED AS FIRST LINE

A group of drugs met the criteria for strong GRADE recommendation for using them as first-line treatment for NeuP (Box 50.1).

High-quality evidence is available for the use of these four groups of drugs. The results have been positive in most clinical trials and the drugs have moderate tolerability.

It is important to note that TCAs as a group appear to have similar effectiveness. However, in adults greater than 65 years of age, TCAs with secondary amine structure (desipramine, nortriptyline) are preferred, since TCAs with tertiary amine structure (amitriptyline, imipramine, and clomipramine), especially at doses exceeding 75 mg/day, are more likely to cause major anticholinergic and sedative side effects and to increase the risk of falls or sudden cardiac death.[18] Despite these safety concerns, TCAs have been effective in most trials, with the lowest combined NNT among first-line interventions. Their low cost and ready availability in most countries justified their selection as a first-line treatment.

TABLE 50.1 Summary of Data Available on Main Pharmacologic Agents for the Treatment of Neuropathic Pain

	Between-Arm Comparisons	Total Number of Participants	Achieved Pain Relief With the Active Drug	Achieved Pain Relief With Placebo	NNT (95% CI)	NNH (95% CI)
Tricyclic antidepressants	15	948	217/473	85/475	3.6 (3.0–4.4)	13.4 (9.3–24)
Serotonin-norepinephrine reuptake inhibitors	10	2541	676/1559	278/982	6.4 (5.2–8.4)	11.8 (9.6–15)
Pregabalin	25	5940	1359/3530	578/2410	7.7 (6.5–9.4)	13.9 (12–17)
Gabapentin (including ER formulation and gabapentin enacarbil)	14	3503	719/2073	291/1430	7.2 (5.9–9.1)	25.6 (15–79)
Tramadol	6	741	176/380	96/361	4.7 (3.6–6.7)	12.6 (8.4–25)
Strong opioids	7	383	211/426	108/412	4.3 (3.4–5.8)	11.7 (8.4–19)
Capsaicin 8%	6	2073	466/1299	212/774	10.6 (7.4–18.8)	NA (single treatment)
Botulinum toxin A	4	137	42/70	4/67	1.9 (1.5–2.4)	NA (single treatment)

ER, *Extended release;* NA, *not applicable;* NNH, *numbers needed to harm;* NNT, *numbers needed to treat.*

BOX 50.1 First-Line Drugs for the Treatment of Neuropathic Pain

FIRST-LINE DRUGS FOR NEUROPATHIC PAIN	COMMENTS
Tricyclic antidepressants (TCAs)	Data based mainly on amitriptyline. Studies with desipramine, maprotiline, imipramine, and nortriptyline suggest a class effect, although some differences among TCAs may exist.
Serotonin-norepinephrine reuptake inhibitors (SNRIs)	Data based mainly on duloxetine; fewer studies available on venlafaxine.
Gabapentin	Data based mainly on gabapentin IR (immediate release). Data from gabapentin extended release (ER) and gabapentin enacarbil studies suggest similar effects.
Pregabalin	All studies performed with IR pregabalin.

DRUGS WITH WEAK GRADE RECOMMENDATIONS FOR USE AND RECOMMENDED AS SECOND LINE

Three groups of drugs are included in this category: oral tramadol, 8% capsaicin patches, and 5% lidocaine patches.

Tramadol has a final moderate quality of evidence with positive trials in NeuP. Compared with strong opioids, tramadol has historically been associated with a lower potential for misuse, abuse, and dependency. However, potential safety concerns have been on the rise in the past decade. An increase in deaths associated with its use and overdose has been reported[19–21]; therefore chronic tramadol should be used with caution until more safety data are available.

Capsaicin high-concentration patches have high final quality of evidence, but a high NNT indicates limited effectiveness compared with placebo. Its simple compliance (single administration) is offset by pain during application. Training is required for patch application, and in some countries, such as France and the United Kingdom, the drug must be administered in a hospital setting.

Lidocaine 5% patches have poor quality of evidence, with effectiveness based mainly on short-term positive studies.[22] However, high values and preferences, excellent balance between desirable and undesirable side effects, and recent positive data[23] warrant its classification as second-line treatment.

DRUGS WITH WEAK GRADE RECOMMENDATION FOR USE AND RECOMMENDED AS THIRD LINE

These include strong opioids (particularly oxycodone and morphine, which are the most studied drugs) and botulinum toxin type A (BTX-A).

Strong opioids have moderate final quality of evidence and demonstrated effectiveness in the short term, but they score low on patient values and preferences in addition to potential safety concerns associated with chronic opioid therapy. Their long-term use may be associated with risk of abuse, particularly with high doses, as well as potential cognitive impairment and endocrine and immunologic changes.[24] There are concerns about a recent increase in prescription opioid-associated overdose mortality, diversion, misuse, and other opioid-related morbidity,[25] particularly in the United States, Canada, and the United Kingdom.

BTX-A has moderate quality of evidence, a very low NNT in published trials, a good safety profile in NeuP, and high patient values and preferences. However, one large unpublished study (without dichotomous data) was negative. BTX-A should be prescribed and administered by specialists.

DRUGS WITH INCONCLUSIVE GRADE RECOMMENDATIONS

This group of drugs includes tapentadol (an opioid receptor agonist and norepinephrine reuptake inhibitor), most antiepileptic drugs (carbamazepine, oxcarbazepine, lamotrigine, lacosamide, topiramate, and zonisamide), capsaicin cream, topical clonidine, N-methyl-D-aspartic acid (NMDA) antagonists, and selective serotonin reuptake inhibitors (SSRIs).

Tapentadol may have lower abuse risk than strong opioids and might have better gastrointestinal tolerability,[26] which probably results in higher values and preferences, but has had inconsistent effects in two trials.

The antiepileptics in this group, as well as capsaicin cream, topical clonidine, SSRIs, and NMDA antagonists have discrepant findings in RCTs and/or low quality of evidence or potential safety concerns, not warranting assigning these to the first three lines of treatment.

Until recently, combination therapy has generally shown discrepant results or weak quality of evidence.[27–29] However, several recent studies have demonstrated that various combinations of antiepileptics and antidepressants (imipramine-pregabalin, nortriptyline-gabapentin, pregabalin-duloxetine) among them or with opioids (gabapentin-morphine and nortriptyline-morphine) are at least as effective and safe as monotherapy.[30–34] Because these drugs are often combined safely in clinical practice, the combination of moderate dosages may be proposed as an alternative to increasing single drug doses for patients not responding to monotherapy. Recent concerns about increased respiratory depression with opioid-antiepileptic combination in the acute pain setting[35] warrant a further look into the potential effect in the setting of chronic pain.

DRUGS WITH WEAK GRADE RECOMMENDATIONS AGAINST THEIR USE

Cannabinoids and valproate have currently weak recommendations against their use, particularly because of generally negative results of clinical trials and potential safety concerns. In particular, the issue of potential misuse or diversion of cannabinoids has to be considered. More than 60% of long-term cannabinoid trials in NeuP have been negative, and epidemiologic data suggest that cannabis use, particularly in adolescents and other susceptible individuals, may be associated with long-term mental health risks, including psychosis and cognitive impairment.[36]

DRUGS WITH STRONG GRADE RECOMMENDATIONS AGAINST THEIR USE

Levetiracetam and mexiletine have strong recommendations against their use in NeuP. Of eight available mexiletine studies, seven were negative, and all five trials of levetiracetam in NeuP have been negative.

OTHER TREATMENT RECOMMENDATIONS

Other national and international treatment recommendations have been published in recent years for the pharmacotherapy of NeuP in general[8,11] or for specific NeuP conditions such as painful polyneuropathies.[7,37] The European Federation of Neurological Societies (EFNS) published its latest guideline in 2010.[6] These guidelines include all NeuP conditions but make separate recommendations for specific etiologies. In addition, the inclusion criteria differed slightly between the NeuPSIG and EFNS studies. Although the NeuPSIG guidelines included randomized double-blind controlled studies of at least 3 weeks' duration, the EFNS also included lower-quality studies (in conditions where no higher-level evidence was available), and had no lower limit for study duration. Both panels included attempts to overcome possible publication bias. The EFNS asked pharmaceutical companies to provide results for studies that were not published, while NeuPSIG recommendations included studies published in the Pharmaceutical Research and Manufacturers of America (PhRMA) Clinical Study Results Database before its closure, and studies with results in primary registries in the World Health Organization Registry Network and the ClinicalTrial.gov website.

The first-line treatment recommendations in the EFNS guidelines are TCAs, gabapentin, pregabalin, and SNRIs; tramadol was recommended as second-line treatment for exacerbations of pain. Specifically for PHN–TCAs, gabapentin and pregabalin were recommended as first-line treatments. Topical lidocaine was also recommended as first-line treatment in the elderly and when there are concerns with systemic side effects such as dizziness and drowsiness.

Strong opioids and capsaicin cream were recommended as second-line treatments. Pregabalin, amitriptyline, and gabapentin were recommended as first-line and tramadol as second-line treatments in central pain conditions even though the recommendation for gabapentin was based on evidence in other pain conditions.

The somewhat different inclusion criteria, the year of literature search, sources of studies, and the process of generating evidence-based recommendations are probably responsible for some of the differences between NeuPSIG and EFNS recommendations.

Special Neuropathic Pain Conditions

Two NeuP conditions that seem to be unique in symptoms but also in terms of response to pharmacotherapy are TGN (described more extensively in Chapter 23), and the group of painful channelopathies that include conditions such as inherited erythromelalgia and paroxysmal extreme pain disorder, which have been linked to specific mutations in voltage-gated sodium channels such as Nav1.7 (for review, see Bennett and Woods[38]).

TRIGEMINAL NEURALGIA

In the NeuPSIG guidelines, only one TGN study met the inclusion criteria.[39] The others did not meet inclusion criteria either due to shorter than 3-week duration, lack of placebo treatment, pain intensity not being the primary outcome, or arm size of 10 or fewer subjects.

In 2008, the American Academy of Neurology (AAN) and the European Federation of Neurological Sciences launched a task force to review the available literature and publish guidelines on the treatment of TGN.[15] The task force discussed not only pharmacologic but also interventional approaches to treating TGN, including microvascular decompression, gamma knife, and gasserian ganglion surgeries. From the perspective of pharmacologic management, the task force concluded that carbamazepine has the best available evidence on effectiveness, with NNTs around 1.7–1.8. The effectiveness, however, was compromised by poor tolerability with NNH of around 3.4. Oxcarbazepine was found similarly effective but better tolerated than carbamazepine, although the studies compared oxcarbazepine directly to carbamazepine, rather than to placebo. Additional data were derived from single studies and suggested that baclofen (skeletal muscle relaxant, antispasmodic), lamotrigine, pimozide (tricyclic antipsychotic), and tocainide (sodium channel blocking antiarrythmic) may have effectiveness in TGN.

HEREDITARY CHANNELOPATHIES

Research into the treatment of painful channelopathies is limited, primarily because of the low incidence of these conditions, which limits the ability to perform large studies. Based on case reports and small-scale available studies, inherited erythromelalgia seems to respond better to drugs that work by blocking voltage-gated sodium channels such as carbamazepine and mexiletine, and experimental blockers of specific sodium channel isoforms such as Nav1.7.[40–42]

PHARMACOLOGY OF DRUGS IMPLIED IN THE TREATMENT OF NEUROPATHIC PAIN

ANTIDEPRESSANTS

Tricyclic Antidepressants

Several studies published in the 1980s[43–45] indicate that amitriptyline is effective in treating NeuP due to diabetic neuropathy and PHN irrespective of its antidepressant effect. Although the NeuP literature on the effectiveness of tricyclic antidepressants (TCAs) is primarily based on amitriptyline, studies with other TCAs suggest the probability of class effect, and various TCAs may not differ substantially from each other in terms of effectiveness. This, however, is not to say that lack of response to one TCA precludes a lack of response to another, since there are still some differences among them, as discussed further on. TCAs have been key drugs for the treatment of various NeuP disorders for the past two decades, with a large amount of clinical experience accumulated over the years.

The mechanism by which TCAs exert their action in treating NeuP is not entirely understood but is thought to be contributed primarily by inhibiting the reuptake of serotonin and norepinephrine in bulbospinal neurons, thus enhancing the descending inhibitory serotonergic and noradrenergic controls from the brain stem to the spinal cord dorsal horn.[46,47] TCAs are known to have multiple additional mechanisms. For example, TCAs are reported to act on NMDA receptors, adenosine receptors, $\alpha 2$ receptors, sodium channels (particularly amitriptyline); they also have anticholinergic and antihistaminic effects.[46]

All TCAs share a tricyclic chemical structure, as their name suggests, and can be divided to secondary amines and tertiary amines, depending on the number of methyl ($-CH_3$) groups on the side chain nitrogen. Secondary amine TCAs (nortriptyline, desipramine) result from the metabolism of tertiary amines (amitriptyline and imipramine, respectively), during which one of the nitrogen methyl groups is lost and replaced by hydrogen (the demethylation process). Secondary amines typically have higher affinity to the norepinephrine transporter than the serotonin transporter, while in tertiary amines this ratio is reversed. In addition, secondary amines have lower affinity to muscarinic acetylcholine (mAch) receptors, thus they have a lower likelihood of anticholinergic side effects, especially at low doses. There are some differences among tertiary amine TCAs as well. The affinity of imipramine to the blockage of histaminergic H1 receptors, for example, is lower than that of amitriptyline[48]; therefore it might be less sedating.

TCAs share somewhat similar pharmacokinetic properties: They have excellent oral bioavailability and have long (usually 12–50 hours) plasma elimination half-lives for either the parent compound or the active metabolite, typically allowing once-a-day administration.

TCAs are metabolized by hepatic cytochrome P450 (CYP450) system. CYP450 1A2, 2C19, 3A4, and 2D6 participate in the metabolism of tertiary amine TCAs; secondary amine TCAs, on the other hand, are metabolized almost exclusively by CYP2D6. Subjects with genetic polymorphisms at CYP2D6, resulting in the "slow metabolizer" genotype, are likely to require lower doses of nortriptyline and desipramine (50 mg for depression) versus subjects with the "ultrarapid 2D6 metabolizer" genotype, who are likely to require higher doses of the drugs, around 150 mg/day.[48] Tertiary amines, due to multiple metabolic pathways, are less affected by CYP450-mediated drug interactions or genetic polymorphism affecting a single CYP450 enzyme; however, a substantial intersubject variability still exists in the pharmacokinetics of these drugs and their metabolites.[47,49]

Common side effects of TCAs include drowsiness, dry mouth, urinary retention, constipation, weight gain, and orthostatic hypotension. Other effects can include increased intraocular pressure, increased risks of falls in the elderly, palpitations, QT prolongation, and arrhythmias at high doses. TCAs should not be combined with other QT-prolonging drugs, used in caution with other serotonergic agents to minimize the risk of serotonin syndrome, and used with caution in epileptic patients, as TCAs can reduce the threshold for seizures.

Dosing

Most TCAs can be initiated at 10–25 mg once a day at bedtime and titrated in 10- to 25-mg increments every 1–2 weeks to a target dose of about 75 mg/day, which has been the average dose in clinical trials. Doses can be increased further, up to 150 mg/day, based on tolerability; however, some studies question the benefits of doses higher than 100 mg/day. Although TCA doses are typically titrated to clinical response, plasma concentration monitoring may be helpful in guiding treatment, especially for avoiding toxicity in "slow metabolizers."

Serotonin-Norepinephrine Reuptake Inhibitors

Duloxetine and venlafaxine are currently the two SNRIs recommended for the treatment of NeuP pain, although venlafaxine does not have an FDA-approved indication for treating NeuP and is currently indicated (similarly to desvenlafaxine) for the treatment of depression. Both duloxetine and venlafaxine inhibit the serotonin and norepinephrine transporters, although duloxetine appears to have a higher affinity to both.[50] The mechanism of SNRIs for NeuP is assumed to be similar to that of TCAs in terms of serotonin and norepinephrine reuptake inhibition; however, both duloxetine and venlafaxine have very low affinity to cholinergic, adrenergic, histaminergic, and dopaminergic receptors.

Duloxetine has oral bioavailability of 30%–80%. Its absorption is slow, and takes about 2 hours for plasma concentrations to peak. Taking duloxetine with or after meals further delays the absorption but does not seem to affect the peak plasma concentration substantially.

Duloxetine is metabolized by the liver CYP450 enzymes, primarily CYP 1A2 and 2D6. The metabolites undergo renal excretion. Since CYP1A2 in chronic smokers may be induced, smokers may require about 15%–30% higher doses of duloxetine[51,52]; however, dose change based on smoking status may not be warranted.[53]

Most common side effects include nausea, drowsiness, and dizziness. Gastrointestinal side effects such as constipation, diarrhea, and dry mouth are often reported. Hypertension and orthostatic hypotension have been reported; fatigue and diaphoresis has been reported at higher rates than with placebo. SNRIs, similarly to SSRIs, may affect the effects of serotonin on platelets and increase the risk of (mainly gastrointestinal) bleeding, particularly in patients on chronic anticoagulant, antiplatelet, NSAID, aspirin, or systemic corticosteroid therapy.

The main drug interactions of duloxetine are with other serotonergic drugs (monoamine oxidase inhibitors [MAOIs], SSRIs, tramadol, linezolide, etc.) by increasing the risk of serotonin syndrome, and with drugs affecting coagulation and platelet adhesion by increasing the risk of bleeding. CYP 1A2 inhibitors such as fluvoxamine can cause a substantial increase in duloxetine plasma concentrations.

Dosage is usually 60 mg once a day (it may be started at 30 mg once a day if tolerability concerns exist). Effectiveness in clinical studies has been shown with doses of 60 and 120 mg/day. Duloxetine should not be used in patients with renal impairment (i.e., creatinine clearance below 30 mL/min) and should be avoided in moderate to severe liver disease and cirrhosis.

Venlafaxine is well absorbed orally but undergoes extensive first-pass metabolism, and therefore has only 12%–45% bioavailability depending on the dosage form. Extended-release formulations result in improved bioavailability (Effexor XR product information, Wyeth Pharmaceuticals). Food does not seem to have an effect on bioavailability. Venlafaxine undergoes extensive liver metabolism by the CYP450 2D6 isoenzyme to an active metabolite, N,O-didesmethylvenlafaxine (Effexor product information, Wyeth Pharmaceuticals).

Most common side effects include nausea, sweating, weight loss, dizziness, drowsiness, and headaches. Hypertension has been reported in 3%–13% of subjects, especially with high doses of 375 mg/day. At doses below 225 mg/day, the average increase in blood pressure was less than 2 mm Hg. Palpitation and electrocardiographic abnormalities were reported in 3%–5% of patients. Caution is advised in using high dosages of venlafaxine (>150 mg/day) in patients with cardiac conditions. Abnormal ejaculation/orgasm and erectile dysfunction have been reported with venlafaxine.

Potential drug interaction concerns are with QT-prolonging drugs, serotonergic agents, and drugs that affect coagulation and increase the risk of bleeding.

Dosage: The initial recommended dosage of venlafaxine is 37.5 mg once or twice a day as an immediate-release formulation or 75 mg/day in an extended-release formulation. The doses then can be increased in 37.5- to 75-mg increments every 1–3 weeks to 150 mg/day and, if required, further up to 225 mg/day with appropriate monitoring in cardiac patients.

The dosage should be reduced by 25%–50% in patients with mild to moderate renal impairment and by at least 50% in patients with cirrhosis or mild to moderate liver impairment.

ANTICONVULSANTS

Calcium Channel α2δ Subunit Ligands

Gabapentin and pregabalin are both ligands of α2δ subunit of neuronal voltage-gated calcium channels. The exact analgesic mechanism of these compounds is unknown, but they appear to reduce calcium-dependent release of excitatory neurotransmitters, thus decreasing neuronal hyperexcitability.[54,55] Although gabapentin and pregabalin are structurally related to gamma-aminobutyric acid (GABA), they do not bind to either $GABA_A$ or $GABA_B$ receptors.

Gabapentin has nonlinear oral absorption kinetics, with the percentage of bioavailable drug decreasing with an absolute increase in a dose. For example, approximately 60% of a 300-mg dose is absorbed, whereas a 1200-mg dose results in 30% absorption (Neurontin product Information, Parke Davis). This is due to a narrow absorption window in the proximal small intestine, mediated by gabapentin uptake by saturable transport mechanisms. Taking gabapentin with food slows the rate of passage from stomach to duodenum and can improve absorption. The nonlinear absorption kinetics of gabapentin have led to a variety of pharmaceutical modifications to introduce products such as extended-release formulations[56] and better-absorbable prodrugs such as gabapentin enacarbil for increased and more predictable bioavailability. The half-life of gabapentin is 5–7 hours, and it usually requires three times a day (tid) dosing in immediate-release formulations. Gabapentin is not metabolized by the liver and is excreted unchanged in urine.

Dosing: Gabapentin is typically initiated at 100–300 mg three times a day. It can be increased in 100- to 300-mg increments every 3–7 days to reach target doses. Most studies have utilized 1800–2400 mg/day doses in NeuP, but doses can be increased up to 3600 mg/day. No dose adjustment is required in patients with liver impairment. The dose should be reduced in patients with mild to moderate renal insufficiency, and gabapentin is not recommended in patients with Clcr < 30 mL/min. Dose reduction and post-dialysis dose supplementation are warranted in patients undergoing hemodialysis.

Pregabalin has high oral bioavailability of approximately 90% and linear absorption kinetics. Administration with food may increase the peak plasma concentrations but overall does not have a substantial effect on bioavailability.

Dosing: Pregabalin is typically initiated at 75 mg twice a day and can be increased in 75 mg-increments every 3–7 days to reach target doses of 300–600 mg/day. Although mostly administered twice a day, several clinical trials have employed thrice daily dosing; this approach may be useful in patients who experience side effects related to high peak plasma concentrations soon after drug intake. Similar to gabapentin, pregabalin is almost entirely excreted renally and does not require dose adjustment in hepatic insufficiency.

Both pregabalin and gabapentin have very few drug-interactions, if any. Their absorption may be somewhat compromised by the concomitant intake of antacids.

Most common side effects of both gabapentin and pregabalin include dizziness and drowsiness. Peripheral edema occurs in 3%–10% of patients. Both drugs may cause a variety of neurologic and ophthalmic adverse effects, including ataxia, asthenia (primarily with pregabalin), nystagmus, and diplopia. Weight gain has been reported in 3%–10% of the subjects in clinical trials; fluctuations in blood glucose levels may occur. Severe hypersensitivity reactions, although rare, have been reported with both drugs.

OTHER ANTICONVULSANTS

Carbamazepine and Oxcarbazepine

Carbamazepine is chemically related to TCAs. Its mechanism of action in NeuP is unclear but is probably related to its membrane-stabilizing effect, mediated by blocking voltage-gated sodium channels to reduce hyperactivity in both central and peripheral neurons. A variety of additional effects on calcium and potassium channels as well as on potentiation of GABAergic inhibition[54,55] have been proposed, but their clinical relevance is unclear.

The analgesic effect of carbamazepine was first suggested in TGN by Blom in 1962, and TGN still remains the most useful indication for carbamazepine.

Carbamazepine is well absorbed orally and is extensively metabolized by the liver. Carbamazepine is a potent inducer of liver and gut CYP450 enzymes and can impair the oral bioavailability and increase the clearance of various CYP450 substrates. Importantly, carbamazepine induces its own metabolism. Since enzyme induction process may take 2–3 weeks to peak, this effect may be delayed, requiring individual adjustment of dosing.

Oxcarbazepine is structurally very similar to carbamazepine and has a similar effectiveness profile in epilepsy and NeuP. Although both drugs are eventually metabolized to dihydroxycarbamazepine, one of the main differences is that oxcarbazepine metabolism does not involve the formation of carbamazepine 10,11-epoxide, an important contributor to carbamazepine toxicity and CYP450 enzyme induction.

The NNT (95% CI) for carbamazepine/oxcarbazepine in NeuP was 5.7 (3.4–18), along with an NNH of 5.5 (4.3–7.9), indicating that for each five or six treated patients one will have a good analgesic response but one will discontinue treatment due to adverse effects.

Dosing: Initial doses of carbamazepine typically start at 50 mg 4 times a day of immediate-release formulations or 100 mg twice a day of extended-release formulations. The dose may be titrated in increments of 200 mg/day until target doses of 400–800 mg/day—which have demonstrated effectiveness in clinical trials—are reached. Doses should not exceed 1200 mg/day. Carbamazepine is usually dosed twice a day in extended-release formulations. Some generic formulations of carbamazepine might not be interchangeable for certain patients, resulting in different plasma concentration profiles. This difference has not been observed consistently[57] and is more critical to the anticonvulsant effects of the drug; it is unclear which patients are at risk. No dose adjustment in renal insufficiency is required; dose reduction in liver insufficiency may be warranted.

Oxcarbazepine is typically initiated at 300 mg twice a day; this can be increased in increments of 300 mg every 1–2 weeks up to the therapeutic dose of 1800–2400 mg/day. In patients with severe renal impairment (Clcr < 30 mL/min), the initial dose and the dose increments should be reduced by 50%. Oxcarbazepine should not be administered to patients with severe hepatic impairment.

Most common side effects of carbamazepine and oxcarbazepine treatment are drowsiness, slurred speech, ataxia, hallucinations, nausea, tremor, and blurred vision.

Rare, but serious skin reactions such as toxic epidermal necrolysis, including Stevens-Johnson syndrome, may occur with both drugs. Because blood dyscrasias such as agranulocytosis and aplastic anemia as well as liver failure may also occur with carbamazepine, monitoring is warranted.

Overall, oxcarbazepine appears to have a better safety profile than carbamazepine, with a lower prevalence of liver failure, major skin reactions, and drug-drug interactions based on CYP450 enzyme induction.[58,59] On the other hand, oxcarbazepine results in more hyponatremia than carbamazepine, which is potentially contributed by the drug-induced syndrome of inappropriate antidiuretic hormone (SIADH) secretion.

The presence of the HLA-B*1502 allele[60] has been highly associated with Stevens-Johnson syndrome and toxic epidermal necrolysis following carbamazepine treatment in Chinese and Taiwanese populations, and the FDA now recommends genotyping for the presence of the HLA-B*1502 allele in all Asian patients before initiating carbamazepine or oxcarbazepine treatment. The correlation in Caucasian and other ethnic groups is unclear; HLA-B*1502 is more prevalent in Asian populations, and there might be a genotype-ethnicity combination, which is of importance in this drug toxicity. Currently, there appears to be no apparent value in genotyping non-Asian patients for the allele.[60]

Drug interactions are frequent, primarily based on the CYP450-inducing effect of carbamazepine. Plasma concentrations of drugs undergoing metabolism by CYP450 3A4, 1A2, or 2C19 may be affected. More serious interactions occur with warfarin (warranting close international normalized ratio [INR] monitoring); and drugs such as tacrolimus, for which plasma concentration maintenance within the therapeutic window is critically important to prevent graft rejection.

Lamotrigine

The primary mechanism of action of lamotrigine is thought to be mediated via inhibition of glutamate release by blocking neuronal voltage-gated sodium channels, although the exact mechanism has not been elucidated.[54] Three positive trials have been published (in CPSP, DPN, and HIV sensory neuropathy), but virtually all large trials in NeuP have been negative.

Lamotrigine may cause serious, sometimes life-threatening skin rashes. Dose titration should be performed slowly, by starting at 25 mg/day, with slow increases at 2-week intervals to 50, 100, and then 200 mg/day (up to a maximum 400 mg/day). More rapid dose titration increases the risk of serious skin reactions. It is important to note that the titration schedule is different in patients who are taking other drugs (primary anticonvulsants) that can inhibit or induce the hepatic metabolism of lamotrigine.

Topiramate

The drug appears to have several mechanisms of action, including activation of $GABA_A$ receptors, blockade of AMPA/kainate receptors for glutamate, and blockade of voltage-gated sodium channels. Although positive results were seen in one trial involving DPN,[61] a combined report of three studies in DPN[62] and a study with lumbar radiculopathy[63] were negative.

Topiramate doses up to 400 mg/day have been used in NeuP trials. The dose is typically initiated at 25 mg/day and titrated to analgesic response by increments of 25 mg per dose at weekly intervals. A variety of skin adverse effects are reported with topiramate, including rash, flushing, and alopecia. Hyperammonemia and/or a drop in serum bicarbonate level are frequently reported with topiramate treatment (9%–67% prevalence, but usually mild) and may be dose-related. Topiramate may cause loss of appetite and weigh loss in 10%–24% of patients. Dizziness, somnolence, and a variety of neurologic side effects may occur.

Lacosamide

The exact mechanism of action of lacosamide is unknown. It is a functionalized amino acid and appears to selectively enhance voltage-gated sodium channel slow inactivation, thus reducing neuronal hyperexcitability. As in the case of topiramate, several larger negative trials followed one positive trial, all in DPN. The initial dose of lacosamide is 100 mg twice a day, which can be increased weekly by 50 mg twice a day up to a total daily dose of 400 mg.

Cardiovascular side effects have been reported with lacosamide, including atrioventricular blocks of various degrees, bradycardia, and atrial fibrillation/flutter. Nausea and dizziness are among the most common side effects; ophthalmic side effects such as diplopia and blurred vision may occur in 5%–10% of subjects.

Valproic Acid

Valproic acid (as valproate or divalproex sodium) has shown positive results in three trials (two DPN, one PHN) of relatively poor quality, especially for PHN. Three studies (SCI, DPN, and mixed peripheral neuropathy) have been negative. Valproic acid has multiple mechanisms of action, and those responsible for analgesic effect are unclear. This drug is also a subject of multiple drug interactions by inhibiting the hepatic metabolism of some drugs, being affected by other CYP450 inducers and inhibitors, or additional mechanisms affecting its glucuronidation pathways.[64,65] Valproic acid may cause fatal hepatotoxicity in 1 of 800 children under the age of 2; the incidence in adults is not clear, but appears to be around 1 in 10,000–40,000 patients. Thrombocytopenia has been reported in 1%–30% patients treated with valproic acid. Due to the above safety issues, the treatment for NeuP is usually not recommended. This is particularly true for women of childbearing age because of a twofold to fivefold increase in the rate of birth defects with perinatal exposure to valproic acid.

Levetiracetam

Levetiracetam has an excellent safety profile compared with other anticonvulsants and therefore has been an attractive candidate for testing its effectiveness in NeuP. Unfortunately none of the six RCTs with levetiracetam that met NeuPSIG inclusion criteria showed any difference from placebo in terms of effectiveness. Therefore levetiracetam is currently not recommended for the treatment of NeuP.

TRAMADOL

Tramadol is a weak agonist of mu opioid receptors; it is used for the treatment of mild to moderate musculoskeletal pain but also inhibits the reuptake of serotonin and norepinephrine, somewhat similarly to SNRIs. In doses up to 400 mg/day, it was shown to be effective in seven RCTs, with a combined NNT of 4.7.

Adult doses typically start at 25–50 mg/day (or up to 100 mg/day of an extended-release formulation); they are titrated as tolerated up to 400 mg/day. In elderly patients the initial dose should be low, and titration might need to be slower to prevent excessive drowsiness, dizziness, and falls.

Both the opioidergic and serotonergic-noradrenergic effects of tramadol must be accounted for in considering its potential side effects and drug-drug interactions. A more detailed pharmacology of tramadol appears in Chapter 43.

OPIOIDS

Opioids, primarily oral morphine and oxycodone, have moderate evidence to support their use in NeuP. Despite a reasonable effectiveness profile, the main consideration in discussing NeuP treatment with opioids is focused on long-term safety issues including cognitive and metabolic side effects as well as risk of misuse, aversion, and deaths related to opioid overdose.[24,25] Chapters 42 and 43 address the pharmacology, dosing, and safety considerations of treating pain with opioid medications.

Methadone might theoretically be a suitable opioid for treating NeuP because of its additional mechanisms of NMDA antagonism; however, evidence supporting methadone use in NeuP or chronic noncancer pain in general[66] is lacking, and clinicians who prescribe methadone should be highly familiar with its unique pharmacokinetic properties, which include accumulation due to a long half-life, potential genetic polymorphism of CYP2B6 affecting its clearance and thus plasma levels, as well as induction of its own metabolism (i.e., autoinduction). These all require more frequent patient monitoring and careful dose adjustments.[67,68]

Tapentadol has a unique mechanism of action, as it is a full agonist at the mu-opioid receptor, but also inhibits the reuptake of norepinephrine, similarly to tramadol. The current evidence of its effectiveness in NeuP is unclear,[10] and more data are required to determine whether it is similar to other opioids.

TOPICAL CAPSAICIN

Capsaicin is the active pungent ingredient in chili peppers. Capsaicin binds to the transient receptor potential vanilloid (TRPV1) channel, which is an ion channel also activated by heat and protons.[69] Activation of the TRPV1 channel by capsaicin results in an acute effect, with a burning and painful sensation as well as a peripheral and central sensitization with allodynia and hyperalgesia in and around the area of application. Capsaicin also has a long-term analgesic effect; repeated applications of a low-concentration capsaicin cream or a single application of a high-concentration capsaicin patch are used in the treatment of NeuP. The long-term analgesic effect is thought to be related to desensitization of nociceptors due to the depletion of substance P from small-size sensory primary afferents. High doses of capsaicin cause a reversible reduction in epidermal and subepidermal nerve fiber density. The majority of epidermal nerve fibers regenerate within a few months, but a reduced regenerative rate has been seen in subjects with diabetes.[70] In addition, capsaicin treatment causes a defunctionalization of small fibers due to the temporarily altered transportation of neurotrophic factors and a loss of membrane potential.[71]

Capsaicin Cream

Capsaicin cream is available in low concentrations (0.025%–0.1%) for topical administration. Studies are difficult to blind because of the associated pain and burning upon application, and while some studies have shown effect (particularly in PHN and DPN) other studies have been negative and thus the overall recommendation for using capsaicin cream for NeuP was inconclusive.[10]

Capsaicin cream is applied to the painful skin area and exerts its effect locally, as the systemic uptake is limited. The cream is applied up to 4 to 5 times daily, and it requires a treatment period of approximately 4 weeks until maximum effectiveness is observed.

Side effects are most often related to a temporary burning sensation, pruritus, and erythema at the application site, which typically diminish after repeated applications. Systemic side effects are rare, but irritation in the airways from inhalation of capsaicin particles has been reported. Capsaicin should not be applied to damaged or irritated skin or to mucosal membranes. It is recommended to wash the hands with water and soap immediately after application or to use vinyl gloves for the application process.

Capsaicin 8% Patch

Studies have shown a modest effect of the capsaicin 8% patch in PHN, while studies in HIV-related painful polyneuropathy have been inconsistent. RCTs on capsaicin patches have used an application of a low-dose capsaicin patch, with no expected long-term effect, as the placebo control to preserve blinding. Capsaicin 8% patches are approved by the FDA for PHN and by the European Medicines Agency for peripheral NeuP.

Capsaicin 8% patches are applied by a doctor or nurse and in some countries in a hospital setting. They should be applied on nonirritated and unbroken skin. Up to four patches can be applied at the same time. Topical lidocaine or tramadol premedication can be used because the application is often unpleasant or painful. The patch is applied for 30 or 60 minutes. The treatment may be repeated every 3 months.

Local side effects with erythema and burning pain are common but transient. Throat irritation and skin itching, blisters, and swelling may also occur, and there are reports of first- and second-degree burns. Systemic side effects are rare and of limited duration since there is very limited systemic absorption. There is a potential risk of blood pressure elevation due to the immediate pain caused by the application.[72] The long-term safety of repeated applications in patients has not been clearly established, particularly with respect to the degeneration of epidermal nerve fibers and possible loss of protective sensory function, which may be a concern in, for example, progressive neuropathy. Capsaicin patches have the advantage of high compliance, since the effect may last for 3 months after a single application. There is a low risk for systemic side effects and drug-drug interactions, but the effect size is modest and the treatment is associated with high costs.

TOPICAL LIDOCAINE

Lidocaine is a local anesthetic of the amide-linked class that acts by blocking voltage-gated sodium-channels. Lidocaine produces analgesia by reducing the influx of sodium, thus stabilizing nerve membranes and preventing depolarization, impulse generation, and the conduction of nerve impulses. Lidocaine exerts a use-dependent blockade of sodium channels and inhibits ectopic discharges at doses that do not block nerve conduction.[73] It results in an incomplete and variable degree of small-fiber blockade. Lidocaine is also suggested to exert analgesic effects independent of sodium channel–mediated effects on primary afferent neurons.[74]

Lidocaine-medicated patches are adhesive patches containing lidocaine 5%; they are applied on intact, dry, nonirritated skin. These patches have FDA approval for PHN. Lidocaine may also be applied topically on the skin in a gel or spray form. Lidocaine patches cause a steady release of lidocaine, which penetrates the skin in small amounts and acts near the site of administration. Up to three to four lidocaine 10- by 14-cm patches containing 700 mg lidocaine each can be applied to intact skin. The patches are applied for 12 hours per day with a 12-hour patch-free interval before new patches are applied. The patches may be cut to fit the area of pain. There is minimal (about 3%) systemic uptake when patches are applied to intact skin, with steady-state concentrations being reached in 4 days.[75] Following the application of three patches, the maximum plasma concentration of lidocaine reaches 0.13 (±0.06) μg/mL (Lidoderm product information, Endo Pharmaceuticals Inc.), which is less than 15% of what would be reached from a typical peripheral nerve block (e.g., combined tibial-peroneal nerve block with 2% lidocaine), and less than

5% of what is reached with an intravenous infusion of 5 mg/kg.[76] Lidocaine undergoes hepatic metabolism and is excreted by the kidneys.

There are few side effects of topical lidocaine and they are often mild and related to local skin irritation or discomfort when the patch is taken off. There are usually no systemic side effects and no drug interactions because of minimal absorption and distribution resulting in plasma concentrations well below the levels for toxicity and antiarrhythmic activity. The absorption may be increased in highly vascular areas such as the forehead and mucosal membranes.[75] Lidocaine patches should not be used in patients with known hypersensitivity to local anesthetics of the amide type and used with caution in patients with severe renal or hepatic impairment.

CANNABINOIDS

Cannabinoids are ligands for the cannabinoid receptors and include endocannabinoids (anandamide and 2-arachidonoylglycerol), or naturally occurring compounds found in the plants such as *Cannabis sativa* and structurally related synthetic analogues. Cannabis plants contain several cannabinoids, including Δ-9-tetrahydrocannabinol (THC) with high psychoactive effects and cannabidiol (CBD). Cannabinoid receptors are G protein–coupled receptors. CB1 receptors are expressed in the human brain and along pain pathways in the spinal cord and peripheral nerves, whereas the CB2 receptors are mainly expressed in peripheral tissues and are thought to play a role in immune function.[77]

There is a large variability of available medical cannabinoids in different countries. Dronabinol and nabilone are synthetic analogs of THC available in oral tablet form; nabiximols is the name for a cannabis extract containing THC and CBD, available in some countries as an oromucosal spray. In certain countries, smoked or vaporized cannabis products are available and approved for pain indications.

Smoking cannabis provides a rapid absorption, which is slower with oral administration. Because of first-pass hepatic metabolisms and high lipid solubility, only a smaller amount of administered noninhaled cannabinoids reach the systemic circulation. Dronabinol has an onset of action of 0.5–1 hour and a peak effect at 2–4 hours. With oromucosal nabiximols, the maximum plasma concentration of THC and CBD is reached after 60–150 minutes. The elimination is biexponential; the initial half-life of both THC and CBD is 1.5–2 hours, but the terminal elimination half-life is 24–36 hours, with a large interpatient variation. Cannabinoids are distributed throughout the body and metabolized in the liver. The drugs and their metabolites are excreted in the urine and feces. Both THC and CBD may be stored in the fatty tissues, and subtherapeutic levels of metabolites may be found after several weeks in the urine and feces. Cannabinoid doses are highly variable, depending on the formulation; all should be slowly titrated to response so as to avoid side effects associated with high plasma concentrations.

Cannabis use is commonly associated with dizziness, particularly in the run-in period. Other side effects include drowsiness, increased pulse rate, dry mouth, anxiety, mood changes, disorientation, impaired memory and cognition, constipation, and diarrhea. Studies on smoked cannabis showed similar side effects, with a higher incidence of particular neurocognitive effects—such as dizziness, feeling high or "stoned," concentration difficulties, fatigue, and headaches—as compared with placebo.[78] Cannabinoids should not be used in patients with serious cardiovascular disease and used with caution in patients with a history of epilepsy or seizures and in patients with renal or hepatic impairment. In addition, they should not be used in patients with a history of psychotic or substance abuse disorders, and a careful risk assessment should be carried out.

THC and CBD are metabolized by the cytochrome P450 system, particularly CYP2C9, CYP2C19, and CYP3A4.[79] Potential CYP-mediated drug interactions exist, but current research in this area is quite limited, and it is unclear which interactions are clinically important. A precaution must be taken in coprescribing cannabinoids with other psychoactive drugs with sedative or neurologic side effects.

A few RCT studies showing a positive effect of smoked or inhaled cannabis in NeuP are available,[80–82] but all are of very short duration and none of them met the criteria of inclusion in NeuPSIG guidelines. The evidence is inconsistent for other medical cannabinoids for NeuP. Because of the short duration of RCTs in NeuP, the long-term psychoactive and neurocognitive side effects of cannabis are unknown.[78] Observational studies show that recreational cannabis use is associated with substance dependence and serious adverse effects, such as impaired cognitive and motor function, changes in brain function as well as risk behavior, and motor vehicle accidents.[36,83] In addition, the long-term effects on pulmonary function are unsettled.[84] Two recent studies of medical cannabis treatment for a mixed group of neuropathic and non-NeuP pain patients with 7–12 months of follow-up[85,86] demonstrated a reasonable safety profile; however, serious side effects were seen in 1%–2% of patients, and the concerns regarding long-term respiratory, cognitive, and psychiatric effects of cannabis cannot be ruled out. Long-term effectiveness and safety of medical cannabinoids in NeuP need to be addressed in larger studies before making changes in treatment recommendations. Other cannabinoids and drugs that potentiate endocannabinoid effects are under development.

BOTULINUM TOXIN

BTX-A is a neurotoxin produced from the bacterium *Clostidium botulinum*. BTX-A binds to receptors on presynaptic cholinergic nerve terminals and blocks the release of acetylcholine. Intramuscular injections of BTX-A is used for focal spasticity and dystonia but also, for example, for overactive bladder, hyperhidrosis, and cosmetic procedures. For the treatment of NeuP, intradermal or subcutaneous injections are used. The mechanisms by which BTX-A exerts analgesic effects are not known in detail. The effect on pain may be related to the inhibition of neurotransmitter and neuropeptide release from primary afferent terminals (e.g., substance P, CGRP [calcitonin-gene related peptide] and glutamate), reduction of TRPV1 and sodium channel activity, decreased local inflammation, or related to central effects via retrograde axonal transport.[87]

The results of BTX-A studies in NeuP are largely positive, but most studies are small and the overall quality of current evidence is weak to moderate. BTX-A is administered by subcutaneous or intradermal injections at multiple points within the area of pain in a total dose of 100–200 IU. Treatment may be repeated every 3 months. Injection into deeper structures and muscles should be avoided. Side effects include local reactions with edema, and pain upon injections. BTX-A injections are sometimes administered under nitrous oxide or other sedation to reduce injections site pain experience. BTX-A is contraindicated in patients with known hypersensitivity to the drug and in patients with myasthenia gravis or Eaton-Lambert syndrome.

N-METHYL-D-ASPARTATE RECEPTOR ANTAGONISTS

NMDA receptors for glutatame have been implicated in the development of NeuP.[88] Therefore, several oral NMDA-receptor antagonist drugs, primarily dextromethorphan and memantine, have been tested for effectiveness in this setting. With dextromethorphan in doses between 400 and 960 mg/day, two of six studies were positive. With memantine in doses between 20 and 55 mg/day, all five studies were negative. Short-term studies with intravenous administration of other NMDA antagonists such as ketamine[89,90] and amantadine have been positive,[91] but more long-term data are needed to assess the applicability of these interventions. The combined NNH with oral NMDA antagonists is around 8.7, suggesting limited tolerability, and there are currently inconclusive recommendations regarding the place of these drugs in the therapy of NeuP.

INTRAVENOUS LIDOCAINE

The NeuPSIG treatment guidelines did not consider intravenous treatment recommendations. However, it may be noted that some studies support the effectiveness of intravenous lidocaine for the treatment of NeuP.[92] Systemic lidocaine presumably works by blocking voltage-gated sodium channels; however, it is unclear whether its primary effect in NeuP is at the primary afferent fibers, or more centrally. Various dosing regimens have been implemented, most of them in the range of 3- to 5-mg/kg infused over 30–60 minutes.

Side effects usually include dizziness, perioral numbness, drowsiness, blurred vision, and (more rarely) cardiac rhythm abnormalities; these are primarily plasma concentration–dependent.

The duration of the analgesic effects is uncertain, with some studies assessing pain relief anywhere between 35 minutes and 6 hours,[93–95] while other studies reporting pain reduction in individual patients for up to 1–2 weeks.[96,97] However, it is unclear which patients are more likely to have long-term effect with this approach, since daily or weekly treatments with intravenous infusions are not a particularly feasible approach for treating chronic pain.

ORAL MEXILETINE

Mexiletine is an orally bioavailable analog of lidocaine, indicated for the treatment of cardiac arrhythmias. Among eight studies of mexiletine in NeuP, only one was positive. Oral mexiletine doses utilized in NeuP studies ranged between 225 and 1200 mg/day. Mexiletine may cause heartburn and nausea and vomiting, with at least one of these occurring in up to 40% of patients. Among common side effects are coordination problems (10%) as well as dizziness and tremor (25% of patients). Infrequent side effects include cardiac rhythm abnormalities, liver enzyme elevation (1%–2% of patients), and blood dyscarsias such as leukopenia or agranulocytosis (1 in 1000 treated patients).

Based on current evidence and risk-to-benefit considerations, the recommendation was against using mexiletine for the treatment of NeuP.

COMBINATION TREATMENTS

Most of the clinical trials address the effectiveness of a single drug—either as monotherapy or as an add-on to an existing regimen. In add-on trials, there is typically a variety of pharmacologic agents the patients may be taking, and none of the trials address how existing additional treatments affect the overall results.

In clinical practice, however, it is very common to try combinations of two or more drugs from different pharmacologic groups to improve treatment outcomes. Several controlled trials addressing combination therapy have been conducted in recent years. The five major ones address the combination of gabapentin with morphine, gabapentin-nortriptyline, nortriptyline-morphine, imipramine-pregabalin, and pregabalin-duloxetine.[30–34]

There were some differences in study designs among these, since some included placebo groups whereas others were head-to-head comparisons or compared low-dose combinations to high-dose monotherapy. In general the current evidence supports combination treatments (with drugs working by different mechanisms) for the treatment of NeuP. The effect sizes do not seem to be very large, but the combinations allow using somewhat lower doses of each drug. This results in comparable or somewhat improved side-effect profiles and in modestly improved pain outcomes.

FUTURE DIRECTIONS

Several drugs are under development for NeuP; they are aimed at a variety of receptors including, but not limited to, angiotensin II receptor type 2, TRPV1 channels, CGRP receptors, specific voltage-gated sodium channel isoforms,[98,99] and other targets. Although the preclinical-to-clinical translation in analgesic drug development has been very disappointing so far, we hope that the currently ongoing refinement in preclinical models[100–102] will help with better translation and the discovery of new NeuP medications in the near future.

Some research effort is focused on identifying patient subgroups that might be more responsive to certain treatments than others, but currently there is no strong evidence to support this approach. Several studies have been published where patients with a certain pain or sensory "phenotype" (i.e., meeting certain criteria based on psychophysical testing) were more likely to respond to treatment with oxcarbazepine,[103] intravenous lidocaine,[96] and duloxetine[104] versus patients without the specific phenotype. At this point, however, none of these approaches has been proved to be robust and reproducible, nor has any drug been approved by the FDA or the European Medicine Agency for such subgroup indications. More research is necessary to determine the feasibility and the generalizability of these personalized approaches.

KEY POINTS

- The probability of NeuP can be determined based on the following three criteria: (a) patient's history of signs, symptoms, and descriptors suggestive of pain related to a neurologic lesion or disease and a pain distribution that is consistent with the suspected lesion or disease; (b) the presence of sensory disturbances in the painful area and with a neuroanatomically plausible distribution; and (c) diagnostic tests that confirm the lesion or disease of the somatosensory nervous system.
- The majority of RCTs have been performed in DPN and PHN. Poorer effectiveness of pharmacotherapy was shown in painful radiculopathy, CIPN, and HIV sensory neuropathy.
- First-line drugs for NeuP include the TCAs, SNRIs, gabapentin, and pregabalin.
- Second-line drugs (weak GRADE recommendations for use) include oral tramadol, 8% capsaicin patches, and 5% lidocaine patches.
- Third-line drugs include strong opioids (particularly oxycodone and morphine, which are the most studied drugs) and BTX-A.
- Drugs with inconclusive GRADE recommendations include the tapentadol, most antiepileptic drugs (carbamazepine, oxcarbazepine, lamotrigine, lacosamide, topiramate, and zonisamide), capsaicin cream, topical clonidine, NMDA antagonists, and SSRI antidepressants.
- Cannabinoids and valproate are drugs with weak GRADE recommendations against their use.
- Levetiracetam and mexiletine have strong GRADE recommendations against their use in NeuP.

REFERENCES

Access the reference list online at ExpertConsult.com.

CHAPTER 51

Nonopioid Analgesics: Nonsteroidal Antiinflammatory Drugs, Cyclooxygenase-2 Inhibitors, and Acetaminophen

Bryan S. Williams, MD, MPH

Nonsteroidal antiinflammatory drugs (NSAIDs) were first developed in the late 19th century, when salicylic acid was formulated by Kolbe and colleagues, and lead to the founding of the Heyden Chemical Company. In 1897 Felix Hoffman and Arthur Eichengrün developed acetylsalicylic acid (ASA), the acetylated form of salicylic acid. This new molecule, "Aspirin," was patented by the Bayer Corporation and became the most widely used medication in the world.[1] The early class of NSAIDs were salicylates (aspirin-like medications), which have been used to treat pain conditions for thousands of years, with the Ebers papyrus recommending the application of a decoction of the dried leaves of myrtle to the abdomen and back to expel rheumatic pains from the womb. In ancient Greece, Hippocrates recommended the juices of the poplar tree to treat eye diseases and those of willow bark to relieve the pain of childbirth and reduce fever. NSAIDs are among the oldest, most successful drugs known to modern medicine in the treatment of fever, pain, and inflammation. Annually, more than 111 million prescriptions were written for NSAIDs in the United States, accounting for approximately 60% of the US over-the-counter (OTC) analgesic market.[2] In the United States it has been estimated that greater than 30 million people use NSAIDs daily. Approximately 43 million adults (19.0%) were regular aspirin users (took aspirin at least 3 times per week for more than 3 months) and more than 29 million adults (12.1%) were regular users of NSAIDs. Compared with 2005, when 12.1% were regular users of aspirin and 9.1% were regular users of NSAIDs. This was an overall increase of 57% in aspirin use and 41% in NSAID use.[3] This volume of use and the increase represent substantial concerns, which are compounded by the results of telephone surveys indicating that up to 26% of nonprescription NSAID users take more than the recommended dose.[4]

NSAIDs are a diverse group of compounds with analgesic, antipyretic, and antiinflammatory activity. In 1971 the molecular mechanism responsible for NSAID activity was discovered when John Vane demonstrated that ASA and other NSAIDs inhibited the activity of cyclooxygenase (COX) enzymes responsible for the conversion of arachidonic acid to prostanoids.[5] The prototypical NSAID, aspirin, has been largely replaced by newer NSAIDs. This class of medications contains compounds that are often chemically diverse but are grouped together based on their therapeutic actions. Many of the NSAIDs used today are available as over-the-counter (OTC) products, with more than 14 million patients using NSAIDs for the relief of symptoms associated with arthritis alone.

MECHANISM OF ACTION

Prostaglandins are important in the regulation and generation of the inflammatory response, but they are also important in the regulation of thrombocyte aggregation, the induction of pain and fever, the regulation of vessel perfusion, and many other processes.[6] These complex activities and interactions promote a range of diverse, and often opposing, physiologic and pathologic processes, including induction and resolution of the inflammatory response, protection of and damage to the gastrointestinal (GI) mucosa, promotion and inhibition of blood clotting and atherosclerosis, and renal control of blood pressure and renal disease.[7–9] Their biosynthesis is significantly increased in inflamed tissue, and they contribute to the development of the cardinal signs of acute inflammation.[10]

The mechanism of action of the NSAIDs is inhibition of prostanoid production from arachidonic acid by either reversible or irreversible acetylation of the COX (Fig. 51.1). COX is present in at least two isoforms (COX-1 and COX-2) and is dispersed throughout the body.[11] COX-1 is necessary for normal functions and is found in most cell types, mediating the production of prostaglandins, which are essential in the homeostatic processes in the stomach (gastric protection), lung, and kidney and in platelet aggregation. The inhibition of COX-1 isoform may be responsible for the adverse effects (AE) related to the nonselective NSAIDs.[12,13] It is the COX-2 isoform that is induced by proinflammatory stimuli and cytokines, causing fever, inflammation, and pain; it is thus the target of antipyresis, antiinflammation, and analgesia by NSAIDs.[11] COX-2, despite being the inducible isoform, is expressed under normal conditions in a number of tissues, which probably include brain, testis, and kidney. In inflammatory states, COX-2 becomes expressed in macrophages and other cells propagating the inflammatory process.[14] The pain associated with inflammation and prostaglandin production results from the production of prostanoids in the inflamed body tissues; these sensitize nerve endings, leading to the sensation of pain.[15]

Research indicates that NSAIDs, originally thought to possess solely peripheral inhibition of prostaglandin production, have peripheral and central mechanisms of action.[16–18] Peripherally, prostaglandins contribute to hyperalgesia by sensitizing nociceptive sensory nerve endings to other mediators (such as histamine and bradykinin) and by sensitizing nociceptors to respond to nonnociceptive stimuli (e.g., touch).[16,19] Peripheral inflammation, as a result of tissue injury, results in the release of inflammatory mediations, inducing a substantial increase in COX-2 and prostaglandin synthase expression

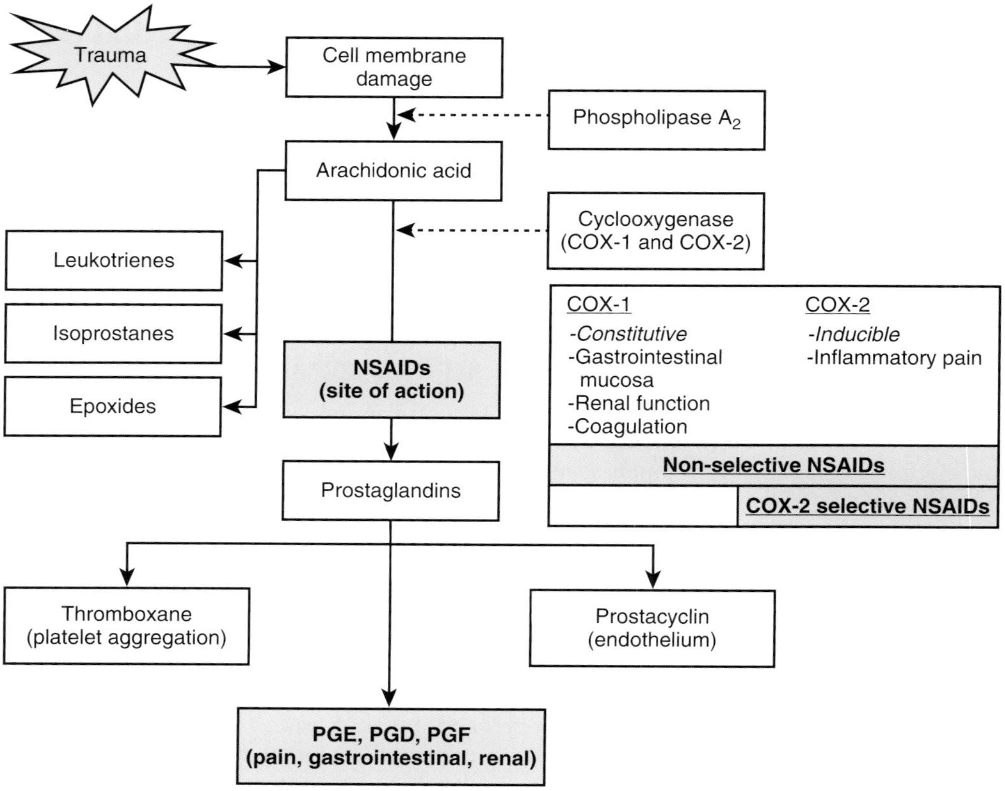

FIG. 51.1 Site of action of nonsteroidal antiinflammatory drugs (NSAIDs). *COX-1*, Cyclooxygenase-1; *COX-2*, cyclooxygenase-2; *PGD*, prostaglandin D; *PGE*, prostaglandin E; *PGF*, prostaglandin F.

in the central nervous system. Centrally, prostaglandins are recognized to have direct actions at the level of the spinal cord enhancing nociception, notably the terminals of sensory neurons in the dorsal horn.[20] Both COX-1 and COX-2 are expressed constitutively in dorsal root ganglia and spinal dorsal and ventral gray matter, but inhibition of COX-2 and not COX-1 reduces hyperalgesia.[21] Additionally, the proinflammatory cytokine interleukin-1beta (IL-1β) plays a major role in inducing COX-2 in local inflammatory cells by activating the transcription factor NF-κB. In the central nervous system (CNS) IL-1β causes increased production of COX-2 and prostaglandin E2 (PGE_2), producing hyperalgesia, but this is not the result of neural activity arising from the sensory fibers innervating the inflamed tissue or of systemic IL-1β in the plasma.[22] Peripheral inflammation possibly produces other signal molecules that enter the circulation, crossing the blood-brain barrier, and act to elevate IL-lβ, leading to COX-2 expression in neurons and nonneuronal cells in many different areas of the spinal cord.[22,23] Evidence suggests that interleukin 6 (IL-6) triggers the formation of IL-1β in the CNS, which in turn causes increased production of COX-2 and PGE_2.[22]

The analgesic effects of NSAIDs are primarily due to inhibition of the COX-2 isoform. Structurally, NSAIDs differ in their intrinsic ability to inhibit COX-1 and COX-2, with individual NSAIDs tending to be more selective for one COX enzyme than the other.[24] The inhibition of the two COX isoforms by NSAIDs may be assessed by calculation of the concentration of a drug causing 50% inhibition (IC_{50}) of the COX-2 and COX-1 and expressing the two values as a ratio. A ratio of 1.0 indicates a nonselective NSAID, whereas a ratio less than 1 is considered more selective for COX-1. NSAIDs with a COX selectivity ratio greater than 1 are considered more potent COX-2 inhibitors. NSAIDs are used therapeutically at doses that produce more than a 50% reduction in prostanoid formation, and the analgesic therapeutic plasma concentration is directly correlated with the IC_{80}.[25] Comparing the COX-2 and COX-1 IC_{50} values as a ratio provides an estimate of an NSAID's selectivity but does not indicate the actual ratio of inhibition of COX-2 to COX-1 achieved in vivo at commonly prescribed NSAID doses.[24] Comparison of the potencies of the NSAIDs against COX-1 and COX-2 at the IC_{80} value therefore appears more appropriate.[13] In fact, IC_{80} values of COX-2 inhibition of 22 different COX inhibitors have been found to correlate directly with the analgesic/antiinflammatory plasma concentrations of different COX inhibitors.[26]

PHARMACOKINETICS

Pharmacokinetic variables such as absorption, distribution, metabolism (biotransformation), and elimination, along with the dose delivered may contribute to plasma concentrations achieved after drug administration. These variables are considered a central determinant of the therapeutic and adverse responses associated with the administration of NSAIDs.[26] NSAIDs are most often delivered enterally, but intravenous (IV), intramuscular (IM), rectal, intraocular, and topical preparations are available. In general, COX inhibitors are lipid-soluble, weakly acid drugs that bind extensively to plasma proteins, with albumin as the major binding protein.[25] NSAIDs comprise a heterogeneous group of compounds in several chemical classes (Table 51.1). This chemical diversity yields a broad range

TABLE 51.1 Chemical Characteristics and Dosage of Nonsteroidal Antiinflammatory Drugs and Acetaminophen

Medication (Generic) Name	Proprietary (Trade) Name	$t_{½}$ (h)	Percent Protein Bound (%)	Usual 24-Hour Adult Dose Range	Adult Daily Dose and Frequency		Comments
					Dosage	Schedule	
Salicylates							
Aspirin	Multiple	2–3	~90	2.4–4 g	600–1500 mg	qid	Irreversible inhibitor of cyclooxygenase, cardioprotective, caution when used in combination with anticoagulants, associated with Reye syndrome in children
Buffered/enteric	Bayer, Bufferin, Ecotrin, multiple others			2.4–4 g	600–1500 mg	qid	
Propionic Acid Derivatives							
Naproxen	Naprosyn, others	14	99	750 mg–1.0 g	250, 375, 500 mg	bid	
Naproxen sodium	Aleve, Anaprox	14	99	550–1100 mg	275–550 mg	bid	—
Ibuprofen	Motrin, Advil, others	6	99	1.2–2.4 g (pain) 2.4–3.2 g (inflammation)	200–800 mg Maximum 3200 mg	qid qid	Available without prescription, parenteral formulation
Parenteral	Caldolor	~2	99	3.2 g	400–800 mg	Every 6 h	
Ketoprofen	Orudis, Oruvail	2–4	99	225 mg	50–75 mg	qid	
Oxaprozin	Daypro	40–60	99	1.2 g	1.2 g	Once daily	
Acetic Acid Derivatives							
Diclofenac	Voltaren	1–2	99	150–200 mg	50 mg 75 mg	bid–qid	Accumulates in synovial fluid, multiple formulations
Diclofenac/misoprostol	Arthrotec	1–2	99	150–200 mg *misoprostol should not exceed 800 μg*	50 mg/200 μg 75 mg/200 μg	bid–qid	Gastroprotective, contraindicated in pregnancy
Gel	Voltaren gel (1%)		99	32 g	2–4 g	qid	Decreased systemic absorption
Patch	Flector patch (1.3%)	12	99	360 mg	1 patch (180 mg)	bid	Decreased systemic absorption
Etodolac	Lodine	7	99	400–1000 mg	200–300 mg	bid, tid	15–20 mg/kg per 24 h
Indomethacin	Indocin Indocin SR, multiple others	~4	90	<200 mg	25–50 mg SR: 75 mg; rarely >150 mg	bid or tid	Limited use because of high side-effect profile in elderly
Ketorolac	Toradol	4–6	99	Oral not >40 mg/day Parenteral 30–60 mg, then 15–30 mg	Oral: 10 mg q6h for not >5 days total	qid	Limit use duration (<5 days), may precipitate renal failure in elderly or hypovolemic patients, efficacious in treating postoperative pain
Nabumetone	Relafen	24	99	1.0–1.5 g	500–750 mg	bid	Gastroprotective prodrug that is converted into the active molecule

Continued

TABLE 51.1 Chemical Characteristics and Dosage of Nonsteroidal Antiinflammatory Drugs and Acetaminophen—cont'd

Medication (Generic) Name	Proprietary (Trade) Name	$t_{½}$ (h)	Percent Protein Bound (%)	Usual 24-Hour Adult Dose Range	Adult Daily Dose and Frequency		Comments
					Dosage	Schedule	
Anthranilic Acid Derivatives							
Mefenamic acid	Ponstel	3–4	99	1.0 g	250 mg	qid	Limit use duration <7 days
Oxicam							
Meloxicam	Mobic	15–20	99	7.5–15 mg	7.5 mg (OA) 15 mg (RA)	bid qd	COX-2 selectivity at 7.5-mg dose
Coxibs (COX-2–Selective NSAIDs)							
Celecoxib	Celebrex	6–12	97	200 mg	100–200 mg 400 mg—acute pain	Once daily or bid	Gastroprotective
Aniline Derivative							
Acetaminophen	Tylenol, others	2	20–50	2–4 g	325–650 mg 650 mg–1 g	q4h qid	Hepatotoxicity in many combination medications; therefore patient education is needed

OA, *Osteoarthritis;* RA, *rheumatoid arthritis;* SR, *sustained release.*

of pharmacokinetic characteristics. Although there are many differences in the kinetics of NSAIDs, they have some general properties in common. All but one of the NSAIDs are weak organic acids as given; the exception, nabumetone, is a ketone prodrug that is metabolized to the acidic active drug.[27]

There are various classifications of NSAIDs including chemical structure (e.g., salicylic acids, acetic acids), the t1/2 delineated by those shorter (<6 hours) or longer half-lives (>10 hours) and following the development of the selective COX-2 inhibitors, the classification into traditional NSAIDs (tNSAIDs) COX-2–selective NSAIDs. Traditional NSAIDs inhibit both COX-1 and COX-2, and COX-2–selective NSAIDs preferentially inhibit COX-2.[28] Initially, only "coxibs" (e.g., celecoxib) were deemed COX-2–selective NSAIDs but the use of blood assays assessing COX-1 activity, thromboxane, COX-2 activity, and prostaglandin levels the degree of selectivity for COX-2 can be expressed in the inhibitory concentration (IC_{50}) ratios for COX-1/COX-2. The aforementioned IC_{50} is a means of comparing NSAID potency; however, more than 50% inhibition is required to achieve analgesia. It has been shown that 80% inhibition (IC_{80}) correlates with plasma levels that produce clinically relevant analgesia and that the IC_{80} may be a better measure of selectivity.[13,25,29] The IC_{80} estimates the actual ratio of inhibition of COX-2 to COX-1 achieved in vivo at commonly prescribed NSAID doses (Fig. 51.2).

ABSORPTION, DISTRIBUTION, AND ELIMINATION

Absorption

Most NSAIDs are rapidly absorbed following oral ingestion, and peak plasma concentrations usually are reached within 2–4 hours. The presence of food tends to delay absorption without affecting peak concentration. Antacids, commonly prescribed to patients on NSAID therapy, variably delay but rarely reduce absorption. Most interaction studies performed with proton pump inhibitors (PPIs) suggest that relevant changes in NSAID kinetics are unlikely.[28] Ketorolac, paracetamol, diclofenac, and ibuprofen are the few NSAIDs approved for parenteral administration, but most NSAIDs are not available in parenteral forms in the United States. Parenteral administration may have the advantage of decreased direct local toxicity in the GI tract, but parenteral ketorolac tromethamine, for example, does not decrease the risk of adverse events associated with COX-1 inhibition. Multiple NSAIDs can be formulated or compounded for transdermal delivery. These topical NSAIDs purport to have the advantage of providing local action without systemic AE. These medications, such as diclofenac in a transdermal patch, gel and topical solution, are formulated to traverse the skin to reach the adjacent joints and muscles and there exert therapeutic activity.

Distribution

The majority of NSAIDs are weakly acidic, highly bound to plasma proteins (albumin), and lipophilic. The relatively low pH of most NSAIDs determines in part their distribution as they are ionized at physiologic pHs. In areas with acidic extracellular pH values, NSAIDs may accumulate (inflamed tissue, GI tract, kidneys). NSAIDs can be classified as acidic or nonacidic based on their chemical structure, and the acidity of the drug can have an effect on its distribution. NSAIDs with acidic functional groups (e.g., diclofenac, ibuprofen, ketoprofen) and with a high degree of protein binding have been shown to selectively accumulate and persist at sites of inflammation, whereas nonacidic

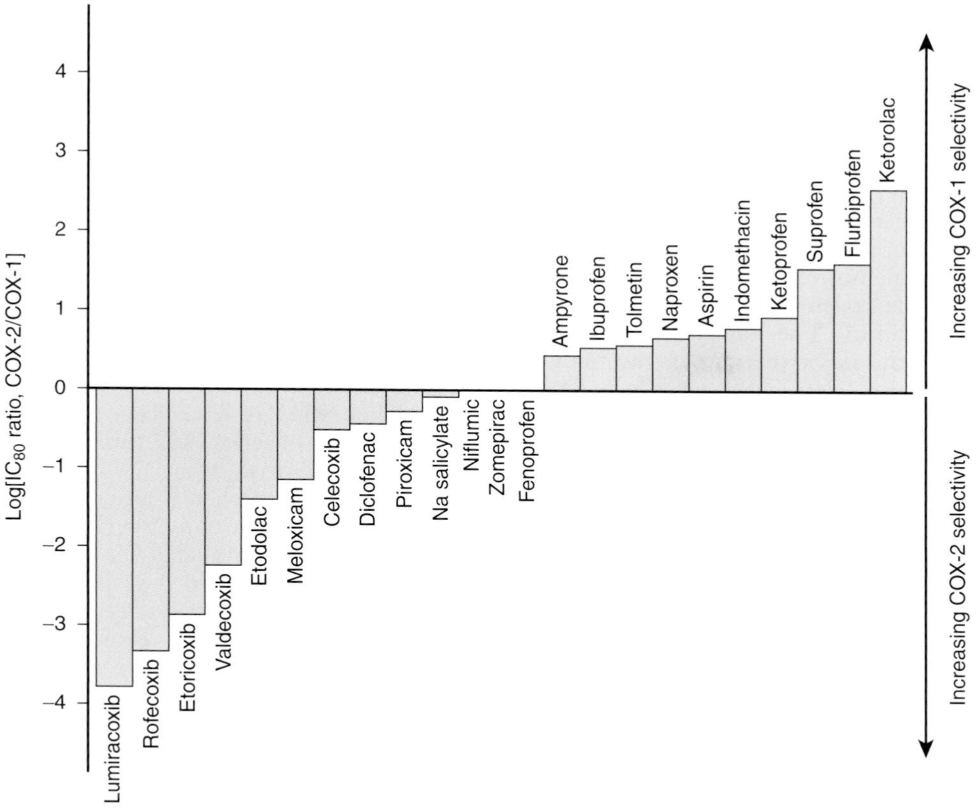

FIG. 51.2 Cyclooxygenase selectivity. (Adapted with permission from Warner TD, Mitchell JA: COX-2 selectivity alone does not define the cardiovascular risks associated with non-steroidal anti-inflammatory drugs. *Lancet.* 371(9608):270-273, 2008.)

NSAIDs (e.g., acetaminophen, celecoxib, rofecoxib) tend to be distributed homogenously throughout the body.[7] The high protein binding (≥90%) of the NSAIDs has particular relevance in the elderly population. The elderly tend to have decreased concentrations of serum albumin, resulting in higher free fractions of NSAIDs in the blood. Although such elevated free fractions may enhance efficacy, they can also increase toxicity.[30] Conditions that alter plasma protein concentration may result in an increased free drug fraction with potential toxic effects. Highly protein-bound NSAIDs have the potential to displace other drugs (e.g., warfarin) if they compete for the same binding sites, resulting in an increased plasma concentration of the displaced molecule.[28]

Elimination

The major metabolic pathway for elimination of NSAIDs is hepatic oxidation or conjugation. The cytochrome P450 (CYP) system is the enzymatic catalyst for the oxidative biotransformation NSAIDs; hepatic biotransformation followed by renal excretion is the principal route of elimination of the majority of NSAIDs.[28] NSAIDs may have active metabolites altering their half-lives, as active metabolites may be present or the metabolite is the active form when liberated from the prodrug. Also, elimination of the NSAID may determine the dosing frequency, as NSAID plasma elimination half-lives vary widely from 0.25 to 70 hours.[31] Acidic NSAIDs with short plasma half-lives (e.g., diclofenac, ibuprofen, ketoprofen) may be associated with tolerability benefits compared with drugs with long plasma half-lives because of their rapid clearance from the plasma and nontargeted tissues, allowing for the recovery of COX activity in other tissues (e.g., production of vasoprotective prostanoids by endothelial COX-2) even while the drug continues to actively inhibit COX-2 at sites of inflammation.[7] The plasma elimination half-lives of NSAIDs vary considerably, from 1 to 4 hours (ibuprofen, diclofenac) to greater than 12 hours (piroxicam, naproxen, and meloxicam). Drugs with short half-lives possess a fast onset of action and short duration of action. Drugs with long half-lives or those formulated for sustained release may have a longer duration of action but may also be associated with increased side effects, such as an NSAID-related gastropathy.[32]

SPECIFIC MEDICATIONS

There are multiple NSAIDs available in the United States and even more are available outside of the United States. Table 51.1 provides information on chemical class, pharmacologic data, and therapeutic dosages. The US Food and Drug Administration (FDA) has strengthened an existing label warning that all nonaspirin NSAIDs have an increased risk for heart attack or stroke. The following included selected representatives of different classes of NSAIDs.

SALICYLATES

Aspirin: This is the most common salicylate. It is an ester derivative of salicylic acid with medicinal properties similar to those of salicylic acid without having the bitter taste or producing the significant GI irritation of the latter. Aspirin competitively and irreversibly inhibits COX activity. This is an important distinction from all the NSAIDs because the duration of aspirin's effects is related to the turnover rate of COXs in different target tissues. The duration of effect of nonaspirin NSAIDs, which competitively inhibit the active sites of the COX enzymes, relates more directly to the time course of drug disposition.[33] The importance of enzyme turnover in relief from the action of aspirin is most notable in platelets, which, being anucleate, have a markedly limited capacity for protein synthesis. Thus this inhibition of platelet COX-1 lasts for the lifetime of the platelet. Aspirin will irreversibly block and permanently arrest the production of thromboxane A2 (TXA_2), thus inhibiting platelet aggregation for the duration of the platelets' life cycle and making aspirin a cardiovascular (CV) protective agent. Salicylates also displace other NSAIDs, such as naproxen and phenylbutazone, from plasma binding sites, thus increasing the free concentrations of those drugs and increasing the risk of toxicity.[30] Of note, salicylates have been associated with Reye syndrome, a potentially lethal pediatric disorder that produces seizures and coma. Therefore salicylates should be avoided in children with viral illnesses and associated fever.

Aspirin has three therapeutic dosage ranges: The low range (<300 mg/day) is effective in reducing platelet aggregation, intermediate doses (300–2400 mg/day) have antipyretic and analgesic effects, and high doses (2400–4000 mg/day) are used for an antiinflammatory effect.[34] The maximum recommended daily dose of aspirin for adults and children above 12 years of age is 4 g. Although aspirin is regarded as the standard against which other drugs should be compared for the treatment of rheumatoid arthritis, many clinicians favor the use of other NSAIDs perceived to have better GI tolerability.[28]

There are other salicylate NSAIDs; these include but are not limited to diflunisal, choline magnesium trisalicylate, and salsalate.

PROPRIONIC ACID

Propionic acid derivatives are traditional nonselective COX inhibitors. This class included ibuprofen, ketoprofen, naproxen, and oxaprozin.

Ibuprofen: Ibuprofen is one of the most widely used NSAIDs and one of the first to be available without a prescription (≤200 mg). It is rapidly absorbed from the upper GI tract with peak plasma levels achieved about 1–2 hours after administration. Ibuprofen is highly plasma protein–bound and has an estimated volume of distribution of 0.14 L/kg. Ibuprofen is primarily hepatically metabolized (90%) with less than 10% excreted unchanged in the urine and bile. The half-life is approximately 2 hours (2 ± ½ hour); the lack of active metabolites, OTC availability, and low toxicity potential support the use of ibuprofen in febrile and mild to moderate pain conditions. As an acidic NSAID with high protein binding, its persistence in the synovial fluid more than in the plasma allows continued antiinflammatory and analgesic activity after plasma levels have declined. Ibuprofen at a dose of 1200–2400 mg/day has a predominately analgesic effect for mild to moderate pain conditions, with a dose of 3200 mg/day recommended only under the continued care of clinical professionals. Even at antiinflammatory doses of more than 1600 mg/day, renal side effects are almost exclusively encountered in patients with low intravascular volume and low cardiac output, particularly in the elderly.[35] The effectiveness of ibuprofen has been demonstrated in the treatment of headache and migraine, menstrual pain, and acute postoperative pain.[36–38] Ibuprofen is available in OTC form, by prescription, and in combination with opioid medications, decongestants, and antihistamines. As a parenteral formulation, it has shown efficacy in postoperative pain reduction in multiple studies.[39] Ibuprofen, consistent with other NSAIDs, has a boxed warning from the FDA for increased risk of serious CV thrombotic events, myocardial infarction, and stroke.

Naproxen: Naproxen is a nonprescription NSAID that first became available as a prescription-only medication but it has now become available OTC. However, a controlled-release tablet (Naprelan) is available by prescription only. Naproxen is fully absorbed after enteral administration and has a half-life of 14 hours. Peak concentrations in plasma occur within 2–4 hours and are somewhat more rapid after the administration of naproxen sodium. It is fully absorbed after enteral administration and has a half-life of 14 hours, but steady-state serum levels require more than 48 hours. Naproxen has a volume of distribution of 0.16 L/kg. At therapeutic levels, naproxen is more than 99% albumin-bound, but this may be increased in the elderly in relation to the decrement in renal function.[28] Naproxen has been formulated in combination, including the fixed-dose combination of sumatriptan/naproxen sodium (Treximet), approved for the acute treatment of migraine-type headaches.[40] In contrast to other tNSAIDS, naproxen has been shown to be unassociated with an increased risk of major vascular events. A meta-analysis of over 600 clinical trials comprising more than 300,000 participants revealed a dose-related risk of major cardiovascular events with NSAIDs (tNSAIDS and coxibs) but not with naproxen.[24,41] An ongoing study (completion 2016), the Prospective Randomized Evaluation of Celecoxib Integrated Safety versus Ibuprofen or Naproxen (PRECISION) study, will provide further data on the comparative CV safety of celecoxib, ibuprofen, and naproxen.

Ketoprofen: The pharmacologic properties of ketoprofen are similar to other propionic acid derivatives, although the different formulations differ in their release characteristics. Peak plasma levels were achieved at about 1–2 hours after oral administration, with a half-life of approximately 2 hours. Ketoprofen has high plasma protein binding (98%–99%) and an estimated volume of distribution of 0.11 L/kg. Ketoprofen is conjugated with glucuronic acid in the liver, and the conjugate is excreted in the urine. The glucuronic acid moiety can be converted back to the parent compound. Thus the metabolite serves as a potential reservoir for the parent drug, which may be important in persons with renal insufficiency. Ketoprofen is available by prescription in multiple dose formulations (i.e., immediate release and extended release). The usual starting dose of ketoprofen is 50 or 75 mg with immediate-release capsules being administered every 6–8 hours or 200 mg with extended-release capsules being given once daily.

The maximum dose is 300 mg/day of immediate-release capsules or 200 mg/day of extended-release capsules. Ketoprofen has a comparatively short half-life, potentially minimizing activity at COX-2, allowing COX-2 recovery; however, ketoprofen is associated with increased side effects (e.g., mild gastropathy).[28] Although not approved by the FDA for transdermal prescription issuance, ketoprofen has been formulated for transdermal application. The topical application facilitates a reduction in systematic concentration while local (site of application) concentrations remain therapeutic. Transdermal application of ketoprofen has provided more efficacy than placebo at reducing pain in patients with a variety of painful soft tissue/musculoskeletal conditions.[42,43]

OTHER PROPIONIC ACID DERIVATIVES

Fenoprofen, flurbiprofen, and oxaprozin are additional propionic acid derivatives. All of these medications except oxaprozin have similar pharmacologic properties, including time to peak plasma levels, protein binding, and half-life. Oxaprozin has a time to peak concentration of 3–4 hours and a half-life of 40–60 hours (see Table 51.1). Oxaprozin diffuses readily into inflamed synovial tissues after oral administration and is capable of inhibiting both anandamide hydrolase in neurons and NF-kappaB activation in inflammatory cells, which are crucial for the synthesis of proinflammatory and histotoxic mediators in inflamed joints.[44–46]

ACETIC ACID DERIVATIVES

Acetic acid derivatives are traditional, nonselective COX inhibitors. This class includes diclofenac, etodolac, ketorolac, tolmentin, sulindac and indomethacin.

Indomethacin: Indomethacin is a potent nonselective COX inhibitor introduced in 1963. It was widely used as an antiinflammatory medication but has fallen out of favor with the advent of safer alternatives. The tendency toward AE of indomethacin compared with other commercially available NSAIDs has limited its indication and duration of use. In the United States it is available only by prescription. Oral indomethacin has excellent bioavailability, with peak concentrations occurring 1–2 hours after dosing. Indomethacin is 90% bound to plasma proteins and tissues. The half-life in plasma is variable, perhaps because of enterohepatic cycling, but averages about 2.5 hours.[28] Complaints associated with GI irritation are common, including diarrhea, and ulcerative lesions are a contraindication to indomethacin use. A meta-analysis of 280 placebo-controlled trials of NSAIDs showed that indomethacin posed an "intermediate risk" of GI irritation, with coxibs posing a lower risk and medications such as ketorolac posing the highest risk.[47] In addition to gastropathy, indomethacin is associated with central nervous system adverse events, with severe frontal headache occurring in 25%–50% of patients who take the drug for long periods. Dizziness, vertigo, light-headedness, and mental confusion may also occur.[28] Indomethacin is available in enteral and parenteral formulation and is indicated for the treatment of acute mild to moderate pain. Parenteral indomethacin has an indication for the closure of persistent patent ductus arteriosus, but its side effect profile limits other uses of the parenteral formulation.

Etodolac: Etodolac has some degree of COX-2 selectivity, conferring less gastric irritation compared with other NSAIDs.[13,28] After oral administration, peak serum concentrations are attained within 2 hours. Etodolac is highly bound to plasma proteins, with an estimated volume of distribution of 0.4 L/kg. It is excreted primarily in the urine, and 60% of a dose is recovered within 24 hours. The half-life of etodolac is 6–8 hours irrespective of dosage form; therefore it attains steady state quickly with only a modest degree of accumulation with chronic administration.[48] Etodolac is available by prescription; in a review of nine studies (1459 participants), etodolac showed usefulness as an analgesic in postoperative pain, with efficacy similar to single dose paracetamol 1000 mg and celecoxib 200 mg.[49] Additionally, in providing relief of postsurgical pain, etodolac 100–200 mg was approximately equivalent to aspirin 650 mg, although etodolac had a longer duration of action.[50] Etodolac 600 mg/day showed substantially better gastroduodenal tolerability than ibuprofen (2.4 g/day), indomethacin (200 mg/day), or naproxen (1 g/day). A review of etodolac safety data from more than 3000 patients enrolled in double-blind and open-label clinical trials and from more than 8000 patients taking etodolac in postmarketing surveillance studies found that the rates of abdominal pain and dyspepsia were similar to those with several other NSAIDs and that GI ulceration occurs in less than 0.3% of patients taking etodolac.[51,52]

Nabumetone: Nabumetone is a ketone prodrug with weak COX inhibitory activity in vitro; in vivo, however, it undergoes hepatic biotransformation to the active component, 6-methoxy-2-naphthylacetic acid (6-MNA), which is a relatively selective COX-2 inhibitor that has antiinflammatory and analgesic properties.[53] Nabumetone is highly bound to plasma proteins and has an estimated volume of distribution of 0.68 L/kg. Nabumetone is excreted primarily in the urine and has a half-life of approximately 20–24 hours, achieving substantial concentrations in synovial fluid.[53] The long plasma half-life of 6-MNA and its persistence in synovial fluid facilitate a once-daily dosage regimen. Compared with other NSAIDs, nabumetone has tended to show efficacy[54] and tolerability in the treatment of arthritis,[55,56] but studies are lacking in the treatment of acute postoperative pain.[57] Nabumetone compares favorably with other NSAIDs with respect to its renal and GI AE profile. The most frequent AE are those commonly seen with COX inhibitors; they include diarrhea, dyspepsia, headache, abdominal pain, and nausea. In common with other COX inhibitors, nabumetone may increase the risk of GI AE, but studies have reported incidents equal to other COX-2 selective inhibitors but considerably lower than for nonselective COX inhibitors. This has been attributed mainly to the nonacidic chemical properties of nabumetone but also to its COX-1/COX-2 inhibitor profile.[58]

Ketorolac: Ketorolac is an NSAID with activity at COX-1 and COX-2 enzymes, thus blocking prostaglandin production. After oral administration, peak serum concentrations are attained within 0.5–1 hour.[59] Ketorolac is highly bound to plasma proteins and has an estimated volume of distribution of 0.28 L/kg. Ketorolac is excreted primarily in the urine and has a half-life of approximately 5–6 hours in healthy subjects. Since its approval, it has drawn more favor as a potent analgesic agent because of its moderately effective antiinflammatory effects.[28] Multiple studies have investigated the analgesic potency of ketorolac; in animal models, the analgesic potency has been estimated to be between 180 and 800 times that of aspirin.[59,60] Compared with morphine, ketorolac 30 mg IM has been shown to be equivalent to IV morphine 2–4 mg, 12 mg morphine IM, and 100 mg meperidine IM.[59,61] Ketorolac is available for enteral, ophthalmic, and parenteral administration. An intranasal formulation (Sprix) is available for use in the United States. This may be more effective than administration by oral routes in providing improved absorption, avoidance of first-pass effects, GI AE, and improved patient compliance.[62,63] It has been observed that the mean values for total body clearance were decreased by about 50% and that the half-life was approximately doubled in patients with renal impairment compared with healthy control subjects.[64] Ketorolac may precipitate or exacerbate renal failure in hypovolemic patients, the elderly, or especially those with underlying renal dysfunction. Ketorolac is recommended for limited use (3–5 days).

Diclofenac: Diclofenac was introduced in 1973 and has become the most widely prescribed NSAID.[5] It is available by prescription in many formulations (enteral, parenteral, transdermal, and ophthalmic). It has COX-2 selectivity and its potency against COX-2 is substantially greater than that of indomethacin, naproxen, or several other NSAIDs; it is similar to celecoxib.[28,65] Diclofenac is rapidly absorbed after oral administration but may vary between different salt formulations. Substantial first-pass metabolism occurs; only about 50%–60% of diclofenac is available systemically.[5,28,66] After oral administration, peak serum concentrations are attained within 2–3 hours but may vary secondary to differences in GI pH, partial precipitation of the dose in the acidic conditions in the stomach, variable timing in gastric emptying, and enterohepatic circulation.[5] Diclofenac is highly bound to plasma proteins and has an estimated volume of distribution of 0.12 L/kg. Diclofenac is excreted primarily in the urine (65%) and as bile conjugates (35%). Uniquely, diclofenac accumulates in inflamed tissues and synovial fluid after oral administration,[66] which may explain why its duration of therapeutic effect is considerably longer than its plasma half-life of 1–2 hours. Diclofenac administered as the sodium salt was detectable in synovial fluid for up to 11 hours following administration of a 50-mg enteric-coated tablet and up to 25 hours following administration of a 100-mg slow-release tablet.[5] Diclofenac sodium, usually distributed in enteric-coated tablets, resists dissolution in low-pH gastric environments, releasing instead in the duodenum.[67] Diclofenac potassium is more water-soluble and was considered to provide more rapid dissolution and faster absorption with the aim of releasing the active drug in the stomach to permit rapid uptake and prompt pain relief. Topical preparations are available with the purpose of limiting systemic exposure, reducing the AE, but providing localized analgesia and pain reduction. Topically, diclofenac has a much smaller total systemic absorption (approximately 3%–5%) than oral diclofenac products and less than 10% of the C_{max} achieved following oral administration.[5,68,69] On the other hand, interstitial concentrations of diclofenac in muscle tissue are usually higher after topical treatment than after oral administration of NSAIDs.[5,68] The injectable formulations of diclofenac have been developed, with Dyloject receiving FDA approval for moderate pain, principally postoperative pain. Diclofenac has been formulated in fixed-dose combinations including diclofenac sodium-misoprostol (Arthrotec), for patients at high risk for developing NSAID-induced gastric ulcers, erosion, or similar complications.

ANTHRANILIC ACID

Mefenamic acid: Arthranilic acid, also known as mefenamic acid, is a weak organic acid. Peak plasma levels are attained in 2–4 hours and its elimination half-life is approximately 2 hours. More than 90% has been reported to be bound to albumin; it has an estimated volume of distribution of 1.06 L/kg.[70,71] The mechanism of action, like that of other NSAIDS, is the inhibition of prostaglandin synthesis. In addition, however, mefenamic acid appears to reduce the activity of prostaglandins, possibly by binding to and blocking prostaglandin receptors on cells in a dose-dependent fashion.[72,73] Mefanamic acid is available by prescription and has potential utility in its ability to affect smooth muscle and decreasing uterine resting pressure. It also has a dose-dependent effect for relaxing tonic uterine contraction.[72] Its use in clinical medicine has declined, since mefenamic acid may offer no clinical advantage over other NSAIDs.[28]

OXICAM

Meloxicam: Oxicam, or meloxicam, is an enolic acid derivative that has relative COX-2 selectivity. Meloxicam has high plasma protein binding (99%) and an estimated volume of distribution of 0.1–0.2 L/kg.[74] Its terminal elimination half-life is approximately 20 hours, making it suitable for once-daily dosing. Its steady-state drug plasma concentrations are reached within 3–5 days.[75] Although there is little evidence for the efficacy of this drug in the postoperative setting (lack of data),[76,77] meloxicam has shown efficacy in the treatment of osteoarthritis.[78] Additionally, an oral formulation of meloxicam (SoluMatrix) has been developed, aimed at decreasing the dose-related risk for serious GI, CV, and renal adverse events associated with NSAIDs.[79]

CYCLOOXYGENASE-2 INHIBITORS

All NSAIDs are COX-2 inhibitors with varying degrees of COX-1 activity. The inhibition of the constitutive COX-1 isoform can be described as a side effect of NSAID use and the inhibition of COX-2 as the purposeful intent. Inhibition of COX-1 can alter homeostatic functions, such as protection of the GI mucosa and platelet activation. The COX-2 inhibitors as a class were developed to decrease the risk of injury to the GI tract associated with the inhibition of COX-1 activity while taking advantage of the COX-2 inhibition resulting in antiinflammatory, analgesic, and antipyretic properties. Approved by the FDA in 1998, celecoxib was the first selective COX-2 inhibitor indicated for the treatment of osteoarthritis, rheumatoid arthritis, ankylosing spondylitis, and acute pain conditions. Two other coxibs were developed and brought to market, but owing to an increased risk of CV side effects, rofecoxib and valdecoxib were withdrawn. To date, celecoxib is the only coxib approved by the FDA for use in the United States, although others are available for use in Europe (e.g., etoricoxib, parecoxib, lumiracoxib).

Celecoxib: Currently celecoxib is the only selective COX-2 inhibitor available in the United States. It is 30-fold more selective for COX-2 than COX-1, compared with 0.5-fold for ibuprofen, 0.7-fold for naproxen, 1.9-fold for indomethacin, 18-fold for meloxicam, 29-fold for diclofenac, and 267-fold for rofecoxib.[80] Peak serum concentrations are attained 2–4 hours after administration. Celecoxib is highly bound to plasma proteins, is excreted primarily by hepatic metabolism, and has a half-life of approximately 11.2 and 15.6 hours.[81] Additionally, NSAID-induced GI complications are among the most common serious drug-related adverse events, but celecoxib preferentially inhibits the inducible COX-2 isoform and not the constitutive COX-1 isoform, thus conferring a gastroprotective effect. When used for a long time, celecoxib has fewer side effects associated with the digestive system than other NSAIDs.[82] There is no evidence to suggest that differences in the selectivity of these agents toward one COX isoenzyme is of importance with respect to analgesia, as currently all drugs used for analgesia are COX-2 inhibitors.[83–85] Additionally there are no clear differences in efficacy for pain relief associated with different NSAIDs, although celecoxib was associated with a lower risk of ulcer complications compared with nonselective NSAIDs.[86] Celecoxib, which has a relatively slow rate of absorption, can be administered at standard doses to effectively treat osteoarthritis pain, but it is "not ideal" for the treatment of acute pain, since it takes considerable time for absorption and often requires a loading dose to achieve clinically meaningful analgesia.[83] Although celecoxib has been shown to be effective in treating acute postoperative pain,[82] its primary indication is for the treatment of osteoarthritis and rheumatoid arthritis.

As stated earlier celecoxib is the sole selective COX-2 inhibitor available in the United States secondary to increased cardiovascular risk associated with the withdrawn rofecoxib and valdecoxib. The Prospective Randomized Evaluation of Celecoxib Integrated Safety versus Ibuprofen or Naproxen (PRECISION) Study assessed the noninferiority of celecoxib compared to two most commonly prescribed traditional NSAIDs (ibuprofen & naproxen) with regard to the primary composite outcome of cardiovascular death (including hemorrhagic death), nonfatal myocardial infarction, or nonfatal stroke. Although the study recorded a high study discontinuation rate (69%), the findings suggest that modest-dose celecoxib was noninferior to ibuprofen or naproxen in regard to cardiovascular safety.[86a]

ACETAMINOPHEN

Acetaminophen (paracetamol, or APAP) is an analgesic and antipyretic medication that produces its analgesic effect by inhibiting central prostaglandin synthesis with minimal inhibition of peripheral prostaglandin synthesis.[28,87] Acetaminophen and NSAIDs have important differences, such as acetaminophen's weak antiinflammatory effects and its generally poor ability to inhibit COX in the presence of high concentrations of peroxides, as are found at sites of inflammation.[28,87] It also does not have AE on platelet function[88] or the gastric mucosa.[87] After oral administration, peak serum concentrations are attained within 0.5–1.0 hour. A small portion of acetaminophen is bound to plasma proteins (20%–50%), and elimination from the body is primarily by the formation of glucuronide and sulfate conjugates in a dose-dependent manner.[28] The half-life of acetaminophen is approximately 2–3 hours in healthy subjects. Acetaminophen is perhaps the safest and most cost-effective nonopioid analgesic when it is administered in analgesic doses.[89]

The maximum daily dose in healthy adults is 4000 mg/day. The FDA has reduced the maximum daily dose of acetaminophen in fixed-dose prescription medications and OTC fixed-dose medications to no more than 325 mg per unit dose, but concern remains for fixed-dose OTC vitamins, minerals, other dietary supplements containing acetaminophen and the potential for toxicity by inadvertent cumulative exposure. In elderly persons, acetaminophen may be recommended as first-line therapy for pain,[26,90] and tNSIADs should be used with caution because drug interactions and AE. Although often labeled as a first-line medication for pain attenuation, acetaminophen has shown minimal efficacy in treating osteoarthritis; it is ineffective in the treatment of low back pain[91] but was shown to offer effective pain relief for about half of participants experiencing moderate to severe pain after surgery.[92]

In 2010, the FDA approved the IV formulation of acetaminophen (OFIRMEV), indicated for the management of mild to moderate pain, management of moderate to severe pain with adjunctive opioid analgesics, and reduction of fever. Prior to the approval of OFIRMEV, propacetamol, a water-soluble prodrug of acetaminophen, was available in Europe as a parenteral form yielding 0.5 g acetaminophen per 1 g of propacetamol.[93] The use of IV acetaminophen has been studied in acute postoperative pain, revealing rapid and effective analgesia in patients with moderate to severe pain after surgery.[94,95] In comparing enteral and parenteral acetaminophen, no clear indication exists for preferential prescribing of IV acetaminophen.[96,97] One of the main clinical and practical advantages associated with IV administration is the faster onset of analgesia relative to an equivalent oral dose. In addition, IV administration is associated with more predictable pharmacokinetic and pharmacodynamic behavior. Another potential advantage of IV administration is avoidance of first-pass hepatic exposure through the portal circulation, which may reduce the potential for hepatic injury.[96]

SAFETY, TOXICITY, AND ADVERSE EFFECTS

Although NSAIDs are the most widely used OTC medications, with a long history of use, research, and medication advancements, NSAIDs remain a source of AE. NSAIDs not only share therapeutic actions but also AE, which include GI ulceration and bleeding, disturbance of platelet function, sodium and water retention, nephrotoxicity, and hypersensitivity reactions.[98] In fact, in 1995, the FDA requested that all prescription medications containing NSAIDs provide a warning of "potential serious adverse CV events and the serious, and potentially life-threatening GI AE associated with the use of this class of

TABLE 51.2 Risk Factors for Nonsteroidal Antiinflammatory Drug–Induced Gastrointestinal and Cardiovascular Complications[4,7]

Risk Factors for Gastrointestinal Side Effects	Risk Factors for Cardiovascular Side Effects
• Age > 65 years	• Unstable angina
• Concomitant *Helicobacter pylori* infection	• Myocardial infarction
• Receiving hemodialysis	• Recent cardiac bypass surgery
• High-dose or multiple NSAID use	• Recent cardiovascular stent placement
• History of upper gastrointestinal injury	• High-dose NSAID use
• Anticoagulant use	• Hypertension
• Oral corticosteroid use; prednisone	• Heart failure
• Selective serotonin reuptake inhibitor use	—
• Cigarette smoking	—
• Alcohol consumption	—

NSAID, *Nonsteroidal antiinflammatory drugs.*

drugs." In 2005, the FDA added a boxed warning ("black box warning") to all prescription NSAIDs, with labeling changes to include a warning, highlighting the potential for increased risk of CV events and the well-described, serious, potentially life-threatening GI bleeding associated with their use. In 2015, the FDA strengthened an existing label warning that nonaspirin NSAIDs increase the chance of a heart attack or stroke, requiring updates to the drug labels of all prescription NSAIDs. Additionally, similar updates to the existing myocardial infarction and stroke risk information for OTC nonaspirin NSAIDs was requested. The most common adverse drug reactions to NSAIDs are GI, renal, dermatologic, and neuropsychiatric.[30,99,100] However, most clinically significant complications involve the GI, renal, hematologic, and hepatic organ systems.[30] Available data from observational studies strongly suggest that GI and CV events and renal failure are related to total daily dose in patients treated with NSAIDs.[24] In particular, as the NSAID dose increased, CV risks increased for all NSAIDs evaluated with the exception of naproxen.[24,41] Also observed is a twofold to threefold increased risk of GI complications with the use of high versus low to medium doses of individual NSAIDs with the exception of celecoxib, for which dose-related effects were not demonstrated.[24,47]

GASTROINTESTINAL EFFECTS

GI bleeding is one of the most frequently reported significant complications of NSAID use occurring with the use of OTC and prescription NSAIDs. GI complications are generally thought to be mediated primarily through inhibition of mucosal COX-1 and resultant suppression of prostaglandin production. However, COX-2 inhibition and other mechanisms, such as changes in the bacterial microbiome in the gut or the generation of free radicals, are also possibly involved.[4] Several factors are associated with increased risk of developing significant GI-related AE (Table 51.2). In addition to patient risk factors, pharmacokinetic properties of the drugs have importance in adverse events. For example, NSAIDs with a long half-life or slow-release formulation are associated with a greater risk of upper GI bleeding/perforation.[26] Also NSAIDs that produce a profound and coincident inhibition of both COX-1 and COX-2 isozymes (which translates into deficiency of prostanoid generation in the GI tract) at therapeutic doses are the most toxic drugs for the GI tract. This is thought to be related to the role that COX-1 and COX-2 play in prostanoid biosynthesis and maintenance of gastric mucosal integrity.[26] The coadministration of NSAIDs with PPIs is a well-documented and effective, although underutilized, approach to reduce endoscopic damage and controlling dyspeptic symptoms associated with the use of NSAIDs.[4] There are several fixed-dose preparations, including NSAID plus PPI, NSAID plus H_2 receptor antagonist, and NSAID plus misoprostol, a synthetic prostaglandin E1 analog. Additionally, the selective COX-2 inhibitor celecoxib can be employed for its gastroprotective properties. Comparisons of coxib versus fixed-dose preparations have shown variability between groups and subgroups.[85,101] For patients with both low GI and CV risks, any tNSAID alone may be acceptable. For those with low GI and high CV risks, naproxen may be preferred because of its potential lower CV risk compared with other tNSAIDs or COX-2 selective inhibitors, but celecoxib at the lowest approved dose (200 mg once daily) may be acceptable. In patients with high GI risk, if CV risk is low, a COX-2 selective inhibitor alone or tNSAID with a PPI appears to offer similar protection from upper GI events. However, only celecoxib will reduce mucosal harm throughout the entire GI tract. When both GI and CV risks are high, the optimal strategy is to avoid NSAID therapy if at all possible.[102]

RENAL EFFECTS

NSAIDs can decrease renal function and cause renal failure. Renal impairment has been reported to occur in as many as 18% of patients using ibuprofen, whereas acute renal failure has been shown to occur in about 6% of patients using NSAIDs.[30,103,104] The proposed mechanism is a reduction in prostaglandin production exacerbating the reduction of renal blood flow with subsequent medullary ischemia.[105] The primary NSAID-related renal abnormalities are fluid and electrolyte disturbances, acute deterioration of renal function, nephrotic syndrome with interstitial nephritis, and papillary necrosis.[106] Acute renal failure may occur with any COX-2-selective or nonselective NSAID.[107] The risk factors for NSAID-induced renal toxicity include chronic NSAID use, the use of high-dose or multiple NSAIDs, volume depletion, congestive heart failure, vascular disease, hyperreninemia, shock, sepsis, systemic lupus erythematous, hepatic disease, sodium depletion, nephrotic syndrome, diuresis, concomitant drug therapy (diuretics, angiotensin-converting enzyme inhibitors, beta-blockers, potassium supplements), and advanced age.[108]

CARDIOVASCULAR EFFECTS

The imbalance between COX-1 and COX-2 inhibition contributes to increased CV risk. COX-2 selectivity, reducing gastropathy, was the basis for the development of the coxibs. Selective COX-2 inhibitors were developed to preferentially inhibit COX-2 and thus afford the gastroprotective effect of COX-1. The inhibition of COX, without selectivity, equally reduces the production of TX and prostacyclin. TX functions as a vasoconstrictor and *facilitates* platelet aggregation. TXA_2, produced by activated platelets, has prothrombotic properties, stimulating the activation of new platelets as well as increasing platelet aggregation. Endothelial-derived prostacyclin (PGI_2) functions in concert with TX, primarily *inhibiting* platelet activation, thus preventing the formation of a hemostatic plug. Nonselective NSAIDs inhibit both COX-1 and COX-2, thus reducing the production of TX and prostacyclin. The imbalance of TX and prostacyclin may lead to a thrombogenic condition. Although selective COX-2 inhibitors have no effect on TxA_2 production, selective COX-2 inhibitors may tip the natural balance between prothrombotic TxA_2 and antiinflammatory PGI_2 by decreasing PGI_2 production, which could potentially increase the possibility of a thrombotic CV event.[109] Individual NSAIDs causing a degree of COX-2 inhibition greater than 90% are associated with a significant increase in nonfatal myocardial infarction.[26] Rofecoxib was 267-fold more selective for COX-2 than COX-1.[80] The VIGOR[110] study compared rofecoxib against naproxen and showed a twofold reduction of GI events in favor of this coxib but a fivefold increase in the incidence of myocardial infarction.[111] In the Cardiovascular Events in Colorectal Adenoma Chemoprevention (APPROVe) trial,[112] the use of rofecoxib was associated with increased myocardial infarctions (46 vs. over 3327 patient-years of follow-up) with a persisting risk up to 1 year after interruption of therapy.[111] In addition to the imbalance in COX inhibition by selective COX-2 agents, the nonaspirin NSAIDs pose an increased CV risk compared with aspirin. Aspirin irreversibly acetylates platelet-dependent COX-1, reducing serum TX levels and platelet aggregation for the life of the platelet. Studies in vivo have shown that 95% suppression of platelet COX-1 activity is needed to inhibit TX A2-dependent platelet aggregation.[113] Although this degree of inhibition is obtained with low-dose aspirin, other nonselective NSAIDs produce variable COX inhibition ranging from 50% to 95% in a reversible time-dependent fashion. This inhibitory pattern may be insufficient to provide cardioprotection throughout the dosing interval and may explain the greater CV protection provided by aspirin; unlike other NSAIDs, aspirin is much less dependent on pharmacokinetics.[111] Naproxen is the exception in that is has shown CV protection by COX-1 inhibition similar to aspirin and superior CV safety than diclofenac, ibuprofen, and high-dose coxib.[111,114] In addition to the pharmacokinetic properties of the individual NSAIDs, additional factors may contribute to the risk of CV events (see Table 51.2).

MEDICATION SELECTION

Many factors determine the selection of an NSAID, and balancing risk versus benefit may influence the choice. The decisive factors may include efficacy, safety, antecedents, and/or GI pathology of the patient; acute or chronic process; and type of inflammatory process.[115] The goal in selection is to obtain a level of efficacy while limiting or mitigating adverse events. The mechanism of action that produces NSAID efficacy (COX inhibition) is the same mechanism that produces an adverse event associated with NSAID use. Exploiting the pharmacokinetic and pharmacodynamic factors of the individual NSAID while considering the patient's potential risk factors can assist in determining the most appropriate NSAID. The IC_{80} estimates the actual ratio of inhibition of COX-2 to COX-1 achieved in vivo at commonly prescribed NSAID doses. IC_{80} concentrations of NSAIDs for COX-2 have been found to correlate with analgesia.[24,25] In addition to IC_{80} concentration, the time to attainment of therapeutic levels/concentration contributes to the rapid amelioration of painful conditions. The pharmacokinetics associated with the time to maximum concentration may be associated with the formulation of the medication (immediate release vs. extended release), and this property of the individual NSAID cannot be overlooked. Diclofenac potassium has a time to maximum concentration substantially shorter (range 0.63–1.26 hours) than that of a diclofenac sodium enteric-coated 50-mg tablet (range 1.13–2.75 hours) secondary to the absorption characteristics.[5] The amount of time needed for the drug plasma concentration to be reduced by half is the elimination half-life, which can be extrapolated to the duration of action. However, this is not always the case, as with diclofenac, which has short half-life of 1–2 hours but maintains durable inhibition at the active site of COX enzymes.[24] Acidic NSAIDs with a high degree of protein binding (diclofenac) may remain in inflamed tissues or synovial fluid for a longer time than in the plasma.[7] As stated, the mechanisms by which NSAIDs have their effect are equally important in AE.

The pharmacokinetic properties and formulations of individual NSAIDs may increase these AE. Drugs with a long plasma half-life and/or slow-release formulations have been associated with an increased risk of upper GI bleeding, likely due to persistent exposure of the GI tract to circulating NSAIDs.[7] Those NSAIDs with half-lives of at least 12 hours were associated with a greater relative risk for developing GI events compared with NSAIDs with half-lives of less than 12 hours.[24] Naproxen, with a half-life of approximately 12 hours, has an increased risk associated with continued use, whereas diclofenac (half-life, 1–2 hours) has a decreased associated risk.[47] Additionally, NSAIDs with half-lives of less than 4 hours did not significantly increase the risk of compromising impaired renal function.[24]

SUMMARY

NSAIDs are a diverse group of compounds that are useful for their analgesic, antipyretic, and antiinflammatory activity. The same mechanisms by which NSAIDs have effect are those by which side effects arise. In an attempt to mitigate GI complications, coxibs were developed; it was the withdrawal of rofecoxib in 2004 that prompted the strengthening of labeling on NSAIDs by the FDA in 2005 because of CV risks associated with NSAID use. NSAIDs are a cornerstone of the attenuation of painful conditions and appropriate medication therapy considers the lowest effective dose necessary for efficacy while also minimizing the risk of adverse events. This chapter has provided an overview of the NSAIDs and acetaminophen. Effective use of the tools in our armamentarium requires knowledge of the tools and how to use them.

KEY POINTS

- Research indicates that NSAIDs have peripheral and central mechanisms of action. Peripherally, prostaglandins contribute to hyperalgesia by sensitizing nociceptive sensory nerve endings to other mediators and by sensitizing nociceptors to respond to nonnociceptive stimuli. Centrally, prostaglandins have direct actions at the level of the spinal cord, thus enhancing nociception, notably at the terminals of sensory neurons in the dorsal horn.
- Parenteral administration of NSAIDs has the advantage of decreased direct local toxicity in the GI tract, but this does not decrease the risk of adverse events associated with COX-1 inhibition.
- Aspirin competitively and irreversibly inhibits COX activity. The duration of aspirin's effects is related to the turnover rate of COXs in different target tissues. In contrast, the duration of effect of nonaspirin NSAIDs relates more directly to the time course of drug disposition.
- Salicylates have been associated with Reye syndrome, a potentially lethal pediatric disorder that produces seizures and coma. Therefore salicylates should be avoided in children with viral illnesses and associated fever.
- Ibuprofen, an acidic NSAID with high protein binding, persists in the synovial fluid more than in the plasma, allowing continued antiinflammatory and analgesic activity after its plasma levels have declined.
- In contrast to other NSAIDs, naproxen has been shown not to be associated with increased risk of major vascular events.
- Ketoprofen is conjugated with glucuronic acid in the liver, and the conjugate is excreted in the urine. The glucuronic acid moiety can be converted back to the parent compound, serving as a potential reservoir for the parent drug. This may be important in patients with renal insufficiency.
- Parenteral indomethacin has an indication for the closure of persistent patent ductus arteriosus, but its side-effect profile limits other uses of the parenteral formulation.
- The analgesic potency of ketorolac has been estimated to be between 180 and 800 times that of aspirin.
- Diclofenac, the most widely prescribed NSAID, has COX-2 selectivity, and its potency against COX-2 is substantially greater than that of indomethacin, naproxen, or several other NSAIDs and is similar to that of celecoxib.
- There is no evidence to suggest that differences in the selectivity of these agents toward one COX isoenzyme is of importance with respect to analgesia, as currently all drugs used for analgesia are COX-2 inhibitors.
- The FDA has reduced the maximum daily dose of acetaminophen in fixed-dose prescription medications and OTC fixed-dose medications to no more than 325 mg per unit dose. Concerns remain for fixed-dose OTC vitamins, minerals, other dietary supplements containing acetaminophen, and the potential for toxicity by inadvertent cumulative exposure.
- In elderly persons, acetaminophen may be recommended as first-line therapy for pain.
- IV acetaminophen has a faster onset of analgesia relative to an equivalent oral dose. It has more predictable pharmacokinetic and pharmacodynamic properties. It avoids first-pass hepatic exposure through the portal circulation, which may reduce the potential for hepatic injury.
- In 2015 the FDA strengthened an existing label warning that nonaspirin NSAIDs increase the chance of a heart attack or stroke and required updates to the drug labels of all prescription NSAIDs.
- In addition to patient risk factors, NSAIDs with a long half-life or slow-release formulation are associated with a greater risk of upper-GI bleeding/perforation. NSAIDs that produce a profound inhibition of both COX-1 and COX-2 isozymes at therapeutic doses are the most toxic drugs for the GI tract.
- The proposed mechanism is reduction in prostaglandin production, leading to increased reduced renal blood flow with subsequent medullary ischemia.
- For patients with both low GI and CV risks, any tNSAID may be acceptable. For those with low GI and high CV risk, naproxen or COX-2 selective inhibitors may be preferred, but celecoxib at the lowest approved dose may be acceptable. In patients with high GI risk, if CV risk is low, a COX-2–selective inhibitor alone or a tNSAID with a PPI appears to offer similar protection. When both GI and CV risks are high, the optimal strategy is to avoid NSAID therapy, if at all possible.

REFERENCES

Access the reference list online at ExpertConsult.com.

CHAPTER 52

INTRAVENOUS INFUSIONS FOR REFRACTORY CANCER AND CHRONIC PAIN STATES

Sheetal K. DeCaria, MD ✪ Magdalena Anitescu, MD, PhD

Unrelenting, severe chronic pain is often difficult to treat, especially when it does not respond to conventional medical management. Among invasive interventions, infusion therapies have emerged as an effective treatment for refractory chronic pain when other noninvasive treatments have been exhausted. Several pharmacologic options for intravenous (IV) infusions for intractable chronic pain states are reviewed here.

LOCAL ANESTHETIC (LIDOCAINE)

Local anesthetic infusions have been used to treat chronic pain for years. IV procaine was given to control posttraumatic pain as early as 1948.[1] Local anesthetic drugs block sodium channels. The activation of voltage-gated sodium channels affects the pathogenesis and maintenance of both neuropathic and inflammatory pain, making local anesthetic infusions a potential therapeutic option for these conditions. Administration of high doses of lidocaine and other local anesthetics, however, may produce allergic reactions, seizure, or toxicity.

After peripheral nerve injury, neuromas and dorsal root ganglia can demonstrate increased spontaneous activity as well as increased sensitivity to chemical and mechanical stimuli.[2] IV lidocaine indiscriminately blocks sodium channels (Na^+), an effect that may reduce neuropathic and other chronic pain conditions. It has been used as a potential treatment in many chronic pain and cancer-pain syndromes, often after other pain modalities have failed. The effectiveness of local anesthetic in chronic pain syndromes is tied to whether deafferentation is a major component of the pain.[3]

In one study of 182 patients with various chronic pain conditions, 83 (46%) responded to IV lidocaine infusions at doses between 1 and 5 mg/kg of 1% lidocaine by infusion pump over periods up to 1 hour. Patients with radicular symptoms had the greatest response rate (75%) with relief that lasted longer than a week. Of those with peripheral neuropathies, 59% responded and 42% had some relief beyond a week. Analgesic response was not consistent in those with sympathetic mediated pain.[4]

A systematic review of 17 randomized controlled trials compared IV lidocaine with placebo.[5] A total of nine studies treated neuropathic pain: three cancer pain, three acute migraine, one fibromyalgia, and one myofascial pain. In nine trials, five different pain conditions were analyzed in 199 patients: peripheral nerve injury, diabetic neuropathy, postherpetic neuralgia, trigeminal neuralgia, and dysesthetic pain after spinal cord injury. IV lidocaine resulted in better pain relief than placebo.[6] In another study, 11 women with fibromyalgia had 50% relief that lasted for 4–7 days.[7] For cancer-related pain from bony metastases and for chemotherapy-induced polyneuropathy- or radiotherapy-induced plexopathy, relief with lidocaine was no different than that with saline.[8,9] An electrocardiogram (ECG) was monitored continuously throughout the infusions. No arrhythmias were noted. A total of 143 lidocaine infusions were given to 134 patients. Adverse effects were experienced during 23 (16%) of the infusions; they included lightheadedness, somnolence, nausea, and perioral numbness. Unfortunately none of these studies examined the long-term efficacy of lidocaine infusions.

When complex regional pain syndrome (CRPS) was studied in 49 patients who received escalating doses of IV lidocaine over 5 days, follow-up lasted 6 months. Blood lidocaine levels were obtained daily and the infusion rate was adjusted to achieve a blood level of 5 mg/L. Infusion doses were increased only if the blood level was below the target 5 mg/L and was decreased or stopped if side effects such as arrhythmias occurred. In most patients, pain relief lasted an average of 3 months. The symptoms of mechanical and thermal allodynia were the most responsive.[10]

IV lidocaine at 5 mg kg^{-1} h^{-1} was more effective than saline in relieving spontaneous neuropathic pain in 32 patients; however, lower doses of lidocaine were no more effective than placebo.[11] IV lidocaine effectively lessened the pain associated with severe headache, chronic daily headache, transformed migraine, and medication overuse headache in 90% of subjects. This effect was maintained at 1 month follow-up. The most common complications were nausea, vomiting, tachycardia, or tremors, which resolved with dose reduction.[12,13]

We showed a sustained reduction of neuropathic pain from central sensitization in a variety of pain conditions with IV lidocaine.[14] We administered an initial bolus of 1 mg/kg lidocaine before an infusion of 2–4 mg/kg over 30 minutes and a recovery period of 30 minutes to 1 hour. All patients were continuously monitored with standard monitors (blood pressure, EKG, pulse oximetry, capnography) and pain scores were obtained by trained anesthesia personnel. Our protocol for outpatient lidocaine infusions is described in Table 52.1.

Yet lidocaine is associated with dose-related side effects, such as tinnitus, sedation, dizziness, and, rarely, seizures and arrhythmias. The studies with IV lidocaine reviewed previously did not note any serious side effects such as seizures and arrhythmias. One limitation to IV lidocaine treatment for pain is the limited sustained benefit and impracticality of infusion as a long-term treatment. Studies are needed to prove its long-term efficacy and ideal dose.

TABLE 52.1 University of Chicago Protocol for Lidocaine Infusion

Consultation
• Obtain baseline EKG and cardiac history • Evaluate the patient for arrhythmias before scheduling procedure
Day of Procedure

• Assess the patient for fasting and alertness
• Determine effects of previous infusion, if any, on
  • Pain reduction
  • Duration of effects
  • Patient function after infusion
  • Decrease in use of pain medication since infusion
• Verify that patient has a companion to accompany him or her home
• Obtain signature on consent form

Procedure

• Apply standard monitors: blood pressure, EKG, pulse oximeter, capnograph
• Start intravenous access and administer 1 mg/kg lidocaine bolus over 3–5 min
• Follow with 4 mg/kg lidocaine (or 2–4 mg/kg) administered slowly over 30 min (or 20–30 min)
• Record at 1, 5, 10, 15, 20, 25, and 30 min the following:
  • Time of administration
  • Blood pressure
  • Heart rate
  • Pulse oximetry
  • Pain score
• Stop the infusion in the event of seizure activity or cardiac instability

Recovery
• Patients recover within 30–60 min after the procedure • Vital signs are monitored over 15 min for a 60-min recovery period • At the end of the recovery period, the patient is discharged from the clinic with the accompanying caregiver
Follow-up
• In 4 weeks, patient returns for evaluation of treatment or repeat infusion • The dose of lidocaine is not increased if the initial infusion was performed with 4 mg/kg over 20 min

KETAMINE

Ketamine acts on both the central and peripheral nervous system and mediates multiple receptor subtypes, including opioid, N-methyl-D-aspartate (NMDA), alpha-amino-3-hydroxy-5-methyl-4-isoxazole propionate, kainite, and gabba-aminobutyric acid (GABA)-A receptors. In chronic pain, the NMDA receptor is thought to be the main receptor mediated by ketamine. When stimulated, primarily via the neurotransmitter glutamate, up-regulation of the NMDA receptor creates central sensitization. Ketamine antagonizes the NMDA receptors. It may decrease opioid tolerance through an interaction between the receptors, the nitric oxide pathway, and μ-opioid receptors.[15]

Ketamine has shown some analgesic efficacy in patients with CRPS, neuropathic pain, cancer pain, fibromyalgia, postherpetic neuralgia, and diabetic neuropathy.[15] It has been most extensively studied as a treatment for CRPS. A growing body of literature supports the use of ketamine in subanesthetic doses as an analgesic. In our retrospective series, conditions that responded favorably to ketamine infusions were most commonly CRPS, intractable headache, and refractory back pain.[15] All chronic pain conditions received analgesic benefit with ketamine for varying durations and half received benefit for 3 weeks. Side effects—including hallucination (10% of patients) and hypertension (12% of patients)—were mild and self-limited. In our pain clinic, patients who receive IV ketamine are pretreated with ondansetron 4 mg by intravenous push (IVP) and midazolam 2 mg IVP. Ketamine 0.3 mg/kg IV is then administered over 30–60 minutes. A recovery period lasts 30–90 minutes postinfusion. All patients are continuously monitored for vital signs, pain, and side effects during the infusion and in the recovery period using American Society of Anesthesiologists (ASA) standard monitors (blood pressure, pulse oximetry, EKG, capnography) by trained anesthesia personnel. Follow-up is approximately 4–6 weeks after the infusion. Depending on the pain scores, the duration of pain relief and the occurrence of side effects, the dose is increased, maintained, or discontinued. Table 52.2 summarizes our clinic's protocol for outpatient ketamine infusions.

In one retrospective review, 33 patients with CRPS were treated with a ketamine infusion.[16] There was complete pain relief in 25 (76%) and partial relief in 6 (18%) patients. All 12 patients who received a second course of treatment experienced complete relief of their CRPS pain. The most common side effect was a feeling of hallucination. Less frequent side effects were lightheadedness, dizziness, and nausea. In a randomized double-blind crossover study of 20 patients with phantom limb pain, IV ketamine infusion (0.4 mg kg h^{-1}) reduced pain.[17] Yet in a different study of 12 patients with neuropathic pain after nerve injury, ketamine had no effect on spontaneous pain.[18] When fibromyalgia syndrome was treated with IV ketamine infusion (0.3 mg/kg given over 30 minutes on two separate occasions a week apart) in 29 patients, ketamine infusion reduced visual analogue scale (VAS) scores of muscular pain at rest as well as local and referred pain compared with placebo.[19] However, others who treated 24 fibromyalgia patients with IV ketamine (0.5 mg/kg over 30 minutes) or placebo found that after an 8-week follow-up visit, pain scores did not improve significantly beyond the immediate postinfusion period.

These last investigators concluded that a short-term infusion of ketamine was not sufficient to produce a long-term analgesic effect in these patients.[20] Ketamine has also been studied in cancer patients whose pain was not relieved by morphine. In 10 patients, a single-day 30-minute IV infusion of ketamine at 0.25 and 0.5 mg/kg was compared with placebo. Pain relief persisted for both doses of ketamine after 180 minutes.[21] In an open-label study, ketamine infusions were administered to 247 patients with refractory headache. Of the 162 patients with refractory migraine enrolled in the study, 93% had a greater than 50% reduction in their pain intensity. All of the 11 patients suffering from debilitating cluster headaches had complete resolution of the pain for an average of 6.4 days.[22,23]

Ketamine carries risks, and these should be kept in mind in utilizing these infusions. It produces a state of dissociative anesthesia, which can be accompanied by visual and/or auditory hallucinations that may persist. There also is a possibility of sympathetic stimulation,

TABLE 52.2 University of Chicago Protocol for Ketamine Infusion

Consultation

- Obtain baseline EKG and cardiac history
- Evaluate the patient for arrhythmias before scheduling procedure

Day of Procedure

- Assess the patient for fasting and alertness
- Determine effects of previous infusion, if any, on
  - Pain reduction
  - Duration of effects
  - Patient function after infusion
  - Decrease in use of pain medication since infusion
- Verify that patient has a companion to accompany him or her home
- Obtain signature on consent form

Procedure

- Apply standard monitors: blood pressure, EKG, pulse oximeter, capnograph
- Start intravenous (IV) access and pretreat with
  - Midazolam 2 mg IV
  - Ondansetron 4 mg IV
- Begin ketamine infusion with 0.3 mg/kg in 100-mL bag for 30–45 min
- Record at 1, 5, 10, 15, 20, 25, and 30 min the following:
  - Time of administration
  - Blood pressure
  - Heart rate
  - Pulse oximetry
  - Pain score
- Depending on the patient's vital signs and pain scores, the infusion may be extended to 60 min
- Stop the infusion in the event of any of the following adverse effects:
  - Hallucinations
  - Blood pressure increase >20% of baseline
  - Severe anxiety
  - Nausea
  - Unmanageable, symptomatic nystagmus
- Most adverse effects disappear when infusion is stopped
- Assess the patient for urgent management

Recovery

- Patients recover within 30–60 min after the procedure
- Vital signs are monitored every 5–15 min for 60 min during recovery or more frequently if needed
- At the end of the recovery period, the patient is discharged with accompanying caregiver

Follow-up

- In 4 weeks, patient returns for evaluation of treatment or repeat infusion
- Infusion doses may be increased to 0.6–1 mg/kg depending on the effect of the infusion on pain scores and patient function or satisfaction with pain relief

including tachyarrhythmias. Although ketamine is available in an oral form, its use has been limited thus far by side effects as well as a low bioavailability. Ketamine is metabolized to norketamine (an active metabolite) on hepatic first-pass metabolism. Norketamine has analgesic properties as well, although it is less potent than ketamine.[24]

In a study of neuropathic pain in cancer patients, seven of nine patients who were given oral ketamine as an adjunct to morphine experienced a decrease in pain score of more than 3 points on a numerical rating scale. They were given ketamine in a dose of 0.5 mg/kg 3 times a day in addition to their existing regimen. However, four individuals experienced nausea, two loss of appetite, and eight sedation. In this small study, patients did not report any visual or auditory hallucinations.[25] However, this study illustrated that low-dose oral ketamine is beneficial in the management of refractory neuropathic pain secondary to cancer.

Patients receiving IV ketamine typically need repeated infusions to provide sustained benefit, which limits its long-term use. The long-term sequelae of ketamine infusions have not yet been elucidated. In current ketamine users, cognitive impairment and depressive symptoms were noted, but not in former ketamine users.[26] The same results were found in another study where frequent ketamine users experienced impairments in working memory, episodic memory, and aspects of executive function as well as reduced psychologic well-being.[27]

BISPHOSPHONATES

IV pamidronate, alendronate, ibandronate, neridronate, and clodronate are all bisphosphonates that have been studied in patients with refractory CRPS. Bone demineralization has been found to accompany advanced stages of this condition. Bisphosphonates have been proposed as a treatment because they inhibit bone resorption, which may contribute to pain. In one systemic review, bisphosphonates had the potential to reduce pain associated with bone loss.[28] Weak evidence supports bisphosphonates for CRPS compared with placebo.[29]

Recent evidence supports the use of IV bisphosphonates in the treatment of chronic low back pain. In a study of escalating doses of pamidronate administered to patients suffering from chronic low back pain with magnetic resonance imaging (MRI) evidence of degenerative disk disease, a cumulative dose of 180 mg IV pamidronate (two doses of 90 mg IV 4 weeks apart) produced significant and sustained decreased daily average pain intensity with the highest effect observed at 6 months postinfusion.[30] Similarly, in a small randomized placebo-controlled study, zoledronic acid infusion was administered to patients suffering from chronic low back pain and with MRI images of Modic I changes consistent with discogenic inflammation. The study group, administered 5 mg IV zoledronic acid, showed improvement of pain intensity at 1 month and less use of nonsteroidal antiinflammatory drugs (NSAIDs) at 1 year when compared with placebo.[31] This property of bisphosphonates may be related to their demonstrated effects on suppression of proinflammatory cytokine (interleukin-1, tumor necrosis factor-alpha, interleukin-6) secretion[32] as well as a reduction in prostaglandin E2 levels.[33]

IV bisphosphonates improve pain and increase quality of life in patients with osteoporosis, an effect related to their antiabsorptive activity (osteoclast inhibition, control of osteoblastic proliferation and differentiation) as well as suppression of the neuropeptide (substance P, calcitonin gene–related peptide) production.[34] Various infusion protocols comprising zoledronic acid, pamidronate, ibandronate, and others are currently used to improve chronic pain in osteoporosis.

Multiple infusions of pamidronate (every 4 weeks) are generally used for the palliative treatment of painful bone metastases and bone-related conditions such as Paget disease or fibrous dysplasia.[35,36] Zoledronic acid infusion has been found to be preferable to oral ibandronic acid in the prevention of skeletal-related events caused by bone metastases from breast cancer.[37] These results were confirmed in a systematic review and meta-analysis of the use of bisphosphonates in the treatment of patients with lung cancer and metastatic bone disease. This study showed that the addition of bisphosphonates to chemotherapy resulted in significantly better pain control than the standard treatments; zoledronic acid, pamidronate, and clodronate used in combination with other modalities of treatment (radiation therapy, chemotherapy, radioisotope therapy) provided better pain control, improved quality of life, and less progression of bone lesions than the other therapies alone.[38]

Addition of IV bisphosphonates infusions to surgical instrumentation and radiation therapy for painful vertebral metastases may lead to better local tumor sterilization and improved pain control.[39] The majority of side effects after bisphosphonate infusion relate to flulike symptoms in the immediate (3–4 days) postinfusion period. However, more severe complications such as osteonecrosis of the jaw have been reported. Known to occur at high doses of therapy, recent evidence suggests that early stages (stage 0) of bisphosphonate-related osteonecrosis of the jaw (BRONJ) can occur with zoledronic acid infusion even in low-dose protocols. Clinical and radiologic signs are needed to confirm the diagnosis of BRONJ. Dental pretherapeutic and follow-up oral-maxillofacial examination, as well as close collaboration between dentists and medical specialists prescribing bisphosphonates, may be necessary for early diagnosis and treatment of this complication.[40]

IMMUNOGLOBULIN

Chronic pain may often have an underlying inflammatory mechanism, particularly states that lead to abnormal sensitivity (spontaneous pain and hyperalgesia). Immune cell therapy might play a crucial role, not only in inflammatory pain but also in neuropathic or centralized pain states. IV immunoglobulins have emerged as a novel treatment modality for refractory pain in CRPS, fibromyalgia, and neuropathic pain.[41] The optimal dosing, duration of treatment, and side effect profile remain to be studied.

MAGNESIUM

Magnesium is the second most abundant cation in the human body. It has been used in the treatment of severe migraines and refractory headaches. Its use as an antimigranous agent stems from the observation that patients with migraines often suffer from hypomagnesemia, especially when the headache is associated with aura. Oral doses of 9 mg/kg per day magnesium were found to reduce the frequency of headaches in children and adolescents with migraine.[42] In another series, 1 g of IV magnesium administered over 30 minutes rendered 86% of patients headache free.[43]

Magnesium is associated with side effects such as diarrhea and flushing; however, IV magnesium sulfate in doses of 0.5–2 mg seems to be well tolerated and effective in the treatment of chronic pain in hospital settings. Because magnesium is a potent vasodilator, coadministration of metoclopramide may worsen therapeutic outcome. When magnesium is administered with calcium channel blockers, it may be effective in the treatment of reversible cerebral vasoconstrictive syndrome.[44]

PHENTOLAMINE

Autonomic nervous system dysfunction frequently accompanies chronic pain. Thus interruption of sympathetic pathways with agents such as phentolamine may alleviate symptoms. For example, phentolamine can be used to treat CRPS, central and peripheral neuropathic pain, orofacial pain, cancer, fibromyalgia, and phantom pain.[45,46] There are limited studies investigating the efficacy of an IV phentolamine infusion for chronic pain, but the infusion has been used in attempts to diagnose sympathetically maintained pain. Twenty patients with hyperalgesia to mechanical and cold stimuli reported pain relief with 20–35-mg doses of phentolamine.[47] Maximum pain relief lasted 20–30 minutes except in four patients who had 3–10 hours of pain relief. In a randomized trial, 37 patients with neuropathic pain were treated with IV phentolamine 35 mg over 30 minutes, and 16 of these patients were subsequently treated with 50 or 75 mg IV phentolamine. Sixteen patients (43%) reported pain relief following at least one infusion and reported that the relief lasted more than a day. In this last group, eight patients experienced at least 1 week of pain relief. There was no difference in pain scores with higher-dosage infusions.[48]

Among the risks of phentolamine infusions are hypotension, tachycardia, and arrhythmias. These risks must be balanced against the limited long-term benefit of the infusion, thus making IV phentolamine a less desirable therapeutic option for chronic pain. It may be useful as a diagnostic tool when the etiology of pain is in question.

In summary, IV infusions may play a role in managing refractory chronic pain. The risks and benefits must be considered, since these infusions may result in toxicity. Additional studies are needed to elucidate the diagnoses that will respond best to each infusion as well as whether these treatments offer sustained benefits that justify their risks.

KEY POINTS

- Local anesthetic infusions work via voltage-gated sodium channels for neuropathic and inflammatory pain conditions.
- Dose-related side effects of lidocaine exist (tinnitus, sedation, dizziness, seizures, arrhythmia).
- Ketamine works via multiple receptors (opioid, NMDA, kainite, and GABA-A, to name a few).
- Ketamine has shown some efficacy in treating CRPS, neuropathic pain, cancer pain, fibromyalgia, postherpetic neuralgia, and diabetic neuropathy.
- Ketamine infusions carry risks (i.e., hypertension, tachyarrythmias, visual and/or auditory hallucinations).

- Oral ketamine is limited due to low bioavailability and side effects.
- Bisphosphonates inhibit bone reabsorption and may help with specific conditions such as CRPS, bony metastasis, and low back pain.
- Most common side effects of bisphosphonate infusions are flulike symptoms.
- Magnesium has been proven effective as an infusion for migraine headaches.
- Phentolamine infusions in chronic pain are limited by lack of long-term benefit and many side effects.

REFERENCES

Access the reference list online at ExpertConsult.com.

CHAPTER 53

Pharmacologic Management of Myofascial Pain

Julie H. Huang-Lionnet, MD, MBA ◎ Haroon Hameed, MD ◎ Steven P. Cohen, MD

Myofascial pain disorders are a heterogeneous group of clinical entities that share features that originate from soft tissue with resultant regional symptomatology. Common examples of myofascial pain disorders include episodic tension-type headache (TTH), myofascial pain syndrome (MPS), temporomandibular disorder (TMD), muscle cramps, and nonspecific low back and neck pain.

MECHANISMS OF MUSCLE PAIN

Muscle pain is thought to occur by two main mechanisms: peripheral and central. Peripheral factors include trauma, dysregulated deep-tissue microcirculation,[1] and altered muscular metabolism and mitochondrial function.[2] Mechanical, thermal, or chemical stimulation can lead to activation of intramuscular group III and group IV nociceptors, which in turn give rise to an inflammatory cascade mediated by immune cells, leading to further recruitment of inflammatory cells and propagation of local inflammation and sensitization. Pain transmission occurs along Aδ and C-fibers into the inner lamina of the spinal cord where complex changes occur, leading to sensitization and chronic pain.

Continuous nociceptive input via these pathways can lead to central sensitization of higher-order neurons, resulting in enhanced sensitivity to painful stimuli via excitatory glutamate- and aspartate-related neurotransmitter release (hyperalgesia),[3,4] reduced thresholds to nonpainful stimuli (allodynia), and increased receptive fields, causing referred pain.[5] Increased expression of the excitatory glutamate- and aspartate-related neurotransmitters and their receptors in the spinal cord[3] is well known to play a role in the development of mechanical hyperalgesia in noninflammatory muscle pain.[4]

Supraspinal mechanisms can also contribute to chronic muscular pain states. These include decreased modulatory activity, hippocampal suppression, and possibly impaired stress responses.[6,7] Once central sensitization occurs, pain becomes autonomous from sensory input from the affected muscle(s).

PAINFUL CONDITIONS WITH MYOFASCIAL INVOLVEMENT

TENSION-TYPE HEADACHE

The International Headache Society classifies TTHs as infrequent episodic (<12 days/year), frequent episodic (12 to fewer than 180 days/year), and chronic (≥180 days/year). Pathophysiologic mechanisms responsible for TTH can be divided into peripheral and central causes. Peripheral mechanisms are demonstrated by increased tenderness of pericranial myofascial tissue compared to a healthy population,[8,9] as well as increased electromyographic (EMG) and algometric pressure recordings. Continuous nociceptive input can lead to central sensitization, thereby converting episodic TTH into chronic headaches.[10] Patients with frequent TTH often demonstrate nociceptive hypersensitivity to various stimuli at both cephalic and extracephalic sites.[11–13] Seventy percent of patients with tension headaches suffer from muscle tightness and tenderness, indicative of peripheral pain mechanisms, with the percentage even higher in individuals suffering episodic headaches.[14] Other studies support roles for increased nitric oxide production, N-methyl-D-aspartate (NMDA) receptor activation,[15] and neurogenic inflammation of the trigeminovascular system.[16] Central pain processing appears to be relatively normal in patients with infrequent episodic headaches where peripheral pain mechanisms probably play a larger role.[17]

TEMPOROMANDIBULAR DISORDER

TMD is a broad term used to describe conditions arising in the jaw joint, muscles of mastication, and associated craniofacial structures.[18] These conditions most commonly include pain, dysfunction, arthritis, and internal derangement.[19] The International Headache Society designates TMD as a subtype of secondary headaches, and the American Academy of Orofacial Pain subclassifies it into articular and masticatory muscle disorders. Many patients also have mixed arthrogenous and myogenous TMD. Myogenous pain has been reported to contribute to up to 50% of temporomandibular joint disorders.[20] TMD is more prevalent in females than males, and mostly affects adults aged 20–50 years. Young patients may be more likely to suffer from myogenous TMD.[21] TMD often coexists with other functional pain syndromes. According to a recent multicenter cohort study, patients with preexisting low back pain (LBP) have a 50% higher, and those with genital pain have a 75% higher incidence of TMD than those without these conditions.[22] EMG recordings have demonstrated altered muscular contraction,[23] as well as increased muscular tone in patients with TMD.[24] Not surprisingly, EMG biofeedback has shown efficacy in TMD.[25] Other evidence suggests that small muscles, such as those involved in mastication, may be more prone to hyperalgesia than larger muscles.[26]

MYOFASCIAL PAIN SYNDROME

Despite the lack of specific objective criteria for the diagnosis of MPS, the work of Travell and Simons characterizes MPS by the presence of loci of hypersensitivity within a tender, taut, palpable band of muscle called a trigger point (TP). TPs are characterized by referred pain on palpation and elicitation of a local twitch response (LTR) with application of mechanical pressure; yet, in spite of these conventionally accepted criteria, studies have shown weak interrater reliability in the identification of TPs.[27,28]

TPs can be classified into active TPs or latent TPs. Active TPs are described as pain in a motor locus associated with spontaneous electrical activity,[29] whereas the more common latent TPs do not cause spontaneous pain, but can be triggered by factors such as mechanical or emotional stressors, dysfunctional postures, changes in weather, and either excessive immobility or the exaggerated use of muscles.[21] It has been suggested that a positive feedback cycle involving disproportionate acetylcholine release, sarcomere shortening, and increased concentrations of sensitizing substances leads to the formation of a TP circuit, which upon connection with other spinal dorsal horn neuronal pathways, activates latent TPs to become an active TP.[30] Some studies have shown that latent TPs are present in the shoulder-girdle muscles of half of asymptomatic young adults and in 5%–45% of lumbogluteal muscles. Other hypotheses suggest that hyperactive muscle spindles and end plates, focal dystonia, and/or psychological morbidity may play a role in the formation of TPs.

LOW BACK PAIN

LBP is a significant public health problem with a lifetime prevalence rate ranging between 50% and 80%.[31] Spine structures serve many functions, including protecting the spinal cord, maintaining posture and truncal stability, and acting as a steadying force for movement of the extremities. Skeletal and ligamentous structures serve as a protective foundation from which attached muscles provide functional motor control, flexibility, and movement coordination. Lumbar muscle function is well known to play an important role in LBP. Correct neuromuscular control and lumbar muscle proprioceptive feedback is essential in preventing LBP and sustaining postural stability.[32] Weakness in the core muscles (lumbo-pelvic-hip complex), unbalanced gait mechanics, or dysfunctional muscular proprioception can lead to tears, strains, sprains, or spasm within the paraspinal musculature. Multiple studies show EMG evidence of increased paraspinal muscle tone in patients suffering from chronic LBP,[33–35] and muscle spasm may be superimposed on primary injuries such as acute disc herniation. However, attributing LBP to solely myofascial pathology requires excluding other causes. Among the three layers of lumbar paraspinal musculature, only the most superficial is palpable. Additional support for muscular dysfunction as the cause of LBP comes from controlled trials demonstrating efficacy for botulinum toxin and a variety of muscle relaxants,[36] as well as the proven effectiveness of neuromuscular reeducation and lumbar stabilization.[37]

NECK PAIN

Neck pain is a common cause of disability, with an annual prevalence rate of about 37%.[38] Among the various causes, myofascial pain comprises a significant percentage of cases, both as a primary and a secondary etiology. Individuals with nonspecific neck pain often manifest delays in the onset of neck muscle contractions, altered patterns of muscle activation, and elevated levels of myoelectric activity. Similar to LBP, posture, body mechanics, sleep patterns, nutrition, psychological stress, and environmental factors play an important role. Cervical dystonia, torticollis, acute whiplash injury, and other etiologies of neck pain may be masked or difficult to distinguish from myofascial pain. Neck pain can also present as referred pain from masticatory muscles, and primary headache conditions such as migraine and occipital neuralgia headaches. Active myofascial TPs in the neck and parascapular region are often superimposed on cervical pathology, including acute cervical disc herniation. A clinical trial of patients with cervical radiculopathy and healthy controls found a significant difference in the distribution of active and latent myofascial TPs. No active myofascial TPs were noted in the control group, while latent myofascial TPs in the upper trapezius muscles were found to be increased in patients with cervical radiculopathy.[39]

MUSCLE CRAMPS

True muscle cramps are painful involuntary skeletal muscle contractions associated with electrical activity.[40] EMG studies show fast rates of repetitive firing in motor units of affected muscles.[41,42] True muscle cramps, which by definition occur in the absence of fluid or electrolyte imbalance, have diverse etiologies. They are more commonly found in patients with well-developed muscles, in the third trimester of pregnancy, and in metabolic disorders such as cirrhosis and renal disease.[43] Other causes of muscle cramps include medications, lower motor neuron disease, hypothyroidism, and hereditary disorders.[40] The precise origin of cramps is the subject of debate, but there is evidence that abnormal discharges come from both central origins and peripheral motor neurons.[44] Arguments in favor of a peripheral origin include the variable EMG morphology of fasciculations,[45] the fact that cramps can be induced by repetitive peripheral nerve stimulation, and their high-frequency discharge rates (>150 Hz). Painful cramps can often be terminated by stretching the cramped muscle.

TREATMENT

TRICYCLIC ANTIDEPRESSANTS

Tricyclic antidepressants (TCAs)—amitriptyline, nortriptyline, desipramine, and imipramine—provide analgesia independent of their antidepressive effects by multiple mechanisms, which include norepinephrine (NE) and serotonin reuptake inhibition in inhibitory descending pathways (Table 53.1). Among the two, serotonergic reuptake inhibition may be less important in analgesia, although combined serotonin–NE reuptake inhibitors are generally better analgesics than selective NE reuptake inhibitors. The former point may explain the comparative decreased efficacy of selective serotonin reuptake inhibitors (SSRIs). Other active mechanisms include blockade of peripheral neural sodium channels, muscarinic and nicotinic acetylcholine receptors, alpha adrenergic receptors, NMDA receptors, dopamine receptors, and decreased substance P release.[46]

TABLE 53.1 Differences in Mechanisms of Action of Tricyclic Antidepressants

Drug	Serotonin	Norepinephrine	Dopamine	Sedative	Antimuscarinic
Amitriptyline	+++	+	—	+++	+++
Nortriptyline	+++	++	—	++	++
Desipramine	—	+++	—	+	+
Imipramine	+++	++	—	++	++

+, *Mild interaction;* ++, *moderate interaction;* +++, *profound interaction.*

Multiple studies have shown TCAs to be effective in reducing the frequency and intensity of TTHs[47–49] and facial pain/TMD.[50–52] The typical doses of amitriptyline in these studies ranged between 20 and 100 mg, which is considerably lower than that required to treat depression. Yet, even at these low doses, their use is limited secondary to myriad side effects, which include dry mouth, constipation, fluid retention, weight gain, difficulty concentrating, and cardiotoxicity.

Multiple systematic reviews have concluded TCAs to be effective at reducing the frequency and intensity of TTH (Table 53.2).[46,53] Of note, a double-blind, placebo-controlled, three-way crossover study in TTH found significant reductions in scalp tenderness and headache intensity with intermediate doses of amitriptyline (75 mg/day) compared with the serotonin-specific reuptake inhibitor citalopram and placebo.[49] For TMD, the evidence appears more modest, with two randomized controlled trials (RCTs) demonstrating efficacy for amitriptyline and a sulfur-containing analog of amitriptyline, dothiepin. One double-blind, RCT assessing the efficacy of dothiepin in chronic atypical facial pain and arthromyalgia found 71% of the 93 patients in the treatment group became pain-free after 9 weeks versus 47% in the placebo group.[50] Sixty-eight (81%) of the 84 patients who elected to continue treatment with dothiepin were pain-free at their 1-year follow-up. A subsequent study found significantly reduced pain intensity in patients with chronic facial pain who received amitriptyline compared with placebo. No dose-response relationship measuring analgesia between low-dose (≤30 mg) and high-dose (≤150 mg) amitriptyline was deemed significant, suggesting either a low ceiling effect or a high percentage of placebo responders.[51]

ANTICONVULSANTS AND CALCIUM CHANNEL ANTAGONISTS

Pregabalin and gabapentin, an analog of gamma-aminobutyric acid (GABA), exert their analgesic effects by acting on the α_2-δ_1 subunit of cellular calcium channels and blocking neurotransmitter release. Their binding to calcium channels results in suppression of abnormal neuronal discharges and an increased threshold for nerve activation. Although generally well tolerated, the most common side effects of gabapentin and pregabalin include dizziness, sedation, lightheadedness, somnolence, and weight gain.

Gabapentin and pregabalin are first-line agents for the treatment of neuropathic pain, but have also demonstrated some effectiveness in conditions characterized by muscle pathology (Table 53.3). A randomized, placebo-controlled study conducted in 133 patients with chronic daily headache, which can involve increased muscle tone,[54,55] demonstrated a modest improvement in the severity and frequency of headaches in gabapentin-treated patients compared to controls.[55] Another recent prospective open-label study performed in patients with myofascial facial pain found that using a two-tiered approach utilizing TCAs and then gabapentin in nonresponders resulted in 54% of patients who obtained a ≥50% decrease in pain scores.[56] This and other studies have led some experts to recommend gabapentin as a first-line treatment for headache prophylaxis. Placebo-controlled studies have also shown benefit for gabapentin in reducing spasticity in patients with multiple sclerosis and spinal cord injury (SCI),[57,58] and for chronic masticatory myalgia.[59]

Weaker evidence supports use of gabapentinoids for other myofascial pain disorders. A retrospective review of gabapentin treatment in patients with neuropathic pain, myofascial pain, and chronic LBP found significant decreases in pain scores in both the neuropathic pain and myofascial groups, but not for LBP.[60] In an open-label study evaluating gabapentin in patients with muscle cramps associated with a variety of different medical conditions, Serrao et al. noted a significant reduction in muscle cramps at the first 2-week follow-up visit after gabapentin treatment. Cramps had resolved in all patients by 3 months, lasting for the 6-month treatment period.[61]

Other membrane stabilizers have been studied in muscle pain. Both placebo-controlled[62] and open-label[63] studies evaluating sodium valproate, an anticonvulsant that acts via a variety of mechanisms including the blockade of T-type calcium and sodium channels, and facilitation of GABA, have shown benefit in TTH and chronic daily headaches. An earlier randomized, placebo-controlled trial also found phenytoin pretreatment to be an effective means of reducing succinylcholine-induced postoperative myalgias.[64]

SKELETAL MUSCLE RELAXANTS

Skeletal muscle relaxants such as cyclobenzaprine (Flexeril), chlorzoxazone (Paraflex), carisoprodol (Soma), methocarbamol (Robaxin, Robaxisal), tizanidine (Zanaflex), and baclofen (Lioresal) are believed to exert their mechanism of action primarily within the brain and, in some cases, spinal motor neurons. Cyclobenzaprine, structurally related to first-generation TCAs, inhibits the reuptake of NE in the locus coeruleus and inhibits descending serotonergic pathways in the spinal cord. The latter effect may have an inhibitory effect on alpha motor neurons in the spinal cord, resulting in decreased firing and a reduction

TABLE 53.2 Tricyclic Antidepressants

Drug	Trade Name	Mechanism of Action	Typical Dose Range, mg/day	Pharmacology	Evidence for Efficacy	Common Adverse Side Effects
Amitriptyline	Elavil, Endep	Inhibits NE and 5HT reuptake, muscarinic acetylcholine receptor antagonist, H1 receptor antagonist, α1 adrenergic receptor antagonist, blocks Na^+ channels	10–150 in evening/bedtime dosing; starting dose 25–75 mg oral; starting dose in elderly 10–25 mg (oral)	Liver metabolism and urine excretion primarily and feces; half-life 10–26 h	Strong—tension headache Moderate—facial pain with myofascial component and TMD	Dry mouth, constipation, fluid retention, weight gain, difficulty concentrating, and cardiotoxicity
Nortriptyline	Pamelor	Inhibits NE and 5HT reuptake, muscarinic acetylcholine receptor antagonist, blocks Na^+ channels	25–150 in evening/bedtime dosing; starting dose 25–50 mg (oral)	Liver metabolism, urine excretion primarily and feces; half-life 18–44 h	Moderate—chronic tension-type headache	Drowsiness, dizziness, nausea, vomiting, insomnia, sweating, dry mouth, tachycardia, pruritus, weight gain, constipation
Imipramine	Tofranil	Inhibits NE and 5HT reuptake, M2 muscarinic acetylcholine receptor antagonist, histamine H1 receptors antagonist, blocks Na^+ channels, enhances dopaminergic activity	25–150, 0.2–3 mg/kg, starting dose 0.2–0.4 mg/kg (oral)	Liver metabolism, urine excretion primarily and bile/feces; half-life 11–25 h	Moderate—tension-type headache	Drowsiness, dizziness, nausea, vomiting, headache, insomnia, sweating, confusion, dry mouth, tachycardia, constipation
Desipramine	Norpramin	Inhibits NE reuptake, muscarinic acetylcholine receptor antagonist, blocks Na^+ channels	25–150; starting dose 25–75 mg daily (oral)	Liver metabolism, urine excretion primarily; half-life 12–27 h	Weak—tension-type headache	Drowsiness, dizziness, nausea, vomiting, blurry vision, diaphoresis, confusion, dry mouth, tachycardia, constipation

5HT, *5-Hydroxytryptamine (serotonin);* NE, *norepinephrine;* TMD, *temporomandibular disorder.*

TABLE 53.3 Calcium Channel Antagonists

Drug	Trade Name	Mechanism of Action	Typical Dose Range, mg/day	Pharmacology	Evidence for Efficacy	Common Adverse Side Effects
Gabapentin	Neurontin	Binds α^2-δ^1 subunit of calcium channels blocking neurotransmitter release	300–3600 in TID dosing; starting dose 100 daily or TID (oral)	Urine excretion; half-life 5–7 h	Strong—neuropathic pain Moderate—spasticity in patients with multiple sclerosis and spinal cord injury, fibromyalgia Weak—chronic daily headache, myofascial pain, low back pain, muscle cramps	Dizziness, sedation, lightheadedness, somnolence, nausea, vomiting, weight gain
Pregabalin	Lyrica	Binds α^2-δ^1 subunit of calcium channels blocking neurotransmitter release	50–450 in BID or TID dosing; starting 50 mg BID (oral)	Negligible metabolism; urine excretion (90%); half-life 6.3 h	Strong—neuropathic pain, fibromyalgia	Dizziness, somnolence, ataxia, weight gain, peripheral edema, headache, dry mouth, blurred vision

in monosynaptic and polysynaptic spinal reflexes. Tizanidine acts as a weak agonist at alpha-2 adrenergic receptors, and enhances presynaptic inhibition at spinal motor neurons. Carisoprodol, a precursor of the sedative-hypnotic meprobamate, is believed to produce muscle relaxation by blocking interneuronal activity in the descending reticular formation and spinal cord. Baclofen activates GABA-B receptors in the brain and reduces the release of excitatory neurotransmitters in both the brain and spinal cord. Baclofen also acts by inhibiting the release of substance P in the spinal cord. In addition to muscle spasm, the muscle relaxants dantrolene, baclofen, and tizanidine have been shown to be effective for spasticity.

Numerous studies conducted over many years have evaluated various skeletal muscle relaxants in conditions associated with muscle pain (Table 53.4). Three separate randomized trials evaluating cyclobenzaprine in patients with cervical and lumbar spinal muscle spasm demonstrated efficacy in short-term follow-up.[65–67] In two of these studies,[66,67] cyclobenzaprine was superior to diazepam. A meta-analysis review found that cyclobenzaprine is more effective than placebo for LBP associated with muscle spasm, especially in the first 4 days of treatment.[68] However, a recent randomized study found that adding cyclobenzaprine or oxycodone/acetaminophen in emergency department patients presenting with acute LBP did not improve function 1 week after discharge.[69] Another randomized, placebo-controlled trial found cyclobenzaprine to be more effective than both placebo and clonazepam in patients with TMD.[70] Of note, two randomized, controlled trials that evaluated dose-response in patients with acute muscle spasm found that 2.5 mg three times per day of cyclobenzaprine was not better than placebo, while 5 mg three times daily was equivalent to 10 mg three times per day.[71]

An extended-release formulation of cyclobenzaprine, which would presumably be better tolerated than immediate-release preparations, was tested in a randomized, double-blind, two period, crossover study that showed sustained plasma concentration levels during a 24-hour dose interval. The main adverse effects included somnolence (10%), dry mouth (58%), dizziness (19%), and headache (17%).[72]

In a double-blind, placebo-controlled trial evaluating carisoprodol treatment in TMD, no difference was found between treatment and control groups.[73] Yet in a more recent multicenter, randomized, double-blind, placebo-controlled, parallel-group study, carisoprodol was found to provide significant pain relief in patients with acute, painful muscle spasm of the lower back when compared to placebo. Another double-blind, placebo-controlled trial reported a significant improvement in subjective feedback in TMD treated with meprobamate, which is a metabolite of carisoprodol.[74]

Two randomized, double-blind studies performed in patients with acute lumbar and cervical paravertebral muscle spasm found that tizanidine provided comparable pain relief to diazepam, but was associated with increased spinal mobility.[75,76] Another placebo-controlled study found tizanidine to be effective for patients with painful muscle spasm following lumbar disk surgery.[77] Studies determining efficacy of tizanidine for treating TTH have yielded conflicting results, with some,[78,79] but not all,[80] demonstrating efficacy.

There is robust evidence supporting the use of intrathecal baclofen in SCI-related spasticity.[81–83] With regard to oral agents for spasticity associated with multiple sclerosis, several controlled studies have shown benefit for oral baclofen.[84] For tizanidine, most, but not all studies have demonstrated efficacy.[84] In a systematic review on the use of muscle relaxants for spasticity and musculoskeletal conditions, Chou et al. concluded that there was fair evidence that tizanidine and baclofen were equally efficacious.[85]

BENZODIAZEPINES

Benzodiazepines enhance presynaptic inhibition in the spinal cord by targeting inhibitory neurotransmitter receptors that are directly activated by GABA. Benzodiazepine receptor binding facilitates GABA-A receptor binding, increasing the influx of negatively charged chloride ions across the cell membrane. The increased membrane conductance leads to hyperpolarization of Ia afferent terminals at neuronal synapses. These changes in membrane polarization lead to inhibition of normal neuronal transmission and reduced motor neuron output. Common side effects include dizziness, somnolence, confusion, memory loss, ataxia, sedation, and physical dependence with sustained use. Psychological effects include paradoxical anxiety, depression, paranoia, irritability, and addiction.

Clinical studies have shown conflicting results regarding the use of benzodiazepines such as diazepam (Valium), clonazepam (Klonopin), alprazolam (Xanax), and midazolam (Versed) in TMD and TTH. The evidence for their effectiveness in muscle spasm is moderate, but their significant adverse effect profile and possible inferiority when compared to traditional muscle relaxants should preclude their routine use (Table 53.5).

Several systematic reviews[86–88] have concluded that benzodiazepines serve a beneficial role in managing TMD. Specifically, clinical trials have demonstrated the efficacy of long-term use of agents such as diazepam and clonazepam in TMD.[89–91] One such randomized, placebo-controlled study showed diazepam to be more effective in treating chronic myofascial orofacial pain when compared with ibuprofen or placebo.[92] Among short-acting benzodiazepines, midazolam and triazolam have been studied. The former was found to exhibit antinociceptive properties in both animal and human studies involving induced-facial pain.[93,94] In a 4-day placebo-controlled trial, the latter was noted to improve sleep but not reduce pain or nocturnal masticatory muscle activity in patients with TMD.[95]

In other studies, benzodiazepines have shown varying degrees of efficacy in relieving TTH. A randomized, double-blind, placebo-controlled crossover study comparing alprazolam to placebo in the treatment of chronic tension headache demonstrated that alprazolam reduced the intensity but not the frequency of headaches.[96] This effect may be related to the fact that alprazolam, in contrast to other benzodiazepines, possesses some antidepressant activity. Several placebo-controlled studies have found diazepam to be effective in muscle contraction headaches.[97,98] In a double-blind, placebo-controlled study comparing frontalis EMG biofeedback, diazepam, placebo pills, and sham

TABLE 53.4 Skeletal Muscle Relaxants

Drug	Trade Name	Mechanism of Action	Typical Dose Range, mg/day	Pharmacology	Evidence for Efficacy	Common Adverse Side Effects
Cyclobenzaprine	Flexeril	Exact mechanism unknown, likely primary action on brain stem (central-acting)	5–30 in divided doses; starting 5 mg daily (oral)	Liver metabolism and urine excretion primarily; half-life 18 h	Strong—cervical and lumbar spinal pain, muscle spasm Moderate—TMD with myofascial pain	Dry mouth, drowsiness, headache, diarrhea, constipation, dizziness, nausea, confusion
Chlorzoxazone	Paraflex, Parafon Forte	Exact mechanism unknown, likely inhibits polysynaptic reflex pathways in spinal cord (central-acting)	750–3000; starting 250 mg TID (oral)	Liver metabolism and urine excretion; half-life 1.1 h	Moderate—acute musculoskeletal pain, back pain, acute lumbosacral muscle strain	Drowsiness, dizziness, headache, lightheadedness, hepatotoxicity, GI upset, malaise, paradoxical CNS stimulation
Carisoprodol	Soma	Exact mechanism unknown, likely interneuronal inhibition in spinal cord and descending reticular activating system (central-acting)	1050–1400; starting 250–350 mg QID (oral)	Liver metabolism and urine excretion; half-life 2.4 h	Moderate—acute musculoskeletal pain, not for spasticity Weak—TMD	Drowsiness, dizziness, headache, ataxia, insomnia, confusion, tremor, irritability
Methocarbamol	Robaxin	Exact mechanism unknown (central-acting)	3000–8000; starting 750 mg Q6H (oral)	Liver metabolism and urine excretion; half-life 1–2 h	Moderate—nocturnal leg cramps, acute muscle spasm	Dizziness, drowsiness, lightheadedness, nausea, rash, headache, somnolence, hypotension
Tizanidine	Zanaflex, Sirdalud	Binds to α2-adrenergic receptors, reducing presynaptic neurotransmitter release (central-acting)	2–36; starting 2 mg (oral)	Liver metabolism and urine excretion (60%) and feces (20%); half-life 2.5 h	Moderate—spasticity, paravertebral muscle spasm Weak—TTH	Dry mouth, somnolence, asthenia, headache, dizziness, hallucinations, hypotension, constipation
Baclofen	Kemstro, Lioresal	Binds to GABA-B receptors, inhibiting neurotransmitter release (central-acting)	15–80; starting 5 mg TID (oral)	Liver metabolism (15%) and urine excretion (70%–80%) and feces; half-life 5.5 h	Strong—spasticity of spinal cord origin Moderate—cervical dystonia, upper motor neuron disease, stiff-person syndrome, acute back pain	Drowsiness, nausea, weakness, somnolence, dizziness, confusion, ataxia, constipation, headache, hypotension, weight gain

CNS, *Central nervous system;* GI, *gastrointestinal;* TMD, *temporomandibular disorder;* TTH, *tension-type headache.*

TABLE 53.5 Benzodiazepines

Drug	Trade Name	Mechanism of Action	Typical Dose Range, mg/day	Pharmacology	Evidence for Efficacy	Common Adverse Side Effects
Diazepam	Valium	Increases inhibitory GABA transmission	2–40; starting dose 2 mg PRN or BID–QID (oral, IM, IV)	Liver metabolism and urine excretion; half-life 30–60 h	Strong—spasticity of spinal cord origin Moderate—chronic orofacial muscle pain, tension-type headache Weak—TMD	Drowsiness, dizziness, ataxia, headache, nausea, somnolence, tremor, sedation
Clonazepam	Klonopin	Increases inhibitory GABA transmission	0.5–4; starting 0.25 mg BID (oral)	Liver metabolism and urine excretion; half-life 20–50 h	Moderate—TMD with myofascial pain, nocturnal muscle spasms	Drowsiness, ataxia, confusion, diarrhea, constipation, dry mouth, fatigue, headache, tremor, dysuria, hypotension
Alprazolam	Xanax	Increases inhibitory GABA transmission	0.75–4; starting 0.25 mg TID (oral)	Liver metabolism and urine excretion; half-life 11.2 h, (elderly) 16.3 h, (alcoholic liver disease) 19.7 h	Moderate—TTH	Lightheadedness, dry mouth, nausea, headache, vomiting, constipation, depression, insomnia, rigidity, hypotension, ataxia, tachycardia
Lorazepam	Ativan	Increases inhibitory GABA transmission	1–10; starting dose 2–3 mg/day; divided BID–TID; starting dose 1–2 mg/day divided BID–TID in elderly (oral, IM, IV)	Liver metabolism and urine excretion; half-life 14 h		Sedation, dizziness, weakness, hypotension, respiratory depression, hypoventilation, local injection site reaction, weakness, unsteadiness

GABA, *Gamma-aminobutyric acid;* IM, *intramuscular;* IV, *intravenous;* TMD, *temporomandibular disorder;* TTH, *tension-type headache.*

EMG biofeedback in patients with chronic muscle tension headaches, both treatment groups were found to be superior to placebo, although only diazepam reached statistical significance.[99] Interestingly, the biofeedback patients experienced a persistent reduction in the frequency and intensity of headaches at 4-week follow-up, while headaches returned to baseline in the diazepam group.

Several studies have compared diazepam to conventional muscle relaxants for cervical and lumbar paravertebral muscle spasm with conflicting results.[66,67,75,76] In two studies comparing cyclobenzaprine to diazepam, one found cyclobenzaprine to be superior to diazepam, which in turn was better than placebo,[67] while the other found no meaningful differences between treatment groups.[66] For the two studies comparing diazepam to tizanidine, both found better range of motion in the lumbar spine in the tizanidine group, but no differences in pain, functional capacity, or self-assessment.[75,76]

NONSTEROIDAL ANTIINFLAMMATORY DRUGS

Nonsteroidal antiinflammatory drugs (NSAIDs) may be used to reduce myofascial pain and associated inflammation while facilitating recovery. NSAIDs are widely considered to be a first-line treatment for acute TTH, though persistent use (greater than 8 times per month) may lead to rebound headaches. In individuals with TMD, systematic reviews have found them to be beneficial, though the evidence is limited by the poor quality of the studies.[100,101] For acute LBP, they have been shown to both alleviate pain and improve function. Several studies have compared topical formulations to placebo. A randomized, double-blind, placebo-controlled study on diclofenac diethylamine 1.16% gel use in acute neck pain showed statistically significant improvement in pain on movement (primary outcome), pain at rest, functional neck disability index, and response to treatment measures. No adverse effects were noted with diclofenac gel.[102] Another randomized, single blind controlled study comparing NSAID patch as monotherapy or with transcutaneous electric nerve stimulation (TENS), heating pad, or topical capsaicin in treating MPS involving the upper trapezius showed no statistical difference among the four different methods on clinical endpoints.[103]

BOTULINUM TOXIN

TP injections are thought to deactivate TPs, one of the prime etiologies of regional musculoskeletal pain. For refractory cases to local anesthetic, botulinum toxin A (Botox) has demonstrated effectiveness with few self-limiting adverse effects. Botox is a purified neurotoxin complex produced from the fermentation of clostridium botulinum type A that inhibits acetylcholine release into the neuromuscular junction, resulting in reduced muscular contraction. Several studies have examined the efficacy of Botox injections for myofascial pain. A randomized, double-blind, placebo-controlled trial assessing Botox type A injection for cervical and shoulder girdle myofascial pain showed significant improvement in average pain scores, number of headaches per week, and brief pain inventory (BPI) interference scores for general activity and sleep for those who received a second dose of Botox type A compared to placebo.[104] Another prospective, randomized, double-blind, placebo-controlled, multicenter study found no significant improvement in proportion of patients with mild or no pain (i.e., responders) at week 5, though significant differences were observed at weeks 8 and 12 with respect to daily pain and patient and physician global assessments.[105] In a systematic review evaluating botulinum toxins for TMD, the authors found the five randomized trials decidedly mixed, with two showing efficacy against placebo, two demonstrating no significant benefit, and one showing equivalent effectiveness compared to facial manipulation.[106] Botox types A and B have been shown in clinical trials to have similar efficacy[107] (see Table 53.6).

OPIOIDS

Opioids are commonly used for the treatment of myofascial pain disorders. However, their long-term side effects, including opioid hyperalgesia, physical dependence, hormonal dysfunction, physical dependence, and addiction, must be carefully considered before a trial of opioids is instituted. Although opioids may provide short-term benefit for certain conditions characterized by myofascial pain such as LBP, they have not been shown to definitively provide long-term benefit, improvement in function, or greater benefit when compared to nonopioid therapy.[108]

TABLE 53.6 Botulinum Toxin

Drug	Trade Names	Mechanism of Action	Typical Dose Range, mg/day	Pharmacology	Evidence for Efficacy	Common Adverse Side Effects
Botulinum Type A and B Toxin	BOTOX, Dysport, Myobloc	Inhibits acetylcholine release from nerve endings, reducing neuromuscular transmission and local muscle activity (neurotoxin)	Follow guidelines for number of units per muscle	Unknown excretion; half-life unknown; clinical effect typically lasts 3 months	Strong—onabotulinumtoxin A in refractory myofascial pain syndrome Weak—Both onabotulinumtoxin A, and rimabotulinumtoxin B in TMD with masseter spasm	Hypersensitivity reaction, anaphylaxis, toxin effect spread, respiratory compromise, autonomic dysreflexia, urinary retention, dysphagia, corneal ulcer, myasthenia gravis exacerbation, retrobulbar hemorrhage, facial paralysis

TMD, *Temporomandibular disorder.*

A recent position paper by the American Academy of Neurology concluded that the risks of long-term opioid therapy outweigh the benefits in the treatment of headache, chronic LBP, and other noncancer pain conditions, and that they should only be used as part of a multifaceted treatment approach with strict surveillance.[109]

OTHER TREATMENTS

Several studies have looked at other topical formulations in the treatment of myofascial pain. An evaluator-blinded, randomized clinical study comparing lidocaine-prilocaine (EMLA) cream phonophoresis with ultrasound therapy on MPS of the trapezius showed a statistically significant improvement with EMLA cream phonophoresis compared to conventional ultrasound therapy in terms of pain and associated neck disability after 15 sessions.[110] Another randomized, double-blind, placebo-controlled study evaluating a 5% lidocaine patch in 60 patients with MPS of the upper trapezius revealed a significant difference in a verbal rating pain scale (VRS) at day 14, but not at day 7 or 28.[111] On the contrary, no significant difference in outcome measures were determined in a double-blind randomized study on the efficacy of 0.1% capsaicin hydrogel patch for myofascial neck pain[112] (see Table 53.7).

CONCLUSION

Myofascial pain is a common, yet underappreciated condition that can occur in isolation, or as a result of biomechanical alterations that accompany primary disorders. In view of the heterogeneity of myofascial pain, multiple mechanisms may exist in different patients, or even within a single patient. This poses serious challenges to pharmacologic management. There are many different medication classes that have been demonstrated to be effective for muscle disorders, with perhaps the strongest evidence supporting TCAs and muscle relaxants. Cyclobenzaprine now has an extended-release formulation for treatment of myofascial pain, which may reduce adverse effects and improve compliance. Topical formulations ranging from local anesthetic combinations such as EMLA cream to topical lidocaine patch have been shown in clinical studies to be effective treatments for MPS. For refractory cases, TP injections with local anesthetics or botulinum toxin type A should be considered. However, the effect size is modest for pharmacotherapy, which underscores the need for a multimodal approach that emphasizes an individually structured exercise program, psychotherapy if indicated, complementary and alternative medicine, and functional restoration. Comparative-effectiveness studies, studies that evaluate therapies that seek to prevent the transition from acute to chronic pain, and large, pragmatic trials evaluating different treatment approaches are needed to identify which patients will respond best to various treatments, and to develop more effective preventive measures.

KEY POINTS

- Muscle pain is thought to occur by peripheral and central mechanisms. Peripheral factors include trauma, dysregulated deep-tissue microcirculation, and altered muscular metabolism and mitochondrial function.

TABLE 53.7 Topical Formulations

Drug	Trade Name	Mechanism of Action	Typical Dose Range, mg/day	Pharmacology	Evidence for Efficacy	Common Adverse Side Effects
Diclofenac gel	Voltaren Gel	Inhibits cyclooxygenase, reducing prostaglandin and thromboxane synthesis	1% Gel; starting dose apply 2–4 g QID; Max 16 g/lower extremity joint and 8 g/upper extremity joint up to 32 g/day total	Urine and bile excretion; half-life 1.9 h (terminal), 37–79 h (plasma)	Moderate—myofascial pain syndrome of trapezius	Hypersensitivity reaction, anaphylaxis, bronchospasm, skin reaction, hypertension, nephrotoxicity, GI bleeding, GI perforation/ ulcer
Lidocaine patch	Lidoderm	Inhibits Na ion channels, stabilizing neuronal cell membranes and inhibiting nerve impulse initiation and conduction (amide local anesthetic)	5% patch; apply up to 12 h/day; Max 3 patches at a time × 12 h/day	Urine excretion; half-life 1.5–2 h	Moderate—myofascial pain syndrome of the upper trapezius	Anaphylactoid reaction, CNS excitation, CNS depression, cardiac arrest, seizures, arrhythmias, coma, familial malignant hyperthermia exacerbation
Lidocaine-prilocaine topical	EMLA	Inhibits Na ion channels, stabilizing neuronal cell membranes and inhibiting nerve impulse initiation and conduction (amide local anesthetic)	2.5%/2.5% cream; apply 1–3 g for 1 h or shortest effective duration; do not apply on open wounds	Urine excretion; half-life 70 min	Moderate—myofascial pain syndrome of the trapezius	Anaphylaxis, respiratory depression, cardiac arrest, seizures, arrhythmias, coma, methemoglobinemia

CNS, *Central nervous system;* GI, *gastrointestinal.*

Supraspinal mechanisms include decreased modulatory activity, hippocampal suppression, and possibly impaired stress responses.
- Seventy percent of patients with tension headaches suffer from muscle tightness and tenderness, with the percentage even higher in individuals suffering episodic headaches.
- Myogenic pain has been reported to contribute to up to 50% of temporomandibular joint disorders.
- Myofascial pain is characterized by the presence of loci of hypersensitivity within tender, taut, palpable bands of muscle called TPs.
- There is increased paraspinal muscle tone in patients suffering from chronic LBP and muscle spasm may be superimposed on primary injuries such as acute disc herniation.
- Individuals with nonspecific neck pain often manifest neck muscle contractions, altered patterns of muscle activation, and elevated levels of myoelectric activity.
- True muscle cramps are painful involuntary skeletal muscle contractions associated with electrical activity. True muscle cramps, by definition, occur in the absence of fluid or electrolyte imbalance, and have diverse etiologies.
- Studies showed TCAs to be effective in reducing the frequency and intensity of TTHs and facial pain/TMD.
- Gabapentin and pregabalin are first-line agents for the treatment of neuropathic pain, but have also demonstrated some effectiveness in conditions characterized by muscle pathology.
- Studies showed varying effectiveness of muscle relaxants compared to other medications.
- Studies have shown conflicting results regarding the use of benzodiazepines in TMD and TTH. The evidence for their effectiveness in muscle spasm is moderate, and their adverse effect profile and inferiority compared to traditional muscle relaxants preclude their routine use.
- NSAIDs are considered to be a first-line treatment for acute TTH, though persistent use may lead to rebound headaches. In TMD, NSAIDs can be beneficial although the evidence is limited by the poor quality of the studies.
- Controlled studies showed botulinum toxin to be effective in myofascial pain.
- Opioids may provide short-term benefit for certain conditions characterized by myofascial pain but they have not been shown to definitively provide long-term benefit, improvement in function, or greater benefit when compared to nonopioid therapy.
- The efficacy of topical treatments in myofascial pain has not been consistently shown.

REFERENCES

Access the reference list online at ExpertConsult.com.

CHAPTER 54

Pharmacologic Management of Complex Regional Pain Syndrome

Rena Beckerly, MD, MBA ⊛ Honorio T. Benzon, MD

The treatment options for Chronic Regional Pain Syndrome (CRPS) have dramatically evolved since Dr. Weir Mitchell first described the disease in 1986. He noted a subset of patients who experienced persistent pain despite healing of their gunshot wounds. Over the past 30 years, the disease has been referred to by several different names: causalgia, Sudeck atrophy, reflex sympathetic dystrophy, and now CRPS. Although hundreds of studies and case reports have been published about CRPS, their utility is limited given the numerous classification systems utilized to diagnose the syndrome. Ultimately, researchers applied the International Association of Pain diagnostic criteria.[1] Recently, the Budapest Criteria was proposed to assist practitioners in diagnosing this challenging disease.[2] While the International Association for the Study of Pain (IASP) criteria offered good sensitivity (1.00), it lacked specificity (0.4). The Budapest Criteria showed high sensitivity (0.99) and improved specificity (0.68). This allowed providers a more accurate tool to diagnose patients properly 88% of the time.[2]

CRPS patients are routinely prescribed a combination of interventional procedures, physical therapy (PT), antidepressants, antiinflammatory medications, antiepileptics, and opiates. However, little has been available to patients when these modalities fail to control their pain. In terms of pharmacologic management, there has been increased interest in the use of ketamine, bisphosphonates, calcitonin, magnesium, and free radical scavengers for CRPS.[3,4] Several studies on these various agents have produced promising results. However, given the lack of consistent diagnostic criteria and treatment algorithms, interpretation of these results is challenging.

A review of the pathophysiology of chronic pain can clarify the roles each agent plays in the treatment of CRPS. Our current understanding of the disease stems from the notion that central sensitization leads to neuropathic pain. Localized trauma causes a release of reactive oxygen particles, inflammatory mediators, and neuropeptides, which create a cascade of events leading to central sensitization or wind up. Local structures, such as C and A-delta fibers, become sensitized and continuously release glutamate, which activate the alpha-amino-3-hydroxy-5-methyl-4-isoxazolepropionic acid receptor (AMPA) via calcium release. As calcium influx occurs, the cell is depolarized and releases the voltage-dependent magnesium block on the N-methyl-D-aspartate (NMDA) receptors. Once magnesium is displaced from the NMDA receptor, signal propagation is activated. The NMDA receptor plays a key role in the induction and propagation of peripheral and central sensitization. This results in an amplified response even to benign peripheral stimuli, known as allodynia or hyperalgesia. It is clear why NMDA antagonists, such as ketamine, may have critical treatment potential. Additionally, calcium plays an integral role in this cascade and its levels are modified through calcitonin and bisphosphonate applications.

INTRAVENOUS KETAMINE

Ketamine has analgesic properties within the central and peripheral nervous system via interactions with several receptor subtypes including NMDA, opioid, and AMPA. Additionally, ketamine plays a role in the inhibition of serotonin and dopamine reuptake.[5] Whereas some studies have shown complete relief of pain with anesthetic doses of ketamine, the utility of this treatment is limited by adverse effects associated with high doses of ketamine and the financial burden of inpatient hospitalization required for the treatment.[6] Subanesthetic doses of ketamine have offered short-term pain relief for a subset of patients.

PHARMACOLOGY

Ketamine is a dissociative anesthetic that offers analgesia and amnesia. It is a phenylepiperidine derivative that is structurally similar to phencyclidine (PCP) with a 2(2-chlorophenyl)-2-(methylamino)-cyclohexane ring. Ketamine has a chiral center that creates two stereoisomers, S(+) and R(−) ketamine. Currently, there are two commercially available forms of ketamine: the S(+) ketamine (S-ketamine or ketanest-S) or the racemic mixture (Ketalar). The S(+) enantiomer is preferable as it has twice the analgesic potency, better cardiovascular profile, and may confer neuroprotective properties.[7]

Intravenous (IV) ketamine has a redistribution half-life of 7–15 minutes, clearance 15 $mg.kg^{-1}.min^{-1}$, and elimination half-life 2–3 hours.[8] Ketamine readily crosses the blood-brain barrier, which allows for rapid onset of acute analgesic effect. It is metabolized in the liver by CYP3A4, CYP2B6, and CYP2C9 to its metabolite norketamine via N-demethylation. Norketamine is produced within minutes of IV ketamine injection and may outlive the parent compound. Ultimately, norketamine undergoes glucuronidation in the liver and is eliminated by the kidneys and bile. Upon discontinuation of ketamine infusion, the concentration of ketamine rapidly drops. However, when utilized for chronic pain, the analgesic effects outlast serum concentrations, likely due to ketamine's neuromodulatory effects on the NMDA receptor (NMDAR).

Ketamine plays a role in both acute and chronic pain but through different mechanisms. Sigtermans et al. performed an observational study investigating the analgesic effects of ketamine in acute experimental pain versus chronic spontaneous pain in CRPS patients.[9] Ten patients with CRPS underwent seven IV low-dose S(+) ketamine infusions in 5-minute infusion periods. Each 5-minute infusion was followed by a 20-minute break before another infusion (of an increased dose) was initiated. Spontaneous pain ratings and visual analogue scale (VAS) to experimental heat stimulation was recorded during the infusion and 3 hours later. Additionally, serum ketamine levels were monitored throughout the infusions. The authors concluded that ketamine produced profound analgesia (VAS decreased from 6.2 ± 0.2 to 0.4 ± 0.3) by the end of the infusion. However, the analgesic effects of ketamine, with experimental thermal pain, ended when the infusion stopped. Pain relief persisted beyond the termination of infusion (175 minutes after infusion) and when ketamine serum levels were very low (<100 ng/mL). Thus, in the acute setting, ketamine's effect on experimental pain is dictated by its pharmacokinetics while its effects on CRPS pain persisted despite lower serum concentrations. The authors concluded that, even with a short-lived infusion, ketamine likely plays a neuromodulatory role in CRPS, possibly via desensitization of the NMDA receptor within the spinal cord or via restoration of inhibitory sensory control within the brain.

MECHANISM OF ACTION

The pathophysiology of CRPS may involve a combination of the following mechanisms: NMDAR phosphorylation and upregulation, loss of descending inhibition, activation of the immune cells within the spinal cord which release proinflammatory cytokines, and plastic changes in the spinal cord. The NMDAR is an excitatory glutamate receptor located at the dorsal horn of the spinal cord and in supraspinal structures. Central sensitization occurs when prolonged nociceptive input causes activation and upregulation of the NMDAR, resulting in amplified signaling of the pain pathway to the brain. Over time, this pathway is continuously activated, regardless of the stimulus, and can contribute to the perseverance of chronic pain states. As a noncompetitive NMDA antagonist, ketamine blocks the NMDAR and decreases neuronal hyperexcitability. Ketamine has traditionally been thought to antagonize the NMDAR but also interacts with opioid receptors, muscarinic, and monoaminergic receptors.[5]

NMDA receptors are highly expressed in the temporal cortex, hippocampus, basal ganglia, cerebellum, and brainstem. Ketamine may also affect the descending inhibitory pathways involved in chronic pain states. In an elegant study, resting-state functional magnetic resonance imaging (fMRI) was performed before, during, and after subanesthetic ketamine infusions. The investigators showed activation of the anterior cingulate cortex, orbital frontal cortex, insula, and brainstem after the infusion; these areas are involved in the descending inhibitory pain pathway.[10]

USE IN CHRONIC PAIN

Pain relief has been reported with anesthetic doses of ketamine. Kiefer et al. conducted an open-labeled phase II study in 20 patients treated with anesthetic doses of ketamine requiring intubation.[11] They noted complete pain relief in all patients at 1 month and in 16/20 patients at 6 months. Additionally, they showed improvement in quality of life, associated movement disorder, and ability to work in the majority of patients. Upon emergence from ketamine anesthesia, the majority of patients reported psychotropic side effects of anxiety, dysphoria, nightmares, and sleep difficulties. Seven patients developed respiratory infections associated with mechanical ventilation. Sixteen patients experienced elevations in their liver function tests, noted on day 5 of the treatment. Unfortunately, similar salutary effects have not been replicated with subanesthetic doses of ketamine. A recent meta-analysis by Collins et al. was not able to show significant pain relief with ketamine infusions in CRPS (–0.65 [CI 95% –1.47, 0.16], $P = .11$). They noted that while the data are encouraging, further studies are necessary.[12]

The majority of the studies on the effects of ketamine included patients diagnosed according to the IASP criteria who were allowed to continue their home medications throughout the trials. Most studies excluded patients with serious medical issues, drug or alcohol abuse, history of psychosis, increased intracranial pressure, major opioid use, pain scores less than 5 on a 0–10 scale, or pregnancy/lactation. Two randomized controlled, double-blinded, placebo-controlled trials[13,14] further investigated the benefits of subanesthetic doses of ketamine in the treatment of CRPS. Both showed significant improvement in VAS scores over the treatment duration and in 3-month follow-up despite varying infusion rates. However, neither showed any improvement in functional capacity.

Sigtermans et al.[13] evaluated 60 patients with severe, long-standing CRPS (up to 9 years' duration of symptoms) where 30 inpatients were treated with ketamine infusions for 4.2 days (1.2 $\mu g.kg^{-1}.min^{-1}$ or 5 mg/hour with up-titration to a maximum of 7.2 $\mu g.kg^{-1}.min^{-1}$ or 30 mg/hour). VAS scores were recorded prior to treatment and then weekly for 11 weeks. VAS scores were dramatically improved within the first week (7.2–2.6) and continued until the 11th week. At 12 weeks, ketamine's treatment effects subsided. However, while patients reported decreased pain scores, their functional capacity did not improve. Interestingly, this study did not find an association with the duration of symptoms and response to ketamine infusion. The ketamine group complained of more nausea/vomiting, psychotomimetic effects, but there were no differences with respect to headache, blood pressure, and liver function when compared to controls.

A similar study was conducted by Schwartzman et al.[14] in an outpatient clinic setting where 19 patients with severe, long-standing, intractable CRPS received ketamine infusions at a rate of 100 mg/4 hours, which was increased halfway through the study to 200 mg/4 hours for 10 days (5 days on, 2 days off, 5 days on). Patients were pretreated with midazolam 2 mg, clonidine 0.1 mg PO, and an additional midazolam 2 mg posttreatment. Follow-up occurred at 2 weeks, and then monthly for 3 months. This study showed statistically significant improvement in pain scores that lasted until the 12-week posttreatment period, with none of the parameters returning to their pretreatment levels. Similarly to the Sigtermans' study, this study was not able to show a statistically significant improvement in activity levels or quality of life. Side effects of ketamine included nausea, headache, tiredness, or dysphoria. None of the patients reported hallucination, delusions, or out-of-body experiences.

Although neither randomized control trial (RCT)[13,14] showed a statistically significant improvement in functional capacity, an open-label prospective study by Goldberg et al. did show improvement in initiation of activity.[15] Forty patients received outpatient infusions of ketamine 40–80 mg/4 hours for 10 days. Similar to Schwartzman's study, patients were pretreated with midazolam 2–4 mg and clonidine 0.1 mg PO. Goldberg et al. reported a significant reduction in pain scores over the 10-day period and showed a statistically significant improvement in movement initiation by the tenth day of infusion. The authors suggested that longer treatment periods may produce a more pronounced effect. Additionally, they reported 10% of patients had return of "worst pain" by 2 weeks, 62% had at least 70% reduction in worst pain at 6 weeks and were back to baseline pain 9 weeks after treatment. Twenty percent of the patients reported greater than 70% reduction in pain for 11–12 weeks; 8% of the patients were pain-free at 15 months.

Although Sigtermans et al.[13] and Schwartzman et al.[14] evaluated the efficacy of ketamine infusions in patients with CRPS, Gustin et al. examined the role of combination therapy using an NMDA antagonist and morphine in alleviating pain in CRPS patients.[10] The rationale for their study was that NMDA antagonism may reduce the body's adaptation to morphine. When morphine binds to the μ-receptor, it can release mediators that bind to the NMDA receptor and enhance pain sensitivity. NMDA antagonism may blunt this response. CRPS patients may exhibit central neuroplastic changes involving an alteration of the representation zones in the somatosensory and motor cortexes. Gustin et al.[10] used fMRI to detect cerebral activity changes while treating patients with combination therapy. This double-blinded, randomized controlled trial included 20 patients randomized to either a group treated with an NMDA antagonist and morphine or a group treated with placebo and morphine. Patients were diagnosed using IASP criteria, had symptoms for greater than 6 months (average 16 months), and had a baseline VAS pain score of at least 3. They excluded patients who were left-handed, had contraindications to fMRI, and who had no demonstrable motor deficits on neurological exam.

All patients underwent a 2-day washout period for existing CRPS medications. Morphine was administered 3 times per day for 56 days (titrated from 10 mg for 5 days up to 30 mg for the remaining 51 days). Memantine was started on day 8 at 5 mg per day and titrated up to 40 mg by the end of the study. They used fMRI during movement of both upper extremities, before and after treatment of 56 days. Only the combination group of memantine/morphine showed a statistically significant reduction in pain at rest and during movement. After 49 days of treatment, MRI findings showed reduced activation of the contralateral primary somatosensory and anterior cingulate when the affected limb was moved but not at rest. These reduced activation areas also correlated to pain relief during the treatment period. Overall, they showed that combination therapy significantly affected the cerebral processing of nociceptive information in CRPS patients. Additionally, patients experienced improvement in mood and disability. Side effects of fatigue, drowsiness, nausea, akathisia, vertigo, head pain, and anxiety were mildly reported.[10]

The results of studies on IV ketamine are in Table 54.1.

SIDE EFFECTS OF KETAMINE

Ketamine exposure has several associated risks that can affect the central nervous, cardiovascular, and hepatic systems. Much of our understanding of ketamine's side effect profile was derived from recreational and chronic ketamine abusers. Given the known risk of central nervous system (CNS) related side effects, it may be prudent to withhold ketamine from patients with schizophrenia, manic depressive disorder, and a history of substance abuse.

CENTRAL NERVOUS SYSTEM EFFECTS

Ketamine is known to have psychotropic or psychedelic effects, which usually occur in a dose-dependent manner. Niesters et al.[32] examined the effects of subanesthetic doses of ketamine on intrinsic functional brain connectivity in a placebo-controlled fMRI trial. They exposed 12 healthy males to a 2-hour infusion of S(+) ketamine (20 mg/70 kg for the first hour, then 40 mg/70 kg for the second hour). They found NMDAR expression to be high in the temporal cortex, hippocampus, basal ganglia, cerebellum, and brainstem, with the highest concentration noted in the cerebellum. The cerebellum is thought to play a critical role in emotional processing (mainly anxiety) and thought coordination. Niesters' study showed alterations in connectivity of the cerebellum, which may be related to the psychedelic side effects during ketamine infusions.[32] fMRI also showed large connectivity changes in the visual cortex and the optic radiation, which may explain the visual hallucinations, blurry vision, and double vision observed with ketamine infusion. These CNS effects resolved within 30 minutes of infusion termination. Blagrove et al.[33] reported that unpleasant dreams could persist for up to 3 days after terminating infusion. Midazolam and clonidine have been critical in tempering these effects but do not completely prevent the occurrence of these unpleasant side effects.

Ketamine administration also offers amnestic properties, which are temporary in ketamine-naïve patients. However, limited data are available on memory impairment with long-term use of low-dose ketamine utilization. Koffler et al. studied the effects of anesthetic doses of ketamine on neurocognitive function following a 4.5-day infusion of ketamine (250–300 μg/dL level), which resulted in a medically induced coma.[6] Nine patients with severe refractory CRPS underwent neuropsychological testing before the treatment and 6 weeks following the infusion. They reported no adverse cognitive effects of extended treatment with anesthetic doses of ketamine.

CARDIOVASCULAR EFFECTS

Ketamine activates the sympathetic nervous system causing systemic release of catecholamines, inhibition of parasympathetic output, and inhibition of norepinephrine reuptake at peripheral nerves. However, it has direct myocardial depressant properties in high doses. Patients undergoing low-dose ketamine infusions may experience tachycardia, increases in pulmonary arterial pressure, systemic blood pressure, and increases in myocardial oxygen consumption. Thus, all patients undergoing ketamine infusion therapy require continuous monitoring of their heart rate,

TABLE 54.1 Randomized Studies on Pharmacologic Management of Complex Regional Pain Syndrome

Study	Type of Study; Medications Compared; Duration of Follow-Up	Outcome Measures	Results	Comments
Ketamine				
Sigtermans et al.[13]; 60 patients with CRPS	DB, PC, parallel group. Ketamine 1.2–7.2 $\mu g.kg^{-1}.min^{-1}$ × 4.2 days. 30 pts per group. 12-week follow-up.	VAS, functional capacity.	VAS improved until 11th week. Treatment effect subsided by 12 weeks. No change in functional capacity.	No association with duration of symptoms and response to ketamine.
Schwartzman et al.[14]; 19 patients with severe, long-standing CRPS	DB, PC. 9 patients received ketamine IV 100 mg/4 h increased to 200 mg/4 h × 10 days vs. 10 patients with placebo (NS IV). 3-month follow-up.	VAS, functional capacity.	Improvement in VAS past 3 months. No change in functional capacity.	Patients pretreated with midazolam 2 mg before and after treatment, Clonidine 0.1 mg PO. No psychotomimetic side effects noted.
Gustin et al.[10]; 20 patients with CRPS	R, DB, PC. 10 patients with memantine 5 mg–40 mg QD + morphine 10–30 mg QD × 8 days. 10 patients with morphine alone. 56-day follow-up.	VAS, fMRI during affected/unaffected hand (before and after treatment) at 49 days for both groups.	fMRI showed reduced activation of contralateral primary somatosensory and anterior cingulate cortexes with affected limb movement. This correlated with improved VAS. Patients had improvement in mood and disability.	NMDA antagonism may reduce the body's adaption to morphine.
Bisphosphonates				
Maillefert et al.[16]; 11 patients with CRPS UE/LE	OL, P. Pamidronate 30 mg in NS 500 mL over 4 h QD × 3 days. Follow-up at 1 and 3 months.	VAS pain scores and physician global assessment based on clinical evaluation (hyperhidrosis, vasomotor changes, joint stiffness), blood cell count, and serum calcium measure	VAS pain scores significantly decreased at 3 months. Global assessment: four patients—no improvement, one patient—moderate improvement, six patients—significant or excellent improvement at 3 months.	Diagnosed by Doury's criteria, duration of symptoms >6 months, refractory to calcitonin and PT.
Robinson et al.[17]; 27 patients UE/LE	PC, R, DB. Pamidronate 60 mg single dose vs. NS. 14 patients given pamidronate vs. 13 patients on placebo.	VAS pain scores, global assessment of disease severity scores, SF-36 at 1 and 3 months.	Overall improvement in VAS global assessment of disease severity score and SF-36 at 3 months.	There was great variability of responses among individuals. Duration of symptoms 3 months–6 years. Used IASP criteria.
Adami et al.[18]; 20 patients with CRPS of foot and hand.	R, DB, PC. 10 patients each received alendronate 7.5 mg in 250 NS IV vs. placebo with NS × 3 days. 2 weeks later all patients underwent open label alendronate infusion. Follow-up 12 months.	Pain, tenderness, improvement in motion.	Diminished pain, tenderness, swelling and improvement in motion noted in alendronate group at 2–4 weeks. Similar results during open label phase of placebo patients treated with alendronate. Statistically significant rise in bone mineral density at 6 weeks. At 12 months 9 patients in remission, 7 relapsed.	10 patients had failed nasal calcitonin therapy. Duration of symptoms 5–34 weeks.
Manicourt et al.[19]; 40 patients with LE CRPS	R, DB, PC. 19 patients received alendronate vs. 19 who received placebo. Alendronate 40 mg tablet × 8 weeks. Optional open label phase.	VAS pain score, joint mobility, LE edema, LE tolerance to pressure, levels of spontaneous pain.	Significant decrease in VAS pain score at 4, 8, 12 weeks. Improved joint mobility. The group that received two courses of alendronate treatments showed further improvement in symptoms without plateau effect.	Mean duration of symptoms was 7 months. Excluded patients with previous bisphosphonate therapy, sympathetic blocks, calcitonin therapy. Allowed PT.

Varenna et al.[20]; 82 patients with CRPS of hand or foot	PC, R, DB: Neridronate 100 mg QID × 10 days vs. NS. 41 patients per group. Open extension phase where placebo group was treated. 20-month follow up.	VAS pain scores, clinical assessment (edema, pain at motion, allodynia, hyperalgesia) SF-36, McGill Pain Questionnaire	Significant decrease in VAS pain scores and improved clinical signs/functional status.	Most patients were in the early phase of the disease.
Varenna et al.[21]; 32 patients with CRPS	R, DB, PC. 15 patients received clodronate 300 mg QD × 10 days vs. placebo (15 patients). After 40-day washout, placebo group received clodronate treatment. Follow-up 180 days.	VAS, clinical global assessment, efficacy verbal score.	Significantly better relief of pain and global assessment.	
Breuer et al.[22]; 9 patients of hand and foot CRPS	Observational; 9 patients ibandroante 6 mg IV QD × 3 days. Follow-up 4 weeks.	VAS, neuropathic pain qualities.	Improvement in average and worst pain scores after 4 weeks. 30% of patients with improvement activity levels.	CRPS for at least 1 month. Used to justify a randomized trial. Hand CRPS more common than foot CRPS.
Magnesium				
Collins et al.[23]; 8 patients CRPS of UE/LE	R, PC. 6 patients received MG++ 70 mg/kg in 50 mL over 4 h × 5 days vs. 2 patients who received NS.	Pain assessment (11-point box scale and McGill Pain Questionnaire at baseline, 1, 3, 6, 12 weeks).	Pain significantly reduced at all measured time points and McGill sensory subscale was significantly improved at 1 week. At 12 weeks, there was a statistically significant improvement in impairment level and quality of life.	All patients continued PT. No change in skin sensitivity and functional limitations. Diagnosis: IASP criteria.
Fischer et al.[24]; 56 CRPS UE/LE	R, PC. 56 patients, 29 patients received MG 70 mg/kg over 4 h × 5 consecutive days. 27 patients received NaCl.	Pain assessment (11-point box scale and McGill Pain Questionnaire at baseline, 1, 3, 6, and 12 weeks).	Statistically significant improvement on level of impairment at 1 week, improvement in McGill pain scores at 6 weeks, improvement in perceived job participation at 12 weeks.	Mean duration of symptoms 16 months.
Gabapentin and Pregabalin				
Serpell[25]; 307 patients with neuropathic pain symptoms (28% with CRPS)	R, DB, PC. 153 patients received gabapentin 2700 mg × 8 weeks vs. placebo (154 patients).	Neuropathic pain symptoms, quality of life via SF-36.	Statistically significant reduction in neuropathic pain.	Participants had a wide range of neuropathic symptoms (28% with CRPS). Used IASP criteria.
Van de Vusse et al.[26]; 58 patients with CRPS of UE/LE	R, DB, Crossover study. 29 patients treated with gabapentin 1800 mg QD × 3 weeks vs. placebo. 2-week washout with crossover to other treatment group. 8-week follow-up.	VAS, allodynia, edema, discoloration, range of motion, quality of life.	No greater pain relief with Gabapentin over placebo. Sensory deficits significantly reversed in Gabapentin users. No change in allodynia, edema, discoloration, range of motion, quality of life.	Used IASP criteria. Interestingly, first half of the study showed a benefit with Gabapentin.
Tadalafil				
Groeneweg et al.[27]; 24 patients with cold LE CRPS	R, DB, PC. 12 patients received tadalafil 10 mg QD × 4 weeks then 20 mg QD × 8 weeks, vs. 12 patients who received placebo.	VAS pain score, temperature change, range of motion, standing, walking.	15% reduction in VAS vs. placebo, small nonstatistically significant improvement in muscle strength over time, walking ability, and reduced need for crutches. No change in temperature.	Diagnostic criteria not defined. Minimal change in blood pressure. Allowed to do PT.
Free Radical Scavengers				
Zuurmond et al.[28]; 32 patients with acute CRPS (secondary to trauma)	P, R, DB, PC. 16 patients treated with 50% DMSO cream (applied five times daily) vs. 17 treated with placebo cream. 2-month follow up.	CRPS symptoms.	Significantly better CRPS symptom improvement than placebo	Diagnosed via Veldman and Dutch criteria.

Continued

TABLE 54.1 Randomized Studies on Pharmacologic Management of Complex Regional Pain Syndrome—cont'd

Study	Type of Study; Medications Compared; Duration of Follow-Up	Outcome Measures	Results	Comments
Perez et al.[29]; 41 patients with CRPS-LE	P, R, DB, PC. 22 patients treated with 10% mannitol in 1 L NS in affected limb over 4 h × 5 days vs. 20 patients treated with placebo NS infusion. 9-week follow-up.	Pain, function level, quality of life at 2, 6 and 9 weeks.	No difference in pain function level, or quality of life.	Diagnosed according to Bruehl criteria. Mean duration of symptoms 6.5 months. PT performed in all subjects. Concluded mannitol maybe more helpful during acute phase when more inflammatory mediators are present.
Perez et al.[30]; 146 patients with CRPS in UE/LE	R, DB. DMSO 50% (5 times per day) vs. NAC 600 mg TID (both combined with placebo) × 17 weeks. 24-month follow-up.	Impairment level sum score, UE/LE skills/function.	NAC and DMSO were equally beneficial but subgroup analysis showed warm extremity CRPS responded better to DMSO while cold extremity CRPS responded better to NAC tablets.	Allowed rescue with Paracetamol 500 mg, Naproxen 250–500 mg and/or Tramadol. Diagnosed according to Veldman and Netherlands WHO collaboration Criteria. CRPS for >1 year. Allowed to do PT.
Tan et al.[31]; 68 patients with CRPS UE/LE	Retrospective, consecutive group of 68 CRPS patients treated with 10% mannitol in 1 L NS per 24 h × 7–10 days.	CRPS symptoms (not specified). Overall improvement defined as <3 of the following symptoms: pain, swelling, edema, temperature, loss of range of motion, and increase in exercise.	24% improvement after 1 week, 30% after 1 month. Warm CRPS may have responded better than cold CRPS.	Diagnosed via Veldman criteria. Median duration of symptoms 129 days with a range of 3–1046 days.

Note: See specific studies for details. Studies on calcitonin are in Table 54.2.

CRPS, *Complex regional pain syndrome;* DB, *double-blind;* DMSO, *dimethyl sulfoxide;* fMRI, *functional magnetic resonance imaging;* IV, *intravenous;* LE, *lower extremity;* NAC, *N-acetylcysteine;* NaCl, *sodium chloride;* NMDA, *N-methyl-D-aspartate;* NS, *normal saline;* OL, *open label;* P, *prospective;* PC, *placebo controlled;* PT, *physical therapy;* R, *randomized;* UE, *upper extremity;* WHO, *World Heath Organization.*

blood pressure, and oxygen consumption. Some studies[7] have utilized clonidine 0.2 mg to blunt the sympathetic effects of ketamine.

HEPATIC EFFECTS

Ketamine-induced liver dysfunction has been reported with prolonged or repeat infusions within a short time frame. Noppers et al.[34] reported six patients with CRPS who were exposed to two 100-hour infusions of S(+) ketamine (10–20 mg/hour) separated by 16 days. Three of the six patients exhibited elevated liver enzymes (up to three times normal values). These levels normalized over the subsequent 2 months. The exact mechanism of injury is unclear but may involve impaired hepatic oxygen delivery, formation of free radicals, or an allergic hepatitis.

BISPHOSPHONATES

Patients with CRPS are believed to have osteoclast hyperactivity leading to localized osteoporosis. Osteoclast hyperactivity and bone marrow swelling may contribute to the ignition of chronic pain in CRPS patients. Bisphosphonates inhibit bone resorption and may play a critical role in pain relief associated with CRPS. There is level 1B+ evidence (one or more RCTs with methodologic weaknesses, demonstrate effectiveness; the benefits clearly outweigh risk and burdens) supporting the use of bisphosphonates in the early stage of CRPS when there are emerging signs of osteoporosis.[3] Hence, early treatment with bisphosphonates may be beneficial in a subset of CRPS patients. Many studies have investigated different bisphosphonates in the treatment of CRPS: neridronate, pamidronate, alendronate. The challenge is identifying the ideal bisphosphonate, dosage, and timing of treatment.

PHARMACOLOGY

Bisphosphonates are a unique class of drugs that all have a common P-C-P structure, and vary at the carbon "R" group attachment. Although these agents share a similar chemical structure, their antiabsorbing capabilities differ dramatically. Bisphosphonates are further classified into nitrogen-containing agents (alendronate, neridronate, ibandronate, pamidronate, risedronate, and zoledronic acid) and nonnitrogen-containing compounds (etidronate and tiludronate).[35] This class of drugs is resistant to enzymatic or chemical breakdown and are poorly absorbed in the gastrointestinal (GI) tract due to their low lipophilicity. Upon entering the systemic circulation, bisphosphonates quickly disappear from the plasma where half the drug is excreted unchanged by the kidney. The remaining drug has a very high affinity for bone tissue and is absorbed onto the bone surface.

MECHANISM OF ACTION

Bisphosphonates preferentially bind to bones undergoing high turnover. Once they are taken into the bone, they are not released until that bone is resorbed. Thus, their half-life can be prolonged (1–10 years) depending on the rate of bone turnover.[35] Bisphosphonates work by two mechanisms depending on their chemical structure. Nitrogen-containing agents will attach to the hydroxyapatite binding site on the resorbed bone surfaces. Osteoclasts will bind to the bone impregnated with bisphosphonate and attempt to resorb it. However, in breaking down the bone, the bisphosphonates are released and prevent the osteoclast from further binding to the bone. More specifically, nitrogen-containing bisphosphonates inhibit the enzyme farnesyl pyrophosphate synthase (FPP), which is involved in creating the cytoskeleton of the osteoclast. Once this process is inhibited, the osteoclast cannot attach to the bone perimeter to resorb bone. The potency of each bisphosphonate is related to its ability to inhibit FPP.

Nonnitrogen-containing compounds (etidronate and tiludronate) are metabolized by osteoclasts and produce by-products that inhibit ATP production, resulting in osteoclast apoptosis. Interestingly, bisphosphonates may also play a role in preventing osteoblast apoptosis. Bisphosphonates may have analgesic effects via modification of inflammatory cytokines (interleukin one [IL-1], prostaglandin E2 [PGE2]) which are involved in sensitizing painful nociceptors and low-threshold mechanoreceptors.

USE IN CHRONIC REGIONAL PAIN SYNDROME

Pamidronate

There is level 1B+ evidence supporting the use of pamidronate, a second-generation bisphosphonate, in CRPS.[3] Two different doses of pamidronate have been evaluated. Pamidronate 30 mg IV infusion was administered for 3 days in an open-label, prospective study[16] of 11 patients with CRPS in their upper or lower extremity for a duration of at least 6 months (mean 14.6 months). Patients reported a decreased VAS pain score (mean VAS 58.8/100–41.1/100) at 1 month, and a mean VAS of 33.8 at 3 months. Additionally, 7 of the 11 patients showed at least moderate improvement in the physician global assessment at 3 months. Side effects included mild symptoms of fever and hypocalcemia. Another study[17] looked at a single pamidronate 60 mg IV infusion, which showed similar results: lower VAS pain scores and improvement on Short Form Health Survey-36 (SF-36) at 3 months when compared to placebo normal saline infusion. They included patients with upper and lower extremity CRPS (according to IASP criteria) with a broad duration of symptoms (3 months–6 years). The authors noted a broad range of variability in responses within the treatment groups. There were minor side effects of flulike symptoms and infusion reaction with erythema/discomfort, which quickly resolved. One confounder of this study was that the pamidronate group had higher pain scores at the beginning of the study.

Alendronate

Level 1B+ evidence supports the use of alendronate in CRPS.[3] Both oral and IV alendronate have been evaluated in clinical studies and show improvement in pain scores, bone mineralization, and joint mobility.

A double-blinded, placebo controlled, randomized controlled trial[18] in 20 patients with CRPS for 5–34 weeks was performed, where half the subjects received alendronate 7.5 mg IV infusion for 3 days. This was followed by an open-label phase where all patients were exposed to the treatment. Interestingly, 10 patients had failed nasal calcitonin therapy, another osteoclastic agent. Patients treated with alendronate showed significant differences with respect to spontaneous pain, tenderness, swelling, and improvement in motion within the first 2 weeks. There was also a statistically significant rise in bone mineral density within 6 weeks. Similar results were seen in the placebo group treated with alendronate during the open-label phase of the study. At the 12-month follow-up, nine patients were in remission (seven were on their second course of alendronate) while seven patients had a relapse in their symptoms (four patients were receiving their initial course of alendronate). The treatment was well tolerated but three patients experienced fever on the day after the infusion.

The evaluation of oral alendronate has shown similar benefits. A double-blind, placebo-controlled trial[19] was conducted in 20 patients with CRPS for a mean duration of 7 months. Patients were treated with alendronate 40 mg PO for 8 weeks, followed by an optional open-label phase of similar treatment. They excluded patients with previous bisphosphonate therapy, sympathetic nerve blocks, and calcitonin therapy, but allowed patients to continue PT. This study showed a significant decrease in VAS pain score by 4 weeks, with further declines at 8 and 12 weeks (33% of placebo at 12 weeks). The mean score for joint mobility was significantly higher in the alendronate group. Additionally, during the open-label portion of the trial, placebo treated patients who were given alendronate showed dramatic improvement in VAS scores for spontaneous pain, pressure tolerance, and joint mobility. The patients previously treated with alendronate experienced further improvement suggesting no plateau effect. Two patients reported GI intolerance with alendronate and discontinued the study.

Neridronate

The utility of neridronate was evaluated in a double-blind, placebo-controlled, randomized trial[20] performed in 82 patients with CRPS of less than 4 months' duration who were exposed to four neridronate 100-mg infusions over 10 days. Similarly to other studies noted, the placebo arm was then exposed to the same intervention after 50 days. Of the studies discussed, this was the first study to diagnose patients according to the Budapest criteria. The mean VAS pain score in the neridronate treatment group was significantly reduced within the first 20 days, more dramatically at 40 days. Patients experienced less allodynia, hyperalgesia, edema, decreased use of rescue medications, and improved range of motion at 40 days. Follow-up data at 7–14 months showed that patients did not relapse and their symptoms improved. Minimal side effects of fever and myalgias were noted.

Clodronate

Level 1B+ evidence supports the use of a nonnitrogen group bisphosphonate, clodronate, in CRPS patients.[3] Thirty-two patients received daily infusions of either clodronate 300 mg IV (15 patients) for 10 days or placebo, in a double-blinded, placebo (17 patients) controlled, randomized controlled trial.[21] After a 40-day washout period, the placebo group was exposed to the same treatment. They noted an overall percentage decrease in VAS pain scores of 93.2% ± 15.6%, with 30 patients reporting significant improvement or being devoid of symptoms.

Ibandronate

Weaker evidence (2C+; effectiveness only demonstrated in observational studies, with no conclusive evidence of beneficial effects, and potential benefits closely balanced with risks and burdens) exists for the use of ibandronate in CRPS patients.[3] An open-labeled trial[22] exposed nine CRPS patients with symptoms for at least 1 month to an ibandronate 6-mg IV infusion for 3 consecutive days. Patients reported improvements in average and worst pain scores after 4 weeks. Thirty percent of patients reported significant improvement in their activity level. Interestingly, patients with hand CRPS benefited more than foot CRPS. The medication was well tolerated despite mild flu-like symptoms.

The results of studies on bisphosphonates are summarized in Table 54.1.

SIDE EFFECTS

The majority of side effects associated with bisphosphonate therapy are mild in nature. One of the most concerning side effects is decreased bone formation as bisphosphonates disrupt the normal balance of bone formation and resorption. There have been case reports of jaw necrosis[36] with exposure to long-term, high-dose, bisphosphonate therapy. The majority of these cases were in cancer patients undergoing aggressive bisphosphonate therapy; only 5% of cases were reported in low-dose bisphosphonate therapy.[36]

Oral formulations of bisphosphonates are difficult to absorb and may cause GI upset in addition to inflammation/erosive esophagitis. The majority of the studies reported mild flulike symptoms with treatment. One study noted slightly decreased calcium levels while another study preemptively treated patients with oral calcium and vitamin D to minimize this risk.[22]

CALCITONIN

Calcitonin is a polypeptide hormone that is produced by the parafollicular cells of the thyroid gland. It opposes the effects of parathyroid hormone and reduces blood calcium levels. Calcitonin can be found in fish, reptiles, birds, and mammals. It has been utilized in the treatment of several bone-related diseases such as postmenopausal osteoporosis, Paget disease, bone metastasis, as well as for hypercalcemia, phantom limb pain, and to provide short-term pain relief for vertebral fractures. Salmon calcitonin is most widely used as it has 40 times higher affinity for the human calcitonin receptor than human calcitonin.[37]

PHARMACOLOGY

Calcitonin is US Food and Drug Administration (FDA)-approved for intramuscular, subcutaneous, or nasal spray application. Nasal spray calcitonin has a short absorption time (10–15 minutes) and elimination half-life (50–80 minutes).

Salmon calcitonin is rapidly absorbed and eliminated, with peak plasma concentrations noted within the first hour of administration. The intramuscular or subcutaneous calcitonin half-life is nearly an hour, with a duration of action of 6–8 hours. After parenteral intake, the kidneys metabolize calcitonin into metabolites with weaker metabolic activity. Better bioavailability is appreciated with subcutaneous and intramuscular injection in humans (71% and 66%, respectively) than with nasal spray (3%–5% relative to intramuscular administration). Plasma protein binding is 30%–40%.

MECHANISM OF ACTION

Calcitonin is believed to counteract the effects of parathyroid hormone which increases calcium levels within the blood. Calcitonin lowers blood calcium levels via four possible mechanisms: inhibition of calcium absorption from the intestines, inhibition of osteoclast activity in bones, stimulation of osteoblast activity in bones, and inhibition of renal tubular reabsorption of calcium so that it may be excreted in urine. Several mechanisms have been postulated regarding the analgesic effects of calcitonin: (1) direct action on specific receptors in the CNS, (2) peripheral antiinflammatory action, (3) release of B-endorphin, and (4) changes in the descending serotonergic modification on the sensory transmission by C afferent fibers.

CLINICAL USE

Medications that inhibit osteoclast activity play a critical role in the treatment of CRPS. In a network meta-analysis of 16 randomized controlled trials, Wertli et al.[38] concluded that bisphosphonates should be the treatment of choice for the early stages of CRPS. However, calcitonin was superior to bisphosphonates as a short-term medication for more chronic stages of CRPS. Given the lack to randomization and blinding in many of the referenced articles, the utilization of calcitonin for CRPS has level 2B– evidence.[4]

In a randomized, double-blind, placebo-controlled randomized controlled trial,[39] Bickerstaff and Kanis exposed 20 patients to nasal calcitonin 400 IU daily for 4 weeks and compared pain levels with saline placebo treatment. They were not able to appreciate any differences among the two groups with respect to pain scores, swelling, or stiffness. Sahin et al.[40] conducted a similar study (randomized, placebo controlled, single blinded) on 18 patients treated with nasal calcitonin 200 IU/day for 2 months, calcium 500 mg/day, stellate ganglion blocks, and PT for 2 months. These patients were compared with CRPS patients treated with paracetamol 1500 mg/day, PT, and stellate ganglion blocks. Both groups showed improvement in pain and clinical assessment but no differences were appreciated between the two groups. They concluded that nasal calcitonin did not offer any benefits over paracetamol 1500 mg/day. Gobelet et al. was able to show a statistically significant difference in a randomized, double-blind, placebo-controlled trial[41] of 66 patients with CRPS. One group was treated with daily calcitonin 100 IU, PT, and transcutaneous electrical nerve stimulation (TENS) unit for 3 weeks. During the 8-week follow-up, patients treated with calcitonin had improved pain, range of motion, and returned to work faster than those treated with placebo. Overall, these studies reveal inconsistent results with nasal calcitonin and further studies are warranted.

Intramuscular calcitonin may offer better results. Hamamci et al. compared intramuscular calcitonin 100 IU daily for 4 weeks (25 patients) to a normal saline control group (16 patients) in 41 patients.[42] They were able to show significantly lower pain scores and improved range of motion/motor function in the treatment group (better shoulder abduction, external rotation, wrist flexion, and metacarpophalangeal extension). The calcitonin intramuscular (IM) group had higher baseline pain scores, which may have been a confounding factor. Gobelet et al. also examined the potential for daily subcutaneous calcitonin 100 IU for 3 weeks in 12 patients who were allowed to do PT.[43] In this randomized controlled trial, the treatment group was compared to a control group of 12 patients treated with PT alone. Pain scores improved in the calcitonin group compared to the control group, although no differences were detected in range of motion, return-to-work, or edema.

The results of studies evaluating calcitonin are summarized in Table 54.2.

SIDE EFFECTS

Calcitonin has been associated with pruritus, headache, epigastric pain, hypocalcemia, and vertigo. Animal studies on salmon calcitonin show that it does not cross the placental barrier and have not shown any embryotoxic, teratogenic, or mutagenic potential. Calcitonin is secreted in breast milk, and animal studies have demonstrated suppression of breast milk production. Two FDA advisory committees have associated salmon calcitonin nasal spray and oral formulations with an increased risk of cancer, including prostate cancer. In March 2014, the FDA published an official warning regarding the increased risk of malignancy with nasal salmon calcitonin utilization. This warning was based on a meta-analysis of 21 randomized controlled clinical trials, which reported a higher rate of malignancies in calcitonin treated patients (4.1%) compared to placebo treated patients (2.9%).[44]

MAGNESIUM

Magnesium plays a critical role in the structure and function of the human body, particularly within the CNS. Magnesium acts as an NMDA receptor cation channel blocker, which stabilizes abnormal nerve transmission involved in central sensitization and hyperalgesia throughout the early postoperative period. Several studies have suggested analgesic benefits from magnesium in acute and chronic pain states.[3]

MECHANISM OF ACTION

Magnesium is a cation with the second highest intracellular and the fourth highest extracellular concentrations. Magnesium is involved in the Na/K ATPase system, which is critical in establishing the electrical potential across cell membranes. Additionally, magnesium levels affect calcium metabolism as magnesium acts as a calcium antagonist via inhibition of influx through the calcium channel. Magnesium is considered to be a CNS depressant, as it decreases

TABLE 54.2 Results of Studies on Calcitonin for Complex Regional Pain Syndrome

Study	Type of Study; Medications Compared; Duration of Follow-Up	Outcome Measures	Results
Bickerstaff et al.[39]; 40 patients with algodystrophy after a Colles' fracture	P, R, DB; 400 IU *nasal* calcitonin daily × 4 weeks vs. nasal saline, 20 patients per group. No other treatment given; 12-week follow-up.	Clinical assessment (pain, vasomotor and sudomotor changes, hand swelling, finger stiffness, grip strength) and blood and urine determinations	Improvements in pain, swelling, and stiffness in both groups with no difference between groups; decrease in serum calcium in calcitonin group
Sahin et al.[40]; 35 patients with stage 1 of CRPS	P, R, SB; 200 IU *nasal* calcitonin with calcium 500 mg/day for 2 months (18 patients) vs. paracetamol 1500 mg/day (17 patients). Patients also received PT, stellate ganglion blocks, and TENS; 2-month follow-up.	Pain, clinical assessments (allodynia, hyperalgesia, trophic changes)	Patients recovered in all parameters, no difference between groups
Gobelet et al.[43]; 66 patients with RSD	P, R, DB; 3 × 100 IU *nasal* calcitonin (33 patients) versus placebo (33 patients). Patients also received PT and TENS; 8-week follow-up.	Pain, range of motion, return to work	Pain, range of motion, and return to work were better improved by calcitonin.
Hamamci et al.[42]; 41 patients with RSD after hemiplegia	*Intramuscular* calcitonin, 1 × 100 IU/day for 4 weeks (25 patients) versus intramuscular saline (1 mL/day). All patients had PT. No comment on randomization or blinding; 4-week follow-up.	Pain score; clinical assessments (edema, tenderness, vasomotor and sudomotor changes, ROM of joints)	Significantly lower pain scores in calcitonin group at 4 weeks; significantly better results with calcitonin in tenderness, shoulder abduction and external rotation, wrist flexion, and metacarpophalangeal extension
Gobelet et al.[41]; 24 patients with RSD of the hands or feet, following trauma	R, C; *subcutaneous* calcitonin, 100 u a day for 3 weeks (12 patients) plus PT versus PT alone (12 patients). Follow-up for 8 (pain edema, range of motion) and 12 weeks (fitness for work).	Pain score; edema, range of movement; blood and urine assays (calcium, parathyroid hormone, phosphate); return to work	Significantly better pain relief with calcitonin; no difference between the two groups in terms of improvement in edema, range of motion, and return to work

Note: The diagnosis of CRPS in all the studies were not based on the IASP or Budapest criteria.
C, *Controlled;* CRPS, *complex regional pain syndrome;* DB, *double-blind;* P, *prospective;* PT, *physical therapy;* R, *randomized;* ROM, *range of motion;* RSD, *reflex sympathetic dystrophy;* SB, *single-blind;* TENS, *transcutaneous electrical nerve stimulation;* u, *units.*
With permission from Benzon HT, Liu SS, Buvanendran A: Evolving definitions and pharmacologic management of complex regional pain syndrome. Anesth Analg. *122:601-604, 2016.*

the release of acetylcholine at the neuromuscular junction by antagonizing calcium ions at the presynaptic cleft. This reduces the excitability of the neuron and decreases action potential propagation. Consequently, magnesium is often considered to be an NMDA receptor antagonist.

PHARMACOLOGY

Nearly half of the body's magnesium is stored in muscle and other soft tissue, with the remaining half residing in bone and erythrocytes. The majority of magnesium is stored intracellularly, with only 1% present in extracellular fluid, though this is the physiologically active form. Approximately one-third of dietary magnesium is absorbed in the small intestines, with most reabsorption occurring in the kidneys. Parathyroid hormone increases magnesium absorption from the small intestines and kidneys. Additionally, magnesium levels affect calcium metabolism and hypomagnesemia is routinely associated with hypocalcemia. IV magnesium has an immediate onset and the effects last about 30 minutes. Intramuscular administration has an onset time of 1 hour and a duration of action of 3–4 hours. Excretion is primarily through the kidneys.

CLINICAL USE

The effects of IV magnesium sulfate on chronic pain and function were studied in two RCTs by the Collins group. The first study[23] exposed eight patients with CRPS (duration 61–176 days) to IV magnesium (70 mg/kg over 4 hours) for 5 days, and two patients were treated with sodium chloride infusions. All patients were allowed to continue PT. Pain assessments were conducted via an 11-point box scale and the McGill Pain Questionnaire at baseline, 1, 3, 6, and 12 weeks. Pain was significantly reduced at all measured points in the magnesium group but the McGill sensory subscale was significantly improved only at week 1. However, at 12 weeks, statistically significant improvements in impairment levels and quality of life were observed. No changes were noted with respect to skin sensitivity and functional limitation. These findings were further corroborated by a subsequent randomized controlled trial[24] by the same group in which 56 CRPS patients (mean duration of symptoms was 16 months) were treated using a similar protocol. The magnesium treated group of 29 patients experienced clinically relevant and statistically significant improvements in level of impairment at 1 week, the McGill Questionnaire at 6 weeks, and perceived job participation at 12 weeks. Overall, the authors concluded that magnesium treatment provided insignificant benefits compared to placebo. Mild side effects of flushing, palpitations, phlebitis, and vasovagal reactions were noted.

SIDE EFFECTS

Magnesium is a fundamental cation in the physiology of many organ systems and cells. Several points should be kept in mind prior to initiating magnesium therapy. Infusions must be administered slowly to avoid hypermagnesemia, with the normal serum magnesium at 1.5–2.5 mEq/L. Any patient with myocardial damage or heart block should be carefully treated with IV magnesium under close physician supervision. Parenteral use in patients with renal failure may result in the accumulation of magnesium as the kidneys are the sole organs responsible for clearance. Magnesium levels should be checked regularly and a thorough physical examination, including reflexes, can help assess clinical response. Additionally, prolonged treatment with magnesium infusions in pregnant women for more than 5 days can cause hypercalcemia and bone abnormalities in the developing fetus. Overall, mild symptoms of flushing and sweating are seen with high frequency.

Magnesium may interact with certain CNS depressants, neuromuscular blockers, and cardiac glycosides. Caution should be exercised when combining magnesium with other CNS depressants such as barbiturates, opiates, and other hypnotics. Oftentimes, the dose of these agents needs to be adjusted to prevent oversedation. Magnesium will potentiate the effects of neuromuscular blocking agents, resulting in prolonged neuromuscular blockage. Lastly, the combination of magnesium and digitalis may precipitate serious conduction abnormalities or heart block.

GABAPENTIN AND PREGABALIN

Gabapentin and pregabalin are unique compounds that display high-affinity binding to the alpha-2 delta protein subunit of the calcium channel throughout the CNS. Calcium channel blockage ultimately inhibits the release of neurotransmitters and confers antinociceptive, anticonvulsant, and anxiolytic-like effects.[45] Although they were initially approved as anticonvulsants, these agents have become first-line treatments for neuropathic pain conditions such as painful diabetic/peripheral neuropathy, CRPS, and postherpetic neuralgia. They effectively treat many symptoms of neuropathic pain such as burning, shooting pain, allodynia, and hyperalgesia. Both agents have similar mechanisms of action and side-effect profiles, but display different pharmacokinetics and pharmacodynamics. Gabapentin was originally approved in the United Kingdom in 1993 and in 2005, pregabalin received FDA approval for neuropathic pain associated with diabetic neuropathy, postherpetic neuralgia, and as an adjunct for treatment of partial seizures.

PHARMACOLOGY

Gabapentin and pregabalin are nonnaturally occurring branched amino acids that are chemical analogues of gamma-aminobutyric acid (GABA). Neither drug interacts with the GABAergic neuronal system. Bockbrader et al. performed a comparison of the pharmacokinetics of the two agents.[45] Gabapentin is absorbed slowly from the GI tract through the LAT1 transporter resulting in dose-limited absorption, possibly due to saturation of the transporter. The maximum plasma concentrations are attained within 3–4 hours and it exhibits nonlinear (zero-order) processes. This makes gabapentin's pharmacokinetics less predictable, since it does not display linear increases in plasma concentrations with increasing oral dosages.

Pregabalin's absorption is mediated by an additional pathway that allows for near-complete, nonsaturable absorption into the blood, usually within 1 hour (threefold faster onset than gabapentin). Approximately 50%–75% of gabapentin doses of 1800–4800 mg/day are not absorbed. Any agent that slows down gastric motility (such as morphine) may enhance the absorption of gabapentin. The absolute bioavailability of gabapentin drops from 60% to 33% as the dose is increased from 900 mg to 3600 mg daily.[45] Pregabalin's bioavailability is consistently greater than 90%, irrespective of dosage. Pregabalin can be dosed up to 600 mg per day. Similar effects are noted with twice per day dosing compared with three times per day treatment. Pain relief has been reported as early as 1 day after pregabalin treatment (300 mg/day). Similar to pregabalin, gabapentin does not bind plasma proteins, does not undergo hepatic metabolism, and is excreted unchanged within 6 hours.

MECHANISM OF ACTION

The exact mechanism(s) of action of gabapentin and pregablin is unclear. However, we do know they have a high affinity for the alpha-2 delta subunit of the calcium channel. Presynaptic calcium channel blockage inhibits the release of neurotransmitters such as glutamate and substance P from primary nociceptive afferents, thereby modulating nociceptive transmission.

SIDE EFFECTS

The main side effects associated with gabapentin and pregabalin are drowsiness, dry mouth, and lower extremity edema. The side effects of both drugs are dose-dependent and reversible. The recommended gabapentin dose range is 1800–3600 mg/day, although doses greater than 1800 mg/day are unlikely to offer additional benefit. Slow titration of gabapentin (100–300 mg/day with gradual increase of 100–300 mg every 1–3 days) may temper the drowsiness associated with the medication. The drowsiness usually abates within 7–10 days after treatment.

CLINICAL USE

There is level two evidence supporting the use of gabapentin in CRPS. Serpell[25] evaluated the effects of gabapentin in neuropathic pain patients, 28% of whom had CRPS. Patients were exposed to gabapentin 2700 mg/day for 8 weeks and showed a statistically significant reduction in neuropathic pain symptoms. In 2004, Van de Vusse et al.[26] conducted a double-blinded RCT crossover study in 58 patients (with upper or lower extremity CRPS diagnosed via IASP criteria) randomized to two groups: treatment (gabapentin 1800 mg/day for 3 weeks) or placebo. Patients underwent a 2-week washout period, and then crossed over to the other group. They concluded that gabapentin did not offer greater pain relief than placebo for the study group as a whole, though patients reported significant pain relief in the first half of the study with gabapentin. Curiously, there was an unexpected increase in VAS pain scores in both groups during the washout period. Sensory deficits were significantly reversed in gabapentin users. No differences were noted with respect to allodynia, edema, discoloration, range of motion, or quality of life. Patients experienced side effects such as dizziness, somnolence, and lethargy.

TADALAFIL

Histopathologic studies on skin samples from CRPS patients have revealed numerous abnormalities in vascular innervation and structure.[27] As CRPS advances to the chronic phase, inflammation signs give way to muscle atrophy, reduced regional blood flow, and reduced skin temperature. Although central sensitization and sympathetic dysregulation have been better studied as mechanisms for CRPS, local ischemia is also suspected to play an integral role. Early in the disease, unilateral inhibition of sympathetic vasoconstrictor neurons manifests as warm extremities. As the disease progresses, CRPS patients experience dysregulation of their microcirculation which leads hypoperfusion, tissue ischemia, and subsequent metabolic acidosis within tissues. Secondary changes in neurovascular transmission lead to increased sensitivity to circulating catecholamines and alpha-1 receptors, resulting in vasoconstriction and cold extremities. The tone of the microcirculation is under neural and endothelial control. Within the endothelium, the PDE-5 inhibitor tadalafil causes vasodilation of the vessels and may therefore be beneficial in CRPS patients.

MECHANISM OF ACTION

Vessel endothelium regulates vascular tone by releasing mediators such as nitric oxide, prostacyclin, bradykinin, endothelium-derived hyperpolarizing factor, endothelin-1 (ET-1), and angiotensin II. Nitric oxide will increase the intracellular concentration of cyclic guanosine monophosphate (cGMP) within the endothelial cell which activates a cascade of reactions resulting in hyperpolarization of the muscle membrane and blockade of calcium influx at the calcium channel. As cytosolic calcium concentrations drop, smooth muscle relaxes, and the vessel vasodilates.[27] cGMP is hydrolyzed by phosphodiesterase type 5 (PDE-5), and thus inhibition of this enzyme (by PDE-5 inhibitors, such as tadalafil) will increase intracellular concentrations of cGMP and promote smooth muscle vasodilation.

PHARMACOLOGY

Tadalafil is absorbed quickly (within 2 hours), has an extended half-life of 17.5 hours, a clearance of 2.4 L/h, and a volume of distribution of 62.6 L. The pharmacokinetics are linear with respect to dose and time but are not affected by food intake. Tadalafil is metabolized in the liver via the CYP3A4 system and undergoes renal elimination. Patients with liver or kidney dysfunction should be treated with lower doses and followed closely by a physician.

CLINICAL USE

Groeneweg et al.[27] investigated the potential benefits of daily tadalafil in a randomized, double-blind, placebo-controlled trial in 24 patients with chronic, cold extremity CRPS. Twelve patients received tadalafil 10 mg daily for 4 weeks, which was then increased to tadalafil 20 mg daily for 8 weeks to avoid tolerance to the medication. Diagnostic criteria were not clearly delineated. This study demonstrated a 15% reduction in VAS pain scores when compared to placebo, and a small, nonstatistically significant improvement in muscle strength over time, walking ability, and reduced need for crutches. They were not able to show a statistically significant change in temperature reduction despite the fact that most patients in the tadalafil group reported warmer extremities. Minimal side effects were reported including fatigue and exhaustion. Blood pressure was minimally affected. Whereas these results may be promising, the authors noted that longer-term treatment may be more beneficial as with treatment of erectile dysfunction, pulmonary hypertension, and Raynaud phenomenon. Further studies are necessary to clarify the role tadalafil plays in CRPS treatment.

SIDE EFFECTS

Tadalafil has been extensively studied in several clinical trials not involving pain management. The most common side effects are headache, GI upset (including pain, indigestion, belching, reflux), backache, myalgia, flushing, and rhinorrhea. Although most of these side effects are short-lived, myalgia and back pain can last for up to 24 hours.

In 2005, a postmarketing analysis showed a possible association between tadalafil and vision impairment due to nonarteritic anterior ischemic optic neuropathy (NAION). The patients who developed the complication had increased risk factors of underlying anatomic or vascular disease including low cup-to-disc ratio, age greater than 50 years, hypertension, coronary artery disease, smoking, and hyperlipidemia. Given the low incidence of NAION and the vast utilization of tadalafil, the FDA did not issue an official warning but did mandate an alert on the medication labeling. Additionally, postmarket analysis showed an increased risk of sudden hearing loss, which is also noted as an alert on the drug packaging.

Tadalafil can cause transient decreases in blood pressure. Groeneweg et al.[27] noted minimal changes in blood pressure over the course of their 12-week study, a mean decrease in systolic blood pressure (SBP) from 142 (±18) to 140 (±19) in the treatment group versus a decrease from SBP 134 (±10) to 130 (±16) in the placebo group. Hypotension can be life-threatening when combined with organic nitrates. Patients on tadalafil should not take nitrates within 48 hours of tadalafil. Patients taking nitrates for angina should seek medical attention with recent use of tadalafil.

FREE RADICAL SCAVENGERS

The symptoms of CRPS are similar to those seen with inflammatory reactions: calor, dolor, rubor, tumor, etc. Although the inflammatory response is localized, CRPS affects a larger than expected area of the extremity. Initially, localized inflammatory reactions may trigger a continuous overproduction of toxic oxygen radicals, leading to surrounding tissue destruction that may trigger CRPS.[28] Free radical scavengers such as dimethyl sulfoxide (DMSO), N-acetylcysteine (NAC), and mannitol have been studied in patients with CRPS. Data on the exact mechanism of action and pharmacokinetics of these agents are limited.

DIMETHYL SULFOXIDE CREAM

Since 1963, DMSO has been studied and applied in almost every specialty of medicine in the treatment of ulcerative colitis, interstitial cystitis, organ transplantation, arthritis, scleroderma, amyloidosis, and increased intracranial pressure. DMSO has antiinflammatory, local anesthetic, weak bacteriostatic, and diuretic effects. However, it is mostly utilized as a topical analgesic for burns, pain, sprains, and healing incisions.

MECHANISM OF ACTION

DMSO reduces inflammation through several different mechanisms including acting as an antioxidant and a free radical scavenger at the site of injury. DMSO 50% is a particularly potent scavenger of the hydroxyl radical and may relieve pain by blocking peripheral C fibers.

PHARMACOLOGY

DMSO is an organosulfur compound that readily passes through membranes depending on the strength of the preparation. DMSO 70%–90% will readily pass through the skin. This permeability allows the drug to enhance the diffusion of other medications across membranes (e.g., morphine sulfate, penicillin, steroids, and insulin). Relief is reported almost immediately and lasts up to 6 hours. This has made DMSO ideal for acute pain in athletes who require immediate pain relief. The agent is quickly eliminated from the body. Chronic pain patients may need to apply DMSO for nearly 6 weeks prior to noticing an effect.

SIDE EFFECTS

The most common side effects of DMSO are headache (especially at higher doses), and rash/skin irritation on contact with the skin. Several severe reactions have caused the FDA to halt clinical trials on DMSO as some studies reported eye damage and life-threatening allergic reactions. The FDA has since allowed clinical trials to resume and has approved DMSO for the treatment of interstitial cystitis. It is currently marketed as an alternative medicine.

DMSO may increase the effects of blood thinners, steroids, cardiac medications, and sedatives. Its extensive permeability may cause contaminants, toxins, and other medications to readily permeate the skin and have unexpected effects. The drug may be neurotoxic at doses lower than 0.3 mg/kg, which is especially concerning in children as this dose is exceeded during bone marrow transplantation. Less concerning is the foul, garliclike odor that is produced with DMSO application.

N-ACETYLCYSTEINE TABLETS

NAC is most widely utilized as an antidote for acetaminophen overdose. However, it has vast applications including treatment of amyotrophic lateral sclerosis, certain forms of epilepsy, chronic fatigue syndrome, Sjögren syndrome, Alzheimer disease, keratoconjunctivitis, and as a mucolytic in patients with chronic obstructive pulmonary disease (COPD)/bronchitis. Additionally, it has been used to prevent alcoholic liver damage, contrast-induced nephropathy, and toxicity associated with chemotherapeutic agents. NAC is available as an inhalation agent, IV injection, ocular solution, and oral tablet. In the United States, the oral tablet is marketed as a nutritional supplement while the IV and inhalation formulations require a prescription. Few studies have been performed evaluating NAC alone.

MECHANISM OF ACTION

NAC has been shown to directly reduce hydroxyl radials, hydrogen peroxide, and hypochlorus acid.[46] Antiinflammatory activity results from reduced release of proinflammatory mediators such as tumor necrosis factor (TNF-alpha) and NF-$_{KB}$.[30] Additionally, NAC is a prodrug to L-cysteine, which is a precursor to the antioxidant glutathione. Glutathione may have endogenous neuromodulatory effects as it binds to the glutamate recognition side of the NMDA and AMPA receptors. NAC may also improve vascular function by promoting endothelium-derived vasodilation.

PHARMACOLOGY

NAC has an onset time of 5–10 minutes when inhaled and 1–2 hours with oral intake. It is extensively metabolized in the liver by CYP450 and renally cleared. Its half-life is 5.6 hours but is prolonged in neonates to 11 hours.

SIDE EFFECTS

The most common side effects of NAC are nausea, vomiting, and diarrhea or constipation. Less common side effects include headache, drowsiness, low blood pressure, rash, fever, and liver problems. Similar to DMSO, NAC has an unpleasant odor associated with utilization. Other concerns include increased risk of bleeding in patients with bleeding disorders, which may pose a risk if taken within 2 weeks of surgery. NAC does cross the placenta and it is unclear if it is transmitted through breast milk. The effects to the fetus are unknown. The effects of nitroglycerin are potentiated by NAC and may cause headache, lightheadedness, and dizziness. NAC can also decrease the absorbing effects of activated charcoal when used to treat acetaminophen overdose. Lastly, anaphylactoid reactions have been noted and may be severe with IV administration.

CLINICAL USE

Some evidence exists for the utilization of DMSO in CRPS, while level 3 data support the use of NAC tablets in CRPS. In 1996, Zuurmond et al.[28] performed a randomized, double-blind trial in 32 patients with CRPS who were treated with 50% DMSO cream applied five times daily. Two-month follow-up revealed significantly better results for CRPS symptoms than placebo. A follow-up study compared the efficacy of DMSO to NAC (600-mg effervescent tablet 3 times per day) in a randomized, double-blind study conducted in 146 CRPS patients with 2-year follow-up.[30] Rescue analgesics such as Paracetamol 500 mg, naproxen 250/500 mg, and tramadol were allowed. Participants were diagnosed according to the Netherlands WHO collaborating center criteria and had symptoms for less than 1 year. Overall, they noted that both radical scavengers were equally beneficial but subgroup analysis revealed warm extremity CRPS responded better to DMSO while cold extremity CRPS benefited more from NAC tablets.

MANNITOL

Mannitol is an osmotic diuretic which is traditionally used for low-output acute renal failure, increased intracranial pressure/edema, increased intraocular pressure, and to promote urinary excretion of toxic material. However, it has been studied in CRPS patients as a free-radical scavenger, being the strongest among the free-radical detoxifiers.

MECHANISM OF ACTION

Mannitol reduces the concentration of free radicals that promote cell membrane lipid peroxidation and ultimately destruction of cellular tissue.[47] It also promotes cerebral blood flow by reducing blood viscosity and microcirculatory resistance.

PHARMACOLOGY

Mannitol, chemically 1,2,3,4,5,6 hexanehexol, is a polyol (sugar alcohol) that is found naturally in marine algae, fresh mushrooms, and exudates from trees. Onset time is fastest with IV infusion for increased intracranial pressure (15–30 minutes). Mannitol undergoes negligible liver metabolism to glycogen, undergoes 90% renal excretion (60%–90% unchanged), and has a biological half-life of 100 minutes. It does not cross the blood-brain barrier. Commercially, mannitol is available in 5%, 10%, 15%, 20%, or 25% in a 500–1000-mL bag. At room temperature, mannitol may crystallize but will dissolve upon heating.

CLINICAL USE

Perez et al.[29] examined the role of mannitol in 41 CRPS patients in a double-blind, placebo-controlled trial. The treatment group received 10% mannitol in 1 L NS (into the affected limb) over 4 hours for 5 consecutive days while the placebo group received normal saline infusion. This study failed to show any difference between mannitol infusion and placebo with respect to pain, function level, or quality of life. The majority of patients in the study had symptoms for less than 1 year, with the mean duration of symptoms in the mannitol group being 6.5 months. It is possible that mannitol may be more beneficial during the acute phase when more inflammatory mediators are present. No serious side effects were noted. These results were confirmed by a follow-up retrospective study[31] in 68 patients with CRPS (median duration of symptoms was 129 days with a range of 3–1046 days) exposed to 10% mannitol/1 L per 24 hours for 7–10 days via the subclavian vein. They did note that patients with warm CRPS experienced more favorable results than cold CRPS.

SIDE EFFECTS

Minimal side effects have been reported with slow, low-dose mannitol infusions for CRPS. However, caution must be taken in patients with renal failure. Mannitol side effects can include pulmonary congestion, chest pain/heart failure, electrolyte abnormalities, acidosis, dry mouth, venous thrombosis/phlebitis, blurry vision, nausea, vomiting, and dehydration. There is an FDA box warning for risks of severe bronchospasm with inhaled mannitol.

CONCLUSION

There has been great progress in the pharmacologic management of CRPS. Whereas health care providers had little to offer patients in the past, there are now an array of medications that can be administered via the oral, IV, intramuscular, subcutaneous, and topical routes (see Tables 54.1 and 54.2). Yet, the efficacy of these drugs has not been definitively established since most of the studies employed nonstringent criteria in diagnosing CRPS.[4] Moreover, some of the drugs are associated with troublesome side effects. Head-to-head comparisons between drugs need to be performed. Finally, the effectiveness of the drugs in relation to the stage of CRPS has to be determined.

KEY POINTS

- The IASP criteria for diagnosing CRPS offer good sensitivity (1.00) but lack specificity (0.4). The Budapest Criteria show high sensitivity (0.99) and improved specificity (0.68), allowing practitioners to more accurately diagnose patients (88% accuracy).
- CRPS patients are routinely prescribed a combination of interventional procedures, PT, antidepressants, anti-inflammatory medications, antiepileptics, and opiates.
- Ketamine has analgesic properties within the central and peripheral nervous systems via interactions with several receptor subtypes including NMDA, opioid, and AMPA. The level of evidence for use of ketamine in CRPS is 1B+ (one or more RCT with methodologic weaknesses demonstrating effectiveness; the benefits clearly outweigh the risks and burdens).
- Ketamine-induced liver dysfunction has been reported with prolonged or repeat infusions within a short time frame. The elevated liver enzymes typically normalize over 2 months. The exact mechanism of injury may involve impaired hepatic oxygen delivery, formation of free radicals, or an allergic hepatitis.
- Bisphosphonates inhibit bone resorption and may play a critical role in pain relief associated with CRPS. The overall level of evidence for IV bisphosphonates is 1B+. This class of medications includes pamidronate, alendronate, neridronate, and clodronate. For ibandronate, the level of evidence is 2C+ (effectiveness demonstrated in observational studies).
- In view of the lack of randomization and blinding in many of the published articles, the utilization of calcitonin for CRPS has level 2B evidence.
- Calcitonin has been associated with pruritus, headache, epigastric pain, hypocalcemia, and vertigo. In March 2014, the FDA published an official warning regarding the increased risk of malignancy associated with nasal salmon calcitonin utilization.
- Magnesium is an NMDA receptor antagonist which stabilizes abnormal nerve transmission involved in central sensitization and hyperalgesia. The level of evidence for its use in CRPS is 2B.
- There is level two evidence supporting the use of gabapentin in CRPS.

REFERENCES

Access the reference list online at ExpertConsult.com.

CHAPTER 55

Pharmacology for the Interventional Pain Physician

Andrea L. Nicol, MD, MSc ◎ Magdalena Anitescu, MD, PhD ◎ Honorio T. Benzon, MD

A comprehensive understanding of pharmacologic agents used by the interventional pain physician is vital for safe and successful patient care. This chapter reviews the clinical pharmacology, therapeutic mechanisms, and side effects of corticosteroids, botulinum toxins (BoNT), radiocontrast agents, and topical antiseptics.

CORTICOSTEROIDS

Naturally occurring corticosteroids are classified into three functional groups: (1) mineralocorticoids, (2) glucocorticoids, and (3) adrenal androgens.[1] Mineralocorticoids maintain normal fluid and electrolyte balance. Glucocorticoids act primarily to enhance the production of high-energy fuel, glucose, and reduce other metabolic activity.[2,3] Injections of glucocorticoids for the relief of vertebrogenic, arthritic, and radiculopathic pains are widely accepted.[4] There are many proposed mechanisms of action that are believed to underlie the therapeutic use of corticosteroids. These actions include antiinflammatory effects, modulation of peripheral nociceptor neurons and spinal cord dorsal horn cells, and direct stabilization of neural membranes.

Corticosteroids are the most potent and effective agents in controlling inflammation through numerous mechanisms, including effects on cytokines, inflammatory mediators, inflammatory cells, nitric oxide synthase, and adhesion molecules. Cytokines are important mediators of inflammation, and the pattern of their expression largely determines the magnitude and duration of the inflammatory response.[5] Steroids have inhibitory effects on cytokine transcription and synthesis, especially the ones relevant in chronic inflammation (interleukin [IL]-1, IL-3, IL-4, IL-5, IL-6, IL-8, tumor necrosis factor [TNF]-α, and granulocyte-macrophage colony-stimulating factor).[6,7] Steroids not only inhibit cytokine synthesis, but also interfere with their activity.[7] Steroids increase the synthesis of lipocortin (annexin) 1, a phospholipase A_2 inhibitor, and thus decrease the production of inflammatory mediators, such as leukotrienes, prostaglandins, and platelet-activating factor.[7,8] Corticosteroids interfere with macrophage activity by impairing phagocytosis, intracellular digestion of antigens, and macrophage release of IL-1 and TNF-α.[2] By inhibiting the expression of chemokines, corticosteroids prevent the activation and recruitment of inflammatory cells, including eosinophils, basophils, and lymphocytes.[9] In addition, steroids cause an expansion in the number of circulating neutrophils secondary to decreased adherence to vascular endothelium (demargination) and stimulation of bone marrow production.[10] Corticosteroids interfere with T-cell-mediated immunity. They inhibit the production of T lymphocytes by downregulating T-cell growth factors IL-1β and IL-2, and inhibit the release of various T-lymphocyte cytokines.[2]

Other mechanisms of action for injected corticosteroids include suppression of spontaneous ectopic neural discharge originating in experimental neuromas.[11] Following peripheral nerve injury, a number of morphologic and biochemical changes occur at the injury site, including the formation of neuromas, which leads to increased electrical excitability. Ectopic discharge from the injury site leads to a persistent afferent barrage, which maintains neuralgic pains and paresthesias. Furthermore, the topical application of methylprednisolone has also been shown to reversibly block transmission of C-fibers but not the A-β fibers.[12] Together, these data support the notion that locally applied corticosteroids suppress afferent ectopic nociceptive discharges, suggesting a direct membrane-stabilizing effect. Lastly, glucocorticoid receptor sites have been found on 5-hydroxytryptamine (5-HT) and noradrenergic neurons within the dorsal horn substantia gelatinosa. These are known pathways of pain transmission, and this suggests that corticosteroids may possibly modulate nociceptive transmission by a direct action on the spinal cord.

Several synthetic steroid preparations are available and widely used for interventional pain procedures. They vary in their antiinflammatory potencies, mineralocorticoid activities, solubility, and durations of action. It should be noted that none of the available preparations have been approved for perineural or epidural administration by any regulatory agency in the United States or internationally.

Short-acting synthetic steroids have durations of action of 8 to 12 hours; these include the active agent hydrocortisone and the inactive cortisone (converted by the liver to the biologically active cortisol). The intermediate-acting steroids, prednisone, prednisolone, methylprednisolone, and triamcinolone, have durations of action of 24 to 36 hours. Prednisone is an inactive agent, which is metabolized to the active agent prednisolone by the liver. The longest acting steroids, dexamethasone and betamethasone, have durations of action longer than 48 hours. Although the choice of steroid used by interventional pain physicians is frequently based upon its antiinflammatory potency and duration of action, the steroid particulate size relative to a red blood cell and whether or not it aggregates has become major determinants of corticosteroid selection given reported catastrophic neurological sequelae as described elsewhere in this text. Table 55.1 provides a summary of the properties of commonly used injectable corticosteroids.

The majority of systemic adverse effects from corticosteroid administration are usually mild and short-lived when they are administered as intermittent injections, as is

TABLE 55.1 Properties of Commonly Used Injectable Corticosteroids

Steroid	Commercial Name	Equivalent Potency (mg)	Relative GC Potency	Solubility	Maximum Particle Size (μm)	Particles > 10 μm (%)	Particle Aggregates
Methypred-nisolone acetate	Depo-medrol, solu-medrol	4	5	0.001	>500	45	Extensive
Triamcinolone acetonide	Kenalog	4	5	0.0002	>500	45	Extensive
Betamethasone acetate, betametha-sone sodium phosphate	Celestone soluspan, betaject	0.75	33	Acetate form: "practically insoluble." Sodium phosphate form:freely soluble	500	35	Some
Dexametha-sone sodium phosphate	Decadron phosphate, adrenocort, decaject	0.75	27	Freely soluble	0.5	0	None

GC, *Glucocorticoid.*
Reproduced and adapted from: MacMahon PJ, Eustace SJ, Kavanagh EC. Injectable corticosteroids and local anaesthetics preparations: a review for radiologists. Radiology. *2009;252(3):647-681 and Benzon HT, Chew TL, McCarthy RJ, et al. Comparison of the particle sizes of different steroids and the effect of dilution.* Anesthesiology. *2007;106(2):331-338.*

common in interventional pain management procedures. This is in contrast to long-term supraphysiologic administration of steroids, where more serious side effects may occur. Side effects from short-term therapy are rare, but may include fluid retention (if higher mineralocorticoid activity steroids are used), hyperglycemia, elevated blood pressure, mood changes, insomnia, menstrual irregularities, gastritis, Cushing syndrome, increased appetite, weight gain, increased infections, delayed wound healing, bone demineralization, and acneiform eruptions.

Sterile meningitis and arachnoiditis have been reported following intrathecal injection of methylprednisolone, but may have been related to the polyethylene preservative.[13] Anaphylactoid and hypersensitivity reactions are rare, but have been reported following intramuscular and soft-tissue injections.[14–16] Any type of anaphylactic reaction warrants prompt and aggressive life-support therapy, including resuscitation of airway, breathing, and circulation, with oxygen support and cardiac life support when indicated.

Most studies showed increased blood glucose levels after an epidural steroid injection of triamcinolone or betamethasone.[17,18] There appears to be no correlation between preinjection hemoglobin A1c levels or patient age with the changes in blood glucose.[17] In most patients, the blood glucose returned to baseline 7 days later.[18] Another study showed a minimal effect of epidural methylprednisolone.[19] The depot steroid preparations used for epidural injections may produce adrenocorticotropic hormone (ACTH) suppression and cushingoid symptoms that can last up to a few weeks.[20] Cushing syndrome has occurred following a single epidural injection of 60 mg of methylprednisolone[21] or triamcinolone,[22] and has been reported in several patients following repeated epidural steroid injections when 200 mg of methylprednisolone was exceeded.[23] Lumbar epidural injection of triamcinolone, 80 mg, caused profound hypothalamic, pituitary, adrenal (HPA) axis suppression for 3 weeks, although a steroid was undetectable in the plasma during this time. Comparable studies of patients who have received intraarticular steroid injections have shown detectable levels in the circulation and HPA axis suppression for up to 4 weeks.[24]

Epidural injection of triamcinolone, 80 mg, caused a marked reduction in insulin sensitivity in patients with normal glucose tolerance and caused fasting hyperglycemia in patients with a preexisting degree of insulin resistance.[25] In this study, insulin sensitivity and fasting glucose levels were normal 1 week after injection. Because patients with diabetes commonly experience increased insulin requirements for several days following the injection, it is suggested that they be given specific advice on the management of their condition following epidural steroid injection.

The overall safety of fluoroscopically guided epidural steroid injections has been confirmed in a retrospective study.[26] However, there have been several reported cases of central nervous system injuries after transforaminal epidural steroid injections, and these complications are discussed in Chapter 63.

BOTULINUM TOXIN THERAPY

BoNTs are produced by the gram-negative anaerobic bacterium *Clostridium botulinum.* They produce flaccid paralysis by preventing the presynaptic release of acetylcholine (ACh) at the neuromuscular junction. There are eight BoNT subtypes—A, B, C_1, C_2, D, E, F, and G.[27] The US Food and Drug Administration (FDA) approved the use of onabotulinum toxin A for the treatment of strabismus, blepharospasm, and hemifacial spasm. In 2000, BoNT B (Myobloc) was approved by the FDA for treating cervical dystonia, and 10 years later the agency approved the use of onabotulinum toxin A (Botox or Botox Cosmetic) in chronic migraine treatment. The type A subtypes appear to be the most potent and has the longest duration of action.

BoNT is synthesized as a single-chain polypeptide, consisting of a heavy (H) chain (molecular weight [MW], 100,000) and a light (L) chain (MW, 50,000). The H chain is responsible for binding to presynaptic cholinergic nerve terminals at the neuromuscular junction, whereas the L chain is the neurotoxic component. The H and L chains are bound together by disulfide bonds, and the toxin is activated by proteolytic enzymes in a cleaving process. It is estimated that the human lethal dose of BoNT-A is about 2800 to 3500 units for a 70-kg adult. The lethal dose of BoNT-B in humans is estimated at 144,000 units.

Two botulinum neurotoxins, types A and B, are used in clinical practice. There are three commercially available type A preparations, Botox, Dysport, and Xeomin. Each vial of Botox (Allergan, Inc., Irvine, California) contains 100 units of onabotulinum toxin A as a sterile, vacuum-dried form without preservative that can be reconstituted with preservative-free sterile saline prior to injection. Dysport (abobotulinum toxin A) (Ipsen, Ltd., Berkshire, UK) is marketed in the form of 500-unit vials. Data from patients treated for cervical dystonia suggest that 1 unit of Botox equals 3 to 5 units of Dysport. Xeomin (Merz Pharmaceutical, Frankfurt AM Main, Germany) is marketed as 100 units of incobotulinum toxin A powder, reconstituted upon use in preservative-free sterile normal saline. Myobloc (Solstice Neurosciences Inc., Malvern, Pennsylvania) is marketed as a sterile liquid formulation of a purified BoNT B (rimabotulinum toxin B).

BoNT A (BoNT-A) in the Botox formulation, the commercially available product in the United States, is inactivated by heat, shaking, excessive dilution, and surface tension from bubbles during reconstitution. Boiling dissolves the disulfide bonds between the H and L chains of BoNT-A, thus rendering the toxin inactive, because neither chain can exert neurotoxicity independently. BoNT-A must be reconstituted with preservative-free sterile normal saline. Dilution of a 100-unit vial may be performed with 1, 2, 5, or 10 mL of 0.9% sodium chloride. This will yield a concentration of 10, 5, 2, or 1 units/0.1 mL, respectively. The higher concentrations are appropriate for larger muscles; for example, hip flexors or piriformis muscles. Lower concentrations are used for facial injections, for example, for the glabella, temporalis, and frontalis muscles.

BoNT-A should be used within 4 hours of preparation and stored at 2°C to 8°C during this time. It has been shown that there is no loss of activity 6 hours after reconstitution at room temperature; however, a 44% loss of activity is observed at 12 hours.[28] Refreezing the toxin after reconstitution causes a 70% reduction in bioactivity at 1 to 2 weeks.

BoNTs act by blocking the presynaptic release of ACh from cholinergic terminals of motor and autonomic nerves. BoNT neurotoxicity occurs in three stages: binding, internalization, and proteolysis.[29] Following activation by proteolytic cleavage, the BoNT H chain binds irreversibly to the presynaptic terminals of cholinergic neurons. The C-terminal region of the H chain binds in a serotype-specific manner to receptors on the motor end plates and at autonomic cholinergic ganglia.

In addition to the pain relief associated with its paralytic effect, BoNT-A has been shown to influence pain processing via reduction in peripheral and central sensitization through a number of different mechanisms. BoNT-A has been shown to inhibit the release of pain peptides, substance P, calcitonin gene-related peptide (CGRP), glutamate, and bradykinin from the trigeminal and dorsal root ganglia.[30–32] This mechanism is modulated by the synaptosomal-associated protein 25 (SNAP-25) located within the cell membrane. In a formalin model of pain, injection of BoNT-A into a rat paw one week prior to formalin injection, reduces the postformalin inflammatory peak of pain in a dose-related manner. Tissue examination of the injected site reveals decreased inflammation and a reduction of local glutamate accumulation compared with controls.[33] Additionally, BoNT-A inhibits a family of G proteins, including Rho guanosine triphosphatase, which is necessary for activation of IL-1, an important proinflammatory cytokine.[34] Finally, BoNT-A has been shown to affect cyclooxygenase-2 expression,[35] impair sympathetic transmission of pain,[36] and reduce allodynia in diabetic rats, suggesting a central analgesic effect of BoNT-A.[37]

The BoNT molecule cannot cross the blood-brain barrier, and therefore does not have any direct central nervous system (CNS) effects.[38] At the neuromuscular junction, BoNTs cause a chemical denervation, thereby inhibiting skeletal muscle contraction. In humans, clinical effects typically appear after 2 to 3 days, but the peak effects are observed at 2 to 6 weeks. BoNT-induced chemical denervation is permanent, so skeletal muscle remains paralyzed until new axons and synapses have formed to reestablish the neuromuscular junction. Functional denervation is observed for 6 weeks up to 6 months following injection, but usually lasts for 3 to 4 months.

Repeated injections of onabotulinum toxin A have been associated with antibody formation, which renders any subsequent onabotulinum toxin A injections ineffective. A study of 32 patients with spasmodic torticollis treated with repeated onabotulinum toxin A injections has revealed that four patients (12.5%) produced antibodies after 2 to 9 months of treatment.[39] It appears that higher toxin doses and frequent injections are the leading factors in the development of neutralizing antibodies.[40]

Reported complications of BoNT injection include injection site reaction, pain at the injection site, headache, fatigue, flulike symptoms, muscle weakness, fever, pruritis, and significant regional sequelae depending on the injection site (i.e., dysphagia, facial paralysis). Muscle weakness occurs if more than 50 units of onabotulinum toxin A are injected into a muscle.[41]

The use of BoNT-A for analgesia in humans has been well studied and extensively reported with regard to the treatment of cervical dystonia. For those with cervical dystonia, BoNT (serotype A or B) significantly reduces neck pain in 60% to 80% of patients.[42] Other prospective and placebo-controlled studies using BoNT in humans reported efficacy and improved pain in patients with myofascial pain syndrome,[43–50] plantar fasciitis,[51] pelvic pain,[52] migraine headaches,[53–55] lateral epicondylitis,[56–59] postherpetic neuralgia,[60] low back pain,[61] and piriformis syndrome.[62,63] Recent studies also showed improvement in neuropathic pain and allodynia associated with

TABLE 55.2 Summary of Levels of Evidence for Use of Botulinum Toxins in Various Painful Clinical Conditions

Level of Evidence	Recommendations	Clinical Condition
A	Established and recommended	Cervical dystonia Chronic migraine Chronic lateral epicondylitis
B	Probably effective, should be considered for treatment	Postherpetic neuralgia Posttraumatic neuralgia Plantar fasciitis Pyriformis syndrome Total knee arthroplasty
C	Possibly effective; can be used at the discretion of the physician	Allodynia in diabetic neuropathy Chronic low back pain Knee osteoarthritis Anterior knee pain with vastus lateralis imbalance Pelvic pain Postoperative pain in children with cerebral palsy Postoperative pain after mastectomy Sphincter spasm and pain after hemorroidectomy
U	Insufficient evidence due to contradictory results	Myofascial pain syndrome Chronic daily headaches

Reproduced from Jabbari B, Machado D. Treatment of refractory pain with botulinum toxins—an evidence-based review. Pain Med. *2011;12:1594-1606.*

painful diabetic neuropathy after intradermal injections of BoNT-A.[64,65]

Jabbari and Machado[66] conducted an evidence-based review in which they used American Academy of Neurology methodology as stated by the guidelines of the society's Therapeutics and Assessment Subcommittee to rate the scientific evidence for the use of BoNTs in clinical practice. They found four levels of clinical evidence in the use of BoNT in painful clinical conditions (Table 55.2).

RADIOGRAPHIC CONTRAST MEDIA

Interventional physicians routinely use radiocontrast media (RCM) agents during various pain procedures; it serves as confirmation of correct needle placement; it also helps the proceduralist with the visualization of the spread of medication during therapeutic or diagnostic injections.[67]

The first contrast agent used in medicine for the study of neural structures was sodium iodide as a 40% solution suspended in the oil of poppy seeds. The product was very insoluble and carried significant side effects, such as severe local irritation, nausea and vomiting, arthralgias, lymph node swelling, and hives, and had a very low radiographic yield. In 1927, the reported concentration of this RCM was reduced to 20% and although still with a low radiographic yield, the physicians were able to diagnose a brain abscess with a reported decrease in side effects from the agent.[68]

The following decades brought some new improvements in RCMs. In the 1950s, sodium iodide was replaced by sodium, calcium, or methylguanine diatrizoic acid salts; those agents had high osmolarity of greater than 1700 mOsm (5 to 8 times that of blood), and were therefore called high osmolar contrast media (HOCM). HOCM have a ratio of 3:2 (iodine to particle) and dissociation of those two components commonly occurred. Adverse events related to HOCM, such as hypertension, cardiac arrhythmias, or fluid overload, were commonly present.[69]

Low osmolar contrast media (LOCM) were not available for clinical use until the late 1970s. Research and ultimate discovery was fueled by goals to increase the safety profile by decreasing the significant and commonly present adverse events with existing RCMs. With an osmolality of less than 850 mOsm and an iodine to particle ratio of 3:1, which allowed for less dissociation, these products were made from benzoic acid side chains. Despite improvements, adverse events such as nausea, angina, and anaphylaxis still occurred.[69,70]

In the 1980s, RCM agents with low osmolar properties, less lipophilicity, and less toxicity were available for use. The improvements were due to the use of monoacid dimers with two benzoic rings containing iodine at positions 2, 4, and 6 bound together to form nonionic compounds.[71]

The only iso-osmolar RCM agent was introduced in the mid-1990s, iodixanol, with an iodine content of 300 mg/mL, which nearly matches that of blood.[70]

Commonly used RCM agents are divided in ionic and nonionic, and each category is subdivided into monomers and dimers. Table 55.3 presents a summary of the physical properties of the commonly used RCMs.

Modern agents used in current interventional pain practice are nonionic, contain hydroxyl and amide groups, and have an improved safety profile with fewer reported side effects, such as arrhythmias and cell membrane electrical disturbances. In addition, improvements in digital technology require less RCM per image. Additionally, less concentrated RCMs are also available; for example, the commonly used iohexol can be used in the concentration of iodine of 140 to 350 mg/mL.

The most feared adverse effect of the use of the RCM in interventional pain practice is a severe allergic reaction to the agent used. The incidence of reactions to RCM varies depending of the type of agent used. While HOCM are associated with an overall incidence of 15% toxic reactions, this number decreases to 3% when LOCM are used.[71,72] There are several risk factors reported to be implicated in the development of severe anaphylaxis in response to RCMs. Among those are history of previous reaction to contrast medium, allergy or atopy, asthma, history of multiple allergies, systemic mastocytosis, and female gender. They were well summarized in the Cardarelli Hospital Radiocontrast Media and Anesthetic Induced Anaphylaxis Prevention (CHRAIAP) scale.[73] Adverse reactions to RCMs depend primarily on the specific properties of those agents[67] and their mechanism of action. Table 55.4 summarizes common pathophysiologic actions, adverse reactions, symptoms, and clinical manifestations that occur in response to RCMs.

If a patient reports a shellfish allergy, this claim needs further investigation. In fact, most of the claimed shellfish

TABLE 55.3 Characteristics and Physical Properties of Commonly Used Contrast Agents

Name	Ionicity/Form	Type	Iodine Concentration (mg/mL)	Osmolality (mOsm/ kgH_2O)
Iodixanol	Nonionic dimer	IOCM	320	290
Iomeprol	Nonionic monomer	LOCM	350	620
Ioxaglate	Ionic dimer	LOCM	350	680
Ioxilan	Nonionic monomer	LOCM	350	695
Iopamidol	Nonionic monomer	LOCM	350	730
Iopromide	Nonionic monomer	LOCM	350	730
Iohexol	Nonionic monomer	LOCM	350	780
Ioversol	Nonionic monomer	LOCM	350	790

IOCM, *Iso-osmolar contrast medium;* LOCM, *low osmolar contrast medium.*
Modified with permission from Newmark JL, Mehra A, Singla AK. Radiocontrast media allergic reactions and interventional pain practice—a review. Pain Physician. *2012;15: E665-E675.*

TABLE 55.4 Common Symptoms, Clinical Manifestations and Pathophysiology of Radiocontrast Media

Type of Reaction	Clinical Manifestations	Agents Involved and Mechanism
Chemotoxicity	Nausea/vomiting, flushing, injection site pain, nephrotoxicity	Low water-soluble agents, highly osmolar with high iodine content
Osmotoxicity	Injection site pain, hypotension, bradycardia, loss of consciousness, pulmonary edema, ventricular arrhythmia Increased vagal tone	Low water-soluble agents, highly osmolar with high iodine content Arrhythmia linked to cellular membrane disturbances from iconicity and low solubility
Iodism	Iodide mumps (swollen parotids, sublingual submandibular, lacrimal), skin rashes, coryza, thyrotoxicosis	High iodine content in ratios of 3:2 iodine to particles
Delayed-type reactions (1 hour to 1 week after RCM exposure)	Fever, pruritus, urticarial, angioedema, flushing, nausea, arthralgia	Usually with nonionic agents High iodine content lead to protein iodination and antibody formation ± Antigen cross-reactivity, entails cellular release of inflammatory substances
Idiosyncratic reactions; can be lethal, clinically similar with allergy/anaphylaxis	Tachycardia, hypotension, tongue swelling, rhinitis, wheezing, laryngeal edema, bronchospasm, dyspnea, palpitation, hives, angina	No prior exposure Cellular release of inflammatory mediators High iodine content lead to protein iodination and antibody formation
Anaphylaxis; within minutes	Tachycardia, hypotension, tongue swelling, rhinitis, wheezing, laryngeal edema, bronchospasm, dyspnea, palpitation, hives, angina, oxygen desaturation, shock, cardiopulmonary arrest, death	± IgE ± Prior exposure ± Antigen cross-reactivity RCM directly stimulates immune cells High iodine leads to anaphylaxis by systemic protein iodination and antibody formation

IgE, *Immunoglobulin E;* RCM, *radiocontrast media.*
Modified with permission from Newmark JL, Mehra A, Singla AK. Radiocontrast media allergic reactions and interventional pain practice—a review. Pain Physician. *2012;15:E665-E675.*

allergies are food intolerances. If a true allergy to shellfish exists, patients should be counseled that they have a 1.5- to 3-fold increased chance of experiencing a hypersensitivity reaction to RCMs, but this value is similar to the risk of the patients that report a history of multiple medication and food allergies.[74] Therefore, an iodine allergy should not automatically be assumed in the presence of a shellfish allergy.

When a true, known, and severe allergy to RCMs exists, proceduralists need to follow a pretreatment protocol. While many protocols do exist, one feasible option is to pretreat patients with oral methylprednisolone 32 mg orally 12 and 2 hours preprocedure or with prednisone 50 mg orally 13, 7, and 1 hour preprocedure. Additional oral administration of diphenhydramine 50 mg and ranitidine 150 mg 1 hour preprocedure may be necessary.[75,76]

In more urgent procedures, high-risk patients may receive intravenously 100 mg hydrocortisone and 50 mg diphenhydramine preprocedure. If more than 2 hours elapses, then the dose may be repeated with the addition of 50 mg intravenous ranitidine.

Gadolinium, for example, gadopentate dimeglumine (Magnevist) may be used in patients who have a history of allergy to the contrast media. The use of gadolinium chelates is discussed in Chapter 77 (fluoroscopy and radiation safety).

SKIN ANTISEPTIC AGENTS

The majority of interventional pain procedures are performed with percutaneous needle placement. The use of

TABLE 55.5 Activity and Clinical Considerations of Common Skin Antiseptic Agents

	Alcohol	Povidone-Iodine	Chlorhexidine Gluconate	Chlorhexidine Gluconate With Alcohol
Mechanism of action	Denatures proteins	Oxidation/substitution with free iodine	Disrupts cell membranes	Disrupts cell membranes and denatures proteins
Gram-positive bacteria	Excellent	Excellent	Excellent	Excellent
Gram-negative bacteria	Excellent	Good	Good	Excellent
Viruses	Good	Good	Good	Good
Speed of action	Excellent	Moderate	Moderate	Excellent
Residual activity	None	Minimal	Excellent	Excellent
Use on mucous membranes	No	Yes	With caution	No
Cautions	Flammable. Optimum concentration 60%–90%	Maximum effectiveness after it has dried. Inactivated by blood. Shellfish allergies are not a contraindication.	Avoid direct contact with cornea, nerves, and meninges	Flammable. Avoid direct contact with cornea, nerves, and meninges

Source: Modified from Schaefer MK, Jhung M, Dahl M, et al. Infection control assessment of ambulatory surgical centers. JAMA. *303:2273-2279, 2010.*

antiseptic solutions is instrumental in preventing infectious complications when performing peripheral and neuraxial pain procedures. At a minimum, the skin at the procedure site should be cleaned and prepped with an antimicrobial agent to reduce the risk of postprocedure infection. There exists no single antimicrobial agent that is effective in killing all microbes, including bacteria, viruses, and spores, on the skin. Important characteristics of an ideal skin antiseptic agent include: (1) effectiveness against a wide array of microorganisms, (2) fast onset of efficacy, (3) long-term effect, (4) lack of inactivation by organic materials (blood, body fluids, and pus), and (5) minimal toxic effects to the skin.[77]

The most common skin antiseptic preparation agents in clinical use include solutions containing iodophors and chlorhexidine gluconate. Additionally, these agents can be further classified as either aqueous-based or alcohol-based. Aqueous-based iodophors, such as povidone-iodine, can be safely used on mucous membrane surfaces. Alcohol-based solutions offer a quicker onset and often more sustained antimicrobial activity. All have the potential for skin irritation with prolonged contact; therefore, it is advisable to remove the residual antiseptic preparation at the end of the procedure and evaluate the patient's skin condition prior to discharge.

Povidone-iodine is a germicidal compound that has good activity against most gram-positive and gram-negative microbes. The bactericidal effect of this compound relies on the continuous release of iodine, which penetrates cell walls and alters or attenuates protein synthesis.[78] Unlike chlorhexidine, this mechanism of action takes several minutes to achieve maximal microorganism reduction; however, the addition of isopropyl alcohol does further increase the release of iodine. There is a limited duration of effect of povidone-iodine, which is a distinct disadvantage of this compound when compared to chlorhexidine. In addition, organic compounds, such as blood or other proteinaceous material, may inhibit or neutralize its antiseptic effect. Acute skin reactions can occur after the application of povidone-iodine, including urticarial, vesicular lesions, or focal erythema. Bacterial resistance can occur, particularly with various strains of *Staphylococcus aureus*.[79]

Chlorhexidine gluconate is a potent broad-spectrum germicide that is effective against nearly all nosocomial bacteria (gram-positive and gram-negative) and yeasts. Resistance to chlorhexidine is exceedingly rare. The compound efficiently alters cell wall permeability, immediately precipitating components of the cytoplasm and cell membrane.[78] The addition of isopropyl alcohol synergistically accelerates these bactericidal effects. A major advantage of chlorhexidine is its ability to adhere to and penetrate the stratum corneum of the skin, which prolongs its duration of action for several hours after its application. Its efficacy is maintained in the presence of organic compounds, such as blood. In general, chlorehexidine induces fewer and milder skin reactions than other skin antiseptic compounds.

It is important to note that the FDA has not formally approved chlorhexidine for skin preparation prior to neuraxial procedures. This is due to the lack of preclinical studies investigating the potential for neurotoxicity of the compound. There are no reported human cases of nerve injury with chlorhexidine; in fact, there are no confirmed cases of human nerve injury with either chlorehexidine or isopropyl alcohol.[80] Multiple investigations have compared the antiseptic effects of povidone-iodine and chlorhexidine under experimental conditions.[78,81–89] Chlorhexidine was shown in all but one study to result in a superior and more rapid bactericidal effect. Therefore, alcohol-based chlorhexidine solutions are recommended by the American Society of Regional Anesthesia and Pain Medicine, the American Society of Anesthesiologists, and the Royal College of Anaesthetists as the skin antiseptic of choice prior to neuraxial or regional anesthetic procedures.[77,90,91] Table 55.5 reviews common skin-preparation antiseptic agents.

Infections associated with percutaneous interventional pain procedures are relatively rare. However, infections related to typical percutaneous interventional pain procedures not only involve skin and subcutaneous tissues, but also the targeted neuraxial structures. This can lead to potentially devastating infectious sequelae, including epidural abscess, discitis, osteomyelitis, and meningitis. The treatment of these serious infections may require hospitalization, prolonged antibiotic therapy, and surgery. Thus, it is imperative to adhere to comprehensive infection-control practices for preprocedure skin antisepsis, regardless of the setting in which the pain procedure is performed. These universal safe practices are applicable to all clinical settings, including hospital operating rooms, ambulatory surgery centers, radiology suites, and outpatient physician offices.

Infection control and aseptic techniques require attention to much more than simply the selection of the skin antiseptic solution. Physicians who perform interventional pain procedures must adhere to *all* infection-control-related practices, including thorough preprocedure hand washing, removal of watches and jewelry, protective barriers (including surgical hat and mask and sterile gloves), skin antiseptic preparation, proper sterile draping techniques, maintenance of a sterile field, and timely antibiotic prophylaxis when indicated. Compliance with these infection control standards will likely significantly reduce the risk of infectious complications associated with interventional pain procedures.

KEY POINTS

- Steroids have inhibitory effects on cytokine transcription and synthesis, especially the ones relevant in chronic inflammation. Steroids increase the synthesis of lipocortin (annexin) 1, a phospholipase A_2 inhibitor, decreasing the production of inflammatory mediators.
- Corticosteroids suppress spontaneous ectopic neural discharge originating in experimental neuromas. The topical application of methylprednisolone has also been shown to reversibly block transmission of C-fibers but not the A-β fibers.
- The inactive cortisone is converted by the liver to the biologically active cortisol. Prednisone, an inactive agent, is metabolized to the active agent prednisolone by the liver.
- BoNTs are produced by the gram-negative anaerobic bacterium *Clostridium botulinum*. They produce flaccid paralysis by preventing the presynaptic release of ACh at the neuromuscular junction.
- In addition to the pain relief associated with its paralytic effect, BoNT-A has been shown to influence pain processing via a reduction in peripheral and central sensitization through a number of different mechanisms.
- The BoNT molecule cannot cross the blood-brain barrier, and therefore does not have any direct CNS effects. Repeated injections of onabotulinum toxin A have been associated with antibody formation, which renders any subsequent onabotulinum toxin A injections ineffective.
- Risk factors to the development of severe allergic reaction to RCM include history of previous reaction to contrast medium, allergy or atopy, asthma, history of multiple allergies, systemic mastocytosis, and female gender.
- The bactericidal effect of povidone-iodine depends on the continuous release of iodine, which penetrates cell walls and alters protein synthesis. It takes several minutes to achieve maximal effect; the addition of isopropyl alcohol increases the release of iodine. It has a limited duration of action, and organic compounds (blood or other proteinaceous material) may inhibit or neutralize its effect.
- Chlorhexidine gluconate is effective against nearly all bacteria and yeasts, and resistance to it is rare. It alters cell-wall permeability, immediately precipitating components of the cytoplasm and cell membrane. Isopropyl alcohol accelerates chlohexidine's bactericidal effects. Chlorhexidine's efficacy is maintained in the presence of organic compounds.

REFERENCES

Access the reference list online at ExpertConsult.com.

CHAPTER 56

ROLE OF CANNABINOIDS IN PAIN MANAGEMENT

Omar I. Halawa, MD ◎ Timothy J. Furnish, MD ◎ Mark S. Wallace, MD

Cannabinoids are a diverse group of herbal, endogenous, and synthetic compounds that bind to specific inhibitory receptors in the body. The most common source of cannabinoids is the *Cannabis* plant, which has been used recreationally, industrially, and medicinally for thousands of years. In modern times, few substances have carried more stigma or ignited more debate. However, over the past 20 years, the public and medical community's attitude towards cannabinoids has been shifting. While it remains illegal federally, multiple US states have loosened state restrictions, including decriminalizing possession, legalizing medicinal use, and approving recreational use. With this changing landscape come many challenging questions from providers and patients: What role do cannabinoids play in alleviating pain? Should physicians recommend cannabinoids for the treatment of pain? What are the risks and side effects? How do patients obtain and use a cannabinoid drug? How should physicians who choose to recommend cannabinoids select appropriate patients and monitor them? What are the legal and regulatory issues that providers and researchers face in dealing with cannabinoids?

HISTORY OF CANNABINOIDS IN MEDICINE

Cannabis is one of the oldest documented herbal medicines, used for at least 5000 years.[1,2] It was initially utilized for its industrial properties to produce paper, textiles, and clothing, and as an important food source of hemp milk, oil, and seed.[3] Around the 1st century, the Chinese pharmacopoeia recommended its use for rheumatic pain, constipation, disorders of the female reproductive system, and malaria.[3,4] The ancient Indians used it to treat headaches, insomnia, gastrointestinal disorders, and pain during childbirth.[5] The West remained isolated from cannabis until the mid-19th century, when an Irish physician serving in the British military force in India documented cannabis's medicinal properties, igniting its spread into Europe and the Americas. In 1845, it was first listed in the United States Dispensatory as a sedative, analgesic, and anticonvulsant.[6–8] Popularity for this herbal remedy continued, and its indications expanded to include: headaches, migraine, eye-strain, menopause, brain tumors, neuralgia, gastric ulcer, uterine disturbances, dysmenorrhea, chronic inflammation, acute rheumatism, tingling, and relief of dental pain.[3,9] As the production of medicines became more commercial in the late 1800s, pharmaceutical companies marketed tinctures and extracts of cannabis leading to increased public consumption.[10]

In the early 20th century, there was an overall decline in herbal remedies—including cannabis—as pharmaceutically synthesized compounds like barbiturates, aspirin, and opioids became the accepted norm.[3,7,9] Additionally, cannabis's psychotropic effects, criminal associations, and lack of regulation led to further decrease in public consumption. In 1937, Congress passed the Marihuana Tax Act restricting and taxing the medical and nonmedical use of the drug. This led to the removal of cannabis from the American Pharmacopeia.[3,7,11] In 1970, the Controlled Substances Act (CSA) classified cannabis as a Schedule I drug, cementing its status as an illegal substance without acceptable medical use. This increasingly restrictive environment contrasted with emerging research into cannabis's pharmacological properties. The 1940s marked the first experiments performed using single cannabinoids. Tetrahydro-cannabinol (THC), the major psychoactive ingredient in cannabis, was isolated in the 1960s by Mechoulam and Gaoni,[7] ushering in a new understanding into the mechanisms and effects of cannabinoids on the central nervous system (CNS).[12–14] This was further solidified in the 1980s and 1990s by the discovery of endogenous cannabinoids (endocannabinoids) and their specific receptor targets, cannabinoid receptor type 1 and 2 (CB1 and CB2).[15]

The 1990s brought about a more permissive view of cannabinoids as US states, like California and Arizona, passed the first *medicinal marijuana* legislation (Arizona's referendum was invalidated 5 months later, but has since been reinstated by voters). Currently, 23 US states (plus the District of Columbia) have approved the medicinal use of cannabis in various forms. Four states have legalized its recreational use, while several others have decriminalized its possession. This legalization trend is likely to continue, with increasing calls for the Federal government to reevaluate its classification of cannabis as a Schedule I drug.[16]

The medicinal cannabinoid debate, specifically relating to marijuana, remains quite polarized. Its supporters argue that the herb contains numerous active constituents making it potentially more clinically effective than any synthetic or single constituent pharmaceutical. Moreover, it has a superior safety profile compared to analgesics like opioids because of its lack of lethal dose or risk of respiratory depression, substantiated by millennia of use. Opponents, on the other hand, argue that because it is a plant, its contents are nonstandardized and thus highly variable. Additionally, cannabis is addictive, impairs cognitive function, and has potential long-term risks, particularly in children and adolescents. Finally, removing the Schedule I classification of cannabis would lead to more widespread availability and recreational use, leading to untold public harm.

CLASSIFICATION OF CANNABINOIDS

The term *cannabinoid* refers to both endogenous and exogenous compounds that bind to specific inhibitory cannabinoid receptors, ultimately decreasing neurotransmitter

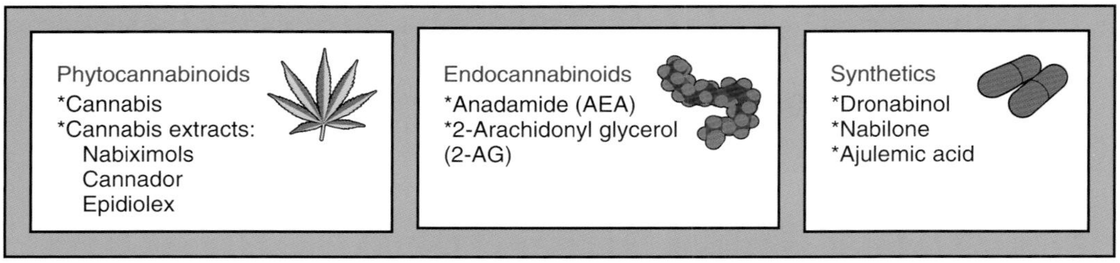

FIG. 56.1 Types of cannabinoids. There are three types of cannabinoids: the phytocannabinoids (plant-based), endocannabinoids (produced by the body), and synthetics (pharmaceutically derived). *AEA*, Anadamide; *2-AG*, 2-arachidonyl glycerol.

release. Historically, it referred to compounds derived from the *Cannabis* plant. With the discovery of human cannabinoid receptors, endogenous cannabinoids, and the development of new synthetic nonherbal compounds with similar effects, the term now applies more broadly to any compound having an interaction with these cannabinoid receptors.[17] Cannabinoids can be divided into three types: phytocannabinoids (compounds derived from cannabis), synthetics (manufactured compounds), and endocannabinoids (compounds produced by the body, which interact with cannabinoid receptors) (Fig. 56.1).

PHYTOCANNABINOIDS (CANNABIS AND ITS DERIVATIVES)

Cannabis is the genus of the family, cannabaceae (hemp). Cannabis is an herb that grows in temperate and tropical climates and has three major subspecies: *Cannabis sativa*, *Cannabis indica*, and *Cannabis ruderalis*. Although there is ongoing taxonomical controversy, it is generally thought that these subspecies are distinct in morphology and origin.[18] Anecdotally, *Cannabis sativa* has more psychoactive features compared to *indica*, though this is a matter of ongoing debate as both have significant levels of THC.[19] These two subspecies are commonly referred to as "marijuana." *Cannabis sativa* is also the most widespread of the species, growing in almost all climates. There are wide varieties of cannabis hybrid plants that combine desired features of each of these subspecies. This has led to a plethora of cannabis strains with unique cannabinoid profiles based on the cultivation conditions, as well as selection and breeding. *Cannabis ruderalis* usually has very low amounts of THC (<1%) but may be a good source of cannabidiol (CBD) extract.

The cannabis plant contains over 400 chemical compounds, of which at least 80 are cannabinoids.[1] Delta-9-tetrahydrocannabinol (Δ 9-THC) is the most well-known and the primary psychoactive compound in cannabis.[17,20–22] It mimics the action of anandamide (AEA), an endogenous cannabinoid in humans, having approximately equal affinity for the CB1 and CB2 receptors. Other cannabinoids include CBD, delta-8-tetrahydrocannabinol (Δ 8-THC), cannabigerol (CBG), and cannabinol (CBN). The concentration of cannabinoids in each cannabis strain can vary tremendously.[20] Due to selective breeding, the concentration of THC in recreational cannabis seized by the Drug Enforcement Administration (DEA) has increased from an average of 3% in the 1980s to 13% in 2009. More recently in medical marijuana dispensaries and recreational cannabis shops, the THC concentrations advertised range from the mid-teens to as high as 34%.[23,24] The majority of these strains contain CBD in very low concentrations, usually under 1%. There are strains with lower THC concentrations available, as well as "high CBD" strains with concentrations generally in the range of 5% to 15%.

CBD is the second most abundant compound in cannabis after THC.[11,20,25] It is thought to have wider medical applications than THC, which has fueled the demand for medical marijuana and pharmaceuticals with higher CBD concentrations compared to recreational marijuana.[26,27] CBD is generally considered to have no psychoactive effects, but clinically it has been reported to reduce seizures, improve muscle spasm, and reduce inflammation.[21,28,29] It has a very low affinity for the CB1 and CB2 receptors, and may act as an inverse agonist/antagonist.[20,28] These interactions with the CB receptors may attenuate some of the psychotropic effects of THC.[28,30,31] The majority of the marijuana strains available in medical marijuana dispensaries and recreational shops contain predominately THC, with CBD in very low concentrations.[32] However, there are low THC strains available, which have higher CBD concentrations ranging from 5% to 15%.[23,24] CBN, a metabolite of THC, is minimally psychoactive and found in only trace amounts in the plant.[33] Δ 8-THC is also minimally psychoactive and present at low concentrations.

In addition to whole-leaf cannabis plants, there is another class of phytocannabinoids collectively referred to as cannabis-based medicine extracts (CBME). These are derived by extracting compounds directly from cannabis plants.[34,35] There are two subtypes of CBMEs. The first are those produced by pharmaceutical companies under well-regulated, controlled conditions, and undergoing rigorous clinical trials. The second are products produced and sold in medical marijuana dispensaries without any regulatory oversight or clinical trials. There is increasing interest in CBD oil extracts for its wide range of medicinal uses. Industrial hemp, which is used in manufacturing thousands of commercial products, has a high CBD content and is used for CBD extracts in other countries. Although industrial hemp contains very low levels of THC (0.3%), legally grown hemp in the United States still falls under Schedule I drug policy so CBD extraction is not allowed. However, CBD extracts from hemp in other countries can legally be sold in the United States as found on websites, health food stores, and dispensaries.

There are three pharmaceutically manufactured CBMEs that have undergone clinical trials. Nabiximols (Sativex) is a sublingual spray with a 1:1 ratio of THC to CBD. Cannador is an oral capsule with a 2:1 ratio of THC to CBD. Epidiolex is a solution of purified CBD.[2,30,34] Nabiximols is currently approved in Canada and Europe for the treatment of spasticity in multiple sclerosis (MS). In Canada, it also has a conditional license as an adjunctive medication for MS-related neuropathic pain and cancer-related pain.[36,37] In the United States it has been studied in clinical trials, which initially showed promising results for advanced cancer pain. However, the most recent phase III trial failed to show superiority over placebo, and thus far it does not have Food and Drug Administration (FDA) approval.[38–40] Cannador has been used in several research studies in patients with MS spasticity and parkinsonian dyskinesia, but is not clinically available.[30] The CBD-based extract Epidiolex is being studied to treat certain rare forms of epilepsy and is currently undergoing phase III trials.

The category of nonpharmaceutically derived CBMEs contains a large variety of products made from the cannabis plant and sold in medical marijuana dispensaries. These include extracts, oils, tinctures, patches, topical creams, and pills. The delivery routes of these cannabinoid products include oral administration, vaporizer inhalation, transmucosal absorption, transdermal delivery, and rectal suppository. Additionally, most dispensaries sell a variety of foods, drinks, and candies infused with cannabinoids. There is wide variation in cannabinoid concentrations in these products, and there are no clinical studies on their effects for pain or other conditions.

SYNTHETIC CANNABINOIDS

There are two FDA-approved synthetic cannabinoid medications, dronabinol (Marinol) and nabilone (Cesamet). Dronabinol is a Schedule III synthetic form of Δ 9-THC, which is marketed in the United States for the treatment of nausea associated with chemotherapy, and as an appetite stimulant for HIV-related wasting syndrome.[28,41] Nabilone is a Schedule II synthetic analogue of Δ 9-THC, which is FDA approved to treat chemotherapy-induced nausea. Both dronabinol and nabilone have been studied for the treatment of chronic pain and spasticity.[21,42] Ajulemic acid is a newer synthetic analogue of the nonpsychoactive terminal metabolite of Δ 8-THC. It is currently being investigated as an antiinflammatory and analgesic agent.[11,43] A newer highly purified version of this molecule (Resunab) is currently under clinical investigation for a variety of inflammatory diseases.[44]

ENDOCANNABINOID SYSTEM

The endocannabinoid system (ECS) refers to the human body's network of cannabinoid neuromodulators (endocannabinoids), enzymes, and receptors. This intricate system is influenced by the phytocannabinoids in cannabis. The ECS is thought to regulate myriad behavioral processes, including pain, mood, memory, learning, addiction, and appetite.[45] Until the cannabinoid receptors were discovered, it was thought that cannabinoid effects in the body were nonspecific, due to lipophilic disruption of the phospholipid membrane. However, discovery of CB1 and CB2 receptors and advances in genotyping and pharmacology in the 1990s led to the understanding of receptor-specific processes.

The two primary endocannabinoids are AEA and 2-arachidonoylglycerol (2-AG).[17] These eicosanoids are synthesized in postsynaptic neurons and act as retrograde signaling messengers. During neurotransmission between a presynaptic and postsynaptic neuron, there are a multitude of excitatory, inhibitory, and secondary messenger systems at play. Endocannabinoids are thought to be produced on-site/on-demand from cell membrane lipid precursors to inhibit the presynaptic release of a variety of neurotransmitters, including acetylcholine, dopamine, gamma amino butyric acid (GABA), glutamate, serotonin, norepinephrine, and endorphins (Fig. 56.2).[46]

Anandamide (AEA), named from the Sanskrit word *Ananda*, meaning *bliss*, is an amide of ethanolamine and arachidonic acid. It is generated from its membrane precursor, *N*-arachidonoyl phosphatidylethanolamine (NAPE) via a multitude of pathways including phospholipase A2, phospholipase C, and phospholipase D.[47,48] 2-AG, on the other hand, is synthesized from diacylglycerol[49] through Ca-dependent pathways including diacylglycerol lipase and phosphatidycholine.[49] AEA is degraded in the postsynaptic terminal primarily by fatty acid amino hydrolase (FAAH), whereas 2-AG is mostly degraded presynaptically by monoacylglycerol lipase (MAG).[28,50] Both of these endocannabinoids are released into the presynaptic space by some combination of simple diffusion and facilitated, carrier-mediated transport.[28,50]

Pharmacodynamically, AEA and 2-AG bind to the G-protein coupled receptors (GPCRs), CB1 and CB2, which are located in the CNS and the peripheral nervous system. The analgesic properties of AEA likely involve its partial agonism (moderate affinity, low efficacy) of the CB1 receptor, which, in turn, decreases the release of excitatory neurotransmitters.[51] It has also been shown to act as a weak agonist at the transient receptor potential vanilloid 1 (TRPV-1) receptors.[47,52] The TRPV-1 receptors are expressed in nociceptive sensory neurons and respond to noxious mechanical, thermal, and chemical stimuli. AEA and capsaicin share the same TRPV-1 binding site, but higher concentrations of AEA are required in order to activate TRPV-1.[47,52] Unlike AEA, 2-AG is found in much higher concentrations in the brain (up to 170-fold) and is thought to be a full agonist (low affinity, high efficacy) of the CB1 receptor.[47,51,52]

PHARMACOLOGY OF CANNABINOIDS

The precise pharmacology of most cannabinoids remains unknown. However, researchers have elicited major mechanisms underlying the active compounds in cannabis including THC, CBD, and CBN. Complicating this is the highly variable absorption due to the plethora of delivery forms and routes. These include inhalation and ingestion, as well as absorption via oral, sublingual, topical, or rectal application.[53] For centuries, the primary means of delivering cannabinoids has been via the inhaled smoke of cannabis or hashish. The variable concentration of THC and other cannabinoids in cannabis, the lack of controlled production and testing in most medical marijuana products, and the diversity of delivery routes makes the prediction of pharmacologic effects difficult.[21,46]

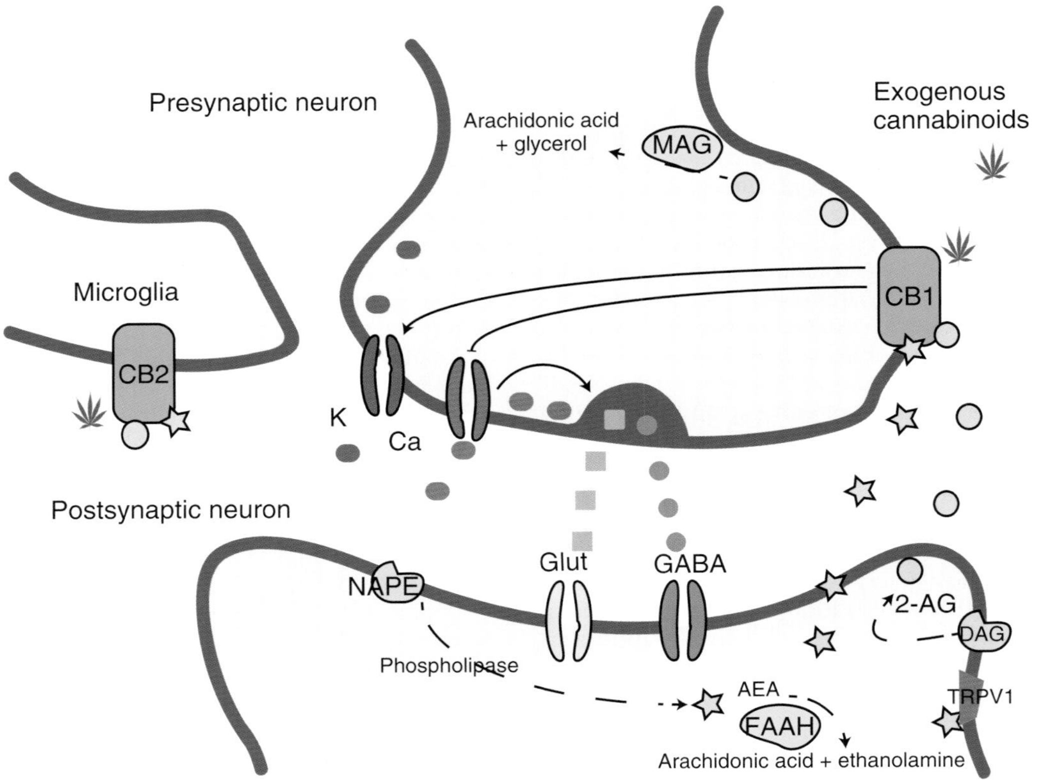

FIG. 56.2 The Endocannabinoid System. Anandamide (AEA) and 2-arachidonyl glycerol (2-AG) are endocannabinoids that activate presynaptic cannabinoid type I (CB1) receptors to inhibit release of neurotransmitters like GABA and glutamate (Glut). This is done via two mechanisms, inhibiting calcium entry into the presynaptic cell and increasing potassium efflux out of the cell. The synthesis of endocannabinoids is initiated by the activation of the glutamate receptor (Glut), which activates the breakdown of diacylglycerol into 2-AG. This endocannabinoid is transported in retrograde fashion into the synaptic cleft where it activates the presynaptic CB1 receptor. AEA is synthesized from N-arachidonoyl phosphatidylethanolamine (NAPE) via multiple phospholipases. Both 2-AG and AEA have endocannabinoid transporters that facilitate their reuptake and subsequent degradation. 2-AG is degraded in the presynaptic neuron by monoacylglycerol lipase (MAG lipase) into arachidonic acid and glycerol. AEA is broken down postsynaptically by fatty acid amino hydrolase (FAAH) into arachidonic acid and ethanolamine. AEA is unique in its activation of transient receptor potential channel 1 (TRPV1).

ACTIVATION DELIVERY AND ABSORPTION OF CANNABINOIDS

Patients who prefer not to smoke are increasingly using cannabis in a multitude of other forms. Cannabis vaporizers, similar to tobacco vaporizers or e-cigarettes, heat the plant material and vaporize the active ingredients (due to the low volatility of cannabinoids) without resulting in combustion or smoke. The use of cannabis-infused foods, candies, and drinks, or "edibles," has surged in popularity due to their slower onset of action and longer-lasting effects. Many of these food products are produced with butter or oil that has been infused with cannabinoids. The buds of the cannabis plant are heated in oil to extract the cannabinoids and decarboxylate the THC into its active form. The ingestion of the raw cannabis plant, without first heating and decarboxylating the THC, has little pharmacologic effect. The delayed onset and variable absorption of edibles often prolongs the clinical effects but increases the risk of overdose. Additionally, many of the commercially produced edibles are sweets and candies, and pose a temptation and risk of children being exposed. Tinctures, oils, and tonics are available in medical marijuana dispensaries, which can be administered sublingually or added to food and drink items. Cannabis topicals, including lotions, sprays, creams, and balms, are marketed to provide local analgesic and antiinflammatory effects. Finally, products such as hash and wax contain very potent concentrations of cannabinoids that can be eaten, smoked, or ingested.

PHARMACOKINETICS

The metabolism of cannabinoids occurs in the liver via the cytochrome P450 (CYP450) systems CYP2C subfamily of isoenzymes, particularly CYP2C9; therefore, this can result in decreased metabolism of other drugs that use the CYP450 system. Some metabolism occurs in the lungs as well as other tissues. Elimination is primarily in the form of acid metabolites both renally and through biliary excretion with only 5% eliminated unchanged.[54] Extensive tissue storage of metabolites results in prolonged elimination, which may explain the lack of or reduced withdrawal symptoms with chronic use and abrupt cessation. The detection of metabolites in urine will fluctuate between positive and negative results for days after last use. For infrequent users, the average time to the first negative urine test is 8.5 days with 12.9 days to the last positive test. For frequent users, the average time to first negative test is 19.1 days with 31.5 days to the last positive test.[55]

Inhaled cannabis, whether smoked or vaporized, is the most popular delivery mechanism. It is easier to titrate than ingestion, producing fast and relatively predictable results. Smoking cannabis results in rapid absorption, delivering into the lungs approximately 50% of its THC content in the inhaled smoke. Fifty percent or more of this inhaled THC is then lost to exhalation and local metabolism in the lung, leaving a bioavailability for the active drug between 10% and 35%.[54,55] Bioavailability varies depending on depth of inhalation, puff duration, and breath-holding with regular users being more efficient. Vaporization is another means of inhaled delivery without burning the cannabis and results in higher bioavailability. The volatile cannabinoids are vaporized when heated air is drawn through the cannabis.[21,56] Alveolar absorption results in maximal plasma concentration within minutes, and psychotropic effects starting within a few seconds and reaching maximal effect within 15 to 30 minutes. Psychotropic effects with inhalation will last 2 to 3 hours.[54]

The oral administration of cannabis produces slow, but relatively high, absorption with peak plasma concentrations at 60 to 120 minutes. However, first-pass metabolism results in a low bioavailability of 6% to 20% with significant variability.[55] The delay in peak blood levels of THC from oral administration makes self-titration more difficult. Psychotropic effects begin within 30 to 90 minutes after oral ingestion, reaching maximal effect after 2 to 3 hours and may last 4 to 12 hours.[54] Absorption of the cannabinoids can be increased with coingestion of a fatty meal.

PHARMACODYNAMICS

The location of the cannabinoid receptors and their respective interactions with these ligands is a field of extensive study. CB1 receptors are located mainly in the CNS at nerve terminals where they mediate inhibition of transmitter release.[17,47,52] In the brain, they are located in the cerebral cortex, hippocampus, caudate-putamen, substantia nigra, pars reticulata, cerebellum, the mesolimbic system, as well as the brainstem and spinal cord.[17,50] The CB2 receptor is found mainly on immune cells including microglia, monocytes, macrophages, and B and T lymphocytes where they modulate cytokine release.[17,47,50] Both CB1 and CB2 receptors are coupled through G proteins, negatively to adenylate cyclase (inhibiting the production of cyclic adenosine monophosphate [AMP]), and positively to mitogen active protein kinase (MAPK).[17,50] Additionally, CB1 is coupled positively to inwardly rectifying and A-type outward potassium channels, and negatively to N-type and P/Q-type calcium channels.[17,50] Within the spinal cord, CB1 receptors have been localized to multiple areas involved in nociceptive processing including the superficial dorsal horn, dorsolateral funiculus, and lamina X.[52] The activation of CB1 receptors in central nociceptive processing regions and primary afferents inhibits the release of neurotransmitters via decreased calcium conductance and increasing potassium conductance, which forms the anatomical basis for the analgesic action of cannabinoid agonists (see Fig. 56.2).[50] Additionally, there are CB1 receptors located in peripheral tissues in adipocytes, liver, lung, reproductive organs, smooth muscle, gastrointestinal tract, immune system, and peripheral sensory nerves.[48]

CB2 receptors play a role in mediating analgesia through reducing inflammation in the periphery. The CB2 receptors are found in the spleen, tonsils, thymus, and other tissues responsible for immune cell production and regulation. Activation of CB2 receptors down-modulates mast cell function with evidence that it can trigger microglial cell migration and regulate cytokine release.[17,52] The effect of CB2 on mast cells may play a role in modulating nerve growth factor (NGF)–driven sensitization of nerve terminals during inflammation, which has been implicated in the development of inflammatory hyperalgesia.[52] There is also evidence that CB2 receptors are located on and play a role in nociceptive regulation of primary sensory neurons.[48]

Emerging research suggests that there might be a third cannabinoid receptor. One possible candidate is the orphan receptor GPR55, based on its sequence homology to CB1 and CB2.[57] This GPCR expressed in the putamen and caudate nucleus responds to cannabinoid ligands particularly the endogenous lysophosphatidylinositol.[58] Further research is likely to yield more cannabinoid and cannabinoid-like receptors and ligands as advanced genetic and pharmacological technologies emerge.

Historically, the study of cannabinoids has focused mainly on THC. Recently, there has been an interest in coadministration of CBD and THC due to evolving research highlighting CBD's neuroprotective and medicinal effects. CBD as a sole agent does not produce any of the psychoactive effects associated with THC, and has a multitude of analgesic, anxiolytic, antiepileptic, antinausea, and antipsychotic actions.[59] Moreover, it is thought to antagonize many of THC's psychotropic and other adverse reactions; however, the associated mechanism remains unclear. This effect of CBD has been shown in a few animal and human studies where it attenuated some of the anxiety, paranoia, mental slowing, and tachycardic effects produced by THC.[3,30,60] Findings like these have supported the surge in low-THC/high-CBD cannabis products that might have more targeted roles for pain and inflammation without some of the adverse psychomimetic features. Even more recently, there has been a shift in drug development to focus on peripheral cannabinoid targets, thereby eliminating the central psychotropic effects completely.[61]

CANNABINOIDS AS ANALGESICS

There are a limited number of randomized, controlled, clinical trials (RCTs) involving cannabinoids for the treatment of pain. Stimulated by the burden of chronic pain globally, and the need to find safer, nonopioid therapeutic targets, the number of studies has been rising. Complicating this area of research, however, are complex federal regulatory issues due to the Schedule I status of cannabinoids, and the lack of standards for cannabinoid form and administration across various studies. The studies differ in the type of cannabinoid (plant, extract, synthetic), route of administration (inhalation, ingestion, mucosal absorption), and dosing that create unique challenges in interpretation. All of the current studies have focused on THC. There are no studies focusing on CBD, although there is increasing interest given its lack of psychoactive properties. To date, all studies that used cannabis supplied by the National Institutes of Health (NIH) had CBD levels of less than 1%. A summary of select RCTs across several pain conditions is highlighted in Table 56.1.

EXPERIMENTAL HUMAN PAIN STUDIES

Studies using experimental human pain models in healthy volunteers are limited and have produced mixed results. Several have shown that cannabis increases the pain threshold suggesting an analgesic effect. Other studies have found either no effect on pain thresholds or a lowering of the pain threshold.[63–68] In one trial of smoked cannabis on capsaicin-induced pain and hyperalgesia, cannabis cigarettes with 2% THC produced no effect on pain, 4% THC significantly decreased pain, and 8% THC significantly increased pain compared to placebo.[62] Another study found that 4% THC had a significant effect on both neuropathic pain and experimental capsaicin-induced pain in HIV patients.[80] CBD levels used in both of these studies were <1%. These studies suggest that there may be a therapeutic window for analgesia from cannabis. Another study of cannabis extracts found a hyperalgesic effect in human experimental models of acute pain.[90]

CLINICAL PAIN STUDIES

A recent meta-analysis of cannabinoids in noncancer pain found that 22 of 29 high-quality RCTs demonstrated modest analgesic effect with minimal side effects.[91,92] Their summary of the evidence for various pain indications showed relatively solid evidence for MS pain and spasticity. Modest efficacy has been reported for certain cannabinoid drugs in other neuropathic pain states and for cancer-related pain. Mixed or limited evidence exists for acute pain, inflammatory, and nociceptive pain states.

ACUTE PAIN

Studies conducted in the postoperative setting and in healthy human volunteers suggest that cannabinoids are least effective in acute pain. In fact, in some cases, their administration was associated with increased pain. Potential limitations to these studies include small sample sizes and possibly inadequate dosing. One multicenter dose escalation study in 30 postoperative patients showed a dose-dependent reduction in pain with administration of the cannabis-based medical extract, Cannador.[69] Contrarily, two studies with the synthetic cannabinoids, dronabinol and nabilone, failed to show any effect on postoperative pain.[70,71]

CHRONIC NONNEUROPATHIC PAIN

A handful of studies have evaluated cannabinoids for nociceptive, musculoskeletal, or inflammatory pain states. One study of dronabinol in mixed etiology chronic noncancer pain found that single daily doses of 10 and 20 mg resulted in a dose-dependent decrease in pain.[74] Nabiximols has been compared to placebo in patients with chronic pain due to rheumatoid arthritis. The nabiximols group experienced significant reduction in pain with movement and at rest, and improved quality of sleep compared to placebo. However, nabiximols did not decrease morning stiffness.[75]

CHRONIC NEUROPATHIC PAIN

Cannabinoids have shown the most promise in the treatment of chronic neuropathic pain. The majority of studies of cannabinoids for neuropathic pain states have been for MS pain and spasticity. However, there are several studies in other types of neuropathic pain. A meta-analysis of cannabinoid medications, including nabiximols, dronabinol, and cannabidiol studied for MS-related and neuropathic pain, found significant evidence of analgesic efficacy.[93]

Nabiximols (Sativex) has been evaluated in studies with various types of neuropathic pain. In a three-arm study, nabiximols and Δ 9-THC were compared to placebo in patients with pain from brachial plexus injury. Both nabiximols and Δ 9-THC produced significant improvements in pain as well as quality of sleep.[94] In unilateral neuropathy patients, nabiximols reduced pain, improved mechanical and punctate allodynia, and improved sleep disturbances.[81]

Two studies have evaluated the effects of inhaled cannabis for HIV-associated peripheral neuropathy.[25,80] Both found a significant effect in pain reduction compared to placebo. In studies of mixed etiology neuropathic pain, higher-dose smoked cannabis (7% to 9.4%) resulted in analgesia when compared to placebo or low doses of smoked cannabis.[79,95] A recent study was published evaluating inhaled cannabis on painful diabetic neuropathy. There was a dose-dependent reduction in pain with the highest dose being most effective. Although there were minimal effects of neurocognitive functioning, there was a dose-dependent increase in euphoria.[77]

Patients with MS have both neuropathic pain and painful spasticity. Both of these symptoms have been targets of cannabinoid therapy studies. A study of patients with MS-related neuropathic pain found a significant improvement in pain and pain-related sleep disturbance with nabiximols.[35] A three-arm trial with 630 MS patients comparing either oral Δ 9-THC, or a cannabis extract (Cannador) containing both THC and CBD versus placebo, found subjective improvement in spasticity and pain for both cannabinoid compounds compared to placebo, but no objective improvement in spasticity on the Ashworth Spasticity Scale. A 1-year continuation study found both THC and THC + CBD improved objective spasticity on the Ashworth scale at 1 year compared to baseline.[96] A multicenter trial of 160 patients with MS compared nabiximols to placebo and found a decrease in pain intensity but not spasticity.[97] Smoked marijuana studies in MS-related pain and spasticity have been small and have produced mixed results.[56,98] A summary of selected published cannabinoid studies is presented in Table 56.1.

The Canadian Pain Society's consensus statement regarding the treatment of neuropathic pain lists cannabinoids as a recommended third-line analgesic ahead of selective serotonin reuptake inhibitors (SSRIs), methadone, and topical lidocaine. Additionally, a systematic review by the American Academy of Neurology's guidelines

TABLE 56.1 Summary of Select Published Cannabinoid Studies on Pain

Pain Model	Drug (Route)	Outcome	Side Effects	Author, Year
Healthy volunteers	Cannabis (smoked)	No effect (low dose) Decreased pain (moderate dose) Increased pain (high dose)	Mild	Wallace et al., 2007[62]
Healthy volunteers	THC (oral)	No effect	Mild	Naef et al., 2003[63]
Healthy volunteers	Cannabis (smoked)	Decreased pain	Mild	Greenwald and Stitzer, 2000[64]
Healthy volunteers	Cannabis (smoked)	Decreased pain	Mild	Greenwald and Stitzer, 2000[64]
Healthy volunteers	Cannabis (smoked)	Decreased pain	Mild	Milstein et al., 1975[65]
Healthy volunteers	Cannabis (smoked)	Increased pain		Clark et al., 1981[66]
Healthy volunteers	Cannabis (smoked)	Increased pain		Hill et al., 1974[67]
Healthy volunteers	THC (oral)	No effect	Mild	Zeidenberg et al., 1973[68]
Acute pain	Cannador (oral)	Decreased pain (dose dependent)	Mild	Holdcroft et al., 2006[69]
Acute pain	THC analogue (oral)	Increased pain	Mild	Beaulieu, 2006[70]
Acute pain	THC (oral)	No effect	Mild	Buggy et al., 2003[71]
Acute pain	Levonantradol (IM)	Decreased pain	Mild	Jain et al., 1981[72]
Acute pain	THC (IV)	Decreased pain (low dose) Increased pain (high dose)	Moderate	Raft et al., 1977[73]
Chronic pain	Nabiximols (SL spray)	Decreased pain	Mild	Narang et al., 2008[74]
Chronic pain	THC/cannabidiol (SL spray)	Decreased pain	Mild	Blake, 2006[75]
Chronic pain	THC (SL spray)	Decreased pain	Mild	Notcutt et al., 2004[76]
Chronic pain	THC/cannabidiol (SL spray)	Decreased pain	Mild	Notcutt et al., 2004[76]
Chronic pain	Cannabidiol (SL spray)	No effect	Mild	Notcutt et al., 2004[76]
Neuropathic pain	Cannabis (smoked)	Decreased pain (dose dependent)	Mild	Wallace et al., 2015[77]
Neuropathic pain	Nabixomols (SL spray)	Decreased pain	Mild	Serpell et al., 2014[78]
Neuropathic pain	Cannabis (smoked)	Decreased pain (high dose)	Mild	Ware et al., 2010[79]
Neuropathic pain	Cannabis (smoked)	Decreased pain (high dose)	2 cases of toxic psychosis	Ellis et al., 2009[25]
Neuropathic pain	Cannabis (smoked)	Decreased pain (high dose)	Mild	Wilsey et al., 2008[31]
Neuropathic pain	Cannabis (smoked)	Decreased pain	Mild	Abrams et al., 2007[80]
Neuropathic pain	Nabiximols (SL spray)	Decreased pain	Mild	Nurmikko et al., 2007[81]
Neuropathic pain	Nabiximols (SL spray)	Decreased pain	Mild	Rog et al., 2005[35]
Neuropathic pain	Nabiximols (SL spray)	Decreased pain	Mild	Berman et al., 2004[82]
Neuropathic pain	Synthetic analog of THC (oral)	Decreased pain	Mild	Karst et al., 2003[83]
Neuropathic pain	Cannador (oral)	Decreased pain	Mild	Zajicek et al., 2003,[84] 2005[40]
Neuropathic pain	Nabiximols (SL spray)	Decreased pain	Mild	Wade et al., 2003[85]
Cancer pain	Nabixomols (SL spray)	Decreased pain (low and middle dose) No effect (high dose)	Mild	Portenoy et al., 2012[38]
Cancer pain	Nabixomols (SL spray) + THC extract	Decreased pain (nabiximols) Increased pain (THC extract)	Mild	Johnson et al., 2010[86]
Cancer pain	Benzopyranoperidine (oral)	Increased pain	Yes (similar to codeine)	Jochimsen et al., 1978[87]
Cancer pain	Benzopyranoperidine (oral)	Decreased pain	Yes (similar to codeine)	Staquet et al., 1978[88]
Cancer pain	THC (oral)	Decreased pain	Yes	Noyes et al., 1975[89]

IM, *Intramuscular;* IV, *intravenous;* SL, *sublingual;* THC, *tetrahydro-cannabinol.*

subcommittee found that oral cannabis extract and smoked marijuana were effective for reducing patient-reported symptoms of spasticity, and that nabiximols were effective at both patient-reported spasticity and objective measures of spasticity.[98] For the treatment of MS-related pain, the same review found oral cannabis extracts effective, and both nabiximols and dronabinol probably effective.[97]

CANCER PAIN

Cannabinoid products have a longer history of use in the cancer population as an adjuvant for chemotherapy-induced nausea and vomiting. For pain, several early studies of oral dronabinol showed it to be effective for cancer pain at higher doses (15 to 20 mg) with efficacy similar to codeine (60 to 120 mg), but with more significant adverse effects than codeine.[89]

In the advanced cancer pain population, nabiximols (THC/CBD sublingual spray) has been studied with mixed results. Initially, there were positive phase II studies showing efficacy of nabiximols as adjuvant therapy with opioids for intractable cancer pain when compared to placebo.[38,86] Specifically, the trials showed greater than 30% pain reduction, but with higher doses being viewed unfavorably by patients due to side effects. However, more recent phase III studies have been reported to be negative, showing no significant differences when compared to placebo.[39] Another synthetic THC compound, benzopyranoperidine, showed positive results over placebo, but sedation was a common side effect.[88] A study on the same compound in cancer pain showed no benefit over placebo.[87]

RISKS AND SIDE EFFECTS OF CANNABINOIDS

As with any potential therapy, cannabinoids carry risks and adverse effects. The most common cannabinoid side effects include sedation, dizziness, dry mouth, and dysphoria. Other significant side effects include cognitive impairment, anxiety, and psychosis. It is important to note that most of the published side effects of cannabis and cannabinoids come from the study of their recreational use.

Use of cannabis can produce perceptual alterations, including euphoria, in addition to other cognitive and psychomotor changes. These tend to last for a few hours depending on the type and method of administration (inhaled, ingested, topical). Physiologic changes include decreased body temperature, muscle relaxation, conjunctival injection, hyposalivation/dry mouth, tachycardia, vasodilation, orthostatic hypotension, and bronchodilation. Acutely, there is also impairment in attention, balance, cognition, memory, judgment, and sense of time.[21,54,98] Less commonly, cannabis can induce unpleasant effects including anxiety, panic, and paranoia.[21,98] In rare cases, cannabis use may lead to acute psychosis involving delusions and hallucinations. There is an association between heavy cannabis use in adolescence and the development of schizophrenia, as well as an association between cannabis use and worsening symptoms in schizophrenia.[54,99] Strains of cannabis with higher CBD content may be associated with a lower risk of adverse psychiatric effects. Contrary to popular belief, cannabis does carry a risk of dependence, approximately 9%, but this is significantly lower than the greater than 20% and 60% for alcohol and tobacco, respectively.[100]

There are no documented deaths from cannabis or cannabinoid-based products.[54] In a systemic review of studies of oral and oral-mucosal cannabis for various medical conditions, the majority of adverse events reports were considered nonserious (96.6%).[101] The nonserious adverse events were significantly more common in the cannabinoid groups compared to placebo, with the most common events being nervous system disorders, such as dizziness and anxiety. The number of serious adverse events was not significantly different than in control groups and involved vomiting, urinary tract infections, respiratory infections, and a relapse of MS.[101] A more recent prospective cohort trial in noncancer chronic pain showed no statistical difference in serious adverse events between the cannabis and noncannabis group.[102] There was, however, an increased risk of nonserious side effects in the cannabis group.

Risk of cannabinoid exposure varies widely across ages. Prenatal exposure to cannabinoids is associated with persistent neurodevelopmental differences in neonates and children.[103] Thus, cannabis should not be used in pregnancy. In adolescence, there are several studies that show early age use leads to persistent cognitive deficits and reduced educational achievement. Adolescent users who started before age 18 tended to become more persistent users. After comparing adolescent and adult-onset users with the total number of cannabis-dependence diagnoses, adolescent-onset users showed greater IQ decline.[99,104,105] Adult-onset cannabis users did not appear to experience IQ decline as a function of persistence of cannabis use. Thus in adolescence, though the studies are mixed, the overall trend suggests that cannabis may have a significant and permanent impact on neurocognition compared to those who begin use in adulthood.[106] Therefore, an extensive risk/benefit analysis should be undertaken prior to initiating cannabinoids in any person younger than 18 years old. In the adult population, a review of 40 articles on the use of cannabis found no consistent evidence for persisting neuropsychological deficits. However, half of the studies reported at least some subtle impairment. Another review of 11 articles covering 623 cannabis users and 409 nonusers or minimal users concluded that there might be decrements in the ability to learn and remember new information, whereas other cognitive abilities are unaffected.[98,107]

Cannabis can induce changes in the cardiopulmonary system. There is evidence of mild tachycardia and orthostatic hypotension, more clinically significant in the elderly due to an increased risk of falls.[108] In chronic heavy smokers of marijuana, there is evidence of an increased risk of bronchitis and other respiratory disorders.[109,110] There is conflicting evidence on long-term pulmonary function. A longitudinal study of 972 tobacco and marijuana smokers found increased forced vital capacity (FVC), total lung capacity (TLC), and functional residual capacity (FRC) independent of the effects of tobacco use.[111] Other studies have failed to find similar associations. A review of 34 articles on cannabis smoking and pulmonary function found no association between long-term use and airflow obstruction; however, it did find increased chronic cough, sputum production, and wheezing.[112] In a study of cannabis-only smokers compared to tobacco-only smokers, the effect on forced expiratory volume (FEV)-1 of one cannabis cigarette was found to be 2.5 to 5 times as pronounced as one tobacco cigarette.[113] This may be, in part, because each inhalation of a cannabis cigarette is typically two-thirds larger, inhaled one-third deeper, and held 4 times longer. Additionally, cannabis cigarettes were found to be 50% higher in tar.[114] Cannabis smoke contains many of the same chemicals and carcinogens as tobacco smoke, including benzene, acetone, and ammonia.[115] Epidemiologic studies have not consistently found an increased risk of lung cancer in chronic marijuana smokers when controlled for concurrent use of tobacco.[99,110] However, some studies have found an increased risk of head and neck cancers in chronic marijuana users.[99,110]

Cannabis withdrawal syndrome has been demonstrated in frequent, heavy users. The syndrome is characterized by increased anxiety, restlessness, anger and aggression, and irritability, with decreased appetite, weight loss, sleeplessness, depressed mood, and stomach pains.[98,116] These symptoms may emerge 2 days after cessation of use and remit in 1 to 2 weeks.[117] Unlike the withdrawal syndromes associated with opioids, alcohol, and benzodiazepines, cannabis withdrawal lacks serious physiological symptoms or effects.[116]

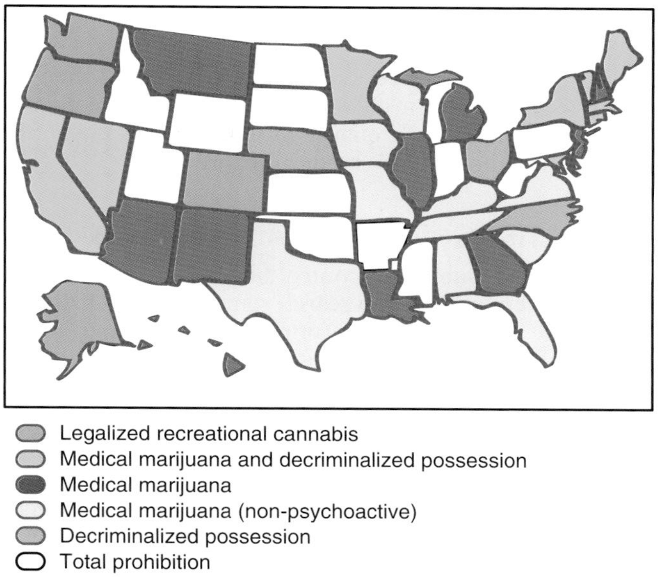

FIG. 56.3 Map of United States Cannabis Laws (2015). This constantly evolving map highlights the varied legal landscape across US states ranging from legalized recreational cannabis to total prohibition.

REGULATORY, PROFESSIONAL, AND LEGAL CONSIDERATIONS

REGULATIONS FOR CLINICAL USE

Possession and use of cannabis remains illegal under federal law. Since 1970, cannabis has been listed by the DEA as a Schedule I drug with "high potential for abuse," "no currently accepted medical use," and "lack of acceptable safety for use under medical supervision." This is in direct contrast to its legal status within many US states for medicinal and recreational use. This has created confusion for many providers and patients.

The FDA has approved two cannabis-based medications: dronabinol and nabilone. It is the FDA's responsibility to ensure that pharmaceutical products are efficacious, safe, and produced under good manufacturing practices to ensure high quality. Neither the FDA nor any other federal regulatory agency currently oversees or regulates the production and distribution of cannabis or the myriad cannabis-based products sold in medical marijuana dispensaries. Moreover, there is no national oversight, and limited state regulation of the labeling, concentration, dosing, or purity of cannabis and cannabis-based products. Thus, it is often left up to the growers, processors, and distributors of medical cannabis, in states where it has been legalized, to self-regulate. This is in contrast to the Netherlands, Canada, and Israel who have successful federally regulated cultivation, production, and distribution of medical marijuana. Lastly, neither cannabis nor any of these products have undergone the large-scale clinical trials necessary for showing clear efficacy for a particular indication.

Efforts are emerging to provide better oversight of herbal marijuana processing and distribution. Oregon recently passed a bill that designates the Oregon Liquor Commission to work with the Department of Agriculture and the Department of Health to oversee the growth, processing, and distribution of marijuana into the marketplace. In addition, laboratories that assay the leaf for cannabinoid concentrations and contaminants are proliferating across the country. These laboratories, however, are currently not under any regulatory oversight and testing fees are often paid by the growers themselves; thus, the accuracy of their results may be questionable.

Marijuana laws vary widely among those states that have passed some form of legalization (Fig. 56.3), and the clinician must be familiar with the state in which they practice. These state laws vary on (1) which medical conditions marijuana can be used for, (2) the type of medical marijuana (any form vs. CBD only), (3) how physicians are certified, (4) physician responsibilities when recommending marijuana, (5) how much marijuana or number of cannabis plants a patient can possess for medicinal use, (6) the legality of possession by designated caregivers, and (7) rules governing the dispensaries. Since marijuana is not FDA approved, no state requires a physician to write a prescription. In 2009, Attorney General Eric Holder stated: "It will not be a priority to use federal resources to prosecute patients with serious illnesses or their caregivers who are complying with state laws on medical marijuana."[118] There has been a push by the American Medical Association (AMA) to enact federal legislation protecting physicians who prescribe cannabis. Since it is not an FDA-approved medication, there are no third-party payers or insurance companies that provide coverage for medical marijuana. Most hospitals will prohibit patients from using any form of cannabinoid, including edibles, tinctures, and extracts while an inpatient. Allowing patients to use a Schedule I substance would potentially jeopardize a hospital pharmacy's DEA license.

Some states provide guidelines for recommending medicinal cannabis. In the absence of guidelines, clinicians who choose to recommend cannabis should manage their patients in accordance with good medical practice. This involves becoming familiar with the safety and efficacy of medical cannabis, and counseling patients on their responsibilities and on the side effects. Patients should then be monitored to assess the clinical effects, adverse effects, and impact on function and quality of life. Appropriate documentation in the patient's medical record should be made.

REGULATIONS FOR CLINICAL RESEARCH

As marijuana is subject to control under Schedule I of the CSA conducting clinical research remains quite challenging. While the federal government currently appears to be forgoing enforcement against patients who may obtain marijuana for medicinal purposes from state dispensaries, research with marijuana is heavily regulated. Marijuana research oversight involves multiple agencies including the DEA,[119] the Department of Health and Human Services (DHHS), the FDA, and the National Institute of Drug Abuse (NIDA). Obtaining a Schedule I DEA license is required in order to conduct marijuana research. This license requires a much more intensive application process than is necessary for obtaining a regular Schedule II license. First, the proposed research must be submitted for review by the Office of Public Health and Science (an interagency review panel within the DHHS). After approval, an Investigational New Drug (IND) application must be filed with the FDA. After IND approval, the study is submitted for further review by NIDA and the DEA. Simultaneous approval must be obtained from the local DEA office. The local DEA will inspect the location of the proposed study and the researchers' practices for storage, safeguarding, and dispensing of marijuana, which have more stringent requirements than for other investigational drugs. Some states have additional review and approval (i.e., California requires all research with Schedule I or II controlled substances to undergo review by the Research Advisory Panel of California, a branch of the Office of the Attorney General in the California State Department of Justice).

Since 1968, the University of Mississippi has been the sole supplier of cannabis for research in the United States through a contract with NIDA. The agency has made cannabis available with different concentrations of THC, with a placebo leaf and with CBD levels typically being very low (<1%). CBD oil for use in research is actively being pursued.

CANNABINOIDS IN THE PAIN CLINIC

Given medical cannabis' illegality under federal law and its quasi-legal status in 23 US states, there are many concerns by providers and patients. Some providers will decide not to recommend cannabinoids due to legality issues under federal law. Others will decline to recommend it due to concerns about lack of clear efficacy data, side effects, and the unregulated and unpredictable nature of marijuana production and distribution. Alternatively, some providers will recommend its use for certain patients due to its long safety record and emerging, albeit modest, evidence for various pain conditions.

As with many therapies, the most challenging issue is appropriate patient selection. Determining an appropriate patient for medical cannabis use requires a thorough pain and social history, physical exam, and clear pain diagnosis with extensive evaluation of risk factors that might place the patient at higher risk for cannabinoid therapy. A synthesis of clinical guidelines on medical cannabis is detailed in Table 56.2. These cover such areas as patient evaluation and selection, where to send patients to obtain the drug and in what form they should administer it, monitoring and coadministration of other controlled substances, and what disclosures are necessary regarding the potential risks of medical marijuana.

TABLE 56.2 Recommendations for Pain Practitioners to Consider Prior to Initiating Cannabinoids

Be aware of United States federal law (Schedule I, illegal as of 2015) and your state law (see Fig. 56.3)
Conduct a comprehensive history, and a physical examination, establishing a pain diagnosis
Does the patient have any medical risk factors that would exclude them from medicinal cannabinoids? (Active substance abuse, psychotic disorder, unstable/serious mood disorder, active cardiac conditions.)
What is the patient's level of interest in medicinal cannabinoids?
Conduct thorough informed consent (risks vs. benefits) based on the patient's pain condition, symptoms, comorbidities. Explain the level of evidence for their type of pain
Refer to a medical marijuana specialist for advice on cannabis strains (high CBD, low THC), route of administration, titration. (Recognizing the lack of regulatory oversight and herbal uniformity.)
Conduct regular monitoring as with any controlled substance: • Timely intervals • Assess control of targeted symptoms, functional status, pattern of use of cannabis of other substances, and medications • Obtain periodic urine drug screens for objective information on substance use
Continue or discontinue based on observed outcomes: • Continue authorization if goals of treatment are met with little harm/risk • Discontinue if not helpful in moving towards goals or if major intolerance or unsafe medication or substance use
Intervene through counseling or referral if harmful use or declining function is apparent
Renew or recommend authorization/certification, or not, based on observed outcomes: • Continuation if goals of treatment being met without harm • Discontinuation if not helpful in moving towards goals or if there is unsafe medication or substance use

CBD, *Cannabidiol;* THC, *tetrahydro-cannabinol.*
Modified from California Medical Board guideline "Marijuana for Medical Purposes." http://www.mbc.ca.gov/Licensees/Prescribing/Medical_Marijuana.aspx and Savage SR, Romero-Sandoval A, Schatman M, et al: Cannabis in pain treatment: clinical and research considerations. J Pain *17(6):654–668, 2016.*

PATIENT SELECTION

There are no published guidelines for risk stratification or patient selection for medical marijuana use. Nabilone (DEA Schedule II) and dronabinol (DEA Schedule III) have some abuse potential, as does cannabis itself. Evaluation of a patient's risk for substance abuse should be a part of the patient selection process. Although there are widely used tools for opioid risk evaluation, such as the Opioid Risk Tool (ORT) or the Screener and Opioid Assessment for Patients with Pain (SOAPP-R), these have not been studied specifically for marijuana abuse risk. Regardless, they may be a good starting point. Those patients who have failed first- and second-line therapies, especially for cancer-related or neuropathic pain, may be the most likely candidates. Those patients with a history of serious mental illness, such as schizophrenia or bipolar disorder, are not acceptable candidates.[120] The tachycardia and blood pressure fluctuations that may occur limit the acceptability of cannabis therapy for the elderly and those with substantial coronary artery disease.

The drugs dronabinol and nabiximols have been evaluated for abuse potential in various studies. Clinical use of dronabinol has not been shown to be associated with significant diversion, drug-seeking, or street value. In studies with recreational marijuana users, both dronabinol and nabiximols were found to have some abuse potential although nabiximols was significantly lower than dronabinol. While dronabinol is known to have significant psychoactive effects, it has been found less desirable than marijuana by regular users due to the higher incidence of dysphoria, the slower onset, and the less flexible titration of effect. Nabiximols has been found to have significantly lower euphoria or psychoactive effects compared to dronabinol.[121]

DISPENSARIES AND ROUTES OF ADMINISTRATION

It is important that practitioners understand the laws regarding medical marijuana within the state in which they practice (noting it is still considered an illegal substance by the federal government). Moreover, clinicians should understand that their role in recommending cannabis also varies by state. Some states require a trial of cannabis prior to long-term initiation; others require a physician to certify a patient with a diagnosis prior to the patient registering for medical use. Even more, states may differ in their requirements for risk/benefit discussions, follow-up, and recertification after the initiation of therapy. States also place limits on the amount of medical cannabis a patient may possess, the amount that can be grown by a patient, and the amount that may be sold by dispensaries, as well as imposing restrictions on the availability and packaging of certain forms, like edibles.

In California, as with most states with legalized medical marijuana, any physician can recommend the use of marijuana to a patient for the treatment of a medical condition. Provision of a letter to the patient verifying this recommendation provides some protections against state and local prosecution for the possession and use of marijuana up to the statutorily prescribed state quantity limits. Such a letter provides no protection against prosecution by federal authorities. In California, patients may take this letter along with proof of identification to their county's program office to obtain a Medical Marijuana Identification Card (MMIC). Subsequently, a patient may possess and obtain medical marijuana for their medical condition.

Each US state differs in its specific medicinal marijuana program, highlighting in detail (often through websites) its requirements for patients prior to their usage. Obtaining a state-issued ID card is optional in several states, but is required in some other states. The registration of an ID card places the patient's name in a database accessible by marijuana dispensaries and law enforcement to aid in identifying those with the required physician recommendations. Medical marijuana dispensaries (in the 23 legalized medicinal cannabis states) sell the drug in various forms. These may include the dried buds of the plant for smoking or vaporizing, oils and tinctures that can be ingested, creams or solutions for topical application, and prepared cookies and other edible products made with marijuana infused oils and fats. Some of the pulmonary adverse effects may be attenuated with the use of a vaporizer device instead of smoking.[120] The potency of marijuana products available in dispensaries will vary considerably. In most locations there will be labeling of THC or CBD content, but without any independent testing of such content. A reputable and knowledgeable dispensary may provide some assistance in educating patients and directing them to lower THC and higher CBD content products than those cultivated primarily for recreational purposes. In 15 of the 23 states with medical marijuana laws, patients or their caregivers may cultivate their own marijuana at home with some limits on the number of plants per patient. The quantity of marijuana an individual patient may possess varies among the 23 states from 1 ounce up to 24 ounces.

Currently, no insurance companies cover medical cannabis; thus it remains an out-of-pocket expense for patients. Prices range depending on cannabis strain, potency, type (buds, tinctures, oils, drinks, and edibles), organic/nonorganic, and location in which it is sold. Cannabis, particularly the bud of the plant, which is smoked or vaporized, is typically sold in grams (~$5 to $20 per gram). Concentrates (oils, waxes) may be more expensive, averaging ~$20 to $60 per gram. The cost and potency of edibles and tinctures will also vary widely. A simple internet search reveals multiple websites with extensive information on the locations of legal dispensaries, as well as the cost and advertised cannabinoid concentrations of their cannabis products.[122] Given the lack of insurance coverage for these products, cost may be a significant obstacle for some patients.

COMBINING MEDICAL MARIJUANA WITH OPIOIDS

Studies in healthy adults have shown an additive or synergistic effect with cannabinoids and opioids in combination.[56] In cancer-related pain, nabiximols was studied as add-on therapy along with opioids. However, the combination of different controlled substances with addictive and psychomimetic effects should be considered with caution. No clear guidelines yet exist regarding the coadministration of opioids and cannabinoids. Cannabis use in patients on chronic opioids has been associated with future aberrant opioid-related behaviors.[120] At minimum, clinicians should exercise careful evaluation of patients' substance abuse risk. There should also be ongoing monitoring for aberrant drug-seeking behaviors, positive analgesic and functional effects, and appropriate use of only the prescribed or recommended drugs via urine drug screening. Some have advocated the use of a medicinal cannabis agreement, analogous to opioid agreements, which outline the various risks and expected responsibilities and behaviors of patients on this therapy.[120]

MEDICAL MARIJUANA RISK DISCLOSURES

There are several risks associated with the possession and use of medical marijuana, which should be part of any patient disclosure prior to recommending the drug. First is the legal risk for possessing and using a controlled substance that is still categorized as Schedule I by the DEA. Accidental pediatric exposures have increased, along with the spread of medical marijuana laws.[21] Cannabis-containing foods and drinks carry a particular risk for pediatric exposures and patients should be warned to keep cannabis-containing products out of reach of children. While likely lower risk for addiction than opioids or alcohol, there remains a dependence, addiction, and withdrawal risk, which should be discussed with patients.[107] The pulmonary and cancer risks of smoking cannabis remain unclear; however, some discussion of potential pulmonary complications is important.[56] Cannabis use impairs the ability to operate a vehicle, and this impairment is exacerbated when combined with alcohol. Patients should be cautioned not to drive while using cannabis or cannabinoid medications, especially those containing THC.[107]

CONCLUSION

A rapidly shifting legislative landscape and accumulating, yet limited, data from clinical trials has renewed interest in the role of cannabinoids in pain management. Though the evidence for efficacy is modest, this may change with increasing research studies looking at various cannabinoid combinations and delivery systems. However, there are significant legal issues, which add complexity to recommending cannabinoids as a therapy for pain. Regardless, pain physicians are increasingly being asked about cannabinoids in their practice, whether or not they choose to recommend medical cannabis or prescribe cannabis-derived pharmaceuticals. This makes it imperative for pain physicians to understand the evidence for and against cannabinoids, and to stay informed regarding the constantly changing legislative environment. Those who choose to recommend cannabis use should employ careful patient selection and informed consent prior to initiating therapy, and engage in appropriate monitoring to ensure that benefits outweigh the associated risks of cannabinoid therapy.

KEY POINTS

- Cannabinoids are a diverse group of herbal, endogenous, and synthetic compounds that bind to specific inhibitory receptors in the body.
- Cannabis, an herbal cannabinoid, has an extensive medicinal, industrial, and recreational history with humans dating back at least 5000 years.
- Secondary to its federal classification in the United States as a Schedule I drug (illegal without acceptable medical use), cannabis continues to elicit many legal and regulatory issues for practitioners, scientists, and patients interested in its medicinal use. This legislative landscape is constantly evolving as multiple US states loosen their restrictions.
- Cannabinoids can be divided into three types: phytocannabinoids (compounds derived from cannabis), synthetics (manufactured compounds), and endocannabinoids (compounds produced by the body, which interact with cannabinoid receptors).
- The cannabis plant contains over 400 chemical compounds, of which at least 80 are cannabinoids. The most well-known compound is Δ 9-THC known for its primarily psychoactive properties. CBD, another cannabinoid, has stronger analgesic properties with limited psychoactive features representing a potential therapy in pain management.
- A review of clinical trials in pain management shows modest efficacy for cannabinoids across a variety of conditions including: neuropathic pain, cancer pain, and spasticity. This level of evidence may change with emerging research studies investigating specific cannabinoid compounds/combinations within different delivery systems.
- Cannabinoids have a very favorable risk/benefit profile showing limited evidence of significant adverse events and minimal issues of dependency.
- Medical practitioners choosing to recommend cannabinoids for pain management must employ careful patient selection and informed consent, taking into account emerging evidence and constantly evolving legal issues.

REFERENCES

Access the reference list online at ExpertConsult.com.

SECTION VII

THERAPEUTIC INTERVENTIONS

SECTION OUTLINE HEAD

CHAPTER 57

Ablative Neurosurgical Procedures for Treatment of Chronic Pain

Joshua Rosenow, MD, FAANS, FACS

The destruction of the nervous system is an irreversible technique to control otherwise intractable pain. However, prior to the development of effective augmentative techniques, such as intrathecal drug delivery and neurostimulation (both peripheral and central), these were the mainstay of neurosurgical pain treatment. Options exist for lesioning the brain and brain stem, cranial nerves, spinal cord, and peripheral nerves. Although the rise of these newer therapies has pushed aside many ablative procedures, several still remain valuable components of the neurosurgical armamentarium.

GENERAL COMMENTS

The interruption of peripheral or central nervous system pathways carrying pain has always seemed the most direct and logical manner to solve the problem of medically intractable pain, whether benign or malignant in origin. The targets for these interventions are myriad, beginning with peripheral nerves and ganglia and extending to the ascending spinothalamic tract and central aspects of the spinal cord, as well as the trigeminothalamic tract (Figs. 57.1 and 57.2). Supratentorial structures such as the thalamus and cingulate gyrus have also been destroyed in the quest for pain control. Unfortunately, the results of these interventions have not been as straightforward as the theories behind their use, once again demonstrating that the physiology underlying the development and maintenance of chronic pain is more complex than we understand.

Several methods have been used to lesion the nervous system. The easiest is simply avulsion/resection of a peripheral nerve or cranial nerve branch. Thermocoagulation (TC) or radiofrequency (RF) lesioning has been most often used in the central nervous system, including the creation of ganglionic, spinal cord, and intracerebral lesions. Cryoablation found some favor in the 20th century but is rarely used nowadays.

Patients selected for these procedures should have chronic pain that has failed to adequately respond to multiple other conservative nonsurgical treatments. These may include rehabilitation, oral medications (antiinflammatory medications, opioids, anticonvulsants, antidepressants), and injections. Given the advances in neurostimulation and intrathecal drug delivery, it is also reasonable to conduct a trial of these therapies prior to considering ablative procedures. This is true both for patients with pain due to late stage malignancies (due to their higher medical risk in undergoing surgery) and those with pain from nonmalignant causes (due to the risk of permanent neurologic morbidity from the procedures).

After the patient is selected, it is just as important to carefully select the correct ablative procedure, considering both the etiology of the pain and its location within the nervous system, so as to maximize the chance of achieving pain relief. For instance, central neuropathic pain will not likely respond well to a peripheral neurectomy or dorsal root ganglion lesion.

This chapter reviews the published experience with several neuroablative procedures, beginning with those that are still most commonly in use. Certain procedures (such as trigeminal ganglionic lesions and spinal facet denervation) are covered elsewhere in this book (Chapters 65, 66, and 82).

DORSAL ROOT ENTRY ZONE LESIONS/ CAUDALIS DORSAL ROOT ENTRY ZONE

The dorsal horn of the spinal cord serves as both a relay center and an integration site for sensory signaling. First performed by Sindou[1] in 1972 (via coagulation) and then Nashold and Ostdahl[2] in 1974 (via RF energy), lesioning of the dorsal root entry zone (DREZ) was seen as a way to remove the portions of the central nervous system that had already undergone central sensitization in response to a peripheral lesion, such as malignancy or nerve injury. The lesions are intended to injure Lissauer tract and preserve fibers subserving proprioception and certain aspects of touch that travel in the dorsal rootlets to the dorsal columns. It continues to have clinical application primarily for the treatment of pain due to traumatic brachial plexus root avulsions.

PROCEDURE

Intradural exposure of the intended anatomic levels is accomplished, followed by microsurgical dissection of the dorsal rootlets to free them from each other. After identifying the correct anatomic levels, either by electrical stimulation or by the presence of avulsed rootlets, lesions are created on the inferolateral aspect of the rootlet entry zone. The small unmyelinated or lightly myelinated fibers that carry pain signals to the dorsal horn enter from the lateral aspect of the DREZ, whereas the medial side contains primarily those fibers destined for the dorsal columns. Lesions are created either by coagulating and opening the pia on the lateral aspect of the dorsal rootlets followed by microbipolar coagulation of the DREZ (Sindou's method) or by using a DREZ RF needle (0.25-mm diameter) to make 1 mm–spaced lesions at 75°C for 15 seconds. Laser[3] and ultrasonically[4] created lesions have also been described.

For the treatment of facial pain, the lesions may be made in the trigeminal nucleus caudalis. This is essentially a cranial continuation of the dorsal horn, extending from the brain stem down into the upper cervical spinal cord, and receives

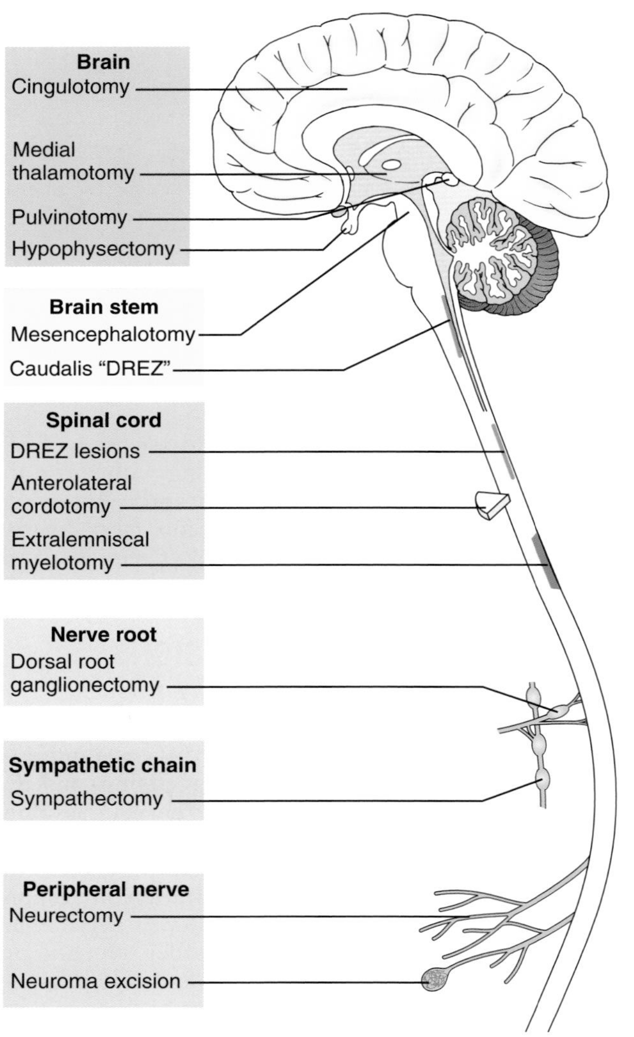

FIG. 57.1 Schematic diagram of the variety of neuroablative procedures available for the treatment of intractable pain. *DREZ,* Dorsal root entry zone.

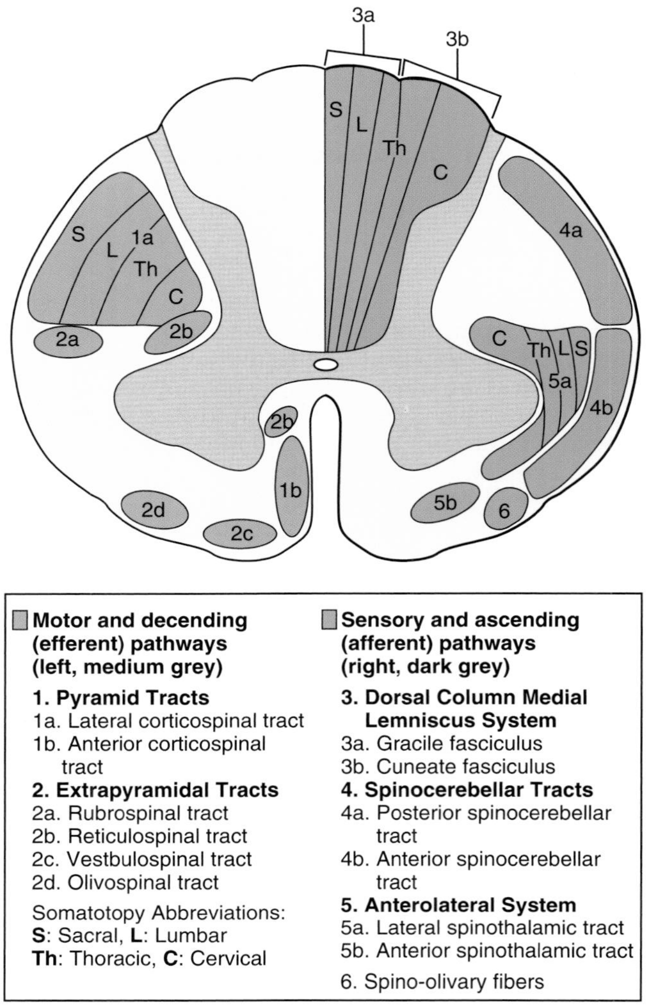

FIG. 57.2 Diagram depicting the ascending and descending tracts of the spinal cord.

much of the nociceptive signaling from the trigeminal system. As pioneered by Bernard et al.[5] these lesions are made from the upper rootlets of C2 to a point just above the obex. In the nucleus caudalis, cells receiving input from the first division are located in a more ventrolateral position, whereas cells receiving input from the third division are located in a more dorsomedial position. Moreover, the third division is represented only in the more cranial aspect of the nucleus, whereas the first division has a much broader extent.

Great care must be exercised in targeting DREZ lesions due to the presence of the corticospinal tract just laterally to the dorsal horn. Moreover, the size and angulation of the DREZ and dorsal horn vary depending on the spinal level, being much thinner in the thoracic region. Moreover, the inherently tenuous vascular supply to the spinal cord must not be disrupted. The incidence of weakness ranges from 0% to 69%.[6]

RESULTS

Larger series show reasonable rates of pain control. Dreval published results of 124 patients with brachial plexus avulsion pain followed a mean of 47.5 months after DREZ and reported an 87% rate of good pain control.[4] Most series for this indication note good pain relief in a majority of patients (usually between 50% and 80% of the cohort). The limited series of results of DREZ lesioning for phantom limb pain show less favorable outcomes (14%–67% good pain relief). This is similar for pain due to spinal cord injury and truncal postherpetic pain.[6] More recent publications[7–10] have shown successful pain reduction (even if not complete) in approximately two-thirds of patients (Table 57.1). Patients do better if the DREZ is not involved in the original injury.[11] A systematic review of the efficacy of REZ in spinal cord injury pain revealed mostly level 4 studies.[9] The DREZ was noted to be effective in segmental pain compared with diffuse pain after spinal cord injury.[9]

Initially, the caudalis DREZ procedure was plagued by a high incidence of postoperative ataxia (up to 90%) due to the location of the nucleus caudalis deep to the spinocerebellar tract. Nashold developed new angled, insulated RF needles specifically for this procedure that protected this pathway from damage during lesioning of the nucleus caudalis, reducing the ataxia complication rate down to 39%.[12] As opposed to spinal DREZ, the best indication

TABLE 57.1 Results of Recent Studies on Efficacy of Dorsal Root Entry Zone

Study	Etiology of Pain; Nature of Study	Results	Comments
Haninec et al. 2014[7]	Brachial plexus injury; retrospective; DREZ over 17 years (1995–2011); 52 patients; 3 groups based on decrease in pain scores: I (>75% decrease of pain), II (50%–75% decrease); III (<50%)	71% had >75% decrease (group I); 21% had 50%–75% (group II)	Group I patients complained of residual nociceptive pain; group II had pain of unclear origin; group III had residual neuropathic pain. Surgery was successful in 92%, unsuccessful in 8%.
Awad et al. 2013[10]	Etiology of pain different (brachial plexus avulsion, spinal cord injury pain); retrospective study; patients who had DREZ from 1986 to 2011; 19 of 101 patients contacted	Seven (37%) had complete relief; six (32%) reported good improvement; three (16%) had mild relief; three (16%) reported poor results.	More than half of patients reported good quality of life.
Ko et al. 2016[11]	Brachial plexus injury; retrospective; patients had DREZ from 1995 to 2012; 27 patients	Initial success rate of 73% which declined to 66% at median follow-up of 62.5 months.	Damage to DREZ or dorsal horn correlated with poorer outcomes. Longer duration of pain before DREZ predicted treatment success.

The study by Chivukula et al.[8] *involved nucleus caudalis and spinal DREZ and was not included. Other studies were published a lot earlier.*
DREZ, *Dorsal root entry zone.*

for caudalis DREZ is postherpetic facial pain (71% excellent to good relief in the Duke series).[13] Newer series[8] have shown approximately 50%–60% pain reduction with this procedure with approximately one-third of patients experiencing recurrence in the first year and overall less than half of patients maintaining relief over 5 years.

PERIPHERAL NEURECTOMY/ GANGLIONECTOMY

Resection of a peripheral nerve found its most significant use in the treatment of trigeminal neuralgia[14–17] and peripheral neuromas.[18,19] Although it is not often used for the former indication, it remains a mainstay of treatment for the latter.

PROCEDURE—NEURECTOMY

Avulsion of the peripheral branches of V1 (supraorbital and supratrochlear nerves) was often used in the treatment of trigeminal neuralgia in this region so as to selectively cause cutaneous anesthesia and spare the corneal anesthesia that often results from RF trigeminal gangliolysis that includes V1. This has also been applied to the V2 and V3 branches in those patients deemed inappropriate candidates for other procedures for relief of trigeminal pain.

Supraorbital neurectomy is most commonly performed via an incision through the eyebrow, whereas infraorbital neurectomy uses an approach to the maxilla via the gingivolabial margin. After the nerve is located, it is wound around a small instrument and avulsed.

RESULTS

In the series of Grantham and Segerberg[20] the average duration of pain relief from these procedures was 33.6 months. Oturai et al.[21] compared RF coagulation and neurectomy and found that only 51% of patients undergoing neurectomy were pain free postoperatively and 78% had pain recurrence, compared with a pain-free rate of 83% of the RF cohort, with only 49% pain recurrence.

Neurectomy has also been used for orbital pain,[22] thoracic pain,[23] shoulder pain,[24] and pelvic pain.[25–27] It is sometimes applied as a treatment for postoperative neuropathic pain that afflicts 5%–8% of people undergoing hernia repair.[28] Among the 26 patients with postherniorraphy pain reported by Zacest et al.,[29] 19 had significant pain improvement after ilioinguinal neurectomy, but 13 had later pain recurrence. Others[30] have also reported results that indicate that the long-term results for this procedure are not durable. Publications that do report better pain relief from this procedure are either small series[31] or more limited in their follow-up time.[32]

PROCEDURE—GANGLIONECTOMY

Ganglionectomy is intended to avoid the issue of peripheral nerve regeneration, which may follow peripheral RF ablation or avulsion. Although selecting patients who will benefit most from the procedure is still a challenge, most investigators agree that diagnostic anesthetic nerve blocks of the prospective target root should produce significant temporary pain relief.

The dorsal root ganglion contains the cell bodies of the sensory neurons whose central projections enter the dorsal horn of the spinal cord. The ganglion itself lies in the lateral aspect of the neural foramen, distal to the termination of the subarachnoid space in the nerve root sleeve. It may be exposed by resection of the lateral portion of the facet joint and inferior aspect of the lamina of the superior vertebral segment overlying the target root. Opening the root sleeve exposes the ganglion, which can be separated from the underlying ventral root and resected.

The C2 ganglion has been resected as a therapy for intractable occipital neuralgia. In this procedure the ganglion is located ventral to the copious venous plexus in between the laminae of C1 and C2. The inferior aspect of the C1 lamina must sometimes be removed to gain access to the ganglion.

RESULTS

Results from ganglionectomy have been highly variable. In Taub's[33] large series of 61 patients who underwent ganglionectomy for persistent radicular pain following lumbar surgery, 59% of patients achieved good pain relief. Strait and Hunter[34] reported that 66% of his patients who had both the L5 and S1 ganglia resected for this same indication were pain free. However, of the 37 patients in a series by Wetzel et al.[35] followed at least 2 years after ganglionectomy, only 19% of patients had durable pain relief from the procedure. North et al.[36] published even more disappointing results, with only 1 of the 13 patients reporting greater than 50% pain relief at 5.5 years postoperatively. There was little effect on medication intake and minimal functional improvement in the cohort.

Despite these issues, ganglionectomy may yet have a role to play. Young[37] and Arbit et al.[38] both published series of patients treated with ganglionectomy for cancer pain. In the latter series, 13 of 14 patients had excellent or good results following thoracic ganglion resection for malignant chest wall pain. However, the median follow-up was only 22 weeks (long 45 weeks), which may provide one explanation for the greater utility of the procedure in cancer pain.

Acar et al.[39] found that the procedure may also be useful for treatment of intractable occipital neuralgia in patients who received good temporary relief from selective C2 and C3 blocks. At final follow-up (mean, 42.5 months), 60% of patients reported either excellent or moderate pain relief. In Lozano's[40] series, 80% of patients with neuropathic occipital pain or a traumatic etiology reported an excellent or good response to the procedure. Not surprisingly, those individuals who had undergone a prior peripheral neurectomy or RF ablation procedure did not obtain additional pain relief from the procedure.

SYMPATHECTOMY

Currently the most common indication for sympathectomy is palmar hyperhidrosis. However, for many decades, interruption of the sympathetic chain has been performed for a variety of pain syndromes, such as complex regional pain syndrome (I and II) and angina pectoris, as well as painful vasospastic disorders such as syndrome X and Raynaud syndrome. Often these conditions are characterized by pain that does not conform to traditional peripheral nerve or dermatomal innervation patterns and whose intensity is out of proportion to the inciting event and/or imaging findings. Vascular and dystrophic changes often accompany the pain.

Roberts[41] proposed the term *sympathetically mediated pain* (SMP) to describe the phenomenon of pain abolition due to cessation (temporary or permanent) of sympathetic transmission. However, there is still a dearth of concrete understanding of the exact mechanisms by which the sympathetic nervous system either generates or maintains neuropathic pain syndromes despite significant research in this area.[42] In determining a patient's candidacy for sympathectomy, a determination must be made as to the relative contributions of SMP and sympathetically independent pain (SIP) to the overall level of pain. Most commonly this is determined by observing the clinical response to local anesthetic sympathetic blocks. Intravenous phentolamine (α_2—adrenergic blockade) and guanethidine Bier (intravenous regional) block, resulting in adrenergic depletion, may also be used. Sympathectomy is offered to those patients with appropriate pain syndromes who have failed other therapies and have demonstrated substantial temporary relief from these injections.

PROCEDURE

Surgical sympathectomy may be performed via several routes, depending on the region of the chain to be disrupted. Thoracic sympathectomy is most commonly performed by resecting the T2 and T3 ganglia for the treatment of upper extremity pain. This region is approached either anteriorly via a small thoracotomy or, most typically, via thoracoscopic approaches. In the thoracoscopic procedure, ports are placed after deflating the ipsilateral lung. After elevating or opening the pleura, the sympathetic chain is identified in the paramedial posterior thoracic wall. The chain is coagulated and sectioned above and below the intended ganglia, and the specimen is removed. Pneumothorax is evacuated with a small red rubber catheter or chest tube prior to closing. It is rare to leave a chest tube following a thoracoscopic sympathectomy. The chain may also be approached posteriorly, via costotransverectomies at T2 and T3. The pleura is dissected away from the underside of the rib heads and transverse processes prior to their resection. The chain is located over the pleura near the lateral vertebral body. This is clipped/coagulated and resected. A similar approach may be conducted in the lower thoracic region for relief of neuropathic visceral pain (such as chronic pancreatitis) that has responded temporarily to splanchnic blockade. For this purpose, the ganglia from T9 to T12 are resected, along with the splanchnic nerves. This most frequently is performed as a bilateral procedure.

Lumbar sympathectomy is performed for relief of pain in the lower extremities. Typically the ganglia at L2 and L3 are resected. This may be approached via an open, muscle-splitting retroperitoneal approach through a flank incision, sweeping the peritoneal sac away from the vena cava or aorta (depending on the side of symptoms). The chain is found at the junction of vertebral body and psoas muscle.

Wilkinson[43] has pioneered RF thoracic sympathectomy. This involves fluoroscopically placing RF needle electrodes at the levels of the T2 and T3 sympathetic ganglia. The ganglion is located near the dorsal half of the vertebral body near the craniocaudal midpoint of the vertebral body. Multiple lesions are created in the craniocaudal direction to ensure appropriate lesioning. Intraprocedural monitoring of limb temperature may be used to determine the procedural endpoint. A 2°C rise in temperature in the ipsilateral limb is considered significant. Complications from thoracic procedures include pneumothorax, Horner syndrome, vascular injury, and intercostal neuralgia. Lumbar sympathectomy carries the risk of ejaculation problems in men. Rarely, patients may experience "postsympathectomy neuralgia," a constant, aching pain in the proximal portion of the targeted limb. This is almost always self limited to several months.

RESULTS

Series of patients undergoing thoracic sympathectomy for pain[44–47] have reported rates of 65%–100% at achieving significant pain relief, at least initially. Success rates for lumbar sympathectomy are similar.[48,49]

Wilkinson[50] performed 37 RF sympathectomies for pain in 27 patients (3 bilateral). Eight were diagnosed with complex regional pain syndrome (CRPS) and 14 with causalgia. Useful pain relief was initially noted in 93% of targeted regions, but this declined to 69% at 1-year follow-up. In his entire series of 110 patients undergoing RF sympathectomy for a variety of indications, there were 6 symptomatic pneumothoraces. Two patients developed persistent Horner syndrome, and seven patients had transient intercostal neuralgia.

CORDOTOMY

The none-too-subtle premise of cordotomy is the interruption of the spinothalamic and spinoreticular pathways in the anterolateral quadrant of the cord carrying pain inputs to the brain from the periphery. These lesions are intended to preserve fine touch and proprioceptive tracts. Within the spinothalamic tract, the sacral fibers are located more dorsolaterally and the cervical fibers more ventromedially. Moreover, at any spinal level, axons composing the spinothalamic tract are primarily projections from cells located in the contralateral cord beginning two to three spinal segments below the specific level. Therefore a lesion should produce pain relief beginning two to three dermatomes below the level of the lesion. However, caution must be taken in lesioning the upper cervical cord, due to respiratory fibers of the reticulospinal tract lying medial to the spinothalamic tract. For this reason, bilateral upper cervical cordotomy is often not performed and patients with tenuous respiratory function are often considered unsuitable candidates. This procedure has found most utility in the treatment of refractory malignant pain. Although open cordotomy was first performed by Spiller in 1912, Mullan[51–53] pioneered the percutaneous approach, which enabled even medically fragile patients with advanced malignancies to undergo the procedure.

PROCEDURE

In the open procedure, intradural exposure is first accomplished, followed by sectioning of the dentate ligament at the appropriate level. Grasping the free end of the dentate ligament allows the surgeon to gently rotate the cord away from the operative side and expose the ventral cord. A cordotomy hook with a 45-degree angle is inserted into the anterolateral quadrant and may be taken to the medial pia before sweeping ventrally. Care is taken to not violate the medial pia and risk injury to the anterior spinal vessels.

Percutaneous cordotomy is often performed in the upper cervical (C1-2) region to treat hemibody pain. This may be done using either computed tomography (CT) or fluoroscopic guidance combined with contrast myelography.[54–56] Following dural puncture from a lateral approach, contrast is instilled into the cerebrospinal fluid (CSF), allowing identification of the dentate ligament and definition of the ventral hemicord. A stimulating/lesioning electrode is advanced through the needle, and impedance mapping is used to signal entry into the cord. Pial penetration is heralded by an increase in the impedance from approximately 300 ohms to more than 500 ohms. Patients may also report pain with this maneuver. Low-frequency electrical stimulation is used to obtain a motor threshold for approximation of the distance to corticospinal tract. High-frequency stimulation should produce contralateral sensations covering the painful region. Serial RF lesions are then created until the area of pinprick analgesia encompasses the patient's area of pain.

RESULTS

The majority of the outcomes literature regarding cordotomy deals with percutaneous procedures. A review of the efficacy of cordotomy is difficult to perform because most publications are retrospective in nature, dealt with small number of cases,[54,55] or combined it with other procedures. Sindou et al.[57] culled 2022 patients from the literature and personal experience who underwent cordotomy for malignant pain and reported a 75% success rate at 6 months and 40% at 1 year. Tasker[58] noted that he could complete the procedure with a single lesion 95.5% of the time, with 94.4% of patients achieving an adequate result, dropping to 84% at last follow-up. The most common complications are ataxia or paresis due to collateral lesioning of the nearby spinocerebellar and corticospinal tracts, respectively. This is transient in a significant percentage of patients (2.9%–100%) but permanent in a minority (1%–20%). Severe respiratory failure was noted in 0.5%–27% of patients, and some[59] have advocated an anterior transdiscal approach in the lower cervical region as a method of avoiding this complication. Modern series[60] have shown excellent immediate pain reduction with results sustained at least over several weeks. In this review of 45 patients who had different cancer diagnosis (mesothelioma, head and neck, bronchial, esophageal, colon, pelvic, rectal) and underwent cordotomy, significant reduction of pain was noted at 2 days (median score: 0, interquartile range [IR]: 0–5) and 28 days (median score: 0, IR: 0–3.3) after the procedure.[60] Adverse events included headache, dysesthesia, motor weakness, and increase in pain, but no serious events were noted.

Cordotomy has also been used in combination with other palliative pain procedures, such as intrathecal neuromodulation.[61] Unfortunately, one particularly devastating complication is the late onset of new pain following cordotomy. Of Nagaro's[62] series of 45 patients who underwent cordotomy, 33 experienced this problem. In 28 patients the new pain was in the mirror-image location of the original pain and could often be abolished by blockade of the nerves subserving the original pain. However, this pain is not always simple to treat.[63] This issue has been reported as affecting 1%–16% of patients in various series. Bowsher[64] suggested that this was due to destruction of pathways providing unilateral inhibition of nociceptive cells with naturally bilateral receptive fields.

Regarding surgical cordotomy, Cowie's[65] report of 56 patients listed a 95% immediate pain-free result, which diminished to 55% at 1-year follow-up. For patients with nonmalignant pain, the success rate was 85% initially, but only 35% at 1 year and 20% at 3 years. Two patients died from respiratory failure. More recent series[66] of open thoracic cordotomy highlight the sometimes problematic nature of the procedure, with new pain, leg weakness, and urinary problems all complicating the outcome.

COMMISSURAL MYELOTOMY

Commissural myelotomy involves severing the fibers of the spinothalamic tract where they cross the spinal cord in the anterior commissure. It is expected that interrupting the flow of nociceptive information in this fashion will produce analgesia at the spinal level of the myelotomy and just below. However, more extensive areas of pain relief are often noted following this procedure. It has been frequently noted that the pattern of postmeylotomy pain relief cannot be predicted on the basis of the traditional maps of the spinal tracts. The exact mechanism behind this phenomenon is not known but likely involves the existence of extralemniscal nociceptive pathways. Given that myelotomy does produce some damage to the dorsal columns, even in the most talented of hands, and that the dorsal columns already carry multimodality sensory information, this procedure may destroy collateral pathways.[67–69] Myelotomy is considered primarily for patients with intractable pain in the lower body and pelvis.

PROCEDURE

The spinal cord is exposed over the spinal neural level (rather than the bony spinal segment) corresponding to the pain. A small probe is inserted just lateral to the fibrous septum in the dorsal midline between the posterior columns. Traditionally, this is then used to carefully section the midline crossing fibers until the anterior cleft of the cord is noted, taking care not to injure the ventrally located anterior spinal artery and other epidural veins. For lower body and pelvic pain, the cord is often exposed via a T9 laminectomy.

Nauta and others[70] have reduced the exposure and depth of dissection required for this procedure. In their technique, which may be performed either openly or stereotactically,[71] a single punctate lesion is made in the dorsal midline of the cord. Given the theory that pain relief from this procedure is due to the lesioning of a dorsal column nociceptive pathway, some surgeons[72] perform bilateral lesions of the paramedian dorsal columns without sectioning of the deeper midline crossing fibers.

RESULTS

Given that the patient population considered eligible for this procedure is rather small (and smaller still in the era of neurostimulation), extant series are all rather small. Most patients are suffering from intractable malignant pain and have a limited life expectancy following the procedure. In Hirshberg's[69] series of eight patients, survival ranged from 3 to 11 months following myelotomy and all had significant pain relief up until death. One patient experienced new leg weakness following the procedure. Nauta's group[70] of six patients who underwent punctate midline myelotomy had similar results. However, in Kim's[73] cohort of eight patients undergoing high thoracic myelotomy for visceral pain from gastric cancer, three developed new pain at other sites (with relief of the preoperative pain) and one developed proprioceptive deficits and paresthesias. A review of 11 patients treated with midline myelotomy at MD Anderson Cancer Center[74] revealed that most patients had good pain reduction but complications such as weakness and urinary retention were not uncommon. Across the published series, the outcomes from punctate and traditional techniques do not differ much.

INTRACEREBRAL LESIONS

Moving the site of lesioning cranially is often intended to accomplish one of several well-defined goals: capture pain involving the face, head, and neck that cannot be treated with spinal ablative lesions, treat a wider area of the body, treat the affective nature of pain, or reduce hormonal drivers of malignancy.

MIDBRAIN TRACTOTOMY

First performed in 1938 by Dogliotti and then reported in 1942 by Walker, sectioning of the spinothalamic tract in the midbrain is intended to produce hemibody analgesia in patients with intractable pain that involves the head and neck.[75] Unfortunately its utility has been severely hampered by disturbing postoperative dysesthesias and other complications, such as auditory disturbances due to the approach through the colliculus. Moreover, the technical difficulty of the exposure was also a hindrance. Wycis and Spiegel described a stereotactic, rather than open, technique for the procedure.[76] This and other series[77,78] report more than 150 patients undergoing the procedure. Pain relief was highly variable and complications plentiful. The most common complications were dysesthesias (15%–40%), gaze palsy, and hemiparesis. Attempts to minimize complications and improve pain relief included moving the lesion more cranially to avoid the auditory and visual problems inherent in lesioning the brain stem near the colliculi. Colombo[79] noted that the disturbing dysesthesias are often associated with abolition of the somatosensory evoked potential (SSEP) signals, indicating unintended lesioning of the medial lemniscal fibers in addition to the spinothalamic fibers. Intraoperative stimulation may help to identify the spinothalamic fibers from the lemniscal fibers by the painful sensations evoked by stimulating the former and the more vibratory or pleasant sensations from stimulating the latter tract. Lesioning includes not only the spinothalamic tract proper but often also a second lesion just medial to the first that includes the periaqueductal gray matter.

THALAMOTOMY

The thalamus serves as the main deep relay nucleus for most motor and sensory functions. Several thalamic nuclei have been targeted, either singly or in isolation, to achieve pain control, including the medial/intralaminar thalamus, ventroacudal (Vc) nucleus, and pulvinar. Cells in the Vc nucleus subserving anesthetic body regions have a higher likelihood of exhibiting an abnormal bursting firing pattern as compared to those Vc cells subserving areas of normal sensation.[80] In the medial thalamus, the central lateral (CL) and centromedian/parafascicular (CM/Pf) complex are most commonly lesioned due to their large input from the spinothalamic tract and diffuse cortical projection.[42] These nuclei are more difficult to identify due to the lack of specific somatotopic physiologic responses evoked with intraoperative stimulation, unlike what is observed when targeting the Vc nucleus. Of 913 patients undergoing medial thalamotomy for pain reported in the literature, 73% had some initial pain relief with a recurrence rate of approximately 25%. Lesioning other nuclei in addition to the medial thalamus did not appear to increase the chance of clinical success.[81] Stimulation of the Vc thalamus produces a paresthetic sensation akin to that of spinal cord stimulation. This is frequently evoked as part of the mediolateral targeting process during surgery to implant thalamic stimulating electrodes in the ventral intermediate (Vim) nucleus for tremor control. Several groups have reported that stimulation of the CM and Pf nuclei may be associated with unpleasant and even painful sensations.[82]

Lesioning the medial thalamic complex (CL or CM/Pf) does not produce sensory deficits. The largest series have been published by Jeanmonod et al.[83] Their initial paper described 69 patients who underwent CL thalamotomy. Two-thirds of these patients achieved at least 50% pain relief. This group later expanded the series to 85 patients, 52% of whom experienced greater than 50% pain relief with a mean follow-up of 3 years.[81] One-third of patients had no pain relief. Interestingly, patients with only constant pain (without superimposed paroxysms) were more likely to fail the procedure. Young et al.[84] performed radiosurgical medial thalamotomy for intractable pain in 19 patients (24 lesions). After a mean of 12 months, four patients were pain free and five others had greater than 50% pain relief. However, in both the series of Urabe and Tsubokawa,[85] as well as that of Sugita et al.[86] approximately 15% of patients had significant postoperative confusion.

Mark et al.[87,88] reported results of Vc thalamotomy in 28 patients. Eighteen obtained good pain relief. They defined several patterns of postoperative neurologic changes. Those patients with "VPL sensory syndrome" exhibited significant hypesthesia but little pain relief. Those with intralaminar or Pf nucleus syndrome had good pain relief without significant sensory changes. Tasker[89] reviewed the literature on Vc thalamotomy for pain and noted significant complications in 32% of patients and only a similar percentage with good pain relief. Postoperative dysesthesias were common. He stated that lesioning this target is not very useful for eliminating burning pain and recommended a trial of neurostimulation in this region rather than lesioning.

Lesions in the pulvinar, located posterior to the CM/Pf complex, have also been created for the treatment of intractable pain. These lesions produce pain relief in a minority of patients and appear to be better for relief of oncologic pain and less so for those with neuropathic pain of nonmalignant origin. As has been noted with other ablative procedures for pain, the clinical benefit tends to substantially fade with time.[90]

HYPOPHYSECTOMY

This procedure was a logical extension of the work by Huggins[91] and others that demonstrated that hormonal deprivation slowed the growth of prostate and breast cancers. Luft and Olivecrona's series[92] of 12 patients was the first demonstration of the utility of pituitary ablation for control of prostate and breast cancer, with relief of severe pain in one patient. Thompson et al.[93] reported results of 47 patients undergoing the procedure for prostate cancer. Interestingly, 60% had significant initial pain relief, whereas only 14% had oncologic control. However, only 16% maintained this pain relief at 1 year postoperatively. Among the 203 breast cancer patients undergoing hypophysectomy in Fracchia's series,[94] 90% had initial pain relief and 101 were still alive and pain free 1 year later. Other series[95] show similar dramatic initial results that often are lost as the cancer progresses. No significant series of the use of this technique for pain have been published in more than 20 years.

The pituitary gland may be ablated via either a standard craniotomy or a less invasive transphenoidal approach. The gland is destroyed either via direct resection, instillation of alcohol into the sella, RF, cryotherapy, or interstitial brachytherapy. Stereotactic radiosurgery may also be considered, but the variable time to onset of clinical effect with this technique may limit its utility in patients with a limited life expectancy and urgent problems. The complications of the panhypopituitarism produced by this technique are not surprising.

CINGULOTOMY

Lesions of the anterior cingulate gyrus target the affective components of pain, rather than the pain transmission itself. Freeman and Watts[96] anecdotally noted that some patients undergoing prefrontal lobotomy for psychiatric indications also experienced significant pain relief. Autopsy studies revealed involvement of the cingulate gyrus. The procedure typically involves bilateral stereotactically placed RF or radiosurgical lesions in the bilateral anterior cingulate gyrus. Foltz and White[97] published the first series of 12 patients undergoing stereotactic (as opposed to open) cingulatomy for pain. Of the 16 patients reported, 4 of 11 with bilateral lesions had an excellent result and 5 of 11 had a fair result. Most reported series are retrospective analyses of small cohorts.[98–104] The largest series is that of Ballantine et al.[105] who reported results on 133 patients undergoing cingulotomy for pain relief. Pain relief was initially obtained by 20 of the 35 patients with malignant pain, but this waned significantly over several months. However, 62% of patients with failed back surgery syndrome obtained significant durable pain relief. Grouping together multiple series, the procedure shows a modest benefit, with slight majorities of patients with malignant (52%) and benign (53%) etiologies obtaining useful pain relief.[106]

CONCLUSION

Although not commonly used, certain ablative neurosurgical techniques continue to have a role in the management of medically intractable pain. Moreover, they all have a role to play in our understanding of the pathophysiology behind the generation and maintenance of chronic pain states. With the rise in neurostimulation as a treatment of many types of neuropathic pain, there is significant concern that some of these valuable treatments will be lost forever. Neurosurgeons and other physicians who treat chronic pain must continue to be educated in these procedures to ensure that they continue to be available for carefully selected patient populations.

KEY POINTS

- Ablative techniques have been used for decades to control intractable pain. Although they continue to have some well-defined indications, they have largely been replaced with neurostimulation procedures.
- The results of ablative procedures for pain relief tend to be highly variable, with a substantial proportion of patients obtaining relief early and then experiencing recurrence of pain.
- Spinal DREZ lesions may be useful in treating neuropathic pain due to brachial plexus root avulsion, if a trial of neurostimulation has failed.
- Ablative procedures such as cordotomy may be useful in treating pain of malignant origin, given the limited life expectancy of these patients.
- Review of the efficacy of neurosurgical ablative procedures is hampered by the lack of recent publications, retrospective nature of studies, and small number of patients.
- The physiology underlying the development and maintenance of neuropathic pain and the mechanism of action/loss of effect of ablative neurosurgical procedure for pain remain to be fully elucidated.

REFERENCES

Access the reference list online at ExpertConsult.com.

CHAPTER 58

PHYSICAL MEDICINE AND REHABILITATION APPROACHES TO PAIN MANAGEMENT

Paul Scholten, MD ◎ Steven P. Stanos, DO ◎ W. Evan Rivers, DO ◎ Heidi Prather, DO ◎ Joel Press, MD

Physical medicine and rehabilitation practitioners use a comprehensive approach to assess and manage acute and chronic pain conditions. The treatment they provide is guided by understanding and then optimizing each patient's functional ability.[1] The philosophic framework in which this is conceptualized for physiatrists throughout their training is the World Health Organization's International Classification of Functioning, Disability and Health (Table 58.1).[2] The goal is to identify and then treat impairments such as weakness or restricted range of motion as well as related psychosocial factors—all of which contribute to activity limitations and participation restrictions in an effort to optimize performance. Therapeutic programs often include medication and exercise for flexibility, strength, and fitness and may use injections, interventional treatments, and cognitive and behavioral treatments. Passive modalities are utilized typically only as an adjunct to these strategies. Treatment programs for acute pain focus on addressing the underlying cause(s) of pain, which can often be accurately determined through a thorough clinical physical examination[3] using temporary relative rest if indicated, and education for stretching, strengthening, fitness, and proper biomechanics. Programs for chronic pain also include active treatments and exercise regimens but often require behavioral and psychologic interventions; direct treatment of a single "pain generator" itself is rarely effective. Physical medicine approaches often include the various techniques and methods provided by physical therapy.[1] Physical therapy includes therapeutic exercise, functional training in home and work activities, manual therapy, prescription and application of assistive devices, and passive modalities. The goals of chronic pain treatment programs vary considerably between patients, but the cornerstones are improving the patient's psychosocial factors (i.e., reducing anxiety, depression, catastrophizing, improving coping, and self-efficacy); returning the patient to the most optimal level of leisure, sport, or work function; and acceptable analgesia.

The purpose of this chapter is to briefly review commonly used physical modalities and therapeutic exercise, discuss the basics of a rehabilitation program for pain, and to introduce the concept of comprehensive interdisciplinary pain management.

OVERVIEW OF MODALITIES

Modalities are methods used by therapists to exchange energy with tissues with the goal of creating a therapeutic response. Passive modalities may include the application of heat, cold, sound waves, electricity, and electromagnetic waves to effect changes in tissue structures such as muscle, fascia, ligament, tendon, capsule, and nerve. Modalities comprise adjunctive treatments included as part of a rehabilitation program; they are rarely used in isolation. Modalities are most useful in treating acute pain where the specific underlying musculoskeletal abnormalities can be matched with an appropriate intervention. For most patients, the long-term use of modalities is discouraged, since they may reinforce passive coping behavior, and strong evidence for their lasting effectiveness in chronic conditions is lacking.

HEAT AND COLD

Therapeutic heat transfer occurs by one or a combination of mechanisms: radiation, conduction, convection, conversion, and evaporation. *Radiation* is the transfer of heat through thermal radiation at the surface. *Conduction* is heat exchange through direct contact. *Convection* is characterized by transfer of thermal energy through movement in a fluid medium, although the therapeutic energy exchange still occurs through conduction. *Conversion* occurs when a different type of energy is converted to heat energy. *Evaporation* results in loss of heat when a liquid on a surface undergoes a phase transition into a gas. These mechanisms may be used alone or in combination to transfer heat to or from tissues, resulting in physiologic changes. Of these

TABLE 58.1 World Health Organization Definitions

Term	Definition	Example
Impairment	Any loss or abnormality of body structure or of a physiologic or psychologic function.	Right dorsiflexion weakness due to an L5 radiculopathy.
Activity	The nature and extent of functioning at the level of the person.	The person has difficulty ambulating and clearing his or her right foot.
Participation	The nature and extent of a person's involvement in life situations in relation to impairments, activities, health conditions, and contextual factors.	The person is unable to play sports or perform activities of daily living owing to restriction of ambulation caused by an impairment in ankle dorsiflexion.

mechanisms, only conversion can be used to transfer heat to structures deeper than several centimeters beneath the surface. Remaining mechanisms are able to provide only superficial exchange of thermal energy.

The application of heat causes improved elasticity of soft tissue as well as increased blood flow, metabolic activity, enzymatic activity, oxygen demand, and capillary permeability.[4] Nerve conduction velocity increases with the application of heat. The heated tissues become suppler, and there are increases in healing cells and nutrients and decreases in metabolic waste. However, heat can also increase edema and bleeding. There is some evidence from animal models that heat improves chronic inflammatory conditions but may aggravate acute inflammation. The target temperature for these modalities is generally accepted to be 40°C–45°C, and the thermal pain threshold is normally about 45°C. Using the patient's pain response to a modality can prevent excessive or even damaging temperatures, as long as the sensorium is intact. Box 58.1 summarizes the indications for heat modalities used for musculoskeletal pain management. Box 58.2 lists general contraindications and precautions for the use of therapeutic heat.

BOX 58.1 Indications for Therapeutic Heat

Muscle spasm
Pain
Contracture
Hematoma resolution
Hyperemia
Increase collagen extensibility
Accelerate metabolic processes

BOX 58.2 Contraindications to Therapeutic Heat

Acute inflammation
Hemorrhage or bleeding disorders
Decreased sensation
Poor thermal regulation
Malignancy
Edema
Peripheral vascular disease
Ischemia
Atrophic skin or scarred skin
Inability to respond to pain

Superficial heat causes the greatest increase in temperature at the surface of the skin, with less heat penetrating to the deep tissues—about 1°C at a depth of 2–3 cm.[4,5] Heat is often applied using hydrocollator packs, a variety of fluid baths, and infrared lamps. Hydrocollator packs are heated to 74.5°C. Several layers of towels are used to prevent burning of the skin and minimize loss of heat to the air. Although heat therapy is often used as an adjunct to rehabilitation programs, the evidence for its effectiveness is mixed and appears to depend on the specific condition being treated, the chronicity of symptoms, and the outcome measure being evaluated. When evidence from three randomized controlled trials involving 179 patients with knee osteoarthritis was reviewed systematically, it was determined that hot packs had no effect on edema compared with placebo or cold application.[6] In looking at the use of heat before isokinetic exercises among women with knee osteoarthritis, heat was found to lead to improved exercise performance, reduced pain, and improved function.[7] When used for low back pain a Cochrane review determined that there is moderate evidence that continuous heat wrap therapy reduces pain and disability in the short term, in a mixed population with acute and subacute low back pain (up to 3 months), and that the addition of exercise to heat wrap therapy further reduces pain and improves function.[8] Immersion of body parts in water of around 40°C is another way of applying superficial heat, which allows for therapy to take place during heating. Paraffin baths are typically used for peripheral limbs, especially the hands and arms. Temperatures around 53°C are used because paraffin transfers less heat than water does. Most commonly this modality is used for rheumatoid arthritis, and while the evidence is insufficient to draw definitive conclusions regarding its efficacy, a recent systematic review did find that it safely relieves pain and stiffness immediately after its application; when followed by exercise it can significantly improve hand function.[9] Superficial heat leads to mild analgesia and a sense of relaxation, but the mechanisms remain unclear and systematic reviews suggest that further well-designed studies are needed to draw definitive conclusions about its effectiveness in the treatment of painful musculoskeletal conditions.

Ultrasound waves, shortwaves, and microwaves can safely penetrate deep into tissues before the energy they carry is converted to thermal energy. Ultrasound diathermy (as distinguished from diagnostic ultrasound) is the only method commonly used at this time. It can easily heat the bone-muscle interface up to 45°C, even in deep structures such as the hip.[4] Ultrasound generators convert electrical energy into vibratory energy through the piezoelectric properties of a crystal transducer. When ultrasound vibrations are directed into tissue, they generate heat based on the water and protein content of the tissue and in areas of transition between tissue densities, such as at the interface between bone and muscle. Tissues that heat poorly due to high water concentration are fat and skin, and tissues that heat well due to high protein concentration are ligament, tendon, muscle, bone, and nerve, with bone and nerve heating the most. Ultrasound is safe for use near metal implants because the heat energy is rapidly conducted away, but caution must be used near prosthetic cements, which do not release heat as easily. Ultrasound may also cause gaseous cavitation and acoustic streaming effects that do not transmit thermal energy but may increase tissue pressures and cellular metabolism and disrupt cell membranes. Duration of treatment is 5–10 minutes and is based on the size of the treatment area. Although ultrasound diathermy has superior deep-heating capability, it does not produce the same degree of analgesia or relaxation as superficial heat modalities. Box 58.3 lists some common uses and Box 58.4 lists precautions for ultrasound.

Despite a long history of clinical use, the evidence for the effectiveness of ultrasound diathermy in the treatment of musculoskeletal disorders is largely lacking. A systematic review of five small trials totaling 341 patients with

BOX 58.3 Common Uses for Therapeutic Ultrasound

Contractures
Tendonitis
Degenerative arthritis
Subacute trauma

BOX 58.4 Precautions for Ultrasound

Malignancy
Open epiphysis
Pacemaker
Laminectomy site
Radiculopathy
Near brain, eyes, or reproductive organs
Pregnant or menstruating uterus
Heat precautions in general
Caution around arthroplasties, methyl methacrylate, or high-density polyethylene

BOX 58.5 Indications for Cryotherapy

Acute trauma
Edema
Hemorrhage
Pain
Muscle spasm
Spasticity
Reduction of metabolic activity

BOX 58.6 Precautions and Contraindications to Cryotherapy

Ischemia
Raynaud disease or phenomenon
Cold intolerance
Insensitivity
Inability to report pain

knee osteoarthritis evaluating a mixture of pulsed and continuous ultrasound found that treatment with this modality compared with control decreased pain by 1.2 cm on a 10-cm visual analog scale and also positively affects function without causing any adverse events. However, the poor quality and heterogeneity among the included studies suggest that further investigations are needed to draw more definitive conclusions.[10] When evaluated in the treatment of soft tissue complaints such as lateral epicondylitis, shoulder pain, degenerative rheumatic disorders, ankle distortions, temporomandibular pain, or myofascial pain, most studies do not support clinical or statistical differences in favor of ultrasound therapy.[11,12] When studied specifically in the treatment of myofascial trigger points, the evidence is mixed, with one study demonstrating that low-dose ultrasound evokes short-term segmental antinociceptive effects[13] and others suggesting that ultrasound provides no reduction in pain in this population.[14]

The application of cold through conduction, convection, or evaporation results in loss of heat from tissues, leading to vasoconstriction followed by vasodilation, decreased local metabolic activity, decreased enzymatic activity, and decreased oxygen demand. Tissues and muscles become stiffer, nerve conduction slows, and the activity of muscle spindles and Golgi tendon organs decreases.[4] Muscle isometric strength increases and the rate of muscle fatigue decreases.[4] Cold also results in analgesia and relaxation. Boxes 58.5 and 58.6 summarize general indications and contraindications for cryotherapy.

Cold is often used during the first 48 hours after an acute musculoskeletal injury to decrease inflammation, edema, and pain. The application of cold should not exceed 30 minutes and should not be placed directly over superficial nerves so as to prevent neurapraxia. Cold is normally applied in ice packs at −12°C with towels layered over the pack to protect the skin. As with the application of superficial heat, the surface of the skin is affected first and most, but after 20 minutes, tissues 2 cm deep are cooled by about 5°C.[4] Although the local application of cold is known to decrease the temperature of the skin as well as superficial and deeper tissues,[5] the evidence to support its use is not strong.[8] A systematic review of cryotherapy in the treatment of acute soft tissue injuries found marginal evidence that ice in addition to exercise is most effective after ankle sprain and postoperatively, with few studies assessing the effectiveness of ice on closed soft tissue injuries.[15] In patients with osteoarthritis, ice massage improved range of motion, function, and knee strength but did not significantly impact pain.[6] Immersion in cold water (5°C–13°C) can be used but is generally poorly tolerated, although muscle temperatures can decrease by about 6°C after 30 minutes of immersion.[4] Vapocoolant spray is used for cutaneous anesthesia and is used by some practitioners in conjunction with passive stretching to treat myofascial pain. Evaporation of the spray induces cutaneous cooling, with postulated cutaneosomatic reflex effects at the level of the muscle spindle.

Cold and heat can be used together in contrast baths, with alternating warm and cold immersion, to cause cyclic vasodilation and vasoconstriction, with beneficial effects hypothesized for pain from rheumatologic and neuropathic conditions.

Thermal modalities should be used in conjunction with exercises for motion and flexibility. The long-term effects of most of these treatments on functional outcomes and range of motion are minimal when used alone.[4,16]

ELECTRICITY

Iontophoresis is the process by which various drugs (i.e., corticosteroids, lidocaine) are introduced into a joint or around periligamentous or tendinous structures via electrical current. Iontophoresis uses electromigration and electroosmosis to increase permeation of charged and neutral compounds. The medicine is applied to the electrode with the same charge, and then the electrical field is set up on the skin surface to push the medicine away from the electrode and toward the target tissue. Topical delivery minimizes systemic side effects and bypasses hepatic metabolism.[4] Iontophoresis is noninvasive and painless and avoids potential side effects and adverse reactions of oral medications or injection therapies (i.e., increasing risk for bleeding, intravenous catheter infiltration, and pump malfunction). Penetration may be particularly intense at sweat glands and areas of skin breakdown. Iontophoresis is commonly used with overuse and chronic conditions such as rheumatoid arthritis, various tendinopathies, and plantar fasciitis.[17,18] When used to deliver steroid treatment to patients under the age of 45 with shoulder tendinopathy, subjects' self-reports of pain improved after treatment, with none of the subjects in the placebo group reporting any benefit.[19] Positive effects in terms of pain reduction using this method to deliver localized doses of steroids have also been found in the treatment of acute Achilles tendon pain[20] and rheumatoid arthritis of the knee.[21]

Electrical fields are also used in transcutaneous electrical nerve stimulation (TENS) to directly affect pain transmission. Suggested mechanisms of pain relief include modulation of the gating mechanisms at the dorsal horn system to decrease pain transmission to the brain and stimulation of endogenous neurotransmitters and opioids. Cutaneous nerve fibers are stimulated using surface electrodes emitting a mild electrical current. The stimulation can vary by type of current, amplitude, pulse width, and frequency. Duration of the treatment and length of each treatment can vary widely, with some protocols calling for continuous treatment. High-frequency, low-intensity stimulation patterns are better tolerated and result in immediate analgesia, whereas low-frequency, high-intensity patterns cause more discomfort and result in longer-lasting analgesia. Despite common clinical usage, a systematic review of five trials with 170 subjects receiving sham-TENS and 251 subjects receiving active TENS found no evidence to support the use of TENS in the treatment of chronic low back pain.[22] Interferential current therapy (ICT) uses electrical current, like TENS, but combines two different high-frequency pulses, so that their interference pattern creates a low-frequency stimulation. The high-frequency stimulation penetrates skin better than low-frequency stimulation, but the treatment results in the longer-lasting effects of low-frequency stimulation.[4,23]

OVERVIEW OF A COMPREHENSIVE REHABILITATION PROGRAM

An individualized therapeutic program aims to correct soft tissue inflexibilities and improve muscle strength deficits and imbalances, endurance, and power to the appropriate muscle groups with the cumulative goal of optimizing performance. Consideration is given to the joints above and below the injured area that are linked together and are referred to as *the kinetic chain*. The program should also include patient education about posture, body mechanics, and proprioception. A patient's return to activity should be monitored in a supervised setting, so that any residual problems can be addressed.

A comprehensive rehabilitation program consists of acute, recovery, and maintenance phases (Table 58.2). During the acute phase, education about how to protect the injured tissue is important. A review of proper body mechanics and activities of daily living should be completed. Relative rest is important, because excessive immobilization results in decreased muscle strength, endurance, and flexibility. Modalities can be used judiciously for symptom control and reduction in swelling. Medications may be used to facilitate the rehabilitation program by decreasing pain and inflammation. Manual therapy techniques may help modify pain by assisting in early controlled motion of the injured tissue. Mechanoreceptor activation can assist in modifying muscle tone and pain. Therapeutic exercise should begin during the acute phase. Once acute inflammation and pain have been addressed, the program focuses on the subacute or recovery phase. Goals of this phase include achievement of full or optimal range of motion with limited or no pain and regaining appropriate strength, balance, and proprioception. Manual techniques should focus on improving soft tissue extensibility that helps promote proper alignment of collagen fibers during healing and remodeling. These techniques may include massage, fascial stretching, traction, and joint mobilization. Myofascial release improves elasticity and motion by applying pressure in shear forces directed by fascial planes and assists with pain control. Mobilization is also used to facilitate motion at specific joints or joint segments. These techniques may facilitate a patient's progress but again should not be relied upon solely because protracted passive treatment places the patient in a dependent role.

TABLE 58.2 Comprehensive Rehabilitation Program

Phases	Therapy Focus
Acute	Education, relative rest, pain control
Recovery	Full or optimal range of motion, strength, balance, proprioception
Maintenance	Return to work- and sport-specific activity, aerobic conditioning

A flexibility program is devised to achieve proper balance and allow the patient to achieve a neutral position, improving posture and reducing pain. While maintaining the posture, exercises progress from static to dynamic. Challenges to the neutral posture are thereafter incorporated by gravity and then by a therapist or assistive device. Activity-specific retraining is initiated first by breaking the motion into components. Training for each component is completed before reassembling the entire motion. Cardiovascular training should be maintained, adapting the method to the specific injury. Aquatic training should be considered if a nonweight-bearing activity is necessary.

The final or maintenance phase is devised as the patient returns to the work- or sport-specific activity to promote continued fitness as well as to prevent reinjury. Education about ergonomics and equipment or adaptive devices should be complete. The patient should be able to perform a home exercise program independently and know how to solve problems that may occur during this last stage of recovery.

THERAPEUTIC EXERCISE

There are three main types of therapeutic exercise: those that improve (1) flexibility, (2) muscle strength, and (3) aerobic capacity. A rehabilitation program to manage musculoskeletal pain and dysfunction will address all three. Education about proper biomechanics and ergonomics customized to specific work or sport activities will also be an important part of the individualized rehabilitation program.

In implementing an exercise program, the specific adaptation to imposed demand (SAID) principle should be applied. This principle states that the body responds to given demands with specific and predictable adaptations. Stronger muscles develop with strength training. Oxidative capacities of skeletal muscles increase with aerobic training. Pliability of connective tissue increases with flexibility exercises.

FLEXIBILITY EXERCISES

Maintaining or regaining muscle flexibility and range of motion is an important part of a rehabilitation program. Connective tissue stretches with a small amount of force and returns to its original length when the force is removed. When the muscle fibers are straightened, more force is required to apply a stretch. Furthermore, if connective tissues are stretched to a certain length and maintained, the tension within the tissue decreases. For best results, stretching should be maintained for 30 seconds with the patient perceiving a pulling sensation rather than pain. Warming an area before stretching improves the elongation of the collagen fibers. Rapid or bouncing stretches promote tissue recoil and a sustained stretch is not achieved. The risk of excessive loading and injury also occurs with bouncing. If too much force is applied with stretching, the patient will experience muscle soreness for more than 24 hours. Joint laxity may result from excessive stretching during healing of tendons and ligaments. With adherence to an appropriately applied stretching program, flexibility should improve within 1–2 months.

STRENGTH TRAINING

Muscle strengthening is a well-accepted part of any rehabilitation program. The practitioner must have a complete understanding of functional anatomy so that the appropriate balance between agonist and antagonist muscle groups is achieved. The amount of resistance to be applied is determined by the muscle's capability and should be assessed for each individual. Improvements in strength observed during the first 2 weeks of resistance training are related to neuromuscular reeducation and more efficient recruitment of muscles. Later gains are due to hypertrophy of muscle fibers and result in increased cross-sectional area. Training is most effective when exercises focus on different muscle groups in rotating sessions. Initially, one to three sets of 8–12 repetitions 3 to 5 times a week is recommended. Resistance should not be increased by more than 10% per week. If progress is not made, the practitioner should evaluate the technique and training intensity and also consider neurogenic weakness.

AEROBIC FITNESS

A therapeutic rehabilitation plan should also include initiating or reestablishing cardiovascular fitness. If the injury or dysfunction prohibits weight bearing, a nonweight-bearing aerobic activity needs to be implemented. To improve aerobic capacity, the oxidative metabolism of the muscle must be stressed. Oxygen consumption (VO_2) increases in proportion to the intensity of the exercise. VO_2 max, the highest level of VO_2 achieved during exercise, is the best indicator of aerobic fitness. Intensity of exercise is the difficulty level of the exercise and is usually used in reference to maximal effort. This is typically at 40%–85% of VO_2 max for aerobic training. The duration for aerobic training is usually greater than 15 minutes of continuous exercise. Frequency of aerobic training is usually 3 to 6 times a week. In prescribing an exercise program, remember that if the activity level is reduced beyond 1 week, aerobic conditioning decreases. Intensity, duration, and frequency parameters must be adjusted in the deconditioned patient. Increases of 10%–20% of VO_2 max can be noted within 8–12 weeks of training. If improvements are not observed, there may be inadequate frequency, intensity, or duration of training.

A wide range of musculoskeletal conditions are amenable to treatment with therapeutic exercise. Some of the most commonly targeted and best-studied conditions (excluding back pain) are osteoarthritis and tendinopathies such as those of the rotator cuff or Achilles tendon. There is high-quality evidence from 23 systematic reviews examining the effectiveness of physical therapy for patients with knee osteoarthritis that exercise and weight reduction reduce pain and improve physical function in this population.[24] When the literature for the treatment of rotator cuff impingement was reviewed, it was found that exercise is effective in reducing pain and improving function and that home exercise programs may be as effective as supervised exercise; yet manual therapy provided by therapists may augment the positive effects.[25] In a systematic review and meta-analysis of 19 studies for the treatment of Achilles tendinopathy, it was found that eccentric exercise should be considered as an initial intervention but that high-quality randomized controlled studies are needed to adequately study outcomes and determine optimal clinical pathways in this population of patients.[26]

TREATMENT INTERVENTIONS SPECIFIC TO SPINE-RELATED CONDITIONS

Treatment approaches for spine-related conditions include stabilization exercises, mechanical diagnosis and treatment (MDT), neurodynamic therapy, and various manual therapy and soft tissue approaches as well as activity and therapeutic exercise as already described. Stabilization exercise training is the most common technique used and emphasizes not only strengthening muscles but also motor relearning of inhibited muscles. Patients are advanced from training in isometric and eccentric strengthening of core muscle groups to include Swiss ball and other dynamic multiplanar exercises and finally gradual return to work- and sport-specific activities. Stabilization exercises reduce the recurrence of low back pain from spondylolysis and spondylolisthesis.[27] Stabilization exercises prevent recurrence and improve pain and function of nonspecific chronic low back pain but do not reduce pain or disability in acute low back pain.[28,29]

Continuation of normal activity seems to be the best approach for acute low back pain.[30] Exercise programs provided after the resolution of acute low back pain can help return patients to normal daily activities and work[31] and reduce the recurrence rate and lengthen the time to recurrence.[32]

More specific exercise programs based on mechanical assessment may add more specificity to the exercise treatment program. MDT or McKenzie therapy is based on diagnosis and treatment directed by a therapist where pain is relieved or changed in pattern with repeated movement, that is, centralizing symptoms—symptoms in distal extremity (arm or leg) moving to a more proximal area along the spine. Most, but not all, patients who "centralize" do so with extension-based movements; others may respond to side bending or flexion of the spine. This treatment approach may be more appropriate for acute discogenic-related pain conditions.[33] Neurodynamic therapy is based on the premise that irritated nerve structures or chronic tension on cervical, lumbar, or peripheral nerves cause ongoing pain and dysfunction. Therapy focuses on decreasing tension on the neural structures by decreasing tension in the perineural tissues (i.e., soft tissue, muscle) and decreasing pain. When data from randomized controlled trials is pooled and reviewed systematically, McKenzie therapy for low back pain has been shown to result in greater decreases in pain and disability in the short term as compared with other standard therapies such as nonsteroidal antiinflammatory drugs (NSAIDs), patient education, and massage.[34]

INTERDISCIPLINARY COMPREHENSIVE PAIN MANAGEMENT

Patients failing to progress in the acute, subacute, and maintenance program may need referral to a more comprehensive interdisciplinary, functional restoration rehabilitation–based program. Patients may continue to report ongoing pain and reduced physical and psychologic functioning. Progress may also be impeded by disturbed sleep, affective distress (i.e., depression, anger, anxiety), fear of movement and reinjury (i.e., fear-avoidance beliefs), and deconditioning. In these cases, treatment of chronic pain may be focused not only on removing an underlying organic disease but also on the reduction of disability through modification of environmental contingencies and cognitive processes. Behavioral interventions, including cognitive-behavioral therapy, relaxation training (i.e., deep breathing, progressive muscle relaxation), and pain education, are key components in interdisciplinary programs.

Pain treatment programs comprising comprehensive interdisciplinary rehabilitation typically involve a number of health care providers including rehabilitation specialists; physical, occupational, and therapeutic recreational therapists; pain psychologists; biofeedback specialists; and nursing education and vocational counselors. This interdisciplinary approach relies heavily on the coordination of services fostered by ongoing communication between team members with the goal of improving patient function at home and/or in the workplace, fostering independence, and improving psychosocial functioning (Box 58.7). The frequency and duration of treatment will vary, depending on the level of impairment, up to 7–8 hours per day for 3–4 weeks for the most impaired patients. Less intense programs may include 3 to 4 treatment hours per session multiple times per week, based on the same biopsychosocial framework. However, effectiveness studies suggest that intensive treatment programs (>100 hours of therapy) are of greater benefit than less intense programs (<30 hours of treatment).[35] At the completion of their programs, patients are encouraged to continue utilizing pain management techniques as they return to previous levels of sport, work, and/or community function. An extensive review of the behavioral treatment for chronic low back pain has shown that it can be an effective treatment for chronic low back pain.[36–38] Systematic reviews support the efficacy of multidisciplinary and interdisciplinary treatment for chronic pain conditions.[35,39–41] Guidelines published by the American Pain Society for the treatment of low back pain support the use of interdisciplinary treatment, when available, for patients with nonspecific low back pain and as a treatment option that should be discussed for patients considering single-level laminectomy for lumbar disc herniation.[42] The National Pain Strategy, a population-based national plan for transforming pain treatment in the United States, strongly supports integration of multidisciplinary and interdisciplinary approaches at the primary care, pain specialist, and tertiary levels of care.[43]

In addition, pharmacologic interventions should include trials of antidepressant medications for depressed mood and medications to help improve disturbed sleep. Lower-dose tricyclic and tricyclic-like antidepressants may help augment serotonin and norepinephrine levels in the brain and improve the quality of sleep. Targeted analgesia may also involve a variety of medications from a number of pharmacologic classes including antiinflammatories, antiepileptics, muscle relaxants, and, in carefully selected patients, opioid medications.[44]

BOX 58.7 Staff Composition of an Interdisciplinary Pain Management Team

Physiatrist/pain medicine specialist
Nurse educator
Pain psychologist
Physical therapist
Occupational therapist
Vocational counselor
Biofeedback therapist
Therapeutic recreational therapist

KEY POINTS

- Pain management is the first step in the restoration of function. Functional improvement is not always synonymous with alleviation of pain.
- Physical modalities (ultrasound, hot packs, cryotherapy, etc.) may be of benefit in acute pain situations. Chronic use of these interventions should be discouraged.
- Exercise treatment is a helpful adjunct in treating patients with all types of pain disorders. Exercise programs should include flexibility, muscle strengthening, and aerobic exercise.

- Referral for comprehensive multidisciplinary and interdisciplinary treatment may be necessary for those patients failing to progress in the acute, subacute, and maintenance-based programs.
- The treatment of chronic pain may shift focus from removing an underlying organic disease to reducing disability through the modification of environmental factors and cognitive processes.

REFERENCES

Access the reference list online at ExpertConsult.com.

CHAPTER 59

Psychologic Interventions for Chronic Pain

Megan Hosey, PhD ◎ Jessica Wolfman McWhorter, PhD, ABPP/RP ◎ Stephen T. Wegener, PhD

Cognitive, affective, and social factors have long been recognized as influencing the experience of pain. Beecher observed that the personal meaning of pain was an important determinant of the pain complaints he observed in soldiers wounded in World War II.[1] Later, the work of Melzack and Wall on the "gate control" theory of pain[2] stimulated much interest in the multidimensional and subjective aspects of the pain experience. The pioneering work of Fordyce et al.[3] detailed the role that social and environmental factors play in the way an individual expresses pain behaviorally. These historical developments, supported by research, influenced the definition of pain promulgated by the International Society for the Study of Pain, which includes both sensory and emotional factors.[4] It has become well accepted that the experience of pain is best conceptualized within a biopsychosocial model.[5,6]

The literature on the role of psychologic factors in the experience of pain was summarized in the seminal work of Turk and colleagues that detailed the application of cognitive-behavioral interventions in the management of chronic pain.[7] More recently, different models of delivery have been explored for efficacy, including internet-based cognitive-behavioral interventions.[8]

The wide acceptance of psychologic interventions as a treatment modality is based on two complementary lines of research. First, early studies of laboratory pain demonstrated the role of psychologic factors in determining the level of reported pain and pain thresholds. Second, the psychotherapy literature demonstrated the positive impact that psychologic interventions can have on many areas of functioning and quality of life. Moreover, it has been proposed that quality of life should be a primary treatment target within chronic pain populations, above and beyond pain intensity.[9] The benefit of psychologic treatments among individuals with chronic pain is particularly clear for anxiety and depression, emotional states shown to influence the experience of pain.

This chapter provides an overview of psychologic interventions utilized for chronic pain, focusing primarily on the interventions that have been empirically tested in clinical trials. Targets for psychologic treatment are listed in Table 59.1. This chapter provides practitioners with an overview of evidence-based psychologic interventions for the management of chronic pain. Specialized training is needed to developing competency in applying these strategies.

BEHAVIORAL INTERVENTIONS

Learning theory, incorporating the principles of operant conditioning (e.g., reinforcement and punishment), provides the theoretical basis for behavioral interventions in persons with chronic pain.[3,10,11] In the case of acute pain, environmental and interpersonal contingencies have limited time to shape the pain experience. However, in the case of chronic pain, the prolonged nature of the experience provides substantial opportunities for pain behaviors to be reinforced and maintained. Many of the behavioral techniques used in pain management are adapted from the strategies used extensively in managing anxiety, depression, and health behaviors.

OPERANT INTERVENTIONS

In an operant model of pain, the primary focus of intervention is the behavior of the patient. Pain-related behaviors are thought to maintain pain past its expected duration.[3] These behaviors can include either verbal expressions of pain (e.g., complaints of pain or requests for medication), gross motor movements that are indicators of pain (e.g., grimacing or limping), or avoidance of potential pain-generating activities. These observable behaviors are subject to the principles of operant conditioning, which state that a given behavior is highly influenced by the consequences of that behavior. Reinforcing consequences increase the likelihood that a behavior will occur in the future and neutral or punishing consequences decrease the likelihood that a behavior will occur. More specifically, these behaviors can be maintained through positive reinforcement (e.g., attention from a loved one), negative reinforcement (e.g., not having to go to an unpleasant job), or a lack of positive reinforcment.[3] For example, when a patient grimaces and a loved one responds by expressing concern, grimacing may occur more frequently in the future when that loved one is present. In this case, the social attention in the form of concern positively reinforces the grimace. Alternatively, pain can serve as punishment (negative reinforcement) for engaging in an activity. If an individual experiences pain during or following standing or walking, this is likely to decrease the frequency of these activities. Furthermore, there has been research to suggest that operant conditioning may play a role in the level of pain-related disability.[12]

TABLE 59.1 Targets for Psychologic Treatment

1. Reducing pain and pain-related disability
2. Treating comorbid mood disturbances, particularly depression
3. Increasing perceptions of control and self-efficacy for pain management
4. Increasing health behaviors—appropriate medication use, exercise/activation, sleep habits
5. Addressing the impact of pain-related psychosocial factors on family functioning and work life

The goal of operant interventions is to decrease learned pain behaviors and replace maladaptive responses associated with the pain and the sick role with more adaptive behaviors.[3] Operant interventions ideally occur in an environment where there is the opportunity to control the social consequences of pain behaviors and shape new, more adaptive behaviors. Historically, most operant pain programs have been based on inpatient units where a level of control is possible; however, operant conditioning interventions can be incorporated into outpatient treatment as well. For example, "as needed" pain medication prescriptions are changed to fixed time intervals to remove the contingent relationship between complaints of pain (i.e., the pain behavior) and pain relief (i.e., the reinforcer). Vocalizations about pain intensity are largely ignored and more adaptive behaviors, including attending physical therapy and increasing activity level, are socially rewarded (i.e., reinforced). The focus of operant interventions is ideally on targeting the behavior and opposed to addressing pain intensity.[9,10] In doing so, the desired outcome is an improved quality of life, above and beyond decreasing pain intensity. The initial phase of any behavioral intervention is a behavioral analysis. Once an understanding of the pain-related behaviors is established, a behavioral plan can be delineated and executed.

Pacing and behavioral activation are important components of operant behavioral pain management programs.[13] When individuals push their activity levels to the point of pain exacerbation, they are more likely to decrease their activity over time. Operant programs designed to avoid this negative pattern have the following three components: (1) Establish a baseline. A specific target behavior is identified, for example, sitting at a desk.[14] A baseline is established by measuring for several days the amount of time the individual can sit at the desk before his or her back pain is exacerbated (e.g., 30 minutes on average). (2) Begin time-contingent activity. Rather than having the individual sit until the pain becomes intolerable and then stop, an initial goal is set at 70%–80% of the baseline level (e.g., 20–24 minutes). The individual would start by sitting not more than 20 minutes, thus avoiding the punishment of pain exacerbation and obtaining the social reinforcement associated with success. (3) Gradually increase the level of the behavior, usually by not more than 5% per week, and instruct the patient to use time, not pain, as an indicator for stopping the activity. Over a period of weeks, the individual would increase the comfortable duration of sitting to perhaps 60 minutes without shifting position or standing up.

This process of gradually increasing the nature, frequency, and duration of a behavior is called "shaping." The goal of such an intervention is to increase the adaptive behavior while managing the consequences, which include removing any punishment (e.g., pain) and introducing reinforcement (e.g., experience of success, social attention). The involvement of the significant other or family members in treatment is desirable so that they can be taught the principles of shaping behavior. Further, inclusion of others (i.e., family, friends, caregivers) in treatment can facilitate the generalization of treatment gains from the inpatient setting to the home environment.

RELAXATION INTERVENTIONS

An extensive literature documents the benefits of developing a relaxation response, particularly in the areas of anxiety and stress management. The potential utility of targeting negative emotions (e.g., stress, anxiety, depression) in managing chronic pain is a key component of treatment given the well-established relationship between one's pain experience and affective state. The goal of most techniques is nondirected relaxation accomplished through two common components[15]: first, repetitive focus on a word, body sensation, or muscle activity and, second, a passive attitude toward thoughts unrelated to the attentional focus.[7,16,17] Common methods used for teaching relaxation include systematically tensing and relaxing specific muscle groups (e.g., progressive muscle relaxation), focusing on breathing and enhancing diaphragmatic breathing, and using guided imagery. A psychophysiologic model of pain, which has received some empirical support,[18] suggests that stress or pain leads to subtle increases in muscle tension, which can exacerbate pain at the site of an injury. A primary goal of relaxation training is to break the cycle between pain and muscle tension. Expert panels[17] and meta-analyses have summarized empirical support for the use of these techniques in pain management and recommended the broad integration of relaxation techniques with biomedical interventions for pain management.[17,19]

BIOFEEDBACK

Biofeedback provides the individual with detailed information about a physiologic process that is typically not within his or her awareness. Through this detailed feedback, the individual can learn voluntary control over usually involuntary processes. Biofeedback for pain management usually entails providing feedback about muscle tension, typically using electromyographic (EMG) feedback from the site of the pain or a standard location such as the frontalis muscles, or feedback about skin temperature, typically using thermistors attached to the fingers. Empirical support for the efficacy of biofeedback for pain management exists for several specific painful conditions, including the Raynaud phenomenon, tension and migraine headaches, vulvar vestibulitis, and low back pain. Although biofeedback is widely used within the field of pain medicine, particularly in conjunction with relaxation training, empirical support for its specific efficacy beyond the general effects of relaxation strategies has not been widely demonstrated except in the treatment of headaches.[16,20] Biofeedback has been demonstrated to have greater efficacy than relaxation alone for tension headaches.[21] For patients who have difficulty recognizing the physiologic changes that may accompany pain or stress, biofeedback may be useful in helping them to recognize these changes. Further, patients who are drawn to technology or who conceptualize their pain experience as a primarily physical phenomenon may prefer a biofeedback approach to relaxation training.

COGNITIVE-BEHAVIORAL INTERVENTIONS

The data showing that cognitive and emotional factors influence the experience of pain have encouraged the application of cognitive-behavioral theory (CBT) and treatment to the management of chronic pain.[18] These interventions typically include components of the behavioral model, particularly relaxation training and some components of operant conditioning. However, emphasis is also placed on cognitive factors, such as attitudes and beliefs that underlie maladaptive emotional and behavioral responses to pain.[22] The efficacy of CBT for treating chronic pain has been evaluated extensively over the past several decades. Expert panels[17] and meta-analyses[19] have found good evidence for the use of cognitive-behavioral interventions for chronic pain management.[23–25] The strongest support is in the treatment of individuals with low back pain, rheumatoid arthritis, and osteoarthritis pain.[23] CBT[26] has been shown to have a positive impact on pain intensity, pain-related interference, disability, health-related quality of life, and depression among individuals with chronic pain.[19] The effect sizes for such studies have recently been noted to be somewhat variable. This may be an issue of research design limitations,[23] given the extensive research that has supported CBT's utility.

COPING SKILLS TRAINING

Coping skills training has been shown to be a useful aspect of CBT with pain populations.[27] Patients engage in a range of coping responses to manage pain and related stressors. Some coping responses (e.g., activity avoidance) are associated with increased distress and suffering, while others (e.g., problem solving)[18] are linked to better emotional and physical functioning. Specific coping skills are highly adaptive and effective for individuals with chronic pain, often including some of the strategies already outlined, particularly relaxation and pacing of activity level. The primary goals of coping skills training are to increase perceptions of pain as a controllable experience and decreasing the use of maladaptive coping strategies. In this approach the emphasis is on skill development and refinement. In the case of skill development, a new skill is introduced and patients are encouraged to develop and refine the skill during low pain periods before attempting to implement the coping skill during an actual period of pain exacerbation. The skill is shaped over time, so that the skill is gradually applied to increasingly challenging (i.e., painful) episodes as the individual becomes more proficient in that skill. A similar approach is taken to the application of many pain coping skills, including cognitive or behavioral distraction, relaxation, pacing of activities, and the appropriate use of social support. Attention is paid to factors that increase or decrease pain and these factors guide the application of pain coping skills.

COGNITIVE RESTRUCTURING

Cognitive restructuring focuses on the role of cognitive factors, such as attitudes, thoughts, and beliefs, in determining emotional and behavioral responses to pain. These interventions challenge negative self-talk, such as catastrophizing (e.g., "I can't stand the pain anymore"), and replace these self-statements with more positive statements that reduce negative affect, emphasize control, and encourage adaptive coping (e.g., "This is a challenge that I have faced before and I can handle it this time"). Catastrophizing is a particularly maladaptive response to pain, which has been shown to correlate with depression and disability.[22] In the context of treatment, patients are frequently asked to monitor their thoughts about their pain or pain-related situations, identify negative thoughts, and generate more accurate, adaptive thoughts to replace the negative thoughts. The emphasis is on balanced thinking, not necessarily positive thinking. This self-monitoring process is supplemented with more in-depth discussions of the underlying attitudes and beliefs contributing to the negative thoughts. The potential utility for cognitive restructuring is highlighted by an exploration of thoughts associated with chronic pain. For example, when an individual's expectations of pain relief are greatly below what they view as beneficial,[28] there may be poor engagement in interventions. Therefore, if one's beliefs and attitudes could be restructured, increased engagement in interventions may lead to improved outcomes.

MINDFULNESS AND ACCEPTANCE-BASED STRATEGIES

As already noted, cognitive-behavioral strategies emerged as a way of changing thoughts, emotions, and behaviors related to pain. More recent strategies have turned attention to mindfulness and acceptance based strategies that place emphasis on awareness, nonjudgment, and meaning-making in pain rather than strategies to control, avoid, or fight pain.[26,29] Mindfulness is defined as nonjudgmental awareness of the present moment, which provides an opportunity to acknowledge and accept difficult physical and emotional sensations.[30] Examples of mindfulness practice include focusing on the breath, engaging in daily activities while attending to the senses in the present moment, and nonjudgmental observation of the environment. Mindfulness interventions have been demonstrated to have small effects on pain intensity, moderate effects on negative affective states such as depression and anxiety, and moderate effects on quality-of-life outcomes.[26,31] It should be emphasized that reduction in pain intensity is not the goal of mindfulness or acceptance-based interventions. The focus is on the appreciation of life in the context of pain.[26,31]

Along these lines, acceptance and commitment therapy (ACT) is a form of behavioral therapy conceptualized in the late 1980s by Hayes and colleagues.[32] This therapy integrates mindfulness with commitment and behavior change strategies.[33] In this approach, patients are asked to describe their values. Next, they are asked to reflect on how to best match their thoughts, feelings, and behaviors with their values. There is a focus on reducing avoidance of emotional and physical pain by using mindfulness strategies.[33] The past decade has seen an increase in the investigation of the utility of ACT in reducing emotional and physical disability related to pain. For example, in a randomized controlled trial (RCT) comparing ACT to CBT, Wetherell and colleagues found that ACT was equally effective in improving pain interference, depression, and pain-related anxiety.[34] Notably, patients rated higher in satisfaction when they were participating in ACT.[34] Similarly, a 3-year longitudinal study of individuals with chronic pain found that participation in an ACT program resulted in stable, medium effect sizes for change in pain-related anxiety, depression, and psychosocial disability at 3 years after intervention. Effect sizes for change in physical disability were small.[35] Overall, ACT appears to be a promising new approach to the management of chronic pain.

HYPNOSIS

Hypnosis is another tool utilized for pain management that targets beliefs and attitudes about pain and helps to increase control over the pain experience. Hypnosis for pain management usually begins with an induction consisting of suggestions for focused attention and relaxation. This is usually followed by specific suggestions designed to alter how the individual views or experiences the pain.[36] Often the treatment will include a posthypnotic suggestion that the benefit experienced during the session—that is, decreased intensity of pain—will last after the session or that the individual will experience greater comfort when engaging in specific behaviors such as taking a deep breath or touching the painful site. The goal in working with people experiencing chronic pain is to teach them self-hypnosis so that they can use the skill to reduce pain and discomfort outside of the treatment session. Hypnosis has been most widely applied and studied with pain due to cancer, and expert panels have concluded that the use of hypnosis is effective in reducing chronic pain due to malignancies.[17] There are also data supporting its efficacy in treating pain due to irritable bowel syndrome, temporomandibular joint disorders, and tension headaches.[37] Recent advances including virtual reality technology and hypnotic induction techniques have been demonstrated to be effective in inducing hypnotic analgesia for persons undergoing painful treatment for burns.[37] Meta-analyses indicate that hypnosis can lead to significant reductions in pain that are similar to those experienced with the relaxation techniques described earlier. It is not clear whether hypnosis is effective beyond what is seen in these treatments.[36]

SELF-MANAGEMENT AND PEER SUPPORT

Self-management (SM) group interventions, based on the principles of CBT, have gained widespread application with chronic conditions marked by pain, distress, and functional impairment. Key elements in SM include developing knowledge about the health condition, self-monitoring progress, acquiring relevant skills, and problem solving.[38] SM interventions have improved outcomes in many conditions, including rheumatologic diseases,[39] fibromyalgia,[40] and depression.[41] Because SM interventions are often provided in a group setting, they incorporate social support and peer interaction that may facilitate behavior change and maintain treatment gains. SM interventions can be provided by professionals, laypersons, or peers. More recently SM interventions using the Internet and telecommunication technologies have demonstrated improvements in pain and health distress and reduced health care utilization among persons with chronic low back pain.[42] Web-based cognitive-behavioral programs have demonstrated effectiveness with individuals with chronic low back pain,[43] older adults with chronic pain,[44] and people with migraine.[45] Regarding telehealth methods, early studies suggest that SM strategies for pain and CBT-based strategies can be taught effectively over the telephone or via closed circuit television.[46] SM interventions are best conceptualized as one component of a multidisciplinary pain treatment plan.

MULTIDISCIPLINARY TREATMENT

Given that chronic pain is best understood within the context of a biopsychosocial model, this model calls for multidisciplinary treatment. There is significant evidence to support the use of multidisciplinary, multimodal approaches that include psychologic intervention versus single-discipline or unimodal approaches, particularly when the focus is on improving long-term outcomes of mood, daily functioning, return to work, health care utilization, and quality of life.[6,23,47] For example, in a RCT for the treatment of chronic-tension headache, combination therapy (stress management with tricyclic antidepressant medication) was superior to any individual intervention.[48]

The use of a multidisciplinary approach may also extend initial treatment gains over several years.[23] Although psychologic intervention is an integral component of multidisciplinary pain management, it may be particularly important to target individuals whose psychologic and behavioral characteristics may prevent them from benefiting from other aspects of the treatment plan. Individuals who are highly distressed, see their pain as uncontrollable, have highly negative life events, perceive themselves to be disabled, and have low readiness to engage in SM are all at high risk for responding poorly to treatment.[49]

Early detection and referral for potential problems is a primary responsibility of physicians and other providers who encounter such patients, since there is evidence that early intervention for psychologic issues enhances outcome.[50] It appears that earlier intervention in a multidisciplinary context improves patient self-efficacy for pain management and function.[51] Along these lines, studies have shown that the early classification of individuals into low-, medium-, and high-risk groups in transitioning from acute to chronic pain is useful for triaging necessary resources and treatment modalities.[14] Classification of risk generally incorporates an assessment of both physiologic (multisite pain, presence of radicular pain) and emotional-behavioral (catastrophizing, kinesophobia, pessimistic expectations, and level of disability) factors.[14] In the STartBack trial, researchers found that by stratifying patients by risk and providing necessary treatment, including both physiotherapy and psychologically informed education about SM, improvements in health and health care cost savings resulted.[52]

Attention to psychosocial health is a responsibility shared by all members of the multidisciplinary pain team, beginning with the patient and family and including clinicians who are not formally identified as mental health providers. Referral to a specific provider, along with an explanation to the patient that places the referral within the biopsychosocial model of pain and indicates how the psychologist may be helpful to the patient, will facilitate follow through. Physicians who are managing chronic pain patients need to have an established relationship with a psychologist who has pain expertise.

TABLE 59.2 Indications for Inpatient Pain Treatment

1. Nonmalignant pain of 6 months or more
2. Major functional disabilities
3. Need for intensive extensive psychologic or behavioral therapy
4. Need for temporary removal from a detrimental home situation to refocus
5. Failure of conventional methods of treatment

INPATIENT VERSUS OUTPATIENT CARE

Although there are data to support the utility of multidisciplinary treatment for chronic pain,[47] there are few data to guide the clinician in determining what patients require or which patients would benefit from admission to an inpatient pain program. The decision to pursue admission to an inpatient program is based on clinical assessment of the patient and his or her environmental circumstances. Inpatient chronic pain programs offer the advantage of increased medical attention, close monitoring of positive and negative health behaviors, and a structured treatment setting. Indications for inpatient care are listed in Table 59.2. As part of admission planning, both medical and psychologic evaluations should be completed on an outpatient basis. Overall, inpatient programs can be of great utility given the controllability of the environment and ability to implement a multimodal approach. Among mixed chronic pain patients, individuals who completed an inpatient program made greater gains, maintained better health, and had lower health care utilization postdischarge relative to their outpatient counterparts.[53] Despite relatively strong evidence for inpatient programs, a very small number of individuals actually receive such treatment.[20]

SUMMARY

A number of psychologic interventions have been empirically demonstrated to reduce pain and suffering in patients with a wide variety of chronic pain syndromes. A typical course of treatment usually includes many of the behavioral and cognitive approaches detailed here and the specific approaches utilized are tailored to the needs of the patient. These interventions are usually part of a multidisciplinary approach and are provided in conjunction with other pain interventions (e.g., medication, physical therapy). Although many patients with chronic pain may benefit from psychologic intervention, certain subpopulations—those who are highly distressed, see their pain as uncontrollable, have highly negative life events, perceive themselves to be disabled, and have low readiness to engage in SM, and have problematic medication use (dose escalation, misuse, or underuse)—are likely to require psychologic intervention to maximize treatment gains. As research develops, there will be a growing emphasis on matching psychologic pain interventions with patient characteristics.[54] Based on the existing literature, certain pain disorders (e.g., headaches) may be highly responsive to specific psychologic interventions such as behavioral approaches, and these treatments should be considered a standard part of medical management. For individuals who are not suitable candidates for a medical or pharmacologic treatment (e.g., chronic opioid therapy for the recovering substance abuser), psychologic treatment may be considered an essential first-line treatment option. Modern pain theory and the existing evidence base indicate that psychologic intervention should be a routine part of chronic pain management rather than a treatment of last resort.

KEY POINTS

- To alleviate suffering, patients can work with a mental health provider with specialized training to change emotional and behavioral responses to chronic pain.
- Psychologic intervention should be a routine part of chronic pain management.
- Psychologic intervention is multifaceted and should be tailored to the needs of the patient and his or her individual experience of pain.
- Attention to psychosocial health is a responsibility shared by all members of the multidisciplinary pain team.

REFERENCES

Access the reference list online at ExpertConsult.com.

CHAPTER 60

ACUPUNCTURE

Eric S. Hsu, MD ✪ Irene Wu, MD ✪ Brian Lai, MD

Acupuncture (*Jin jiu*) is an essential component of traditional Chinese medicine (TCM). The term *acupuncture* comes from the Greek words *acus* (needle) and *punctura* (puncture). Scientific evidence has demonstrated the physiologic effects of acupuncture (AP) and electro-acupuncture (EA) stimulation over the last four decades. AP consists of mechanical stimulation via needle insertion and thermal input by Moxa (a Chinese herb) or by a heat lamp applied over the needles (moxibustion [Mox]).

HISTORY AND THEORIES

The history of AP can be traced back over 3000 years with origin in China. The first written medical text on AP was in the *Huang Di Nei Jing (The Yellow Emperor's Internal Classic)* written by Chi Po around 2nd century BC. AP became well publicized in the Western world thanks to *New York Times'* writer James Reston's article in 1971. He described his first-hand experience of AP during the emergency appendectomy and perioperative care while accompanying President Nixon on a visit to China.

Theories: Taoist philosophy underlies the hypothetical framework of AP. Tao (way) was described by Lao-tse in the *Tao Te Ching* around 500 BC, which assumed nature is constantly changing. Tao is the source of all creation and acts through two opposing but balancing forces: the yin and the yang. Yin refers to dark, cold, rest, passivity, inward, decrease, wet, and female. Yang refers to bright, hot, activity, outward, increase, dry, and male. People exist within the tensions created by these two forces in a dynamic interaction with nature. Illness occurs when yin and yang fall out of balance and harmony. AP restores the balance by promoting yin and yang energy within organ systems.[1]

The concept of qi (vital energy) is fundamental to the practice of classic AP. Qi is the energy that flows through different "meridians" or channels that connect the internal body with the external environment. There are different types of qi that serve functions such as hereditary, protective, and nourishing energy. The network of meridians runs throughout the body while each meridian is associated with an organ system. There are 12 paired principal, 2 unpaired, and 8 extra meridians. Obstruction of qi may result in disequilibrium of yin and yang that may manifest as pain or illness. The meridians emerge at the surface of the body via AP points (acupoints) where external stimulation may modulate the qi.

There are six pathologic factors that cause disease such as wind, cold, heat, dampness, dryness, and fire in TCM. There are four steps in the assessment of a patient's symptoms: observation; listening and smelling; palpation; and history taking. The goal is to assess balance of yin and yang, and to gain insight into other symptoms. There are eight diagnostic principles for classifications of symptoms including yin or yang, external or internal, cold or hot, and deficiency or excess.[2]

There are more than 361 established AP points (acupoints) that distribute along the meridians. Acupoints are sites of low skin resistance and are accessible for stimulation. Acupoint is identified by its meridian, a Chinese name, and number. Acupoints are located through anatomic landmarks such as bony structures, muscles, and external features. The "cun" is a defined unit of measurement to locate acupoints via specific landmarks. "Cun" is the distance between the joint creases of interphalangeal joints of a patient's flexed middle finger or equivalent to the width of a patient's thumb.

MERIDIANS, ACUPOINTS, AND MYOFASCIAL TRIGGER POINTS

Melzack et al. reported a remarkably high degree (71%) of correlation between myofascial trigger points and acupoints on the basis of two criteria: spatial distribution and the associated pain pattern. This close correlation suggests that trigger points and acupoints for pain, though discovered independently and labeled differently, represent the same phenomenon and can be explained in terms of the same underlying neural mechanisms.[3] Dorsher updated references and confirmed the conceptual comparison of trigger points to acupoints in pain and clinical correspondence was likely 95% or higher. Although separated by 2000 years, the AP and myofascial pain traditions have fundamentally clinical similarities in the treatment of pain disorders.[4]

Dorsher examined whether myofascial referred-pain data can provide independent physiologic evidence of AP meridians. Trigger point regions were subdivided from previously validated trigger point region-classical acupoint correspondence results into subsets according to the 12 AP organs and their anatomically corresponding acupoints. For all 12 subsets of trigger point regions, their summed referred pain patterns accurately predicted the distributions of corresponding AP meridians, particularly in the extremities. Dorsher demonstrated that myofascial referred pain data may provide the physiologic evidence of AP meridians.[5]

TECHNIQUE

No consensus exists about which technique of needle insertion in AP is most favorable or efficacious. Positions of patients may include prone or supine to allow adequate access and optimal comfort. A lateral decubitus or sitting

BOX 60.1 Mechanisms of Acupuncture Analgesia

1. Manual acupuncture (MA) caused suppression of mRNA expression of pain-related genes (fos, opioid receptor-like 1, tachykinin receptor 1, mu-opioid receptor, and 5-hydroxytryptamine receptor 2A) in spinal cord and enhanced antinociceptive effect on formalin-induced pain in a rat model.
2. Gate-control theory (Melzack and Wall) of pain describes the modulation of sensory nerve impulses by inhibitory mechanisms in the central nervous system.
3. Electro-acupuncture (EA) of 2 Hz accelerates the release of encephalin, beta-endorphin, and endomorphin, while EA of 100 Hz selectively increases the release of dynorphin.
4. EA may modulate pain via activation of bioactive chemicals (monoamines such as serotonin and norepinephrine in addition to opioids) through peripheral, spinal, and supraspinal mechanisms.
5. MA induced specific "de qi" response and its association with distinct nerve fibers via functional magnetic resonance imaging (fMRI) study in contrast to sham control with tactile stimulation.
6. Acupuncture (AP) yielded broad deactivation in limbic system, pain status, and default mode network (DMN) and evoked activations in attentional and somatosensory systems via fMRI study in subjects with acute low back pain (LBP).
7. AP induced more deactivations and less activation via fMRI study as compared with sham control. AP may modulate multiple brain networks beyond somatosensory-guided mind-body therapy according to fMRI study in subjects with acute LBP.
8. AP restored less connectivity within the DMN in the dorsolateral prefrontal cortex, medial prefrontal cortex, anterior cingulate gyrus, and precuneus via fMRI study in chronic LBP subjects. The reductions in clinical pain were correlated with increases in DMN connectivity.

position may also work. The skin is wiped with an alcohol pad and stretched prior to needle insertion to minimize discomfort. Tubular guides can assist needle insertion. The usual angle of insertion is perpendicular or oblique. More horizontal insertion is often used over face and chest.

The selection of acupoints may follow various schools of AP. Tender or trigger points are used as local acupoints. Distal points are selected according to involved meridians. The insertion of the needle is usually accompanied by "de qi" (obtaining qi) described as soreness, heaviness, and numbness around the site. There is a feedback as if surrounding tissue were grabbing and holding the needle that confirms accurate placement. The disposable stainless steel needle consists of a body or shaft with a handle. Common sizes are 30–32 gauge with lengths ranging from 20 to 125 mm. Manipulation of the needle depends on either excess or deficiency state of the qi. AP stimulation can be accomplished manually or with EA stimulators. Mox or a heat lamp may be applied over needles. Patients need to avoid strenuous activities since generalized fatigue occurs in the beginning of AP treatment.

MECHANISM OF ACUPUNCTURE ANALGESIA

There are three domains (neurohumoral, neuromodulation, and neuroimaging) of scientific evidence (Box 60.1).[6]

NEUROHUMORAL AND NEUROMODULATION DATA

Pomeranz proposed that AP appears to cause release of various endorphins and monoamine neurotransmitters in both peripheral and central nervous systems (CNS). AP activates sensory nerve fibers in muscles and sends signals to the spinal cord. This activates other centers in midbrain and the hypothalamic–pituitary axis that cause release of neuropeptides. Enkephalin and dynorphin are released at the level of the spinal cord and may block afferent pathways. Enkephalin produced at midbrain may stimulate the inhibitory raphe descending system and release the monoamines serotonin and norepinephrine. These neurotransmitters may further modulate pain transmission in the spinal cord. Beta-endorphin released from the hypothalamic–pituitary axis may result in analgesia through both systemic circulation and cerebrospinal fluid.[7]

To apply appropriate AP stimulation, different needle manipulation techniques are required. These manipulations are performed in many ways such as twirling the needle or varying the insertion angle. Kim et al. designed a study to evaluate the antinociceptive effect of these manipulations to acupoint ST36 on formalin-induced pain in rats.[8] Several pain-related gene expressions were investigated in the spinal cord using reverse transcriptase-polymerase chain reaction analysis. Needle manipulation suppressed the mRNA expression of pain-related genes such as fos, opioid receptor-like 1, tachykinin 1, tachykinin receptor 1, mu-opioid receptor, and 5-hydroxytryptamine receptor 2A in the spinal cord. The authors proposed that needle manipulation enhanced analgesia by suppression of the transcription of pain-related genes.[8] The growing popularity of the gate-control theory of pain by Melzack and Wall led to electrical stimulation therapies and development of the transcutaneous electrical nerve stimulation (TENS) unit. Electrical stimulation has been frequently employed for needle stimulation in EA and related techniques.[9] Han et al. demonstrated that EA of 2 Hz accelerates the release of enkephalin, beta-endorphin, and endomorphin, while EA of 100 Hz selectively increases the release of dynorphin. A combination of the two frequencies produced simultaneous release of all four opioid peptides resulting in maximal therapeutic effects.[10] Zhang et al. summarized that EA activates the nervous system differently in health and in various pain conditions, alleviates both sensory and affective inflammatory pain, and inhibits inflammatory and neuropathic pain more effectively at 2 and 10 Hz than at 100 Hz.[11] They suggested that EA may modulate pain by activating a mixture of bioactive chemicals (opioids, serotonin, and norepinephrine) through peripheral, spinal, and supra-spinal mechanisms.[11]

NEUROIMAGING DATA

Updates in biophysiologic and imaging techniques offer enhanced evaluation of the sequential events following AP-induced stimulation. Functional magnetic resonance imaging (fMRI) is a noninvasive technique that depends on differences in relative concentration of oxygenated to deoxygenated hemoglobin within the brain in response to stimuli. AP stimulation elicits "de qi," a composite of unique sensations that are essential for clinical efficacy according to TCM. Manual acupuncture (MA) was performed in randomized order during fMRI in 42 AP naïve healthy adult volunteers. The most significant differences in de qi sensations between AP and tactile stimulation (sham) control were observed with aching, soreness, pressure, and dull pain. Hui et al. provided scientific data on the characteristics of de qi response in AP and its association with distinct nerve fibers.[12] Shi et al. presented network response to AP in models of experimental acute low back pain (a LBP).[13] As compared with the baseline, the pain state had higher regional homogeneity (ReHo) values in the pain matrix, limbic system, and default mode network (DMN) and lower ReHo values in frontal gyrus and temporal gyrus. AP yielded broad deactivation in subjects, including nearly all of the limbic system, pain status, and DMN, and also evoked numerous activations in the attentional and somatosensory systems. AP induced more deactivations and less activation in the subjects compared with sham. Shi et al. proposed that AP may modulate multiple brain networks beyond somatosensory-guided mind-body therapy.[13] Li et al. studied 4-week AP in chronic low back pain (c LBP) with fMRI. Less connectivity within the DMN was found in c LBP than controls, mainly in the dorsolateral prefrontal cortex, medial prefrontal cortex, anterior cingulate gyrus, and precuneus. The DMN connectivity after AP was restored almost to the control levels. Reductions in clinical pain were correlated with increases in DMN connectivity. Li et al. proposed that imaging of the DMN may offer objective assessment of AP analgesia in c LBP.[14]

INDICATIONS

The National Institute of Health (NIH) organized a conference of experts to evaluate the available literature in 1997. AP was widely practiced for treatment of postoperative and chemotherapy-related nausea and vomiting, and dental pain. Other promising results were seen in headache, low back pain (LBP), asthma, menstrual cramps, fibromyalgia, and myofascial pain.[15] Wang et al. critically examined prospective randomized controlled trials (RCTs) and suggested that AP and stimulation were effective in the short-term management of LBP, neck pain, and osteoarthritis (OA) of the knee.[16] Another group evaluated the Cochrane reviews that were concerned specifically with the effectiveness of AP for pain management. Four reviews concluded that AP is effective for migraines, tension-type headaches, neck disorders, and peripheral joint OA; one review failed to demonstrate effectiveness of AP for rheumatoid arthritis; and three reviews were inconclusive for shoulder pain, lateral elbow pain, and LBP.[17]

ADVERSE EFFECTS, COMPLICATIONS, AND MEDICAL CONSENT OF ACUPUNCTURE

Witt et al. conducted a prospective AP study for OA pain of the knee or hip, LBP, neck pain or headache, allergic rhinitis, asthma, or dysmenorrhea.[18] A total of 229,230 patients received an average of 10 AP treatments. There were 8.6% of patients who reported at least one adverse effect and 2.2% reported one that required treatment. Common adverse effects were bleeding or hematoma (6.1%), pain (1.7%), and vegetative symptoms (0.7%). Two patients experienced a pneumothorax and the longest duration of a side effect was 180 days. There was a proposed medical consent that consists of five modules: Introduction to AP and Mox, Risks of AP treatment, Conditions that can increase the risk, Doctor's statement, and Consent. Witt et al. concluded that AP is a relatively safe treatment and a more detailed consent form could support both patients and professionals.[18] Other investigators analyzed AP-related complications and adverse events in case reports published between 1980 and 2013 in China. There were 182 incidents identified in 133 relevant papers. Internal organ and nerve injury were the main complications of AP, especially pneumothorax and CNS injury. Adverse effects may also include syncope, infections, hemorrhage, allergy, burn, aphonia, hysteria, cough, thirst, fever, somnolence, and broken needles (Box 60.2). The investigators proposed to standardize the practice of AP to minimize adverse events and to promote global popularity of AP treatment.[19]

BOX 60.2 Complications of Acupuncture

1. Bleeding/hematoma
2. Syncope
3. Somnolence
4. Aphonia
5. Hysteria
6. Central nervous system injury
7. Pneumothorax
8. Infection
9. Broken needles

PRECAUTIONS AND RELATIVE CONTRAINDICATIONS

Pregnancy is a relative contraindication due to potential induction of premature labor. Bleeding diathesis and anticoagulant therapy may result in bleeding and hematoma formation. Steroids should be discontinued prior to therapy if possible due to attenuation of AP effects. Heavy meals and alcohol prior to AP is imprudent due to the risk of vasovagal symptoms. Caution should be exercised when performing AP over the thoracic region and avoid electromagnetic interference associated with EA and a pacemaker.

CLINICAL RESEARCH DATA ON ACUPUNCTURE TREATMENT

HEADACHE

Linde et al. studied all randomized trials in tension headache with a postrandomization observation period of at least 8 weeks that compared the clinical effects of AP intervention with a control (treatment of acute headaches only or routine care), a sham AP intervention, or another intervention in patients with episodic or chronic tension-type headache. Eleven trials with 2317 participants met the inclusion criteria. Linde et al. concluded that AP could be a valuable nonpharmacologic tool in patients with frequent episodic or chronic tension-type headaches.[20] The group also reviewed 22 trials in migraine with 4419 participants who met the inclusion criteria. AP was associated with slightly better outcomes and fewer adverse effects than prophylactic drug treatment in these trials of migraine.[21] They reported consistent evidence that AP provided additional benefit to treatment of acute migraine attacks only or to routine care. The investigators suggested that AP was

TABLE 60.1 Efficacy of Acupuncture in Various Conditions

Condition	Efficacy	Comments
Headache	Effective in both prevention and treatment of tension-type and migraine headache	Better outcomes and fewer adverse effects than routine care in migraine headache
Neck pain	More effective than sham treatments and on wait list	Combination with stretching exercise improves outcome
Low back pain	Short term benefit as adjunct to conventional therapies	AP or sham both had similar improvement on acute LBP
Osteoarthritis	AP and NSAID are more effective than sham or NSAID	AP is among the list of more effective physical treatments
Postoperative pain	AP and EA delayed the need and reduced the doses for IV PCA in postoperative pain	Intraoperative AP resulted in improved pain and earlier return of diet postoperatively
Abdominal pain	EA was more effective for constipation in IBS, while moxibustion worked better for diarrhea in IBS patients	EA led to higher activation at insula, pulvinar, medial nucleus of thalamus as compared to sham treatment
Primary dysmenorrhea	AP is as effective as NSAID treatment in dysmenorrhea	AP may avoid hormone side effects with oral contraceptive
Cancer pain	Reduce postsurgical nausea, vomiting and gastroparesis; help chemotherapy neuropathy	Adjunct integrative oncology for symptomatic relief of cancer and pain syndrome
Neuropathic pain	Improve VAS, sleep, motor and sensory function in DPN	Incorporate AP in treatment of acute herpes zoster patients

AP, *Acupuncture;* DPN, *diabetic peripheral neuropathy;* EA, *electro-acupuncture;* IBS, *irritable bowel syndrome;* IV, *intravenous;* LBP, *low back pain;* NSAID, *nonsteroidal antiinflammatory drug;* PCA, *patient-controlled analgesia.*
Please review efficacy, comment, and reference for conditions in each section.

at least as effective or more effective than prophylactic drug treatment for migraine, and had fewer adverse effects.[21] Wang et al. conducted an RCT in 50 patients with frequent migraines.[22] At the end of the 20-week treatment, the AP group reported significantly less migraine days, less severe migraine, more responders, and increased pressure pain thresholds when compared with the sham group. Group differences were maintained at the end of the 3-month period, but not at the 1-year follow-up. The authors recommended AP as an effective and safe treatment for short-term relief of frequent migraine (Table 60.1).[22]

NECK PAIN

Trinh et al. reviewed 10 trials that studied AP for chronic neck pain and concluded that there is moderate evidence that AP relieves neck pain better than some inactive treatments; sham treatments and wait-list control at short-term follow-up.[23] For chronic neck disorders with radicular symptoms, there was moderate evidence that AP was more effective than a wait-list control. There was limited evidence that AP was more effective than massage.[23] A quantitative meta-analysis confirmed the short-term efficacy of AP as compared to control in neck pain.[24] Wilke et al. evaluated the effectiveness of AP plus stretching in neck pain and reported increased mechanical pain threshold (MPT) and significantly improved range of motion (ROM).[24] AP plus stretching could therefore be a treatment option to improve ROM and reduce myofascial pain in the short term.[25]

LOW BACK PAIN

Sherman et al. found little evidence for the existence of subgroups of patients with c LBP that would be especially likely to benefit from AP.[26] They noted that patients who had more severe baseline dysfunction due to LBP had the most short-term benefit from AP. Lam et al. summarized that AP had a clinically meaningful reduction in levels of self-reported pain when compared with sham, and improved function when compared with no treatment in nonspecific LBP. When AP was compared with medications (nonsteroidal antiinflammatory drugs [NSAIDs], muscle relaxants, and analgesics) and usual care in LBP, statistically significant differences were observed between the control and the intervention groups.[27] Another group of investigators appraised systematic reviews and concluded that AP provided short-term improvements in c LBP when either used alone or as an adjunct to conventional therapy. There was inconsistent evidence that AP had a more favorable effect than sham, and whether AP or sham had a similar effect on improving function in a LBP.[28]

OSTEOARTHRITIS

Selfe et al. summarized 10 RCT trials involving 1456 participants and provided updated evidence that AP or EA was an effective treatment for pain and physical dysfunction associated with knee OA.[29] Mavrommatis et al. compared AP plus pharmacotherapy with etoricoxib, sham AP plus etoricoxib, and etoricoxib alone in knee OA.[30] The primary efficacy variable was the Western Ontario and McMaster Universities (WOMAC) index. Secondary efficacy variables included the WOMAC index and visual analog scale (VAS), and the Short Form 36 version 2 (SF-36v2) health surveys. AP plus etoricoxib exhibited statistically significant improvements in primary and secondary outcome measures, except for Short Form mental component, compared with the other treatment groups. AP plus etoricoxib was more effective than sham AP plus etoricoxib, or etoricoxib alone for chronic pain due to knee OA.[30] Corbett et al. conducted a meta-analysis of 114 trials with 22 treatments and 9709 patients with knee OA.[31] AP was noted to be statistically significantly better than muscle-strengthening exercise.

The group proposed that AP can be considered as one of the more effective physical treatments (interferential therapy, TENS, pulsed electrical stimulation, balneotherapy, aerobic exercise, and muscle-strengthening exercise) for alleviating knee OA pain in the short-term. However, much of the evidence in this area of research was of poor quality, including the uncertainty about the efficacy of many physical treatments in OA.[31] Another meta-analysis in OA compared AP to sham, no treatment, and usual care.[32] The authors concluded that AP was associated with statistically significant improvements in pain intensity, functional mobility, and health-related quality of life in OA.[32]

POSTOPERATIVE PAIN

Wu et al. recruited 60 women who had spinal anesthesia during cesarean section and randomly assigned to the control, AP, and EA group.[33] After the operation, the subjects received either AP or EA on bilateral acupoints, San Yin Jiao (Sp6), and patient-controlled analgesia (PCA). The results revealed that the AP and EA group could delay the time of requesting morphine up to 10–11 minutes when compared with control. The total dose of PCA used within the first 24 hours was 30% less in the AP and EA group when compared with the control. The investigators demonstrated that the application of AP and EA could definitely delay the time of requesting pain medication after cesarean section and decrease the requirement of PCA within the first 24 hours.[33] Another study looked at preoperative EA for lower abdominal surgery and demonstrated that low-EA (2 Hz) and high-EA (100 Hz) can both reduce postoperative analgesic requirements and associated side effects.[34] In another study, AP was added to conventional treatment in 60 children aged 3–12 who underwent tonsillectomy.[35] There was less pain, less analgesic consumption, and higher patient and parent satisfaction in the study group without adverse effects.[35] Finally, a study on the effect of intraoperative AP on posttonsillectomy pain in 59 patients aged 3–12 demonstrated that intraoperative AP was feasible, well tolerated, and resulted in improved pain and earlier return of diet postoperatively.[36]

ABDOMINAL PAIN

Chu et al. studied the effect of EA with fMRI on brain activation during noxious rectal distension in irritable bowel syndrome (IBS) randomized to true EA or sham. Rectal distension induced significant activation of the anterior cingulated cortex, prefrontal cortex, thalamus, temporal regions, and cerebellum at baseline. During and immediately after EA, increased cerebral activation from baseline was observed in the anterior cingulated cortex, bilateral prefrontal cortex, thalamus, temporal regions, and right insula in both groups. True EA led to significantly higher activation at right insula, as well as pulvinar and medial nucleus of the thalamus when compared to sham. The authors hypothesized that pain modulation of AP in IBS by two actions: (1) modulation of serotonin pathway at insula, and (2) modulation of mood and affection in higher cortical center via ascending pathway at the pulvinar and medial nucleus of the thalamus.[37] Another study compared the impacts of EA and Mox on IBS patients. Both EA and Mox improved the total VAS-IBS scores. While EA was more effective in relieving constipation, Mox worked better for diarrhea.[38]

DYSMENORRHEA

Sriprasert et al. compared the efficacy of AP and combined oral contraceptive (COC) pill in treating moderate-to-severe primary dysmenorrhea.[39] Both treatments resulted in significant improvement over baseline in all outcomes including maximal dysmenorrhea pain scores, days from suffering from dysmenorrhea, amount of rescue analgesic used, and quality of life. AP did not cause any hormone-related side effects, as did oral contraceptives. AP can therefore be an alternative option for relieving dysmenorrhea, especially when oral contraceptives are not a favorable choice.[39] Other investigators reported that AP was as effective as NSAID in primary dysmenorrhea after 1 month's treatments.[40]

CANCER PAIN

Cancer pain is one of most prevalent symptoms in cancer treatments. The National Comprehensive Cancer Network guidelines for adult cancer pain recommends AP, as one of several integrative interventions, in conjunction with pharmacotherapy as needed. Lu et al. presented evidence regarding the use of AP in cancer pain conditions that may include postoperative cancer pain, postoperative nausea and vomiting, postsurgical gastroparesis syndrome, opioid-induced constipation, opioid-induced pruritus, chemotherapy-induced neuropathy, aromatase inhibitor-associated joint pain, and neck dissection-related pain and dysfunction.[41] Other experts recommended AP as adjunct management for cancer symptoms after retrospectively reviewing the satisfaction ratings of 90 patients receiving AP at an integrative oncology clinic. There was reduction in prevalence rates of fatigue, pain, anxiety, physical distress, emotional distress, and poor quality of life.[42]

NEUROPATHIC PAIN

Tong et al. compared AP with sham to observe the effects on nerve conduction velocity and variety of subjective symptoms associated with diabetic peripheral neuropathy (DPN).[43] There were statistically significant improvements in motor and sensory function, and vibration perception threshold differences. AP was more effective for the treatment of numbness, spontaneous pain, and alterations in temperature perceptions after a 15-day treatment.[43] Garrow et al. enrolled 45 DPN patients for a 10-week course of real or sham AP. There were statistically significant improvements in VAS and sleep problem scale in the true AP group without major side effects.[44] Other investigators performed 4-week AP or standard treatment in herpes zoster (HZ) and reported no significant differences in response rates, mean reduction of VAS and McGill Pain Questionnaire scores, and incidence of PHN after 3 months.[45] The authors suggested AP for the treatment of acute HZ.[45] A meta-analysis showed that AP had a beneficial effect on neurological recovery, motor function, and functional recovery in spinal cord injury.[46]

UPDATES SINCE THE NIH CONSENSUS STATEMENT

A systemic review noted the different effects of MA, EA, and sham on CNS. Only studies comparing MA or EA with sham were eligible for this review: 17 fMRI, 6 electroencephalography (EEG), 5 evoked potentials (EP), and 5 positron emission tomography (PET) studies.[47] The authors proposed that verum (true) AP elicited either more or different modulations on neurological components than sham AP based on evaluation of the very heterogeneous results.[47]

The Society for Acupuncture Research (SAR) hosted an international conference in 2007 for the tenth anniversary of the landmark NIH Conference in 1997. The conference reported that the mechanistic models for AP effects were focused on the nervous system, muscles, and connective tissue. It advocated for future research models that could lead to a better understanding of manual AP (MA) and electrical AP (EA) effects.[48]

SUMMARY

Despite current data showing AP providing only temporary benefits, AP continues to play an important role as an adjunct to multimodal pain management by lowering analgesic dosages and risk of debilitating adverse effects. Most of the current literature on AP consists of anecdotal and biased information from case reports to clinical studies with suboptimal designs. The systematic review and meta-analysis of RCTs should be interpreted in the context of the identified limitations, particularly in relation to the heterogeneity in the study characteristics and the low methodological quality. Small sample size, scarcity of studies for comparison, and lack of ideal sham control all weaken the level of evidence and clinical implications. There is an enormous demand for future RCTs to explore the integration of AP to conventional pain medicine and to differentiate EA from MA and implications for clinical practice. Translational and clinical studies on AP based on recent basic publications will undoubtedly advance the role of AP in pain medicine.

KEY POINTS

- AP modulates pain by activating a mixture of bioactive chemicals (opioids, serotonin, and norepinephrine) through peripheral, spinal, and supraspinal mechanisms, and potentially reversing of neuroplasticity in animal models.
- EA of 2 Hz accelerates the release of enkephalin, beta-endorphin, and endomorphin, while EA of 100 Hz selectively increases the release of dynorphin.
- EA activates the nervous system differently in health and in various pain conditions, alleviates both sensory and affective inflammatory pain, and inhibits inflammatory and neuropathic pain more effectively at 2 and 10 Hz than at 100 Hz.
- Current data regarding the clinical efficacy of AP and related techniques has provided only short-lasting benefits in chronic pain management.
- The integrative medicine using EA maximized treatment efficacy by lowering conventional analgesic dosages and minimized the risk of debilitating adverse effects.
- AP is most likely to provide benefit in patients with neck pain, tension headache, migraines, OA of the knee, and LBP.
- Promising but less definitive data supports AP for myofascial pain, fibromyalgia, postoperative pain, dental pain, and functional bowel disorders.
- AP and related techniques may be considered in women's health for premenstrual syndrome, dysmenorrhea, and pregnancy-related conditions and early stages of labor.
- There is insufficient evidence for AP in neurological conditions, mental health, and rheumatoid arthritis.
- Nausea, pallor, dizziness, and syncope are vasovagal responses to AP. Drowsiness and generalized fatigue are common, especially in the beginning.
- Bleeding, hematoma, and needle discomfort may occur in AP; pneumothorax could be a serious complication requiring vigilant and timely treatment.
- There is no current standard of care in frequency, number, or optimal duration of AP treatment to determine success or failure in pain management.

REFERENCES

Access the reference list online at ExpertConsult.com.

CHAPTER 61

TAI CHI AND CHRONIC PAIN

David Flamer, MD, FRCPC ◎ Philip Peng, MBBS, FRCPC, Founder (Pain Med)

INTRODUCTION

Tai Chi is an ancient Chinese martial art and exercise that combines deep breathing and relaxation with slow and gentle movements.[1] It has been reported that Tai Chi has beneficial effects in a variety of physical and psychological health conditions, including specific chronic pain disorders.[2] The National Centre for Health Statistics in the United States estimates that up to 57% of Americans with chronic pain report significant ongoing limitation of their daily activities.[3] In addition to conventional medical therapies, complementary and alternative treatment options have become increasingly common.[4] Complementary and alternative medicine (CAM) practices are often grouped into two broad categories that include natural products and mind-body medicine (which is the category associated with Tai Chi). A number of investigators have examined the role of Tai Chi in various chronic pain conditions. This chapter will examine existing and recent literature on Tai Chi as it relates to chronic pain management.

PHILOSOPHY, HISTORY, AND DEVELOPMENT OF TAI CHI

The practice of Tai Chi is also referred to as Tai Chi Chuan, Taiji, or Taiji Quan.[2] The terms Chuan and Quan both translate to "fist," and the resulting term Tai Chi translates to "supreme ultimate fist." The practice of Tai Chi is rooted in both Confucianism and Taoism. Tai Chi is believed to be the driving force of the universe, and is composed of the two opposing forces—Yin and Yang—which form the symbol of the practice (Fig. 61.1). Ill health is viewed as an imbalance between Yin and Yang, and Tai Chi is believed to help rebalance such energy disturbances. The practice of Tai Chi involves the constant, slow transfer of body weight that reflects the simultaneous separation and merging of Yin and Yang energies. In Chinese culture, this internal energy of the body is referred to as *qi*, and Tai Chi aims to achieve a balance of *qi* in an effort to maintain balance and harmony.[5,6]

It is believed that Tai Chi was developed in the 12th century by Master Zhang San Feng, a Taoist priest. However, more recent historical sources assign the origin to Master Chen Wang Ting in the 17th century. As it evolved, Tai Chi differentiated into five main styles: Chen, Yang, Wu (Hao), Wu, and Sun. These styles share similarities in foundation, but vary regarding the approach to posture, pace, and order of movements.[7] The traditional art form is complex, and many simplified forms have been developed. In 1956 the Chinese government developed an abbreviated version of Tai Chi as an exercise that could be taught to the masses, which included 24 postures that could be performed in 4–5 minutes.[8,9]

Tai Chi has become a popular exercise worldwide. It is low cost, with no specific equipment or facilities needed. Requirements include a flat area of 4 m^2, loose clothing, and flat-heeled shoes. It can be practiced alone or in a group, and in an indoor or outdoor setting.[7]

TAI CHI HEALTH BENEFITS

PHYSICAL HEALTH BENEFITS

Physical Fitness, Musculoskeletal Strength, Balance

Tai Chi is considered an aerobic exercise of mild to moderate intensity, with considerable variations depending on training approaches, style, posture, speed, and experience of the practitioner.

The peak oxygen uptake is believed to be the best indicator for aerobic capacity and is one of the strongest predictors of the risk of death among normal subjects and patients with cardiovascular disease.[10] A study by Lan et al.[11] found that elderly Tai Chi practitioners had 18%–19% higher VO_{2peak} when compared with sedentary controls. Furthermore, a recent meta-analysis in 2008 found that Tai Chi may significantly improve aerobic capacity, with the greatest gains among middle-aged and older women.[12]

Tai Chi practice involves continuous weight shifting and body rotation, which increases the load on the lower limbs. As a result, Tai Chi has been shown to improve overall muscle strength and balance.[13–15] Jacobson et al.[13] found that subjects between ages 20 and 45 who practiced 3 times per week for 12 weeks had significantly increased strength of the knee extensors. Long-term Tai Chi has also shown to significantly decrease the latency of semitendinosis muscle.[16] The prevention of falls in the elderly depends on the timely initiation of a postural response, and it is believed that the improved muscle strength and response can contribute to improved overall balance. This is an important

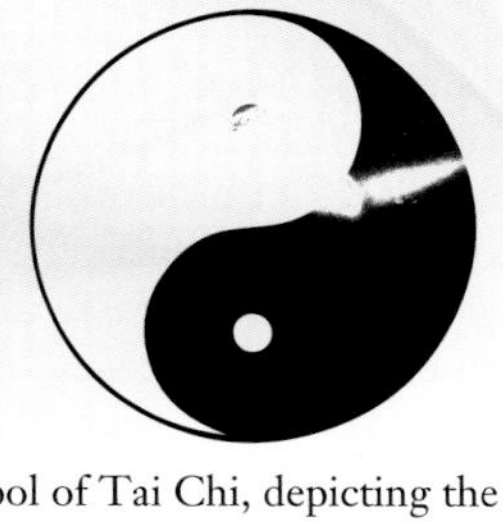

FIG. 61.1 The symbol of Tai Chi, depicting the close relationship of Yin and Yang.

health issue, as approximately 30% of community-living people aged 65 years and older experience a fall at some point in their lives, with approximately 20% of those requiring medical attention.[17] A recent systematic review and meta-analysis by Leung et al.[18] found that Tai Chi was effective in improving balance of older individuals, but its superiority to other interventions remains equivocal. Future research in this area is required.

PSYCHOLOGICAL BENEFITS

Mind-Body Control

It is well known that higher cognitive centers play an important role in nociception and pain perception.[19] *Attention* is a mechanism by which nociceptive information is processed and enters our awareness. Neurocognitive models postulate two distinct modes of attention ("top-down selection" and "bottom-up selection"), both of which are discussed in further detail outside of this chapter.[2,20,21] It is believed that the practice of Tai Chi may help an individual exert *executive control* over this nociceptive input, thus enhancing one's ability to cope, by improving either the top-down or bottom-up selection processes. Similarly, this concept may help an individual exert *executive control* over anticipated (or expected) nociceptive input that may arise. The use of imagery techniques and meditation strategies are some of the methods employed by Tai Chi for this purpose.[22,23]

Tai Chi is an excellent exercise for training the mind-body interaction. The fundamental teachings of Tai Chi emphasize the interrelationship of the mind and body: consciousness *(yi)* leads to the movement of energy *(qi)*, which in turn leads to the movement of the body.[24,25] Tai Chi demands synchronized and harmonious movements of the body. This requires concentration, focus, and awareness of both self and environment. When practiced correctly, the practitioner aims to feel the internal movement of energy *(qi)* like water flowing across the body. The use of visual imagery ("grasp the bird's tail" or "white crane spreads its wing") can help the user achieve this goal.

Emotional Well-Being

Epidemiologic and clinical studies have demonstrated a high prevalence of psychological comorbidities in patients with chronic pain.[26–31] A World Health Organization (WHO) survey of nearly 26,000 patients found that chronic pain sufferers exhibit a fourfold increase in the odds of having an anxiety or depressive disorder compared to those without chronic pain.[27] Tai Chi is a useful practice because it is safe to perform, with low physical and emotional risk, and allows patients to take a more active role in their care.[32]

A systematic review and meta-analysis by Wang et al.[33] evaluated the role of Tai Chi and psychological well-being. This review included 17 randomized controlled trials (RCTs) and approximately 3800 subjects. Tai Chi was found to be associated with reduced stress, anxiety, depression, and mood disturbance, and increased self-esteem. These improvements are thought to be related to both the mind-body interaction and the physical therapy components, which help amplify the psychological benefits.[34–36]

TAI CHI BENEFITS IN CHRONIC PAIN CONDITIONS

OSTEOARTHRITIS

Background

Osteoarthritis (OA) is one of the most common causes of pain and disability in older adults in Western countries.[37–38] OA causes pain and stiffness in the affected joint, and often results in significant limitation of daily activities and loss of independent function with progression over time.[39] Treatment modalities include pharmacologic, nonpharmacologic, and surgical options. Nonpharmacologic strategies focus on the importance of weight loss, exercise routines, and self-management programs that aim to improve pain, function, and psychological well-being.[40] Various exercise modalities have been investigated as potential treatment options, including walking, resistance training, and hydrotherapy.[41,42] Tai Chi has gained increasing popularity for patients with OA. A growing number of randomized controlled trials have evaluated its role in the OA population, and more recently, the American College of Rheumatology (ACR) guidelines have listed Tai Chi as a conditional recommendation for managing knee OA.[43]

Review of Evidence

The quality of studies reviewed in this chapter was evaluated using the Jadad score (Table 61.1), a validated tool assessing the study design and quality of reporting. The level of evidence was assessed with evidence statements and grades of recommendations from the US Department of Health and Human Services Agency for Health Care Policy and Research (Table 61.2). Seven RCTs (Table 61.3) have evaluated the efficacy of Tai Chi on patients with OA.[39,44–49] The duration of Tai Chi practice ranged from 6 to 20 weeks. As the practice of Tai Chi cannot be blinded, the maximum Jadad score achieved was 3. Out of the seven included RCTs, six reached a score of three, with the most recent RCT being of lower quality and achieving a score of 1. Five out of seven studies included patients with OA limited to the knee, and four of these five studies demonstrated a reduction in pain.

In summary, the results of these studies indicate that there is good evidence to suggest Tai Chi as a beneficial technique to reduce pain in the management of knee OA (level 1b, recommendation A). Other possible benefits include reduced stiffness, improved function, and enhanced mobility. Evidence is limited regarding the efficacy of Tai Chi in the management of patients with OA of other joints.

RHEUMATOID ARTHRITIS

Background

Rheumatoid arthritis (RA) is a systemic, chronic inflammatory disorder that has an incidence of 25–50 cases per 100,000 people.[50] RA can lead to considerable joint damage and disability, particularly if poorly managed. Treatment utilizes a multimodal approach, with goals to address pain, inflammation, disease progression, physical function, and psychological well-being.[51,52] Many of the novel

TABLE 61.1 Jadad Score

Study Characteristic	Score
Was the study described as randomized (this includes words such as randomly, random, and randomization)?	0/1
Was the method used to generate the sequence of randomization described and appropriate (table of random numbers, computer generated, etc)?	0/1
Was the study described as double-blind?	0/1
Was the method of double-blinding described and appropriate (identical placebo, active placebo, dummy, etc.)?	0/1
Was there a description of withdrawals and dropouts?	0/1
Deduct one point if the method used to generate the sequence of randomization was described and it was inappropriate (patients were allocated alternately, or according to date of birth, hospital number, etc.).	0/−1
Deduct one point if the study was described as double-blind but the method of blinding was inappropriate (e.g., comparison of tablet vs. injection with no double dummy).	0/−1

The first five items are indications of good study quality; a point is added for each criteria met. The last two items indicate poor study quality; a point is subtracted for each criteria met. The Jadad score therefore ranges from 0 to 5.
From Jadad AR, Moore RA, Carroll D, et al. Assessing the quality of reports of randomized clinical trials: is blinding necessary? Control Clin Trials. *17(1):1-12, 1996.*

TABLE 61.2 Key to Evidence Statements and Grades of Recommendations

Statements of Evidence	
Ia	Evidence obtained from meta-analysis of RCTs
Ib	Evidence obtained from at least one RCT
IIa	Evidence obtained from at least one well-designed controlled study without randomization
IIb	Evidence obtained from at least one other type of well-designed quasiexperimental study
III	Evidence obtained from well-designed nonexperimental descriptive studies, such as comparative studies, correlation studies, and case reports
IV	Evidence obtained from expert committee reports or opinions and/or clinical experiences of respected authorities
Grades of Recommendations	
A	Requires at least one prospective, randomized controlled trial as part of a body of literature of overall good quality and consistency addressing the specific recommendation (evidence levels Ia and Ib)
B	Requires the availability of well-conducted clinical studies, but no prospective, randomized clinical trials on the topic of recommendation (evidence levels IIa, IIb, III)
C	Requires evidence obtained from expert committee reports or opinions and/or clinical experiences of respected authorities; indicates an absence of directly applicable clinical studies of good quality (evidence level IV)

Source: US Department of Health and Human Services Agency for Health Care Policy and Research.

pharmacologic agents have minimized the rate of disease progression, but can have limited efficacy and numerous adverse effects.[52] Tai Chi is expected to be helpful in RA because of its known beneficial effects on muscle strength, bone health, and stress reduction.[53]

Review of Evidence

The evidence in support of Tai Chi for RA is less robust when compared to OA. To date, two RCTs have been published.[54,55] Both of these studies are of low quality (Jadad score 2), small sample size, and do not identify a reduction in pain. More recently, there have been two nonrandomized studies that have demonstrated positive findings.[56,57] Waite-Jones et al.[56] demonstrated an improvement in psychological well-being in those who practiced Tai Chi, with specific reductions in anxiety, depression, and self-esteem. Uhlig et al.[57] found improvements in lower limb muscle function at the completion of 12 weeks of Tai Chi practice.

In summary, there is limited evidence to support the role of Tai Chi as a beneficial technique to reduce pain in the management of RA. Further high-quality RCTs are necessary.

FIBROMYALGIA

Background

Fibromyalgia (FM) is a chronic, multisymptomatic pain illness with significant functional limitations.[58] The global prevalence of FM has been estimated at 2.7%.[59] The range of symptoms can include widespread musculoskeletal pain, fatigue, poor sleep, and associated mood disorders. Furthermore, studies show that patients with FM have a decreased efficacy of descending pain inhibitory mechanisms—diffuse noxious inhibitory control (DNIC) or conditioned pain modulation (CPM).[60,61] DNIC is important, as it can act to modulate ascending nociceptive signals through opioid or nonopioid receptors.[61] The treatment approach is multidisciplinary and involves a combination of pharmacologic therapy for specific symptoms, as well as nonpharmacologic options such as lifestyle changes, exercise, patient education, and self-help.[62–64] The goals of therapy are to restore function and improve both psychological and somatic symptoms.[62] Tai Chi may have benefit in treating FM through three distinct mechanisms: (1) an exercise component to address physical function, (2) mind-body control to address the deficit in DNIC that may exist, and (3) as a meditation/breathing component to address psychological well-being.

Review of Evidence

There are two RCTs evaluating the beneficial effects of Tai Chi in FM.[58,65] Both assess the effects of a 12-week course of Tai Chi compared with control groups of education alone or education combined with stretching (Table 61.4). Both of these studies demonstrated significant improvement in the Tai Chi groups in various domains, including reduction in FM Impact Questionnaire Scores, reduced Brief Pain Inventory (BPI) severity scores, improved patient and physician global assessment in pain, and improved physical and mental components of SF-36 (36-item Short Form Health Survey). Wang et al.[65] found that these effect sizes were even larger than those from FDA-approved pharmacotherapy, including antidepressants, gabapentoids, and milnacipran.

More recently, two nonrandomized studies have demonstrated beneficial effects in patients with FM.[66,67] Romero-Zurita et al.[66] found that a 28-week course of Tai Chi could improve pain, functional capacity, and psychological

TABLE 61.3 Published RCTs for Tai Chi Intervention in Osteoarthritis

First Author/Year	Osteoarthritis Regions; Total Number of Patients Randomized/Analyzed	Jadad Score/ AC/Blind Assessor	Tai Chi Intervention	Control	Pain Outcome	Other Outcomes	Remarks
Hartman/2000	Multiple; 35/33	3/–/–	Yang; 2/week/12 weeks	Routine care and usual physical activity	NS—ASE	↑ Arthritis self-efficacy ↑ Satisfaction general health (AIMS) ↓ Tension (AIMS)	Baseline ↑ Arthritis pain in TC group
Song/2003	Knee: 72/43	3/+/–	Sun; 3/week; 12 weeks	Routine treatment	↓ Pain-K-WOMAC	↓ Stiffness, ↑ physical functioning K-WOMAC ↑ Balance	
Brismee/2007	Knee; 41/39	3/–/+	Yang; 3/week for 6 weeks; home Tai Chi 6 weeks	Attention control program[a]	↓ Overall and maximum pain-↓ VAS	↑ Overall and physical function in WOMAC	
Fransen[b]/2007	Hip/knee; 97/97[c]	3/+/+	Sun; 2/week; 12 weeks	Wait list	NS-WOMAC	↑ Physical function in WOMAC; better timed stair climb	Three groups in comparison with hydrotherapy
Wang/2009	Knee; 40/40[c]	3/+/+	Yang; 2/week; 12 weeks	Attention control program[a]	↓ Pain-WOMAC	↑ Physical function in WOMAC, patient, and physician global VAS; ↑ balance, SF-36 PCS; ↓ CES-D	
Tsai/2012	Knee; 28/27[c]	3/+/+	Sun; 3/week; 20 weeks	Attention control Program[a]	↓ Pain-WOMAC (From week 9)	↓ Stiffness-WOMAC (from week 17) NS-function-WOMAC and MMSE	
Wortley[d]/2013	Knee; 39/31	1/–/–	Yang; 2/week; 10 weeks	Usual physical activity	NS—WOMAC	↑ Mobility	Additional third group with resistance training

[a]*Attention control program: referred to lectures in health topics in Brismee's study and to wellness education and stretching exercise in Wang's study, health education, culture-related and social activities in Tsai study.*
[b]*In Fransen's study, the third group (hydrotherapy group) was not included.*
[c]*Intent-to-treat statistical analysis.*
[d]*In Wortley's study, the third group (resistance training group) was not included.*
AC, *Allocation concealment;* AIMS, *arthritis impact measure scales;* ASE, *arthritis self-efficacy, questions are scored on a Likert scale from 0 to 100, with higher scores representing greater self-efficacy;* CES-D, *scores on the Centre for Epidemiologic Studies—Depression index ranging from 0 to 60, with higher scores indicating more dysphoria;* K-WOMAC, *WOMAC in Korean;* MMSE, *mini-mental state examination—a 30-point questionnaire to screen cognitive impairment;* NS, *no significant difference;* PCS, *physical component summary of SF-36;* SF-36, *medical outcomes study 36-item short-form health survey is a self-administered, 36-item questionnaire that assesses the concepts of physical functioning, role limitations due to physical problems, social function, bodily pain, general mental health, role limitations due to emotional problems, vitality, and general health perceptions (scores range from 0 to 100, with higher scores indicating better health status);* TC, *Tai Chi; Universities Osteoarthritis Index, scores are standardized to a 0–100 range, with higher scores indicating greater pain or physical disability;* VAS, *visual analog scale;* WOMAC, *Western Ontario and McMaster.*
Adapted with modification from Peng PWH: Tai Chi and Chronic Pain. Reg Anesth Pain Med. *37(4):372-382, 2012.*

TABLE 61.4 Published RCTs on Other Pain Conditions

Diagnosis: Patients Randomized/ Analyzed	First Author/ Year	Jadad Score/ Allocation[a]/ Blind Assessor	Tai Chi Intervention	Control	Pain Outcome[b]	Other Outcomes	Remarks
Fibromyalgia: 66/66[c]	Wang/2010	3/+/+	Yang; 2/week; 12 weeks	Wellness education and stretching exercise	↓ FIQ	↑ Sleep (PSQI), SF-36 (MCS, PCS), global assessment by patient and physician; mood (CES-D), CPSS	All improvement maintained at 24 weeks except CPSS
Fibromyalgia: 101/98[c]	Jones/2012	3/+/+	Yang; 2/week; 12 weeks	Education intervention	↓ FIQ	↓ BPI-pain severity and BPI-pain interference ↑ Self-efficacy. ↑ Functional variables: • static balance • dynamic balance • timed get up and go	
Rheumatoid arthritis: 20/20	Wang/2008	2/–/+	Yang; 2/week; 12 weeks	Wellness education and stretching exercise	VAS, HAQ-NS	↑ Mood (CES-D), ↑ vitality (SF-36); ↓ disability (HAQ)	
Rheumatoid arthritis: 42/31	Lee/2005	2/–/–	Sun; 1/week; 6 weeks	Usual activity	VAS-NS	↑ Mood (profile of mood state)	
Low back pain:160/160[c]	Hall/2011	3/+/–	Sun; 2/week for 8 weeks, 1/week for 2 weeks	Wait list	↓ Pain bothersome	↓ PDI, RMDQ, QBPDS, PSFS	
Low back pain; 320/304	Weifen/2011	3/+/+	Chen; 5/week; 24 weeks	Exercise and usual activity	↓ VAS at 3, 6 months (not when compared with swimming subgroup)		Exercise group subdivided into backward walking, jogging, and swimming groups
Tension-type headache: 47/30 [176]	Abbott/2007	2/–/–	Yang; 2/week; 15 weeks	Wait list	↓ HIT-6	↑ SF-36-MCS	

[a] *Allocation concealment.*

[b] *In certain pain conditions, the principal outcome measurement is not by the pain intensity but a well-validated composite score such as FIQ in fibromyalgia and HIT-6 in tension-type headache.*

[c] *The study was analyzed based on the intent-to-treat analysis.*

BPI, *Brief pain inventory;* CES-D, *Centre for Epidemiology Studies-Depression index;* CPSS, *Chronic Pain Self-efficacy Scale;* FIQ, *fibromyalgia impact questionnaire;* HAQ, *health assessment questionnaire and includes pain in the past week (15-cm VAS that is scored 0–3);* HIT-6, *Headache Impact Test - 6;* MCS, *mental component summary of SF-36;* NS, *no significant difference;* PCS, *physical component summary of SF-36;* PDI, *pain disability index;* PSFS, *Patient-Specific Functional Scale;* PSQI, *Pittsburgh Sleep Quality Index;* QBPDS, *Quebec Back Pain Disability Scale;* RMDQ, *Roland-Morris disability questionnaire;* SF-36, *medical outcomes study 36-item short-form health survey;* VAS, *visual analog scale.*

Reproduced with permission from Peng PWH: Tai Chi and Chronic Pain. Reg Anesth Pain Med. *37(4):372-382, 2012.*

outcomes (FIQ and SF-36). Likewise, Segura-Jimenez et al.[67] demonstrated decreased levels of acute pain in patients who participated in a 12-week course of Tai Chi. Overall, evidence suggests that Tai Chi is an effective modality in FM patients not only for pain relief but also for improving physical function and optimizing emotional well-being (Level Ib, Recommendation A).

CHRONIC LOW BACK PAIN

Background

Chronic low back pain is the most prevalent musculoskeletal disorder.[3,68] It is estimated that greater than 80% of adults have suffered from low back pain at least once in their lives.[69] Treatment strategies are multidisciplinary. A variety of nonpharmacologic options are recommended, with the exercise components of stretching and strengthening as being the most predictive for positive outcomes.[70] The low-impact and moderate intensity exercise of Tai Chi has been found to improve muscle strength and joint flexibility, and for these reasons it has been recommended as a CAM modality for patients suffering from chronic low back pain.[71]

Review of Evidence

There are two RCTs evaluating the role of Tai Chi in patients with chronic low back pain,[72,73] and one RCT involving subjects with acute low back pain.[74] The study published by Hall et al.[72] was well-conducted and included 160 patients that were randomized to either 10 weeks of Tai Chi or to the wait-list group. There was improvement in back pain symptoms, as well as health-related quality of life, mood, and cognition (Rolland-Morris Disability Questionnaire, Pain Disability Index, Quebec Back Pain, and Patient-Specific Functional Scale). The second RCT evaluating chronic low back pain was of poor quality and involved a population of 320 "retired athletes" who were randomized to either Tai Chi or exercise control groups.[73] Results indicated improved pain scores in the Tai Chi group compared with the majority of exercise subgroup controls.

Cho et al.[74] evaluated the effects of Tai Chi in 40 young males with acute low back pain (duration of symptoms not defined). Subjects were randomized to 4 weeks of Tai Chi or a stretching control group. Results indicated improved pain scores in the Tai Chi group, indicating a role for Tai Chi in this patient population.

Overall, although there are limited quality studies evaluating the role of Tai Chi in chronic low back pain, evidence suggests that it can improve pain and disability (Level 1b, Recommendation A).

TENSION-TYPE HEADACHE

Background

Tension-type headache (TTH) represents approximately 78% of all headaches.[75] Symptoms include a tightening bandlike sensation around the head, with associated pressure and pain, and are generally bilateral. Treatment options include pharmacotherapy (muscle relaxants, analgesics) and nonpharmacologic modalities (relaxation, massage, biofeedback, stress reduction).[76] It is believed that the mind-body interaction of Tai Chi may help enhance relaxation and improve headache-related disability.

Review of Evidence

One RCT has evaluated the role of Tai Chi in patients with TTH.[76] Abbott et al.[76] randomized subjects to receive either 15 weeks of Tai Chi or to the wait-list control group. Participation after randomization was low, with only 30 of 47 patients completing the study. Of those involved, the Tai Chi group demonstrated significant improvements in Headache Impact Test 6 score and the pain, energy/fatigue, social functioning, emotional well being, and mental health survey summary scores in the SF-36.

Overall, definitive conclusions regarding the beneficial effects of Tai Chi in the headache population cannot be made based on available literature. More high-quality studies are recommended.

LIMITATIONS OF EVIDENCE

The practice of Tai Chi poses inherent challenges in designing a scientific study.[77] When designing a study that involves mind-body interaction, one must consider the ability to perform a double-blinded assessment. This technique is impractical, as participants will be aware of which group they are assigned to. Furthermore, designing a "sham" Tai Chi practice, where a researcher may attempt to separate the mind-body interaction, will undoubtedly affect the integrity of the study. Another significant challenge lies in the heterogeneity of the various Tai Chi practice styles. Intensity, posture, and duration of practice are all important factors that will influence outcome comparisons. Finally, instructors or masters will each have vastly different experiences and teaching styles, which will also influence the therapeutic outcomes.

FUTURE RESEARCH

The interest in the role of Tai Chi in treating various health conditions, including specific chronic pain disorders, has grown considerably. There continues to be an expanding body of research aimed at investigating its beneficial effects. However, the amount of high-quality studies is limited, with many of the RCTs being associated with a high risk of bias. Given the inherent challenge in performing double-blind trials, well-conducted single-blind studies are reasonable. Developing a standardized protocol of Tai Chi practice that could be used for comparative studies would be worthwhile.

Recently, a systematic review about the safety of Tai Chi practice was conducted by Wayne et al.[78] There were a total of 153 eligible RCTs identified, with only 18 of these trials reporting an explicit adverse event monitoring protocol. It is reassuring to both practitioners and patients alike that no serious intervention-related adverse events were found. Future studies on this topic are encouraged and should be extended to other common chronic pain conditions, such as neuropathic pain and neck pain.

CONCLUSION

Tai Chi is an ancient Chinese martial art that integrates mind-body interaction with gentle, coordinated movements of the upper and lower limbs. Previous literature supports the role of Tai Chi in physical health promotion, with improvements in muscle strength, coordination, balance, and bone density. The psychological components of Tai Chi are associated with reduced stress, anxiety, and depression, and an improved self-esteem. Aside from minor musculoskeletal aches and pains, it is unlikely to result in serious adverse events. High-quality evidence supports the effectiveness of Tai Chi in OA, FM, and chronic low back pain. Evidence for its role in other chronic pain conditions is limited, and future high-quality trials are required.

KEY POINTS

- Tai Chi is an ancient Chinese martial art that combines gentle physical movements of the upper and lower limbs with meditation and breathing.
- Tai Chi is practiced as a mild to moderate aerobic exercise and has become a popular CAM practice.
- Aside from minor musculoskeletal aches and pains, the practice of Tai Chi is unlikely to result in serious adverse events.
- Evidence supports the role of Tai Chi in physical health promotion, with improvements in muscle strength, coordination, balance, and bone density.
- Psychological benefits of Tai Chi include reduced stress, anxiety, depression, and an improved self-esteem.
- High-quality evidence supports the effectiveness of Tai Chi in OA, FM, and chronic low back pain.

REFERENCES

Access the reference list online at ExpertConsult.com.

SECTION VIII

INTERVENTIONAL TECHNIQUES FOR PAIN MANAGEMENT

SECTION OUTLINE HEAD

CHAPTER 62

Interlaminar Epidural Steroid Injections

Indy Wilkinson, MD ◎ Steven P. Cohen, MD

INTRODUCTION

Back pain is the leading cause of disability worldwide,[1] with an estimated financial burden exceeding $100 billion annually in the United States alone.[2] Most cases of back pain seen in the primary care setting are acute and axial, attributable to muscular and ligamentous strain and spasm. But patients who are referred to the pain medicine specialist typically suffer from pain that is chronic and more complex in nature. Chronic spine pain arises from an array of often overlapping etiologies and, in many cases, exhibits a radicular component, with epidemiologic studies estimating approximately 40% to be predominantly neuropathic in nature.[3] Although randomized, controlled studies have demonstrated that epidural steroid injections (ESIs) may alleviate axial spine pain,[4–8] it is widely acknowledged that it is most effective in the treatment of radicular pain, particularly pain arising from a herniated disc.[3]

Radicular pain, also known by the ambiguous and misleading term *sciatica*, can be caused by several distinct conditions, but by far its most common causes are herniated disc and spinal stenosis. Disc herniation, or the extrusion of disc material from the nucleus pulposus beyond the limits of the intervertebral disc space, results in the liberation of inflammatory mediators near spinal nerve roots.[9] A combination of chemical and mechanical factors may serve to irritate adjacent exposed nerve root(s), causing radiating pain that is often described as tingling, burning, or electrical in nature. The prevalence of disc disruption in patients with chronic low back pain is high and has been reported to be near 40%.[10–12] Whereas 95% of all disc herniation occurs in the lumbar spine at L4-5 or L5-S1, the cervical spine can also be affected, most commonly at C6-7.[13]

Spinal stenosis, or the progressive narrowing of the spinal canal, may occur alone or in conjunction with disc herniation. Spinal stenosis can be congenital (i.e., short pedicles) but is most frequently caused by degenerative changes of the spinal anatomy, which may include thickening and buckling of the ligamentum flavum, facet hypertrophy, osteophyte formation, or a combination of these conditions.[14] A narrowed central spinal canal results in compression-induced ischemia of the spinal cord (in the neck) and/or cauda equina.[15] The incidence of spinal stenosis increases with age, with the prevalence among patients aged 60–69 years documented to be as high as 47% for mild to moderate stenosis and 19% for severe stenosis (defined as a spinal canal anteroposterior diameter of less than 12 mm).[16] The most common vertebral levels affected by spinal stenosis are L4-5 in the lumbar spine[17] and C5-6 in the neck.[18]

Physicians have performed therapeutic epidural injections for well over 100 years in an effort to treat a wide scope of conditions.[19] Until the first epidural injection of corticosteroids was performed in 1952, these procedures utilized an injectate of plain local anesthetic (LA) solution.[20] In this case study published by Robecchi and Capra,[20] hydrocortisone was injected through the S1 posterior sacral foramen in an effort to treat lumbar radicular pain. Since that time, the procedure has evolved, and the sacral route, though still utilized,[21] has largely been supplanted in favor of the more targeted and accessible caudal, lumbar, and cervical techniques.[22,23] Today, ESIs are the most frequently performed procedures by interventional pain physicians worldwide and have been the subject of dozens of reviews and guidelines.[3] Despite its extensive study, the resulting body of data has been largely conflicting in terms of procedural efficacy, polarizing health care professionals on its utility and casting a shadow on the future of the procedure.

TECHNIQUE

The performance of interlaminar ESI (ILESI) requires directing a needle at the midline or paramedian interlaminar space closest to the site of pathology. The needle must pass through the skin, subcutaneous fat, supraspinous ligament, interspinous ligament, and ligamentum flavum to enter the epidural space. The loss-of-resistance (LOR) technique, where manual pressure is applied to the plunger as the needle is advanced through the spinous ligaments, exploits the palpable difference in resistance between the thick fibrous ligamentum flavum and the vacuous potential epidural space. Typically, a 17- or 18-gauge Tuohy needle is used. Smaller 20-gauge needles have been advocated to optimize patient comfort and decrease the risk of spinal headache, but they have been found to be more technically difficult to use and less accurate than their larger counterparts.[24]

Studies analyzing the accuracy of epidural needle positioning have found that extradural injection occurs in up to 30% of patients in whom blind placement is attempted, even in the hands of experienced proceduralists,[25,26] compared with very accurate and precise placement using confirmatory fluoroscopy.[27] A multicenter, retrospective analysis of cervical epidurograms by Stojanovic et al. observed a 53% rate of false LOR during the first attempt to enter the epidural space and determined that the use of epidurography can improve the accuracy of needle placement and medication delivery.[28] Whereas blind ESI is still performed in some places, the use of fluoroscopic guidance has been found to provide superior accuracy and safety and has become the standard of care.[29,30]

Even without the use of real-time fluoroscopic guidance, the inherent margin of safety of lumbar ILESI is relatively high due in part to the diameter of the lumbar epidural space (4–7 mm)[31] and the free mobility of the cauda equina (Fig. 62.1). However, at the cervical level the small diameter of the cervical epidural space (1–4 mm) and other factors increase the risk for catastrophic complications associated with inadvertent dural puncture.[32,33] The 2015 Multi-society Pain Workgroup guidelines state that cervical ESI should not be attempted above C6-7.[34] Because of this consideration, some physicians employ the “hanging drop” or “infusion drip” technique. In this method, whereby a column of saline is attached to the epidural needle via intravenous tubing, entry into the epidural space is theoretically confirmed when the negative pressure of the potential space causes the meniscus of the hanging fluid to drop into the tubing.

Despite the notional advantages of this technique, studies have not borne out any evidence of increased safety as compared with LOR.[35,36] This finding may stem from the fact that the epidural pressure on which this technique depends is not intrinsically negative. A study comparing 30 cervical epidural pressures found them to be highly dependent upon patient positioning, with the vast majority being positive in both the sitting and prone positions.[37]

In the neck, the ligamentum flavum is incompletely fused at the midline, with an incidence of gaps between C3 and T2 of 83%–100%.[38,39] The absence of this fibrous harbinger of the epidural space has been theorized to account for incidents of inadvertent subarachnoid puncture even with proper use of the LOR technique.[40] A prospective, randomized comparative study by Joo and colleagues compared the pressure changes throughout the pathway to the cervical epidural space between the midline and paramedian approaches.[41] The investigators found that an abrupt pressure decrease at the moment of exiting the ligamentum flavum was more frequently observed when the paramedian approach was being used and concluded that this is a superior technique when employed for cervical ESI[41] (Fig. 62.2).

The caudal technique involves introducing a needle at the sacral hiatus via the sacrococcygeal ligament into the epidural space (Fig. 62.3). The hiatus may be located by palpation or lateral fluoroscopic imaging, and the needle is advanced until it is felt to penetrate the membrane that encloses the hiatus with an abrupt LOR. Advantages attributed to this approach are its ease of use, particularly in cases of altered anatomy, and a decreased risk of dural puncture and consequent intrathecal injection.

Because of the distance from the site of injection to the site of lumbar pathology, caudal injections require a substantially larger volume of fluid to be injected as compared with lumbar ESI. Whereas historical volume recommendations vary from 10 to 64 mL,[42–44] a study by Kim and colleagues used fluoroscopy to determine that 10 mL of injectate was sufficient to reach the L3-4 interspace.[45] The investigators observed that after the initial injection of 10 mL, serial injections of up to 40 mL achieved additional spread of only one level cephalad. Despite the purported ease of the caudal technique, studies evaluating the accuracy of landmark-guided injections have demonstrated failure of the injectate to reach the epidural space in up to 35% of cases,[46,47] signifying the need for fluoroscopic guidance with this technique as well. Each of the three ESI methods is associated with unique advantages and disadvantages that must be understood and tailored to the individual patient (Table 62.1).

INJECTATE COMPOSITION

The most commonly employed and best-studied steroids used in ESI are methylprednisolone and triamcinolone

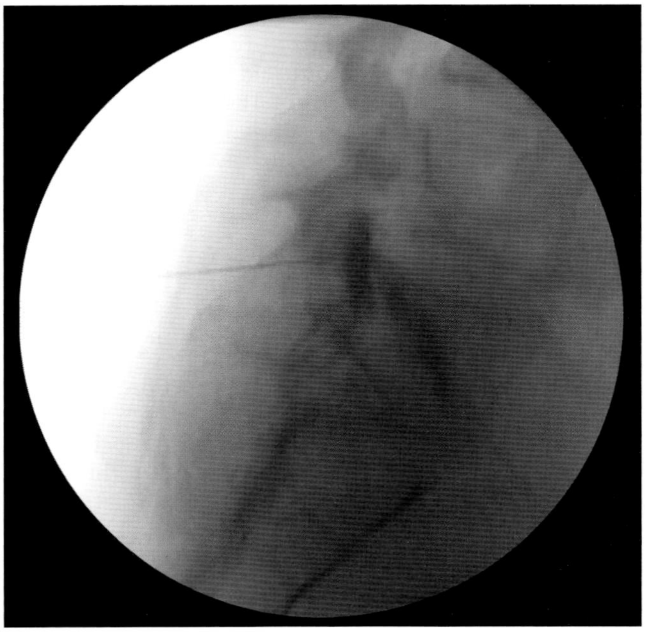

FIG. 62.1 Lateral fluoroscopic view demonstrating contrast spread during an L5-S1 interlaminar epidural steroid injection.

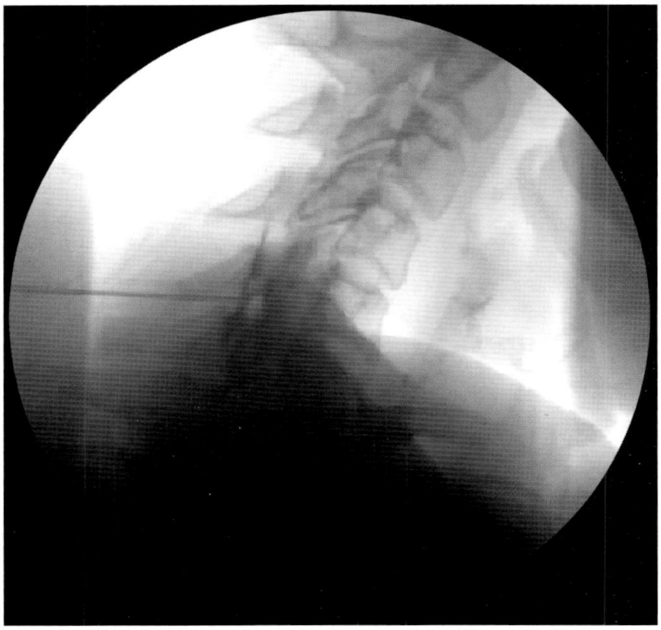

FIG. 62.2 Lateral fluoroscopic view demonstrating contrast spread during a C5-6 cervical epidural steroid injection. For safety concerns and because of the increased spread in the cervical epidural space compared with the lumbar region, higher levels (e.g., C6-7 and C7-T1) should generally be targeted.

diacetate. The therapeutic ESI dose range for both medications is typically 40–80 mg, although three randomized trials comparing 40 mg with 80 mg all found no difference in effectiveness.[48–50] No large-scale studies have been performed comparing triamcinolone and methylprednisolone, although one small, nonrandomized study found methylprednisolone to be more effective.[51] An area of intense interest, especially for transforaminal (TF) ESI, centers around the use of nonparticulate steroids. Although some studies have found comparable benefit between depo-steroids and soluble dexamethasone, the two largest studies have demonstrated greater effectiveness for depo-steroids.[52,53] The reduced risk of embolic phenomenon[54] and damage to the blood-brain barrier[55] cited for the use of nondepo-steroids does not apply to interlaminar injections, and the Multi-Society Pain Workgroup guidelines endorse the use of depo-steroids as a first-line treatment for interlaminar ESI.[56]

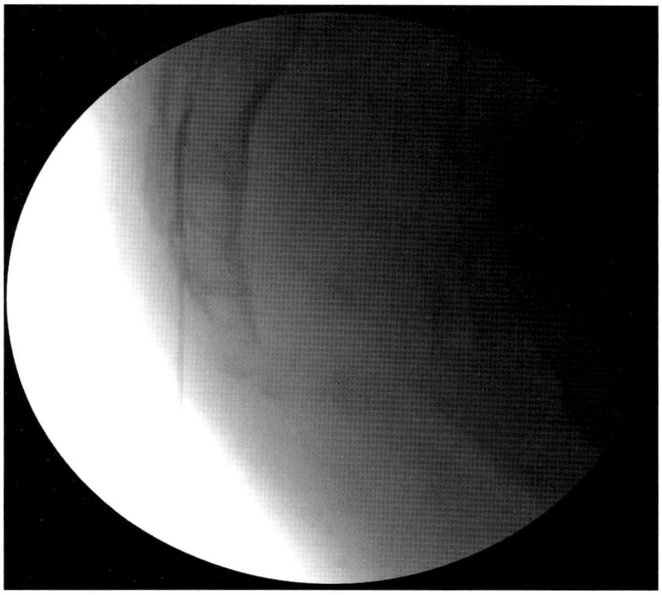

FIG. 62.3 Lateral fluoroscopic view demonstrating caudal epidural steroid injection. The caudal approach is often employed when an epidural steroid injection is performed after low back surgery to reduce the risk of dural puncture and in performing epidural lysis of adhesions.

Although one might surmise that higher injectate volumes may dilute the steroid concentration from epidural injections targeted to the level of pathology and result in inferior outcomes, this is not the case. A systematic review by Rabinovitch et al. found that higher volumes resulted in significantly better outcomes in the short (6 weeks to 3 months) and intermediate (3 months to 1 year) terms than lower volumes, controlling for the dose of steroid.[57] Studies evaluating the spread of lumbar ILESI injectate have found that volumes of 3–5 mL reach a median of two vertebral levels.[58–60] A study of cervical ESI by Stojanovic et al. found that a 2-mL injectate achieved an average spread of 3.14 vertebral levels.[28] The greater degree of spread observed is likely a result of the smaller volume of the cervical epidural space compared with that of more caudal levels. Goel and colleagues found that the injection of 2–4 mL in the cervical epidural space resulted in an average spread of 3.75 vertebral levels,[61] whereas a study by Lee et al. found that injecting contrast volumes of 2.5, 5, and 10 mL resulted in spread to 8.3, 11, and 13.6 levels, respectively.[62] If a caudal route is selected, larger volumes (approximately 10–20 mL) should be used to ensure adequate spread to the levels of pathology.[63] In a study of caudal epidural flow patterns by Cleary et al., an injectate volume of 20 mL reached a median segmental level of L3 with a range of T9 to L5,[64] leading investigators to conclude that the caudal route should not be recommended for the treatment of disease pathology above L3.

MECHANISM(S) OF ACTION

Numerous theories have been proposed to explain the analgesic mechanism of action of ESI. The oldest and best supported among these attributes epidural analgesia to the antiinflammatory properties of corticosteroids. Inflammation and nociception share two key biochemical pathways, the lipoxygenase and cyclooxygenase pathways, which result in the formation of leukotrienes, prostaglandins, and

TABLE 62.1 Differences in Approaches to Epidural Steroid Injection

Transforaminal	Caudal	Interlaminar
Direct deposition near ventral epidural space at affected level	Inject through sacral hiatus, far from pathology	Inject at affected level in dorsal epidural space
Risks high, especially in cervical and thoracic regions	Lowest risks; only for radiculopathy	Low risks, most likely to result in spinal headache; can be used anywhere
Requires fluoroscopy	Fluoroscopy may be helpful but not necessary	Fluoroscopy assures correct level and spread
Greater risks and challenges in FBSS, especially fusions and instrumentations	Surgery has no effect on anatomy; used for epidural lysis of adhesions in FBSS	Difficult and increased risk with prior surgery
Used for unilateral symptoms	Unilateral or bilateral symptoms	Unilateral or bilateral symptoms
Low volumes used and often sufficient	Requires high volumes	Intermediate volumes; higher volumes associated with better outcomes
More expensive; can bill for more than one level despite no evidence supporting this	Single injection sufficient	Single injection sufficient
Higher efficacy	Efficacy similar to ILESI	Efficacy similar to caudal

FBSS, *Failed back surgery syndrome;* ILESI, *interlaminar epidural steroid injection.*

thromboxanes, respectively. These biochemical mediators serve to promote both direct nociception and inflammation-induced pain. The inflammatory enzyme phospholipase A2 converts membrane phospholipids into arachidonic acid, an important substrate in both pathways that is found in high concentrations in intervertebral discs.[65] This finding could explain why conditions causing the extrusion of disc contents result in an inflammatory-mediated chronic pain syndrome.

Exogenous glucocorticoids directly inhibit the lipoxygenase pathway, resulting in diminished downstream formation of leukotrienes. In addition, cells exposed to glucocorticoids release lipomodulin, a phospholipase A2-inhibitory glycoprotein that downregulates the formation of arachidonic acid and consequently its downstream pronociceptive and inflammatory metabolites. Steroid preparations inhibit the inflammatory process at a step antecedent to that blocked by nonsteroidal antiinflammatory drugs (NSAIDs). This has a theoretical advantage in patients with a chemical rather than a mechanical radicular pain syndrome and negative radiologic studies.

In addition to the antiinflammatory theory, several alternate or complementary mechanisms of action have been postulated. Corticosteroids have been found to directly suppress the ectopic discharge of injured neurons.[66,67] Indirectly, exogenous glucocorticoids have been shown to reduce collagen deposition and its subsequent scar formation.[68,69] A lower scar tissue burden has the theoretical benefit of reducing mechanical pressure on posttraumatic nerve roots. The addition of LA, which has been utilized in the majority of clinical trials evaluating epidural steroids, may alleviate pain by enhancing blood flow to ischemic nerve roots, which may be particularly important in individuals with neurogenic claudication.[70] In addition, as noted earlier, high volumes of injectate may alleviate pain by washing out inflammatory mediators such as cytokines and chemokines.

Another documented effect of steroid administration is the reduction of capillary wall permeability, leading to a reduction in the formation of edema.[71] On the genomic level, glucocorticoids bind to an intracellular receptor, forming a glucocorticoid-receptor complex that translocates to the cell nucleus and transcriptionally activates (transactivation) or represses (transrepression) genes involved in the inflammatory pathway.[72] This mechanism has been shown to impact the expression of more than 6500 genes.[73]

EFFICACY

Despite extensive study of the efficacy of ILESI, the literature has failed to produce a consensus opinion on the subject. Even when studies that are retrospective, unblinded, and/or lacking a control group are excluded, efficacy data remain frustratingly variable (Table 62.2). The lack of unanimity can be at least partially attributed to the enormous challenges investigators face in designing protocols.

Even in higher-quality studies, patient populations are often poorly defined and lack homogeneity. Subjects suffering from acute, chronic, and postsurgical back pain secondary to various etiologies are often pooled into collective cohorts without controlling for their significant differences. Treatment protocols, measurement tools, follow-up observations and outcome criteria all lack standardization, so interpretation of the mixed data often falls to expert opinion.

This too is fraught with uncertainty, as different investigators reviewing the same literature have come to contradictory conclusions. In some cases, this discrepancy can be accredited to bias, such as the fact that those with an interventional background are 3 times more likely to ascribe success to the procedure than those who do not perform ESI.[3,90] In other cases, efficacy determination is closely tied to the reviewer's definition of procedural success.

Pain relief, though the primary goal of ESI, is but one measure of efficacy. Other surrogate markers include functional capacity, opioid reduction, return to work,[91] and prevention of surgery. Studies evaluating improvement in functional capacity have met with mixed results, and those finding relative improvement in ESI groups showed that patients with the worst self-reported health-related quality of life had the greatest improvement.[92,93] Investigators searching for a reduction in opioid intake following ESI have also found conflicting data, as both ESI and control groups have been shown to experience a decline in analgesic intake.[94]

In controlling for etiology, randomized studies of comparative effectiveness have generally found that ESI reduces opioid consumption for within-group but not between-group comparisons in patients suffering from herniated disc,[95,96] failed back surgery syndrome,[75,97] discogenic spine pain,[98,99] and lumbosacral spinal stenosis.[85,100,101] Whereas a majority of clinical trials have failed to report a significant difference between return-to-work rates or missed work days when ESI and control groups are compared,[81,83,89,102] some studies suggest that in well-selected patient groups, ESI may improve work status.[80,103,104] In a review of 26 randomized controlled trials (RCTs), moderate evidence was found in support of ESI as a surgery-sparing intervention for up to 1 year but not thereafter.[105]

Comparative-effectiveness studies are more clinically relevant than efficacy studies and are a cornerstone of the Affordable Care Act's research priorities. In a randomized double-blind comparative efficacy study, ESI performed via the IL and TF routes were found to be superior to gabapentin in some outcome measures—such as a reduction in worst leg pain at 1 month—but the differences were modest thereafter.[106] In an open-label, comparative-effectiveness study comparing a series of cervical ILESIs, conservative treatment consisting of first-line adjuvants and physical therapy or a combination of the two approaches in patients with cervical radiculopathy, the combination group fared better than the two stand-alone treatments for up to 6 months.[107] Whereas all randomized trials that occurred before 1999 focused solely on IL procedures, many subsequent studies feature either solely TFESI or a combination of the two.[108]

Wilson-MacDonald and colleagues performed a randomized, controlled trial evaluating 93 patients with radiologic evidence of disc herniation, spinal stenosis, or a combination of the two.[84] The experimental group received ILESI of 40 mg bupivacaine 0.5% with 80 mg methylprednisolone, while the control group received

TABLE 62.2 Randomized Studies Evaluating the Efficacy of Interlaminar and Caudal Epidural Steroid Injections

Study	Design	Patients	Treatments	Results
Stav et al. (1993)[5]	Randomized descriptive	50 patients with chronic neck and arm pain of greater than 6 months' duration	Treatment group, 1–3 cervical ILESI of 80 mg methylprednisolone and 5 mL 1% lidocaine; control group, intramuscular injection of 80 mg methylprednisolone and 5 mL 1% lidocaine	68% had good to very good relief after cervical ESI vs. 12% after intramuscular injection at 1-year follow-up
Castagnera et al. (1994)[74]	Randomized controlled	24 patients with chronic cervical radicular pain without nerve root compression of greater than 12 months' duration	Treatment group, single cervical ILESI of an equivalent volume of 0.5% lidocaine plus triamcinolone acetonide (10 mg/mL) plus 2.5 mg morphine sulfate; control group, single cervical ILESI of an equivalent volume of 0.5% lidocaine plus triamcinolone acetonide (10 mg/mL)	Success (visual analogue scale pain score reduction by at least 51%) rate was 78.5% (11/14) in the control group and 80% (8/10) in the treatment group at 12 months; no added benefit of morphine sulfate was noted.
Manchikanti et al. (2012)[75]	Randomized double-blind	120 patients with cervical spinal stenosis	Treatment group, cervical ILESI with 4 mL 0.5% lidocaine mixed with 6 mg nonparticulate betamethasone; control group, cervical epidural injection of 5 mL 0.5% lidocaine	Significant pain relief (greater than 50% reduction in NRS or NDI scores) was seen in 73% of patients in the treatment group and 70% of patients in the control group at 12-month follow-up. No statistical significant difference was noted between the treatment and control groups.
Dilke et al. (1973)[76]	Randomized double-blind	100 patients with lumbar nerve root compression	Treatment group, single lumbar ILESI of 80 mg methylprednisolone in 10 mL normal saline; control group, interligamentous injection of 1 mL normal saline	60% vs. 31% initial pain relief; at 3 months, the treatment group had 33/36 return to work vs. 21/35 in the control group along with a statistically significant decrease in analgesic consumption.
Snoek et al. (1977)[77]	Randomized double-blind	51 patients with lumbar nerve root compression of 12 days' to 36 weeks' duration	Treatment group, single lumbar ILESI of 80 mg methylprednisolone; control group, lumbar epidural injection of 2 mL normal saline	25%–70% improvement in multiple outcome measures in ESI group vs. 7%–43% in placebo group (not significant) with a follow-up of 14 ±6 months.
Cuckler et al. (1985)[78]	Randomized double-blind	73 patients with lumbar radicular pain	Treatment group, lumbar ILESI with 80 mg methylprednisolone and 5 mL 1% procaine; control group, lumbar epidural injection of saline and procaine	No statistically significant difference was observed between the control and experimental groups through 20 months.
Ridley et al. (1988)[79]	Randomized double-blind	39 patients with history of sciatica	Treatment group, ILESI with 80 mg methylprednisolone and saline; control group, interspinous saline injection	Significant difference in pain relief favoring the steroid group at 2 weeks that disappeared before 6 months.
Rogers et al. (1992)[80]	Randomized single-blind	30 patients with sciatica	Treatment group, lumbar ILESI with 14 mL 2% lidocaine with 80 mg methylprednisolone acetate; control group, lumbar interlaminar injection of 14 mL 2% lidocaine with 6 mL normal saline	LA and steroid group had significantly better results at 1-month follow-up.
Carette et al. (1997)[81]	Randomized double-blind	158 patients with sciatica secondary to herniated lumbar nucleus pulposus	Treatment group, up to three lumbar ILESI of 80 mg methylprednisolone acetate in 8 mL normal saline; control group, lumbar epidural injection of 1 mL normal saline	The treatment group exhibited less sensory deficits and leg pain at 6 weeks; functional disability and incidence of surgery were equivalent after 3 months.
Valat et al. (2003)[82]	Randomized double-blind	42 patients with sciatica	Treatment group, series of three lumbar ILESI with 50 mg prednisolone acetate; control group, series of three epidural injections with saline	Epidural steroids provided no additional improvement compared with the control injection through 35-day follow-up.
Arden et al. (2005)[83]	Randomized double-blind	228 patients with unilateral sciatica of 1–18 months' duration receiving either three lumbar ILESI with triamcinolone or interligamentous saline	Treatment group, series of three lumbar ILESI with 80 mg triamcinolone acetate and 10 mL 0.25% bupivacaine; control group, series of three injections of 2 mL interligamentous saline	Treatment superior to control at 3 weeks but not thereafter.

continued

TABLE 62.2 Randomized Studies Evaluating the Efficacy of Interlaminar and Caudal Epidural Steroid Injections—cont'd

Study	Design	Patients	Treatments	Results
Wilson-MacDonald et al. (2005)[84]	Randomized controlled	93 patients characterized as potential surgical candidates due to lumbar radiculopathy	Treatment group, lumbar ILESI with 8 mL 0.5% bupivacaine and 80 mg methylprednisolone; control group, intramuscular injection of 8 mL 0.5% bupivacaine and 80 mg methylprednisolone	Significant difference in pain relief between the two groups at 35 days with the treatment group faring better.
Manchikanti et al. (2012)[85]	Randomized double-blind	120 patients with lumbar central spinal stenosis	Treatment group, lumbar ILESI of 5 mL 0.5% lidocaine mixed with 1 mL nonparticulate betamethasone; control group, lumbar epidural injection of 26 mL 0.5% lidocaine	Significant pain relief (≥50%) was demonstrated in 55% to 65% of the patients at 12 months and functional status improvement with 40% reduction in ODI scores in 55%–80% of the patients with an average efficacy time of 40.8 ± 11.7 weeks. There was no statistically significant difference between the treatment and control groups.
Meadeb et al. (2001)[86]	Randomized controlled	47 patients with postdiscectomy sciatica	Treatment group 1, 3 caudal injections of 125 mg prednisolone acetate; treatment group 2, series of 3 forceful caudal injections of 20 mL saline after 125 mg prednisolone acetate; control group, series of 3 forceful caudal injections of 20 mL of saline alone	Caudal prednisolone acetate produced a statistically significant pain reduction at 30 days and a nonsignificant improvement at 4 months compared with control treatment.
Matthews et al. (1987)[87]	Randomized double-blind	53 patients with lumbar nerve root pain and unilateral neurologic deficit	Treatment group, three caudal injections of 80 mg methylprednisolone acetate in 20 mL bupivacaine; control group, three normal saline injections into the sacral hiatus	At 1 month, recovery was noted in 14/21 in the treatment group versus 18/32 in the control group (not statistically significant). At 3 months, the treatment group had significantly more pain-free patients using the 6-point horizontal VAS ($P < 0.05$).
Manchikanti et al. (2008)[88]	Randomized double-blind	72 patients with lumbar discogenic pain without disc herniation or radiculitis	Treatment group, caudal injection of 9 mL lidocaine with 6 mg betamethasone; control group, caudal injection of 10 mL 0.5% lidocaine	Significant pain relief (≥50%) was demonstrated in 72%–81% of patients and functional improvement in 81% at 1-year follow-up. There was no statistically significant difference between the treatment and control groups.
Sayegh et al. (2009)[4]	Randomized double-blind	183 patients with history of severe chronic low back pain and sciatica	Treatment group, caudal injection of 12 mL 2% lidocaine and 1 mL of betamethasone dipropionate and betamethasone phosphate (2+5) mg/dL betamethasone; control group, caudal injection of 12 mL 2% lidocaine and 8 mL water	Patients receiving caudal injection with steroid experienced faster relief, but the difference disappeared at 1 month.
Iversen et al. (2011)[89]	Randomized double-blind	116 patients with lumbar radiculopathy >12 weeks	Treatment group, caudal injection of 40 mg triamcinolone acetonide in 29 mL normal saline; control group 1, caudal injection of 30 mL normal saline; control group 2, subcutaneous sham injection of 2 mL normal saline	No significant difference in leg pain, back pain, or sick leave between the groups at 6, 12, and 52 weeks.

ESI, *Epidural steroid injection;* ILESI, *interlaminar epidural steroid injection;* LA, *local anesthetic;* NDI, *neck disability index;* NRS, *numeric rating scale;* ODI, *Oswestry disability index.*

the same injectate as an intramuscular injection. Patients randomized to the ILESI group experienced a statistically significant improvement in nerve root symptoms at up to 35 days, but long-term relief and reduction in need for surgery was not demonstrated at 2-year follow-up.

In another randomized, controlled study by Arden et al. in which 228 patients with unilateral sciatica were randomized to receive a series of three ILESIs consisting of either 80 mg of triamcinolone acetonide and 10 mL of bupivacaine (at weeks 0, 3, and 6) or placebo injections with 2 mL normal saline, patients in the experimental group showed significant improvement in functionality as compared with the placebo group at 3 but not 6 weeks.[83] In studies comparing caudal or conventional ILESI to epidural saline injection,[81,109] a similar short-term improvement in symptoms has been found. In treating radiculopathy associated with spinal stenosis, results suggest that patient symptom improvement is optimized when ILESI is performed at the intervertebral level of maximal stenosis.[3,54,110,111]

ILESI VS. TFESI

Controversy continues regarding the most effective method of ESI. Despite the wealth of literature dedicated to ESI, few randomized trials have compared the two methods head to head. Most studies have been retrospective or technically focused and have yielded conflicting data. Yet the preponderance of evidence gleaned from these studies seems to favor TFESI over ILESI for short-term pain reduction in patients with disc herniation and spinal stenosis.[112–114]

A recent randomized, double-blind outcome study by Gharibo and colleagues on 42 patients with nonstenotic radicular pain generated data suggesting that patients may experience greater subjective relief, as determined by the postinjection numeric rating scale (NRS), from TFESI but that more objective and subacute therapeutic effects (disability, activity, opioid use) are similar at the 10–16-day follow-up period.[115] In another nonblinded prospective, randomized study of 64 patients with chronic radiculopathy by Rados et al., the investigators compared ILESI and TFESI in patients with chronic unilateral radicular pain. They found that using both routes of epidural injections provided significant improvements in patient function and pain relief, but no statistically significant difference could be found between the two techniques at 24 weeks.[116]

A systematic review evaluating five prospective and three retrospective studies comparing transforaminal and interlaminar approaches found that both ILESI and TFESI were effective in reducing pain. At 2 weeks, data from the combined prospective studies favored the TFESI group by a little more than 10%, with no differences noted at 6 months. For functional improvement, there were no clinically meaningful differences between the different routes of epidural steroid administration.[117] In a large, systematic review and meta-analysis by Chou et al., 38 placebo-controlled studies were analyzed; the authors found that ESIs for radiculopathy were associated with immediate reductions in pain and improvement in function, but the results were small and not sustained.[118] Data suggested no differences between TFESI and ILESI based on limited evidence and no clear benefits for spinal stenosis.

The common use of epidurography in performing ESI has allowed practitioners to become more mindful of the pattern of injectate spread, which is sometimes used as a surrogate outcome measure for improvement. Although the TFESI technique has been touted to deposit injectate more closely to the site of unilateral, single-level pathology (i.e., the ventral epidural space of the affected nerve root), the use of ILESI allows for bilateral spread to multiple spinal levels.[59,119] Of note, the use of a parasagittal approach has been shown to both increase the incidence of ventral epidural spread[120,121] and improve treatment outcomes in a randomized double-blind comparative effectiveness trial[122] compared with the traditional, midline interlaminar approach.

A review of the literature reveals that a disproportionate percentage of ESI complications are related to the transforaminal approach, with the greatest risk occurring with cervical TFESI.[123,124] The TFESI method, especially when particulate steroids are used, carries certain unique risks and has been implicated in permanent, severe complications such as spinal cord infarction, paralysis, and inadvertent disc injection in the presence of lateral disc herniations.[125,126] Although the incidence of postdural puncture headache is reduced by the TFESI approach, it does not decrease the risk of many other complications compared with ILESI. In fact, the risk of many complications, including catastrophic embolic events, is increased in using the TFESI method; some feel that ILESI should therefore always be used as a first-line treatment.[56]

COMPLICATIONS

Complications associated with ILESI can be separated into those that are secondary to procedural technique and those associated with the injectate utilized. Complications related to injected drugs can be further subdivided into those related to the uptake and metabolism of corticosteroid and those associated with that of LA. The remaining category of complications covers those that are generically associated with performing an injection of any type (Table 62.3).

GENERIC COMPLICATIONS

Whenever the protective integumentary system is disrupted during the course of a procedure, there is a tangible risk of infection. Although historically infectious complications have been exceedingly rare,[134] two widespread outbreaks of fungal meningitis occurred in 2002 and 2012–2013.[135] Although these caused the procedure to gain a degree of national infamy, both episodes originated from unsterile techniques in drug compounding. This practice, intended to prevent the inclusion of neurotoxic preservatives in medications, occurs before the medications arrive at the clinical setting; thus it is difficult to address at the interventionalist level. The practice of compounding medications, an often less expensive way of obtaining steroid preparations, does not require approval from the US Food and Drug Administration (FDA), and no steroid preparation to date has received FDA approval for spinal injection (Centers for Disease Control and Prevention, multistate fungal meningitis outbreak). ESI is an elective procedure

TABLE 62.3 Incidence Rates for Complications Stratified by Type and Region of Epidural Steroid Injection

	Interlaminar											
	Cervical			Thoracic			Lumbar			Caudal		
Complications	**%**	**No./Total**	**Ref.**	**%**	**No./Total**	**Ref**	**%**	**No./Total**	**Ref**	**%**	**No./Total**	**Ref**
Bleeding	0.7	16/2376	127	1.3	4/301	127	0.8	11/1450	127	0.2	Nov-85	127
Vascular injection	4.2	100/2376	127	4	12/301	127	0.5	7/1450	127	7.9 13.1	122/3985	127
Nerve damage	0	0/2376	127	0	0/301	127	0	0/301	127	0	0/301	127
Intradiscal injection						128	0	1/4623	128	0.2, 0.2, 12.4		
Vasovagal reaction	0.0, 8.4, 1.7, 0–4	1/2376, 21/249, 6/157	127,129,130,131	0.3	1/301	127	0	0/1450	127	0.1, 0.8	0/3985, 2/123	127,132
Dural puncture	0.3, 0.8, 1.0	1/157, 2/249, 24/2376	127,129,133	1.3	4/301	127	0.1	2/1450	127	0, 0.8	1/3985	127
Postdural puncture headache	8.3	2/24	127	25	1/4	127	9	1/11	127	0	0/1	127
Paresthesias/radicular pain	0.3, 7.2	6/2376, 18/249	127,129	0.3	1/301	127	0.3	4/1450	127	4.6, 13.2	0/3985	127
Flushing	0.1, 1.5, 1.6–9.2	2/2376, 5/157	127,130,131	0.3	1/301	127	0.1	2/1450	127	11.3, 0.2	0/3985	127

Modified and reproduced with permission from Pain Management as agreed by Future Science Ltd.
Bicket MC, Chakravarthy K, Chang D, et al: Epidural steroid injections: an updated review on recent trends in safety and complications. *Pain Manag.* 5:129–146, 2015.

for which infection at the injection site is an absolute contraindication; however, standard sterile technique should prevent most infectious complications.[136]

PROCEDURAL COMPLICATIONS

Complications associated with the ESI technique are typically due to tissue disruption by the needle tip either along or near its intended path. Affected structures in this vicinity are either vascular or neurologic. Whereas most bleeding associated with ILESI is minor and self-limited, the development of a hematoma in the epidural space is a potentially catastrophic complication. An expanding epidural hematoma has the potential to compress the spinal cord and/or nerve roots against unyielding bony structures, resulting in ischemia and cell death. Though exceedingly rare, the severity of sequelae from an epidural hematoma makes ESI a high-risk neuraxial procedure.[137] Risk factors for epidural hematoma include abnormal hemostasis, difficult or traumatic needle placement, blind injection, the use of a large-bore needle, anatomic variation, increased age, and female gender.[138,139]

Whereas strict adherence to the American Society of Regional Anesthesia and Pain Medicine (ASRA) guidelines for performing neuraxial procedures in the setting of anticoagulation[138] reduces the risk of bleeding complications, it does not completely eliminate it.[140] It is critical to weigh the risks versus the benefits of withholding anticoagulation therapy for an elective procedure sure as ESI (see Chapter 85, on anticoagulants). Patients are typically prescribed these medications as a result of a higher-than-normal risk of thrombosis, and a large survey of interventional pain physicians reported that the number of thromboembolic events was 17 times greater when anticoagulants were withheld.[141]

Indirect neurologic injury as a result of embolized particulate steroid is a feared complication that has been linked to stroke and spinal cord injury. This complication, however, is almost exclusively observed with TFESI due to the technique of passing the epidural needle laterally and near vessels like the ascending cervical and vertebral arteries (for cervical ESI) (Fig. 62.4). Because of the absence of major vessels along the needle path used for ILESI, this complication is not discussed in this chapter.

A complication that may be more common with the IL technique is that of arachnoiditis, which has been theorized to result from the inadvertent injection of particulate steroid into the intrathecal space. This condition, referring to the inflammatory process resulting from irritation of the leptomeninges and underlying neural structures, presents via a wide array of clinical pathoanatomic manifestations.[142] Patients suffering from arachnoiditis may have minimal symptoms or may present with significant pain, which has been described as burning in nature, radiating down the extremities.[143]

Direct damage to nervous tissue can happen as a result of improper needle placement. TFESI has been shown to be associated with a greater than 10-fold increase in injury to the nerve roots.[127] Because injection into the nerve root itself has been implicated in this complication, patient feedback in a setting of minimal to no sedation can help to minimize its risk. Direct trauma to the spinal cord, causing severe morbidity, has also been reported. Although rare, this complication occurs most frequently in patients who received either general anesthesia or sedation strong enough to render them unresponsive.[144]

Whereas intradiscal injection is far more common in TFESI than with the IL technique,[128] it has been observed in both approaches. Flow of contrast into the disc space may occur despite correct placement owing to the existence in some patients of tracts that communicate between the intravertebral disc and the epidural space.[145] The use of real-time fluoroscopy during injection should provide early detection and minimization of this complication.

Inadvertent dural puncture can be associated with postdural puncture headache, with rates varying by needle type and size. This complication is uncommon and occurs at rates similar to that of continuous epidural placement.[127] Higher rates are associated with young patients, women, large-bore needles, needles with cutting tips, and blind injections.[3]

PHARMACOLOGIC COMPLICATIONS

Although the intended site of action of epidural corticosteroids is the ventral epidural space or affected nerve root, either direct or delayed systemic uptake can result in complications associated with medication effects elsewhere in the body. Exogenous steroids affect osteoblast and osteoclast activity such that bone resorption is increased and bone deposition decreased, respectively, resulting in an increased risk of pathologic fractures.[146,147] Trabecular bone sites are affected disproportionately, and vertebrae and pelvic bones, already damaged in much of the demographic population receiving ESI, are at particular risk.[148] An understanding of this pathophysiology is of particular importance in evaluating patients for ESI, as its use in high-risk populations such as postmenopausal women and those with a history of osteopenia, osteoporosis, and pathologic fractures should entail a judicious risk/benefit analysis.[149]

In addition to bone demineralization, the administration of glucocorticoids results in dysregulation of the hypothalamic-pituitary-adrenal (HPA) axis. Exogenous corticosteroids act on the adrenal gland to initiate a negative feedback loop suppressing corticotropin releasing hormone and corticotropin secretion, resulting in decreased production of endogenous cortisol and growth hormone.[150] Once thought to be a complication exclusive to long-term systemic glucocorticoid use, a single ESI can cause a patient to develop Cushing syndrome.[151] Even if a patient does not develop the signs and symptoms of Cushing syndrome, subclinical HPA suppression can last from 3 weeks[92] to 3 months.[152] Many experts advocate for patients scheduled to undergo surgery within 14 days of ESI to have a cosyntropin stimulation test to evaluate the need for stress-dose steroids. Alternatively, stress-dose steroids can be given intraoperatively if the patient shows signs of HPA suppression.

Glucocorticoids increase hepatic glucose production, induce insulin resistance and hyperinsulinemia, and inhibit glucose transport into cells—all of which serve to raise glucose concentration of the blood.[153] In diabetic patients, doses of exogenous glucocorticoids given during ESI result in clinically significant elevations in plasma glucose levels. These elevations occur immediately after injection[154] and

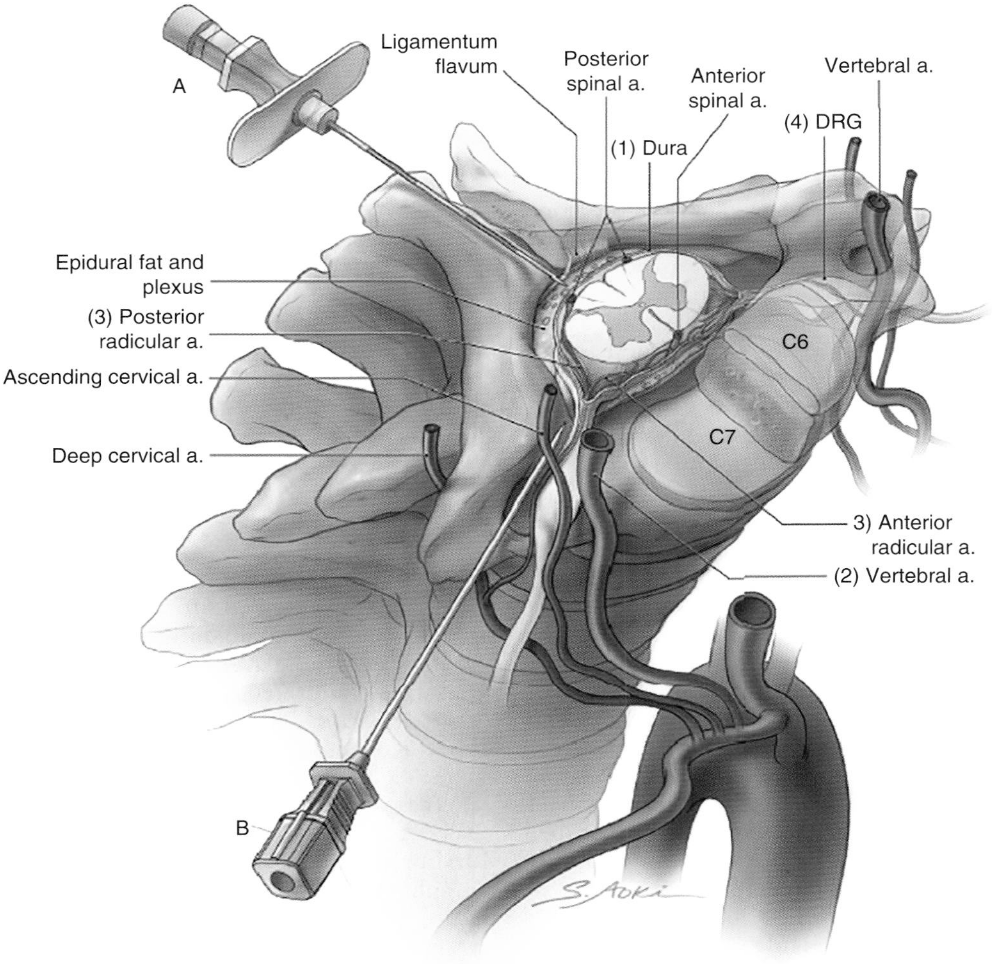

FIG. 62.4 Interlaminar (A) and transforaminal (B) epidural injections at the C6-7 spinal level. (1) Violation of the dura may lead to high or total spinal anesthesia, spinal cord injury, postdural puncture headache, or pneumocephalus. High volumes or rapid injection into the epidural space can cause blindness. (2) Injection of local anesthetic and particulate steroids into the vertebral artery or injury to the artery may cause seizures (local anesthetic) and stroke. (3) Injection of particulate steroid into or injury to a radiculomedullary artery may result in spinal cord infarction. (4) Injury or injection into a dorsal root ganglion can cause nerve damage and neurologic symptoms. *DRG*, Dorsal root ganglion. (Drawing by Shizuka N. Aoki-Anatomize I Medical Media. Reproduced with permission from Pain Management as agreed by Future Science Ltd. Bicket MC, Chakravarthy K, Chang D, et al: Epidural steroid injections: an updated review on recent trends in safety and complications. *Pain Manag.* 5:129-146, 2015.)

may persist for 2–6 days.[155,156] Diabetic patients should be informed of this effect so that they can adjust their diet and/or hypoglycemic medications to compensate for it.

Although the aforementioned antiinflammatory effects of epidural steroids are considered to be the major factor in reducing radicular pain, the disruption of inflammatory pathways also inhibits the immunologic system, impairs wound healing,[157] and increases infection risk. Exogenous corticosteroids suppress B cells, T cells, and macrophages by disrupting the binding of interleukins to B cells, thus interfering with the production of cytokines critical to T-cell proliferation and downregulating the expression of Fc receptors on macrophages.[158–160] Infection risk following ESI is increased in patients with preexisting immunosuppressive conditions.[134]

If LA is used as the diluent for ESI, complications associated with this class of medications can be observed. Allergic reactions to amide LAs are typically associated with the use of preservatives that are not found in neuraxial preparations and thus are exceedingly rare in ESI. LA toxicity is rarely seen with the small LA doses used for ESI, and while seizures from injection of LA into the vertebral artery have been reported, this complication is generally associated with the TF technique.

CONCLUSION

ILESI has been safely used for decades to provide short-term relief of back and neck pain caused by a variety of conditions. Although surrogate efficacy markers have been examined in lieu of pain relief, studies have yielded conflicting results. Recent efficacy data suggest that TFESI may provide superior pain relief; however, the more favorable safety profile along with the relative technical ease of ILESI have caused some experts to recommend its use as a first-line treatment, reserving TFESI only for those patients who have failed an ILESI trial. Novel variations of ILESI, such as the parasagittal technique, attempt to improve injectate deposition into the ventral epidural space while avoiding the lateral arteries found near the path of TFESI, but more studies are needed.

KEY POINTS

- The mechanisms of action of ESI include its antiinflammatory and antinociceptive effects. Other mechanisms include reduction of collagen deposition with less scar formation, enhancement of blood flow, and washout of inflammatory mediators.
- Compared with small volumes, large volumes of injectate are associated with better results in short- and intermediate-term outcomes.
- Based on limited evidence, there appears to be little difference in the efficacy between IL and TFESI.
- The TF approach is associated with the catastrophic complication of paraplegia, probably from embolization of the particulate steroid through the radicular artery accompanying the nerve root, ascending cervical and deep cervical arteries, and the vertebral artery.
- A working group has recommended against the use of particulate steroid in cervical TFESI and for the initial use of nonparticulate steroid in lumbar TFESI.
- The injection of contrast and minimal sedation has been recommended for ESIs.
- The working group recommended that cervical ILESI should not be above C6-C7 because of smaller dimensions above this level and a higher frequency of gaps in the ligamentum flavum.

REFERENCES

Access the reference list online at ExpertConsult.com.

CHAPTER 63

Transforaminal Epidural Steroid Injections and Selective Nerve Root Blocks

Mark C. Bicket, MD ◌ Honorio T. Benzon, MD ◌ Steven P. Cohen, MD

INTRODUCTION

Transforaminal epidural steroid injections (TFESI) and selective nerve blocks provide an alternative interventional approach to address radicular pain, in comparison with interlaminar epidural steroid injections (ILESI; as reviewed in Chapter 62). The rationale for using the former routes of injection compared with the latter is that the delivery of medications occurs directly onto the nerve root(s) using the transforaminal approach. This permits maximal concentration of medication delivered to the site of suspected pathology. The distinction between TFESI and selective nerve root blocks may involve some overlap given anatomical considerations. Upon exiting the epidural space, spinal nerves transition in their covering from the dura mater to the fascial sheath in a continuous fashion. Consequently, medication injected adjacent to the spinal nerve may enter the epidural space irrespective of whether the needle tip progresses through the intervertebral foramen or not. Both transforaminal injections and selective nerve root blocks describe injections of medication adjacent to spinal nerves, but differ in the final location of the needle tip. The term *selective nerve root block* typically describes an injection adjacent to the spinal nerve root, with the needle tip remaining outside of the intervertebral foramen. In contrast, the term *transforaminal injection* describes an injection with the needle tip that resides within the intervertebral foramen.

The role of epidural steroid injections (ESI) in the treatment of lumbosacral radicular pain and other disorders has generated significant discussion and debate since its first description. Historically, the first publication describing ESI reported on the transforaminal or selective nerve root approach in 1952. Robechhi and Capra published a case study on the periradicular injection of hydrocortisone to the first sacral nerve root via the S1 sacral foramen for the treatment of lumbosacral radicular pain,[1] and additional reports detailing treatment outcomes for radicular pain using the transforaminal approach soon followed.[2] Alternate approaches then supplanted transforaminal injections in the following decades, including the use of intrathecal injections of steroids in the 1960s, which was later abandoned due to complications such as arachnoiditis.[3–5] Use of the interlaminar technique was more frequent in practice, likely as a result of the procedure being performed by anesthesiologists who were most accustomed to the "blind" loss-of-resistance technique for interlaminar injections. The transforaminal technique received renewed attention for the management of radicular pain in 1992, when Derby et al. described fluoroscopically guided selective nerve root blocks as a predictive tool before lumbar disc surgery.[6] The following decade bore witness to a significant rise in the use of interventional pain procedures, including TFESI, which were associated with a concomitant rise in rare, catastrophic neurological complications.[7,8] A renewed outlook on transforaminal and selective nerve root injections incorporates safeguards to prevent such complications.[9]

Among the different approaches for ESI, the transforaminal injection shares many commonalties with the interlaminar approach, including similar use of medications composing the injectate, a shared mechanism of action (see Chapter 62, Mechanism(s) of Action), overlapping indications for treatment, and improved accuracy with use of fluoroscopic guidance. In contrast to the interlaminar and caudal approaches, transforaminal injections require the navigation of more complex anatomy to place a needle within the neural foramen, mandate the use of fluoroscopic guidance including appropriate image interpretation, and involve greater risks.[8] Yet transforaminal injections increase the possibility of ventral epidural spread of the injectate,[10] carry a lower risk of inadvertent dural puncture,[11] and appear more likely to provide positive patient outcomes relative to interlaminar (or caudal) injections.[12] Consequently, every patient deserves a close examination of the clinical need for the specific type of epidural injection and an informed discussion of the potential benefits and risks of the planned approach.

TECHNIQUE

SELECTIVE NERVE ROOT BLOCK

The techniques of TFESI and selective nerve root blocks share similar anatomical considerations, given that the approach to the spinal nerve root is the same. The term *selective nerve root block* fails to acknowledge the continuous nature of the spinal nerve root sheath with the dura mater, which typically permits injectate volumes as low as 0.5 mL to spread to other nerve roots.[13] A technically perfect selective nerve root block with the needle verified to be outside of the foramen as viewed fluoroscopically may nevertheless result in epidural spread of the injectate.[14] Despite this shared space, a selective nerve root block more selectively targets the spinal nerve root than the interlaminar approach, which permits these injections to be used diagnostically to isolate symptoms, and prognostically to predict surgical outcomes, when multilevel vertebral pathology is present.

Evidence for the diagnostic and prognostic characteristics of selective nerve root injections to improve surgical outcomes is weak but positive. The ability of different nerve blocks to localize an anatomical source of radicular pain was examined by North et al. in a randomized controlled trial of 33 patients with lumbosacral radicular pain, which revealed that most patients noted significant pain relief with selective nerve root, sciatic nerve, and facet blocks.[15]

Injectate volumes delivered in the study consisted of a relatively larger volume of local anesthetic (3 mL), which likely resulted in blockade of other nerve roots besides those targeted. As a result, positive responses to diagnostic selective nerve root blocks were unable to identify those with true nerve root involvement beyond other types of nerve blocks, and positive responses to nerve blocks lacked specificity. On the other hand, negative responses to diagnostic blocks appeared clinically informative.

The lack of specificity of selective nerve root blocks may be partially attributable to the inadvertent spread of small injectate volumes through the epidural and nerve root space, as established in a study by Castro et al. that tracked the spread of injectate to nearby nerve roots with various injectate volumes during L4 selective nerve root blocks.[13] Using the smallest 0.5-mL volume to block L4 nerve roots, epidural and L3/L5 nerve root spread was fluoroscopically verified in 48% and 27% of injections, respectively. Additionally, spread of local anesthetic to the psoas muscle, situated in close proximity to the lumbosacral plexus, occurred in 12% of 0.5-mL injections and 71% of 2-mL injections. The unrestrained flow of local anesthetic injectate in selective nerve root blocks may partially explain the lack of specificity.

As past studies suggest, higher volumes of injectate contribute to worse specificity of selective nerve root blocks. In a quantitative evaluation of lumbosacral contrast flow patterns, Furman et al. injected 0.5-mL increments of contrast and examined fluoroscopic images for evidence of contrast spread in areas other than the single, ipsilateral nerve root.[16] Using 0.5 mL of contrast, 30% of injections were no longer specific to the targeted nerve root. Specificity was further reduced with higher volumes, as injections of 1 mL and 1.5 mL of contrast were no longer specific in 67% and 87% of injections, respectively. A study by Anderberg et al. that compared injection volumes of 0.6, 1.1, and 1.7 mL in the cervical region illustrated a similar lack of specificity in the distribution patterns.[17] The authors found that distribution patterns using 0.6 mL of contrast demonstrated sufficient nerve root specificity, though epidural spread was still documented, even at this low volume. At higher volumes, spread was noted in the epidural space or adjacent nerve roots in more than 50% of cases. The authors concluded that the diagnostic selectivity of a selective nerve root block is unreliable with volumes in excess of 0.5–0.6 mL.

Other factors that can influence the interpretation of selective nerve root blocks besides volume of injection include patient characteristics, such as preexisting sensory changes. Using sensory examinations before and after injections, Wolff et al. documented significant variability in pain reduction experienced by patients, even when dermatomal changes in sensation were obtained.[18] Low volume selective nerve root blocks elicit paresthesias and more consistently result in hypesthesias (i.e., diminished sensation) of the affected dermatomes than actual pain reduction.[19] Consequently, the validity of selective nerve root blocks may be reduced in patients with long-standing sensory changes and sensory changes that occur in nondermatomal patterns. When preexisting sensory changes are present, eliciting pain and paresthesias in the target dermatome(s), and producing hypesthesias on examination, can best be achieved when overlapping dermatomes of the target nerve root(s) are taken into consideration.

Reports on the accuracy of selective nerve root blocks vary based on spinal region. Yeom et al. evaluated the accuracy of selective nerve root blocks in 47 patients with single-level lumbosacral radicular pain using a series of 1 mL local anesthetic injections to block the symptomatic level, as well as an adjacent level as a control.[20] A threshold of 70% pain reduction demonstrated the best discriminative ability, with the overall accuracy being 73%. False-positive findings resulted from spread of the injectate to the nearby epidural or nerve root space, with the authors reporting a sensitivity of 57%. The specificity of the injections was 86%, with the injectate failing to spread to the nerve root, insufficient infiltration, and injection within the epineural sheath resulting in the majority of false-negative results. In the cervical region, selective nerve root blocks using 1 mL correctly identified 19 of 20 patients with single-level pathology on magnetic resonance imaging (MRI).[21] Among the 18 patients who underwent surgery, all noted resolution of pain. With more diffuse, two-level pathology, selective nerve root blocks correlated with the level of worst degeneration identified via MRI in 60% of cases, with neurological examination in 27% of cases, and with dermatomal mapping in 23% of cases.[17] Agreement among selective nerve root block, MRI imaging, and neurological examination was rare, and no randomized trials exclusively compared selective nerve root block to MRI imaging. Overall, the accuracy of selective nerve root blocks appears to be moderate.

Selective nerve root blocks may not always contribute as a cost-effective method to the standard diagnostic workup prior to lumbar decompression surgery, based on economic modeling that placed the incremental cost per quality-adjusted life-year in excess of £1.5 million.[22] The overall conclusions, including finding low-specificity for the blocks, relied on few studies with varying methods and overall poor quality. In addition to the relative costs of blocks and surgeries, and how well patients are selected (i.e., poor surgical selection is likely to make prognostic blocks more cost-effective), technical factors and patient characteristics such as discordant clinical symptoms and imaging all influence the cost-effectiveness of selective nerve root blocks.

In summary, the question of whether selective nerve root blocks improve surgical outcomes is answered with weak, positive evidence suggesting they do. Selective nerve root blocks remain appropriate in a number of clinical situations. Discrepancies among the patient's clinical presentation and/or various diagnostic examinations (i.e., electromyography, MRI) raise the utility derived from a selective nerve root block. Patients with unusual extremity pains, anatomical variations such as transitional vertebrae or conjoint nerve roots, or with previous back surgery and atypical extremity pain, may also benefit from information provided from selective nerve root blocks.

TRANSFORAMINAL EPIDURAL INJECTIONS

The approach to transforaminal injections varies based on region of the spine, with regional variations in vertebral, vascular, and neural elements influencing the desired placement of the needle and final location of the needle tip. Multiplanar fluoroscopic guidance with use of contrast dye to verify the trajectory and confirm the location of the needle tip is necessary prior to injecting particulate steroid. This helps minimize the risk of involving nearby critical elements not directly visualized via fluoroscopy, such as the arterial supply to the spinal nerve root and/or the spinal cord or the spinal nerve root itself. Digital subtraction angiography is the reference standard for detecting cases of inadvertent vascular access prior to injection, with one study showing that real-time fluoroscopy has a sensitivity of 71%.[23]

ANATOMY

The cervical transforaminal injection approach differs from that of the thoracic and lumbar because the angle of the vertebral foramen and exiting spinal nerve is anterior in the cervical region, and posterior in the thoracic and lumbar region. Consequently, patient positioning is supine or lateral, with the former position modifying the fluoroscopic image to a postero-anterior (PA) view instead of an antero-posterior (AP) view. The lateral position facilitates injection at C1–C4 levels, while the supine position facilitates views without shoulder tissue at C4–C8 levels. After identification of the appropriate vertebral level, rotation of the C-arm axis obliquely 45–65 degrees optimizes the cervical vertebral foramen to permit clear visualization of surrounding structures. From this perspective, various bony borders outline the cervical vertebral foramen: The superior vertebral body resides anteriorly, the pedicle from the same level resides superiorly, the facet column formed by the inferior and superior articular processes resides posteriorly, and the pedicle from the inferior vertebral body resides inferiorly.

Critical vascular structures include the vertebral artery, which courses within the periodic protection of the transverse foramen but remains mostly unprotected along the anterior aspect of the cervical vertebral foramen (Fig. 63.1). The blood supply of the spinal cord consists of one anterior and two posterior spinal arteries. Spinal radicular arteries,

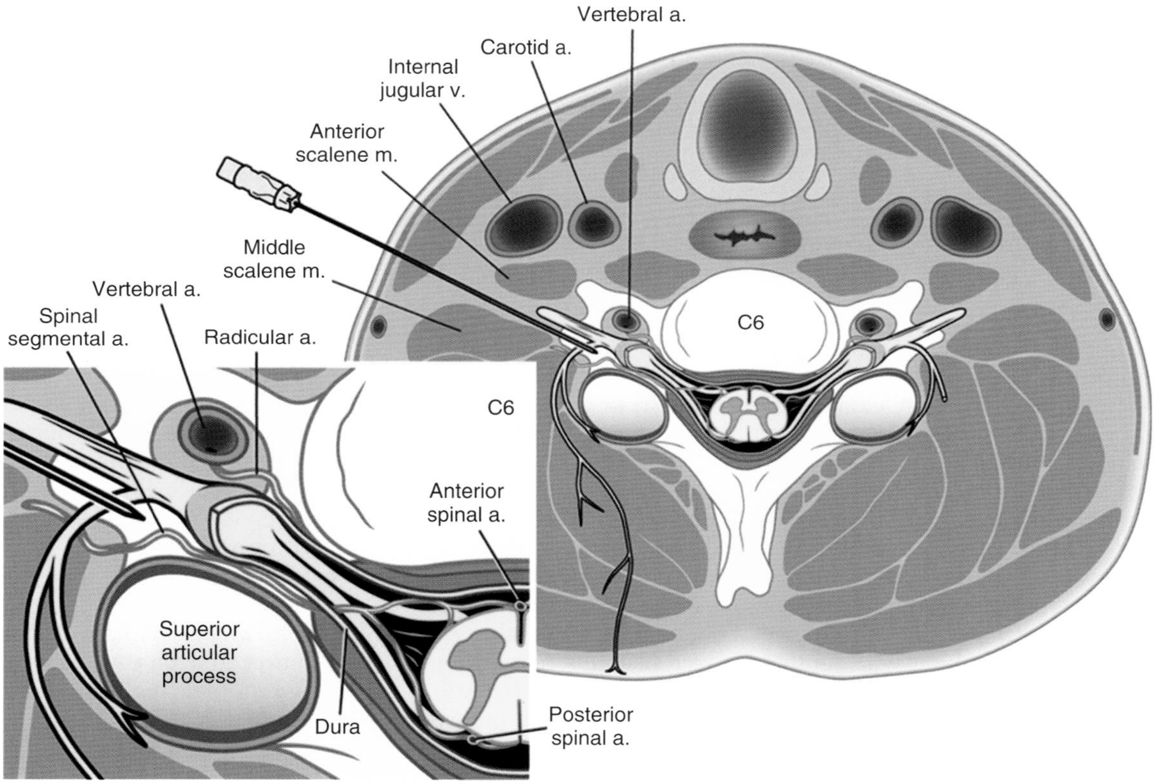

FIG. 63.1 Axial view of cervical transforaminal injection at the level of C6. The needle has been inserted along the axis of the foramen and is illustrated in its final position within the posterior aspect of the foramen. Insertion along this axis avoids the vertebral artery, which lies anterior to the foramen, and the spinal nerve root, which lies within the foramen angled anteriorly toward the interscalene groove. Spinal segmental arteries arise from the deep or ascending cervical artery, enter the foramen at variable locations, and often course through the foramen, penetrate the dura, and join the anterior or posterior spinal arteries that supply the spinal cord *(inset)*. Likewise, arterial branches arise variably from the vertebral artery to supply the nerve root itself (in this illustration, a branch to the nerve root or "radicular" artery is shown); similar branches from the vertebral artery often penetrate the dura to join the anterior or posterior spinal artery. There is great anatomic variation in the vascular supply in this region. The anatomic variant illustrated is shown to demonstrate how a needle can be placed within a small artery that provides critical reinforcing blood supply to the spinal cord during cervical transforaminal injection. Injection of particulate steroid directly into one of these vessels can lead to catastrophic spinal cord injury. *(Adapted from Rathmell JP:* Atlas of Image Guided Intervention in Regional Anesthesia and Pain Medicine, *ed 2. Philadelphia: Lippincott Williams & Wilkins, 2012 and Rathmell JP, Benzon HT, Dreyfuss P, et al: Safeguards to prevent neurologic complications after epidural steroid injections: consensus opinions from a multidisciplinary working group and national organizations.* Anesthesiology. *122(5):974-984, 2015.)*

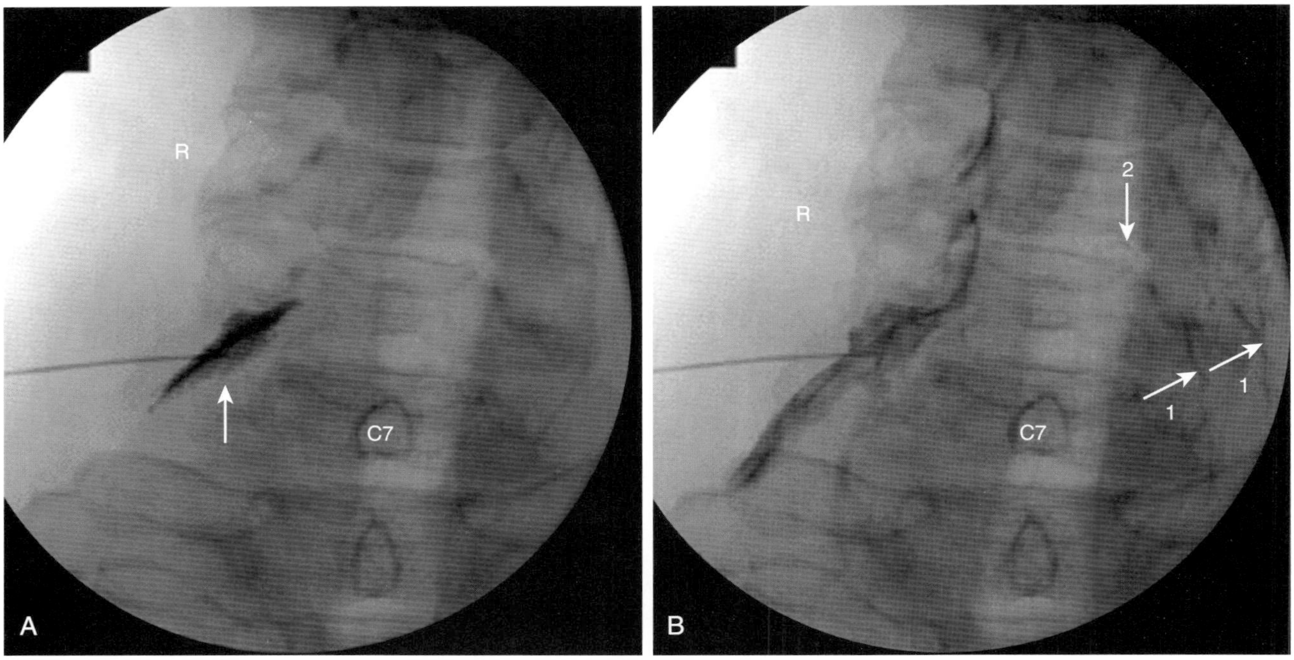

FIG. 63.2 Cervical transforaminal epidural steroid injection (A). (A) An anteroposterior (AP) fluoroscopic view of the cervical spine demonstrating a needle tip within the right C6–7 intervertebral foramen. The C7 vertebral level is identified on the image. Contrast medium outlines the C7 spinal nerve root. (B) An AP fluoroscopic view of the cervical spine demonstrating the injection of contrast medium into C6–7 intervertebral foramen, and following injection of local anesthetic. *White arrows* identify contrast spread into small vertebral veins on the patient's contralateral side *(1);* and the faint outline of a vessel within the vertebral canal opposite the C5–6 disc space *(2). R,* Right side of the cervical region. *(Adapted from Karasek M, Bogduk N: Temporary neurologic deficit after cervical transforaminal injection of local anesthetic,* Pain Med. *5(2):202-205, 2004.)*

which pass out of the foramen and continue as radicular arteries adjacent to the spinal nerve roots, demonstrate a variable anatomical location.[24] Consequently, the most inferior and posterior portion of the foramen is desired as the initial target to minimize the risk of entering or injuring the vertebral artery anteriorly. Introducing the needle via a coaxial fluoroscopic technique followed by contact with the superior articular process posteriorly provides for an additional margin of safety. Upon contact with the posterior portion of the foramen, the needle may be advanced anteriorly into the foramen. The importance of obtaining a lateral image to ascertain the needle depth and avoid inadvertent penetration of the spinal cord should be highlighted. Injection of contrast medium via conventional fluoroscopic imaging in the PA view should then demonstrate an outline of the desired nerve root. If appropriate spread outlining the nerve root or epidural distribution is not noted, slight advancement may be made followed by reassessment with contrast medium. Typically advancement of the needle occurs up to the "redline" of the facet joint, which anatomically serves as an approximate safety limit, depending on the degree of oblique angulation of the image intensifier (i.e., how far the facet column is situated within the vertebral body). Once appropriate needle positioning is confirmed, slow injection of medications is performed (Fig. 63.2).

The lumbar and thoracic transforaminal injection approaches start with the patient prone, which permits an appropriate fluoroscopic view of the vertebral foramina that project in a posterior direction. Although the lumbar and lower thoracic approaches may be performed in a lateral position, most practitioners prefer prone. After identification of the appropriate vertebral level, rotation of the C-arm axis obliquely optimizes the vertebral foramen to permit clear visualization of surrounding structures. In the lumbar region, the degree of angulation of the image intensifier affects the final needle position, and consequently the tendency for epidural versus nerve root spread, when a coaxial approach is used. For example, steeper angulation (>35 degrees) results in a more medial needle position and a greater proportion of epidural uptake, whereas less acute angles are used to obtain more nerve root spread. Caution to avoid overrotation beyond 20 degrees in the T1–T8 thoracic regions is needed, given the increased possibility of the needle trajectory causing a pneumothorax (Fig. 63.3). An optimized oblique image arranges the various bony borders and relevant landmarks of the vertebral foramen in a silhouette that mimics a Scottish terrier in the "scotty dog" position: The superior articular process outlines the dog's ear, the transverse process projects over the vertebral body as the nose, the inferior articular process serves as the dog's front leg, the pedicle overlaps the region of the dog's eye, and the spinous process mimics the dog's feet.

Consensus regarding optimal needle positioning, which permits the delivery of medications without perturbation of the adjacent spinal nerve or injection into nearby vascular structures, continues to be deliberated.[25] Traditionally, the "safe triangle" or subpedicular approach recommended needle placement within the fluoroscopic region posterior to the vertebral body, defined by the lateral aspect of the

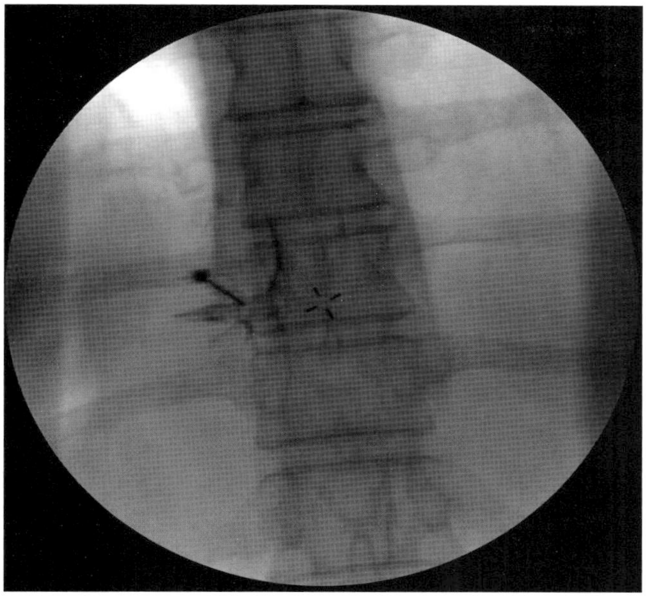

FIG. 63.3 Thoracic transforaminal epidural steroid injection. An anteroposterior fluoroscopic view of thoracic spine demonstrating the needle tip within T11–12 foramen, with contrast medium outlining the T11 nerve root and lateral epidural spread.

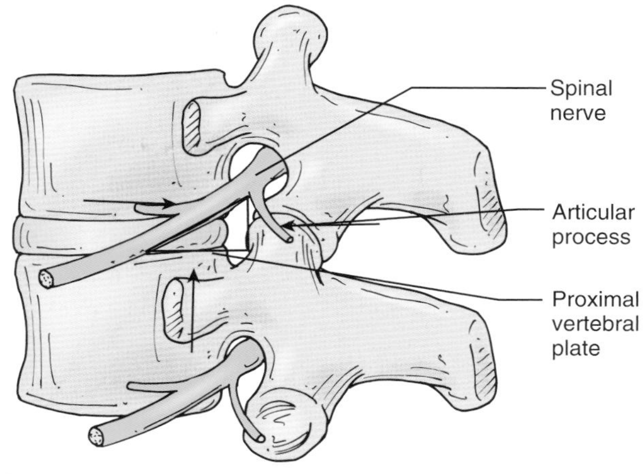

FIG. 63.4 Kambin's triangle. A drawing of an oblique view of the lumbar vertebrae demonstrates Kambin's triangle at the area overlying the posterolateral intervertebral disc. The triangle is bounded by the superior aspect of the vertebral body (base, denoted by vertical arrow), the traversing nerve root or dura medially (vertical leg, denoted by the arrow pointing left), and the inferior aspect of the exiting spinal nerve root (hypotenuse, denoted by the arrow pointing right). *(Adapted from Park JW, Nam HS, Cho SK, et al: Kambin's triangle approach of lumbar transforaminal epidural injection with spinal stenosis,* Ann Rehabil Med. *35:833-843, 2011.)*

inferior pedicle (i.e., below the pedicle) and the superior border of the imagined nerve root that courses from the vertebral foramen inferiorly and laterally.[6] Critics of the subpedicular approach note that the primary advantage of the technique, avoiding needle contact with the spinal nerve, fails to incorporate variability in nearby vascular anatomy (i.e., radicular arteries and the artery of Adamkiewicz), which increases the risk of inadvertent intravascular injection.[8,25] An alternative approach targets Kambin's triangle, a region described in the context of accessing intervertebral discs for surgery in 1972 by Kambin and Sampson.[26] Kambin's triangle describes an area overlying the posterolateral disc that is bounded by the inferior vertebral body at its base, the exiting spinal nerve root at the hypotenuse, and the traversing nerve root or dura at the vertical leg (Fig. 63.4). Kambin's triangle may offer advantages in comparison to the subpedicular approach regarding inadvertent vascular injection, spinal nerve contact, and intradiscal injection, but no one approach for transforaminal injections fully eliminates risk.[27,28]

Critical vascular structures in the thoracic and lumbar regions include similar spinal arterial branches, which were described in the cervical region (Fig. 63.5). However, the largest spinal arterial branch, the artery of Adamkiewicz, typically enters through the left intervertebral foramen in the thoracic or upper lumbar region but may be present on either side from T5 to S1.[29] Besides vascular structures, the ribs, pleura, and mediastinum may be at risk of penetration during the thoracic approach. Using a similar coaxial fluoroscopic technique as described previously, the ideal needle position for the subpedicular approach is slightly inferior to the pedicle and lateral to the pars interarticularis, above the superior articular process inferiorly. The needle is advanced in the superior and posterior aspect of the vertebral foramen to avoid the spinal nerve. An AP fluoroscopic view provides context for the mediolateral location of the needle. Alternatively, the inferolateral aspect of the pars interarticularis may serve as a depth marker from which the needle may be walked off. Unexpected bony resistance along the path is likely from contact with the pars interarticularis, and redirection inferiorly, anteriorly, and medially should permit further advancement. Once the needle tip is located inferior to the medial aspect of the pedicle, a lateral fluoroscopic view permits visualization of the needle tip being advanced into the foramen. The ideal needle tip position resides in the anterior one-third of the foramen, slightly inferior to the pedicle. An ideal trajectory to Kambin's triangle may target the area over the intervertebral disc, slightly lateral to the superior articular process. Contact with the lateral lower aspect of the superior articular process may serve as a depth marker, after which the needle may be directed laterally a few millimeters. Ideal final positioning demonstrates the needle located medially within the upper pedicle using an AP view and at the posteroinferior aspect of the vertebral foramen using a lateral view (Fig. 63.6).

Injections of the L5 nerve root may require modifications to this technique in the presence of an overriding iliac crest that obstructs an oblique view of the vertebral foramen. Aligning the inferior vertebral end plate of L5 by positioning the C-arm in a more cephalad direction adjusts for this anatomical issue. This position creates a triangular area formed by the iliac crest, the superior articular process of S1, and the inferior border of the L5 transverse process.

For S1 nerve root injections, prone patient positioning permits access to the posterior sacral foramen. Slight C-arm axis rotation 5–15 degrees in an ipsilateral, oblique direction may optimize the relevant anatomy and reduce the incidence of intravascular injection. A randomized study comparing transforaminal injections at S1 randomized using two different angles of approach demonstrated intravascular uptake in 29% of injections using the AP

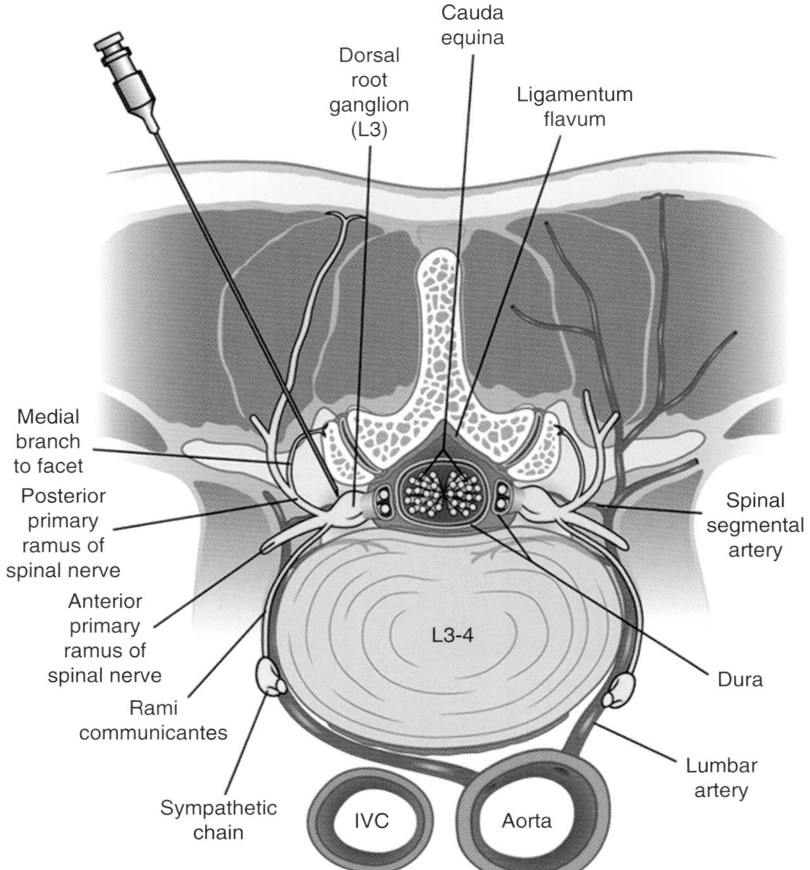

FIG. 63.5 Axial view of lumbar transforaminal injection at L3–4. The anatomy and proper needle position (axial view) for right L3/L4 transforaminal epidural injection. *IVC,* Inferior vena cava. *(Adapted from Rathmell JP:* Atlas of Image Guided Intervention in Regional Anesthesia and Pain Medicine, *ed. 2. Philadelphia: Lippincott Williams & Wilkins, 2012; Rathmell JP, Benzon HT, Dreyfuss P, et al: Safeguards to prevent neurologic complications after epidural steroid injections: consensus opinions from a multidisciplinary working group and national organizations.* Anesthesiology. *122(5):974-984, 2015.)*

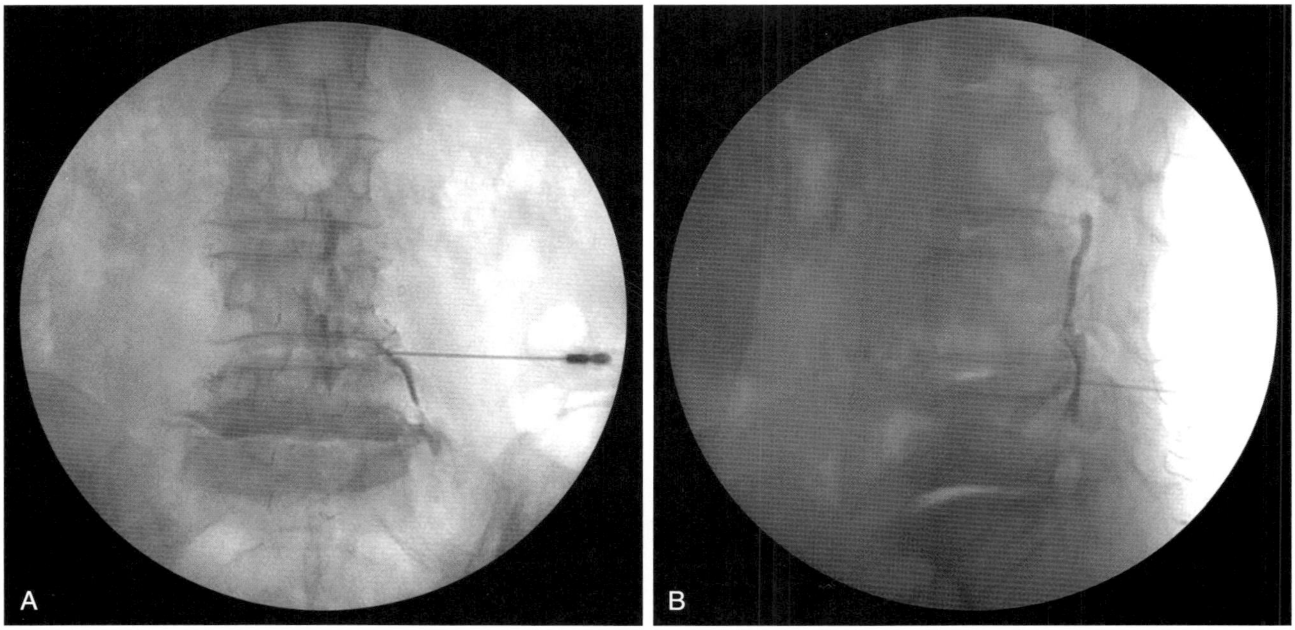

FIG. 63.6 Lumbar transforaminal epidural steroid injection A. (A) An anteroposterior fluoroscopic view of the lumbar spine demonstrating the needle tip within intervertebral foramen at L4–5, with contrast medium outlining the L4 nerve root. Epidural spread of contrast medium is present, as evidenced by darker regions over the central portions of mid-vertebral bodies at midline. (B) A lateral fluoroscopic view of the lumbar spine showing a well-demarcated line of contrast medium indicative of ventral epidural spread from the mid-body of L5 to the inferior body of L3.

view, in contrast to 11% with an oblique view.[30] A small caudocranial rotation (toward the patient's head) may result in an improved view of the S1 foramen given that the sacral foramina project in a slight cephalad direction. Needle advancement toward the sacral foramen may then proceed. Obtaining a lateral view is necessary to confirm the needle tip remains at or above the level of the caudal epidural space and avoids trespassing into the pelvic region.

During the transforaminal approach, the patient may experience paresthesias. Although pain may result from perturbation of the nerve root, other structures such as the facet joint, periosteum, and annulus fibrosus may cause referred pain to the leg. Regardless of the etiology, onset of paresthesias indicates an appropriate time to withdraw the needle slightly. Paresthesias must terminate prior to injection of contrast medium. Additionally, verifying needle tip placement in two views is critical during a transforaminal injection at any region of the spine. Inadvertent penetration of structures such as the spinal cord or vasculature cannot be excluded using only one view. After negative aspiration of blood and cerebrospinal fluid, contrast medium should be injected, which may confirm anterior epidural spread. A pattern of spread in the ventral epidural contrast flow is desirable, given the pattern's association with increased pain relief.[10] Careful examination of the images should ensure the absence of intravascular uptake. Vascular injection is reported to occur in up to 12%–14% of transforaminal injections, and may occur in all spinal regions but is most likely to happen in the cervical region.[8] Inadvertent intravascular injection may be missed without the use of digital subtraction angiography in up to one-third of all cases.[23,31] Because it significantly enhances the ability to detect vascular uptake of contrast medium, digital subtraction angiography was recently endorsed by a multispecialty workgroup, though it is not mandated before injection of steroid.[9] To optimize the image quality of digital subtraction angiography, the patient may be requested to hold their breath. After intrathecal and intravascular injections have been excluded, the medication may be injected.

INJECTATE COMPOSITION AND DELIVERY

A typical injectate for transforaminal injections and selective nerve root blocks may include a combination of local anesthetic, saline, and/or steroid. Characteristics of the injectate may impact patient outcomes. The volume of injectate in the transforaminal region typically ranges from 1.0 to 4.0 mL, lower than volumes for interlaminar and caudal ESI. Because similar volumes result in less segmental spread compared with interlaminar ESI, transforaminal ESI are ideally utilized in individuals with well-delineated, well-localized pathology.[32] In a randomized, double-blinded dose-comparison study evaluating triamcinolone for transforaminal injections, no difference in efficacy was found among triamcinolone doses of 10 mg, 20 mg, and 40 mg.[33] However, 5 mg failed to provide similar levels of benefit. A similar randomized, double-blinded dose comparison study evaluating dexamethasone transforaminal injections found no difference in efficacy among dexamethasone doses of 4 mg, 8 mg, and 12 mg.[34]

Comparisons of particulate and nonparticulate steroids have demonstrated mixed results, although all of these studies have been underpowered. Randomized comparative-effectiveness studies of transforaminal injections have found a statistically significant difference favoring particulate steroids,[35] a nonsignificant benefit favoring particulate steroids,[36] and no difference.[37,38] For these randomized trials, transforaminal injections in the lumbar region were performed in three studies,[35,37,38] while the cervical region was examined in one study.[36] Randomized studies of the interlaminar and caudal approach show similar results, finding significant[39] and nonsignificant differences[40] favoring particulate steroids.

Combining the data for the six randomized studies comparing particulate to nonparticulate epidural injections, three of which involved transforaminal injections, revealed that 71% of participants allocated to receive particulate steroids experienced a positive, early categorical outcome, compared with 55% of those who received dexamethasone.[35–40] Retrospective comparative-effectiveness studies generally parallel these findings with most,[41–44] but not all,[45,46] studies, suggesting that particulate steroids may provide longer-lasting relief than nonparticulate steroids. A recent retrospective intraindividual comparison of particulate and nonparticulate epidural steroids reported longer injection-free intervals with particulate steroids, a result that was more robust when particulate steroids were given via transforaminal compared with other routes.[44] It is important to recognize that whereas particulate steroids have been demonstrated to provide efficacy for radicular pain in a majority of placebo-controlled studies, there have been no randomized, double-blind studies evaluating the benefit of nonparticulate corticosteroids.

The inclusion of local anesthetic with the injectate offers advantages including improved perfusion to ischemic nerve roots, suppression of ectopic discharges from damaged nerves, and interruption of nociception.[47,48] In transforaminal injections, the risk of injection into the intrathecal or intravascular space introduces the possibility of neurological complications such as high spinal or seizure,[8] but comparisons of low and high doses of local anesthetic injections (i.e., 0.125% lidocaine vs. 1% lidocaine) have demonstrated similar effects regarding pain score reduction and overall pain ratings at short- and long-term follow-up.[49]

In most regions of the spine, 22- or 25-gauge spinal or blunt tip needles of 3.5-inch length are sufficient to reach the vertebral foramen in a patient of average build, although 5- or 7-inch needles may be required in obese patients when performing injections in the lumbar region, especially at L5–S1. Randomized trials of blunt tip needles demonstrate significant reductions in the incidence of inadvertent intravascular injection, with reductions ranging from 8.2% to 10.4%.[50,51]

EFFICACY

TFESI generally demonstrate improved pain outcomes in comparison to ILESI, although significant heterogeneity obscures a simplified summary of the existing evidence.[12] The cervical and thoracic regions for TFESI remain less studied than the lumbar region. Evidence for cervical radicular pain includes one randomized trial with positive results that lacked a control group,[52] one negative study,[53] and several randomized studies demonstrating short- and long-term benefit.[43,54,55] Thoracic TFESI have generally been limited to case series reporting only short-term outcomes.[56] The successful treatment of postherpetic neuralgia using transforaminal corticosteroids has been described in a single case report.[57] Systematic reviews for radicular symptoms from lumbar disc herniation generally report good evidence for short-term relief and mixed evidence favoring long-term benefit.[58–61] Reviews examining low back pain secondary to lumbar spinal stenosis, postsurgical pain, and axial pain without disc herniation demonstrate fair or limited evidence regarding treatment with TFESI.[61]

The level of pathology and placement of medication relative to the dorsal root ganglion influence the efficacy of transforaminal epidural injections. For example, a patient with L4–L5 paracentral disc herniation causing L5 radicular pain raises the clinical question of whether superior pain relief is conferred by administering medication at the location of the symptomatic nerve root (i.e., L5–S1, termed "ganglionic") or at the site of pathology adjacent to the intervertebral disc level (i.e., L4–5, termed "preganglionic").[62] A retrospective examination of 33 patients by Lee et al. suggested injections at the site of pathology (termed *preganglionic*) provide more effective pain relief at short-term follow-up.[63] A randomized controlled trial of 239 patients by Jeong et al. confirmed that transforaminal injections performed at the site of pathology (preganglionic) provided superior short-term pain relief compared with injections at the symptomatic nerve root (ganglionic).[64]

A summary of evidence regarding comparisons of the different routes of injection supports the conclusion that TFESI is likely superior to interlaminar or caudal epidural steroid injection, which concurs with the general consensus among most pain practitioners (Table 63.1). Transforaminal injections were found to afford better pain relief and functional improvement compared with interlaminar injections in many[65,68,72,73,75–78] but not all studies[32,66,67,69–71,74,79,80] that directly compared the two routes.

COMPLICATIONS

Complications from TFESI and selective nerve root blocks may be organized by the three main components of the procedure: placement of the needle, delivery of the injectate, and the specific component of the injectate.[8]

NEUROLOGIC INJURY

Catastrophic but rare neurological complications have been associated with cervical TFESI. The cardinal neurological complications for transforaminal injections are infarctions of vital neurologic tissue within the spinal cord, brainstem, cerebrum, and cerebellum.[8,9] Spinal cord injury, nerve damage, and temporary blindness have also been reported following transforaminal injections. Although a majority of reports involved the cervical region, reports in the thoracic and lumbar region have been fewer but of similar severity. A variety of postulated mechanisms for these devastating complications include embolization of the injectate, dissection of the vertebral artery, and trauma or spasm of the nearby artery. Routes of embolization include the periradicular artery that exits the neural foramen and accompanies the nerve root to the spinal cord. In the cervical intervertebral foramina region, the anterior cervical and deep cervical arteries are very close to the nerve root. These arteries send segmental medullary arteries to the anterior spinal artery, and embolization of the particulate steroid can result in spinal cord infarction.[81] Neurologic injuries including cortical blindness and lower extremity paralysis from nonparticulate injectates (contrast and local anesthetic) were temporary, while injuries from the particulate steroids were permanent.[82] This reinforces the assumption that the injuries were secondary to infarction from embolization of the particulate injectate. Given these concerns, the US Food and Drug Administration created a Safe Use Initiative in 2009 to address preventable medication risks associated with ESI. Among 17 clinical considerations aimed at improving safety, 8 directly related to the conduct of TFESI (Table 63.2).

OTHER COMPLICATIONS

Other complications of transforaminal injections may include intradiscal injection, with an incidence ranging from 0.17% to 2%, which is higher than for interlaminar procedures, and bleeding, which creates the potential for an expanding volume to compress the spinal cord and/or nerve roots against nearby bony structures. Withholding anticoagulation medication to perform an epidural steroid injection may lower the risk of periprocedural bleeding complications, but may increase the risk of thromboembolic events. Communication with the patient and the prescriber of the anticoagulation medication while following guidelines regarding neuraxial procedures is essential prior to performing a TFESI.[83] Infectious risks with ESI received national attention due to contamination from compounding pharmacies, which resulted in outbreaks of fungal infections that occurred in 2002 and 2012–2013.[84,85] Other physiologic effects common to ESI include bone demineralization, suppression of the hypothalamic-pituitary-adrenal axis, immune suppression, and hyperglycemia (see Chapter 62, Interlaminar ESI, Complications).

KEY POINTS

- ESI demonstrate efficacy for patients with lumbosacral radicular pain. The mechanism through which steroids facilitate pain reduction occurs through antiinflammatory and antinociceptive effects, including the inhibition of phospholipase A_2. Methylprednisolone inhibits the transmission of impulses through C-fibers but not Aβ fibers.
- Transforaminal injections and selective nerve root blocks share similar approaches regarding needle trajectory, and their difference in the final location of the needle tip may be obviated due to the continuous nature of fascial sheath with the dura mater. By convention, placement of the needle tip within the intervertebral foramen is needed for transforaminal injections, whereas the needle tip remains outside but adjacent to the nerve for selective nerve root blocks.
- The response to selective nerve root blocks may include reduction in pain, elicitation of paresthesias, or generation of hypesthesias. The overall low specificity

TABLE 63.1 Studies Comparing Transforaminal, Interlaminar, and Caudal Epidural Steroidal Injection

Study	Design	Subjects	Interventions	Results	Comments
Ackerman and Ahmad 2007[65]	Randomized evaluator blinded	90 patients with S1 from HNP	TF: 40 mg triamcinolone + 4 mL normal saline IL: 40 mg triamcinolone + 4 mL NS C: 40 mg triamcinolone + 19 mL NS	TFESI > ILESI or caudal ESI at 24 weeks	Patients with ventral epidural spread, more common in TFESI group, had better outcomes
Candido et al. 2008[32]	Randomized	60 patients with unilateral radicular pain from HNP and DDD	TF and IL: 80 mg methyl-prednisolone + 1 mL NS + 1 mL 1% lidocaine	No difference between TFESI and ILESI up to 6 months	Study underpowered
Choi et al. 2015[66]	Randomized	62 patients with cervical radicular or axial pain from HNP or stenosis	TF: 5 mg dexamethasone + 2 mL of 0.18% ropivacaine IL (modified paramedian): 5 mg dexamethasone + 5 mL of 0.18% ropivacaine	No difference between TFESI and modified ILESI up to 3 months	More patients with ventral epidural spread in modified IL group. Dexamethasone used.
Ghai et al. 2014[67]	Randomized evaluator blinded	62 patients with lumbosacral unilateral radicular pain with confirmatory MRI findings	TF and IL: 80 mg methyl-prednisolone + 2 mL NS	No difference between TFESI and modified ILESI up to 12 months	Single center trial. Cointerventions not avoided
Gharibo et al. 2011[68]	Randomized	42 patients with unilateral radicular pain from disc disease <1 year	TF: 40 mg triamcinolone + 1 mL 0.25% bupivacaine IL: 80 mg triamcinolone + 2 mL 0.25% bupivacaine	TFESI > ILESI at 2 weeks follow-up for pain but not function	TF contained half the steroid dose and LA. Short follow-up period.
Hashemi et al. 2015[69]	Randomized evaluator and patient blinded	64 patients with LBP and lumbosacral unilateral radicular pain with confirmatory MRI findings	TF and IL: 80 mg triamcinolone + 2 mL bupivacaine + 6 mL NS	No difference between TFESI and ILESI up to 4 months	Large volume of injectate in both groups.
Karamouzian et al. 2014[70]	Randomized	30 patients with lumbar radicular pain with recurrent HNP after discectomy	TF: 40 mg methylprednisolone + 1 mL bupivacaine + 1 mL 2% lidocaine C: 40 mg methylprednisolone + 1 mL 2% lidocaine + 1 mL 0.25% bupivacaine + 7 mL distilled water	No difference between TFESI and C at 2 and 6 months	Large difference in injectate volumes. Study underpowered.
Kolsi et al. 2000[71]	Randomized	30 patients with sciatic or femoral neuralgia	TF and IL: 3.75 mg cortivazol + 2 mL 0.5% lidocaine	No difference between TFESI and ILESI up to 4 weeks	TFESI > ILESI for initial mean pain score decrease
Kraemer et al. 1997[72]	Randomized	182 patients with LBP	TF, IL, and paravertebral injections not described	TFESI > ILESI > paravertebral local anesthetic up to 3 months	Intramuscular steroid injection added in saline group
Lee et al. 2009[73]	Randomized evaluator blinded	192 patients with axial LBP due to HNP or SS	TF: 20 mg triamcinolone + 4 mL 0.5% lidocaine IL: 40 mg triamcinolone + 8 mL 0.5% lidocaine	TFESI > ILESI up to 4 months	TF injections received half IL dose on each side. Differences between groups greater for SS patients.
Rados et al. 2011[74]	Randomized	64 patients with chronic unilateral lumbar radicular pain	TF: 40 mg methylprednisolone + 3 mL 0.5% lidocaine IL: 80 mg methylprednisolone + 8 mL 0.5% lidocaine	No difference between TFESI and ILESI through 6 months	TF contained half the steroid dose and >50% less LA

Continued

TABLE 63.1 Studies Comparing Transforaminal, Interlaminar, and Caudal Epidural Steroidal Injection—cont'd

Study	Design	Subjects	Interventions	Results	Comments
Thomas et al. 2003[75]	Randomized	31 patients with lumbosacral radicular pain from HNP <3 months	TF and IL: 5 mg dexamethasone in 2 mL solution	TFESI > ILESI up to 6 months	Fluoroscopy used for TFESI, while ILESI done blindly
Lee et al. 2009[76]	Retrospective	233 patients with lumbosacral radicular pain from SS or HNP	TF small volume: 40 mg triamcinolone + 2 mL 0.5% lidocaine TF large volume: 40 mg triamcinolone + 8 mL 0.5% lidocaine IL: 40 mg triamcinolone + 8 mL 0.5% lidocaine C: 40 mg triamcinolone + 15 mL 0.5% lidocaine	Satisfaction and pain scores: TFESI and ILESI > caudal ESI up to 2 months Function: TFESI > ILESI > caudal ESI	Functional benefits of TFESI more pronounced at 2 weeks. Injectate volumes not standardized, with C > TF > IL.
Manchikanti et al. 1999[77]	Retrospective case control	225 patients with low back and leg pain	TF: 1.5–3 mg betamethasone + 1 mL 1% lidocaine IL: 120 mg depo-methylprednisolone + 10 mL 0.5% lidocaine, with 80 mg methylprednisolone on subsequent injections C: 80 mg depo-methylprednisolone + 1-mL 0.5% lidocaine	TFESI and caudal ESI > ILESI at 1–3 months' follow-up, but no difference between groups at 3–6 and 6–12 month follow-up	Longer pain duration in caudal ESI group. Variable steroid dose in TFESI and variable follow-up period.
Schaufele et al. 2006[78]	Retrospective case control	40 patients with lumbosacral radicular pain from single-level HNP	TF: 80 mg methylprednisolone + 1–2 mL 2% lidocaine IL: 80 mg methylprednisolone + 2–3 mL 1% lidocaine	TFESI > ILESI; variable follow-up period averaging 3 weeks	Higher baseline pain scores in ILESI group. Short follow-up period.
Smith et al. 2010[79]	Retrospective case control	38 patients with lumbosacral radicular pain from SS	TF: 80 mg methylprednisolone + 1–2 mL 2% lidocaine IL: 80 mg methylprednisolone + 2–3 mL 2% lidocaine	No difference between TFESI and ILESI; variable follow-up averaging 4–6 weeks	Study underpowered
Mendoza-Lattes et al. 2009[80]	Retrospective case control	93 patients with mostly lower lumbar radicular pain	C: Up to 3 injections of 2 mL of 40 mg/mL depo-methylprednisolone or 3 mL of 6 mg/mL betamethasone. TF: Up to 3 injections of a 1:1 solution containing 1.5–2 mL of bupivacaine 0.25% mixed with depo-methylprednisolone or betamethasone.	C = TF through 2-year follow-up	16 patients lost to follow-up. Equivalent rates of surgery between groups. Low volumes used for caudal injections. Included some patients with stenosis and spondylolisthesis.

C, *Caudal;* DDD, *degenerative disc disease;* ESI, *epidural steroid injection;* HNP, *herniated nucleus pulposus;* IL, *interlaminar;* ILESI, *interlaminar epidural steroid injection;* LA, *local anesthetic;* LBP, *low back pain;* MRI, *magnetic resonance imaging;* SS, *spinal stenosis;* TF, *transforaminal;* TFESI, *transforaminal epidural steroid injection.*

Adapted from Cohen SP, Bicket MC, Jamison D, et al: Epidural steroids: a comprehensive, evidence-based review. Reg Anesth Pain Med. *38(3):175-200, 2013.*

TABLE 63.2 Safeguards to Prevent Neurologic Complications After Epidural Steroid Injections: Multidisciplinary Working Group Consensus Opinions for Transforaminal Epidural Steroid Injections

1. Transforaminal ESI using particular steroid is associated with a rare risk of catastrophic neurovascular complications.
2. Cervical transforaminal ESIs should be performed by injecting contrast medium under real-time fluoroscopy and/or digital subtraction imaging, using an AP view, before injection of any substance that may be hazardous to the patient.
3. Particulate steroids should not be used in therapeutic cervical transforaminal injections.
4. Lumbar transforaminal ESIs should be performed by injection contrast medium under real-time fluoroscopy and/or digital subtraction imaging, using an AP view, before injection of any substance that may be hazardous to the patient.
5. A nonparticulate steroid (e.g., dexamethasone) should be used for the initial injection in lumbar transforaminal epidural injections.
6. There are situations when particulate steroids could be used in the performance of lumbar transforaminal ESIs.
7. Extension tubing is recommended for all transforaminal ESIs.
8. Transforaminal ESIs can be performed without contrast in patients with documented contraindication to use, but in these circumstances, particulate steroids are contraindicated and only preservative-free, particulate-free steroids should be used.

AP, *Anteroposterior;* ESI, *epidural steroid injections.*
Adapted from Rathmell JP, Benzon HT, Dreyfuss P, et al: Safeguards to prevent neurologic complications after epidural steroid injections: consensus opinions from a multidisciplinary working group and national organizations. Anesthesiology. *122(5):974-984, 2015.*

decreases with injection volumes higher than 0.5–0.6 mL, while accuracy decreases in the setting of preexisting sensory changes of long duration and nondermatomal distribution.

- Transforaminal injections require the use of fluoroscopic guidance, and increase the likelihood of ventral epidural spread of medication, but have a higher risk of complications compared with interlaminar injections. Kambin's triangle (defined by the inferior vertebral body, the traversing nerve root or dura, and the exiting spinal nerve) may be preferred to the subpedicular region (defined by the lateral aspect of the inferior pedicle and the superior border of the nerve root), although no target fully mitigates risk of inadvertent vascular injection.
- TFESI demonstrate improved pain outcomes in comparison to interlaminar and caudal ESI. The strongest evidence exists for lumbosacral radicular pain from disc herniation, for which there is good evidence for short-term relief and mixed evidence favoring long-term benefit.
- The rise in rare but devastating neurological injury associated with TFESI has accompanied a sustained rise over the past decade of interventional pain procedures. Multispecialty consensus considerations to improve the safety profile of epidural injections include eight statements directly related to transforaminal injections.
- Critical vascular structures that may be encountered with transforaminal injections include radicular arteries that perfuse the spinal cord and the artery of Adamkiewicz, which typically enters via the left vertebral foramen in the lower thoracic or upper lumbar region but varies in location on either side from T5 to S1.
- Cardinal neurological complications for transforaminal injections include infarctions of vital neurologic tissue such as the spinal cord, brainstem, cerebrum, and cerebellum. Spinal cord injury, nerve damage, and blindness have also been reported following transforaminal injections.

REFERENCES

Access the reference list online at ExpertConsult.com.

CHAPTER 64

Antitumor Necrosis Factor-α Drugs and Disease-Modifying Antirheumatic Drugs for Low Back Pain

Khalid Malik, MD, FRCS

INTRODUCTION

Low back pain (LBP) is a major source of pain and suffering in industrialized nations.[1,2] The collective cost of LBP, comprising both direct and incidental expenses, exceeds billions of dollars every year in the United States alone.[3] Despite the vast resources utilized, treatments for LBP continue to be suboptimal, and substantial dissatisfaction exists among both patients and treating physicians. A comprehensive assessment of novel and innovative treatments for LBP is therefore imperative. In recent years, a range of potent antiinflammatory drugs, including disease-modifying antirheumatic drugs (DMARDs), have become available. In this chapter, a broader range of antiinflammatory drugs, outside of the more commonly utilized nonsteroidal antiinflammatory drugs (NSAIDs) and steroids, is explored.

ROLE OF INFLAMMATION IN LOW BACK PAIN

Among the myriad causes of LBP, syndromes affecting the various spinal elements are the most prevalent. Most notable of these spinal pain syndromes are herniated and degenerated discs and stenosis and arthritic changes of the spine.[4] These spinal lesions can cause pain either directly or indirectly by affecting the neural components housed within the spine.[4,5] First described in 1934, compression of the contiguous nerve root by a herniated disc has traditionally been regarded as a prominent cause of LBP.[6] However, substantial evidence (listed as follows) has accumulated recently that implicates local inflammation as a key factor in LBP.[7,8]

- A herniated nucleus pulposus is highly inflammatory in nature.[9,10]
- Intervertebral discs that cause pain (i.e., are positive for concordant pain on discography), produce high levels of inflammatory mediators.[11,12]
- Tumor necrosis factor-α (TNF-α), a major inflammatory cytokine, is found in high concentrations at the site of the nucleus pulposus-induced nerve injury.[13,14]
- In animal studies, TNF-α is known to cause nerve damage[15] and neuropathic pain behavior,[16] and its blockade at the nerve injury site reduces pain, local edema, and thrombus formation.[17]
- A significant number of patients with LBP have no demonstrable compressive lesion on imaging studies.
- A number of LBP patients continue to have pain despite relief of the presumptive injurious lesion.[18]

Based on these observations, it can be concluded that chronic inflammation plays a key role in the etiology of LBP, and antiinflammatory drugs may have an important role in its treatment.

A BRIEF INTRODUCTION TO ANTIINFLAMMATORY DRUGS

Plant extracts have been used for the treatment of fever and aches since ancient Egyptian and Roman times. The era of antiinflammatory drugs, however, began with the extraction of aspirin from willow bark in the early 19th century.[19,20] The second wave of innovation for the treatment of inflammatory diseases came in the mid-20th century with the discovery of phenylbutazone, indomethacin, and ibuprofen—a group of drugs commonly referred to as NSAIDs.[19,20] Although aspirin and NSAIDs successfully alleviated pain and fever, they were ineffective in preventing disease progression. Glucocorticoids, introduced in the 1950s, had disease-modifying characteristics and revolutionized the treatment of numerous chronic inflammatory conditions. However, long-term glucocorticoid therapy at high doses, often required to treat these chronic disabling conditions, can lead to major metabolic and nonmetabolic adverse effects.[19–21] Consequently, an extensive search for safer antiinflammatory and disease-modifying drugs ensued, and a range of biological and nonbiological DMARDs were introduced.[19–21] Biological DMARDs, often referred to as "biologics," are a homogenous group of recombinant monoclonal peptides or fusion proteins. However, a large group of nonbiological DMARDs are diverse in structure and characteristics, and include drugs such as sulfasalazine, cyclosporine, levamisole, and methotrexate, among others.

Normal inflammatory response is mediated by an array of cytokines, which are peptides released by a variety of cells in order to augment the function of other similar cells.[20,21] The various cytokines typically act synergistically at extremely low concentrations; therefore blockade of one can interrupt the entire inflammatory cascade.[20,21] Biological DMARDs are antibodies to several cytokines, specifically TNF-α, interleukin-1 (IL-1), and IL-6, and their antiinflammatory properties are due to the targeted inhibition of these key cytokines.[20,21] Given that their targets are primarily extracellular, biological DMARDs have few metabolic consequences, and their primary side effect is increased susceptibility to infections. In comparison, nonbiological DMARDs have diverse mechanisms of action. They are frequently potent antimetabolites and suppress cellular replication and inflammatory response. Consequently, nonbiological DMARDs often cause serious immunosuppressive and metabolic adverse effects in a dose-dependent manner. DMARDs are being used increasingly for the treatment of a host of chronic inflammatory and autoimmune conditions such as rheumatoid arthritis, Crohn disease, inflammatory bowel disease, psoriasis, and ankylosing spondylitis. DMARD use in these conditions is characterized by a protocol-driven approach, and a typical DMARD regimen often consists of a combination of one or two biological drugs along with a nonbiological DMARD.[22]

ANTITUMOR NECROSIS FACTOR-α DRUGS AND DISEASE-MODIFYING ANTIRHEUMATIC DRUGS FOR LOW BACK PAIN

The use of antiinflammatory drugs for LBP is not novel. Aspirin and NSAIDs are routinely given orally, parenterally, or applied topically for several LBP syndromes. Steroids, given orally or injected into the epidural space, have been a mainstay of treatment for LBP for the past several decades.[23] However, despite a range of antiinflammatory drugs and DMARDs becoming available in recent years, their use for LBP has exclusively been investigational in nature and limited to only four drugs (Table 64.1). Of these, only two biological drugs (etanercept and infliximab) have been used with any regularity, and the use of two remaining drugs (adalimumab and tocilizumab) is limited only to one study group each (see Table 64.1).

ETANERCEPT

There are six randomized controlled trials (RCTs) evaluating etanercept use for LBP,[24–29] of which four involved epidural route of administration (see Table 64.1).[24–27] Three such trials were in patients with lumbar radicular pain secondary to disc herniation.[24–26]

- A trial of 24 patients (four groups in 3:1 ratio) compared two epidural injections, given 2 weeks apart, of escalating etanercept doses (2, 4 or 6 mg) to placebo (normal saline). It reported efficacy of epidural etanercept at all three doses compared with placebo.[24] This was a well-randomized and blinded trial; however, unblinding occurred at 4 weeks, and therefore only short-term results could be ascertained.
- A trial of 49 patients received two epidural injections 2 weeks apart of either etanercept (0.5, 2.5, or 12.5 mg) or placebo.[25] The results reported efficacy of etanercept relative to placebo for up to 6 months, but only in patients receiving the lowest etanercept dose (0.5 mg). Almost 40% of the randomized patients were excluded from the final analysis, and the results of this trial were therefore not robust.
- The third trial compared epidural etanercept to similarly administered steroids and placebo.[26] Eighty-four patients in three equal groups received two epidural injections 2 weeks apart of etanercept (4 mg), methylprednisolone (60 mg), or placebo (normal saline). One month posttreatment, the steroid group experienced better pain relief and functional improvement than the etanercept and saline groups (the results were similar for the etanercept and the saline groups), with no significant differences reported at 3 months. Even though this study was well conducted and followed patients out to 6 months, those that failed to derive benefit were unblinded after 1 month.

Consequently, with these conflicting results, no valid conclusions can be drawn regarding the efficacy of epidural etanercept in patients with lumbar radicular pain from a herniated disc. Only one trial involving epidural etanercept examined its efficacy in patients with *radicular pain from spinal stenosis*, comparing it with similarly administered steroids.[27] Eighty patients in two equal groups received a single epidural injection of etanercept (10 mg) or dexamethasone (3.3 mg), and relative efficacy of etanercept was reported at 4 weeks. This trial was not blinded, was inadequately randomized, and based on its results, *routine use of epidural etanercept in patients with radicular pain from spinal stenosis could not be recommended.*

Intradiscal etanercept was studied in a single trial of patients with LBP from suspected intervertebral disc pathology.[28] Thirty-six patients in six groups received either escalating doses of etanercept (0.1, 0.25, 0.5, 0.75, 1.0, 1.5 mg) or placebo (sterile water). No difference was observed between the groups at 1 month, so this study did not provide *evidence to substantiate the use of intradiscal etanercept for LBP.*

Subcutaneous etanercept administration has been studied in a single trial of 15 patients with lumbar radicular pain due to herniated disc.[29] Either a single subcutaneous "perispinal" injection of etanercept (25 mg, $n = 8$) or placebo (saline, $n = 7$) was given. No difference in outcomes between the groups was reported at 3 months. The trial was inadequately randomized, not blinded, and only 15 patients were recruited over a 4-year period, with a dropout rate of nearly 20%. It therefore provides *no evidence to substantiate the use of subcutaneous "perispinal" etanercept in patients with lumbar radicular pain from herniated disc.*

Overall, etanercept as used in the treatment of LBP is most frequently administered by epidural injection. The dose used has been substantially lower than the typical subcutaneously administered recommended dose for rheumatologic conditions of 25 mg twice-weekly injections. The doses administered in these LBP studies ranged from 0.1 to 25 mg, usually less than 5 mg, and often only one or a maximum of two injections were given. A typical justification for this substantially lower epidural etanercept dose is the lower dose of epidural opioids compared with their parenteral dosage,[24,26] even though no relationship exists between opioids and biological DMARDs. When administered by the recommended subcutaneous route, etanercept was still usually given well below the recommended frequency, oftentimes only as a single injection.[29]

INFLIXIMAB

Infliximab, normally given by intravenous infusion of 3–5 mg/kg, repeated at 2, 6, and 8 weeks, is the second most commonly used DMARD for LBP. It has been administered exclusively by the intravenous route in all studies examining its effect on LBP, and almost always via a single infusion. The controlled study of infliximab use for LBP is limited to one clinical trial involving a single group of patients with lumbar radicular pain from a herniated disc. The results of this study cohort are reported at 3 months and 1 year in two separate publications.[30,31] Forty patients received a single intravenous infusion of infliximab (5 mg/kg given over 2 hours, $n = 21$) or placebo (saline, $n = 19$). No differences in outcomes were reported at 3 months[30] or 1 year.[31] *The results of this trial therefore did not support the use of intravenous infliximab in patients with lumbar radicular pain from herniated disc.*

TABLE 64.1 Randomized Controlled Trials of Disease-Modifying Antirheumatic Drugs for Low Back Pain

Study	Methodology	Outcomes	Limitations
Cohen et al. 2009[24]	24 patients with radicular pain from herniated disc in four groups received two epidural injections of either escalating doses (2, 4, or 6 mg) of etanercept or saline in 3:1 ratio	Significant improvement in all etanercept groups compared to saline injections at 1 and 6 months	Not blinded after 1 month. Small trial of 24 patients with four study groups.
Freeman et al. 2013[25]	49 patients with radicular pain from herniated disc in four groups received two epidural injections of either etanercept (0.5, 2.5, or 12.5 mg) or placebo	Significant pain relief in only 0.5 mg etanercept group at 2 weeks to 6 months	Etanercept efficacious in only 1 group with lowest etanercept dose. Multiple small groups. High dropout rate of almost 40%.
Cohen et al. 2012[26]	84 patients with radicular pain from herniated disc in three equal groups received two epidural injections of either 60 mg methylprednisolone, 4 mg etanercept, or saline	Pain and disability scores lower at 1 month in steroid group but results not statistically significant	Inconclusive results. Short-term follow-up.
Ohtori et al. 2012[27]	80 patients with radicular pain from spinal stenosis in two equal groups received epidural injection of either 10 mg etanercept or 3.3 mg of dexamethasone	Significant improvement in pain and disability scores in etanercept group at 4 weeks	Nonblinded. Short follow-up.
Cohen et al. 2007[28]	36 patients with back pain from disc pathology received intradiscal injection of escalating doses (0.1, 0.25, 0.5, 0.75, 1.0, or 1.5 mg) of etanercept or sterile water in 5:1 ratio	No difference in pain and disability between the groups at 1 month	Not blinded after 1 month. Short-term results. Small trial of 36 patients with six study groups.
Okoro et al. 2010[29]	15 patients with radicular pain from herniated disc received subcutaneous injection of either 25 mg etanercept (n = 8) or saline (n = 7) in perispinal area	No difference in pain and disability between the groups at 3 months	15 patients recruited over 4 years. High dropout rate of 20%. Poorly randomized. Nonblinded.
Korhonen et al. 2005[30]	40 patients with radicular pain from herniated disc received one intravenous infusion, over 2 h, of either infliximab 5 mg/kg (n = 21) or saline (n = 19)	No significant difference between the groups at 3 months	Inadequate randomization and blinding. Small-sized trial.
Korhonen et al. 2006[31]	40 patients with radicular pain from herniated disc received one intravenous infusion, over 2 h, of either infliximab 5 mg/kg (n = 21) or saline (n = 19)	No significant difference between the groups at 1 year	Inadequate randomization and blinding. Small-sized trial.
Genevay et al. 2010[32]	61 patients with radicular pain from herniated disc received two subcutaneous injections 1 week apart of either adalimumab 40 mg (n = 31) or placebo (n = 30)	Lower pain scores in adalimumab group but only at 6 months	No difference in pain scores between the groups except at 6 months
Ohtori et al. 2012[33]	60 patients with radicular pain from spinal stenosis in two equal groups received epidural injection of either 80 mg to cilizumab or 3.3 mg of dexamethasone	Significant improvement in pain and disability scores in tocilizumab group at 4 weeks	Inadequate randomization. Nonblinded. Short-term results at 4 weeks.

ADALIMUMAB

There is only one published controlled trial of adalimumab use for LBP. Sixty-one patients with lumbar radicular pain from herniated disc received two subcutaneous injections, 1 week apart, of either adalimumab (40 mg, n = 31) or placebo (saline, n = 30).[32] The primary outcome (pain score in the leg) was similar in both groups at all time points, with the exception of the 6-month time point, at which point the pain scores were lower for patients in the adalimumab group. Although the trial was well conducted, it provided *inconsistent evidence of the efficacy of subcutaneous adalimumab* in this group of patients. Additionally, the recommended dosing of adalimumab is 40–80 mg, given indeterminately by subcutaneous injection every 2 weeks, but the investigators in this study administered a course of only two 40-mg subcutaneous injections separated by 1 week.

TOCILIZUMAB

Tocilizumab was also evaluated in only one trial involving patients with radicular pain from lumbar spinal stenosis.[33] Sixty patients in two equal groups received either a single epidural injection of tocilizumab (80 mg in 2 cc of lidocaine) or dexamethasone (3.3 mg). The patients in the tocilizumab group had lower pain and disability scores for up to 4 weeks. This trial was not blinded and inadequately randomized. Based on this, despite the positive results, *tocilizumab is not considered an approved treatment for patients with radicular pain from lumbar spinal stenosis.*

Overall, the current use of DMARDs for LBP can be summarized as follows[34]:

- Use for investigational purposes only
- Exceedingly narrow empiric selection of the drugs
- Significant variation from the recommended drug doses, frequency, and routes of administration
- Lack of any nonbiological DMARD use
- Use of substantially lower cumulative drug dosages
- Lack of any studies evaluating combination drug therapy

EPIDURAL DMARD ADMINISTRATION FOR LOW BACK PAIN

The epidural route has been a frequent choice of DMARD administration for LBP. This selection naturally follows common practice of epidural steroid injections for LBP.[23] However, notwithstanding steroids, only biological DMARDs were administered in the epidural space. It should also be noted that biological DMARDs are highly soluble and biodegradable drugs that do not have a depot formulation, which may limit their duration of action. It is unclear if administration of these exceedingly water-soluble drugs in the highly vascular epidural space has any added advantage over their intravenous administration. Frequent administration of biological DMARDs in the epidural space, as would be necessitated by their pharmacokinetic profile, is impractical. In contrast, steroids given in the epidural space are often in the form of sustained release formulations that prolong their local antiinflammatory activity, and the epidural dose is similar to their parenteral dose.[23] In addition, steroids are potent antiinflammatory drugs that inhibit genetic expression of almost all proinflammatory cytokines. It is therefore unclear if epidural injection of biological DMARDs, especially in small doses or as a monotherapy, would be superior to epidural steroid injections.[34] Epidural steroid injections are generally well tolerated, and the safety of this route of administration is well established.[23] In one randomized study that compared epidurally administered steroids to etanercept and saline, steroids resulted in better outcomes on some measures than the etanercept and control groups.[26] Despite the fact that no serious adverse effects of epidural injection of biological DMARDs have been reported, their potential for neurotoxicity, especially if given in larger doses, or more frequently and if nonbiological DMARDs are used, remains unknown.

SYSTEMIC DMARD USE FOR LOW BACK PAIN

Similar to epidural DMARD use, systemic use of DMARDs for LBP has been characterized by: (1) isolated use of single biological drugs, (2) low cumulative doses, (3) absence of any nonbiological drug use, and (4) lack of combination DMARD therapy.[34] Consequently, the lack of benefit reported in many of the studies evaluating systemic DMARD use for LBP may have been due to inadequate treatment. Combinations of biological and nonbiological DMARDs, despite the significant risk of side effects, is regularly offered early in the course of many rheumatologic conditions in order to prevent the progressive deformities that often characterize the natural history of the disease.[22] Patients undergoing combination DMARD therapy should be monitored for systemic infections, blood dyscrasias, and metabolic abnormalities. In contrast to the many progressively disabling rheumatologic disorders, chronic LBP is often self-limiting, with only a small percentage of patients progressing to a debilitated state.[35] Therefore the routine use of potent combination DMARD therapy is likely unwarranted, and the prudent pain physician should only use this strategy in patients with disabling LBP unresponsive to traditional therapies. If used, systemic DMARD therapy should be modeled after well-established treatment protocols for other rheumatologic disorders, using recommended drug doses and a combination of both biological and nonbiological DMARDs.[22]

ADVERSE EFFECTS OF DMARD USE FOR LOW BACK PAIN

As a result of their primarily extracellular site of action, biological DMARDs have minimal metabolic adverse side effects, and their major limitation is increased susceptibility to infection.[21,22] Biological DMARDs are therefore contraindicated in patients with known infections and those who are otherwise immunocompromised, and their long-term use requires surveillance for chronic indolent infections such as tuberculosis. There are minimal to no adverse effects reported in the literature from the use of biological DMARDs for LBP patients. The likely explanation for this is the low cumulative drug doses, lack of concomitant or prior treatment with other DMARDs, and the fact that LBP patients otherwise possess normal immune function. It is possible that if combination DMARD therapy is used for LBP, the incidence of infections and other complications would rise, and monitoring for chronic infections may become necessary.

CONCLUSION

The current use of DMARDs for LBP, excluding steroids, is exceedingly narrow in scope and nonadherent to standardized protocols. The evidence for the efficacy of the drugs used is either inconclusive or has demonstrated only short-term benefit. Consequently, until further evidence is available, the use of DMARDs for LBP remains largely experimental in nature.

KEY POINTS

- Chronic inflammation plays a robust role in the etiology of many LBP syndromes.
- Despite the availability of a range of potent antiinflammatory drugs and DMARDs in the past few decades, the use of these drugs for LBP syndromes is limited predominantly to the administration of steroids and NSAIDs.

- The current use of nonsteroidal DMARDs for LBP is exceedingly narrow in scope and nonadherent to standardized protocols.
- Current evidence for the efficacy of these drugs is either inconclusive or demonstrates only short-term benefit.
- Until further evidence is available, the use of DMARDs (except steroids) for LBP remains largely experimental in nature.

REFERENCES

Access the reference list online at ExpertConsult.com.

CHAPTER 65

FACET SYNDROME

Julie H. Huang-Lionnet, MD, MBA ✪ Chad Brummett, MD ✪ Steven P. Cohen, MD

Spine pain is one of the leading causes of medical disability in the world. Most people will experience some type of neck and/or back pain throughout their life, with lifetime prevalence estimates as high as 84% for back pain[1] and 67% for neck pain.[2] Among all musculoskeletal disorders, low back pain (LBP) is the number-one reason patients seek medical attention and is the leading cause of disability; neck pain ranks as the fourth most common cause of years lost to disability. Between 2002 and 2004, the overall estimated financial costs for spine conditions, including lost wages, were estimated at over $200 billion.[3] This ranks only behind joint pain as the most expensive musculoskeletal medical condition.*

The causes of neck pain and LBP are complicated and often difficult to diagnose. The etiology is usually multifactorial, including muscles, ligaments, discs, nerve roots, and zygapophysial (facet) joints. The zygapophysial joint is a potential source of neck, shoulder, middle and lower back, and leg pain. It is also a potential source of headaches. Interventions for facet joint pain are second only to epidural steroid injections as the most commonly performed pain procedure in the United States. In 2006, interventions for facet pain represented approximately 37% of all pain interventions from Medicare, a 624% increase from 1997.[4]

ANATOMY AND FUNCTION

The facet joints are paired structures that reside posterolaterally to the vertebral body; along with the intervertebral disc, they compose the three-joint complex. This complex works together to stabilize the joint and allow for different movements depending on the level. Facet joints are true synovial joints formed from the superior articular process of one vertebra and the inferior articular process of the vertebra above. The volume capacity of the joints is 1–1.5 mL and 0.5–1.0 mL in the lumbar and cervical regions, respectively.[5]

The position of the joint relative to the sagittal and coronal planes helps determine the role that the joint plays in the restriction of motion. The lumbar facets vary in angle but are aligned lateral to the sagittal plane, with the inferior articular process facing anterolaterally and the superior articular process facing posteromedially.[6] In the lumbar region, the higher joints tend to be oriented in more of a sagittal plane (26–34 degrees), providing resistance to axial rotation, while the lower lumbar facet joints are more coronally oriented, offering protection to injury incurred by flexion and shearing forces.[7] The thoracic facets are the most vertically oriented joints, allowing for lateral flexion without axial rotation. In the cervical region, the shape and orientation of the joint also differ between the upper and lower joints.[8] The C2–C3 joint, perhaps the most frequent cervical facet pain generator, is aligned approximately 70 degrees from the sagittal plane and 45 degrees from the axial plane, which inhibits rotation and anchors the C2 vertebra as a rotational pivot for the atlantoaxial joint (C1–C2). The area of greatest mobility in the cervical spine is at C5–C6, the second most affected cervical facet joint, which is where the cervical facets transition to their posterolateral position.

The medial branch is the terminal division of the posterior ramus, which provides sensory innervation to the facet joint (Fig. 65.1). This smaller posterior division of the nerve root is divided into lateral, intermediate, and medial branches. The lateral branch in the lumbar region provides innervation to the paraspinous muscles, skin, and sacroiliac joint, while the small intermediate branch innervates the longissimus muscle. The medial branch is the largest of the divisions. It innervates the facet joint, multifidus muscle, interspinal muscle and ligament, and periosteum of the neural arch. Each facet joint is innervated by two medial branches, the medial branch at the same level and that at the level above (i.e., the L4–L5 facet joint is innervated by the L3 and L4 medial branches) (Fig. 65.2).

The position of the medial branch in the lumbar spine does not vary significantly. It divides from the posterior primary ramus and wraps around the transverse process of the level below at the junction of the transverse process and superior articular process (i.e., the L3 medial branch lies on the transverse process of L4). The nerve traverses the dorsal leaf of the intertransverse ligament of the transverse process and courses underneath the mamilloaccessory ligament, splitting into multiple branches as it crosses the vertebral lamina (see Fig. 65.2). The mamilloaccessory ligament can become calcified and be a source of nerve entrapment, especially at L5. The main variation in the lumbar spine is at L5, where it is the primary dorsal ramus itself that is amenable to blockade.[9]

The thoracic spine is generally similar to the lumbar spine in terms of innervation, with each joint being supplied by two medial branches, although some anatomic studies have shown that the dorsal ramus may send branches directly to the facet joint before dividing. In the upper and middle thoracic regions, two medial branches are present, including a cutaneous branch that is absent at lower thoracic levels. In the thoracic spine, medial branches assume different courses depending on the level.[10] At lower thoracic levels, the optimal blockade site is similar for lumbar medial branch blocks. At higher levels, the nerve swings

*National Center for Health Statistics. ftp://ftp.cdc.gov/pub/Health_Statistics/NCHS/Dataset_Documentation/NHIS/2008/srvydesc.pdf; Last accessed on November 29, 2009.

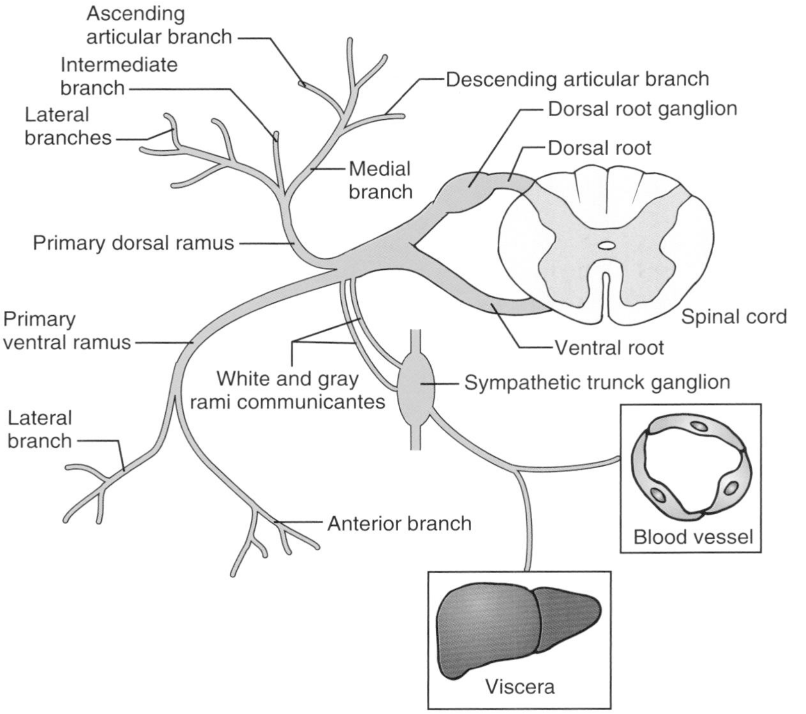

FIG. 65.1 Spinal cord and segmental spinal innervation. The medial branch can be seen branching from the dorsal primary ramus, along with the intermediate and lateral branches. *(From Cohen SP, Raja SN: Pathogenesis, diagnosis and treatment of lumbar zygapophysial [facet] joint pain,* Anesthesiology. *106(3):591-614, 2007.)*

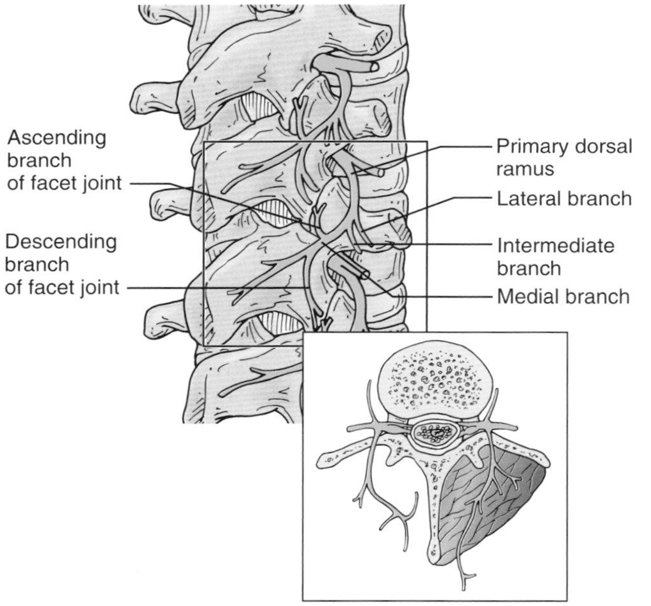

FIG. 65.2 Lumbar facet innervation. A right lateral oblique figure demonstrating the medial branches innervating the facet joints, along with paraspinous muscle innervation. *(From Cohen SP, Raja SN: Pathogenesis, diagnosis and treatment of lumbar zygapophysial [facet] joint pain,* Anesthesiology. *106(3):591-614, 2007.)*

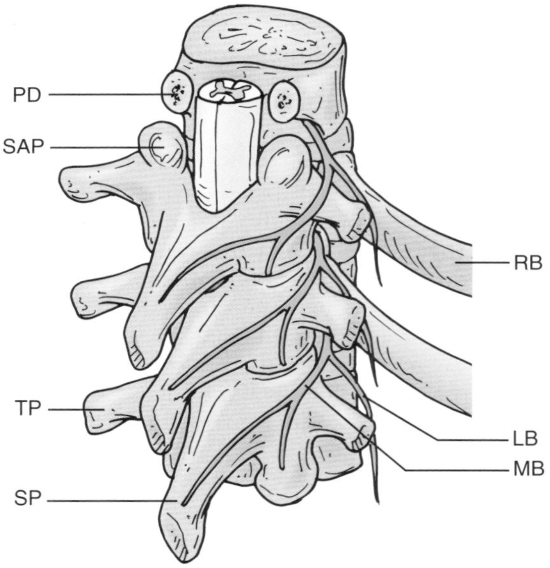

FIG. 65.3 Thoracic facet innervation. The commonly accepted target point of the medial branch is seen along the superolateral portion of the transverse process. *LB*, Lateral branch; *MB*, medial branch; *PD*, pedicle; *RB*, rib; *SAP*, superior articular process; *SP*, spinous process; *TP*, transverse process. *(From Chua WH, Bogduk N: The surgical anatomy of thoracic facet denervation,* Acta Neurochirugia. *136(3-4):140-144, 1995.)*

laterally to circumvent the multifidus muscle, thereby removing multifidus contraction as a means of needle confirmation prior to denervation. From T4 to T8 in some specimens, the medial branch courses somewhere in the intertransverse space without making contact with bone, making medial branch blocks challenging. At the middle and upper thoracic levels, the superolateral corner of the transverse process is the most consistent point for blockade (Fig. 65.3A and B).

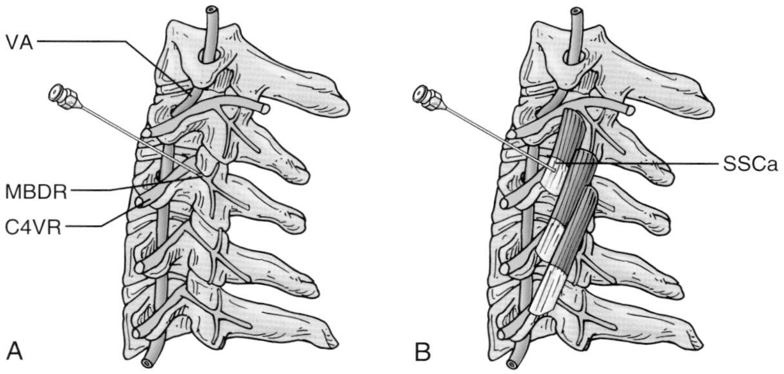

FIG. 65.4 (A) In these posterolateral sketches of the cervical region, the medial branch can be seen crossing the articular pillars. (B) The semispinalis capitis (SSCa) lies over the medial branch, which may hold the local anesthetic in place after a diagnostic block. *VA*, Vertebral artery. *(From Barnsley L, Bogduk N: Medial branch block are specific for the diagnosis of cervical zygapophysial joint pain.* Reg Anesth. *18(6):343-350, 1993.)*

The innervation of the cervical facets is more varied and complicated. There are eight cervical nerve roots, which exit above the corresponding vertebral bodies. Similar to the lumbar and thoracic regions, the C3–C4 through the C7–T1 joints receive innervation from the medial branches at the same level and the level above. The nerves curve around the waist of the articular pillars except at C7 and C8, where the anatomy is more variable.[11] Medial branches at higher levels adhere tightly to the periosteum with tight fascia and the tendons of the semispinalis, which makes positioning more predictable (Fig. 65.4A and B). The majority of the innervation of the C2–C3 joint comes from the dorsal ramus of C3. The C3 dorsal ramus divides into two separate medial branches, the larger of which is known as the third occipital nerve. The C2 dorsal ramus divides into up to five branches, the largest of which is the greater occipital nerve.[12] Pathology involving branches of the C2 and C3 dorsal rami is a common source of occipital headaches. In some people, dual medial branches are present at a single level, which is most common at C4 (27%) and C5 (15%).[13]

The facet joints contain a rich supply of encapsulated, unencapsulated, and free nerve endings.[14] Previous work has established the presence of substance P and calcitonin gene–related peptide reactive nerve fibers in cadaveric facets.[15] Inflammatory mediators, including prostaglandins, interleukin-6, and tumor necrosis factor-α, have been demonstrated in the facet cartilage of patients undergoing surgical therapy for degenerative lumbar disease.[15] Studies have demonstrated that leakage of these cytokines through the ventral joint capsule may be partially responsible for radicular symptoms in lumbar spinal stenosis.[16] In addition, subchondral bone and intraarticular (IA) inclusions of facet joints have nerve endings, signifying that structures besides the joint capsule may be potential pain generators.[17]

PATHOPHYSIOLOGY

With the exception of whiplash injuries and major spine trauma,[18–20] facet arthropathy and facet-mediated pain are infrequently due to acute injury. In a study performed in trauma patients, Levine et al. reported that bilateral facet dislocation occurred in 11% of cases requiring surgical stabilization, with the mechanism of action being "flexion-distraction" in 29 of 30 cases.[21] Instead, years of repetitive strain, intervertebral disc degeneration, and minor trauma are more commonly implicated. Similar to other degenerative joint diseases, there is a poor correlation between pain and the degree of inflammation or degeneration. Facet arthropathy is known to occur more commonly in the elderly, which is consistent with the concept of a degenerative disorder.[22,23]

CADAVERIC AND ANIMAL STUDIES

Cadaveric studies have demonstrated that the greatest degree of motion and strain in the lumbar spine occurs in the lowest two facet joints (L4–L5 and L5–S1).[24] At these joints, strain is maximized by forward flexion. In the middle joints (L3–L4), the greatest degree of strain is observed with contralateral bending, whereas the opposite was seen at the most cephalad joints (L1–L2 and L2–L3). Fusion of an intervertebral level has been shown to accelerate degeneration at adjacent levels.[25,26]

Whereas facet joint pain is not normally considered an active inflammatory state, chronic strain and repetitive stimulation can lead to fluid collection and joint distention.[27] If the intervertebral foramen is already narrowed from other pathology (intervertebral disc herniation, osteophyte formation, etc.), a hypertrophied facet joint may further compress the nerve root, thereby manifesting in radicular pain. In some cases, spasm of the paraspinous musculature can be superimposed.[28]

HUMAN STUDIES

The presence of facet arthropathy is more common in the elderly. The intervertebral disc and facets work in concert, such that degeneration of the intervertebral disc creates additional strain on the facet joints and vice versa.[29] The two most caudal facet joints (L4–L5 and L5–S1) are associated with the greatest degree of degenerative disc disease, with L5–S1 being the most common clinically affected joint and L4–L5 being the most frequently radiologically affected joint. Intervertebral discs degenerate at an earlier age than facet joints, although one cadaveric study found that 93% of cadaver specimens between 40 and 49 years of age had evidence of facet arthrosis.[30] Less common causes of facetogenic pain include inflammatory arthritis and pseudocysts.

As already noted, facetogenic pain can occasionally result from trauma, especially rapid deceleration injuries. In one study, capsular and articular damage was observed in 77% of facet joints in people who died in motor vehicle accidents.[31] The most common presentation of trauma-induced facet pain is whiplash injury, which may account for over 50% of cases of chronic neck pain following motor vehicle accidents.[32] However, trauma still only accounts for a relatively small portion of cervical facetogenic pain (13%–23%).[33]

PREVALENCE

The prevalence of facet pain is a source of controversy. The lumbar facet joints are the most commonly affected due to the high frequency of LBP in the general population and the greater load borne by these joints. However, the cervical facet joints account for a higher percentage of chronic neck pain than the lumbar facet joints do in patients with chronic LBP. One limiting factor in determining the true incidence of facet pain is that the diagnosis cannot be made by history, physical examination, or radiologic findings; hence there is no reference standard according to which the sensitivity and specificity of diagnostic injections can be judged. The most reliable method for determining facetogenic pain is with image-guided medial branch (facet joint nerve) or IA facet joint blocks.[34]

The prevalence of lumbar facet pain varies widely in the literature, with the best estimates ranging between 10% and 15%.[35,36] Although comparative medial branch blocks (MBBs) have been endorsed as a diagnostic standard, the other branches of the dorsal primary ramus will also invariably be blocked when local anesthetic is injected, which may overestimate the prevalence.[37–39] Another source of error is that most epidemiologic studies evaluating the prevalence of lumbar facet joint pain exclude patients with radicular symptoms, despite the fact that facet arthropathy can cause neuroforaminal stenosis and may occur concurrently with radicular pain.[40]

Estimating the prevalence of cervical facet pain is equally challenging, with some of the most elegant clinical studies conducted exclusively in patients with whiplash injuries.[18,20] However, the best studies using double blocks have generally reported prevalence rates ranging between 49% and 60% in patients with chronic, nonradicular neck pain. Among patients with chronic middle- and upper-back pain (BP), the estimated prevalence varies between 40% and 50%. Not surprisingly, reviews performed for lumbar facet joint and sacroiliac joint pain have generally found that studies using lower cutoffs (e.g., 50%) as the threshold for a positive response and those using single blocks report higher prevalence rates than studies that use higher cutoff values and employ double blocks.[41–43]

DIAGNOSIS

HISTORY AND PHYSICAL EXAMINATION

Many studies have investigated the ability to predict response to diagnostic facet blocks on the basis of history and/or physical examination. Although clinical symptoms and pain referral patterns can help guide physicians, the specificity is very poor. The terms *lumbar facet syndrome* and *facet loading* were coined from a small, poorly designed retrospective study of 22 patients done in 1988.[44] Subsequent larger and methodologically sound studies failed to validate these findings.[33,45–47] Yet, many pain physicians continue to rely on misguided signs and symptoms as being diagnostically significant. Tenderness to palpation in the cervical and lumbar paraspinous regions was found to be a positive predictor of radiofrequency (RF) denervation outcome in two large retrospective studies, but such findings need to be confirmed prospectively.[45,46]

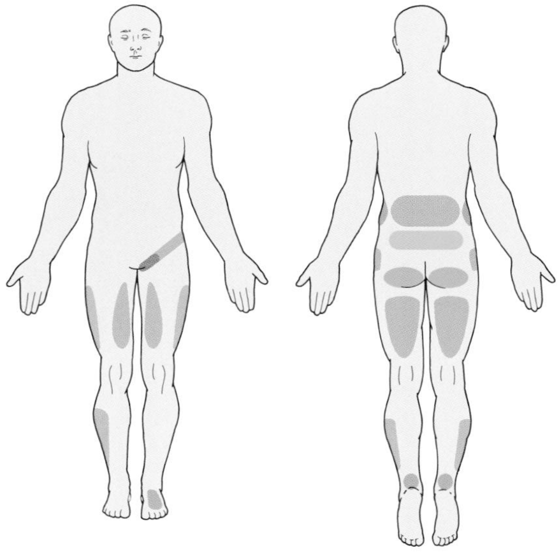

FIG. 65.5 The referral patterns for lumbar facets are shown from the most common areas in the low back (darkest regions) to the less common areas in the flank and feet (lightest regions). Although some facet joints are associated with particular patterns, there is a great deal of overlap between the levels. Therefore a particular level cannot be identified by referral patterns. *(From Cohen SP, Raja SN: Pathogenesis, diagnosis and treatment of lumbar zygapophysial [facet] joint pain,* Anesthesiology. *106(3):591-614, 2007.)*

Pain referral patterns can provide clues to diagnosis. Studies have been conducted by provoking pain in healthy volunteers (i.e., distending the joint capsule and stimulating medial branches) and investigating pain patterns in patients whose symptoms are relieved by diagnostic blocks. Similar to other sources of spinal pain, the referral patterns associated with facet pain tend to be variable and overlapping.[33,35]

Although there is a great deal of overlap between different spinal levels and different structures (i.e., facet joints and discs) at the same level, when the results of provocation and analgesic studies are combined, some patterns emerge (Figs. 65.5 and 65.6). In the lumbar region, the upper facet joints tend to refer pain to the flank, hip, and upper lateral thigh.[33] For lower levels, pain is generally experienced in the posterolateral thigh and occasionally the calf. In the cervical spine, upper facet arthropathy usually manifests as pain felt in the posterior upper neck and occipital region.[35] Pathology involving middle cervical facet joints tends to radiate into the lower neck and supraclavicular region, while lower cervical facetogenic pain typically causes pain in the base of the neck and scapular region.

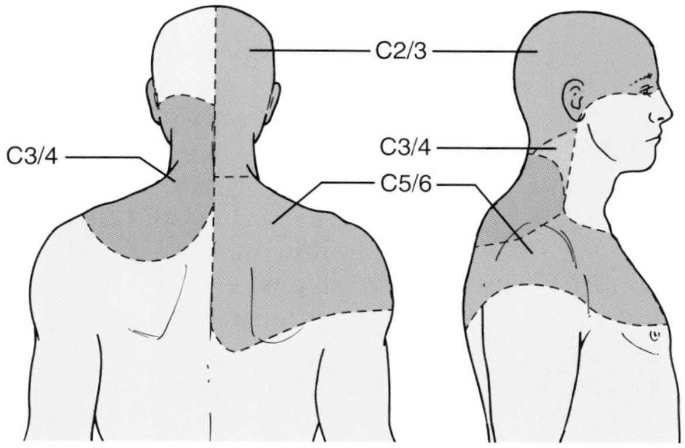

FIG. 65.6 Cervical facet pain referral patterns. The upper cervical facet joints are associated with upper neck and head pain, whereas the lower levels tend to be associated with pain in the lower neck and scapula. *(From Bogduk N, Marsland A: The cervical zygapophysial joints as a source of neck pain,* Spine. *13(6):615, 1988.)*

RADIOLOGY

Although it is common for patients with chronic spinal pain to undergo multiple imaging studies, radiologic examination has limited utility in the diagnosis of facet-mediated pain. Whereas the lumbar facet joints account for a small percentage of chronic LBP cases, the prevalence of facet pathology on computed tomography (CT) scans is between 40% and 85%, with the rate increasing significantly with age.[48,49] Similar rates of abnormal findings have been found in asymptomatic volunteers who undergo cervical and thoracic magnetic resonance imaging (MRI).[50,51] Studies using MRI, CT, and other imaging studies to predict response to facet blocks have been decidedly mixed, with most showing a poor correlation.[45,46]

Although fluoroscopic guidance for facet joint injections is the standard, use of ultrasound guidance is acknowledged as another modality for medial branch and facet joint injections. For RF denervation, ultrasound does not enable one to place electrodes parallel to the course of the target nerves, which limits its use in this context. It has also been shown to be less accurate in obese patients.[52] Ultrasound was shown in a randomized feasibility clinical trial to provide significant differences in visual analog scale (VAS) pain scores and pain remission rate for facet joint injections when compared with blind injection without ultrasound.[53] Ultrasound-guided facet joint injection in the middle and lower cervical spine has been shown to be comparable to CT guidance in VAS pain relief in addition to resulting in significant reduction in procedure duration without any exposure to radiation.[54]

DIAGNOSTIC BLOCKS

The inability to predict facet pain from history, physical examination, or radiologic study has led to the widespread use of medial branch and IA facet blocks for diagnosis. Although diagnostic MBBs have been used in multiple studies,[55–57] some technical and anatomic considerations limit their diagnostic utility. Studies have demonstrated that volumes as small as 0.5 mL spread out over 6 cm^2 of tissue. Hence the intermediate and lateral branches are likely to be anesthetized with typical injection volumes, thereby blocking afferent transmission from portions of the paraspinous musculature and sacroiliac joint. A randomized study has demonstrated a clinically relevant improvement in specificity without undermining sensitivity when 0.25 mL of local anesthetic was used for cervical MBBs compared with 0.5 mL.[58] The use of IA facet injections can reduce issues related to the inadvertent spread of local anesthetic, but they can be technically challenging, with a failure rate exceeding 33%.[59]

Furthermore, excessive volumes of local anesthetic solution can rupture the joint capsule, leading to spread into the intervertebral foramen, epidural space and paraspinous musculature.[27,57,60] Studies that have used MBBs have generally shown better results than those that used IA injections as prognostic procedures. A multicenter case-control study was performed to determine which prognostic facet block, IA injections or medial branch block, was a better predictive tool for analgesic response to RF denervation. The findings from this retrospective study suggest that MBBs are a superior prognostic tool for RF denervation outcomes compared to IA blocks.[61] However, the major reason for treatment failure is poor patient selection (e.g., greater disease burden, psychosocial pathology), which should be taken into consideration when designing clinical trials.

FALSE-POSITIVE DIAGNOSTIC BLOCKS

Both MBBs and IA blocks are associated with high rates of false-positive results. False-positive rates have ranged from 25% to 40% in the lumbar spine[33] and from 25% to 30% in the cervical spine.[62,63] Although some experts have advocated comparative local anesthetic blocks as an alternative to "placebo controls," this paradigm is not without limitations. A randomized, double-blind study of cervical MBBs in 50 whiplash patients with neck pain using normal saline, lidocaine, and bupivacaine in random order found comparative blocks (serial lidocaine and bupivacaine injections) to be highly sensitive (88%) but only marginally specific (54%).[63]

Potential causes of false-positive blocks include placebo response, sedation, excessive superficial local anesthesia, and the spread of local anesthetic to other pain-generating structures.[64] It is our belief that the use of sedation for diagnostic blocks should be limited, as even benzodiazepines can lead to muscle relaxation and interfere with a patient's ability to assess pain relief. However, this assumption has been challenged by some, who argue that using a more stringent pain relief threshold (≥80%) mitigates against a higher false-positive rate when sedation is administered.[65] Prospective and retrospective studies performed in the lumbar spine have found no difference in RF denervation outcomes between those patients who experience 50% or greater relief and higher thresholds.[47,66] Moreover, a prospective crossover study evaluating the effect of sedation on diagnostic specificity found that even light sedation significantly increased the rate of positive blocks.[67]

Several steps can be taken to negate or minimize the role of other factors in false-positive blocks. Dreyfuss et al. found that for lumbar MBB, targeting a lower point midway between the upper border of the transverse process and mamilloaccessory ligament significantly reduced epidural and foraminal spread compared with the conventional target point at the superomedial border of the transverse process.[9] Cohen et al. showed that reducing the volume of injectate from 0.5 to 0.25 mL for cervical MBB resulted in a greater than 50% decrease in spread to adjacent pain-generating structures.[58] In a randomized, double-blind study, Ackerman et al.[68] found that injecting superficial lidocaine down to the facet joint or medial branch resulted in a greater than five-fold increase in positive blocks in the first of two blocks than when patients received superficial saline; this effect was not observed in the second block. One way to reduce the need for superficial injection is to use a single-needle technique, which was demonstrated in a randomized crossover study to decrease the amount of superficial lidocaine by 40% while providing comparable pain relief and contrast spread compared with the traditional multiple-needle technique.[69] Recommendations to limit false-positive blocks are listed in Table 65.1.

FALSE-NEGATIVE BLOCKS

False-negative blocks have garnered less attention than false positives, but they can be a source of misdiagnosis and failure to select appropriate candidates for treatment. A study conducted in which 15 volunteers underwent MBBs with local anesthetic or saline followed by capsular distention estimated the incidence of false-negative blocks to be 11% based on the inability of local anesthetic infiltration to block the pain from facet joint capsular distention.[70] A probable cause was deemed to be "aberrant innervation," which would account for some cases of failed RF denervation in IA block responders. One of the principal causes of false-negative blocks is thought to be vascular uptake. This has been reported to range between 6% and 30% per level,[70,71] with one study finding rates of 3.9% at cervical levels, 3.5% at lumbar levels, and 0.7% at thoracic levels.[72] One study found that when vascular uptake occurs, even if the needle is repositioned, analgesia will be obtained only half the time.[70] The most reliable means of detecting vascular uptake is with digital subtraction angiography, which has been shown to enhance the detection rate.[73] Other potential causes of false-negative blocks are failure to discern between baseline and procedure-related pain and missing a target nerve or nerves.

SELECTION CRITERIA: 50% VERSUS 80% RELIEF, SINGLE VERSUS DOUBLE MEDIAL BRANCH BLOCKS

A great deal of debate has centered on the selection of patients for denervation, with the two primary arguments revolving around the percentage of pain relief and the number of blocks. The thresholds for pain relief studied are somewhat arbitrary, as previous research has determined a two-point or 30% decrease in pain to be clinically meaningful.[74] Multiple retrospective analyses have found no difference in results between using 50% and 80% relief as the cutoff for a positive block.[45–47,75,76] A multicenter prospective correlation study by Cohen et al. set out to evaluate the influence of pain relief after MBBs on RF outcome and determine an optimal "cut-off" threshold for diagnostic lumbar facet blocks. Their study showed no significant differences in RF outcomes based on any MBB with a pain relief cutoff threshold above 50%. No optimal threshold for designating a diagnostic block as positive, above 50% pain relief, could be calculated.[66]

The issue of how many blocks should be performed is also the subject of considerable controversy. The argument in favor of double blocks is bolstered primarily by the high false-positive rate of uncontrolled blocks, whereas those who advocate single blocks point to time and cost constraints, the comparable complication rate between diagnostic blocks and RF denervation, and the fact that confirmatory diagnostic procedures are not used to select patients for intradiscal procedures, surgery, and other more invasive interventions. Multiple retrospective studies evaluating outcomes for lumbar facet, cervical facet, and sacroiliac (SI) joint RF denervation have failed to find a difference in success rates between patients selected with one and two diagnostic blocks.[33,35] In a large, multicenter, randomized study comparing the cost effectiveness of zero, one, and two blocks before lumbar facet RF denervation, although the RF success rate was highest in the double-block group (64%), the overall success rate was 50% higher in the zero-block group (33% vs. 16% vs. 22%, respectively). In the cost-benefit analysis, the cost per effective treatment was $6054 in the zero-block group, $16,236 in the single-block group, and $14,238 in the double-block group.[77]

However, this treatment paradigm remains controversial. A prospective, single-blind, triple-crossover study evaluating the diagnostic validity of facet joint injections in 60 patients with chronic LBP showed that a single IA facet block with local anesthetic provided pain relief comparable to that from a placebo injection or a sham procedure (needle placement outside the facet joint with no injection and was not useful as a diagnostic tool. The authors asserted that the only reliable means to identify a painful facet joint was to use double or triple controlled blocks with at least one placebo injection. However, the patients in this study were not prescreened by diagnostic blocks; it is therefore likely that only a small number of these patients suffered from facet arthropathy.[78]

TABLE 65.1 Techniques to Reduce False-Positive Rates for Lumbar Medial Branch Blocks

1. Avoid the use of sedation and analgesics.
2. Use injectate volumes ≤0.5 mL.
3. Limit the volume of superficial local anesthesia.
4. Aim for lower target point on transverse process.
5. Use a single-needle approach.
6. Consider use of comparative local anesthetic or placebo-controlled blocks.
7. Properly educate patients regarding correct use of pain diary.

TREATMENT

PHARMACOTHERAPY AND NONINTERVENTIONAL TREATMENT MODALITIES

The focus of treatment for spinal pain has become heavily weighted toward interventions. Despite the lack of high-quality studies comparing pharmacologic and alternative therapies to interventions, a reasonable approach is to start with conservative management. There is strong evidence for the use of nonsteroidal antiinflammatory drugs in treating spinal pain, although the effect size is small. A recent meta-analysis on the effectiveness of acetaminophen for LBP concluded that it was not beneficial.[79] Antidepressants and muscle relaxants have also been shown in controlled trials to be effective for nonspecific spinal pain; however, the evidence for muscle relaxants is much stronger in the acute setting where muscle spasm is present.

Similar to other pain conditions, physical activity and weight loss are likely to benefit BP patients. Exercise and yoga programs have been shown to decrease relapses in BP and seem to be more beneficial in patients with chronic pain. Spinal manipulation is superior to sham treatment for acute and chronic spinal pain, but the long-term benefits remain to be proven. Acupuncture also appears effective for spinal pain but has not been shown to be superior to other treatments or sham acupuncture. Comorbid depression, anxiety, and other psychological disorders are common in patients with chronic spinal pain and have been shown to predict poor response to treatment. Therefore a multidisciplinary approach that includes psychotherapy, if indicated, is essential to optimize outcomes.[80]

INTRAARTICULAR CORTICOSTEROID INJECTIONS

Despite the conceptual appeal of IA steroid injections, study results are mostly negative. In addition to other methodologic flaws, many clinical trials failed to preselect patients with diagnostic blocks prior to allocating them to treatment. Several uncontrolled studies have found that patients with an active inflammatory process, as demonstrated by positive single photon emission computed tomography (SPECT) scans, may obtain intermediate-term relief following facet joint steroid infiltration.[33] Two very well designed studies published in the *New England Journal of Medicine* evaluated lumbar and cervical facet IA facet injections in patients prediagnosed with facetogenic pain based on diagnostic screening blocks; both studies failed to demonstrate a significant difference between steroid and saline or local anesthetic injections.[81,82] More recently, however, a randomized controlled trial assessing the effectiveness of IA facet joint injection (six lumbar facet joints) compared with systemic steroid (intramuscular injection of six lumbar paravertebral points) in facet joint syndrome showed improvements in the experimental group compared with the control group on several outcome measures. Improved outcomes were observed on diclofenac intake, quality of life in the 36-item Short Form Health Survey, improvement percentage scale in the Roland-Morris disability questionnaire, and response to treatment as assessed by the Likert scale.[83]

RADIOFREQUENCY DENERVATION OF THE MEDIAL BRANCHES

The most commonly performed treatment for facet-mediated pain is RF denervation. There have been 12 controlled studies for lumbar facet pain and 2 for neck pain (Table 65.2). Some of these studies failed to appropriately select candidates through diagnostic blocks,[84] while others failed to use optimal technique (i.e., placing the electrode parallel to the nerve), making the results difficult to interpret.[84,85] Overall, however, the results argue favorably for the use of denervation in well-selected patients. Several randomized studies have also examined pulsed RF in the treatment of facet joint pain. Although one unblinded study that selected patients based on pain relief 5 minutes after a diagnostic block found pulsed RF to be superior to medial branch blocks done with steroid,[86] two double-blind studies by Tekin et al.[87] and Kroll et al.[88] failed to demonstrate significant efficacy.

TABLE 65.2 Outcomes of Randomized Controlled Trials of Lumbar and Cervical Medial Branch Denervation

Author, Year	Patients Studied	Duration of Follow-Up (months)	Methodologic Scoring	Results	Notes
Lumbar Spine					
King and Lagger, 1976	60 patients with LBP/leg pain and paraspinous tenderness. Three groups: (1) RF of primary posterior ramus, (2) RF of muscle at area of maximal tenderness (myotomy), (3) stimulation but no RF	6	MQ = 2 CR = 5	Group 1, 27% with relief; Group 2, 53% with relief; Group 3, 0% with relief	No diagnostic blocks prior to randomization; included patients with sciatica; used three 120-s lesions without electrical stimulation to determine appropriate placement
Gallagher et al., 1994	41 patients with "clear-cut" (30 patients) or "equivocal" (11 patients) relief after lumbar intraarticular facet injection with local anesthetic and steroid; Randomized to RF or sham	6	MQ = 2 CR = 6	In patients with "clear-cut" response to intraarticular block, RF improved pain scores compared with sham; no difference between groups in patients with "equivocal" response to intraarticular block	Did not define "clear-cut" or "equivocal"; poor description of anatomic landmarks; not blinded; RF needle placed perpendicular to medial branch

Continued

TABLE 65.2 Outcomes of Randomized Controlled Trials of Lumbar and Cervical Medial Branch Denervation—cont'd

Author, Year	Patients Studied	Duration of Follow-Up (months)	Methodologic Scoring	Results	Notes
van Kleef et al., 1999	31 patients with ≥ 50% relief after lumbar MBB; randomized to RF or sham	12	MQ = 5 CR = 8	At 3-mo follow-up, 9/15 in RF group vs. 4/16 in sham group reported ≥50% relief At 12-mo follow-up, 7/15 in lesion group and 2/16 in sham group reported ≥50% relief	Diagnostic blocks with 0.75 mL of local anesthetic; placed RF probe perpendicular to the medial branch for denervation
Sanders and Zuurmond, 1999[100]	34 patients with chronic LBP with ≥50% relief after a single lidocaine intraarticular block; half received medial branch denervation and the other half had intraarticular facet denervation	3	MQ = 1 CR = 6	Both groups improved; however, the intraarticular RF group improved more	Diagnostic blocks with 1 mL RF of medial branch done at inferolateral aspect of facet capsule and upper border of transverse process; three intraarticular lesions done
Leclaire et al., 2001[101]	70 patients with chronic LBP with ≥24 h of "significant" relief after intraarticular lidocaine plus steroid; compared RF with sham procedure	3	MQ = 4 CR = 8	RF group with modest improvement in Roland Morris (P = .05) and VAS (P = ns) scores at 3 mo; no change Oswestry score or other outcomes	Did not define "significant relief" for diagnostic block; greater than 24-h relief not consistent with lidocaine pharmacology Landmarks not noted for RF and needle not placed parallel to medial branch
Tekin et al., 2007	60 patients with chronic LBP with ≥50% relief from single MBB at either L1–L3 or L3–L5 received either sham, pulsed RF, or RF denervation	12	MQ = 4 CR = 8	Continuous RF > pulsed RF and sham for pain; nonsignificant difference between pulsed RF and sham; for ODI, continuous RF and pulsed RF > sham	Used 0.3 mL for diagnostic blocks; proper technique for blocks and RF; study not powered to detect differences between treatment groups
Nath et al., 2008[102]	40 patients with chronic LBP who obtained ≥80% relief from 3 LA blocks	6	MQ = 4 CR = 6	RF group > control group in all outcome measures, although the benefits were modest	40 patients randomized out of 376 screened; created six empirical lesions without stimulation
Van Wijk et al., 2005	81 patients with chronic LBP with ≥50% relief from two-level intraarticular facet block with LA; RF compared with sham	12	MQ = 5 CR = 7	No differences at 3 mo between groups for combined score of pain, physical activity, and analgesic intake; global perceived effect greater in RF compared with sham at 3 mo	Blinding ended at 3 mo with patients with persistent relief followed for 12 mo; placed electrodes perpendicular to nerve
Hashemi et al., 2014	80 patients with degenerative spondylolisthesis randomized to pulsed RF or injections with steroid (triamcinolone) and bupivacaine	12	MQ = 5 CR = 9	Pulsed RF with reduced pain scores at 6 mo compared with steroid and bupivacaine resulted in lower Oswestry Disability Index (ODI) % at 12 weeks and 6 mo; proportion of patients who did not require analgesics was significantly higher in PRF group	Patients selected based on ultrasound-guided MBB done with unspecified volumes and no set cutoff for a positive block, which was assessed 5 min postprocedure; unclear rationale for using pulsed RF for mechanical pain

TABLE 65.2 Outcomes of Randomized Controlled Trials of Lumbar and Cervical Medial Branch Denervation—cont'd

Author, Year	Patients Studied	Duration of Follow-Up (months)	Methodologic Scoring	Results	Notes
Lakemeier et al., 2013[103]	56 patients with lumbar facet joint–related pain randomized to intraarticular facet joint steroid injections or radiofrequency denervation of L3–L4. L4–L5 and L5–S1 segments	6	MQ = 5 CR = 8	No significant difference between groups for pain and function, with both groups experiencing improvement	Did not position electrodes in a parallel orientation to nerves; cointerventions permitted
Civelek et al., 2012[104]	100 patients with chronic LBP and suspected lumbar facet syndrome randomized to lumbar MBB with local anesthetic and steroid injection or radiofrequency denervation	12	MQ = 4 CR = 7	RF superior to medial branch blocks between 1 mo and 12 mo for pain relief, quality of life, and satisfaction	Did not prescreen patients with diagnostic injections
van Tilburg et al. 2016[105]	60 patients with axial low back pain and ≥2-point decrease in pain score after 3-level medial branch blocks.	6	MQ = 4 CR = 6	No significant differences between treatment groups for pain or global perceived effect.	Placed electrodes perpendicular rather than parallel to nerves. Only 22 of 104 patients had negative diagnostic block.
Cervical Spine					
Lord et al., 1996	24 patients with neck pain ≥3 mo after MVA that failed conservative therapy; diagnosed through placebo-controlled (saline vs. LA) MBB; compared 80°C RF vs. 37°C control between C3–C7 medial branches	3 (12 mos in patients with persistent relief)	MQ = 5 CR = 8	Time to return of 50% of predenervation pain was 263 days in RF group vs. 8 days in placebo group ($P < .04$); At 27 wk, 7/12 patients in RF group and 1/12 in placebo group remained pain-free	Excluded patients with exclusively C2-3 pain; 5 patients in RF group had numbness in skin associated with denervated area
Stovner et al., 2004	12 patients with unilateral cervicogenic HA who underwent comparative blocks of medial branches; compared cervical medial branch RF vs. sham	24	MQ = 4 CR = 7	At 3 mo, 4/6 in RF group vs. 2/6 in sham group with meaningful improvement (30% improvement); no differences at 6 mo	Response to diagnostic blocks not used as an inclusion criterion; RF group with better response to diagnostic blocks; recruited only 12 patients in almost 2.9 years; excluded patients with active litigation

Notes: Methodologic quality (MQ) score based on 5-point scale previously described. A score ≥3 indicates high MQ as described by Jadad et al.[98]
Clinical relevance (CR) score based on patient selection parameters and RF technique description (0–9 scale) as described by Geurts et al.[99]
HA, *headache;* LA, *local anesthetic;* LBP, *low back pain;* MBB, *medial branch block;* MVA, *motor vehicle accident;* NS, *nonsignificant;* ODI, *Oswestry Disability Index;* pulsed RF, *pulsed radiofrequency;* pts, *patients;* RF, *radiofrequency;* VAS, *visual analog scale.*
Source: Modified and updated from Brummett CB, Cohen SP: Pathogenesis, diagnosis, and treatment of zygapophyseal (facet) joint pain. In: Benzon HT, Rathmell JP, Wu CL, Turk DC, Argoff CE, Hurley RW, editors: Raj's Practical Management of Pain, *ed 5, London, 2013, Mosby Elsevier, pp. 816–845.*[35]

The medial branch is ablated by placing the active tip of a RF needle at the location of the nerve. For the lumbar region, the active tip is optimally positioned at the junction of the transverse process and lateral neck of the superior articular process in an orientation parallel to the nerve. In the cervical region, the active tip should be placed along the center of the articular pillar at most levels. Sensory stimulation is usually performed prior to denervation, with most experts recommending a threshold of no more than 0.5 V. Motor stimulation is considered a safety measure to ensure adequate distance from motor fibers, although the elicitation of multifidus muscle contraction has also been used to guide needle placement.[89,90] Prior to denervation, local anesthetic is usually injected to reduce procedure-related pain and enhance lesion size; postdenervation, steroids can be given to reduce the incidence of neuritis. The duration of analgesia following RF denervation varies widely between studies, with most demonstrating relief lasting for 6 months to 1 year.[19,87,89,91] Although data are limited, repeat denervation in both the cervical and lumbar regions appears to provide relief comparable to that of the initial procedure.[92]

SURGERY

Surgery is occasionally done for facet pain despite the absence of convincing data to support it.[33] Some surgeons purposefully or inadvertently transect the medial branch during pedicle screw placement, which can provide some pain relief. However, when all data are synthesized, surgery is not recommended as a treatment for facetogenic pain.

COMPLICATIONS FROM MINIMALLY INVASIVE INTERVENTIONS

The most feared risk of RF denervation is thermal damage to the ventral nerve root due to incorrect needle placement, which is rare when motor stimulation is used. Postdenervation neuritis is the most common complication, but significant postprocedural pain occurs in less than 10% of cases. It can be reduced even further with the prophylactic administration of corticosteroid.[93] Some patients describe transient numbness or dysesthesias, which are usually minor and self-limiting.[94] Rarely, breaks in insulation or equipment malfunction can lead to burns.[33,95] Infectious complications are very infrequent and appear to be even less common with RF than with diagnostic blocks.[96]

A prospective, nonrandomized observational study of complications of fluoroscopically directed facet joint nerve blocks showed no major complications with common minor side effects.[97] Overall, there was a 17.4% incidence of adverse effects or complications (7500 total episodes involving 43,000 facet joint nerve blocks with 3370 episodes in the cervical region, 3162 in the lumbar region, and 950 in the thoracic region). Side effects and complications observed included:

1. Overall intravascular penetration in 11.4% of episodes, with 20% in the cervical region, 4% in the lumbar region, and 6% in the thoracic spine
2. Local bleeding in 76.3% of episodes, with the highest rate in the thoracic region and lowest rate in the cervical region
3. Oozing in 19.6% of encounters, being most frequent in the cervical region and lowest in the lumbar region
4. Local hematoma, observed in 1.2% of patients
5. Others—profuse bleeding, bruising, soreness, nerve root irritation, and vasovagal reactions, observed in less than 1% of cases

CONCLUSION

Pain arising from the facet joints is a common source of disability. With the exception of whiplash, facet pain is usually due to chronic degeneration resulting from repetitive stress. There are no historical or physical examination findings pathognomonic for diagnosis, but clinical assessment is important for ruling out other sources of pain and selecting candidates for interventions. IA blocks or MBBs remain the "gold standard" for diagnosis but are characterized by a high false-positive rate and lack of specificity. Studies that have used MBBs have generally shown better results than those that used IA blocks as prognostic procedures. The major reason why people fail treatment is poor patient selection (e.g., psychosocial issues), so these should be taken into consideration for clinical trials. Most, but not all, studies have shown RF denervation to be safe and effective. In carefully selected patients, it can provide significant relief for 6 months to 1 year.

REFERENCES

Access the reference list online at ExpertConsult.com.

CHAPTER 66

Sacroiliac Joint Pain

Steven P. Cohen, MD

ANATOMY, FUNCTION, AND INNERVATION

The sacroiliac (SI) joint complex is the largest spinal joint the body, averaging 17.5 cm^2 in size. It is most frequently classified as an auricular-shaped diarthrodial joint because it contains a fibrous joint capsule filled with synovial fluid, cartilaginous surfaces, and an intricate set of ligamentous connections. The SI joint differs from other synovial joints in that it is not readily mobile, there is discontinuity in the posterior capsule, and the thinner iliac articulation is composed of fibro- instead of hyaline cartilage.[1,2]

The SI joint is supported by a network of myofascial structures that help promote movement, support, and stability. These structures include the gluteus maximus and medius, biceps femoris, piriformis, latissimus dorsi via the thoracolumbar fascia, and erector spinae. The joint is primarily designed for stability and weight bearing, although small degrees of rotation (≤3 degrees) and translation (≤2 mm) occur.[3,4] Previous attempts to establish a causative relationship between pain and motion abnormalities have been unsuccessful.[5]

The nerve supply of the SI-joint complex is very variable and a subject of great relevance for interventional pain practitioners. To summarize the literature, the lateral branches of the S1 and S2 dorsal rami innervate the posterior joint and the surrounding ligaments in nearly all individuals, giving off between one and four branches.[6,7] There is a contribution from S3 in most but not all individuals, with again up to four branches being noted in some people.[6,7] Whereas some cadaveric dissections indicate that people receive innervation from L5,[7,8] most studies have found this to be absent or infrequent.[6,9] For S4, the literature is similarly mixed, with some studies demonstrating a neural connection in most individuals[10,11] but others finding contributions to be rare.[6,9] Anatomic studies have also found anastomoses to be common between segmental spinal levels. Some people receive sensory input from the SI joint through the superior gluteal nerve in addition to the lateral branches.[7]

The innervation of the ventral SI joint is less clinically relevant but no less controversial. Whereas some cadaveric studies have reported nerve filaments stemming from the ventral rami of L4–S2,[12] other experts cite contributions from levels as cephalad as L2.[13] Surprisingly, some anatomic studies have failed to find any ventral neural contribution to the SI joint.[14]

Both intraarticular and extraarticular structures can be sources of SI joint pain. Clinical studies have reported benefit from both intraarticular and extraarticular injections, with one study finding no difference in benefit between the two.[15] An electrophysiologic study performed in cats identified mechanoreceptors in both the joint capsule and adjacent muscles, with most (26/29) residing within the capsule.[16] Among these receptor units, 28 were classified as nociceptive and 1 proprioceptive. Broken down by region, 16 were found in the proximal third, 11 in the middle third, and two in the distal third. Immunohistochemical studies in human cadavers have also found evidence of calcitonin gene–related peptide and substance P immunoreactive nociceptors in both capsular and interosseous ligaments.[17] Clinical studies have documented pain provocation in patients and asymptomatic volunteers with both capsular distention and ligamentous provocation (Figs. 66.1 and 66.2).[18–22]

EPIDEMIOLOGY

Several problems are inherent when ascertaining the prevalence of SI joint pain. These include but are not limited to the lack of any "gold standard" for diagnosis, perspective (i.e., interventional pain specialists generally attribute a greater proportion of low back pain [LBP] to SI joint pathology than surgeons do), the population studied, and method of diagnosis.

Several studies have utilized "double blocks" with lidocaine and bupivacaine to identify a painful SI joint. These studies have generally evaluated only patients without signs of radiculopathy whose predominant pain complaint was below L5. In the five studies using the reference standard of concordant pain relief with lidocaine and bupivacaine as the diagnostic criterion,[23–27] the reported prevalence rates for SI joint pain ranged between 10% and 45%, with the incidence of false-positive results varying between 0%[26] and 43%.[27] One flaw with these studies is that all based their criterion response on intraarticular injections, which likely excluded individuals with predominantly extraarticular pathology (Table 66.1). As already noted, these studies also excluded patients with radiculopathy. In one study that examined the prevalence of SI joint pain in patients with symptoms of radiculopathy and a herniated disc confirmed by magnetic resonance imaging (MRI), over two thirds of patients had SI joint dysfunction as identified by anatomic and pain-provocation tests.[31] This suggests that SI joint pain often coexists with other forms of pathology.

Studies using different diagnostic criteria have yielded similar results. Schwarzer et al.[22] conducted a prevalence study in 43 consecutive patients with chronic LBP predominantly below L5 using fluoroscopically guided intraarticular SI joint injections. The authors diagnosed SI joint pain based on three criteria: pain relief following intraarticular local anesthetic infiltration, ventral capsular tear on post-arthrography computed tomography (CT) scanning, and concordant pain provocation during capsular distension. With analgesic response as the sole criterion for diagnosis,

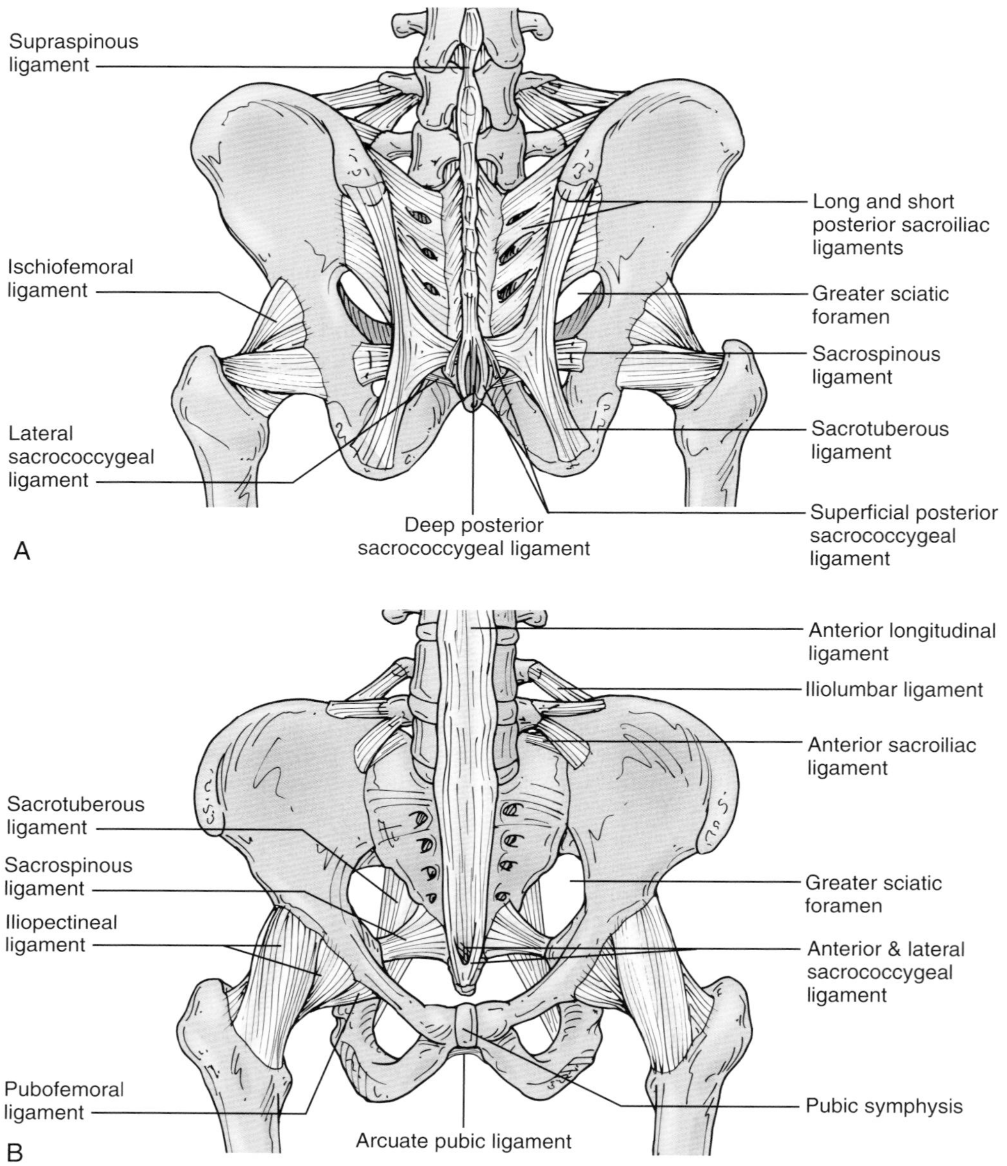

FIG. 66.1 Posterior view of the articulations and associated ligaments of the sacroiliac joint and surrounding structures. (A) The posterior ligaments surrounding the sacroiliac joint. (B) The ventral ligamentous connections. Drawing by Jee Hyun Kim. *(From Cohen SP: Sacroiliac joint pain: a comprehensive review of anatomy, diagnosis and treatment.* Anesth Analg. *101:1440-1453, 2005.)*

the prevalence of SI joint pain was found to be 30%. When 75% or more pain relief combined with a ventral capsular tear was used as the diagnostic criterion, the prevalence rate dropped to 21%. Only seven patients satisfied all three diagnostic criteria, for a lower-limit prevalence rate of 16%. Overall, SI joint pathology appears to be the primary generator in between 15% and 30% of patients with chronic axial LBP below L5, being more common in females and the elderly.[32]

ETIOLOGY

The mechanism of injury to the SI joint complex is frequently described as a combination of axial loading and abrupt rotation.[1] On an anatomic level, injury or pathology involving the myriad structures comprising the SI joint can lead to nociception. These include capsular or synovial disruption, ligamentous injury, myofascial pain, hypomobility or hypermobility, extraneous compression or shearing forces, cysts, abnormal joint mechanics, microfractures or macrofractures, chondromalacia, soft tissue pathology and inflammation. In patients with persistent nociceptive input, central sensitization can play a contributing role (Table 66.2).

Mechanistically, there are numerous reported etiologies for SI joint pain. These causes can be classified into intraarticular and extraarticular sources. Arthritis and the spondyloarthropathies are two examples of intraarticular causes of SI joint pain. Extraarticular sources include enthesopathy, fractures, ligamentous injury, and myofascial pain. The evidence in support of different etiologies

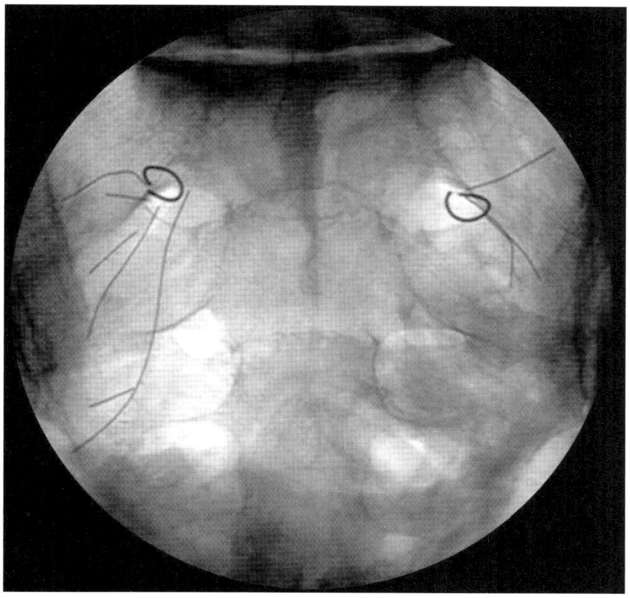

FIG. 66.2 Fluoroscopic image with drawings showing the lateral branch nerve converging on the S1 foramina. *(From Yin W, Willard F, Carreiro J, et al: Sensory stimulation-guided sacroiliac joint radiofrequency neurotomy: technique based on neuroanatomy of the dorsal sacral plexus.* Spine. *28:2419-2425, 2003.)*

includes the fact that clinical studies have demonstrated significant pain relief following both intraarticular and periarticular SI joint injections.[33–36] In one of these studies, periarticular injections were found to provide benefit in patients with spondyloarthropathy, suggesting that the two etiologies may overlap.[35]

Distinguishing between intraarticular and extraarticular pain generators may be clinically relevant in deciding on treatment options. A recent study by Dreyfuss et al. found that multisite lateral branch blocks were more effective at blocking pain from ligamentous probing than for the discomfort elicited during capsular distension.[20] This indicates that lateral branch radiofrequency (RF) denervation may be more likely to be effective in individuals with extraarticular pathology. In contrast to intraarticular pathology, extraarticular pain is more likely to be unilateral, to occur in younger individuals, to present with more prominent tenderness, and to be associated with a specific inciting event or biomechanical etiologies.

Numerous factors can predispose a person to develop SI joint pain. Risk factors that operate by increasing the stress borne by the SI joints include obesity, true and apparent leg-length discrepancy, gait abnormalities, persistent strain/low-grade trauma (e.g., jogging), scoliosis, pregnancy, and surgery, especially fusion of the sacrum. Spine surgery may cause postprocedural SI joint pain by increasing load bearing, weakening the surrounding ligaments, iatrogenic violation of the SI joint complex, and postsurgical hypermobility.[1] In one study that compared presurgical and postsurgical CT scans in fusion patients and matched controls, the investigators found an almost twofold increase in SI joint degeneration in the surgical patients compared with the control subjects (75% vs. 38.2%), with the highest incidence noted with fusions that extended to the sacrum.[37] Studies evaluating the response to diagnostic injections following spinal fusion have reported prevalence rates ranging from 32% to 43%.[38]

Pregnancy predisposes women to SI joint pain via the combination of increased weight gain, exaggerated lordotic posture, the mechanical trauma of parturition, and hormone-induced ligamental laxity. In one large study evaluating over 300 pregnant women between 12 and 18 weeks' gestation, 62% reported LBP, with 54% of these experiencing pelvic girdle pain situated around the SI joints and another 29% describing combination pelvic girdle and lumbar pain.[39] Infrequently, SI subluxation may also occur during pregnancy.

Between 40% and 50% of patients with injection-confirmed SI joint pain cite a specific inciting event. In investigations by Chou et al., Schwarzer et al., and Cohen et al., the leading precipitating events in descending order for trauma-induced SI joint pain were motor vehicle collisions, falls, cumulative strain, and pregnancy.[22,40,41]

DIAGNOSIS AND PRESENTATION

HISTORY AND PHYSICAL EXAM

SI joint pain can be difficult to distinguish from other sources of LBP. Numerous studies have established that no single historical report or sign on physical exam can reliably diagnose a painful SI joint.[21,22,25] Several reviews have sought to evaluate the validity of a battery of physical exam tests in establishing the SI joint as the primary pain generator. These reviews have generally shown that mobility and alignment tests are inadequate in identifying SI joint–mediated pain.[1,42] For provocative maneuvers, the results have been mixed. Whereas some reviews have determined that a combination of provocative maneuvers can accurately discriminate between pain from the SI joint and other sources of spinal pain,[43,44] others have reached equivocal[39,45,46] or negative[47] conclusions.

Nevertheless, clinical studies suggest that a comprehensive history and physical exam can provide important clues to etiology and inform further diagnostic workup. Some of the more common findings used to select candidates for SI joint blocks are pain predominantly localized below L5, pain exacerbated by rising from a sitting position, and tenderness overlying the joint. Several studies and reviews have found that when the area of maximal tenderness is situated close to the posterosuperior iliac spine, there is a high likelihood that the primary pain generator is the SI joint.[18,19,48,49] In contrast to other causes of mechanical LBP, such as myofascial, facetogenic, and discogenic pain, SI joint pain is more likely to be unilateral and occur after a specific inciting event (Table 66.3).[22,40,41]

PAIN REFERRAL PATTERNS

Several investigators have sought to determine pain referral patterns emanating from SI joints. In a provocative study conducted in 10 asymptomatic volunteers, Fortin et al.[18] found that all subjects experienced pain in the ipsilateral buttock, which sometimes radiated into the posterolateral upper thigh. In a retrospective review by Slipman et al.[50] conducted in 50 patients with

TABLE 66.1 Characteristics of Diagnostic Prevalence Studies Using Double Blocks as the Reference Standard

Authors	Subjects	Interventions	Diagnostic Criteria	Results
Maigne et al.[25]	54 patients with chronic unilateral LBP with or without radiation to posterior thigh	Intraarticular blocks using 2 mL of lidocaine and bupivacaine on separate occasions. Authors avoided anesthetizing periarticular ligaments.	≥75% pain relief, with the bupivacaine block lasting ≥2 h.	Prevalence rate 18.5%. False-positive rate 17%.
Manchikanti et al.[24]	20 patients with chronic LBP without neurologic deficits	Intraarticular blocks with unspecified volume of lidocaine and bupivacaine on separate occasions.	Not noted.	Prevalence rate 10%. False-positive rate 20%.
Irwin et al.[27]	158 patients with chronic LBP with or without lower extremity pain	Intraarticular blocks with 2 mL of lidocaine and 2 mL bupivacaine and steroid on separate occasions.	≥70% pain relief, with the bupivacaine block lasting ≥4 h.	Prevalence rate 27%. False-positive rate 43%.
Laslett et al.[26]	48 patients with buttock pain with or without lumbar or lower extremity symptoms, without signs of nerve root compression	Intraarticular blocks with <1.5 mL of lidocaine plus steroid and bupivacaine on separate occasions.	≥80% pain relief with lidocaine and bupivacaine.	Prevalence rate 26%. False-positive rate 0%.
van der Wurff et al.[23]	60 patients with chronic LBP below L5 with or without lower extremity symptoms, without neurologic symptoms	Intraarticular blocks with 2 mL lidocaine and bupivacaine on separate occasions.	≥50% pain relief with lidocaine and bupivacaine, with the bupivacaine block lasting ≥4 h.	Prevalence rate 45%. False-positive rate 12%.
Liliang et al.[28]	150 patients with chronic LBP, no neurologic deficits, and positive provocative SI joint tests	Intraarticular blocks with 2 mL lidocaine or bupivacaine mixed with steroid on separate occasions.	≥50% pain relief lasting at least 6 weeks.	Prevalence rate 33%. False-positive rate 16%.
Liliang et al.[29]	52 patients with chronic LBP who had previously undergone lumbar or lumbosacral spinal fusions, pain below L5 and positive provocative SI-joint tests	Intraarticular blocks with 2 mL lidocaine or bupivacaine mixed with steroid on separate occasions.	≥75% pain relief lasting between 1 and 4 h.	Prevalence rate 40%. False-positive rate 10%.
Cohen et al.[30]	39 patients with chronic LBP below L5 with tenderness over the SI joint and positive provocative tests	Intraarticular blocks with 2 mL bupivacaine mixed with steroid on separate occasions.	≥50% pain relief lasting ≥3 h.	Prevalence 41%. False-positive rate 10%.

LBP, *Low back pain.*

TABLE 66.2 Causes of Intraarticular and Extraarticular Sacroiliac Joint Pain

Intraarticular	Extraarticular
Arthritis (e.g., osteoarthritis, rheumatoid)	Trauma/fractures
Spondyloarthropathy	Ligamentous injury
Trauma	Myofascial pain
Infection	Enthesopathy
Cystic disease	Pregnancy
	Cystic disease

injection-confirmed SI joint pain, the authors found the most common referral patterns to be focal pain in the buttock (94%) and lower lumbar region (72%) and extension into the ipsilateral lower extremity (50%), groin area (14%), upper lumbar region (6%), and abdomen (2%). Despite the widely held view that only radicular pain extends into the lower leg, 28% of patients experienced pain radiating below the knee, with 12% reporting foot pain. Cohen et al.[41] examined pain referral patterns in an analysis of SI joint RF denervation outcome predictors conducted in 77 patients with positive screening blocks. Of these, 43% experienced symptoms localized to the buttock and lower lumbar region, with 35% noting pain referred to the thigh(s). Consistent with Slipman et al.,[50] the authors also noted a high percentage of unusual pain patterns, with 23% reporting lower leg pain and 20% complaining of extension into the groin. Lower back or buttock pain that is referred into the groin was also described by Schwarzer et al.[22] as being the only pattern that distinguished SI joint pain from that due to other pain generators, suggesting that it may indicate ventral joint involvement.

Because the SI joint is the largest axial joint in the body, the radiation pattern may be a by-product of the part of the joint affected. In a clinical study performed in 50 patients with injection-confirmed SI joint pain, the authors found that the upper part of the joint was most frequently associated with pain in the posterosuperior iliac spine, the middle aspect of the joint tended to be associated with pain in the midbuttock, and pain emanating from the inferior portion of the joint was most likely to be experienced in the lower buttock region. In those individuals who experienced groin pain, local anesthetic injections into the upper and middle parts of the joint were more likely to result in pain relief than injections into the lower joint.[55] A previous study conducted in discogenic pain also suggested that the greater the magnitude of nociceptive stimulation, the more distal in the extremity the evoked pain will extend (Fig. 66.3).[56]

TABLE 66.3 Studies Evaluating Historical and Physical Findings in Sacroiliac Joint Pain

Author	Patients	Findings Suggestive of Sacroiliac Joint Pain
Fortin et al.[18,19]	10 volunteers and 16 patients with SI joint pain.	Point of maximum discomfort within 10 cm caudal and 3 cm lateral to PSIS.
Murakami et al.[48]	38 patient responders to periarticular injections	Point of maximum discomfort within 3 cm from PSIS.
Schwarzer et al.[22]	43 patients with axial LBP.	Radiation to groin.
Dreyfuss et al.[21]	85 patients with axial LBP.	None.
Slipman et al.[50]	50 patients with axial LBP.	94% had buttock, 72% lumbar, 28% lower leg, and 14% groin pain.
van der Wurff et al.[23]	60 patients with axial LBP.	None.
Jung et al.[51]	160 patients with SI joint arthropathies.	Buttock pain alone, extending into posterolateral thigh or into groin.
Laslett et al.[26]	48 patients with axial LBP.	Noncentralization or peripheralization of pain.
DePalma et al.[32]	127 responders to IA SI joint blocks.	Lateral midline pain.
Young et al.[52]	102 patients with nonradicular LBP.	Pain rising from sitting, nonmidline pain below L5
Liliang et al.[29]	130 patients evaluated for SI joint pain after fusion.	Unilateral pain, 3 or more provocative maneuvers, postoperative pain different than preoperative pain.
Ostgaard et al.[53]	855 pregnant women.	Pain in the pubic symphysis.
LaPlante et al.[54]	153 patients with axial LBP.	None.
Kurosawa et al.[55]	50 patients with axial LBP who responded to periarticular SI-joint injections.	Pain from the upper joint most commonly noted near posterior superior iliac spine; pain from middle joint most commonly noted in midbuttock, pain from lower joint noted in lower buttock; 44% of patients had groin pain, which was associated with upper joint involvement.

IA, *Intraarticular;* LBP, *low back pain;* PSIS, *posterior superior iliac spine;* SI, *sacroiliac.*

RADIOLOGIC IMAGING

Results of studies correlating radiologic findings with the results of diagnostic blocks have been inconsistent. Studies by Slipman et al.[57] and Maigne et al.[58] found sensitivities of 13% and 46%, respectively, for the use of radionuclide bone scanning in the identification of an injection-confirmed painful SI joint. Despite the greater than 90% specificities in these studies, the low sensitivities indicate that bone scanning is a poor screening tool for SI joint pain (i.e., it will fail to detect most cases). The lack of a strong association between symptoms and diagnostic injections has also been noted for CT and x-ray stereophotogrammetry.[5] In a retrospective analysis by Elgafy et al.,[59] CT imaging was found to be 57.5% sensitive and 69% specific in diagnosing SI joint pain.

MRI is the reference standard for detecting SI joint involvement in patients with spondyloarthropathies. Studies have shown over 80% sensitivity in detecting chronic sacroiliitis, including sclerosis, joint space abnormalities, and ankylosis, with contrast-enhanced and short tau inverted recovery (STIR) providing the highest sensitivity.[60,61] However, MRI pathology does not seem to correlate well with clinical findings.[61] Whereas MRI may be a more sensitive test for detecting active inflammation and concomitant structural changes, CT remains the reference standard for disease processes in which bone destruction or ossification can occur.

INJECTIONS

It is widely acknowledged that an analgesic response to an SI joint injection is the most accurate means of diagnosing a painful SI joint complex. However, without another reliable means to diagnose SI joint pain, this is impossible to prove. In studies and reviews that have sought to determine the predictive value of historical reports and physical exam signs, etiologies, and referral patterns, pain relief in response to low-volume (≤2 mL) SI joint blocks has generally been used as the reference standard. The same criteria have been used in screening patients for more invasive procedures, such as surgery and RF ablation.[62,63] In almost all cases, these injections have been intraarticular. Although some of the injectate may extravasate into adjacent ligaments and muscles, diagnostic capsular injections may underestimate the true prevalence of pain from the SI joint complex by failing to anesthetize the surrounding soft tissues.

The false-positive rate of uncontrolled SI joint blocks is around 20%.[64] This has led some experts to recommend using "double blocks" (also known as comparative local anesthetic blocks) with two local anesthetic drugs having different half-lives, or placebo-controlled blocks, as the best way to identify a painful SI joint. The main problem with this paradigm is that the correlation between the duration of benefit and the pharmacokinetics of local anesthetics is weak and inconsistent.[65] A study performed in patients with suspected cervical facet joint pain using double comparative blocks found that this diagnostic paradigm may be associated with a significant false-negative rate, which means that many patients with the index condition would be misdiagnosed.[66] The double-block diagnostic paradigm has also been found not to be cost-effective in selecting candidates for RF denervation.[67,68] Whereas one might expect higher success rates for RF denervation when candidates are selected based on their response to double compared to single diagnostic blocks, clinical studies have not found this to be the case.[38] A randomized, crossover study also found that the use of sedation during diagnostic SI joint blocks may increase the false-positive rate.[69]

TREATMENT

CONSERVATIVE

The initial treatment of SI joint pain should focus on conservative measures, ideally addressing the underlying

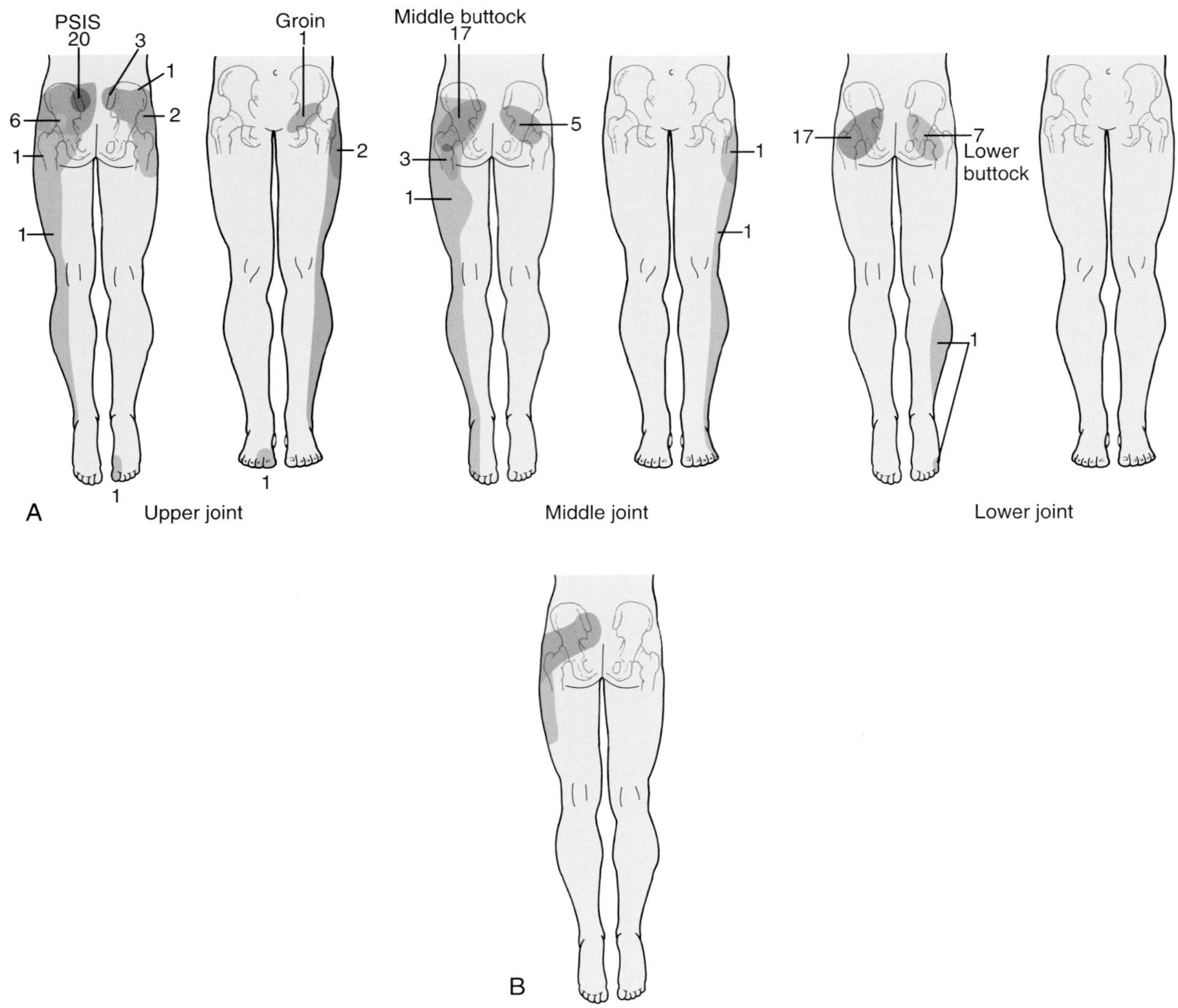

FIG. 66.3 Referral patterns for (A) extraarticular and (B) intraarticular sacroiliac joint pain. *PSIS*, Posterosuperior iliac spine. *([A] From Kurosawa D, Murakami E, Aizawa T: Referred pain location depends on the affected section of the sacroiliac joint.* Eur Spine J. *24:521-527, 2015. [B] From Fortin JD, Dwyer AP, West S, et al: Sacroiliac joint: pain referral maps upon applying a new injection/arthrography technique. Part I: asymptomatic volunteers.* Spine. *19:1475-1482, 1994.)*

etiology. True and functional leg-length discrepancies can be treated with shoe lifts and physical therapy, respectively. True leg-length discrepancies result in increased stress and abnormal force vectors on the ipsilateral lower extremity, which may then extend to the contralateral leg. Since these occur in a large percentage of asymptomatic individuals and many people already compensate for a lower extremity length difference by altering their gait or posture, most experts recommend starting out with inserts that correct only half the incongruity and implementing them gradually. In one study conducted in 798 patients with chronic low back or hip pain and 359 controls, Friberg[70] found that 75% of pain patients had leg length asymmetries of at least 5 mm, versus 43.5% of the asymptomatic cohort. Functional leg-length discrepancies usually occur as a result of muscle weakness or inflexibility at the pelvis or ankle. Specific causes include pelvic obliquity, adduction or flexion contractures of the hip, and genu valgum and varum. The treatment of apparent leg-length discrepancies entails aggressive physical therapy that targets the underlying etiology. If malalignment is suspected, osteopathic or chiropractic manipulation has been reported to be of value,[71] though prospective controlled studies are lacking. For patients with spondyloarthropathies, immunomodulating agents such as cytokine inhibitors and methotrexate may reduce disease progression, alleviate pain, and improve function.

Reviews and guidelines have found exercise to be beneficial for chronic LBP, but few studies have been performed in those with predominantly SI joint pain.[72] Biomechanical models have shown contraction of the transversus abdominis muscle to be associated with reduced laxity of the SI joint and suggest that isolated contraction of transversely oriented musculature (e.g., pelvic floor muscles and the piriformis) can stabilize the joint.[73] In their study, Mooney et al.[74] found five women with injection-confirmed SI joint pain who had electromyographically documented hyperactivity of the ipsilateral gluteus muscles and contralateral latissimus muscle. After a 2.5-month exercise program, all five achieved a reduction in pain and return of electromyographic patterns to normal. In another study evaluating three different physical therapy regimens in pregnant women clinically diagnosed with SI joint pain, no difference was noted between the use of a nonelastic SI belt, home exercise, and a structured exercise program, with all groups demonstrating improvement between the end of gestation and 12-months postpartum.[75]

In patients who do not have a correctable etiology, pharmacotherapy should be considered as part of an interdisciplinary treatment regimen, though no studies have specifically evaluated medications in individuals with SI joint pain. In persons with acute nonneuropathic back pain, both nonsteroidal antiinflammatory drugs (NSAIDs) and muscle relaxants may be effective. In patients with chronic LBP, there is weak evidence supporting the use of tricyclic antidepressants and selective norepinephrine serotonin reuptake inhibitors.[76] For opioids, there is some evidence of short-term benefit, but reviews have generally found minimal evidence to support long-term effectiveness, improvement of function, or superiority over NSAIDs and antidepressants for LBP.[77]

INJECTIONS

Injections with local anesthetic are the reference standard for determining whether or not someone has SI joint pain; but when steroids are added, they may also confer therapeutic benefit. There have been four randomized trials (three of which were placebo-controlled) evaluating the effectiveness SI joint steroid injections, and all demonstrated benefit.[33,35,36,78] Three were performed in patients with spondyloarthropathies[33,35,36] and one was conducted in children.[78] Two studies by the same group of investigators evaluated periarticular injections in patients with spondyloarthropathy, which by definition involves joint pathology.[35,36] However, only one of the placebo-controlled studies followed patients longer than 2 months (albeit in an open-label extension); this study enrolled only 10 patients.[33]

A major issue surrounding the use and evaluation of SI joint injections is whether the primary source of pain is intraarticular, extraarticular, or mixed. Intraarticular SI joint pain is more likely to occur in the elderly and to be bilateral, whereas extraarticular SI joint pain is more likely to be unilateral, to occur in younger individuals, and to be associated with a specific inciting event.[49] There have been few attempts to examine the relative benefit of intraarticular versus extraarticular SI joint injections. A retrospective study by Borowsky and Fagen[79] including 120 patients found that combination intraarticular and extraarticular injections were superior to intraarticular injections alone, although even at 3 weeks postinjection less than half of the patients had experienced over 50% pain relief (42.5% for combination injections vs. 27.5% for intraarticular blocks). Murakami et al.,[80] in a nonrandomized comparative-effectiveness study, found that extraarticular injections guided by pain provocation with hypertonic saline provided better pain relief 5 minutes after treatment than intraarticular injections. However, the lack of any long-term follow-up, myriad methodologic flaws, and the 100% success rate in the extraarticular group indicate the need for caution in interpreting these findings. In another study evaluating the accuracy of ultrasound guidance for SI joint injections in patients with active sacroiliitis, Hartung and colleagues[81] found that there was no difference in treatment outcomes between the 12 patients who received intraarticular injections and the 8 whose injections were situated outside of the joint, with both groups experiencing almost 50% pain relief at 4-week follow-up.

There have been a host of uncontrolled studies evaluating the long-term effects of SI joint injections. In four observational studies conducted in over 100 patients with spondyloarthropathy, when data were combined, over 85% of the subjects obtained significant pain relief lasting for an average of 10 months.[82–85] Comparable results have been obtained in patients without spondyloarthropathy[86,87] and with repeat injections.[88]

Whereas good results have been anecdotally reported with "blind" injections,[89] studies examining the "accuracy" of landmark-guided SI joint blocks have found that only between 12% and 22% of injections end up being intraarticular.[90,91] Yet as alluded to earlier, it is not clear whether intraarticular or extraarticular pathology is more common or which type of injection is more beneficial. A clinical trial is currently under way to answer these questions (ClinicalTrials.gov Identifier: NCT02096653; Tables 66.4 and 66.5; Fig. 66.4).

NEUROABLATION

RF denervation of the SI joint has become the treatment of choice for many patients who fail to respond to conservative treatment. The first report describing SI joint denervation was by Ferrante et al.,[93] who used a bipolar setup to sequentially leapfrog electrodes in the posteroinferior aspect of the SI joint at less than 1-cm intervals. In this small retrospective series, only 12 of 33 patients reported 50% or greater pain relief lasting at least 6 months. Considering that only a small portion of the joint was denervated, these findings are not surprising. Others have attempted intraarticular phenol injections with better results, but the inherent risks involved with uncontrolled neurolysis (e.g., paralysis, incontinence) curtail the widespread use of this modality.[94]

Subsequent attempts at RF ablation targeting the lateral branches of the primary dorsal rami have met with more auspicious results, with most studies reporting sustained relief lasting at least 6 months in over 60% of subjects.[95–98] However, these studies have utilized widely dissimilar selection criteria and targeted different nerves, ranging from the all-inclusive L4–S4 levels to S1–S3. One study targeted only the L5 dorsal ramus but created additional lesions in the posterior interosseous ligaments,[99] whereas another group selected nerves based on concordant sensory stimulation.[97] The uniformly high success rates in uncontrolled studies using disparate methodology have raised many questions regarding selection criteria, technique, and the validity of the results.[100]

Anatomic studies have demonstrated that the lateral branches, which provide nociceptive and proprioceptive

TABLE 66.4 Randomized, Controlled Studies Evaluating Sacroiliac Joint Injections

Author, Year	Study Design	Subjects	Interventions	Results	Comments
Fischer et al., 2003[78]	Randomized, controlled	89 children with juvenile spondyloarthropathy; 56 were responders to NSAIDs (control group) and 33 were nonresponders (treatment group).	Treatment group received steroid without LA injections plus NSAIDs. The control group was continued on NSAIDs alone.	87.5% who received injections reported decreased pain complaints over the 20-month follow-up (VAS pain score decreased from 6.9 to 1.8). The control group showed similar improvements in pain scores, with no difference between groups.	Dx made clinically and by MRI evidence of sacroiliitis. One-third of patients who received injections demonstrated continued joint destruction.
Luukkainen et al., 2002[36]	Randomized, controlled	24 patients without spondyloarthropathy.	All patients underwent unilateral periarticular injections. 13 patients received steroid and LA, with 11 patients receiving saline and LA.	At 1-month follow-up, VAS pain scores decreased significantly more in the steroid group than in the saline group.	Injections were periarticular, not intraarticular. Dx made by PE. No patient had radiologic evidence of sacroiliitis.
Maugars, 1996[33]	Placebo-controlled double-blind	10 patients with spondyloarthropathy, 13 joints.	13 total joints injected. 6 intraarticular injections were performed with steroid and LA and 7 with saline. 6 of 7 placebo patients were reinjected with steroid at 1 month.	5 steroid joints had good or very good pain relief at 1 month vs. 1 in the placebo group. Overall, 12/14 SI joints had good or very good results at 1 month; 8/13 at 3 months and 7/12 at 6 months.	Dx made by PE and radiologic studies. One patient developed radicular pain that lasted 3 weeks.
Luukkainen et al., 1999[35]	Randomized, controlled	20 patients with seronegative spondyloarthropathy received steroid and LA; 10 patients rec'd saline and LA. All patients had unilateral blocks.	All patients underwent unilateral periarticular injections. 10 received corticosteroid without LA; 10 rec'd normal saline with LA.	At 2-month follow-up, VAS pain scores decreased significantly in the steroid group but not in the saline group.	Injections were periarticular, not intraarticular. Dx made by PE and radiologic studies.
Visser et al., 2013[92]	Randomized, comparative-effectiveness	51 patients with SI-joint pain.	Patients rec'd either high-velocity manual manipulation of SI joint, physical therapy, or intraarticular injections with LA and steroid.	At 12 weeks, manual therapy was successful in 72% of patients, SI-joint injections in 50%, and physical therapy in 20%.	Dx based on PE. Injections varied in volume. Evaluators blinded to treatment.

Dx, *Diagnosis;* MRI, *magnetic resonance imaging;* LA, *local anesthetic;* NSAIDs, *nonsteroidal antiinflammatory drugs;* PE, *physical examination;* SI, *sacroiliac;* VAS, *visual analog scale.*

TABLE 66.5 Alternative Treatments for Sacroiliac Joint Pain

Viscosupplementation
Acupuncture
Craniosacral therapy
Spinal manipulation
Alternative exercise programs (e.g., yoga/tai chi)
Cognitive-behavioral therapy/relaxation techniques
Neuromodulation
Proliferative therapy (prolotherapy)

input from the SI joints, vary in number and location from patient to patient, from side to side, and from level to level, with up to four nerves entering the foramina at each spinal level.[97] This precludes the use of sensory stimulation to ensure ablation of all nociceptive input. It also makes capturing all afferent nerve fibers using conventional RF techniques—wherein the typical lesion diameter ranges between 3 and 4 mm in a single plane—technically challenging. There are many ways to enhance lesion size and overcome this obstacle, including fluid modulation (i.e., injecting electrolytic solutions before ablation to reduce impedance and increase power output); heating for longer time periods (>2 minutes); utilizing higher temperatures; using bipolar technology or very large, internally cooled electrodes, or "splayed" electrodes that increase the lesion's surface area; placing prearranged tracks of electrodes (i.e., multilesion probes) along the long axis of the sacrum; and replacing RF electrodes with cryoprobes.[63,101–105] The only two randomized controlled trials evaluating SI-joint denervation both used cooled RF technology, demonstrating significant pain relief and functional improvement lasting between 6 months and 1 year in over half of the treated individuals.[63,106] However, the large, aggressive lesions effected by cooled RF and other lesion-enhancing techniques may increase the rate of postprocedural neuritis, which one study found occurred in close to

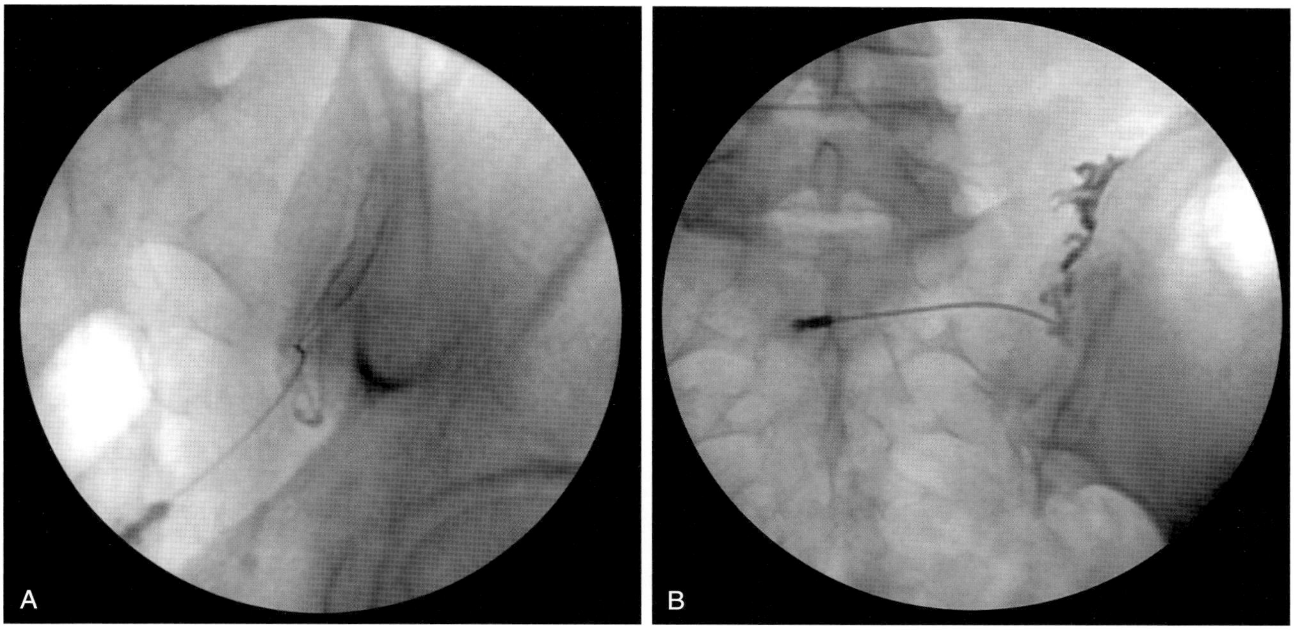

FIG. 66.4 Anteroposterior fluoroscopic images demonstrating (A) intraarticular and (B) extraarticular sacroiliac joint injections.

10% of individuals.[107] For cryoanalgesia, which preserves more of the nerve architecture than heat ablation, the main downside is the shorter duration of benefit.[102]

RF denervation may not be a good treatment option for everyone. Targeting the posterior nerve supply does not address pain emanating from the ventral aspect of the joint, and Dreyfuss et al.,[20] in their study, found that lateral branch blocks were more effective at preventing pain secondary to extraarticular (i.e., ligamentous) stimulation than from capsular distension, suggesting that such treatment may be less effective in patients with arthritis. In an effort to better identify those patients most likely to respond to SI joint RF denervation, Cohen et al.[41] conducted a multicenter study evaluating demographic and clinical factors affecting outcomes in 77 patients. Overall, 52% of the 77 patients continued to experience 50% or greater pain relief 6 months postprocedure. Not surprisingly, patients 65 years of age or older (perhaps because elderly patients are more likely to have intraarticular pathology) had higher preprocedural pain scores, opioid usage, and pain extending below the knee; these factors were associated with treatment failure. Although this study found an association between a positive outcome and the use of cooled RF probes, another study failed to find a difference between the use of cooled and conventional RF ablation (Fig. 66.5).[108]

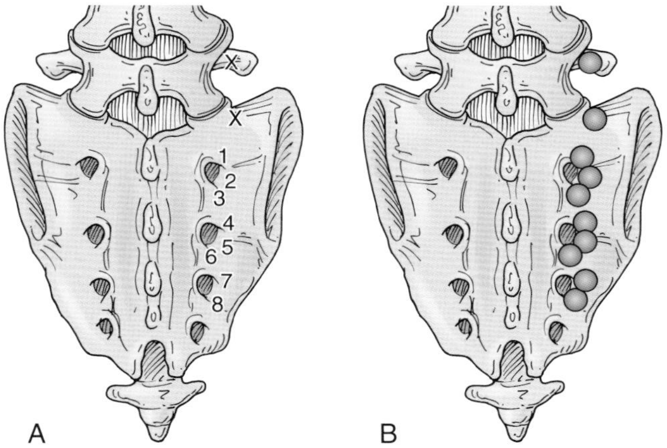

FIG. 66.5 Schematic diagram illustrating (A) target points for right-sided conventional (L4 and L5) and cooled (S1–S3) radiofrequency denervation at the junction of the L5 superior articular and transverse processes (L4 primary dorsal ramus), the sacral ala (L5 primary dorsal ramus), and S1–S3 foramina (lateral branches). (B) Anticipated lesions at each of the target points. *(From Cohen SP, Hurley RW, Buckenmaier CC III, et al: Randomized, placebo-controlled study evaluating lateral branch radiofrequency denervation for sacroiliac joint pain.* Anesthesiology. *109: 279-288, 2008.)*

SURGICAL STABILIZATION

SI joint arthrodesis has been used for decades to treat fractures, instability/dislocations, and pain secondary to degenerative changes. Among these indications, SI joint arthropathy is one of the most controversial, with the available studies being confounded by poor selection criteria and diverse outcome measures. Until recently, the results of these studies have been limited to small, mostly retrospective studies that have yielded mixed results.[109,110] However, in the past few years new minimally invasive technology has yielded more promising results, including a comparative effectiveness study that demonstrated superiority over open SI-joint fusion and a large, multicenter study that found fusion to be more effective than nonstandardized conservative care in patients with either degenerative sacroiliitis or SI joint disruption.[111–113] The rationale behind this technology in the context of arthropathy is that it may reduce strain on the joint in individuals with intraarticular pathology while minimizing the extensive tissue trauma associated with previous hardware placement.

KEY POINTS

- SI joint pain is a common cause of chronic axial LBP, accounting for between 15% and 30% of cases. It typically presents as unilateral pain situated below L5 that often radiates into the posterolateral thigh and occasionally below the knee.
- There is weak positive evidence that a battery of provocative maneuvers can identify a painful SI joint; the reference standard for diagnosis remains diagnostic blocks. However, uncontrolled blocks are associated with a significant false-positive rate.
- SI joint pain is a heterogeneous condition that can be categorized into intraarticular and extraarticular causes. For both, treatment represents a significant challenge.
- When a specific, remediable cause of SI joint pain can be identified (e.g., leg-length discrepancy or muscle weakness), treatment should be based on correcting the underlying pathology.
- Both intraarticular and periarticular corticosteroid injections may provide intermediate-term relief in well-selected patients, but the evidence for long-term benefit is mainly anecdotal.
- There is moderate evidence supporting lateral branch RF denervation to treat SI pain, particularly in individuals with extraarticular pathology.
- In individuals with intraarticular pathology who respond to diagnostic intraarticular injections, there is a growing body of evidence to support minimally invasive arthrodesis.

APPENDIX 66.1 TESTS FOR SACROILIAC JOINT DYSFUNCTION

CRANIAL SHEAR TEST

With the patient prone and the pelvis immobilized through the hip, pressure is applied to the coccygeal end of the sacrum. This test may be positive in patients with SI joint pain.

EXTENSION TEST

The patient is placed in the prone position, with one of the examiner's hands on the thigh of the affected side and the other over the opposite iliac crest. As the examiner exerts downward pressure on the iliac crest while pulling slightly on the anterior thigh, the occurrence of SI joint pain indicates pathology.

FLAMINGO TEST

The patient is asked to stand on the involved leg and hop. Pain in the SI region is indicative of SI joint dysfunction.

GAENSLEN TEST

The patient lies supine on the examining table with both knees drawn to up to the chest. He or she is then asked to shift over to the edge of the table, so that the leg being tested hovers over the edge. The examiner then presses down on the affected side, hyperextending the hip. Generally considered a sign of SI joint pain, a positive Gaenslen test may indicate hip pathology as well.

GILLET TEST

With the patient standing with feet approximately 12 inches apart, the examiner sits behind the patient and palpates the S2 spinous process with one thumb and the posterior superior iliac spine with the other. As if taking a large marching step, the patient then flexes the knee and hip of the side being tested. If the posterosuperior iliac spine fails to move posteroinferiorly with respect to S2, the test is positive. A positive Gillet test indicates SI joint dysfunction.

PELVIC COMPRESSION TEST

This test compresses the pelvis by the application of lateral pressure to the uppermost iliac crest directed toward the opposite iliac crest. It is believed to stretch the posterior SI ligaments and compress the anterior part of the joint.

PELVIC DISTRACTION TEST

For this test, the examiner applies pressure directed posteriorly and laterally to both anterosuperior iliac spines. This is alleged to stretch the anterior SI ligaments.

PELVIC ROCK TEST

With the patient lying supine, the examiner cups both hands around the iliac crests so that the thumbs are on the anterior superior iliac spine and the palms on the iliac tubercles. He or she then forcibly compresses the pelvis toward the midline of the body. Complaints of pain may indicate pathology in the SI joint.

PATRICK TEST

The patient is positioned supine with the foot of the involved side against the opposite knee. The SI joint is then stressed by pressing simultaneously against the flexed knee and contralateral anterosuperior iliac supine. Although this procedure is mainly used to test for SI joint dysfunction, pain in the inguinal or hip area may indicate hip pathology as well. Since this test involves *flexion*, *ab*duction and *e*xternal *r*otation of the hip, it is also called the FABER test.

SACROILIAC SHEAR TEST

With the patient lying prone, the examiner crosses both hands over the sacrum. The overlying hand delivers a posteroanterior thrust, while the underlying hand is used to detect motion in the joint.

THIGH THRUST TEST

This test applies a posterior shearing stress to the sacroiliac joint through the femur.

REFERENCES

Access the reference list online at ExpertConsult.com.

CHAPTER 67

PIRIFORMIS SYNDROME

Dost Khan, MD ◎ Ariana Nelson, MD

Although piriformis syndrome (PS) was first described in 1947,[1] leg pain originating at the ischium was thought to derive from sciatic nerve irritation as early as the 15th century and was termed "sciatica."[2] PS is an uncommon and often misdiagnosed cause of buttock and leg pain,[3–5] with reported prevalence rates typically ranging between 5% and 8%, but it sometimes is cited as high as 36% among patients with low back pain.[3,4,6,7] In this section, the following topics are discussed: (1) the anatomy of the piriformis muscle and anatomic abnormalities that cause PS, (2) etiologies of the syndrome, (3) signs and symptoms associated with the syndrome, and (4) treatments of the syndrome.

ANATOMY OF THE PIRIFORMIS MUSCLE AND THE SCIATIC NERVE

The piriformis muscle is pyramidal in shape and originates from the anterior surface of the S2–S4 sacral vertebrae, the capsule of the sacroiliac joint, and the gluteal surface of the ilium near the posterior surface of the iliac spine.[8] It runs laterally through the greater sciatic foramen, becomes tendinous, and inserts into the piriformis fossa at the medial aspect of the greater trochanter of the femur (Fig. 67.1). Ventral rami of the S1 and S2 spinal nerve course into the deep surface of the piriformis muscle to innervate it.[9] The main function of the piriformis muscle is abduction and external rotation of the femur.[10] The sciatic nerve, posterior femoral cutaneous nerve, gluteal nerves, and the gluteal vessels pass below the piriformis muscle.

With a typical diameter of 2 cm, the sciatic nerve is formed by the ventral rami (L4–S3) of the lumbosacral plexus and exits the pelvis through the greater sciatic foramen. As it is a mixed nerve, it contains both motor fibers, which supply the posterior thigh, hip and knee, and sensory fibers that supply the entire surface of the leg distal to the knee with the exception of the anteromedial calf and medial aspect of the foot.[11] The sciatic nerve typically passes inferior to the piriformis muscle and then divides into the tibial nerve and the peroneal nerve, which ordinarily occurs at the superior angle of the popliteal fossa.

Anatomical variants between the sciatic nerve and piriformis muscle have been described in the literature with prevalence rates anywhere from 6.4% to 16.9%.[12,13] There is a correlation between anatomical variations of the sciatic nerve and increased variability of other morphometric measurements of the lower limbs.[4] The clinical significance of variant anatomy remains disputed, as there was no difference in rates of aberrant anatomy in a surgical case series of patients with PS versus cadaveric dissections (16.2% vs. 16.9%), questioning its importance in the pathogenesis of PS.[13]

Six possible anatomic variants have been described between the sciatic nerve and the piriformis muscle and have been classified by the Beason and Anson Classification system (Table 67.1).[14] Anomalies of the piriformis muscle and the sciatic nerve can cause true sciatica. The compression usually occurs between the tendinous portion of the muscle and the bony pelvis. An abnormal course of the sciatic nerve or the smaller divisions, which are not as durable as the large caliber and well-sheathed sciatic nerve, are more susceptible to compression from muscle hypertrophy.[15] A study of 250 cadavers revealed an anatomical variation in the relationship of the nerve and muscle in 11.7%[16] of the population. The proportion of individuals with aberrant anatomy has previously been described as ranging anywhere between 8%[11] and 21%,[15] further demonstrating that a significant minority of the population exhibits this anatomic risk factor, which is a possible etiology of PS. However, as noted above, the clinical significance of variant anatomy remains disputed.[13]

PATHOPHYSIOLOGY, SIGNS AND SYMPTOMS, AND TREATMENT

The clinical presentation of PS may be due to both somatic and neuropathic pain. Myofascial pain of the piriformis muscle itself is the primary etiology of the somatic component of pain. Etiologies and predisposing factors of the syndrome include trauma to the pelvis or buttock,[3] hypertrophy or spasm of the piriformis and/or adjacent gemelli muscles,[8] female gender, pregnancy, anatomic abnormalities of the piriformis muscle or the sciatic nerve,[8,17] true or apparent leg-length discrepancies (a minimum of half an inch difference in leg lengths),[18] obesity, cerebral palsy secondary to hypertonicity, lumbar hyperlordosis, infection,[19] and rarely a mass effect from space occupying lesions.

Microtrauma to the piriformis muscle may occur from overuse injuries as observed in athletes or individuals performing heavy manual labor. A history of trauma is usually elicited in approximately 50% of the cases.[20] The trauma is usually not dramatic and may occur several months before the initial symptoms. Trauma to the gluteal musculature leads to inflammation and spasm of the muscle. Inflammatory mediators such as prostaglandins, histamine, bradykinin, and serotonin are released from the inflamed muscle and may irritate the sciatic nerve resulting in a pain–spasm–inflammation–irritation–pain cycle.[15,21] The stretched, spastic, and inflamed piriformis muscle may compress the sciatic nerve between the muscle and the bony pelvis.[22]

Other investigators consider PS to be a form of myofascial pain syndrome. Isolated involvement of the piriformis

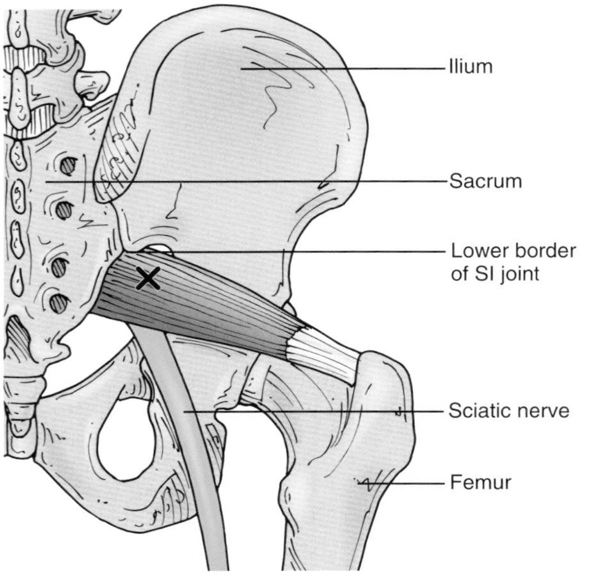

FIG. 67.1 Posterior view of the sacrum, ilium, and greater trochanter of the femur, illustrating the course of the piriformis muscle, sciatic nerve, and the site of injection (marked "X"). *SI*, Sacroiliac. *(Source: Benzon HT, Katz JA, Benzon HA, et al: Piriformis syndrome: anatomic considerations, a new injection technique, and a review of the literature.* Anesthesiology. *98:1442-1448, 2003, with permission.)*

TABLE 67.1 Beason and Anson Classification (14) for the Anatomic Relationship Between the Sciatic Nerve (n.) and Piriformis Muscle (m.)

Beason and Anson Classification		
Normal anatomy	Type 1	Undivided sciatic n. passes inferior to undivided m.
Proximal division	Type 2	One division passes through and one inferior to m.
Aberrant route	Type 3	One division passes inferior and one superior to m.
	Type 4	One division passes inferior and one superior to the m.
Normal division	Type 5	Sciatic n. passes through the m.
Aberrant route	Type 6	Sciatic n. passes superior to the m.

muscle is uncommon and usually occurs as a part of soft tissue injuries resulting from rotation and/or flexion movements of the hip and torso.[4] For this reason, some authors now favor the term "deep gluteal syndrome" instead of PS to describe gluteal sciatic nerve entrapment.[23] In addition to the piriformis muscle, pathology involving the superior and inferior gemelli muscles and the obturator internis can lead to buttock pain with or without lower extremity radiation.

The differential diagnosis of PS includes the myriad causes of low back pain and radiculopathy. Facet syndrome, sacroiliac joint dysfunction, trochanteric and ischial bursitis, myofascial pain syndrome, pelvic tumor, endometriosis, and conditions irritating the sciatic nerve should be considered in the differential diagnosis of PS. These conditions can be ruled out by a complete medical history and physical examination. Diagnosis of PS is usually arrived at only after exclusion of these possibilities.[15]

In a review of 55 studies, the most common features of PS identified were[24]:

- Buttock pain
- External tenderness over the greater sciatic notch
- Aggravation of the pain on prolonged sitting
- Augmentation of the pain with maneuvers that increase piriformis muscle tension

Patients with PS usually complain of buttock pain with or without radiation to the ipsilateral leg.[3] The buttock pain usually extends from the sacrum to the greater trochanter because of the muscle's insertion on the medial aspect of the greater trochanter.[3,4,15] Gluteal pain radiating to the ipsilateral leg is usually present if the piriformis muscle irritates the sciatic nerve.[15] The pain is aggravated by prolonged sitting, as in driving or biking, or when getting up from a seated position.[3,4] Pain can occur with bowel movements due to the proximity of the piriformis muscle to the lateral pelvic wall, and is worse after sitting on hard surfaces.[3]

Physical examination of the patient may reveal a pelvic tilt or tenderness in the buttock.[3] On palpation the contracted piriformis may feel like a spindle/sausage-shaped mass in the buttock, and there may be piriformis tenderness on rectal and pelvic examinations.[4] The pain is aggravated by hip flexion, adduction, and internal rotation. However, when hip flexion exceeds 90 degrees, the piriformis muscle is elongated with external rotation and this heel-contralateral knee maneuver (HCLK) may reproduce pain.[16] Neurologic signs are usually absent, although there may be numbness in the lower leg or foot from compression of the sciatic nerve by the piriformis muscle. The straight leg raise test may be normal or limited with numbness occurring when the sciatic nerve is irritated. The physical examination signs found in Table 67.2 may be helpful in confirming the presence of PS.

The diagnosis of PS is made predominantly on clinical grounds, although electromyography (EMG), computed tomography (CT), and magnetic resonance imaging (MRI) may show abnormalities. EMG may detect myopathic and neuropathic changes including a delay in the H-reflex with the affected leg in a flexed, adducted, and internally rotated (FAIR) position as compared with the same H-reflex in the normal anatomic position.[25] The peroneal H-reflex may serve as a more useful tool than that of the tibial nerve in detecting electrophysiologic changes of the sciatic nerve in those with PS. Electrodiagnostic studies were performed on 13 patients with suspected PS. The results showed that only 3 of 13 patients tested demonstrated prolonged latencies of the tibial H reflex, whereas 7 out of 7 patients noted disappearance of the H-reflex of the peroneal nerve when the affected leg was placed in the painful position of adduction and internal rotation.[26] The prolongation of the H-reflex by three standard deviations has been recommended as the physiologic criterion for diagnosing PS. CT and MRI of the soft tissues of the pelvis may show an enlarged piriformis muscle,[21] although imaging often is negative. Magnetic resonance neurography (MRN), an imaging technique that enhances visualization of peripheral nerves, may permit better detection of peripheral nervous system pathology.[27] MRN performed in two patients with PS identified signal changes of the sciatic nerve under the hypertrophied piriformis.[28]

TABLE 67.2 Tests and Signs Used in Diagnosis of Piriformis Syndrome

Diagnostic Test	Performance of Test	Positive in PS
Pace sign	Pain/weakness with seated abduction of hip against resistance	30%–74%[24]
FAIR test	Flexion, abduction, internal rotation causing pain	—
Lasègue sign	Pain with voluntary flexion, adduction, and internal rotation of the flexed hip	NR
Freiberg sign	Pain with forced internal rotation of the extended hip	32%–63%[24]
Palpation of piriformis line	Trigger point tenderness to palpation with extended thumb on the lateral third of the piriformis line with patient in Sims' position	59%–92%[5,24]
Beatty maneuver	Reproduction of buttock pain when painful leg is flexed and knee is elevated several inches off the table	NR[44]
Hughes test	Pain caused by maximal internal rotation of the painful limb followed by maximal external isometric rotation	NR
Atrophic changes	Gluteal atrophy, shortening of the limb on affected side	NR
Internal palpation	Pain with palpation of medial end of PM by rectal or vaginal exam. Examiner may also palpate a mass along lateral pelvic wall.	100%
External palpation	Tenderness to palpation over the piriformis muscle	38.5%[5]
HCLK (heel contralateral knee)	Hip flexion > 90 degrees with lateral rotation may reproduce buttock and sciatica symptoms after several seconds	NR

NR, *Not reported.*

The treatment of PS includes physical therapy combined with the use of antiinflammatory drugs, analgesics, and muscle relaxants to reduce inflammation, spasm, and pain.[3,4] Physical therapy involves stretching of the piriformis muscle with flexion, adduction, and internal rotation of the hip followed by pressure applied to the piriformis muscle.[3,4] Using computer modeling, conventional piriformis stretches were compared with hip flexion, adduction, then external rotation (adduction [ADD] stretch) and hip flexion, external rotation, then adduction (ExR stretch). ADD and ExR stretching routines increased piriformis muscle length by greater than 30%–40% compared with conventional stretching routines. ADD and ExR stretching comparably elongated the piriformis muscle by 12% and may be more comforting to patients because of the increased emphasis on hip flexion.[29] Abnormal biomechanics caused by posture, pelvic obliquities, and leg length inequalities should be corrected. Early treatment with nonsteroidal antiinflammatory drugs, physical therapy, and injections is effective in 75%–80% of patients.[2] Patients who do not respond to conservative therapy are candidates for piriformis muscle with or without perisciatic nerve injections. Local anesthetic and steroid are routinely administered during the injection, but a study by Misirlioglu observed no difference in numeric rating scale (NRS) and Likert analog scale (LAS) scores in a group of 47 patients divided into local anesthetic only versus local anesthetic + corticosteroid piriformis injection.[30]

TECHNIQUES OF PIRIFORMIS MUSCLE AND PERISCIATIC NERVE INJECTIONS

Initial studies evaluating piriformis muscle injections were done blindly. Current techniques involve identification of the piriformis muscle with ultrasound, muscle EMG, fluoroscopy, or with the use of CT or MRI guidance. In the technique of Fishman et al., fluoroscopy and EMG are used to identify the piriformis muscle. Correct needle placement is confirmed electrophysiologically with muscle EMG and radiographically by injection of contrast media.[31] In the CT-guided approach, the muscle is identified and insertion of the needle is guided radiologically.[32] Local anesthetic with steroid is injected into the muscle, which may be replaced by the injection of botulinum toxin type A (BTX-A) if spasm or hypertrophy is noted. In long-term follow-up of 13 patients treated with CT-guided local anesthetic/corticosteroid injection versus 10 controls, those treated with local anesthetic/corticosteroid had reduced visual analog scale (VAS) pain scores at 2, 3, 6, and 12 months ($P < .001$).[33] One advantage of the CT-guided approach is that it may better facilitate injections targeting the tendinous insertions of the external rotators of the hip (e.g., piriformis, gemelli, obturator internus muscles); however, the ionizing radiation exposure to the patient and personnel has led to reduced utilization of this technique.

Another technique uses the lower border of the sacroiliac joint as the landmark.[15] The patient is placed prone and the lower border of the sacroiliac joint, greater sciatic foramen, and the head of the femur are identified by fluoroscopy. An insulated needle connected to a nerve stimulator is inserted 1–2 cm lateral and 1–2 cm caudal to the lower border of the sacroiliac joint (see Fig. 67.1). The needle is advanced perpendicularly until a motor-evoked response of the sciatic nerve is obtained and is pulled back 0.3–0.5 cm to avoid intraneural injection, after which corticosteroid (40 mg triamcinolone or methylprednisolone) mixed with 5–8 mL saline is injected. Injection of steroid perisciatically is recommended even in the absence of signs of sciatic nerve entrapment, because nerve inflammation is common in this condition. The needle is then pulled back an additional 1.0 cm so that the tip of the needle lies in the belly of the piriformis muscle, contrast is administered to confirm position, and additional local anesthetic and steroid (5–8 mL 1% lidocaine and 40 mg triamcinolone or methylprednisolone) are given (Fig. 67.2). Some patients experience sustained relief of several months' duration with the local anesthetic–steroid injections.[15]

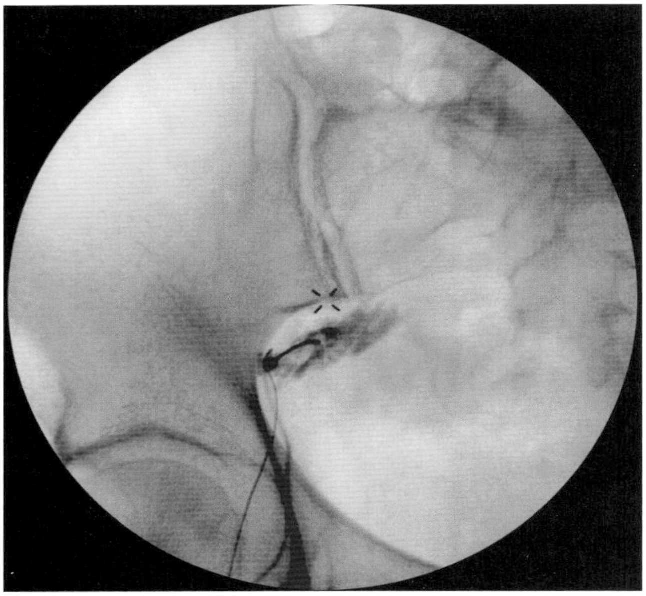

FIG. 67.2 Fluoroscopic image of the insulated needle in the piriformis muscle with the muscle being outlined by the injected radiopaque dye.

Increased utilization of ultrasound in regional anesthesia and musculoskeletal medicine has led to the advent of ultrasound-guided piriformis injections. Ultrasound offers the advantage of direct visualization of the muscle, without contrast and radiation exposure, whilst not sparing accuracy. A cadaveric study comparing the accuracy of ultrasound-guided versus fluoroscopically guided piriformis injection found the ultrasound technique to be more accurate.[34] In the study, a senior interventionalist performed both ultrasound-guided and fluoroscopically guided piriformis injections using different colored latex dye on 20 cadavers. A blinded dissection of the muscles was then performed, which found that 19/20 (95%) ultrasound-guided injections correctly placed dye within the piriformis muscle versus 6/20 (30%) fluoroscopically guided injections. The bulk of incorrectly placed dye was found in the gluteus maximus musculature.

Several ultrasound techniques have been reported, but most rely upon the common identification of the inferior/lateral border of the sacrum. In the technique reported by Chen et al., with the patient in the prone position, the ultrasound probe is walked off the sacral hiatus towards the greater trochanter to identify the piriformis muscle at the inferior/lateral border of the sacrum. The muscle is identified as a hyperechoic mass deep to the gluteus maximus with the sciatic nerve resembling an ovoid structure adjacent to or embedded within the substance of the muscle.[35] A varying technique reported by Smith and colleagues requires identification of prominent bony landmarks, such as the posterior superior iliac spine (PSIS) and the posterior inferior iliac spine (PIIS), to inferiorly move the ultrasound probe off the lateral sacrum and into the greater sciatic notch plane. Upon identification of the piriformis muscle, using a medial to lateral approach, a spinal needle is advanced into the sheath of the muscle followed by deposition of local anesthetic and steroid

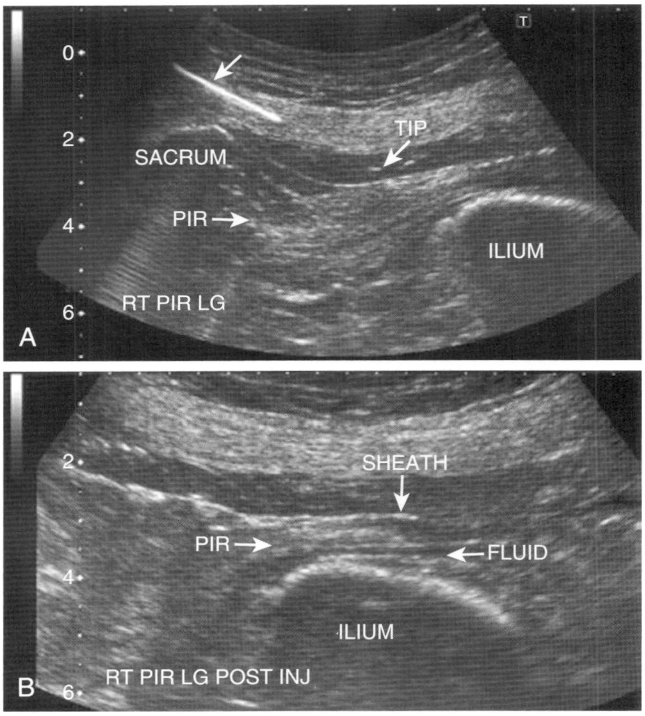

FIG. 67.3 (A) Longitudinal ultrasound view of the piriformis during needle placement using a medial-to-lateral approach parallel to the long axis of the transducer. The proximal end of the needle has been digitally enhanced to highlight needle trajectory. (B) Postinjection tenogram at the level of the greater sciatic foramen. Anechoic injectate (FLUID) within the piriformis tendon sheath lies superficial and deep to the hyperechoic tendon. *RT PIR LG*, Right side, piriformis, longitudinal view; *TIP*, needle tip. *(Source: Smith J, Hurdle MF, Locketz AJ, et al: Ultrasound-guided piriformis injection: technique description and verification.* Arch Phys Med Rehabil. *87:1664-1667, 2006.)*

(Fig. 67.3).[36] In a comparative trial of 28 patients with PS randomized to ultrasound-guided versus fluoroscopic-guided injection, no statistically significant difference was identified in pain scores and patient satisfaction between the cohorts.[37]

Botulinum toxin (100 mouse units of botulinum toxin type A or 5000–10,000 units for botulinum toxin type B) may be injected into the muscle if the patient has a transient response to steroid and local anesthetic.[32] Botulinum toxin, previously administered under CT guidance or fluoroscopy, is now being administered under ultrasound guidance.[38] Botulinum toxin blocks the release of acetylcholine at the neuromuscular junction, resulting in prolonged relaxation; recovery duration depends on neuromuscular sprouting and reinnervation of the muscle. A randomized study compared BTX-A with methylprednisolone in patients with "myofascial piriformis pain." The patients in both groups showed marked reduction in their pain scores 30 days after the injection, with no statistically significant difference observed. However, the patients who received botulinum injections had significantly lower pain scores 60 days after the injection.[32] Radiographically, patients who received botulinum toxin showed increased fatty infiltration of the piriformis muscle with a concomitant reduction in thickness and volume of the muscle.[28,39] These changes may account for the prolonged pain relief seen in patients receiving botulinum toxin. Reported complications from botulinum toxin include plexopathy, polyradiculoneuritis, and local psoriasiform dermatitis.[39,40]

Surgical release, entailing resection of the distal piriformis tendon at its femoral insertion site to decompress the sciatic nerve, may be entertained in recalcitrant cases of PS or in the setting of aberrant anatomy. The obturator internus, gemelli, and quadratus femoris muscles share common functions with the piriformis muscle and can compensate for the loss of piriformis muscle function. Newer surgical techniques using arthroscopy in the deep gluteal region are emerging.[41] Surgical management can lead to improvement, with resumption of patients' daily activities and return to work, in approximately 75% of patients.[42] Recurrent symptoms following surgical release have been attributed to incomplete piriformis tendon release and/or scar/hematoma formation.[43]

KEY POINTS

- The pain of PS is located in the buttock and radiates to the ipsilateral hip. It may radiate to the leg if the sciatic nerve is compressed or irritated.
- Physical examination signs to confirm PS include the Pace, Lasègue, and Freiberg signs.
- The diagnosis of PS is usually made by the presence of the above symptoms and positive provocative tests.
- Perisciatic and piriformis muscle injections of steroid and local anesthetic may result in relief that lasts several months. If the relief is transient, injections of botulinum toxin may provide longer relief.

REFERENCES

Access the reference list online at ExpertConsult.com.

CHAPTER 68

PULSED RADIOFREQUENCY, WATER-COOLED RADIOFREQUENCY, AND CRYONEUROLYSIS

Khalid Malik, MD, FRCS

BACKGROUND AND TECHNIQUE

PULSED RADIOFREQUENCY

The use of radiofrequency (RF) electrical currents to create quantifiable and predictable thermal lesions has been practiced since the 1950s.[1] The first reported use of RF in the treatment of intractable pain appeared in the early 1970s, which involved the use of conventional radiofrequency current (CRF) to create thermal lesions.[2] The CRF lesions for pain control are created by the passage of RF currents through an electrode positioned adjacent to a pain pathway in order to interrupt the nociceptive impulses and provide the needed pain relief. Application of RF current imparts energy to the tissues surrounding the electrode tip, raising the local tissue temperature while the electrode is heated passively. The RF current is switched off once the desired tissue temperature is reached, and repetition of this cycle maintains the selected temperature. Temperatures above 45°C have been known to be neurodestructive, though the time required to achieve neurolysis decreases in conjunction with rising temperatures.[3] Even though selective destruction of unmyelinated C and A-delta fibers has been suggested at lower temperatures,[4] further studies showed that all nerve fiber types were damaged equally during thermal RF application.[5] Hence, during CRF application tissue, temperatures selected are typically above the neurodestructive range but below the point of gas formation—typically from 65°C to a maximum temperature of 80°C–90°C. In order to avoid motor nerve damage causing weakness, and worsening pain secondary to local neuritis, neuroma formation, and deafferentation pain, the use of high-temperature CRF is generally reserved for nonneuropathic pain (e.g., facet joint, sacroiliac joint, and knee arthritis), whereby the target nerves do not contain motor fibers or carry nonpain sensory information. In order to avoid these complications, lower temperatures in the range of 55°C–70°C were arbitrarily selected in a study of CRF application to the dorsal root ganglia (DRG).[6] In another study evaluating DRG lesioning, no difference in clinical results was found between CRF lesions created at 40°C or 67°C.[7] The authors of the latter study hypothesized that the electrical currents rather than temperature resulted in this outcome. This observation generated immense interest, as the risks of weakness and deafferentation pain could theoretically be obviated, and the indications for RF broadened immensely, by the use of lower temperatures.

Pulsed radiofrequency (PRF) was introduced to maximize the delivery of electrical currents by the use of higher voltages, while the risk of thermal tissue injury was concomitantly minimized by maintaining the tissue temperatures well below the neurodestructive range—below 42°C. Because the use of CRF inevitably results in nerve damage (i.e., neuroma), and nerve damage is a requisite for neuropathic pain, the use of PRF is primarily limited to neuropathic pain states. The conflicting goals of PRF, high voltage, and nonneurodestructive temperatures are achieved by applying the RF currents in a pulsatile manner, allowing time for the heat to dissipate in between RF pulses.[8] By using mathematical calculations, the authors showed that the high-density electrical currents generated at the electrode tip could stress the cellular membranes and cause altered cellular function and cell injury.[8] Later investigators suggested a combined role of electrical and thermal tissue injury from PRF application.[9,10] They ascertained that the slow response time of temperature measuring devices used during PRF may not reliably exclude the possibility of brief temperature spikes causing thermal tissue injury. Laboratory studies have shown neuronal activation,[11,12] cellular stress,[13] and cellular substructure damage[9] after PRF application. However, other experimental studies show that the observed cellular injury from PRF application is predominantly a function of thermal injury, thereby undermining the role of electrical currents.[14,15] Although the exact mechanism of PRF application remains unclear, there is a growing body of evidence in the form of randomized controlled preclinical and clinical trials that suggests it may be efficacious in individuals with neuropathic pain.[16–19]

PRF is applied similar to CRF by placing an electrode in the vicinity of the target nociceptive nerve. Although the orientation and size of the electrical field affected by PRF is similar to CRF, whether or not the electrode should be placed parallel to the nerve or at a different orientation is not known. During classic PRF application, RF currents are applied for 20 milliseconds, at 2 Hertz, for a total duration of 120 seconds. Thus for the majority of lesioning duration (480/500 milliseconds) no RF current is applied. The voltage is controlled in a manner such that the maximum electrode temperature achieved remains below 42°C.[8] Variations from this PRF protocol have been infrequent, with the exception of longer treatment duration. PRF has been applied for 4, 8, and 20 minutes by some investigators,[20] and there is evidence from preclinical and clinical studies that longer treatment cycles may be associated with increased effectiveness.

WATER-COOLED RADIOFREQUENCY

Water-cooled radiofrequency (WCRF) ablation has been in clinical use for some time, used primarily in cardiac electrophysiology[21] and for tumor ablation[22]; however, its use in pain medicine is fairly recent. The basic principle of WCRF application is similar to CRF application: A thermal lesion is created by placing an

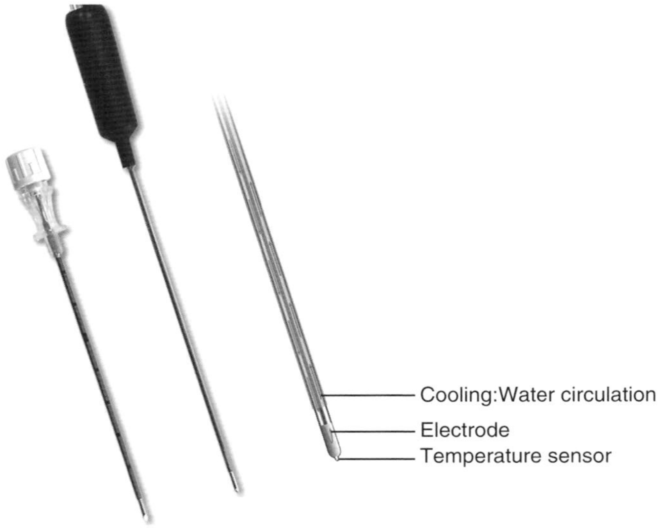

FIG. 68.1 Multichannel water-cooled electrode. *(Courtesy Halyard Health Inc.)*

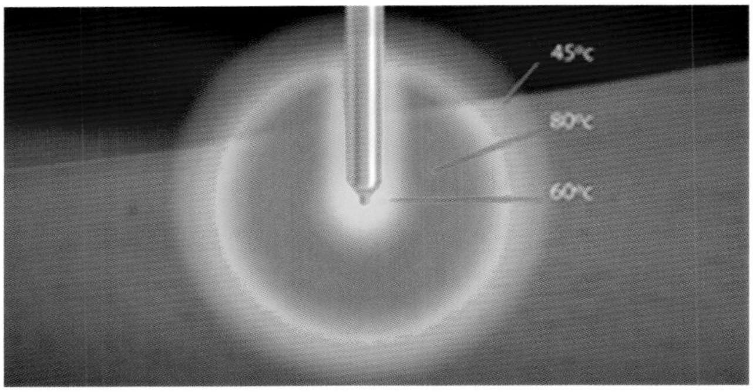

FIG. 68.2 Morphology of water-cooled radiofrequency lesion. *(Courtesy Halyard Health Inc.)*

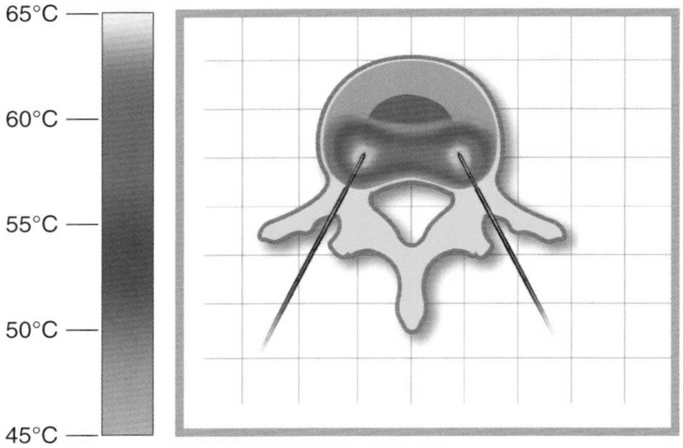

FIG. 68.3 Water-cooled radiofrequency application for discogenic pain. *(Courtesy Halyard Health Inc.)*

electrode in the vicinity of a target neural structure. However, WCRF is applied by using a specialized multichannel electrode that is actively cooled by continuous flow of water at ambient temperature (Fig. 68.1). The active cooling prevents the electrode from acquiring the high surrounding tissue temperature and allows the continued flow of current and consequent heating of a larger tissue volume, thus creating a larger thermal lesion.[21–23] The WCRF thermal lesion is composed of a few millimeters of cooled tissue immediately surrounding the electrode, followed by spherical isotherms of increasing tissue temperature that are surrounded by lower temperature isotherms (Fig. 68.2).[24] Similar to the CRF lesion size, the size of lesion created by WCRF application depends on the probe size, electrode temperature, and duration of current applied. If a 60°C isotherm is used as the measure for the lesion's peripheral extension, a 17-gauge electrode with a 4-mm active tip, and an electrode set temperature of raised to 55°C–60°C for 150 seconds achieves adjacent tissue temperatures of >80°C and would create a thermal lesion of 8–10 mm in diameter.[23–25] Even though a spherical area of tissue heating is expected,[25] several factors influence the symmetry of the WCRF lesion in vivo.[24] Active heat sinks, such as cerebrospinal fluid and blood, which are present in the thecal sac and epidural venous plexus, respectively, and passive heat-sinks, such as osseous and muscular spinal structures, help determine the eventual shape and size of the thermal lesion.[24]

A larger area of tissue damage with WCRF application increases the probability of successful denervation of a pain generator with numerous and/or variable nociceptive innervation.[23,25] The clinical use of WCRF in pain medicine employed two distinct forms of WCRF techniques, monopolar and bipolar lesioning, limited primarily to the treatment of sacroiliac joint dysfunction (SJD) and discogenic pain (DP), respectively. Additional studies are emerging however on the use for treating chronic knee pain. For the treatment of SJD unipolar WCRF is applied to the L5 dorsal ramus and S1, S2, S3, and sometimes S4 lateral branches, which range in number from 1 to 4, and three monopolar lesions are created lateral to each respective sacral foramen (Fig. 68.3).[26,27] Using a 17-gauge specialized electrode with a 4-mm active tip, the RF current is applied for 150 seconds with a set temperature of 60°C. The set temperature of 60°C creates adjacent tissue temperatures >80°C. Due to the larger anticipated lesion size, the introducer needle is typically kept at a "safe distance" from the sacral nerve roots—8–10 mm from the lateral edge of posterior sacral foramen.[27] To avoid injury to the segmental spinal nerve, WCRF is generally not applied to the L5 dorsal ramus, and CRF is used instead.[26] For the treatment of DP, bipolar WCRF is applied to the posterior-lateral disc annulus by placing two 17-gauge introducer needles and specialized RF electrodes (Fig. 68.4).[28,29] The electrode temperature is raised to 55°C over 11 minutes, and this temperature is maintained for an additional 4 minutes.

CRYONEUROLYSIS

Cryogenic nerve injury is not generally associated with neuroma formation, hyperalgesia, and deafferentation pain, attributes typical of neuronal injury caused by other physical modalities such as surgical nerve sectioning, thermal RF lesioning, or chemical neurolysis. Trendelenburg first demonstrated that freezing of peripheral nerves caused nerve disruption without the risk of neuroma formation.[30]

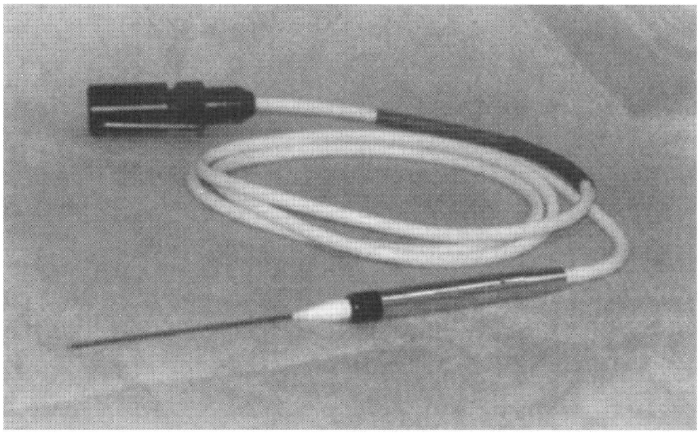

FIG. 68.4 Cryoprobe needle.

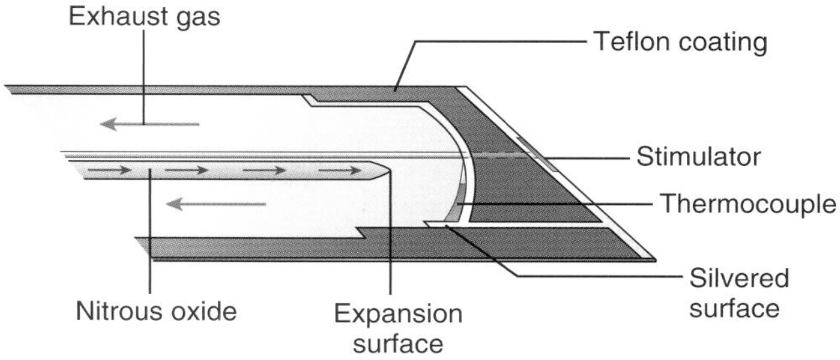

FIG. 68.5 Schematic design of cryoprobe needle.

Later, Carter et al.[31] and Beazley et al.[32] showed that the peripheral nerve injury from extreme cold caused axonal and myelin sheath disintegration and lead to Wallerian nerve degeneration, without disruption of endoneurium, perineurium, and epineurium. The mechanism of cryogenic nerve injury appears to emanate from damage to the vasa nervorum, resulting in endoneural edema, increased endoneural pressure, and consequent axonal disintegration. Autoimmune response triggered by the release of sequestered neural elements has also been implicated in the long-term effects of cryoablation.[33] The spared connective elements and Schwann cell basal laminae provide ready substrate for nerve regeneration from intact proximal axons. The axonal regeneration typically occurs at a rate of about 1–1.5 mm/week, and the duration of analgesia from cryoablation consequently depends on the time taken by the proximal axons to reinnervate the end organs, typically ranging from weeks to months.[34]

Although the local anesthetic-like properties of cold have been known since ancient Egyptian times,[35] tissue temperatures must be lowered to critical levels for adequate duration in order for the disintegrative nerve changes to occur—a distinction analogous to the difference between cold and numb fingers and frostbite. The critical temperature required to cause such disintegrative nerve changes has been shown to be minus 20°C.[36] In addition, the degree and the duration of analgesia is proportional to the severity of the cryogenic nerve damage.[37] It is therefore crucial that the tissue temperatures are maintained below the critical levels for an adequate duration during cryolesioning. The extent of freezing and the likelihood of the target nerve injury therefore depend on the probe size, probe proximity to the target nerve, freezing duration, and number of freeze cycles applied. Repeat freeze and thaw cycles increase the size of the eventual ice ball formed.

The first cryoneedle, developed in 1962, used liquid nitrogen as the refrigerant and lowered the needle tip temperature below minus 196°C.[38] In 1967, the currently used cryoprobe needle (see Figs. 68.4 and 68.5) was developed, using the Joule-Thompson enclosed gas expansion principle and lowering the probe tip temperature to between –ve 50° and –ve 70°C.[39] The contemporary cryoprobe is a double lumen aluminum tube that connects to a gas source by flexible tubing, and either nitrous oxide or carbon dioxide is delivered at a pressure of approximately 42 kg/cm^2 (600 lb/in^2—psi) to the inner cryoprobe lumen. The gas under pressure escapes through a small orifice from the inner lumen near the cryoprobe tip and returns to the console through the outer cryoprobe lumen. The drastic drop in the pressure at the probe tip—from 600–800 psi to 10–15 psi—allows gas expansion and consequent cooling. Heat absorbed from the tissues surrounding the probe tip lowers the temperature and creates an ice ball around the probe tip. Currently available cryoprobe sizes include a 14-gauge (2-mm) probe that roughly forms a 5.5-mm ice ball, and an 18-gauge (1.4-mm) probe that forms a 3.5-mm ice ball.

Meticulous localization of the target nerve is necessary to increase the likelihood of nerve disruption. Most currently used cryoprobes are therefore equipped with a built-in nerve stimulator function that allows both motor (2 Hz) and sensory (100 Hz) testing. The probe also has a thermistor incorporated in the tip to precisely monitor the target tissue temperatures. The console unit is equipped with nerve stimulator controls and temperature and gas pressure gauges, and has a gas regulator switch that allows precise control of gas flow. To ensure safe and effective cryoablation, gas flow must be precisely regulated—inadequate gas flow is ineffective in lowering tissue temperatures below critical levels, while excessive gas flow may lead to tissue freezing proximally along the probe length and cause unintended freeze lesions such as skin burns. The cryoprobe should be withdrawn only after the ice ball has thawed, since withdrawing the probe with the ice ball still present may cause local tissue injury and avulsion of a nerve segment. The use of an introducer, such as a large gauge intravenous catheter, is often recommended during cryoprobe placement. A sharp introducer tip facilitates the placement of the less rigid cryoprobe and affords additional skin protection during cryolesioning of the superficial nerves. Typically, a 12-gauge intravenous catheter is used for the 2.0-mm probe, and a 14- to 16-gauge catheter is used for the 1.4-mm probe.

CLINICAL USES

PULSED RADIOFREQUENCY

Even though PRF has been employed in the clinical practice fairly recently, its use is relatively widespread, and it is used for both painful and some nonpainful conditions.[20] The growing popularity of PRF is likely due to its perceived safety and clinical efficacy, particularly for neuropathic pain. PRF should be considered when further injury to the nerve(s) should be avoided in patients predisposed to neuropathic pain, while thermal RF (ablation) should be a choice for mechanical pain (e.g., facet joint, SI joint, knee arthritis). PRF has been applied to the DRG at all spinal levels in the treatment of multiple pain syndromes, including radicular pain (RP) from a herniated disc, postherpetic neuralgia, postamputation stump pain, occipital neuralgia, and inguinal herniorrhaphy pain.[20] It is applied to a range of peripheral nerves for multiple pain syndromes such as suprascapular nerve (SSN) for shoulder pain, intercostal nerves for postsurgical thoracic pain, lateral femoral cutaneous nerve for meralgia paresthetica, pudendal nerve for pudendal neuralgia, dorsal penile nerves for premature ejaculation, splanchnic nerves for chronic benign pancreatic pain, sciatic nerve for phantom limb pain, obturator and femoral nerves for hip pain, glossopharyngeal nerve for glossopharyngeal neuralgia, occipital nerve(s) for occipital neuralgia, and genitofemoral, ilioinguinal, and iliohypogastric nerves for groin pain and orchialgia.[20] It has also been applied to various peripheral and autonomic ganglia, including the gasserian ganglion (GG) for trigeminal neuralgia (TN); sphenopalatine ganglion for head, neck, and facial pain; and to the lumbar sympathetic chain in the treatment of complex regional pain syndrome.[20] In some reports the target neural structure for PRF application is unclear, such as myofascial trigger points for myofascial pain, scar neuromas for postsurgical scar pain, spermatic cord for testicular pain, and intraarticularly for arthrogenic pain.[20]

WATER-COOLED RADIOFREQUENCY

The use of WCRF is currently limited to pain syndromes where the pain generator is considered to have numerous and variable sources of innervation. WCRF is used mainly for the treatment of SJD[26,27] and DP.[28,29] However, due to its ability to accurately deliver thermal energy to larger tissue volumes, WCRF may be effective when more traditional forms of neuroablation have failed, and its use may be extended to other pain syndromes.

CRYONEUROLYSIS

The reported use of cryoablation in the literature is most prevalent for the treatment of postthoracotomy pain.[40–55] Cryolesioning for this clinical indication is typically performed intraoperatively under direct vision, on individual intercostal nerves in the intercostal grove. All the intercostal nerves likely involved in mediating a patient's pain, from 1 to 2 segments above the upper limit of the incision to 1 to 2 below the lower limit of the incision or the chest drain, are typically treated. The cryoablation experience with postthoracotomy pain led to its use for other chronic pain conditions of the chest wall, such as postoperative neuroma formation, costochondritis, postherpetic neuralgia, and rib fractures.[56–58] In the head, neck, and facial region, cryolesioning of several regional nerves have been reported in multiple studies. The nerves included were inferior alveolar, mental, lingual, buccal, inferior dental, auriculotemporal, supraorbital, and infraorbital nerves.[58–70] The painful head, neck, and facial conditions treated with cryoablation included TN, postherpetic neuralgia, atypical facial pain, and various postsurgical neuralgias. In the majority of these studies, the craniofacial nerves were exposed by open dissection for cryolesioning. In a few studies, the cryoprobe was placed using a closed technique, either percutaneously or transmucosally. There is one study evaluating cryoablation in posttonsillectomy patients, where the exact targeted neural structure was less clear.[70] Cryoablation has also been used for the treatment of spinal and extremity pain. Its use is reported frequently for the treatment of lumbar facet syndrome (FS), where it is applied to the lumbar MBs.[71–73] For extremity pain, it is used in the intermetatarsal space for the treatment of Morton's neuroma.[74] Cryolesioning of the ulnar, median, sural, occipital, palmar branch of the median, and digital nerves has been performed for traumatic nerve injuries and carpal tunnel syndrome.[75] Cryoablation has also been used for the treatment of several painful conditions involving the abdomen, pelvis, and perineum. The most frequent application in this region has been for the treatment of postinguinal herniorrhaphy pain, where it is applied to iliohypogastric and ilioinguinal nerves.[76–79] It has been applied to the lower sacral nerve roots for intractable perineal pain,[80] to ilioinguinal and iliohypogastric nerves for corresponding neuralgiform chronic abdominal pain,[81] and to the ganglion impar for intractable rectal pain.[82] Its use has been described in many forms for pregnancy-related and postpartum pain in women. These include cryolesioning of the ilioinguinal nerve for late pregnancy abdominal pain,[83] application to the sacral extradural canal for severe postpartum sacrococcygeal pain,[84] and to the symphysis pubis for pregnancy-associated symphysis pubis diastasis pelvic pain.[85] Cryolesioning of the iliac crest has also been performed for donor site pain.[86]

CLINICAL EFFICACY

PULSED RADIOFREQUENCY

Radicular Pain

There are five trials of PRF application to the affected DRG for RP (Table 68.1): four in the lumbar and one in the cervical region.[8,18,87–89] The first trial of PRF use by Sluijter et al. reported its efficacy in a group of 36 patients with RP, comparing it with CRF at 42°C at 6 weeks.[8] This trial was limited by its size, vaguely described study population, lack of adequate randomization and blinding, inadequate outcome measures (only patient satisfaction scores were used), absence of long-term follow-up, and lack of a placebo group. It also compared PRF with nonstandard CRF (CRF at 42°C), which is not routinely used in clinical practice. A trial consisting of 76 patients with lumbar RP compared PRF with combined PRF and CRF applied with the DRG, and reported no advantage of adding CRF.[87] This trial used a nonconventional form of CRF, applying current to a maximum tolerated temperature that created a burning sensation extending from the low back to the foot; the average temperature was 54°C for 60 seconds. One trial performed in 100 patients with back pain, with or without RP, compared PRF/DRG with electroacupuncture and conservative treatment, reporting relative efficacy of the PRF treatment.[88] This trial contained significant limitations that included a poorly defined study

TABLE 68.1 Controlled Trials of Pulsed Radiofrequency for Radicular Pain

Study	Methodology	Outcomes	Analysis and Limitations
1998 Sluijter et al.[8]	Nonrandomized controlled trial 36 patients with chronic RP compared PRF with CRF at 42°C	Reported efficacy of PRF at 6 weeks compared with CRF at 42°C. Authors concluded PRF was an effective treatment modality.	Small size (36 patients) Vague study population No randomization or blinding No pain scores, used only patient satisfaction Short-term results at 6 weeks No placebo group Compared PRF to thermal RF at 42°C, which is not routinely used in clinical practice
2008 Simopoulos et al.[87]	RCT 76 patients with lumbar RP, 37 had PRF of DRG, 39 had combined PRF and CRF (maximally tolerated temperatures)	Similar decline in VAS scores between the 2 groups at 2 months. Similar loss of analgesic effect between 2 and 4 months and return of pain to baseline by 8 months. Authors reported PRF of DRG was safe and resulted in short-term benefit; addition of CRF did not offer added benefit.	Use of nonconventional form of thermal RF not routinely practiced. Thermal RF to maximum tolerated temperature that created a burning sensation in low back to the foot. Average temperatures was 54°C for 60 s.
2010 Lin et al.[88]	RCT 100 patients with back pain with or without RP. Compared PRF to DRG with electroacupuncture and conservative treatment.	Reported relative efficacy of the PRF treatment compared to electroacupuncture and conservative treatment	Inadequately defined study population. No description of number and levels of DRG treated. No prior diagnostic nerve blocks performed. Unknown nature of the treatments provided in conservatively treated group. Inadequate description of blinding or randomization techniques. Only short-term results reported.
2014 Shanthanna et al.[89]	RCT, DB, PCT 32 patients with LRP	No difference between PRF and sham treatment at 3 months	Small trial—32 patients Short-term results—3 months
2007 Van Zundert et al.[18]	RCT, DB, PCT 23 patients with cervical RP, 11 had PRF at one level DRG, 12 had ST	Significant improvement reported in 9/11 (82%) patients in the PRF group and in 4/12 GPE (33%) and 3/12 VAS (25%) in the ST group.	This study provides evidence of short-term efficacy of PRF for cervical radicular pain. Limitations: Small size—23 patients Short-term results—3 months

Overall Efficacy of PRF for Radicular Pain Summary:
5trials of PRF-DRG use for RP.
Overall: Either small in size, reported short-term results, and/or compared PRF to unconventional treatments.
Potential efficacy of PRF-DRF for radicular pain essentially unknown.
AU, *Analgesic usage;* CRF, *conventional radiofrequency;* DB, *double-blinded;* DRG, *dorsal root ganglia;* GPE, *global perceived effect;* PCT, *placebo controlled trial;* PRF, *pulsed radiofrequency;* PSS, *patient satisfaction scale;* RCT, *randomized controlled trial;* RP, *radicular pain;* ST, *Sham treatment;* TN, *trigeminal neuralgia;* VAS, *visual analogue scale.*

population, no description of the number and level(s) of DRG treated, no diagnostic nerve blocks performed prior to the DRG treatment, nonstandard treatment in the control group, poor description of blinding and randomization techniques, and the assessment of only short-term results. There are two randomized, double-blinded trials comparing PRF/DRG with sham treatment—one in the cervical and one in the lumbar region.[18,89] Even though these two trials were reasonably well-conducted, both were small in size and reported only modest, short-term efficacy relative to the placebo. Currently, there is only little support of PRF/DRG for the treatment of RP in the literature.

Facet Syndrome

There are three trials evaluating PRF application to the MBs for FS, all in lumbar region (Table 68.2).[90–92] A trial of 60 patients with FS compared PRF, CRF, and sham treatment in three equal groups and reported superior efficacy of CRF and PRF compared with the sham treatment, but only at 6 hours after the treatment.[90] Although patients in the CRF group continued to experience superior pain relief and improved function at 6 and 12 months, those in the PRF and sham-treated groups had similar outcomes at these time points. A similar trial involving 50 patients compared PRF with CRF (lacking a placebo group) and reported no significant differences between the two groups at 3 months. Within-group differences were observed within the CRF group, but not the PRF group over the course of the study.[91] This trial was limited by a high dropout rate, short follow-up, and insufficiently described methods. A more recent trial performed in 80 patients compared PRF with MBs injections (steroid and local anesthetic), reporting relative efficacy of PRF for up to 6 months.[92] In summary, there is insufficient evidence to recommend PRF for facet arthropathy.

Shoulder Pain

Among the four trials assessing PRF of the SSN for shoulder pain, three compared PRF with another treatment modality of uncertain efficacy, and one compared it with sham treatment (Table 68.3).[93–95] A single-blind study of 50 patients, in two equal groups, compared intraarticular steroid injections with fluoroscopically directed PRF of the SSN, and reported relative effectiveness for intraarticular injections at 3 months.[93] A trial performed in 40 patients compared

TABLE 68.2 Randomized Controlled Trials of Pulsed Radiofrequency for Facet Syndrome

Study	Methodology	Outcomes	Study Analysis and Limitations
2007 Tekin et al.[90]	RCT, DB, PCT 60 patients with LFS, 20 had thermal RF, 20 had PRF and 20 had ST	At 6 h significantly lower VAS and ODI scores in thermal and PRF groups compared with ST. However, at 6 months and 1 year, the lower scores were maintained only in thermal RF group. The authors concluded thermal RF and PRF were both useful.	This trial only provides evidence of the efficacy of PRF at 6 h after lumbar facet RF neurotomy.
2008 Kroll et al.[91]	RCT, DB 50 patients with LFS, 13 had thermal RF and 13 had PRF	No significant difference between the thermal RF and PRF groups in relative improvements in either VAS or ODI scores at 3 months.	High dropout rate, short follow-up, and insufficiently described methods. Only 26 of 50 patients available for analysis No difference in the results of PRF and thermal RF at 3 months for facetogenic pain
2014 Hashemi et al.[92]	RCT, DB 80 patients with LFS had either PRF to MBs or steroid and local anesthetic injections	Relative efficacy of PRF for up to 6 months.	Well-conducted DB, RCT

Clinical efficacy of PRF of MBs for Facet Syndrome—Summary.
Two well conducted trials (Tekin and Hashemi) reported opposing results.
Efficacy of PRF of MBs for lumbar FS remains unclear.
No trials of PRF of MBs for treatment of facet syndrome in cervical region.
DB, *Double-blinded;* LFS, *lumbar facet syndrome;* ODI, *Oswestry Disability Index;* PCT, *placebo controlled trial;* PRF, *pulsed radiofrequency;* RCT, *randomized controlled trial;* RF, *radiofrequency;* ST, *Sham treatment;* VAS, *visual analogue scale.*

TABLE 68.3 Controlled Trials of Pulsed Radiofrequency for Shoulder Pain

Study	Methodology	Outcomes	Study Analysis and Limitations
2010 Eyigor et al.[93]	RCT 50 patients in 2 equal groups. Compared intraarticular steroid injections with fluoroscopically directed PRF of the SSN	Relative efficacy of intraarticular steroid injections reported at 3 months	A single-blinded study Short-term results
2010 Korkmaz et al.[94]	RCT 40 patients with chronic shoulder pain. Compared TENS applied to the shoulder joint (20 min 5 times a week for 20 sessions) to fluoroscopically directed PRF of the SSN.	No difference in outcomes between the two groups at 3 months	Randomized controlled, double-blinded Short-term results
2014 Wu et al.[95]	RCT 60 patients with shoulder pain. Compared 12 weeks of PT alone to 12 weeks of PT and single ultrasound-guided PRF of the SSN	Reported relative efficacy of combined treatment at 12 weeks	Randomized controlled, double-blinded Only 42/60 patients completed the study Short-term results
2013 Gofeld et al.[96]	RCT, placebo controlled 22 patients with shoulder pain. Compared PRF of SSN with similarly performed sham procedure (lidocaine injection).	Reported similar efficacy of PRF and placebo at 6 months	Small size Slow recruitment (22 patients recruited over 3 years) High dropout rate (9 of the 22 patients dropped out of the study at 6 months)

PRF of SSN for Shoulder Pain—Summary.
Three trials reported variable efficacy of PRF of SSN when compared to different pain relieving modalities (IA injections, TENS, PT).
One severely limited trial reported its lack of efficacy.
The true value of PRF of SSN for shoulder pain remains essentially unknown.
IA, *Intraarticular;* PRF, *pulsed radiofrequency;* PT, *physical therapy;* RCT, *randomized controlled trial;* SSN, *suprascapular nerve;* TENS, *transcutaneous electrical nerve stimulation.*

transcutaneous electric nerve stimulation (TENS) applied to the shoulder joint (for 20 minutes, 5 times a week, for 20 sessions) and fluoroscopically directed PRF of the SSN. At 3 months, no difference in outcomes was reported between the groups.[94] A trial conducted in 60 patients (only 42 of whom completed the study) compared 12 weeks of physical therapy alone to 12 weeks of physical therapy and a single ultrasound-guided PRF treatment of the SSN, finding relative effectiveness for the combined treatment at 12 weeks.[95] The only placebo-controlled trial evaluating PRF of the

SSN reported similar effectiveness at 6 months between the treatment group and a lidocaine injection, with sham PRF.[96] This trial was limited by its size (only 13 patients were available for analysis at 6 months), so its results were inconclusive. Consequently, with three trials reporting variable benefit for PRF of the SSN compared with disparate pain-relieving modalities of indeterminate effectiveness, and one flawed trial reporting a lack of efficacy, the true value of PRF of SSN for shoulder pain remains unknown.

Cervicogenic Headache

Only one trial evaluated the efficacy of PRF of GON in patients with cervicogenic headache. In this trial, 30 patients divided into two equal groups received either PRF or local anesthetic blocks of the GON. No differences were observed between the groups at 3 and 9 months.[97] This trial was limited by its small size and lack of blinding.

Postherpetic Neuralgia

Only one trial evaluated the efficacy of PRF in patients with PHN affecting thoracic dermatomes.[98] Ninety-six patients were randomized to receive either PRF or sham PRF of the DRG. The study found significant improvements in pain scores and quality of life that persisted throughout the 6-month follow-up period.

Trigeminal Neuralgia

There are three trials evaluating PRF application to the GG for the treatment of TN. A randomized, double-blind trial in 40 patients with TN reported lack of PRF effectiveness compared with CRF at 3 months, and recommended against its use.[99] Another randomized, double-blinded trial performed in 60 patients compared CRF at 75°C for 2–3 minutes, CRF at 75°C for 4–5 minutes, and PRF for 10 minutes combined with CRF at 75°C for 2–3 minutes, and reported no differences between the groups at 1 year.[100] A third randomized, double-blinded study done in 60 patients (53 completed the study) compared standard-voltage (36.30±5.57) with high-voltage (71.52±7.97) PRF, applied for 4 minutes. It reported greater effectiveness for high voltage PRF.[101] Because all the trials assessing PRF of the GG for TN evaluated various combinations of PRF and CRF and did not contain a control group, the effectiveness of PRF remains unknown.

PRF is used extensively in clinical practice for a range of painful and even some nonpainful syndromes. Yet its exact mechanism of action is ambiguous, and based on the variable results reported in a range of clinical trials, the true value of its clinical utility, though certainly auspicious, remains unclear.

WATER-COOLED RADIOFREQUENCY

In addition to the isolated reports of its use for neuromas and superficial nerves,[102,103] WC-RF is currently being used primarily when the potential pain generator has abundant and variable innervation, as is the case for SJD and DP.[19,24,29]

CLINICAL EFFICACY

There are two trials evaluating WC-RF use for the treatment of SJD.[26,104] The first was a double-blind trial of 28 patients, with typical SJD symptoms and a positive response to a single diagnostic sacroiliac joint injection.[26] The patients were randomized in two equal groups, to receive WC-RF (L4–L5 primary dorsal rami and S1–S3 or S4 lateral branches) and sham treatment (local anesthetic blocks with placebo denervation). At 1 month, 11/14 (79%) patients in the RF group and 2/14 patients (14%) in the placebo group had successful outcomes (50% pain relief and significant functional improvement). The second trial, also blinded and randomized, was composed of 51 patients with SJD symptoms and a positive response to dual lateral branch blocks.[104] The patients, randomized in a 2:1 ratio (34 patients in the RF and 17 in the sham group), received either WC-RF (applied to S1–S3 lateral branches and L5 dorsal ramus) or sham treatment (identically performed except for RF application). Unblinding occurred at 3 months, at which time patients were allowed to crossover to the RF group; there were no dropouts at 3 months. Significant improvements in pain (NRS, SF-36BP-Bodily Pain), physical function (SF-36 PF-Physical Functioning), disability (ODI), quality of life, and treatment success (Global Perceived Effect) were reported for the treatment group at 3 months. Hence the two well-conducted trials reported short-term efficacy for WC-RF for SJD. The only trial evaluating WC-RF use for discogenic low back pain was a double-blinded trial performed in 59 well-selected patients with chronic low back pain who reported reproduction of their pain on provocative discography.[105] The patients were randomized to receive either intradiscal biacuplasty (IDB) to the affected discs (n = 27, one level; n = 16, two levels; n = 11) or sham treatment (n = 30, identical procedure except that the probe was not placed in the disc and RF energy was not delivered). The patients in the IDB group exhibited significant improvements in physical function (SF-36), pain (NRS), disability (ODI), and reduced opioid usage for up to 6 months. An open-label extension of this same study found that the benefit of biacuplasty persisted for at least 1 year. But whereas this small, randomized trial and open-label extension study suggest that some individuals may benefit from IDB, this evidence must be weighed against the mixed evidence for intradiscal electrothermal therapy (another intradiscal procedure that utilizes heat ablation) and the possibility that annular puncture may result in enhanced disc degeneration in some individuals.

CRYONEUROLYSIS

The randomized controlled trials (RCTs) evaluating cryoablation pertain mostly to its use after thoracic surgery for the relief of postoperative pain.[40–50] Although the majority of these trials were published in the 1980s and 1990s, some were published as recently as 2008.[49] The comparisons made in these trials varied significantly, comparing cryoablation to no intervention,[40–44] local anesthetic blockade,[40] continuous intravenous narcotic infusion,[45,46] and epidural analgesia.[47–49] Of the five trials that compared cryoablation with no intervention, three[40,41,44] reported statistically significant reduced narcotic usage and pain scores after cryoablation, while two showed no advantage.[42,43] The two trials that compared cryoablation to intravenous narcotic infusion showed no advantage for cryoablation.[45,46] There are three trials comparing epidural analgesia with cryoablation.[47–49] The results of one trial showed that patients in the epidural analgesia group had significantly better pain scores and pulmonary function tests compared with the cryoanalgesia group.[47] Results of the other two trials showed that while cryoablation provided postoperative analgesia comparable to epidural analgesia, it increased the incidence of postthoracotomy neuropathic pain; hence the authors recommended against its use.[48,49] In one controlled trial with four treatment groups, cryoablation was compared with epidural analgesia, continuous narcotic infusion, and intrapleural analgesia.[50] The results of this trial showed epidural analgesia provided the best relief of postoperative pain; however, due to the insufficient number of patients enrolled, the results failed to reach statistical significance. Overall, of the 11 available controlled studies pertaining to the use of cryoablation for the relief of postthoracotomy pain, only three favored its use.[40,41,44] This relative lack of efficacy for intercostal nerve cryoablation has been attributed to unaltered sensitivity of the visceral pleura and the large thoracic wall muscles, such as the latissimus dorsi and serratus anterior.[43]

Although multiple reports of cryoablation in the head, neck, and facial regions have been published,[51–70] only one study is a controlled trial.[70] In this RCT, cryoablation was applied to the tonsillar fossa after tonsillectomy. It reported statistically significant reduced postoperative pain scores in patients receiving cryoablation without evidence of serious complications.

There are three controlled trials assessing cryolesioning for postoperative pain after herniorrhaphy.[77–79] In two trials, isolated cryolesioning of the ilioinguinal nerve was performed at the end of the hernia surgery.[77,78] One of these trials reported reduced postoperative analgesic usage in the cryoanalgesia group,[77] while the other trial reported no difference in pain scores and analgesic consumption between the treatment and the control groups.[78] In the third trial, cryolesioning of both the ilioinguinal and iliohypogastric nerves was performed intraoperatively, and no statistically significant difference in pain scores and analgesic usage was reported between the treatment and the control groups.[79] This trial also reported an increased incidence of sensory disturbances in treatment patients, prompting the authors to recommend against its use for postherniorrhaphy pain.

SIDE EFFECTS AND COMPLICATIONS

Although bleeding, infection, and nerve damage from needle placement, and burns from incorrect placement of the grounding pad, have been reported,[106] no noticeable side effects or complications have been directly attributable to PRF use.

Apart from local transient postprocedural discomfort, none of the four clinical studies of WCRF reported any significant complications.

Despite the theoretical claims of reduced risk of neuroma formation and nerve regeneration after cryoneurolysis, the most frequently reported significant adverse effect of cryoneurolysis has been neuropathic pain characterized by hypersensitivity and allodynia.[48,49,79] Other reported complications from cryoneurolysis are rare and include local tissue injury from the placement of the large gauge introducer, catheter, or cryoprobe needle. Patients may report numbness in the territory of the involved nerve, which is sometimes distressful. A diagnostic local anesthetic block performed prior to the cryoneurolysis allows the patient to experience this numbing effect and judge its tolerability. Alopecia and depigmentation or hyperpigmentation at the lesion site have also been reported, and may be of greater concern when cryolesions are performed in proximity to the face.[107]

CONCLUSION

RF and cryoablation techniques attempt to provide pain relief by interrupting nociceptive pathways. Even though the technique of various RF modalities appear similar, they should not be construed a single treatment modality. Of the three available RF techniques, only thermal and WCRF create a demonstrable tissue lesion. Thermal RF is the most enduring RF technique; however, due to the potential for increased postprocedural pain and sensorimotor dysfunction, its use is limited to few specific pain syndromes. Although the exact mechanism of PRF remains unclear and no demonstrable tissue lesion is created, its use is widespread and a growing body of evidence suggests that it may be efficacious in certain neuropathic pain conditions. WCRF creates a larger thermal tissue lesion and is currently used primarily for pain syndromes where the pain generator has numerous and variable sources of innervation. Cryoablation is a time-honored technique; however, despite being an ablative technique that creates a reversible lesion, with limited postprocedural pain augmentation or dysfunction, its use has declined over the years.

KEY POINTS

- RF and cryoablation attempt to interrupt nociceptive pathways to provide pain relief.
- RF application for pain should not be construed as a single treatment modality.
- Thermal RF creates distinct thermal tissue lesion, but due to the potential for postprocedural increased pain and dysfunction, its use is limited to few specific pain syndromes.
- PRF does not create a distinct tissue lesion; however, its use is widespread, and it may be efficacious in certain neuropathic pain conditions.
- WCRF creates a larger circumscribed thermal lesion, and it is currently used for pain syndromes where the pain generator has numerous and variable innervation.
- Cryoablation creates reversible lesions with less risk for increased postablation pain or persistent dysfunction, and can be applied where there is greater risk of neuritis or deafferentation pain.

REFERENCES

Access the reference list online at ExpertConsult.com.

CHAPTER 69

DISCOGRAPHY

Steven P. Cohen, MD

Discography has been called a "test in search of an indication" and a "solution in need of a problem." Originally employed as a diagnostic tool for herniated discs in the era prior to the advent of advanced imaging, its use in this capacity has been almost completely supplanted by safer, cheaper, and more sensitive modalities such as magnetic resonance imaging (MRI). Over the intervening years, discography continued to be used, evolving from a defunct imaging tool to the only ostensible means to correlate imaging with symptoms. As a diagnostic and prognostic tool, disc stimulation remains one of the most controversial interventional pain procedures, with many physicians and, more importantly, third-party payers refusing to perform it or to authorize its use. Yet new research published since the last edition of this book has demonstrated that at least in some cases, discography may improve surgical outcomes.

OVERVIEW OF SPINAL PAIN

Pain originating from the spine commonly manifests as pain in the low back and neck and less frequently as pain in the midback. Although many components of the spine are capable of generating pain, its exact source is often elusive. Several factors make the identification of spinal pain generators challenging. First, back pain can originate not only from various spinal column components but can also be referred from structures adjacent to the spine, such as abdominal or pelvic viscera, sacroiliac joints, and so on. Second, pain can be difficult to localize due to multisegmental innervation with resultant convergence in the spinal cord. The diagnosis of spinal pain is further complicated by the concurrent presence and overlapping clinical features of various spinal disorders, especially degenerative conditions. The lack of diagnostic tests that can reliably identify a spinal pain generator further adds to these challenges. Currently available tests, often based on high-resolution imaging, frequently show abnormal findings in asymptomatic individuals at all spinal levels.[1-3] Because of the frequent spontaneous resolution of symptoms, the high incidence of benign abnormal findings, and the rarity of serious spinal disorders, indiscriminate diagnostic testing of patients with spinal pain can lead to inappropriate diagnoses and poor treatment results.

MECHANISMS OF DISCOGENIC PAIN

Although the role played by a herniated nucleus pulposus (NP) in causing spinal pain is well known, the concept of pain originating from the disc itself is less understood. The term *internal disc disruption* (IDD) has been used since the early 1970s to describe a disc that is considered the main source of a patient's pain but appears functionally intact on spinal imaging.[4] However, degenerative disc changes seen on spinal imaging are nearly ubiquitous, especially with advanced age.[3] These myriad changes are collectively referred to as *degenerated disc disease* (DDD) and may represent normal age-related phenomena.

Isolated degenerative disc pathology, where one or two discs show profound degeneration in the presence of other relatively normal-appearing discs, is less common and more frequently encountered in younger individuals. Whether IDD and DDD are distinct pathologic entities or represent pathologic progression of the same disease entity is unknown. The terminology surrounding pain stemming from intervertebral discs can be confusing, with one systematic review finding that DDD is most commonly used in studies evaluating surgical treatments.[5] The term *discogenic pain* (DP) describes a clinical state where the disc is considered the main source of spinal pain. For the present discussion, this term seems most appropriate, as it emphasizes the disc as the primary source of a patient's pain irrespective of pathology.

A basic understanding of normal disc physiology is imperative to understand the mechanisms responsible for DP. A normal disc is grossly compartmentalized into its NP and annulus fibrosus (AF). Interspersed in abundant intercellular matrix in the two disc compartments are sparsely present cells. The cells populating the NP are chondrocyte-like, while those comprising the AF more closely resemble fibrocytes.[6] The intercellular matrix in the NP is a "jelly-like" substance containing high concentrations of water and proteoglycans, while the matrix in the AF consists predominantly of type I and II collagen fibers. These fibers are arranged as 10–20 interlacing, concentric lamellae, which are firmly attached to the adjacent vertebral bodies.[6] The compressive forces applied to the disc are directly borne by the NP and are distributed as a tensile force to the annular collagen. The incompressibility exhibited by a normal NP is due to its high water content, which in turn is maintained by the hydrostatic pressure generated by proteoglycans. The normal NP proteoglycan content is a function of the delicate balance between anabolic and catabolic enzymatic activities.

The vascularity of a normal intervertebral disc is limited to the outer one-third of the AF. In addition, the disc is separated from the vascular vertebral body by avascular cartilaginous end plates.[6] Consequently the metabolic needs of the NP and inner AF are met almost entirely by diffusion from the capillary plexuses in the adjacent vertebral bodies and outer AF. This process is facilitated by circadian changes in intradiscal pressure; lower nighttime pressure facilitates the flow of fluids into the disc, while higher daytime pressure forces the fluids out of the disc. The end products of the

NP cellular metabolic activities are also removed by diffusion. However, the disc lacks scavenger cells, so that degradative products tend to accumulate over time, which can interfere with normal homeostatic functions.[7]

The presence of nerve fibers in the normal disc is predominantly limited to the outer one-third of the AF. Disc innervation is mostly in the form of mechanoreceptors, which originate from plexuses along the anterior and posterior longitudinal ligaments. The posterior plexus receives its input from the sinuvertebral nerve and gray rami communicans, while the anterior plexus receives contributions mainly from gray rami communicans. These rich autonomic connections may contribute to the vague, poorly localized pain characteristic of IDD.

As discs begin to lose their water content and degenerate, nerve ingrowth occurs, which increases the density of nociceptive nerve fibers and their penetration toward the NP. The mechanisms by which this occurs may include angiogenesis and alterations in the cellular matrix (e.g., influx of inflammatory cytokines) and function.[8,9] Whether or not axial pain arising from degenerated intervertebral discs could be a form of neuropathic pain is a subject of controversy, but one study suggests that 12% of patients with axial low back pain (LBP) had neuropathic components, with higher numbers reported in those patients who had previously undergone disc surgery.[10]

DDD has been associated with both genetic and acquired factors, such as vascular disease, smoking, lifestyle, and obesity.[11–13] It is most likely a consequence of a combination of factors, including a decline in the number and function of viable disc cells, enhanced matrix metalloproteinase (MMP) activity, and increased activity of discal cytokines and other proinflammatory mediators.[13,14] These metabolic derangements can result in a reduction of nuclear proteoglycans and loss of discal water content. The diminished NP hydrostatic pressure leads to increased NP compressibility, which exposes the AF to direct compressive forces. In addition to mechanical stress, the AF also undergoes degenerative changes similar to those of the NP. In young patients with nondegenerated spines, most of the load bearing is borne anteriorly by the intervertebral discs; but as degeneration occurs, the posterior neural arch assumes an increased burden.[15] Collectively these changes result in the loss of annular collagen, mechanical failure, and the development of annular fissures that spread outward toward the periphery.

Annular fissures are a hallmark of DP. These tears are zones of highly vascularized and richly innervated granulation tissue. On T2-weighted MRI these may be seen as "high-intensity zones." The two different types of nerve fibers found in these granulation zones are vasoregulatory nerves, which accompany neovascularization, and free nerve endings high in substance-P concentration.[16] In addition, annular tears are abundant in mononuclear cell infiltrates, which release nerve growth factors that contribute to nerve ingrowth and accelerated degeneration. Disrupted discs also contain high concentrations of proinflammatory mediators, which serve to sensitize nerve endings and maintain a state of hyperalgesia. This state has been linked to the painful response associated with minimal pressure elevation during discography, a term denoted as "chemically sensitized."[17] Owing to limited

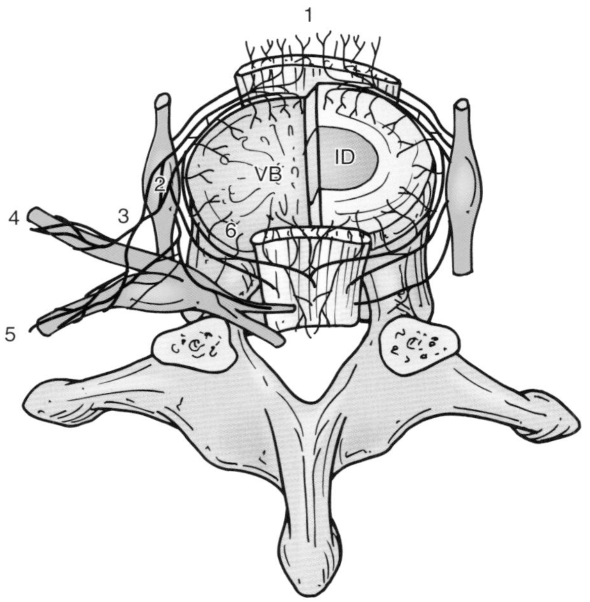

FIG. 69.1 Schematic drawing of the nerve plexi surrounding the vertebral body (VB) and intervertebral disc (ID). The anterior and posterior plexuses are represented by 1 and 6, respectively. The deep, extensive penetration of the nerves indicates that degeneration has occurred. *2*, Sympathetic trunk; *3*, rami communicantes; *4*, ventral ramus of the spinal nerve; *5*, dorsal ramus; *6*, sinuvertebral nerves. *(From Cohen SP, Larkin TM, Barna SA, et al.: Lumbar discography: a comprehensive review of outcome studies, diagnostic accuracy, and principles,* Reg Anesth Pain Med. *30:163-183, 2005. Drawing courtesy of Specialist Jennifer Sempsroft, US Army.)*

repair capacity, a painful disrupted disc may remain a longstanding source of disability.

In the long term, changes in disc morphology may alter spinal mechanics, increase stress on adjacent spinal structures, and result in osteophyte formation, sclerosis, and autofusion.[18] This can, in turn, lead to further degeneration of the disc and vertebral end plate, sacroiliac and facet joint pathology, and spinal stenosis (Fig. 69.1).

PREVALENCE

Epidemiologic studies evaluating the incidence of spinal pain vary greatly, as the conditions producing back and neck pain are often poorly defined. This is especially true for DP. The lifetime prevalence rate for LBP varies between 50% and 80%.[19] For neck pain, the annual prevalence rate generally varies between 15% and 50%,[20] with one systematic review reporting a mean prevalence rate of 37.2%.[21]

Epidemiologic studies for DP are uncommon. In an oft-cited study by Schwarzer et al.[22] conducted in 92 patients with chronic, nonradicular LBP and no previous surgery, the authors reported a 39% prevalence of IDD using exact pain reproduction, abnormal computed tomography (CT)–discography imaging, and a negative adjacent control disc as the criteria. In a large-scale study performed in 127 patients with axial LBP who failed facet interventions, Cohen et al.[23] reported a prevalence rate of 65%. More recently, a systematic review that included three prevalence studies determined that the prevalence of DP, as assessed by radiographic abnormalities and concordant pain provocation, varied between 39% and 42%.[24]

Studies conducted in the cervical spine tend to yield widely disparate results. In a prospective observational study evaluating 173 cervical discograms, Grubb and Kelly[25] reported at least one positive level in 86% of patients. In a smaller (*n* = 31) retrospective study, Connor and Darden[26] found that 84% of patients experienced provocative concordant symptomatology; these were considered positive. Neither study required a control disc. Another retrospective study performed in 143 individuals with chronic neck pain reported the prevalence rate of DP to be 16%.[27] A systematic review published in 2013 evaluating the accuracy and utility of cervical discography found prevalence rates ranging between 16% and 53%.[28]

THE CONTROVERSY SURROUNDING DISCOGRAPHY

RATIONALE

The rationale for discography is based on three factors: the high prevalence of spine pain, the high prevalence rate of abnormal MRI findings at asymptomatic levels, and the low success rate of surgical interventions for degenerative spondylosis. The lifetime prevalence of serious LBP episodes ranges from 50% to 80%[19]; for neck pain, the annual prevalence rates range from 16% to as high as 50%.[21] Confounding matters is that MRI studies conducted in asymptomatic volunteers have consistently demonstrated that a majority of people have abnormalities in the lumbar, thoracic, and cervical spine regions, with the proportion increasing with age.[1–3]

Having an inexpensive, safe, and reliably effective bridge to natural recovery is therefore paramount, yet none exists. Based on systematic reviews, it is clear that surgery performed for axial spine pain is associated with a high rate of failure and significant complications and that most patients recover without procedural interventions.[19,20] The high prevalence rates for spine pain and coincidental imaging abnormalities, coupled with the absence of any reliable interventional treatment for IDD, augur in favor of an accurate means of correlating symptoms with imaging results.

FALSE-POSITIVE AND FALSE-NEGATIVE RESULTS

The principal criticism surrounding provocation discography is the high rate of false-positive (FP) results. The first study to quantitatively question the validity of lumbar discography was performed by Holt over 40 years ago[29]; he reported an FP rate of 37% in 30 asymptomatic prisoners. Over 20 years later, Walsh et al.[30] performed CT-discography in 10 asymptomatic male volunteers and 7 "control" patients with chronic LBP. In the asymptomatic subjects, CT-discograms were interpreted as abnormal in 17% of the 35 discs injected and half of the 10 subjects. However, none of these patients experienced concordant pain associated with pain-related behavior during the injections.

The bulk of the work on FP discography was done by Carragee and colleagues in the late 1990s and early 2000s. In general, these studies have found high FP rates for lumbar discography in patients who had undergone previous iliac crest bone grafting, those with failed back and neck surgery, individuals with psychopathology (especially somatization disorder), and those with secondary gain issues.[31–33]

The Carragee studies have been criticized on several accounts. The first is that modern provocation discography requires that the evoked pain must be concordant with a patient's baseline pain, which is not possible in asymptomatic subjects. Another flaw is that pressure readings were not a determining factor in the designation of a positive disc.

To control for some of these factors, Derby et al.[34] performed 43 discograms in 13 volunteers with either no history or infrequent episodes of LBP. In the subjects with occasional back pain, 35% of injected discs were painful, versus 52% in volunteers without LBP. Most discs required high pressures before pain was provoked. No relationship was noted between painful disc injections and radiologic or discographic abnormalities. Controlling for the intensity of response and the pressures at which pain was elicited, the authors concluded that the incidence of FP discograms was less than 10%.

Wolfer et al.[35] performed a systematic review reanalyzing data from five previous studies including those of Carragee et al. based on the criteria of the International Association for the Study of Pain (IASP) and International Spinal Intervention Society (ISIS) for a positive lumbar discogram. The authors found an overall FP rate of 9.3% per patient and 6.0% per disc. In patients without back pain or confounding factors, the FP rates declined to 3.0% per patient and 2.1% per disc. Patients with chronic pain were found to have FP rates per patient and disc of 5.6% and 3.9%, respectively. The highest FP rates per patient and disc were for postdiscectomy patients (15% and 9.1%, respectively) and those with somatization disorder (50% and 22.2%, respectively).

Fewer studies have examined the incidence of FP discograms in the cervical and thoracic regions. In a study by Schellhas et al.,[36] none of 40 cervical discograms done in 10 asymptomatic volunteers elicited reported pain or facial expressions indicative of pain. In a later study done in the thoracic region, the same group of investigators reached slightly different conclusions[37]; that is, 3 of 40 discs injected in 10 asymptomatic volunteers provoked intense (≥7/10) pain, with 2 positive responses occurring in one subject. One possible cause of inaccurate or FP discography results is that pressurization of a disc during fluid injection results in increased pressure in adjacent discs, which may undermine the specificity.[38]

The issue of "false-negative" discograms has received far less attention but can lead to inaccurate diagnoses, unnecessary interventions, and the withholding of beneficial treatment from otherwise good candidates. There are several reasons for this phenomenon, including failure to detect an inadequate rise in intradiscal pressure because of the lack of pressure monitoring, injecting too slowly, excessive sedation, overzealous use of local anesthetic, and extensive contrast extravasation in severely degenerated discs. The failure to elicit pain in a degenerated, ostensibly painful disc may be more likely to occur in elderly patients.[39] In a review by Cohen et al.,[40] the authors estimated that

TABLE 69.1 Clinical Studies Evaluating False-Positive Discography

Study, Year	Region	Subjects	Criteria	Results
Holt, 1964[42]	Cervical	50 male volunteer inmates, 148 discs	Pain provocation + contrast extravasation	All injections provoked severe pain; contrast extravasation noted in all pts, 93% of discs
Massie and Stevens, 1967[43]	Lumbar	52 male subjects, 156 discs	NR	FP rate not reported but stated "injection only occasionally produced symptoms"
Holt, 1968[29]	Lumbar	30 male volunteer inmates, 70 discs (20 failed injections)	Pain provocation	60% FP rate per subject, 37% per disc
Walsh, 1990[30]	Lumbar	10 male volunteers, 30 discs	3/5 pain provocation + 2/5 pain-related behaviors	0% FP rate per subject and disc
Schellhas, 1996[36]	Cervical	10 volunteers, 40 discs	7/10 pain provocation + facial expressions	0% FP rate per subject and disc
Wood, 1999[37]	Thoracic	10 volunteers, 40 discs	7/10 pain provocation + facial expressions	20% FP rate per subject, 7.5% per disc
Carragee, 1999[31]	Lumbar	8 males who had undergone recent iliac crest bone grafting for problems unrelated to low back pain, 24 discs	3/5 "concordant" pain provocation (to previous iliac crest pain), + 2/5 pain-related behaviors	50% FP rate per subject, 38% per disc
Carragee, 2000[32]	Lumbar	6 subjects with somatization disorder, 10 with failed neck surgery, and 10 control pts with no pain after successful cervical spine surgery; 78 discs	3/5 "concordant" pain provocation (to previous iliac crest pain), + 2/5 pain-related behaviors	FP rate per subject: 83% for somatization, 40% for failed neck surgery, and 10% for "control" group; FP rate per disc: 33% for somatization, 23% for failed neck surgery, and 3% for control group
Carragee, 2000[33]	Lumbar	47 subjects who underwent a single-level discectomy. 20 subjects were "symptom-free," while 27 pts continued to have back and/or leg pain; 138 discs	3/5 pain provocation + 2/5 pain-related behaviors	FP rate per subject: 40% for asymptomatic subjects and 56% for pts with failed back surgery; FP rate per disc: 15% in asymptomatic group
Derby, 2005[34]	Lumbar	13 volunteers, 43 discs	Criteria not noted; used 0–10 pain rating and 0–4 pain behavior scales along with manometry	Using 6/10 as criterion for a (+) disc, 0% FP rate; using 4/10 pain at ≤ 50 psi, FP rate 23% per subject and 9% per disc

FP, *False positive;* NR, *not reported.*

between 15% and 25% of degenerated discs fail to elicit concordant pain provocation during stimulation. The proportion of these occurrences that represent false-negative versus true negative responses is a question that remains to be answered.

In summary, FP discograms can occur in all regions of the spine but are infrequent in unoperated individuals with no confounding factors. A careful consideration of the risks and benefits of discography should be done when discography is being considered for individuals at high risk for FP results since many of these factors are also associated with treatment failure. If discography is conducted in high-risk individuals, one should consider obtaining two adjacent control discs and correlating reported pain with more objective measures such as an increase in heart rate and/or change in facial expression.[30,41] Other factors that may increase the risk of FP discograms include extreme anxiety, performing disc stimulation before allowing previously provoked pain to return to baseline, inadvertent annular injection, contrast-induced irritation of nervous tissue, end-plate deflection resulting from suboptimal needle placement, and rapid or excessive pressurization (Table 69.1).[40]

CORRELATION BETWEEN MAGNETIC RESONANCE IMAGING AND DISCOGRAPHY

Several attempts have been made to correlate imaging with discography results. In one of the earliest studies comparing MRI, the most sensitive test for disc pathology, with lumbar discographic findings, Gibson et al.[44] found agreement in 88% of 50 discograms. Among the six discs in which a discrepancy was observed, evidence of IDD was missed in five discograms and one MRI. Correlation in this study was based solely on radiographic findings and not provocation results. Collins et al.[45] reported similar results. The authors found that discographic and MRI imaging characteristics correlated in 89% of 73 lumbar discograms. Of the eight discordant discs, four revealed early evidence of disc degeneration on discography but were normal on MRI and four were discographically normal but demonstrated mild degeneration on MRI. All discs that provoked concordant symptoms were degenerate on both discography and MRI. In a study by Schneiderman et al.,[46] the correlation between MRI and discographic morphology was 99%, with the only discrepancy being noted in a 13-year-old.

However, the more relevant question is whether provocation results can be predicted by radiologic imaging. Yoshida et al.[47] investigated the relationship between provocation discography and MRI in 56 discograms from 23 patients. The authors found the sensitivity, specificity, positive predictive value, and negative predictive value of T2-weighted, gadolinium-enhanced studies in detecting symptomatic discs to be 94%, 71%, 59%, and 97%, respectively. These findings compared favorably with T1-weighted images. In another study, Aprill and Bogduk[48] found that the presence or absence of a high-intensity zone in 118 discograms had a sensitivity, specificity, and positive predictive value for concordant pain provocation in 97%, 63%, and 95% of levels, respectively. Even stronger correlations have been found by others.[49,50]

Not all studies have demonstrated positive results. Zucherman et al.[51] reported a case series of 18 patients with normal MRI and positive discography. In a retrospective study, Sandhu et al.[52] found a poor correlation between changes in vertebral end-plate signal observed on MRI and the results of provocation discography. In an observational study conducted in 25 patients, Horton and Daftari[53] concluded that discrepancies between findings on MRI and discography necessitated that both be used in surgical planning. Finally, in a small study ($n = 26$) that correlated the results of provocation discography, anesthetic discography, and MRI, Putzier et al.[54] found no correlation between the three parameters and the presence of high-intensity zones, or Dallas and Pfirmann scores, and only a weak correlation between anesthetic discography and Modic changes.

To date, there have been few correlative observational studies performed in the cervical spine. In a study performed in 52 patients (104 discs), Parfenchuk and Janssen[55] found that the sensitivity, specificity, FP and false-negative rates between MRI and pain provocation to be 73%, 67%, 33%, and 27%, respectively. Schellhas et al.[36] later sought to correlate MRI with disc provocation results in 10 asymptomatic volunteers and 10 patients with chronic neck pain. In the asymptomatic cohort, half of the 40 discs were morphologically abnormal on MRI versus 88% that exhibited abnormalities on discography. However, none of the abnormal discs provoked concordant pain during stimulation. In the symptomatic patients, 29 of the 40 discs exhibited some degree of abnormality on MRI. Among the 11 normal discs, 10 were found to have annular tears discographically, with 8 of these shown to be painful when injected. In summary, whereas a significant correlation between concordant pain provocation and MRI findings has been demonstrated, the high FP and false-negative rates suggest the need for a reliable means to ascertain which abnormalities are pain generators.

EFFECT OF SURGICAL OUTCOMES

SPINAL ARTHRODESIS

Although uncontrolled studies evaluating the impact of preoperative discography on surgical outcomes have been mixed, the largest, most recent, and best-designed study suggests that discography may improve arthrodesis when used to screen patients before arthrodesis.

In one of the earliest studies to examine this question, Colhoun et al.[56] found a strong association between disc stimulation findings and fusion results. Among the 137 patients with nonradicular LBP in whom disc stimulation provoked concordant pain, 89% had a favorable outcome at the mean follow-up period of 3.6 years. In contrast, only 52% of the 25 patients whose morphologically abnormal discs failed to elicit symptoms experienced significant benefit. Whereas some investigators cite this as evidence supporting provocation discography as a surgical screening tool, the absence of a comparator group that received MRI and the relatively high success rate in the negative provocation group limit the generalizability of the findings.

Later, uncontrolled studies failed to replicate even these equivocal results. Esses et al.[57] retrospectively examined the influence of discography in predicting external fixation and fusion results in 32 patients with refractory LBP, finding that neither concordant pain provocation nor morphologic abnormalities predicted pain relief. The main flaw in this study is that it was not designed to assess the influence of discography on surgical outcomes. The next attempt to correlate discographic findings with spinal fusion outcomes was by Madan et al.[58] who performed a retrospective analysis in 73 patients with chronic LBP. At the minimum 2-year follow-up, no difference in any outcome measure was noted between the two matched groups. In another retrospective study evaluating the value of discography as a preoperative screening tool, Derby et al.[17] found that patients with chemically sensitized discs experienced better outcomes following interbody/combined fusion than after other treatments.

A recent randomized controlled trial supports the use of discography as a surgical screening tool. Margetic et al.[59] randomized 310 patients with chronic LBP being evaluated for surgery in a 2:1 ratio to receive provocation discography with fusion done only in those with a positive test or fusion performed without discographic screening. In the discography group, 158 subjects had a positive discogram and negative screening for depression and somatization; they proceeded to surgery. At 1-year follow-up, the change in Oswestry disability index scores in the discography group was 29.7%, which compared favorably with the 24.6% improvement in the control group ($P = .12$). When only those with degenerative disc disease were considered ($n = 127$), the difference favoring the treatment group became statistically significant (35% vs. 22% improvement in function; $P < .001$).

In the cervical spine, only one study has evaluated the predictive value of discography in selecting surgical candidates. Kikuchi et al.[60] performed a retrospective study in the pre-MRI era evaluating surgical outcomes on 138 patients with either mechanical ($n = 41$) or radicular ($n = 97$) neck pain who underwent anterior discectomy and fusion based on discography results. One year postprocedure, 80% were either pain-free or experienced only mild discomfort that did not interfere with work. In a control group who underwent cervical fusion without the benefit of discography, 60% had favorable outcomes. Similar to the findings of Colhoun et al.,[56] the lack of MR imaging and the high success rate in the control cohort limit the relevance of these findings.

DETERMINING OPERATIVE LEVELS

Two studies have examined the effect of discography in identifying treatment levels in patients already selected

TABLE 69.2 Comparative Studies Evaluating the Effect of Discography on Fusion Outcomes

Author, Year	Spine Region	Study Design	Patients	Results
Colhoun, 1988[56]	Lumbar	Prospective observational	162 pts with nonradicular LBP	89% of 137 pts with a positive discogram had a favorable outcome vs. 52% of pts in whom discography did not provoke pain; mean follow-up (f/u) 3.6 years
Esses, 1989[57]	Lumbar	Retrospective study evaluating effect of ESF before spinal arthrodesis	35 pts with chronic LBP, 32 of whom underwent preop discography	Discography results not predictive of ESF or arthrodesis results; f/u period not noted
Derby, 1999[17]	Lumbar	Retrospective	96 surgical candidates with chronic LBP	In pts with chemically sensitized discs (concordant pain at <15 psi above opening pressure), success rates were higher (89%) for interbody/combined fusion than other operations or no surgical treatment; mean f/u 28 months
Madan, 2002[58]	Lumbar	Retrospective	41 pts who underwent fusion without discography and 32 who had surgery based on (+) discography	81% of pts who had surgery without discography had satisfactory outcome vs. 76% of pts who underwent arthrodesis based on (+) discography; mean f/u 2.4 years in discography group and 2.8 years in MRI/clinical group
Carragee, 2006[63]	Lumbar	Prospective observational	32 pts with nonradicular LBP and a single (+) low-pressure discogram who underwent spinal fusion	Approximately 43% of discography patients obtained a "satisfactory" outcome vs. 91% of a matched control group with single-level unstable spondylolisthesis who did not undergo discography; f/u period 2 years
Willems, 2007[62]	Lumbar	Prospective observational	82 pts with equivocal indication for fusion who were operated on based on (+) ESF	No difference in outcomes between pts with (+) discogram at an adjacent segment and those with a negative discogram; mean f/u 80 months
Ohtori, 2009[64]	Lumbar	Randomized comparative	42 pts with axial LBP were randomized to provocative discography vs. anesthetic discography	The 15 pts who underwent fusion based on anesthetic discography had better outcomes than the 15 who were fused based on provocative discography; f/u 3 years
Margetic, 2013[59]	Lumbar	Randomized, controlled	310 pts with LBP scheduled for fusion randomized in 2:1 ratio to receive discography and fusion, if positive, or fusion without discography	Decrease in ODI of 30% in pts screened with discography vs. 25% in surgical pts without discography at 1 year; in those with degenerative disc disease (n = 127), the difference favoring the treatment group was more pronounced (35% vs. 22%)
Kikuchi, 1981[60]	Cervical	Retrospective	138 pts with cervicobrachial pain underwent single-level disc excision and anterior fusion	80% of pts improved 1 year after surgery vs. 39% success rate in 54 pts who underwent fusion without discography
Hubach, 1994[61]	Cervical	Prospective observational	193 pts with cervical radiculopathy and/or myelopathy who underwent anterior discectomy and fusion	12 of 156 pts who had fusion based on intraoperative discography developed adjacent segment pain vs. 35% of the 23 pts who underwent fusion without discography; mean f/u 10.4 years

DDD, *Degenerative disc disease;* ESF, *external spinal fixator;* f/u, *follow-up;* LBP, *low back pain;* ODI, *Oswestry disability index score;* Pts, *patients.*

for spinal fusion. In a prospective study conducted in 193 patients with neck pain and neurologic symptoms, Hubach[61] evaluated the use of intraoperative discography to select operative levels. In the initial group of patients (n = 23) who were fused without discography, 35% developed juxtafusional pain at long-term follow-up. In the ensuing 156 patients in whom the operative levels were based on discography, only 12% developed pain at an adjacent segment. Yet in a later prospective study conducted in the lumbar spine, Willems et al.[62] failed to demonstrate a benefit for discography in determining fusion levels. In summary, the evidence favors the use of discography as a screening tool to identify candidates for lumbar spinal fusion, but results are equivocal concerning the cervical spine and regarding whether discography should be used to identify the levels of arthrodesis (Table 69.2).

DISC REPLACEMENT

Initially reported on in the 1960s, disc replacement has been employed to treat lumbar discogenic LBP in Europe since the 1980s and in the United States since the early

2000s. The indications for lumbar disc replacement include one- or two-level mechanical discogenic back pain without radiculopathy or significant facet pathology. Dozens of studies have been published evaluating the outcomes of lumbar disc replacement in various populations; these contain wide variations in selection criteria, outcome measures, and follow-up periods. The success rates in these studies range from less 50% to upward of 90%. Compared with fusion, nearly all randomized trials demonstrate noninferiority, with most also showing improved range of motion and faster onset to benefit.[65] Although discographic screening was previously considered a selection criterion for lumbar disc replacement, numerous postmarketing studies have been published that have not required preoperative discography. Whereas no study has directly compared operative results between surgical candidates selected based on clinical presentation alone and those in which patients were chosen using discography results, indirect comparisons have failed to demonstrate any significant differences in outcomes.[40,66]

Unlike the indications for lumbar disc replacement, cervical discs are implanted in patients with or without neurologic symptoms. In the dozens of studies evaluating cervical disc arthroplasty, over two-thirds of patients generally achieve success at follow-up periods ranging between 1 and 3 years.[67] Some surgeons have advocated cervical discography as a surgical screening tool before disc replacement[68] but no study has routinely used provocation discography in this context; therefore no conclusions can be drawn regarding the predictive value of the procedure.

ALTERNATIVES TO PROVOCATION DISCOGRAPHY

In an attempt to find a less invasive replacement for discography, Yrjama and Vanharanta proposed the bony vibration test (BVT), wherein a blunt, vibrating object is compressed against the skin overlying successive spinous processes to provoke pain. In several studies, the authors found the test to have high sensitivity and specificity compared with provocation discography and radiologic imaging.[69] When patients with complete annular tears, herniated discs, and failed back surgery syndrome are excluded, the sensitivity rises above 90%. Later, the authors found that the addition of ultrasonic disc imaging could further enhance accuracy.

Similar to diagnostic tests for other types of spinal pain, some investigators have proposed "anesthetic" or "analgesic" discography in lieu of or to supplement to disc provocation. In their study, Kotilainen et al.[70] found that over 80% of LBP patients who received intradiscal bupivacaine experienced short-term symptomatic improvement, thus providing a conceptual basis for the technique. Osler[71] and Roth[72] found that relying on pain relief following the intradiscal injection of local anesthetic resulted in good or excellent results in over 80% of patients who underwent anterior cervical fusion, which compared favorably with selecting patients by provocation testing. In a more recent randomized study comparing conventional discography to analgesic discography with 0.75 mL of 0.5% bupivacaine in patients being screened for anterior discectomy and interbody fusion, Ohtori et al.[64] found that the 15 patients selected for surgery based on analgesic discography fared better than an equal number selected based on conventional discography.

The purported advantage of anesthetic discography is that it can reduce the high incidence of FP results obtained with provocation discography, but the results from studies evaluating this are mixed. Whereas some studies have reported that anesthetic discography results in a lower proportion of positive discograms than provocation discography,[73] others have either failed to find a difference between the two techniques[74] or reported a higher proportion of positive results using analgesic response to the local injection of anesthetic.[54]

INTERPRETATION

EVOKED PAIN OR ANALGESIC RESPONSE

The patient's subjective response to intradiscal injection is the most important aspect of discography. Discography is predicated on the fact that normal discs are sparsely innervated, while disrupted discs are relatively richly innervated and have been rendered hyperalgesic from nociceptor exposure to inflammatory mediators. The foundation of provocation discography is based on three premises. The first is that painful stimulation of any kind can provoke symptoms in a patient suffering from chronic pain with central sensitization and psychosocial overlay, including pressurization of a nonpainful disc. Therefore to diagnose DP, a control level must be obtained. A true control disc is present only when pressurization fails to elicit a typical pain response in a nontargeted disc. Both the IASP and the Spine Intervention Society (SIS) consider the presence of two control disc levels in conjunction with one painful disc level to be highly indicative of DP. Pain reproduction in multiple discs with a single positive control disc level is considered to be marginal evidence for DP. When pain is provoked in a suspected disc in the absence of any control level, the presence DP cannot be proven.

The second assumption is that pain caused by stimulation of a nonpainful disc will be different than the patient's usual pain. Thus, only when an evoked pain response is the same or similar (i.e., concordant) to a patient's typical pain can a disc be considered a source of pain. Third, it is assumed that "minor" or nondebilitating pain can be evoked from stimulation of a nonpainful disc. Hence, only generation of significant pain is considered evidence of DP. Such thresholds have arbitrarily been set between 6 and 7 on a pain scale of 0–10.[40] However, there are several flaws with this premise. The foremost is that it fails to take into account a patient's baseline pain. For example, reproducing 5/10 pain in a stoic, debilitated patient who rates his pain as 4/10 at baseline would be considered a "negative" discogram, whereas a somatically focused patient with a baseline pain of 10/10 could be classified as having a positive discogram when disc stimulation provokes a similar pain of 6/10. A second limitation is that discography is often done in a sedated patient in a nonfunctional recumbent position, wherein the distinction between concordant and discordant and significant and insignificant pain can be difficult to discern.

In addition to the quality and magnitude of the evoked response, the amount of pressure needed to evoke pain is considered pivotal to diagnosis. The key rationale behind discography is that pain can be evoked by minimal pressurization of a disrupted disc (akin to allodynia or hyperalgesia), whereas higher intradiscal pressures would be painless in a normal disc. It is important to note that the rate of rise of intradiscal pressure can also influence results (i.e., too rapid an increase can increase FP results).[75] To standardize lumbar disc stimulation, manometric discography was introduced. The intradiscal pressure at which the contrast flow is first observed in the disc is the *opening pressure*, whereas the maximum pressure achieved during a disc injection is referred to as the *peak pressure*. Physiologic variations in disc pressures, however, are significant—intradiscal pressures are higher in upright and lower in recumbent positions. Since intradiscal pressures are typically lower in disrupted discs, the generation of high pressures in severely degenerated discs may not be feasible. Manometery essentially quantifies intradiscal pressures at key events (i.e., opening pressure, pain provocation pressure, pressure at which leakage is noted), so that if concordant pain is evoked below a certain threshold, the discogram is considered "positive."

According to most guidelines, asymptomatic lumbar discs are highly unlikely to evoke pain at pressures below 15 psi.[17,40] Therefore pain evoked at pressure below this level is considered highly suggestive of lumbar DP (i.e., a chemically sensitive disc). At the other end of the spectrum, even a normal disc can provoke pain when the peak pressure is raised too high (i.e., above 90 psi). The implications of pain reproduced at pressures between 15 and 90 psi are less clear. Pain reproduced at pressures between 15 and 50 psi above the opening pressure is considered a likely pain generator in the presence of an adjacent control disc; however, the existence of other pain generators cannot be excluded. This is sometimes referred to as a mechanically sensitive disc.[17,40] A disc in which pain is reproduced between 50 and 90 psi is unlikely to be positive, but its contribution to pain cannot be excluded (i.e., an indeterminate disc). Studies evaluating the effect of treatments and patient outcomes based on pressure discography are lacking. In one retrospective study, the results of interbody/combined fusion surgery were superior when the positive discography level(s) was interpreted as a chemically sensitive disc(s).[17] Pressures above 100 psi are considered detrimental to disc integrity, so that a potential advantage of pressure discography is the avoidance of disc injury.

In the cervical and thoracic spine, manometry is not commonly used. In a cadaveric study, Menkowitz et al.[76] found the median opening pressure to be 30 psi, with the median pressure required to rupture a disc varying between 36.5 psi (in C4–7 discs) and 53 psi in C2–3, C3–4, and C7–T1 discs.

The use of anesthetic discography has not gained a strong foothold as a standalone technique but is sometimes used as an adjunct to disc stimulation. In studies evaluating anesthetic discography, the pain relief required to designate a disc as "positive" has ranged from a three-point reduction to almost complete pain relief.[54,73] One of the inherent dilemmas in interpreting anesthetic discography is how to reconcile analgesic response with the evaluation of multiple discs, as pain relief following local anesthetic infiltration may last for hours or even weeks (Fig. 69.2).

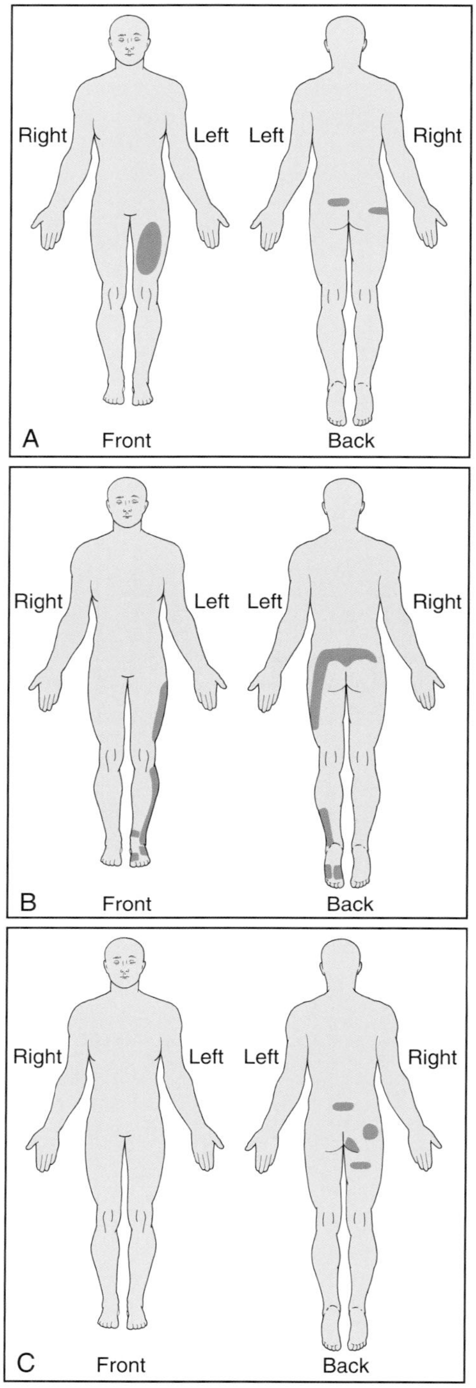

FIG. 69.2 Pain referral patterns from symptomatic L3-4 (A), L4-5 (B), and L5-S1 (C) intervertebral discs. *(Modified from Ohnmeiss DD, Vanharanta H, Ekholm J: Relation between pain location and disc pathology: a study of pain drawings and CT/discography.* Clin J Pain. *15:210-217, 1999.)*

VOLUMETRIC MEASUREMENTS

The volumetric measurements made during discography include the amount of contrast injected and the various endpoints. Normal lumbar discs typically accept less than 1 mL of contrast before firm resistance is reached—a firm endpoint. In cervical and thoracic discs, these volumes are approximately 0.25 and 0.5 mL, respectively. Degenerated

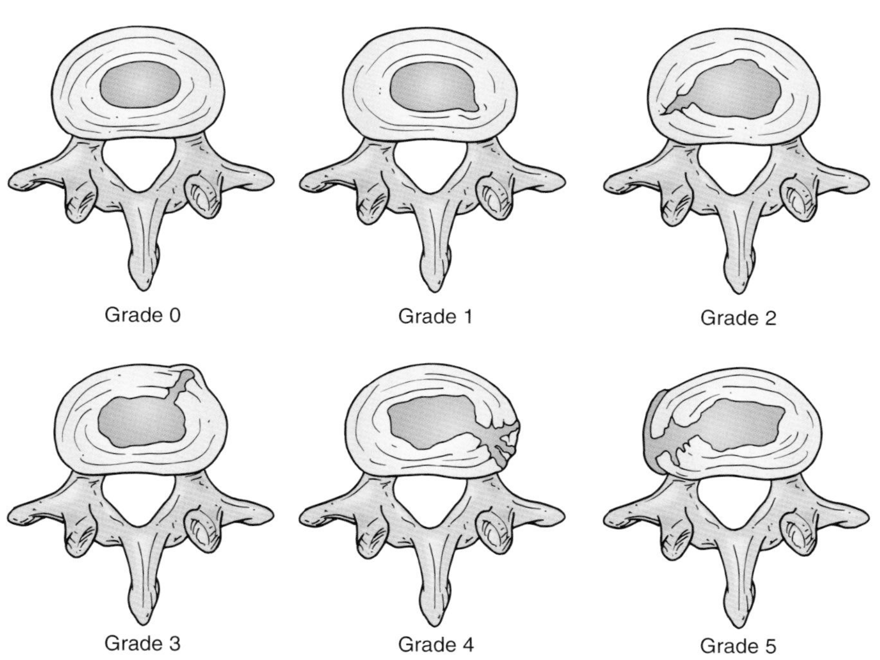

FIG. 69.3 Modified Dallas discogram scheme for the classification of annular tears by CT-discography. *(From Modified from Sachs BL, Vanharanta H, Spivey MA, et al. Dallas discogram description. A new classification of CT/discography in low-back disorders.* Spine *12(3): 287-94; 1987.)*

discs typically accept larger contrast volumes with only moderate resistance—a lower pressure or soft endpoint. In the presence of a complete annular tear where the disc communicates with the epidural space, a nearly unlimited volume of the contrast may be injected under certain circumstances with little or no resistance and minimal pain—a volume endpoint. Provocation of significant pain should result in cessation of any disc injection—a pain endpoint.[40]

MORPHOLOGIC DISC EVALUATION

Morphologic patterns of contrast spread in normal and degenerated discs can be visualized by plain fluoroscopy or CT discography. In contrast to fluoroscopy, CT discography allows for the visualization of internal disc abnormalities not apparent with fluoroscopy or MRI. The intradiscal contrast spread as seen on CT discography has been well described by several authors. In one such rating, which has since been revised,[40,77] grade 0 describes a normal lumbar disc in which contrast is limited to the NP; grades 1–3 designate discs in which contrast extends to the inner, middle, and outer third of the AF, respectively; grade 4 describes a diffusely degenerated disc in which several annular tears extend to the periphery of the annulus; and grade 5 depicts a large tear that results in contrast extending circumferentially to more than 30% of the disc circumference. The pain reproduced on discography has generally but not always been well correlated to the extent of the annular disruption seen on CT discography. Grade 3 tears usually provoke concordant pain, grade 2 disruptions reproduce pain infrequently, and grade 0 and 1 discs rarely evoke pain.[78] Both IASP and SIS guidelines require the presence of a significant annular tear in order for a diagnosis of DP to be rendered (Fig. 69.3 and Table 69.3).

COMPLICATIONS AND DISC INJURY

The avascular nature of the disc renders it vulnerable to the iatrogenic inoculation of bacteria. This is difficult to treat with antibiotics, making discitis the most feared complication of discography. Whereas procedure-related pain is not uncommon, any patient who experiences a new neurologic finding or continues to complain of persistent pain 1 week postprocedure warrants reevaluation. At minimum, the postdiscography workup should include a focused history, physical examination, and laboratory screening tests that include erythrocyte sedimentation rate, C-reactive protein, and white blood cell count.[40] If the erythrocyte sedimentation rate is equal to or greater than 50, a high-resolution MRI focusing on the end plates is needed.

Reviews have been conducted with the aim of determining the incidence of the iatrogenic discitis and whether or not preprocedure antibiotics should be routinely administered. In a review of 12,770 lumbar discograms performed in 4891 patients without prophylactic antibiotics, Willems et al.[79] found a discitis rate of 0.25% per patient and 0.09% per disc. The authors concluded that there was not enough evidence to support the routine use of prophylactic antibiotics. Similar conclusions were reached by Sharma et al.[80] and Kapoor et al.[81] In a review evaluating 14,133 cervical discograms done in 4804 patients, Kapoor et al.[81] found the rate of infection to be 0.44% per patient and 0.15% per disc. Among the 21 reported cases, the time to presentation ranged between 3 days and 3 months. If administered, prophylactic antibiotics can be given either parenterally or intradiscally, with studies suggesting comparable efficacy.[82]

Another controversy surrounding discography is whether the acute elevation of intervertebral disc pressure

TABLE 69.3 Interpretation of Discography

Diagnosis	Alternate Diagnosis	Manometeric Disc Pressure Where Pain Is Evoked	Rating of Pain Intensity	Location of Pain Response	Contrast Spread on PDCT	Control Level Injection	Interpretation
Discogenic pain	Unequivocal discogenic pain/Chemically sensitive disc	<15 psi above the open pressures	>6–7/10	Concordant to patient's usual pain	>Grade 3 annular tear	No pain at >2 control disc levels	The disc is likely the main source of pain
Presumptive discogenic pain	Probable discogenic pain/Mechanically sensitive disc	Between 15 and 50 psi above the open pressure	>6–7/10	Concordant to patient's usual pain	>Grade 3 annular tear	No pain at >1 control discs *or* <5/10 discordant pain at >1 control disc	The disc is likely a source of pain; however other sources cannot be excluded
Remote discogenic pain	Indeterminate disc	Between 50 and 90 psi	>6–7/10	Concordant to patient's usual pain	>Grade 3 annular tear	No pain at >1 control disc *or* <5/10 discordant pain at >1 control disc at >50 psi	The disc is unlikely a source of pain; however its presence cannot be excluded
Normal disc	—	>90 psi	0/10 pain	—	—	—	Normal disc
Iatrogenic disc injury	—	>100 psi	—	—	—	—	These pressures should be avoided to prevent iatrogenic disc injury

PDCT, *Postdiscography computed tomography*; psi, *pounds per square inch*.

can worsen back pain or injure the disc. In a biochemical model tested in 69 cadavers, Iencean[83] found that the pressure needed to effect disc herniation was inversely proportional to the degree of degeneration and ranged from 108–188 psi. This is consistent with the pressure limit of 100 psi imposed by many discographers. A cadaveric study in the cervical spine found that the median pressure required to rupture a disc was 40 psi.[76] However, caution should be exercised even when manometry is used, as there are reports of discography-induced lumbar disc herniation occurring at lower pressures.[84]

The literature is not uniform with regard to whether disc stimulation can have long-term adverse effects. Animal models clearly show that annular puncture can evoke disc degeneration,[85] but its effect in humans remains unknown. In early studies evaluating the clinical and anatomic sequelae of discography, multiple investigators found no evidence that discography causes damage to intervertebral discs.[40] However, only one of these studies used MRI to discern interval disc pathology,[86] and the mean follow-up period in this analysis was only 72 days.

A well-cited study by Carragee et al.[87] contested the assumption that discography is not associated with long-term sequelae. The authors evaluated repeat MRI scans in 52 asymptomatic or minimally symptomatic individuals who underwent discography 7–10 years earlier and 50 matched control subjects. Upon repeat imaging, they found that those who underwent discography were more likely to have greater disc degeneration and a 2.5-fold increased likelihood of disc herniation in injected discs than subjects who had not undergone discography. In an earlier study, the same group of authors found that painful disc injections and annular disruptions were poor and weak predictors of subsequent LBP in patients without preexisting back symptoms, respectively.[88]

A more recent, small prospective study done by Ohtori et al.[89] contradicts the findings of Carragee et al.[87] The authors compared the results of 36 patients who underwent either provocation (n = 18) or anesthetic discography (n = 10) with the results of 10 control patients. They evaluated range of motion and MRIs done before and 5-years postprocedure, finding no differences between groups. However, the smaller numbers and shorter follow-up period make it difficult to draw definitive conclusions. Other complications of discography include headache, convulsions attributed to contrast, nausea and vomiting, severe back pain, hematoma, meningitis, arachnoiditis, nerve root injury, paravertebral muscle spasm, vasovagal reactions, and allergic reactions.[40]

SUMMARY

Discography is the only test that purports to correlate symptoms with pathology. In view of the cost, complications, and high failure rate associated with spine surgery, there is a strong need to refine selection criteria. In recent years, evidence has emerged suggesting that discography may improve outcomes of lumbar fusion in patients with DP. Although the use of anesthetic discography has been advocated as a means of reducing the FP rate associated with disc stimulation, this has not been borne out in clinical studies. More research is needed to confirm whether discography can improve surgical outcomes, particularly with disc replacement and minimally invasive procedures, and whether it can cause clinically relevant disc injury.

KEY POINTS

- Discography purports to be the only means of connecting disc pathology with symptoms, but without a reference test, this is impossible to prove.
- Discography is associated with a high FP rate in select individuals; for a test to be positive, at least one negative control disc must be present.
- The interpretation of discography should consider pain elicitation, concordance, disc morphology, and other factors (e.g., facial expressions, changes in heart rate, presence of a control disc or discs).
- There is weak evidence that discography may improve surgical outcomes.
- There is some evidence that discography may accelerate disc degeneration.
- The search for alternatives to provocation discography continues but remains elusive.

REFERENCES

Access the reference list online at ExpertConsult.com.

CHAPTER 70

VERTEBROPLASTY AND KYPHOPLASTY

Haroon Hameed, MD ◌ Mariam Hameed, MD ◌ Steven P. Cohen, MD

INTRODUCTION

Vertebroplasty (VP) and kyphoplasty (KP) are interventional techniques that utilize the placement of various polymers (e.g., acrylic-based cement) within a vertebral body for the correction of a vertebral compression fracture (VCF), and/or replacement of lost intramedullary bone secondary to neoplastic lesions. In KP, a cavity is also created within the vertebral body through the use of instrumentation consisting of a balloon, osteotome, or other method prior to instilling the acrylic-based cement, which is commonly a barium sulfate containing polymethylmethacrylate or other polymer. Barium sulfate is usually present within these cement mixtures because it is radiopaque.

Initially, correction of a VCF using an acrylic-based cement was described as an open surgical procedure and has been clinically used since at least the 1970s.[1] In 1987, Galibert et al. published the first description of percutaneous VP for vertebral hemangioma in a painful C2 hemangioma.[2] Since then, there have been significant refinements in the indications and technique of performing these procedures, as well as the development of several versions of acrylic-based cement polymers. Although various versions of barium sulfate containing polymethylmethacrylate are most frequently utilized, there are nonacrylic cement polymers commercially available and in various stages of development.

INDICATIONS

The clinical indications for the performance of VP and KP have become controversial. Nevertheless, both modalities have been reported as being useful in the treatment of symptomatic VCF due to a broad range of causes in the published literature.

Osteoporosis is the most common cause of VCF, with multiple myeloma, metastatic disease, painful vertebral body hemangiomas, and others (e.g., Kümmell disease) comprising "secondary" indications for vertebral augmentation procedures. Although osteoporosis has been a somewhat controversial indication since the publication of two negative articles in the *New England Journal of Medicine* in 2009, it remains the most common reason people undergo vertebral augmentation procedures.

OSTEOPOROSIS

Osteoporosis is a disease of bone, which itself is a connective tissue, responsible for hematopoiesis, mechanical and structural support, and mineral storage of inorganic salts and organic material. It is broken down and rebuilt constantly to optimally provide for skeletal support and other functions. Bone loss occurs once the balance of bone turnover favors bone resorption, and after peak bone mass is achieved by about 35 years of age, bone mass continues to decrease until death. Osteoporosis is a common and sometimes debilitating metabolic bone disease that occurs when an increase in bone resorption and a decrease in new bone formation lead to a chemically normal but reduced bone mass per unit volume. This, in turn, results in decreased skeletal function and elasticity, progressive spinal deformity, and vulnerability to fractures.

EPIDEMIOLOGICAL CHARACTERISTICS

- Osteoporosis affects more women than men, as women possess 10% to 25% less total bone mass at maturity.
- Caucasian and Asian women are at highest risk of developing an osteoporotic fracture due to low bone mineral density (BMD).[3–5]
- In the United States, 35% of women over the age of 65 years and 15% of Caucasian postmenopausal women are osteoporotic.[6]
- In the United States, this debilitating disease causes fractures in 1 million individuals per year with $14 billion spent for treatment.[7]
- Hip and vertebral fractures occur in women at a rate of 250,000 and 500,000 cases per year, respectively, and an additional 250,000 fractures are experienced by men every year.[8–9]
- Vertebral fractures in women increase as menopause approaches, and in old age, with a ratio of 2:1 compared to men.[10]

Due to various endocrine-related factors (e.g., decline in estrogen production), women lose 3% to 7% of BMD around the onset of menopause, followed by a 1% to 2% annual decline in the postmenopausal period. Although men also lose trabecular bone as they age at rates similar to postmenopausal women, they continue to increase cortical bone through periosteal deposition until the age of 75 years.[11–12]

There are three main types of osteoporosis, which can be categorized as primary, secondary, and iatrogenic. The two types of primary osteoporosis, as noted by Riggs and Melton, are postmenopausal and senile (Table 70.1).[13] Before making a diagnosis of primary osteoporosis, secondary and iatrogenic causes must be excluded (Table 70.2).[9] Common causes of iatrogenic osteoporosis include prolonged corticosteroid administration, furosemide, thyroid supplements which suppress thyroid-stimulating hormone (TSH) production, anticonvulsants, heparin, lithium (by causing hyperparathyroidism), and cytotoxic agents.[9]

TABLE 70.1 Types of Primary Osteoporosis

Type I	Type II
Postmenopausal	Senile
Primarily trabecular bone	Primarily cortical bone
6:1 female-to-male ages 51–65 years	2:1 female-to-male of age ≥75 years
No calcium deficiency	Calcium deficiency, decreased vitamin D, and increased parathyroid hormone activity
Estrogen deficiency	No estrogen deficiency
Vertebral and Colles' fractures prevalent	Pelvic, hip, proximal tibia, and proximal humerus fractures prevalent
Risk factors: low calcium intake, low weight-bearing regimen, cigarette smoking, and excessive alcohol consumption	Related to low calcium intake

TABLE 70.2 Secondary Causes of Osteoporosis

Paget's disease
Malabsorption syndrome
Hyperparathyroidism
Multiple myeloma
Hyperthyroidism
Prolonged drug therapy
Osteomalacia hypogonadism

DIAGNOSIS AND INITIAL EVALUATION

- Medical evaluation to determine whether or not someone suffers from osteoporosis requires performing a thorough history and physical examination, including family and past medical history.
- Secondary causes or coexisting diseases may be the catalyst for, or exacerbate, bone loss.
- A complete blood cell count, serum chemistry, and a urinalysis including a pH count should be performed.
- Consider obtaining thyrotropin, a 24-hour urinary calcium excretion, erythrocyte sedimentation rate, parathyroid hormone and 25-hydroxyvitamin D concentrations, dexamethasone suppression test, acid-base studies, serum or urine protein electrophoresis, bone biopsy and/or bone marrow examination, and an iliac bone biopsy as appropriate.
- The American Association of Clinical Endocrinologists recommend routing dual-energy X-ray absorptiometry (DXA)[14] screening of the lumbar spine and proximal femur for:
  All women 65 years and older;
  Any adult with a history of fracture not caused by severe trauma;
  Younger postmenopausal women with clinical risk factors for fracture.
- Plain radiographs are an option, but changes are usually not detectable until there is more than 30% loss of bone mass, suggesting this is not a sensitive screening tool.[6]

In 1994, the World Health Organization (WHO) established diagnostic criteria to designate the presence of osteoporosis based on DXA measurements.[15] Normal individuals possess a BMD of one standard deviation of the mean for young adults. Osteopenia is indicated if the standard deviation of BMD is between 1.0 and 2.5 below the mean of a young adult population. If BMD measures 2.5 or more standard deviations below the mean of a young adult population, then osteoporosis is present.

Severe osteoporosis is noted when one or more accompanying fragility fractures are present. Low body mass index has been associated with an increased likelihood of developing a fracture.[3–5] Based on these criteria, it is estimated that 38% of white females in their mid-seventies will have osteoporosis, and low bone mass will characterize 94% of that population.[11,16–18] These criteria were established by the WHO for the purposes of establishing prevalence, and are not intended as guidelines for therapy.

PREVENTION

Antiresorptive therapy and preventive measures are indicated to manage and prevent osteoporosis, respectively. Numerous factors must be considered before administering an appropriate regimen of preventive and therapeutic measures to combat osteoporosis. Potential options are:

- Calcium and vitamin D supplementation[19]
- Bisphosphonates[20–25]
- Calcitonin[26]
- Selective estrogen receptor modulators[27]
- Parathyroid hormone or analogs (e.g., teriparatide)[28,29]
- Sodium fluoride[30–33]
- Exercise
- Modifiable risk factors, such as cigarette smoking, excessive alcohol consumption, and treatment of potential secondary causes (see Table 70.2)

OTHER FRACTURES

Multiple myeloma is the most common primary malignant tumor of the bony spine, and it rarely affects the posterior elements.[34–36] These tumors have an incidence rate of 2 to 3 per 100,000 people, and tend to be radiosensitive, and in some cases chemo-sensitive. The disease is usually multifocal in nature, and surgical consolidation with vertebrectomy and strut grafting is not usually necessary; nevertheless, a single-level lesion can be treated with some success by vertebrectomy. Initially, symptomatic patients with VCFs may report severe pain that is poorly responsive to analgesic therapy.

Vertebral augmentation offers a viable route for immediate pain relief, bone strengthening, and mobility. Although vertebral augmentation may restore the mechanical integrity of a vertebral body and provide pain relief, tumor growth is not prevented. Therefore, radiotherapy and/or chemotherapy accompanying augmentation are appropriate because they do not affect the properties of the bone cement, they may inhibit tumor growth, and they can complement pain relief and promote spine strengthening.[37] A recent systematic review evaluating VP and KP for VCFs caused by multiple myeloma found equally significant improvement in pain scores and analgesic use at less than

1 week, 1 week to 1 year, and greater than 1 year for both interventions.[38] Oswestry Disability Inventory scores also showed a trend towards improvement at all time periods in both groups. Although cement leakage occurred in 11% to 29% of patients, it did not have any effect on postprocedural pain scores.[38]

Hemangiomas are benign bony spine lesions whose detection is usually incidental because of their asymptomatic disposition. They are often detected during the evaluation of back pain and subsequent routine imaging. Soft tissue extension of the lesion may compress the spinal cord and nerve roots, producing neurologic symptoms and even epidural hemorrhage.[39,40] If extensive growth of the hemangioma occurs, vertebral integrity may be compromised, resulting in a fracture with associated pain at the level of the lesion. Hemangioma aggressiveness can be determined by both clinical symptoms and radiological evaluation. Vertebral collapse, neural arch invasion, and soft tissue mass extensions are signs of aggressive lesions, and may signify appropriateness for vertebral augmentation. Patients with lymphomas and eosinophilic granulomas also may be candidates for vertebral augmentation.

Approximately 10% of patients with metastatic tumors develop malignant lesions in the spine in the United States.[41] Per year, 10% to 15% of 120,000 new patients with metastatic lesions to the spine develop VCFs. The most common location is the thoracic spine, but all levels can be affected, and usually more than one level is involved. Every kind of malignancy has been described to spread to the spine, with the most common culprits being breast, lung, and prostate cancers.[41]

CONTRAINDICATIONS (TABLE 70.3)

TABLE 70.3 Contraindications to Vertebral Augmentation

Absolute	Relative
Uncorrectable coagulation disorders	Young age
Allergy to polymethylmethacrylate or contrast	Loss of vertebral height ≥80% (vertebroplasty)
Spinal instability	Posterior wall destruction
Pregnancy	≥20% retropulsion with spinal stenosis
Active site infection or sepsis	Previous spinal stenosis
Pain unrelated to fracture	Vertebra plana, fractured pedicles, and burst fractures
Solid tissue or osteoblastic tumor	Multiple previous surgeries
	Poor pulmonary status
	Greater than three compression fractures

VERTEBROPLASTY AND KYPHOPLASTY TECHNIQUE

Only experienced physicians with appropriate training should perform vertebral augmentation procedures. Requirements for these procedures include: intravenous (IV) access, sedation or general anesthesia, image guidance, IV antibiotic prophylaxis (e.g., cefazolin 1 g or clindamycin 600 mg within 60 min prior to incision), and sterile precautions.

Both VP and KP are similar in the early stages of the procedure with regard to local anesthetic and imaging approach. There are two principal techniques for placing the introducer trocar: transpedicular and parapedicular. For the transpedicular approach, two methods can be utilized: an anteroposterior (AP) approach maintaining visualization of the medial and lateral cortices of the pedicle versus a coaxial approach. Regardless of approach, cranial tilt and lateral fluoroscopic views should be utilized to determine the accurate angle of entry toward the vertebral body.

For the AP approach, the target trocar site is the superior and lateral portion of the pedicle, sometimes described as the 10 o'clock or 2 o'clock for the left and right pedicle on AP view, respectively. If utilizing the coaxial view, the trocar should ideally be placed in the center of the pedicle (Fig. 70.1), but lateral paracentral placement is acceptable for narrower pedicles. Local anesthetic is infiltrated to the periosteum of the pedicle. Then, a small incision is made with an 11-blade scalpel. The trocar is advanced to the pedicle using either a screwdriver technique or gentle tapping with an orthopedic hammer (Fig. 70.2). Once properly engaged, AP and lateral views are obtained to confirm that the medial, superior, and inferior walls of the pedicle remain intact (Fig. 70.3). For VP, the trocar is advanced into the anterior third of the vertebral body, and for KP into the posterior third (Fig. 70.4).

The parapedicular approach involves placing the trocar lateral to the edge of the pedicle and advancing along the surface of the pedicle directly into the vertebral body. The vertebral body to pedicle junction will appear more anterior on lateral imaging. This method is useful when there is poor visualization or a fracture of the pedicle. More central placement of the trocar in the vertebral body, obviating the need for a second trocar, is more frequent with this approach (Fig. 70.5).

Trocar placement for KP is similar to the VP approach except that the trocar is not advanced past the posterior one-third of the vertebral body, and trocar size may be slightly larger. After entering the posterior aspect of the vertebral body, the introducer is removed leaving the cannula in place. A hand-operated drill is advanced to the anterior quarter of the vertebral body in lateral imaging, taking care not to violate the anterior margin. Ideal placement on AP imaging is in the midline. The drill is removed and a negatively pressurized and deflated

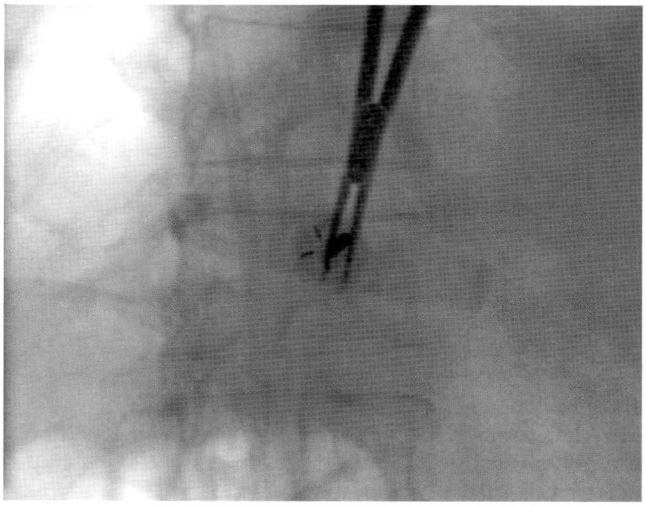

FIG. 70.1 When using a transpedicular coaxial approach, the introducer needle is directed toward the center of the pedicle.

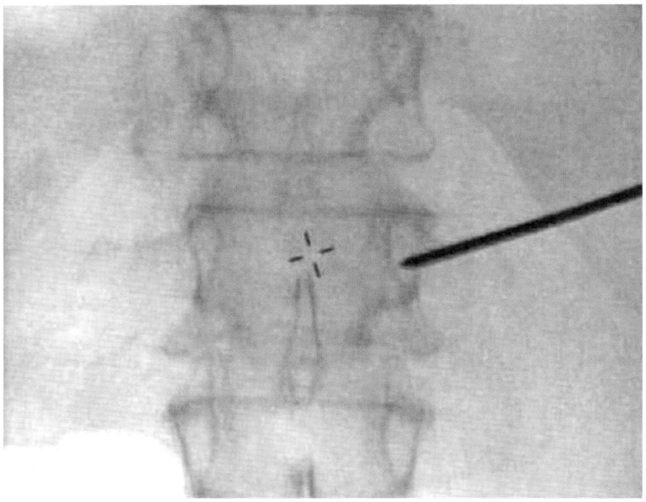

FIG. 70.2 In the anteroposterior (AP) view during transpedicular vertebral augmentation, either with an AP approach, or with intermittent AP views with a coaxial approach, care is taken to ensure the medial border of the pedicle is not violated until the trocar is within the pedicle on a lateral view.

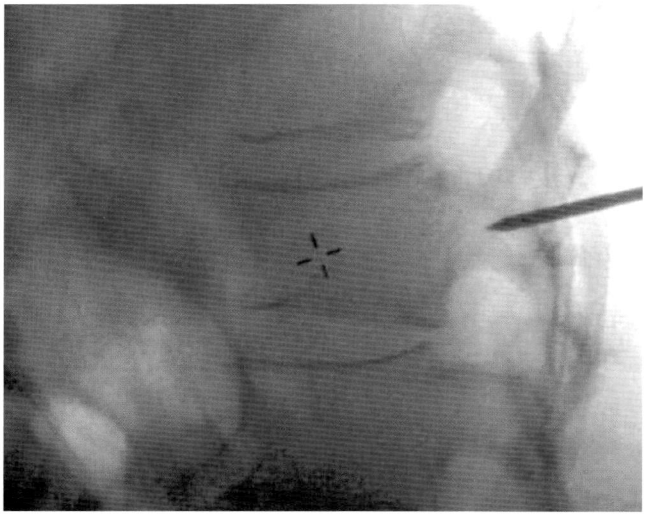

FIG. 70.3 Once the needle is secured within the pedicle, lateral views are obtained to ensure the trajectory of the trocar is accurate, and the superior and inferior walls of the pedicle, and superior and inferior endplates of the vertebral body will not be violated.

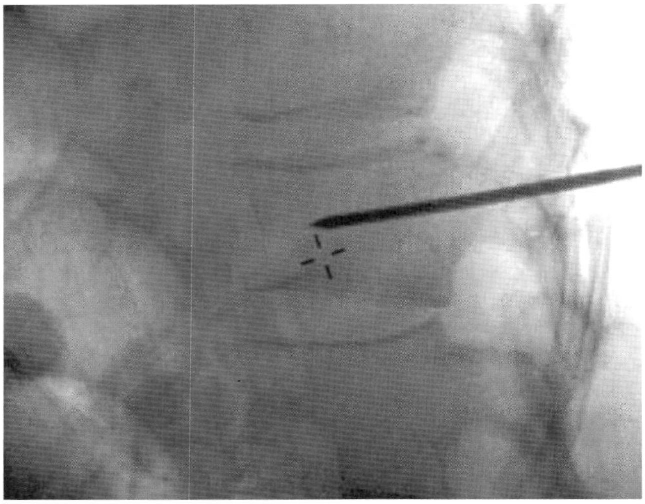

FIG. 70.4 In the lateral view, the needle is advanced into the anterior one-third of the vertebral body during a vertebroplasty procedure.

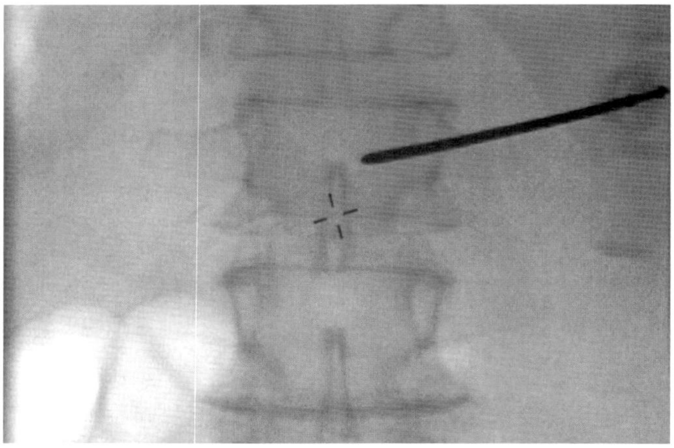

FIG. 70.5 Ideal location of a vertebroplasty trocar is close to the midline. Utilization of the parapedicular approach can result in a more central placement.

balloon is advanced through the cannula into the vertebral body. If a bilateral approach is used, a second introducer and balloon should be placed on the opposite side in a similar fashion. Each balloon is slowly inflated with iodinated contrast via a locking syringe with a manometer to measure pressure, or until the balloon tamp reaches a cortical margin. The balloon is then deflated and removed (Fig 70.6).

Polymethyl methacrylate (PMMA) is prepared by adding normal saline to a powdered phase containing barium. After all ingredients are mixed, there is usually a short working time that varies with the room temperature and formulation. There is also a somewhat more dense bioactive glass ceramic polymer (e.g., Combeite) commercially available as an alternative to PMMA with similar reported efficacy.[42]

With use of either formulation, a cannula is connected to the trocar and the cement is slowly injected under live fluoroscopy beginning in the lateral position, but with frequent AP views to avoid lateral leakage through fracture lines. The injection is stopped when the posterior one-third to one-fourth, or a cortical margin, is reached. If undesirable spread is observed, waiting a few minutes to allow the cement to harden or adjusting the cannula before resuming injection may prevent further spread into unwanted areas. The stylet is replaced into the cannula before extraction to avoid cement leakage back toward the pedicle or toward neuraxial structures (Fig. 70.7).

Although some experts have anecdotally reported that the volume of cement instilled does not correlate with success, a recent study evaluating the SWISSspine national registry found that instillation of greater than 4.5 mL total cement fill during KP was a strong predictor of pain relief.[43,44]

COMPLICATIONS[45–49] (TABLE 70.4)

Among others, complications include infection, bleeding, and cement emboli into perivertebral segment vessels, and the aorta, heart, and lungs. Although pulmonary emboli may occur in up to 25% of patients undergoing VP, they usually lack clinical significance.

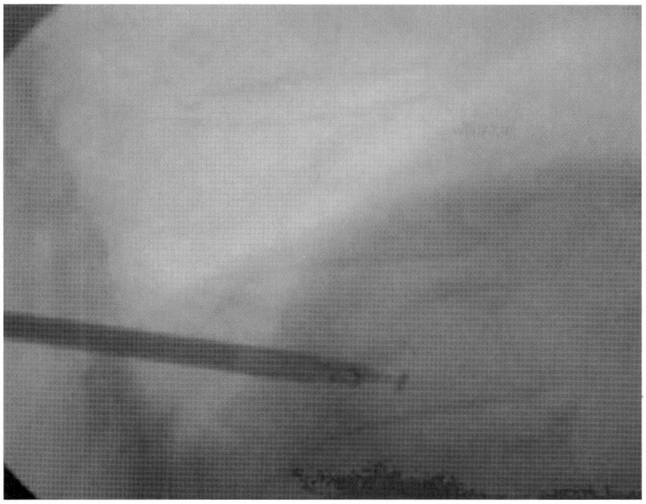

FIG. 70.6 Ideal placement of a kyphoplasty trocar is in the posterior third of the vertebral body. The balloon is advanced into a canal that was previously created with a reaming tool. Both the distal and proximal balloon markers must be within the vertebral body before inflating the balloon with a contrast dye.

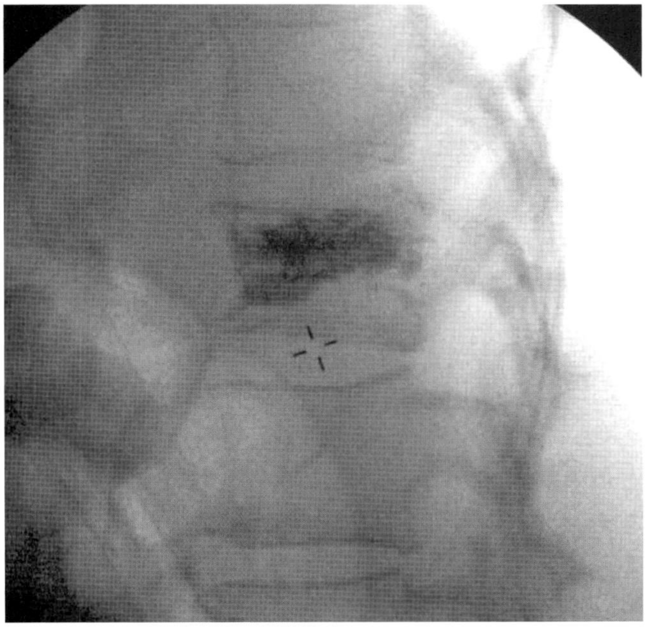

FIG. 70.7 Postaugmentation lateral view of a vertebral body.

CLINICAL EVIDENCE FOR KYPHOPLASTY AND VERTEBROPLASTY FOR THE TREATMENT OF VERTEBRAL COMPRESSION FRACTURES

PROSPECTIVE STUDIES COMPARING VERTEBRAL AUGMENTATION TECHNIQUES AND CONSERVATIVE CARE

There have been several prospective, nonrandomized, studies comparing the effectiveness of VP and KP. Such open-label prospective studies comparing VP and conservative care have consistently found significant improvements in visual analogue scale (VAS) pain scores and measures of function in the short-term, which often persist for more than 6 months.[50–51] Prospective studies comparing KP to conservative care have similarly shown significant improvements in pain scores and function that are sustained, compared to noninterventional treatments.[52–54]

A meta-analysis of these prospective cohort studies found balloon KP and VP to be superior to nonsurgical management with respect to pain relief and fewer subsequent fractures.[55] KP was found to be significantly superior to VP in terms of quality of life (QOL) gains, but only marginally better in disability improvement. In addition, KP resulted in both greater correction of kyphosis and lower risk for cement extravasation.[55]

TABLE 70.4 Complications of Vertebral Augmentation

Complications
Osteomyelitis
Hematoma (paraspinal or epidural)
Rib fracture
Adjacent vertebral fracture
Pedicle fracture
Pulmonary embolus of PMMA
Hypotension
Spinal cord compression
Epidural abscess
Neurologic complications
Allergic reaction to contrast or PMMA

PMMA, *Polymethyl methacrylate.*

RANDOMIZED CONTROLLED TRIALS COMPARING VERTEBRAL AUGMENTATION TO CONSERVATIVE CARE (TABLE 70.5)

There are six high quality, randomized controlled trials (RCTs) comparing VP to conservative care. All six studies reported superiority of VP to conservative care for pain relief at varying time points ranging from 1 week to 1 year.[56–61] Some of these studies also showed an improvement in function ranging from 1 year up to 36 months.[59–61]

Two RCTs that utilized the visual analogue pain scale as a primary outcome measure reported that KP was superior to conservative care for 1 to 2 years.[62–64] With respect to QOL, these studies found KP to be superior to conservative care at follow-up periods ranging from 6 months to 2 years.[62–65] A third RCT also reported better improvement in the kyphotic index for the treatment group at 2 years.[65]

In contrast, two sham controlled studies comparing VP to sham found sham to be equivalent to VP for pain relief, function and QOL, though one study had a statistically higher crossover rate from sham to the treatment arm.[66,67]

PROSPECTIVE AND RANDOMIZED STUDIES COMPARING VERTEBROPLASTY AND KYPHOPLASTY (TABLE 70.6)

Similar to VP, KP employs the use of acrylic cement, but in addition, it makes use of a balloon or other instrumentation for both the creation of a cavity for the cement as well as the reduction of the compression fracture, which can lead to improved pulmonary function. Ultimately, the main goal of VP and KP is restoration of function after the failure of conservative treatment for at least 4 weeks.

TABLE 70.5 Randomized Controlled Trials Comparing Vertebral Augmentation to Conservative Care

Author, Year	Author Specialty	Patients (Number)	Outcome Measures	Results
Voormolen et al., 2007[56]	Interventional Radiology	VP (18) CC (16)	VAS, RM, QUALEFFO	VP > CC at 2 weeks
Rousing et al., 2009[57]	Orthopedic Spine Surgery	VP (26) CC (24)	VAS, SF-36	VP > CC at 1 month
Wardlaw et al., 2009[62]	Orthopedic Surgery	KP (149) CC (151)	VAS, RM, SF-36, EQ-5D	KP > CC by VAS score KP > CC by ODI through 1 year KP > CC by SF-36 up to 6 months KP > CC by EQ-5D up to 1 year
Buchbinder et al., 2009[66]	Rheumatology and Epidemiology	VP (38) Sham (40)	VAS, RM, AQoL, QUALEFFO, EQ-5D	VP equivalent to sham through 6 months
Kallmes et al., 2009[67]	Interventional Neuroradiology	VP (68) Sham (63)	VAS, RM, EQ-5D, SF-36	VP equivalent to sham at 1 month
Klazen et al., 2010[58]	Radiology	VP (101) CC (101)	VAS, RM, QUALEFFO, EQ-5D	VP > CC through 1 year
Farrokhi et al., 2011[59]	Neurosurgery	VP (40) CC (42)	VAS, ODI	VP > CC for pain at 6 months and function through 36 months
Berenson et al., 2011[64]	Hematology/Oncology	KP (70) CC (64)	RM, SF-36, NRS, PCS	KP > CC at 1 month
Boonen et al., 2011[63]	Medicine—Bone Disease	KP (149) CC (151)	RM, EQ-5D, VAS, SF-36	KP > CC for pain up to 2 years, and for QOL for 6 months
Blasco et al., 2012[60]	MD, Interventional Neuroradiology	VP (47) CC (48)	VAS, QUALEFFO-41	VF > CC for pain at 2 months. VF > CC for QOL through 6 months
Van Meirhaeghe et al., 2013[65]	Orthopedic Spine Surgery	KP (149) CC (151)	SF-36 PCS	KP > CC through 2 years
Chen et al., 2014[61]	Orthopedic Surgery	VP (46) CC (43)	VAS, ODI, RM	VP > CC through 1 year. No difference in fracture rate

CC, *Conservative care;* EQ-5D, *Euro QOL 5-dimension questionnaire;* KP, *balloon kyphoplasty;* NRS, *numeric rating scale;* ODI, *Oswestry Disability Index;* PCS, *short form-36 physical component score;* QOL, *quality of life;* QUALEFFO, *quality of life questionnaire by the European Foundation for Osteoporosis;* RM, *Roland Morris disability questionnaire;* SF-36, *short form-36;* VAS, *visual analogue scale pain score;* VP, *vertebroplasty.*

TABLE 70.6 Randomized Controlled Trials Comparing Vertebroplasty and Kyphoplasty

Author, Year	Specialty	Patients	Outcome Measures	Results
Liu et al., 2010[73]	Neurosurgery	KP (50) versus VP (50)	VAS, kyphotic angle correction	KP > VP in kyphotic angle correction. KP = VP for VAS improvement through 6 months
Dohm et al., 2014[74]	Orthopedic Surgery	VP (190) KP (191)	New VF, VAS	KP = VP for pain, disability scores, and new VF up to 24 months. KP > VP for kyphosis correction, longer fracture-free survival, and less cement extravasation at 2 years
Vogl et al., 2013[75]	Radiology	VP (28) KP (49)	Cement leakage	KP > VP grp for cement leakage through 12 months

CC, *Conservative care;* KP, *balloon kyphoplasty;* VAS, *visual analogue scale pain score;* VF, *vertebral fracture;* VP, *vertebroplasty.*

Although most prospective studies comparing VP and KP have shown no difference in pain relief and function for up to 1 year, others have reported better results with KP.[68,69] Restoration of vertebral body height is generally acknowledged to be an advantage of KP compared to VP or conservative treatment, with only two comparative studies demonstrating the equivalence between the two forms of vertebral augmentation.[70,71] Studies (FREE investigators) found that patients with a greater kyphotic angle correction experienced greater QOL gains, and another study showed improved pulmonary function.[62,72] Both of the RCT studies evaluating the degree of kyphotic angle correction found KP to be superior to VP, though both types of vertebral augmentation procedures (VAP) were equivalent in the extent of pain relief.[73,74] KP has also been found to be safer with respect to reduced cement extravasation when compared to VP.[74,75]

TABLE 70.7 Recent Systematic Reviews Comparing Vertebral Augmentation to Conservative Care

Author, Year	Number of Studies	Treatments Compared (n)	Results
Papanastassiou et al., 2012[55]	27	KP VP CC (1923)	KP and VP > CC for improvement in pain and QOL scores up to 7 weeks
Shi et al., 2012[76]	9	VP, KP, Sham, CC (886)	VP = Sham for VAS up to 180 days with significant improvement in both groups. VP > Sham for RM and QUALEFFO scores at 30 days. VP = Sham by RM at 90 days, and by EQ-5D at all time points. VP = Sham by new VF. Some included trials did not separate patients by indication
Anderson et al., 2013[77]	6	VP, KP, CC, Sham (877)	VP > CC for VAS, RM, and ODI in <12 weeks up to >26 weeks
Song et al., 2014[78]	13	VP, KP, CC (1459)	VP = KP = CC for incidence of fractures at 12 months
Buchbinder et al., 2015[103]	12	VP, CC (1320)	Trends toward VP > CC for pain scores, disability, QOL, self-assessed treatment success, and new VCFs (by 6%) at 1 month, although the authors concluded that VP = CC as results did not reach statistical significance

CC, *Conservative care;* EQ-5D, *Euro QOL 5-dimension questionnaire;* KP, *balloon kyphoplasty;* ODI, *Oswestry disability index;* QOL, *quality of life;* QUALEFFO, *quality of life questionnaire by the European Foundation for Osteoporosis;* RM, *Roland Morris disability questionnaire;* VAS, *visual analog scale;* VCF, *vertebral compression fracture;* VP, *vertebroplasty.*

SYSTEMATIC REVIEWS COMPARING VERTEBRAL AUGMENTATION TO CONSERVATIVE CARE (TABLE 70.7)

Most, but not all, systematic reviews have concluded that VP and KP provide greater pain relief and improved QOL than conservative care.[55,76–77] Most systematic reviews have also concluded that the risk of fracture recurrence after VP or KP is not greater than with conservative care.[76,78–79]

CONTROVERSIES

The controversy surrounding the effectiveness of VP and KP has grown over the past several years, as alluded to above. There has been considerable debate over the degree of pain relief and improvement in disability provided by these interventions compared to conservative care following the highly publicized negative studies published by Buchbinder et al. and Kallmes et al.[66,67] Whereas most prospective comparative studies and RCTs demonstrated greater improvement with vertebral augmentation compared to no surgical intervention, these two RCTs showed no relief with VP when compared to an active sham.[50–67] Multiple authors have outlined a critical interpretation of their data.

Criticism of these two RCTs noted that they were underpowered to assess pain relief and improvement of activities of daily living (ADLs), contained inherent selection bias, utilized active sham groups (e.g., blockade of the facet joints, which have been shown to provide significant, long-term pain relief following VCF), and questioned whether the acuity of the fracture(s) was appropriate.[66,67,80–82] The authors who questioned the patient selection in these studies also cited the very low percentage of patients who agreed to participate in their studies.[81,83] The Buchbinder et al. study reported that 78 of 219 eligible patients agreed to participate, while in the Kallmes et al. study, only 131 of 431 eligible patients were enrolled.[66,67] Perhaps more importantly, most patients in both studies did not have acute or subacute fractures. Other criticisms concluded that the high crossover to the treatment group in one study degraded its scientific validity, and that other potential pain generators (e.g., the facet joints and reflex muscle spasm) were not sufficiently excluded and might have responded to the local anesthetic injected at the pedicle, which could explain the high response rate in the control group.[80,81] It is interesting to note that these two negative studies reported similar pain reductions in the VP groups when compared to positive industry-sponsored RCTs studying vertebral augmentation.[62,66–67]

Different factors have been implicated in increasing the risk of VCFs, such as kyphotic angle deformity and the degree of osteoporosis.[84,85] Some studies have suggested that there may be relative propensity for adjacent segment vertebral fractures when cement extravasates through the vertebral endplate(s) into the disc space.[85–88] Others have attributed the possible increased fracture risk with VP to differences between cement elasticity and stiffness, and biologic tissue.[89] However, the majority of prospective studies have found either a reduced incidence of fractures after VAP, or no difference compared to conservative management.[89] To date, no study has shown that VAP increases the rate of adjacent segment or remote VCFs when measured as a primary endpoint.

There is no consensus on the optimal window for correction of VCFs.[89] An analysis of resolution of pain in patients with conservative care (CC) based on data from the VERTOS II study showed that most patients experience resolution of pain within 3 months, leading these authors to recommend fracture correction only after 3 months of failed CC.[90] A retrospective review involving 321 patients found no difference in outcomes between acute, subacute, and chronic VCFs.[91] Other authors recommend performing VP or KP after a 2 to 6 week trial of conservative treatment, since earlier intervention may lead to unnecessary surgery, and late intervention could mitigate the benefits of VAPs. One intermediate position reserves early intervention only for high-risk fractures (e.g., significantly collapsed or burst fracture), and recommends a trial of conservative therapy for between 3 and 6 weeks in lower-risk fractures.[89]

One retrospective study reported that patients receiving VP or KP had a survival rate that was 10% higher compared to those who only underwent conservative treatment.[92] Another study found a 3-year survival rate of 59.9% in individuals who received KP, which favorably compared to survival rates of 49.7% and 42.3% in people who received VP or conservative treatment, respectively.[93] The authors attributed this to improved pulmonary function. However, some experts have attributed this difference to selection bias, and reported similar mortality rates between vertebral augmentation and CC after propensity score matching.[94]

IMPLICATIONS

According to the Department of Health and Human Services, in 2008 the total inpatient admissions for the now obsolete ICD-9 code 733.13 (VCF) were 133,647[95]; 40,800 KPs,[96] and 16,970 VPs[97] were performed on these inpatients. In 2013, there were 108,190 inpatient admissions for VCF[98] in the United States. Among these patients, only 23,870 patients underwent KP,[99] and 8025 underwent VP.[100] The sharp decline in utilization may herald a diminution in the perception of morbidity and the need for urgency in rendering treatment of symptomatic VCFs following the highly publicized negative studies mentioned earlier. Alternatively, these statistics may also indicate a decrease in debilitating VCFs, as a result of improved prophylaxis and treatments for osteoporosis and osteopenia, and earlier detection of malignancies.

A retrospective analysis of vertebral augmentation utilization patterns in the Medicare population demonstrated a 42.6% reduction in VP procedures from 2006 to 2010, and no significant change in utilization.[101] Overall, health care utilization costs have been shown to be similar between patients who undergo vertebral augmentation and those who opt for conservative care for up to 4 years, making vertebral augmentation procedures an economically viable option for the management of VCFs.[102]

CONCLUSION

A large majority of prospective studies, RCTs, and meta-analyses favor the use of both KP and VP for the treatment of subacute (3 to 6 months) VCF-related pain and disability. The evidence suggests that KP may be superior to VP with regard to restoration of vertebral height, improved pulmonary function, and reduced cement extravasation. There is a small but influential subset of publications on vertebral augmentation that contradict the larger body of evidence. The greater influence of these negative studies and reviews within the context of contemporary reimbursement models has propagated a movement toward denial of coverage for vertebral augmentation. Similar to most other procedures, the niche that these therapies ultimately occupy in patient care will be determined by guidelines set forth by federal and commercial payers, indicating a strong need for large, well-designed, pragmatic, clinical trials.

KEY POINTS

- VP and KP are effective techniques for relieving pain related to vertebral compression fractures.
- Their primary indications include painful vertebral compression fractures secondary to osteoporosis, multiple myeloma, and other malignancies.
- Advantages of using KP over VP include less cement extravasation, the potential for restoration of vertebral body height, and improved pulmonary function.
- Despite the large impact of widely publicized negative RCTs, the overwhelming body of literature supports the effectiveness of VP and KP in improving pain and function in patients with painful vertebral compression fractures.

REFERENCES

Access the reference list online at ExpertConsult.com.

CHAPTER 71

Neurolytic Sympathetic Blocks

Sandy Christiansen, MD ⊛ Michael Erdek, MD

Pain associated with cancer may be somatic, visceral, or neuropathic in origin, and approximately 50% of all cancer patients have a combination of pain types at the time of diagnosis. When viscera are stretched, compressed, invaded, or distended, a poorly localized noxious pain is reported. Patients experiencing visceral pain often describe the pain as vague, deep, squeezing, crampy, or colicky in nature. Other signs and symptoms include referred pain, such as shoulder pain due to diaphragm invasion by tumor, nausea, and vomiting.

Visceral pain associated with cancer may be relieved with oral pharmacologic therapy that includes combinations of nonsteroidal antiinflammatory agents, opioids, and coadjuvant therapies. Neurolytic blocks of the sympathetic axis are also effective in controlling visceral cancer pain. Thus neurolysis of the sympathetic axis should be judged as an important adjunct to pharmacologic therapy for the relief of severe cancer-related pain. These blocks rarely eliminate cancer pain, however, due to coexisting somatic and neuropathic pain. Thus oral pharmacologic therapy must often be continued, albeit at lower doses. The goal of performing a neurolytic block of the sympathetic axis is to (1) maximize the analgesic effect of opioid and nonopioid analgesics, and (2) reduce the dosage of these agents to alleviate untoward side effects.

Neurolytic techniques are not without risk. Thus sound clinical judgment and complete patient understanding are essential to minimize undesirable effects. The detailed description of the techniques for these blocks is beyond the scope of this review. Thus the reader is directed to other publications for this purpose.[1,2]

CELIAC PLEXUS BLOCK

The celiac plexus is situated retroperitoneally in the upper abdomen. It is at the level of the T12 and L1 vertebrae, anterior to the crura of the diaphragm. It surrounds the abdominal aorta and celiac artery. The plexus continues inferiorly to form the superior and the inferior mesenteric plexus.

The celiac plexus is composed of a network of nerve fibers, both from the sympathetic and parasympathetic systems. It contains one to five large ganglia, which receive sympathetic fibers from the three splanchnic nerves (greater, lesser, and least). The thoracic splanchnic nerves lie above and posterior to the diaphragm, anterior to the T12 vertebra. The celiac plexus also receives parasympathetic fibers from the vagus nerve, and provides autonomic innervation to the liver, pancreas, gallbladder, stomach, spleen, kidneys, intestines, and adrenal glands, as well as to the blood vessels.

INDICATIONS

Neurolytic blocks of the celiac plexus have been used for malignant and chronic nonmalignant pain. In patients with acute or chronic pancreatitis, it has been used with significant success.[3] Likewise, patients with cancer in the upper abdomen who have a significant visceral pain component have responded well to this block.[4]

TECHNIQUE

There are multiple posterior percutaneous approaches to block nociceptive impulses from the viscera of the upper abdomen. These include the splanchnic nerve block that is accomplished using a retrocrural approach and the celiac plexus block, which uses the anterocrural (or transcrural) approach, which may be transaortic. For the retrocrural approach, the two needles are inserted bilaterally at the level of the first lumbar vertebra, 5–7 cm from the midline. The tip of the needle is then directed toward the vertebral body of T12, or more commonly L1 for the retrocrural and anterocrural approaches. The left needle is positioned just posterior to the aorta, and the right needle can be advanced 1 cm deeper. If a transdiscal retrocrural approach is used, then a single needle approach may be positioned so it ultimately lies at midline of the vertebral body. Similarly, for the anterocrural approach, unilateral needle insertion with the needle tip's final position at midline is often adequate, although a bilateral needle approach may be used as well. As the name indicates, for the anterocrural approach, the needle(s) must be advanced through the diaphragm. This is relatively straightforward on the right side, but more difficult on the left side, due to the proximity of the aorta. Thus, on the left side, the use of a single-needle transaortic technique allows the operator to confirm, using aspiration, passage through the aorta. Regardless of whether the approach is retrocrural or anterocrural, fluoroscopy should reveal spread of contrast posterior to the diaphragm and anterior to the vertebral body.

In addition to the fluoroscopic guidance techniques,[5,6] computed tomography (CT) scan[7] and ultrasound[8] use for percutaneous celiac plexus block have also been described. For the posterior percutaneous CT-guided approach, unilateral or bilateral approaches may be employed, where the left needle is inserted closer to the midline and placed anterolateral to the aorta or through the aorta. Figs. 71.1–71.3 illustrate the final position of the needles and the expected spread of contrast medium after successful placement. Pain specialists also perform neurolysis of the celiac plexus using a transabdominal approach with the assistance of CT[7] and/or ultrasound[8] guidance. This approach is frequently used when patients are unable to tolerate either the prone or

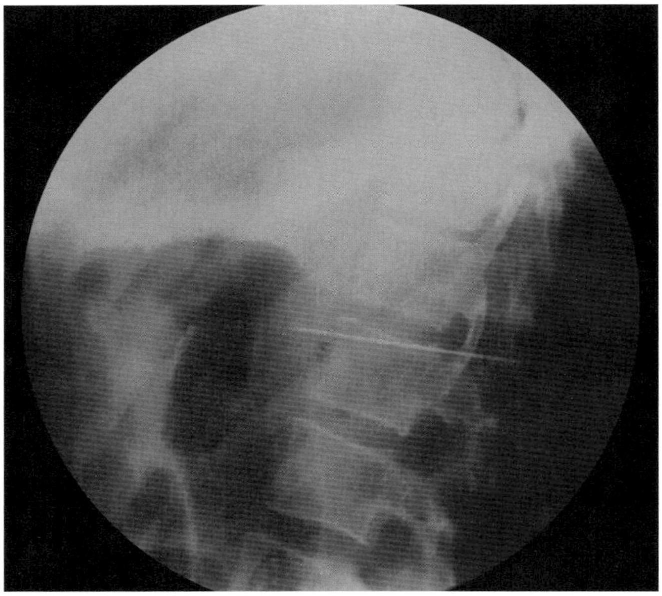

FIG. 71.1 Lateral radiograph showing placement of the needle tip 1.0–1.5 cm anterior to the body of the L1 vertebra.

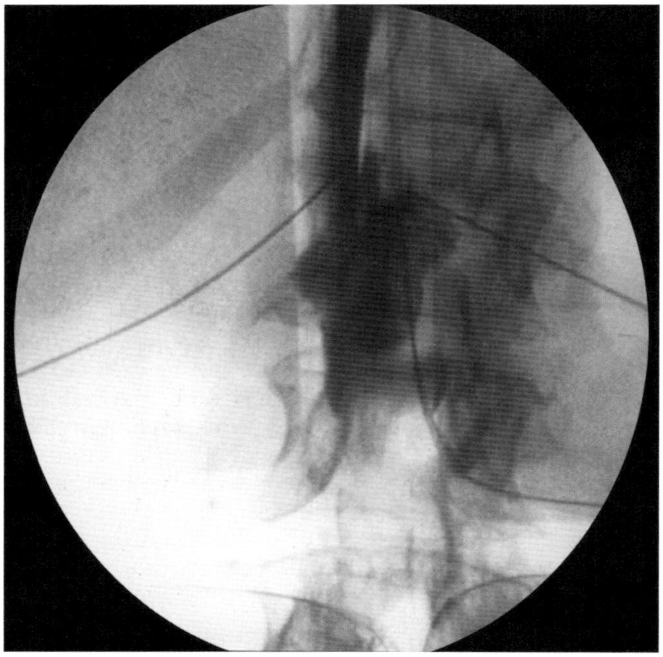

FIG. 71.2 Posteroanterior radiograph showing bilateral caudad spread of contrast medium through the right-sided needle, which is anterocrural, and unilateral cephalad spread through the needle on the left side, which is retrocrural.

lateral decubitus position, or when the liver is so enlarged that a posterior approach is not feasible.

DRUG AND DOSING

For neurolytic blocks, 50%–100% alcohol, 7–15 mL per side, is utilized. The smaller volumes are more appropriate for retrocrural approaches. When injected by itself, alcohol can produce severe pain; thus it is recommended

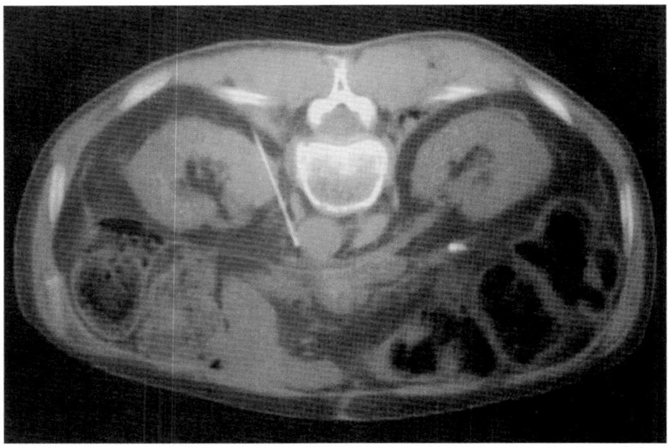

FIG. 71.3 Computed tomographic scan showing the needle adjacent to the lateral wall of the aorta, anterior to the crura of the diaphragm.

to first inject 5–10 mL of a mixture of 2% lidocaine and 0.25%–0.5% bupivacaine 5 minutes prior to the injection of alcohol, or to dilute the 100% alcohol by 50% with local anesthetic (0.25%–0.5% bupivacaine). Phenol in a 10% final concentration may also be used, and has the advantage of being painless on injection. Both agents appear to have similar efficacy.

COMPLICATIONS

Complications associated with celiac plexus blocks appear to be related to the technique used: retrocrural, transcrural,[5,9] or transaortic.[6] In a prospective, randomized study of 61 patients with cancer of the pancreas, Ischia et al.[4] compared the efficacy and the incidence of complications associated with three different approaches to celiac plexus neurolysis (CPN). Orthostatic hypotension was more frequent in patients who had a retrocrural (50%) or splanchnic nerve block technique (52%) than those who underwent an anterocrural approach (10%). In contrast, transient diarrhea was more frequent in patients who had a transaortic celiac plexus block (65%) than those having a bilateral chemical splanchnicectomy (5%), but not the retrocrural approach (25%). The incidence of dysesthesia, interscapular back pain, hiccoughing, or hematuria was not statistically different among the three groups.

The incidence of complications from neurolytic celiac plexus blocks was recently evaluated by Davis[10] in 2730 patients having blocks performed from 1986 to 1990. The overall incidence of major complications, such as paraplegia and bladder and bowel dysfunction, was 1 in 683 procedures. However, the report does not describe which approaches were utilized for the performance of the blocks.

IMPORTANT ASPECTS IN THE DIAGNOSIS AND MANAGEMENT OF SPECIFIC COMPLICATIONS

1. Malposition of the needle should always be ruled out with radiographic or radiologic imaging prior to the injection of a neurolytic agent, as the needle's tip may be intravascular, in the peritoneal cavity, or in a viscus. Imaging techniques currently used include biplanar

fluoroscopy, CT, or ultrasound guidance. Wong and Brown[11] suggested that the use of radiologic imaging does not alter the quality of the block or the incidence of complications, based on a retrospective study of 136 patients with pancreatic cancer pain treated with a celiac plexus block done with or without radiologic guidance. However, it is not clear how many of those patients had radiologic imaging. Assuming that half of the patients did not, the upper 95% confidence limit for complications is 5%, arguably too high not to routinely employ imaging.[12] Erdek et al. compared fluoroscopy versus CT-guided celiac plexus block and found that patients who underwent the procedure under CT guidance were more likely to experience a positive outcome ($P = .06$).[13]

2. Orthostatic hypotension may occur in 1%–3% of patients after the block for up to 5 days. Treatment includes bed rest, avoidance of sudden changes in position, and fluid replacement. Once compensatory vascular reflexes are fully activated, this side effect disappears. Wrapping of the lower extremities from the toe to the upper thighs with elastic bandages has been used with success in patients who developed orthostatic hypotension and needed to ambulate during the first week after the block.
3. Backache may result from (a) local trauma during the needle placement, at its worst resulting in a retroperitoneal hematoma; (b) alcohol irritation of the retroperitoneal structures; or (c) injury to the lumbar plexus. Retroperitoneal hemorrhage is rare but has been reported. Thus, in patients who present with orthostatic hypotension, one must rule out hemorrhage before assuming that it is a physiologic response to the block. Likewise, patients with a persistent backache should have hematocrit measurements checked. If there is a decrease in the hematocrit, radiologic imaging is indicated to rule out a retroperitoneal hematoma. A urinalysis positive for red cells suggests renal injury. A surgical consult should be obtained if necessary.
4. Diarrhea may occur due to sympathetic block of the bowel. Treatment includes hydration and antidiarrheal agents. Oral loperamide is a good choice, although any anticholinergic may be used. Matson et al.[14] have reported near-fatal dehydration from diarrhea after this block. Thus, in debilitated patients, diarrhea must be treated aggressively.
5. Abdominal aortic dissection has also been reported.[15,16] The mechanism of aortic injury is direct damage with the needle during the performance of the block. As expected, the anterocrural approach is more frequently associated with this complication. This approach is best avoided if there is evidence of extensive atherosclerotic disease of the abdominal aorta.
6. Paraplegia and transient motor paralysis have occurred after CPN.[17–23] Current thinking is that these neurologic complications may occur due to spasm of the lumbar segmental arteries that perfuse the spinal cord.[21] In fact, canine lumbar arteries undergo sustained contraction when exposed to both alcohol and phenol.[24] The magnitude of the response to phenol was directly related to concentration, while the alcohol-induced response was inversely related to concentration. Low concentrations of ethanol produce significant contractile effects in human aortic smooth muscle cells by increasing the intracellular concentration of ionized calcium.[25] One might therefore consider avoiding alcohol in the presence of significant atherosclerotic disease of the aorta, as this suggests that the circulation to the spinal cord may also be impaired. However, there is also a report of paraplegia after phenol use,[16] suggesting that other factors, such as direct vascular or neurologic injury, or retrograde spread to the spinal cord, may also play a role. These complications further support the necessity of radiologic imaging during the performance of the block.

EFFICACY

There are six randomized controlled trials designed to ascertain the efficacy, safety, or adverse effects of CPN for pancreatic cancer in adults.[26] One of the studies evaluated CPN versus analgesic therapy with nonsteroidal antiinflammatory drugs (NSAIDs) and morphine on improving quality of life in 21 patients.[27] In this study, CPN patients used less opioids and had quality of life scores that did not deteriorate as quickly as the NSAID and morphine group during the survival period. The second study compared the procedure with oral pharmacologic therapy in 20 pancreatic cancer pain patients. The author found that CPN resulted in an equivalent reduction in visual analogue scale (VAS) pain score compared with therapy with an NSAID–opioid combination.[28] However, opioid consumption was significantly lower in the neurolysis group. Moreover, the incidence of side effects was greater in the group of patients receiving oral pharmacologic therapy. The third randomized controlled trial also compared the CPN with drug therapy in 24 patients with pancreatic cancer.[29] In this study, CPN was associated with better short-term pain relief, transient diarrhea, and hypotension compared with the drug therapy group. Although CPN patients did not demonstrate persistent analgesic benefits when compared with drug therapy patients, the CPN patients had lower analgesic consumption and fewer side effects, such as nausea, vomiting, and constipation. The fourth controlled study evaluating 100 patients with unresectable pancreatic cancer randomized to CPN versus sham injection showed that at 6 weeks, there was a significant decrease in pain in those who received CPN. No differences in opioid use, opioid adverse effects, quality of life, or survival were appreciated.[30] The randomized, controlled, double-blinded study by Lillemoe et al. found improvement in survival in 137 patients with unresectable pancreatic cancer who received chemical splanchnicectomy during surgery with alcohol over the follow-up period of 2-month intervals until death.[31] These findings may be the result of less opioid use in the group of patients randomized to neurolysis, resulting in (1) better preserved immune function, and (2) lower incidence of side effects, such as nausea and vomiting, that affords the patients improved appetite. Finally, the sixth study by Zhang et al. studied 56 pancreatic cancer patients and concluded that participants who received the CT-guided CPN had significantly lower VAS pain scores than those in the pharmacotherapy group; however, in contrast to the Lillemoe et al. study, CPN did not confer a survival benefit.[32]

A Cochrane review of celiac plexus procedures for pancreatic cancer pain in adults found that in 358 patients studied, a statistically significant difference was noted in VAS pain scores at 4 weeks after CPN, with a corresponding decrease in use of analgesic therapy until death in the experimental group.[26] In this meta-analysis, there were no major complications, and the main adverse effect was constipation in the analgesic therapy groups. The review was unable to evaluate the comparative effectiveness of different techniques for the CPN due to a lack of studies.

In addition to the randomized controlled trials, there are also several retrospective studies that further elucidate the benefit of CPN. A recent retrospective statistical analysis showed that patients receiving a morphine equivalent dose of less than 250 mg/day and not receiving sedation for the prognostic procedure were more likely to achieve successful outcome from celiac or splanchnic neurolysis.[13] The results of a meta-analysis that evaluated 21 retrospective studies containing 1145 patients concluded that adequate to excellent pain relief can be achieved in 89% of the patients during the first 2 weeks after the procedure.[33] Partial to complete pain relief continued in approximately 90% of the patients who were alive 3 months postprocedure and in 70%–90% until death, even beyond 3 months after celiac plexus block. The efficacy was similar in patients with pancreatic cancer and in those with other malignancies involving the upper abdomen. It is important to recognize that these results are based on retrospective evaluations, which may not yield reliable information and is subject to publication bias. In addition, statistical techniques used for the analysis must account for the heterogeneity produced by patient selection criteria, technical differences in the performance of the blocks, choice of neurolytic agents and doses, diversity in the tools for the evaluation of pain, and goals of therapy.

The efficacy of CPN may be related to the site and extent of pancreatic tumor involvement. Rykowski and Hilgier demonstrated that sustained, effective pain relief occurred in 92% (33 of 36) of patients, with cancer limited to the head of the pancreas, but in only 29% (4 of 14) of patients with cancer involving the body and tail of the pancreas.[34] Block failure in 13 patients appeared to be explained by the extent of tumor growth around the celiac axis, which was confirmed by CT scan.

As previously discussed, oral pharmacological therapy with opioids, NSAIDs, and coadjuvants is frequently used for the treatment of cancer pain. However, there is evidence to suggest that chronic use of high doses of opioids may have a negative effect on immunity.[35] Thus analgesic techniques that lower opioid consumption could have positive effects on patient outcomes.

SUPERIOR HYPOGASTRIC PLEXUS BLOCK

Cancer patients with tumor extension into the pelvis may experience severe pain unresponsive to oral or parenteral opioids. Moreover, some patients may complain of excessive sedation or other side effects that limit the acceptability and usefulness of oral opioid therapy. In these individuals, a more invasive approach may be needed to control pain and improve quality of life.

The superior hypogastric plexus is situated in the retroperitoneum, bilaterally, extending from the lower third of the fifth lumbar vertebral body to the upper third of the first sacral vertebral body. Both pelvic pain associated with cancer and that observed with chronic nonmalignant conditions may be alleviated by blocking the superior hypogastric plexus.[36–39] A study of 32 patients designed to evaluate which patients would benefit from a superior hypogastric plexus neurolysis found that older patients, patients with pain localized outside of the pelvis, and patients with bladder cancer were more likely to experience positive outcomes, which was defined as greater than or equal to 50% pain relief lasting at least 1 month.[40] Analgesia to the organs in the pelvis is possible because the afferent fibers innervating these structures travel with the sympathetic nerves, trunks, ganglia, and rami, and are accessible for neurolytic block. A sympathectomy for visceral pain is analogous to a peripheral neurectomy or dorsal rhizotomy for somatic pain. Another study has suggested that, even in advanced stages, visceral pain is an important component of the pain syndrome experienced by patients with cancer of the pelvis.[37] Thus it appears that percutaneous neurolytic blocks of the superior hypogastric plexus should be offered more frequently to patients with advanced stages of pelvic cancer.

TECHNIQUE

Patients are placed in the prone position with a pillow under the pelvis to flatten the lumbar lordosis. Local infiltration of the intervening muscle planes can be performed. Needle insertion sites are 5–7 cm lateral to the midline, depending on patient's height and girth, at the level of the L4–L5 interspace. Two 7–9-inch, 22-gauge short beveled needles are inserted with the bevel directed medially, 45 degrees mesiad and 30 degrees caudad, so that the needle tips lie anterolateral to the L5–S1 intervertebral space. Aspiration is important to avoid injection into the iliac vessels. If blood is aspirated, a transvascular approach can be used.

Biplanar fluoroscopy is used to verify accurate needle placement. Anteroposterior (AP) views should reveal the tip of the needle at the level of the junction of the L5 and S1 vertebral bodies. Lateral views will confirm placement of the needle tip just beyond the vertebral body's anterolateral margin. The injection of 2–3 mL of water-soluble contrast medium is used to verify accurate needle placement and to rule out intravascular injection. In the AP view, the spread of contrast should be confined to the midline region. In the lateral view, a smooth posterior contour corresponding to the anterior psoas fascia indicates that the needle is at the appropriate depth. Figs. 71.4 and 71.5 show adequate needle placement and contrast medium spread prior to neurolysis of the superior hypogastric plexus. A transdiscal approach has been described through the L5–S1 disc, which studies have found to be as equally effective as the extradiscal technique. An approach similar to that used for L5–S1 discography is used, but the needle is advanced just anterior to the disc.

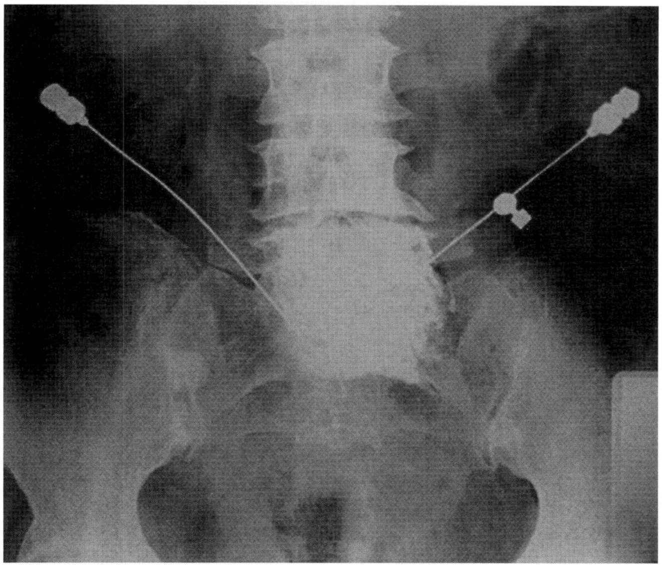

FIG. 71.4 Posteroanterior radiograph demonstrating bilateral correct needle placement and adequate spread of the contrast medium.

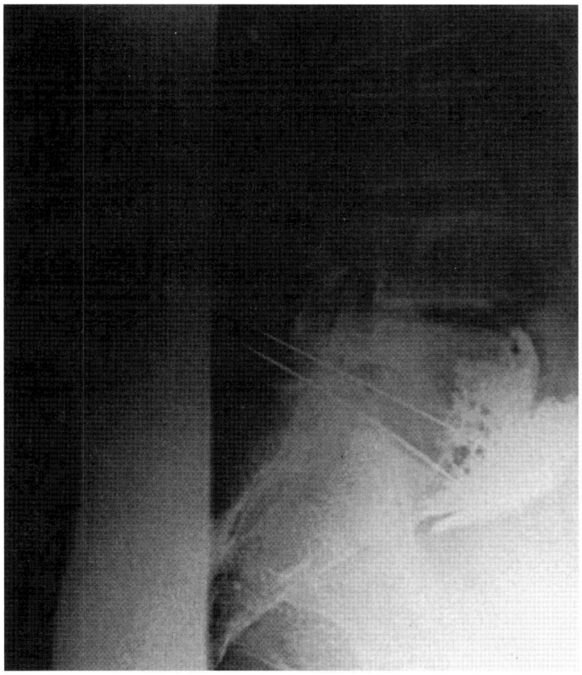

FIG. 71.5 Cross-lateral radiograph demonstrating correct needle placement and adequate spread of the contrast medium.

For a prognostic hypogastric plexus blockade, a volume of 6–8 mL of 0.25% bupivacaine through each needle is recommended. Lower volumes may be sufficient for a transdiscal approach. For therapeutic purposes, a total of 6–8 mL of 10% aqueous phenol or 80%–100% alcohol can be injected through each needle, with the volumes utilized during the prognostic block used to guide those for neurolysis.

COMPLICATIONS

Potential complications relate to the anatomical location of the hypogastric plexus. These include formation of retroperitoneal hematoma, injury to exiting nerve roots or spinal cord, damage to the pelvic viscera including the ureters, inadvertent intravascular, epidural, subdural, or subarachnoid injection, trauma to the intervertebral disc, discitis, and acute ischemia of the foot, due to the dislodgement of an atherosclerotic plaque from the iliac vessels. Also, the superior hypogastric plexus is the only major innervation of the urogenital system; thus injuries of the superior hypogastric plexus have been associated with retrograde ejaculation, which typically is transient.[41] Despite all of the previously noted potential complications, the combined experience of more than 200 cases from the Mexican Institute of Cancer, Roswell Park Cancer Institute, and M.D. Anderson Cancer Center has failed to detect neurologic complications associated with this block.[38] There are also no reports of discitis, disc herniation, or disc rupture with the transdiscal approach to the superior hypogastric plexus block.[42,43]

EFFICACY

The effectiveness of the block was originally demonstrated by documenting a significant decrease in pain scores via a VAS. In this study, Plancarte et al. showed that this block was effective in reducing VAS pain scores in 70% of the patients with pelvic pain associated with cancer.[36] The great majority of the patients enrolled had a diagnosis of cervical cancer. In a subsequent study, 69% of the patients experienced a decrease in VAS scores. Moreover, a mean daily morphine dose reduction of 67% was seen in the success group (736 ± 633 to 251 ± 191 mg/day), and 45% in the failure group (1443 ± 703 to 800 ± 345 mg/day).[37] In a recent multicenter study, 159 patients with pelvic pain associated with cancer were evaluated. Overall, 115 patients (72%) had satisfactory pain relief after one or two neurolytic procedures. Mean opioid use decreased by 40% from 58 ± 43 to 35 ± 18 equianalgesic mg/day of morphine, 3 weeks after treatment in all the studied patients. The decrease in opioid consumption was significant for both the success group (56 ± 32 to 32 ± 16 mg/day) and the failure group (65 ± 28 to 48 ± 21 mg/day).[38] Success was defined in these two studies as the ability to reduce opioid consumption by at least 50% in the 3 weeks following the block and a decrease in the pain scores below 4/10 on the VAS.[37,38] Thirty patients randomized to either transdiscal versus classic posterior approach showed the transdiscal group to have a significantly shorter procedure time (24.4 vs. 67.9 minutes). There was no difference in pain scores or morphine consumption between the groups, and the transdiscal group showed no evidence of discitis or disc herniation.[42] Finally, a recent randomized controlled trial analyzed the efficacy of the anterior ultrasound-guided approach for superior hypogastric plexus neurolysis in pelvic cancer patients and found it to be an effective technique for decreasing VAS scores compared with oral morphine alone.[39]

Three important conclusions may be drawn from the results of these studies. First, reductions in pain scores and in opioid consumption are significant, even in advanced stages of pelvic cancer. This suggests that visceral pain may be an important component of cancer pain, even in the late stages of the disease, when differentiation of somatic pain from visceral pain is very difficult. Second, neurolysis is not as effective in the presence of significant retroperitoneal lymph node involvement (20% vs. 70% response rate).[37] This lack of success may reflect involvement of nerve tissue or tumor spread to somatic structures within the pelvis. However, patients with extensive retroperitoneal pelvic involvement who showed a confluence of contrast material in the midline, on AP fluoroscopic views, experienced good results in one of the studies.[37] Third, use of this neurolytic block early in the management of pelvic visceral pain associated with cancer may be economically sound, based on the opioid reduction experienced by patients in both the failure and the success groups.[37,38]

In a case report, Rosenberg et al. described the effectiveness of this block in a patient with severe chronic nonmalignant penile pain after transurethral resection of the prostate.[44] Although the patient did not receive a neurolytic agent, a "diagnostic" block performed with 0.25% bupivacaine and 20 mg of methylprednisolone acetate was effective in relieving the pain for more than 6 months. However, the usefulness of this block in chronic benign pain conditions has not been adequately documented.

GANGLION IMPAR BLOCK

The ganglion impar is a solitary retroperitoneal structure located at the level of the sacrococcygeal junction. This ganglion marks the end of the two sympathetic chains.

Visceral pain in the perineal area associated with malignancies may be effectively treated with neurolysis of the ganglion impar, also known as the ganglion of Walther.[45,46] Patients likely to benefit from this blockade will frequently present with vague and poorly localized pain, which is burning in character and frequently accompanied by sensations of urgency. However, the clinical value of this block is not as clear as for celiac plexus and superior hypogastric plexus blocks, as the published experience is limited.

TECHNIQUE

This block may be performed with the patient in the left lateral decubitus position with the knees flexed, in the litothomy position, or in the prone position. The originally described technique employs a 22-gauge, 3.5-inch spinal needle that is manually bent to facilitate placement of the needle tip anterior to the concavity of the sacrum and coccyx. The needle is introduced through the anococcygeal ligament with its concavity oriented posteriorly and, under fluoroscopic guidance, is directed along the midline to contact bone at or near the sacrococcygeal junction (Fig. 71.6). Contrast dye confirms retroperitoneal spread; on the lateral view, it is shaped like a comma.

A very popular alternative, transcoccygeal approach is performed with the patient in the prone position. This approach has been reported to be both effective and safe.[47,48] A 20-gauge, 1.5-inch needle is inserted through the sacrococcygeal ligament in the midline. The needle is then advanced until the tip is placed posterior to the rectum. Another less common approach involves inserting two bent needles lateral to the sacrococcygeal junction, such that the tips curve medially just anterior to sacrococcygeal ligament. For diagnostic blocks, 4–8 mL of 1% lidocaine or 0.25% bupivacaine is selected, and for neurolytic block 4 (to 8) mL of 10% phenol or 80%–100% alcohol is used. Although the technique is relatively straightforward, care is needed to prevent perforation of the rectum and injection into the periosteum.

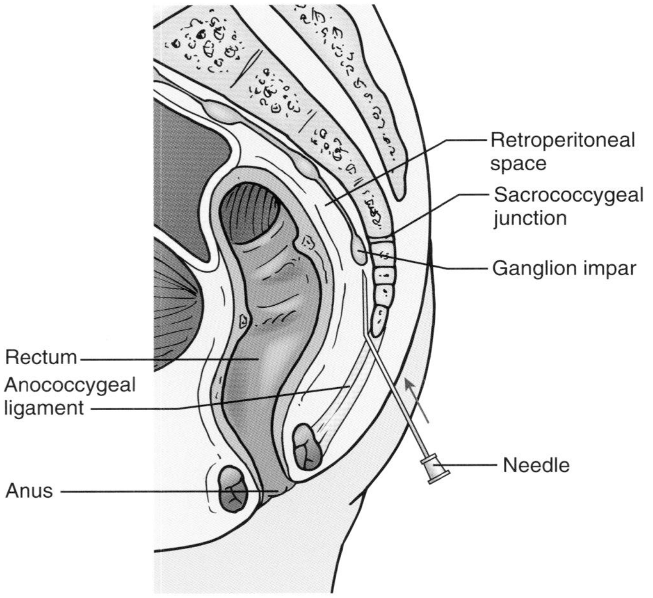

FIG. 71.6 Lateral schematic view of correct needle placement for blockade of the ganglion impar.

COMPLICATIONS

No complications or side effects have been reported with this block, though the proximity of the rectum can lead to infection if the lumen is penetrated.

CONCLUSION

Neurolysis of the sympathetic axis is a safe and cost-effective way to treat visceral pain associated with cancer. The benefits are not limited to improved analgesia but can also include a decrease in opioid consumption and an improved quality of life. These results may have both economic and clinical implications, due to the effects high-dose chronic opioid therapy have on the immune and gastrointestinal systems. A comparison of the indications, complications, and efficacy of the different techniques is in Table 71.1. The knowledge and refined techniques currently used to perform these blocks allow patients to undergo these procedures in a safe and expeditious manner. Pain practitioners would do well to consider them as adjuvant therapy for the successful treatment of cancer pain.

TABLE 71.1 Comparison of Various Sympathetic Blocks

	Level of Evidence	Indications (Origin of Pain)	Anatomical Level of the Block	Complications	Comments
Celiac plexus block	Cochrane review found significant difference in VAS scores in 358 patients with pancreatic cancer	Pancreas, abdominal vessels, esophagus to transverse colon, liver, adrenals, ureters	T12–L1	Orthostatic hypotension, back pain, diarrhea, abdominal aortic dissection, paraplegia and transient motor paralysis	Repeat CPB effective in one-third of people; tumors limited to the head of the pancreas associated with higher response rate
Superior hypogastric plexus block	Few randomized controlled trials	Uterus, ovaries, vagina, bladder, prostate, testes, descending and sigmoid colon, seminal vesicles	L5	Retroperitoneal hematoma, injury to exiting nerve roots or spinal cord, damage to pelvic viscera including the ureters, trauma to intervertebral disc, discitis, retrograde ejaculation	SHP may be more effective for older patients, patients with pain localized outside of the pelvis, and patients with bladder cancer
Ganglion impar block	Limited to small case series	Perineum, rectum, anus, vagina, distal urethra, vulva	Coccyx	Perforation of the rectum, infection, intravascular injection	Patients likely to benefit from this blockade frequently present with poorly localized pain, which is burning and accompanied by sensations of urgency

CPB, *Celiac plexus block;* SHP, *superior hypogastric plexus block;* VAS, *visual analogue scale.*

KEY POINTS

- Neurolytic blocks of the sympathetic axis are an important adjunct to pharmacologic therapy for the relief of severe visceral pain experienced by cancer patients. The goal of performing these blocks is to maximize the analgesic effect of opioid and nonopioid analgesics while reducing their dosage to alleviate untoward side effects.
- Neurolytic celiac plexus block for patients with pancreatic cancer pain results in excellent analgesia, reduced opioid utilization, and decreased side effects such as nausea, vomiting, and constipation when compared with systemic analgesic therapy.
- Patients with nonresectable cancer of the pancreas receiving splanchnic neurolysis had longer survival rates in one study. This may result from their lower opioid use, resulting in preserved immune function, as well as improved nutrition due to fewer opioid side effects.
- Complications of neurolytic celiac plexus block include diarrhea, postural hypotension, back pain, aortic injury, hemorrhage, and paraplegia.
- Neurolytic superior hypogastric plexus block has proven effective, with minimal complications, in reduction of pain and opioid consumption in patients with advanced pelvic cancer, suggesting that a significant component of visceral pain is present even with advanced disease.

REFERENCES

Access the reference list online at ExpertConsult.com.

CHAPTER 72

Central and Peripheral Neurolysis

Kashif Saeed, MD ◎ Meredith C. B. Adams, MD, MS ◎ Robert W. Hurley, MD, PhD

INTRODUCTION

Chemical neurolysis is a modality that has been used for pain control for almost a century. Multiple agents have been evaluated through the years, but only a few are still clinically relevant. Glycerol is used for the treatment of trigeminal neuralgia. Phenol and ethyl alcohol are the only two agents commonly used in the epidural or intrathecal space, as well as for neurolysis of the sympathetic chain, celiac plexus, and splanchnic nerves. The decision to use neurolytic agents usually is made after many other modalities have failed to provide benefit. Chemical and surgical neurolysis potentially have very serious side effects. Their use is primarily limited to patients with pain associated with terminal malignancies. These procedures provide the most benefit in the oncology patients in whom more conservative measures were unsuccessful or possessed too high a side-effect burden. In patients *in extremis*, neurolysis represents a palliative measure to provide pain relief while maintaining the patient's ability to interact with family and friends in their final days to months of life. It can improve pain control in patients who have developed tolerance and hyperalgesia or severe side effects from high-dose opioids. Neurolysis is an alternative to allow patients the ability to control their pain with less systemic medication, significantly improving their quality of life.

PATIENT SELECTION

After a patient is deemed to have a pain pattern or pathology that is appropriate for neurolytic therapy (Table 72.1), it is imperative to clearly explain the specific goals and expectations. Neurolysis can provide substantial analgesia and will usually allow a significant reduction of systemic pain medications. The limitations and complication profile of this modality are not insignificant and are an important part of the decision process for the patient and provider. Although neurolysis can provide analgesia in the nerve distribution affected by the block, it will not necessarily provide pain relief from an expanding tumor or new metastasis. In addition, the effects of this therapy can be temporary and will diminish over time, requiring readministration of the neurolytic agent. Although these agents usually provide good to excellent pain relief, sometimes the level of analgesia is inadequate to meet patient expectations or the duration of pain relief is too short. There have also been reports of limb weakness and loss of bowel or bladder tone. Typically, the patient subset chosen for epidural or intrathecal neurolysis has been escalated through the rungs of the World Health Organization (WHO) analgesia ladder (Fig. 72.1A) without relief, and they are experiencing pain that cannot be adequately controlled by standard analgesics, or the analgesic doses are producing intolerable side effects. These patients will also fall into a category in which advanced interventional pain medicine strategies have been tried, but without inadequate analgesia, or the patient possesses contraindications to these procedures (see Fig. 72.1B). Patients with complaints of neuropathic pain will typically not get the desired results compared with those with visceral or somatic pain. Due to the nature of neurolytic administration, it is ideal for controlling unilateral pain in the trunk that is focused to a few adjacent dermatomes. However, in the presence of an intraspinal tumor, the effectiveness of these techniques will decrease, making these patients unsuitable candidates. Neuraxial neurolytic therapy is ideal for patients with advanced or terminal malignancy and unilateral somatic pain.[1]

PATIENT PREPARATION

Prior to attempting any neurolytic block, it is essential to have a clear and accurate pain diagnosis and the location needs to be accurately mapped with a dermatomal chart (Fig. 72.2). Multiple modalities are available to achieve an accurate diagnosis and should be used to ensure an effective block that is appropriate for the underlying condition.[2] After a definitive plan is established, informed consent should be obtained from the patient, outlining all the risks associated with the particular procedure in detail. A thorough neurologic examination before any invasive techniques are attempted is vital not only for assessing the effectiveness, but also in providing a baseline assessment in the event of any potential complications. In an ideal treatment scenario, a member of the patient's multidisciplinary cancer team will perform these blocks, with all providers aware of the status and progression of the primary and

TABLE 72.1 Intrathecal Neurolysis: Indications for Neurolytic Spinal Blockade

Intractable cancer pain (advanced or terminal malignancy)
Failure of medical and interventional analgesic therapy
Intolerable side effects of current therapy
Unilateral pain
Pain restricted to one to four dermatomal levels
Pain located in the trunk, thorax, abdomen
Primary somatic pain mechanism
Absence of intraspinal tumor spread
Effective analgesia with local anesthetic block
Informed consent of patient
Realistic expectations and family support

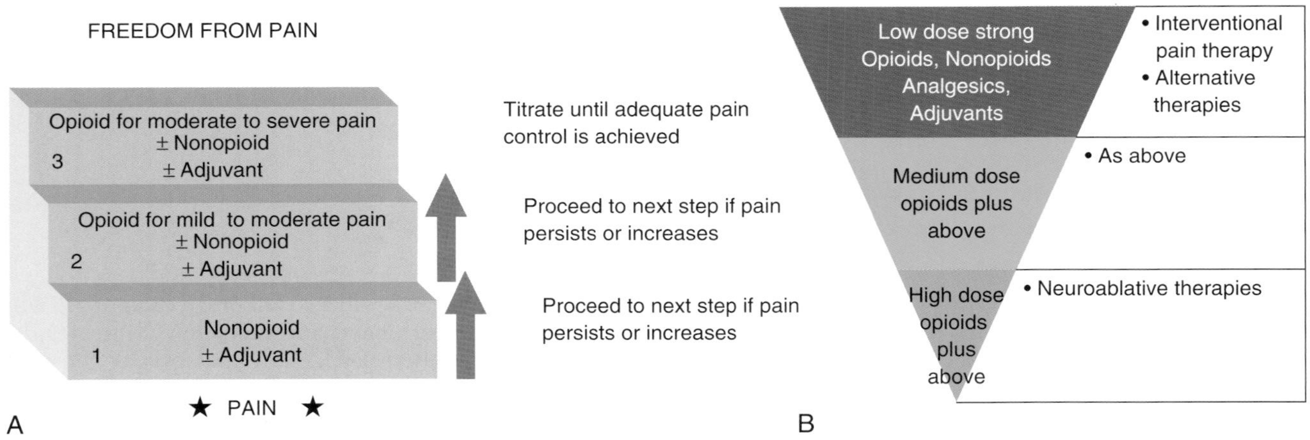

FIG. 72.1 Adapted from WHO Cancer and Palliative Care 2011. In (A), escalation of treatment is represented by moving up the figure, whereas in (B) escalation of treatment is represented by moving down the diagram.

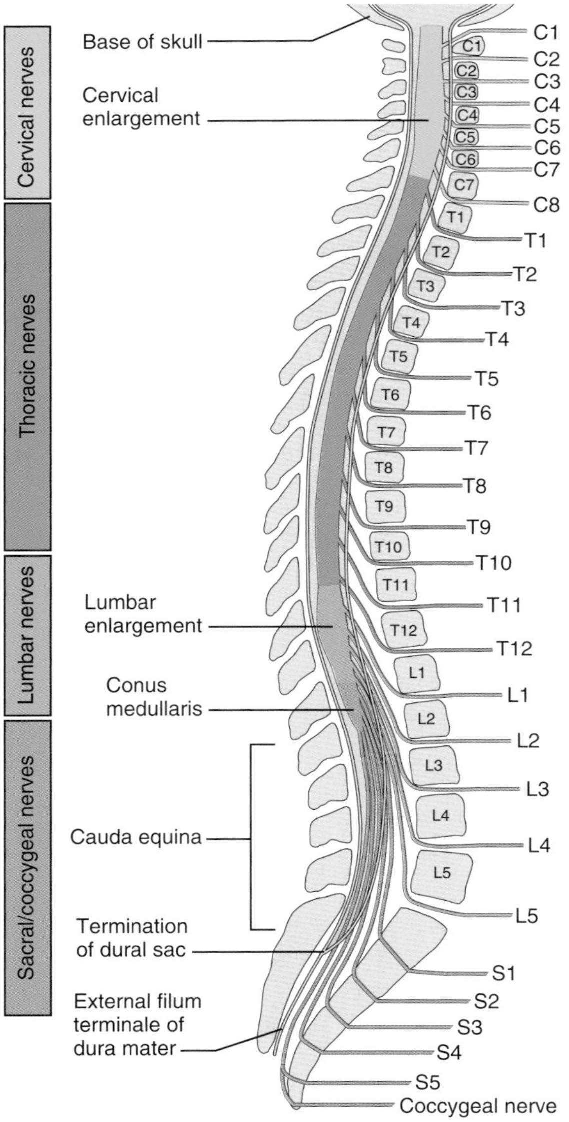

FIG. 72.2 Lateral, midline view of the spinal cord, vertebral bodies, and nerve roots.

metastatic malignancies throughout the treatment period. The patient and primary oncology team should be aware that in cases of rapidly growing tumors, expanding tumor growth may compromise the efficacy of a block. Before any neurolytic agents are used, it is advisable to perform a prognostic blockade with a local anesthetic that reproduces the planned intervention. This "diagnostic" maneuver helps to confirm needle placement and can provide information about the level of effectiveness of the neurolysis.[3] The patient and practitioner should be aware that the agents used for neurolysis have a longer time to onset of pain relief compared with local anesthetics and that the effects may not be as profound or immediate. The choice of neurolytic agent is based upon the location of needle placement, the ability of the patient to get in the required position, and the volume of injectate required (Table 72.2). Baricity may play a role in determining which neurolytic agent to use for the patient. Phenol is a hyperbaric agent that would be more appropriate for intrathecal and saddle blocks compared with a hypobaric agent such as ethanol.

NEUROLYTIC AGENTS

ALCOHOL

Ethyl alcohol (ethanol) is one of the classic neurolytic agents and was first reported by Dogliotti in 1931 for intrathecal injection.[4] Anhydrous ethyl alcohol is commercially available in the United States in undiluted (100% concentration) 1- and 5-mL ampoules. Although commercial preparations are undiluted, exposure to the atmosphere will cause dilution via absorption of water.

Ethyl alcohol injections administered perineurally are associated with burning dysesthesias running along the course of the nerve. This sensation is often extremely unpleasant for the patient and can last from a few minutes to a few weeks. To alleviate this known effect, most practitioners inject a local anesthetic preceding the use of ethyl alcohol. The use of this initial dose of local anesthetic can also provide guidance on the correct location of the injectate.

TABLE 72.2 Characteristics of Neurolytic Agents

	Alcohol	Phenol
Physical properties	Low water solubility	Absorbs water on air exposure
Stability at room temperature	Unstable	Stable
Concentration	100%	4%–7%
Diluent	None	Glycerin
Relative to cerebral spinal fluid	Hypobaric	Hyperbaric
Patient position	Lateral	Lateral
Added tilt	Semiprone	Semisupine
Painful side	Uppermost	Most dependent
Injection sensation	Burning pain	Painless, warm feeling
Onset of neurolysis	Immediate	Delayed (15 min)
Cerebrospinal fluid uptake ends	30 min	15 min
Full effect	3–5 days	1 day

The neurolytic action of alcohol is produced by the extraction of neural cholesterol, phospholipids, and cerebrosides, and the precipitation of mucopeptides.[5] These actions result in sclerosis of the nerve fibers and myelin sheath, leading to demyelination.[1] The basal lamina of the Schwann cell sheath remains intact, allowing for new Schwann cell growth, thereby providing the framework for subsequent nerve fiber growth. This framework encourages the regeneration of axons but only if the cell bodies of these nerves are not completely destroyed.[6] The pathway of degeneration is nonselective and can be observed in peripheral nerves and spinal nerve roots following intrathecal injection. Areas of demyelination can be seen in posterior columns, Lissauer tract, and the dorsal root, followed by wallerian degeneration to the dorsal horn.[7] Intrathecal alcohol injection results in rapid uptake of alcohol and variable injury to the surface of the spinal cord.

Ethyl alcohol is quickly absorbed from the cerebrospinal fluid (CSF) so that only 10% of the initial dose remains in the CSF after 10 minutes and only 4% after 30 minutes.[8] The rapid spread from the injection site means larger volumes are required than for phenol, which in turn may result in local tissue damage.[9] In the case of celiac plexus blocks, alcohol is rapidly absorbed into the bloodstream. It has been shown that serum ethanol levels up to 54 mg/dL can occur after a celiac plexus block, which may be high enough in some people to result in psychomotor effects.[10] However, following intrathecal administration of alcohol, it is unlikely that there will be significant vascular uptake.

The use of ethanol as a neurolytic agent has been associated with a disulfram-like effect due to the inhibition of the enzyme acetaldehyde dehydrogenase. Case reports include patients taking moxalactam, a β-lactam antibiotic that inhibits aldehyde dehydrogenase, and another taking 1-hexyl carbamoyl-5-fluorouracil, an anticancer drug, who experienced similar symptoms.[11] The patients experienced flushing, hypotension, tachycardia, and diaphoresis within 15 minutes of alcohol administration. The symptoms resolved 4 to 6 hours later, and efforts were undertaken to stabilize hemodynamics. Both cases occurred after celiac plexus blocks. It is important for the pain practitioner to recognize medications that may cause disulfiram-like effects, such as chloramphenicol, β-lactams, metronidazole, tolbutamide, chlorpropamide, and disulfiram, before peripheral neurolytic blocks performed with alcohol.[12]

Ethyl alcohol has a specific gravity of less than 0.8, and CSF has a specific gravity of slightly greater than 1.0. Within the CSF, alcohol is hypobaric and will move against gravity, "floating" upwards. Therefore positioning of the patient is an extremely important factor to consider when planning their procedure.

The administration of ethanol for the purpose of neurolysis can have catastrophic consequences. It has been associated with both transient and permanent paraplegia in both celiac plexus and intrathecal blocks. It has been postulated that these effects are secondary to vasospasm of the spinal arteries by the direct action of alcohol.[9] In the case of transient effects, paraplegia developed within 22 minutes and resolved within 90 minutes. The patient had good pain relief for several weeks after his injection, suggesting appropriate needle placement, and frequent negative aspirations during injection indicated that no significant intravascular injection of the alcohol had occurred. In the permanent paraplegia case the patient received an intrathecal block, and symptoms did not develop until 12 hours after the procedure. This patient also had good pain relief; however, she did not regain the use of her lower extremities. She died several weeks later secondary to her primary condition.[13]

PHENOL

Phenol is a benzene ring with one hydroxyl group substituted for a hydrogen atom. It is usually prepared by the hospital pharmacy because it is not commercially available in premixed liquid form. Phenol is poorly soluble in water and, at room temperature, forms only a 6.7% aqueous solution. Consequently, phenol is frequently prepared with contrast dyes and either sterile water, saline, or glycerin. When phenol is exposed to room air, it undergoes oxidation and turns a reddish color; however, it has a shelf life of approximately 1 year if refrigerated and shielded from light exposure. When phenol is prepared with glycerin, it has limited spread, and hence injections are well localized. In rats the aqueous solution of phenol has a greater ability to penetrate the perineurium and produce greater endoneurial damage than glycerin preparations, but there is no difference in results following intraneural injection.[14] Unlike alcohol, phenol injection has an initial local anesthetic effect. It is not associated with localized burning but instead creates a sensation of warmth and numbness. The distribution of this sensation can help the practitioner to verify proper needle placement. Concentrations of 4%–10% are typically used for neurolysis. When phenol is prepared in glycerin, it has a specific gravity of 1.25, making it hyperbaric. Preparations of phenol in glycerin are highly viscous, which may make administration through a spinal needle difficult. Warming the injectate in a heated water bath before drawing it up into a tuberculin syringe may facilitate the ease of injection.[15] Careful patient positioning to allow phenol to settle into the desired location is important and contrary to the concepts associated with patient positioning for alcohol neurolysis.

Putnam and Hampton first used phenol as a neurolytic agent in 1936. Mandl used it for a sympathetic ganglion block in animals in 1947.[16] Phenol was first used as a medication in an intrathecal injection in humans in 1955.[17] Originally, it was surmised that phenol had a selective effect on small-diameter nerve fibers, such as unmyelinated C-fiber afferents and Aδ afferents. Subsequent studies have shown that phenol concentrations determine the type and extent of nerve disruption. Dilute intrathecal phenol can produce a transient local anesthetic blockade, whereas increased concentrations can produce significant neural damage.[18] Phenol concentrations have a direct correlation with the extent of neural damage. At concentrations less than 5%, phenol instigates protein denaturation of axons and surrounding blood vessels. At concentrations greater than 5%, phenol can produce protein coagulation and nonselective segmental demyelination.[9] The nonselective effects of phenol were confirmed by Nathan et al. using histologic studies combined with evidence of electrophysiologic changes to Aα and Aβ fibers.[19] Smith has shown that intrathecal phenol injections in cats and humans primarily destroyed axons in dorsal rootlets and in the dorsal columns of the spinal cord. It was also noted to exert some effects on ventral root axons.[20] Maher and Mehta noted that motor blocks by phenol were possible at concentrations greater than 5%, whereas intrathecal injections of less than 5% produced mostly sensory blocks.[21] At higher concentrations, the extent of damage can increase quite significantly, with the potential for axonal nerve root damage and spinal cord infarcts. Injections of high-concentration phenol have also been associated with arachnoiditis and meningitis.[22]

When compared with alcohol, phenol seems to facilitate axonal regeneration in a shorter period of time. Electrophysiologic studies comparing peripheral nerve destruction in cats showed that those patients injected with phenol had returned to normal by 2 months, whereas at the end of the same time period, those injected with alcohol still demonstrated depression of compound action potentials.[23] However, another study by Smith suggests regeneration is not completed until approximately 14 weeks after the administration of phenol.[20]

It was once believed that phenol's neurolytic effects might be due to local ischemia because of its greater affinity for vascular tissue compared with neural tissue.[24,25] Racz et al. found that unlike epidural injection, tissue destruction resulted after intrathecal injection even though the vasculature remained intact in the areas of spinal cord destruction.[26] This finding points towards direct neurotoxic effects rather than effects secondary to local ischemia. It is possible that phenol's effects may be a combination of direct neurotoxic and ischemic effects.[27]

Romero-Figuero and colleagues demonstrated that vascular thrombosis is likely due to a caustic effect of phenol on the endothelium.[28] The vascular effects of any of the neurolytic agents are salient, particularly when these agents are injected in close proximity to prosthetic vascular grafts. The effect of neurolytic agents on prosthetic grafts seems to depend on the type of graft itself. Gore-Tex grafts appear to be able to withstand exposure to neurotoxic agents unharmed, whereas Dacron grafts show diminished tensile strength after a 72-hour exposure to either 6% phenol or 50% alcohol.[29] Systemic doses of phenol in excess of 8.5 g are associated with toxic side effects. These effects initially are convulsions, followed by central nervous system (CNS) depression, and, finally, cardiovascular collapse. Intravascular injection at lower doses can also produce systemic toxicity. Chronic long-term exposure may be associated with renal toxicity, skin lesions, and gastrointestinal effects. However, phenol is not classically used in long-term settings, and the customary doses of less than 100 mg are unlikely to produce any systemic effects.[1]

NEUROAXIAL NEUROLYSIS

INTRATHECAL ALCOHOL

The nerve root level of the spinal cord does not correspond to the bony vertebral level; therefore a neurolytic intrathecal block should be performed at the level where the target dorsal root leaves the spinal cord and not at the level where it passes through the intervertebral foramen. An accurate determination of the level to be blocked should be evaluated according to dermatome and sclerotome charts, as well as selective local anesthetic blockade.[30] The patient should be positioned laterally so that the rootlets (dorsal root entry zone [DREZ]) are above the injection site.[15] This positioning is necessary given that alcohol is hypobaric compared with the CSF, as previously described.[31] It is not uncommon for the patient to have difficulty moving into the correct position and maintaining it without undue levels of pain. The judicious use of pillows, towels, tape, and maximizing table positioning are prudent to ensure the patient is not at a level of discomfort that would require movement before the block is completed. The patient should also be turned 45 degrees toward the prone position. This will raise the DREZ horizontally so it will be superior to the ventral nerve rootlets.[15]

After proper patient positioning, correct needle depth must be obtained. A short, beveled needle is placed into the predetermined location slowly until arriving at the epidural space. This is best confirmed using loss of resistance to air. Due to patient positioning, the hanging drop technique may be difficult to perform. After ascertaining

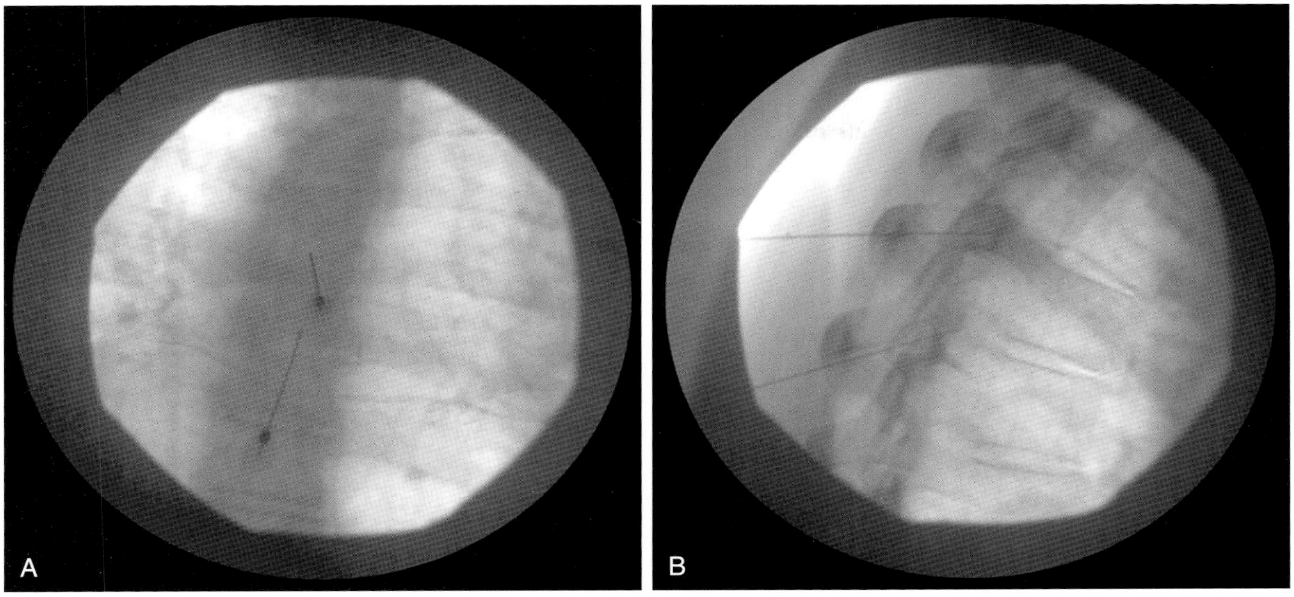

FIG. 72.3 Anterior/posterior (A) and lateral (B) fluoroscopic images of needle placement for neurolysis.

that the epidural space has been reached, the needle should be advanced slowly while aspirating continuously until it reaches the intrathecal space. Once the needle is in the intrathecal space, adjust the bevel so it is anterior to the arachnoid mater.[32] Depending on the institution and practitioner, placement may be verified with radiographic imaging (Fig. 72.3A and B) and contrast dye administration. The practitioner may then inject the alcohol, or it may be preceded by a low-volume injection of local anesthetic. Without the use of local anesthetic, significant discomfort can occur during the procedure. Whether needle placement is confirmed by local anesthetic or by the burning sensation of the alcohol injection, if the patient reports pain areas that are not covered by the primary needle placement, additional adjustments may require local anesthetic. Using a tuberculin syringe, the alcohol is injected in 0.1-mL increments, with at least 60-second intervals (preferably 90 seconds) between repeat administrations. Total alcohol volume should not exceed 0.5 to 0.7 mL.[32] After injection, the patient should remain in the same position for 15 to 30 minutes. This immobilization allows the alcohol to exert its maximal effect at the desired location, with minimal spread to adjacent levels. After the 30-minute time period, a neurologic exam should be performed. Three to 5 days after the alcohol injection, the patient's pain should be reassessed to evaluate the effectiveness of the technique and determine whether repeat injections are required.

INTRATHECAL PHENOL

The considerations that should be taken into account prior to the injection of alcohol also apply to the administration of phenol. The pain location should be determined with dermatome and sclerotome mapping and preferably isolated with a diagnostic injection of local anesthetic or contrast dye under fluoroscopy. The site must be cleaned thoroughly and standard sterile techniques applied. There are two fundamental differences between alcohol and phenol administration. When using phenol, the patient's targeted anatomy must be facing down with the patient leaned 45 degrees supine, and the spinal needle diameter must be larger due to the increased viscosity.

The hyperbaric nature of phenol in glycerin requires positioning much different than with intrathecal alcohol administration. The "sinking" of phenol into its area of effect requires the targeted rootlets to be under the site of administration. Although positioning can be challenging, a common technique involves elevating the head of the bed slightly, with the bed under the target flexed, and the patient turned 45 degrees supine. Turning the patient optimizes the dependent positioning of the nerve rootlets. As with the use of alcohol, it is imperative to optimize the patient's comfort once the desired position has been achieved. Using support devices such as pillows, towels, and foam can facilitate a reasonable level of comfort to prevent failure of the technique due to patient movement. Close monitoring of the patient as the neurolytic agent takes effect and throughout the cycle are essential because of the serious complications associated with these procedures. The feeling of warmth from the phenol is fleeting and may provide some pain relief, but neurolysis is slower to manifest than with alcohol. The phenol can take 15 minutes before it starts to exert its effect. Although there is less outward diffusion with phenol compared with alcohol, the patient should be maintained in position for 30 minutes after phenol administration. The full effect of phenol manifests over approximately 24 hours; if the block is incomplete, the injection can be repeated. A short, 20-gauge needle should allow the thick phenol solution to be injected in most situations. However, if this proves difficult, heating the injectate in a warm water bath before drawing may ease the flow of the injection. Similar to alcohol, phenol is injected in 0.1 mL increments, with 60 to 90 seconds between subsequent injections. Phenol is injected up to a total volume of 0.5 to 0.7 mL.

EPIDURAL NEUROLYTIC BLOCK

An epidural neurolytic block provides bilateral pain relief, although its analgesia effects may not be as complete as intrathecal neurolysis. Epidural neurolysis is used for abdominal cancer pain of both visceral and mixed somatic and visceral origin.[33] Epidural neurolysis remains popular, not only due to its increased safety index and the ease for repeated injections, but also for its greater efficacy on thoracic and cervicothoracic junction pain. Although the traditional technique is described later, a study demonstrated that the use of a transforaminal approach when indicated provided excellent results.[33] However, care must be taken to avoid intravascular injection into a radicular artery.

Selecting the appropriate size needle depends on the agent used. The use of phenol in glycerin requires a large bore needle, whereas the use of aqueous phenol, phenol in saline, or alcohol permits the use of a much smaller needle, in which case an epidural needle or catheter may be used. With an epidural catheter, repeated injections can be performed without accessing the epidural space multiple independent times; however, the catheter can be a nidus for infection. The catheter is a soft, nonkinking, styletted device that can be maneuvered with precision and allows confirmation of position with the injection of a small amount of local anesthetic.

Unlike the intrathecal administration of neurolytic agents, needle or catheter tip location should be chosen near the vertebral levels that correspond to the dermatomal levels manifesting in the patient's pain area to deposit the medication over the appropriate nerve roots. The injections should be performed under sterile conditions. Many expert providers recommend repeated injections over the course of several days, based on the assumption that making a consistent location choice can improve efficacy and outcome.

After needle and patient positioning have been established, the use of contrast-enhanced fluoroscopic imaging and a local anesthetic test dose can be performed to confirm proper needle depth and location. The appropriate volume of injectate depends on the level of the neurolysis being performed. Doses ranging from 2 to 5 mL are usually adequate, with doses increasing as location moves more caudally. As stated earlier, recommendations are that injections be performed daily until satisfactory results are achieved. Racz and colleagues endorse daily injections until noticeable changes in pain levels no longer occur or the patient is pain-free after 24 hours. For up to 3 days after the initial placement of an epidural catheter 3 to 5 cm into the epidural space, ethyl alcohol can be injected daily. Before each daily administration, placement was reaffirmed with a local anesthetic test dose, which also reduced the negative sensations associated with alcohol.[34] Using 0.2 mL increments, they dosed the catheter with 3 to 5 mL of alcohol over a period of 20 to 30 minutes.

Although initial relief was achieved in all cancer patients, results are less significant in patients with chronic nonmalignant pain.[35] In four studies, the results of thoracic epidural neurolysis revealed significant improvement of cancer pain.[6] Pain relief, ranging from 65% to 100%, was achieved in 80% of patients. Pain relief varied among populations and reflected the severity of disease; nonetheless, many patients were pain-free until the time of their death. In the patients who survived, the duration of pain relief varied from less than 1 month to in excess of 3 months.

Although ease of administration is a factor, there does not appear to be an increased margin of safety of epidural neurolysis versus intrathecal neurolysis. A study done by Katz et al. showed that 2 weeks after the lumbar epidural injection of phenol in a group of primates, predominant posterior nerve root damage was noted, in addition to anterior nerve root and spinal cord damage. These test subjects also demonstrated lower extremity motor weakness on physical examination.[36] In a patient who died 24 days after a series of three thoracic epidural alcohol injections by Hayashi et al., the laminar structure of the outer one-third of the dura was destroyed. However, there were no abnormalities noted in the spinal nerve roots or the spinal cord.[37]

COMPLICATIONS ASSOCIATED WITH INTRATHECAL AND EPIDURAL NEUROLYSIS

Complications with neurolysis range in frequency between 1% and 14% and in severity between incomplete block to limb weakness or bladder/rectal paresis.[1] Like most interventional pain procedures, the most common complication is failure of the procedure to provide significant pain relief. Poor pain relief can have numerous etiologies. It is not unusual for patients to have high expectations for pain relief and have those expectations not met by neurolysis. Therefore it is important for the pain practitioner to have clear communication with the patient prior to the procedure to prevent these disappointments. Another cause of inadequate pain relief may be as simple as an incomplete block that can be remedied with a repeat dose. If tumor growth is extensive or crosses several dermatomes, neurolysis may be less effective. Unfortunately, there is always the possibility that the block works well but that local spread of the neurolytic agent may have produced peripheral damage.

There are complications due to entry into the anatomic space where these medications are administered. They include postdural puncture headaches, meningitis, arachnoiditis, and neural damage due to trauma. Postdural headaches usually resolve quickly, within 1 to 5 days. Complications related to neurolytic agents include loss of motor function due to neurolysis of the ventral rootlets, loss of touch and proprioception, and loss of sphincter tone. Among these potential complications, loss of bowel or bladder sphincter tone is relatively common. The complications due to the neurolytic agents are usually transient. According to Gerbershagen, who observed the duration required for resolution of neurolytic complications, 28% resolved within 3 days, 23% within 1 week, 21% within 1 month, 9% within 4 months, and 18% took longer than 4 months.[38] Complication rates appear to be similar between alcohol and phenol as shown by Swerdlow, who analyzed complications in a series of 145 patients.[39]

Complications can be specific to locations along the spine where the neurolysis is performed. At the cervical level, damage can occur to the brachial plexus, most often manifesting as limb paresthesias. Complications at the thoracic level are less common relative to the cervical and lumbar levels. Below the L1 spinal level, injections may travel into the cauda equina, where anterior and posterior roots are not separated. This factor may make the degree of motor or sensory effects difficult to predict.

Hollis et al. documented that patients with complete obstruction of the intrathecal space have different risks of neurological deterioration, depending on the location of penetration. Punctures performed above the site of complete obstruction at C1–2 were not associated with neurologic deterioration, whereas punctures below the site of obstruction in the lumbar region resulted in neurologic deterioration in 14% of patients.[40] This complication may be due to downward spinal coning after the removal of CSF below the lesion and should be considered when performing neurolytic blocks.

Changes in opioid use may occur after a neurolytic block. Patients who have typically been on high doses of opioids for long periods of time will have reduced requirements for pain control with a successful block. Rapid discontinuation of opioids will cause withdrawal side effects; without pain as a stimulus, preneurolysis opioid doses may produce excessive sedation and respiratory depression. Careful observation of the patient in the hours to days post successful neurolysis can circumvent these problems.

PERIPHERAL NEUROLYSIS

Peripheral neurolysis is a controversial subject. Although some argue that it has no real use in cancer pain management, others have a found a role for them in intercostal neurolytic blocks to treat cancer and infrequently noncancer somatic pain. The use of peripheral neurolysis follows successful diagnostic blocks using local anesthetics. Peripheral neurolytic blocks can result in postinjection neuritis and deafferentation pain. Although these complications are unpleasant, they may be preferable to the patient's current pain, or the patient may succumb to their primary disease before these complications fully manifest.[3]

NEUROLYTIC INTERCOSTAL NERVE BLOCKS

Neurolytic intercostal blocks may help with pain that originates from the thoracic wall, abdominal wall, or parietal perineum. Intercostal blocks are performed by "walking the needle off" the inferior border of the rib. Proper needle placement should be verified using fluoroscopy demonstrating a neurogram, and/or paresthesias. Typically, phenol is the agent of choice. Phenol is injected in 1- to 2-mL doses of 5% phenol. Its effects are notable, and repeat dosing over several days is common. Most complications are associated with the agent or the location. As noted before, neuritis, dysesthesias, and pain are relatively common side effects. Pneumothorax is a potential complication but can be minimized by careful technique. Case reports described paraplegia following intercostal nerve neurolysis with alcohol and phenol.[41,42] This is most likely caused by proximal spread to the subarachnoid space.

OTHER NEUROLYTIC BLOCKS

A case report of a neurolytic paravertebral block for cancer-related thoracic spine pain in two patients has been reported.[43] In addition, neurolytic medial branch neurotomy has been described in a randomized control trial versus repeat thermal radiofrequency ablation in the treatment of noncancer-related thoracolumbar facet–mediated joint pain.[44] After 24-month follow-up, the patient cohort who underwent alcohol ablation had longer periods of pain relief based on the Numeric Rating Scale (NRS) and better quality of life reported on the Oswestry Disability Index (ODI), as compared with repeat radiofrequency neurotomy. The rationale behind radiofrequency ablation is that it is a "controlled" lesion; however, when injecting a neurolytic agent such as alcohol or phenol, this control is lost. The medication spread can be more extensive and therefore, it substantially increases the risk for adverse effects such as inadvertent root spread. For refractory sacroiliitis, phenol ablation was described in a case series of 10 patients who had prolonged pain relief.[45] There are no studies that have demonstrated efficacy for neurolysis in facet-mediated cervical spine pain, although neurologic complications have been reported with this technique.

Several other neurolytic blocks have been reported; however, evidence in the literature is sparse. These include pudendal nerve blocks and superior hypogastric plexus blocks for pelvic pain, transversus abdominis plane blocks for abdominal wall pain, cancer pain, distal caudal saddle blocks for rectal pain, and ganglion impar blocks for perineal pain.

ADDITIONAL TECHNIQUES OF NEUROLYSIS

The techniques on cryoanalgesia and surgical approaches to pain management are discussed in other chapters.

KEY POINTS

- Neurolytic therapy should be considered only after other pain modalities have been exhausted. These therapies are usually reserved for patients with terminal disease. Very clear therapeutic goals and limitations need to be communicated between patient and practitioner.
- Neurolytic blocks can offer patients the ability to decrease their systemic pain medications that can improve their quality of life and allow them the opportunity to clearly communicate with loved ones during difficult times.
- Alcohol and phenol are the primary agents used in intrathecal and epidural neurolysis. Alcohol is associated with burning upon injection so it is preceded by local anesthetic injection. Phenol injection is relatively painless and is associated with a feeling of warmth.
- Pain location should be pinpointed with sclerotome, dermatome mapping, and radiologic survey. Patient positioning for injection is determined by patient comfort and by which agent is to be injected. Alcohol is hypobaric and "floats" in CSF, whereas phenol is hyperbaric and "sinks" in CSF.
- A common result is inadequate pain relief. Proper location is paramount. Often, pain relief may require several injections.
- Complications related to intrathecal or epidural neurolytic blocks are loss of motor function, loss of touch or proprioception, and loss of bowel or bladder sphincter tone.

REFERENCES

Access the reference list online at ExpertConsult.com.

CHAPTER

73 Spinal Cord Stimulation

Shravani Durbhakula, MD ✪ Khalid Malik, MD, FRCS

INTRODUCTION

Chronic pain poses a serious burden in American healthcare that ranks among cancer, heart disease, and diabetes. An estimated 100 million adults suffer from persistent pain at any point in time, leading to striking estimates ranging from $100 billion to $300 billion in annual economic losses.[1] As opioids forfeit their place in the evidence-based treatment algorithms for neuropathic pain, pharmacotherapies available to chronic pain providers and patients become increasingly limited, and interventional approaches are more important than ever. Neuromodulation represents an essential, evolving approach to treating the chronic pain patient.

Interestingly, the concept of alleviating pain with electrical stimulation is not new and dates back to 2500 BC, when the ancient Egyptians attempted to treat pain by applying electrogenic fish to painful sites.[2] However, the first written medical reports of this practice came from the ancient Romans, who credited the black torpedo fish with relieving pains through electrical discharges.[2]

In 1965 Melzack and Wall proposed the gate control theory of pain, which links the central and peripheral nervous systems in the complex perception and processing of pain. It hypothesizes that Aδ fibers, C fibers, and Aβ fibers all synapse at the dorsal horn,[3] where they must wrestle to pass through a single-lane physiologic "gate."

Aδ fibers and C fibers transmit pain signals from mechanical, thermal, or chemical nociceptive inputs.[4] Aδ fibers are myelinated and medium diameter, whereas C fibers are unmyelinated and small diameter. Thus Aδ fibers transmit pain more quickly than C fibers (40 mph vs. 3 mph),[4] creating two stages in the pain perception separated by a brief interval. The immediate, sharp pain felt by an individual after touching a hot stove is the result of Aδ-fiber firing, whereas the deeper throbbing pain that persists after the hand is withdrawn is attributed to C-fiber conductance. Meanwhile, Aβ fibers are involved in transmission of touch, pressure, and proprioception and do not conduct pain.[4]

Gate theory explains why rubbing over the site of a soft tissue injury or an insect bite may alleviate pain. If the "gate" is overwhelmed with nonpainful input from the Aβ fibers, it should fail to transmit input from the nociceptive Aδ and C fibers. Although the aforementioned description may be oversimplified, Melzack and Wall's theory laid the foundation for spinal cord stimulation (SCS).

In 1967, 2 years after their theory was published, Norman Shealy successfully implanted a monopolar SCS lead in the intrathecal space near the dorsal column.[5] The patient's impressive neuropathic pain improvement brought neuromodulation into the limelight, and the field has evolved significantly ever since.

MECHANISM OF ACTION

The mechanism of SCS is only partially understood at this time, and more research is needed. SCS is used for a variety of indications, ranging from neuropathic pain to angina, and it has the ability to impact multiple organ systems by inducing changes in either the local autonomic nervous system or viscerosomatic reflexes.[6] It is likely that the mechanism of pain relief varies according to the pathology being treated. For instance, SCS may work differently to relieve neuropathic pain than it does for ischemic pain. In neuropathic pain the suppression of central excitability is likely the key.[6] However, for ischemic pain, vasodilation and inhibition of sympathetic outflow are more likely factors.[6]

Animal studies of SCS have allowed for some hypotheses on pathophysiology. Because neuropathic pain is the most common current indication for SCS, animal model findings regarding neuropathic pain and SCS are detailed next.

- Hyperexcitability of dorsal horn wide dynamic range (WDR) neurons after nerve injury has been found to be due to dysfunction of the local spinal gamma-aminobutyric acid (GABA) system and increased release of excitatory neurotransmitters in the dorsal horn (i.e., glutamate).[6]
- SCS inhibits dorsal horn WDR neuron excitability, increases release of GABA, and decreases release of glutamate.[6]
- SCS increases concentrations of serotonin, norepinephrine, and adenosine in the dorsal horn.[6]
- Segmental hypothesis: SCS requires the participation of only a few spinal segments, with minimal additive inhibitory signals from the brain.[6]
- Supraspinal hypothesis: A supraspinal pathway is activated. Dorsal horn neurons are inhibited by descending antinociceptive pathways.[6]

PATIENT SELECTION AND PREOPERATIVE CONSIDERATIONS

Appropriate patients for neurostimulation implant must meet the following criterion: (1) the patient has a diagnosis amenable to this therapy, (2) the patient has failed conservative therapy for at least 6 months, (3) all significant psychological issues have been ruled out, (4) a history of illicit drug abuse is not present, and (5) a trial has demonstrated pain relief.[7] However, pure neuropathic pain syndromes are relatively less common than the mixed nociceptive/neuropathic disorders, including failed back surgery syndrome (FBSS) (Fig. 73.1). In addition, many patients with chronic pain will have some depressive symptomatology, and psychological screening can be extremely helpful to avoid implanting SCS in patients with major psychological disorders. An interesting study by Olson and colleagues

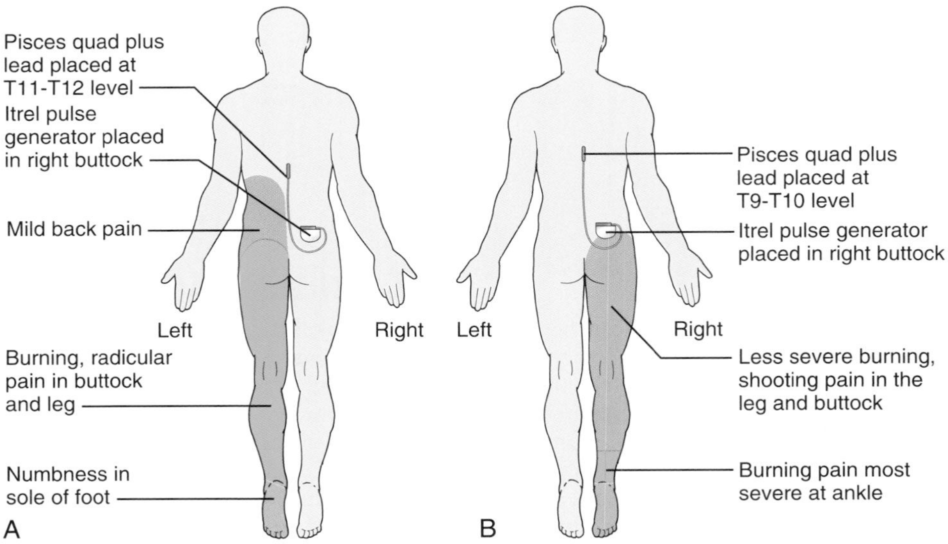

FIG. 73.1 (A and B) Ideal candidates: failed back surgery syndrome/complex regional pain syndrome. Note the radicular versus axial pain pattern. *(Courtesy Medtronic Inc.)*

revealed a high correlation between many items on a complex psychological testing battery and favorable response to a trial of SCS.[8] It is recommended that extensive risk/benefit discussion and support for patients are ensured prior to implementing an invasive procedure.

To maximize the probability of improvements in functional outcomes as well as pain, part of the preoperative evaluation is establishment of functional goals. Doing so will reinforce to the patient that improvement in pain is not the primary endpoint, but rather it is the return of functional activity.[9] Patients are often fearful that pain is indicative of damage, and this belief may limit their rehabilitation even after pain improves.[10] Counseling on functional goals has the potential to question or even break a detrimental belief system.

Preoperatively, images should be reviewed carefully for optimal procedure planning. Consideration should be given to anatomic changes in the spine and variations. Epidural scarring, previous laminectomy, age-related changes, degenerated discs, and tight interlaminar spaces have the potential to vastly complicate the placement of percutaneous leads—and in some cases may even make it impossible.[11] Severe spinal stenosis or the presence of surgical hardware may result in an obliterated epidural space, increasing the risk of complications from stimulator implant, including cord compression from an implanted lead.[11]

EQUIPMENT

SCS is a technically challenging interventional/surgical pain management technique. It merits extensive training and understanding of neuroanatomy, surgical technique, and perioperative patient care. Collaboration between the pain physician and spine surgeon is advocated for optimal success with neurostimulation. SCS involves the placement of platinum alloy electrodes into the posterior epidural space to electrically stimulate the dorsal columns of the spinal cord. It is important for the interventional pain physician to understand the equipment options available.

The SCS electrodes are of two types: percutaneous leads versus paddle electrodes (Fig. 73.2). Percutaneous leads are flexible, cylindrical polyurethane catheters characterized at the distal tip by platinum alloy electrode contacts[4] of variable numbers, lengths, and spacing patterns (depending on model and make). These leads are placed into the epidural space via needle insertion under fluoroscopy and are popularly placed by interventional pain physicians because they are minimally invasive when compared with surgical paddle leads. Percutaneous leads generally range from 8 to 16 contacts. Due to their cylindrical design, they generate circumferential current flow. This may cause stimulation of dorsal structures, such as the ligamentum flavum, and thereby lead to uncomfortable sensations.[4]

The paddle leads are flat, wide, and rectangular at the distal end. They have insulation on one side and electrical pads on the other, with up to 32 electrode contacts. Current flow is unidirectional towards the cord. Therefore the electric field generated by paddle leads is more efficient than that of percutaneous leads, and paddle leads may avoid dorsal structure stimulation.[4] However, these leads require a more invasive approach and are placed under direct visualization into the epidural space after a laminotomy or laminectomy by the spine surgeon. They have been linked in a large retrospective survey by Rosenow and colleagues to increased complications, fractures, and infections when compared with percutaneous leads.[12] However, no adequate prospective studies comparing the percutaneous and paddle leads have been performed to date. Paddle leads may be chosen when anatomy, postsurgical changes, or epidural scarring make percutaneous lead placement difficult.[13] In addition, paddle leads should be considered if lead revision is needed because of lead migration, if the patient experiences undesirable positional stimulation, or if more lead stability is required.[13]

There are three types of power source options: primary cell implantable pulse generators (IPGs), rechargeable IPGs, and radiofrequency (RF) units (Fig. 73.3). RF units, the first of implantable SCS devices, are not limited by battery life but require an external power source. The patient

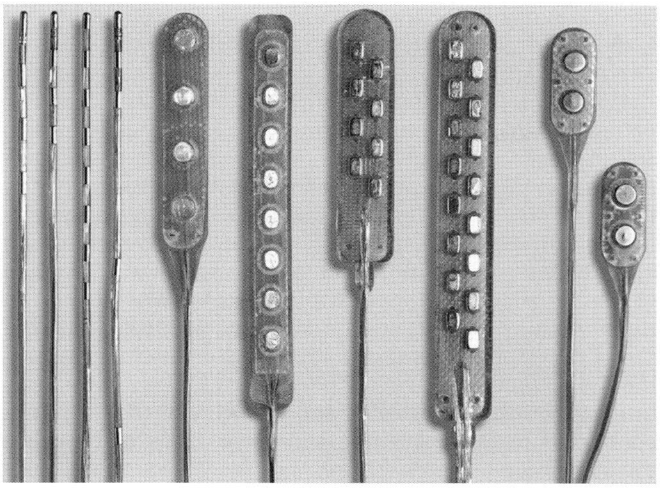

FIG. 73.2 Neurostimulator leads: (left to right) percutaneous type to paddle type. *(Courtesy SJM Inc.)*

must tape an antenna to the skin on top of the device receiver. This is inconvenient and may result in skin irritation.[13] Thus RF units are rarely used nowadays. Primary cell IPGs were introduced in 1980, based on pacemaker technology. Although they tend to be larger and have a shorter life span of 3–4 years, they are low maintenance because they do not require charging or interfere with daily activities. Rechargeable IPGs have been introduced and contain lithium ion cells with a life span of 9 years.

PROCEDURE

An SCS trial is conducted using fluoroscopy, under sterile conditions, and typically one or two leads are placed percutaneously. Prophylactic antibiotics are advocated for infection prevention, and the current recommendation is a cephalosporin, such as cefazolin.[4] Clindamycin is recommended when the patient is allergic to β-lactams, and vancomycin is the agent of choice if the patient is

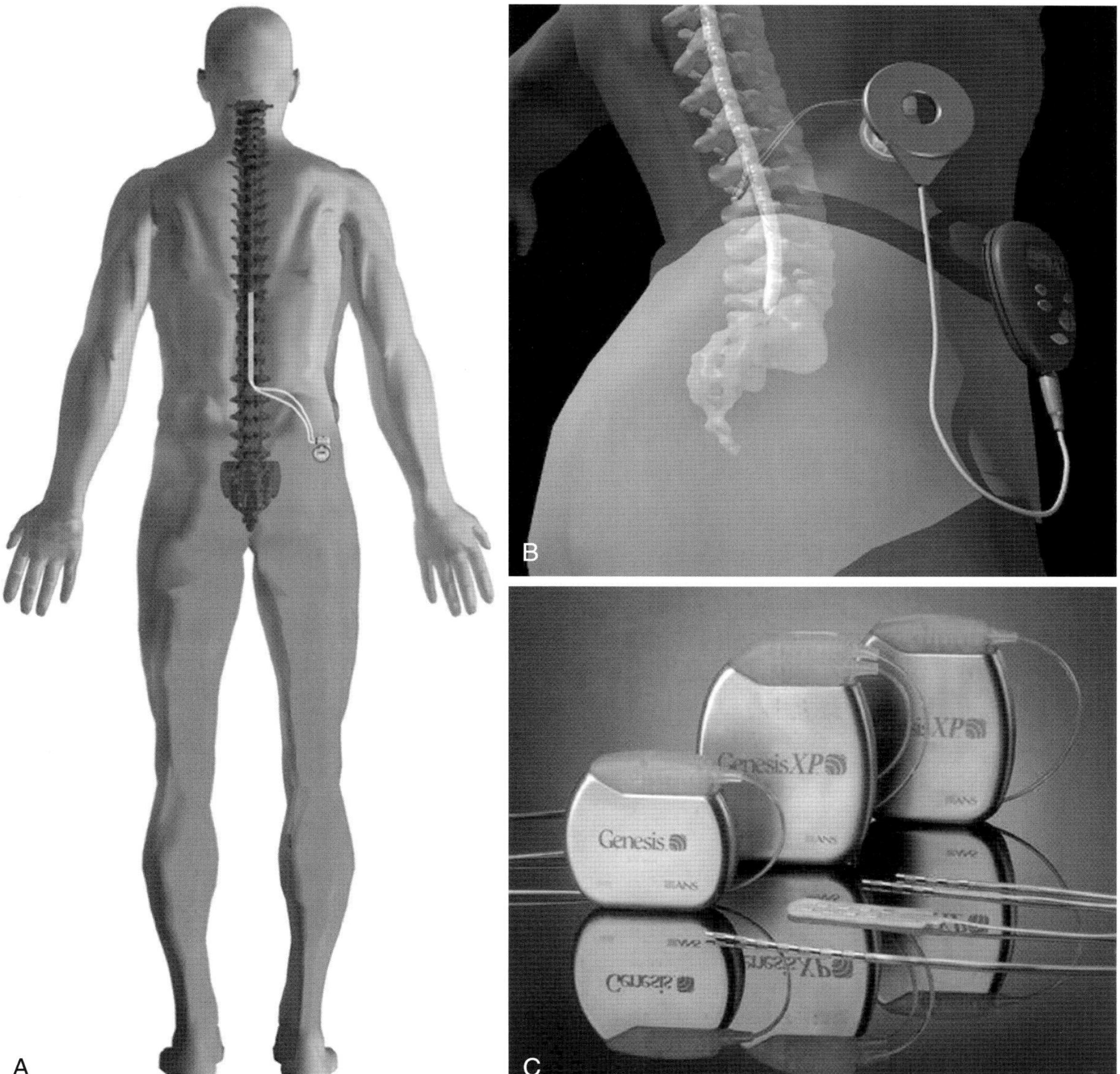

FIG. 73.3 (A) Schematic view of an implanted pulse generator system. *(Courtesy Medtronic Inc.)* (B) Schematic view of an implanted radiofrequency spinal cord stimulation system. *(Courtesy SJM Inc.)* (C) Representative implanted pulse generator neurostimulation units with leads. *(Courtesy SJM Inc.)*

methicillin-resistant *Staphylococcus aureus* (MRSA) positive.[4] After a 14-gauge 9-inch Tuohy introducer needle, supplied with the kit, is percutaneously placed in the dorsal epidural space, using the standard loss of resistance technique, the SCS lead is introduced into the epidural space through the epidural needle (Fig. 73.4). Once in the epidural space, the SCS lead is steered under fluoroscopic guidance into the posterior paramedian epidural space up to the desired anatomic location. Although two SCS leads, juxtaposed in the posterior epidural space, are most common and give superior stimulation options, single lead placement may suffice if adequate coverage of the painful area is achieved. For traditional SCS (excluding high-frequency SCS), short-acting sedatives are preferred, so that the patient can be readily awakened after the lead placement for evaluation of paresthesia coverage over the area of pain. After the successful epidural lead placement, the epidural needle is carefully withdrawn avoiding any lead migration. After the final lead position is confirmed by fluoroscopy, the lead is firmly anchored to the skin using nonabsorbable sutures and/or proprietary anchoring device and a sterile dressing is applied.

When the patient returns after a trial of percutaneously placed leads, the dressing is removed, the sutures are clipped, and the leads are removed and discarded. If the trial is successful, new leads are placed and connected to an implanted IPG when the patient returns for the SCS implantation.

Alternatively, SCS trial leads can be placed through an open wound, over the dorsal spine, using the technique similar to percutaneous lead placement. However, while the original SCS leads are buried subcutaneously, only the tunneled extensions exit the skin. In this circumstance, if the trial is successful, during permanent implantation, only the extensions are discarded and the original trial leads are connected to the implanted generator. This method has the advantage of retaining the same lead position in a successful trial, but it adds an incision at the time of the initial trial, which increases postoperative pain confounding

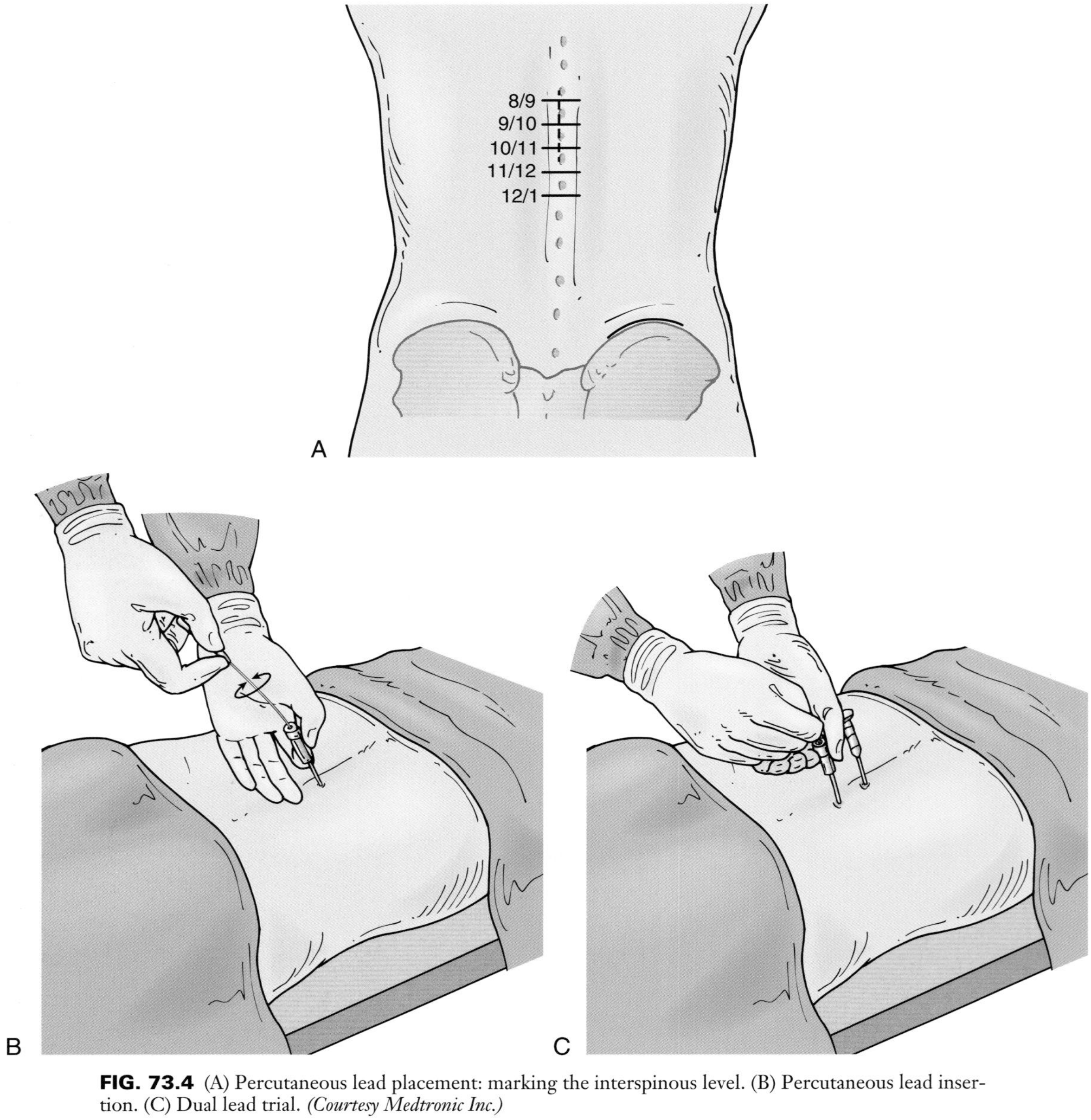

FIG. 73.4 (A) Percutaneous lead placement: marking the interspinous level. (B) Percutaneous lead insertion. (C) Dual lead trial. *(Courtesy Medtronic Inc.)*

the trial interpretation. Furthermore, trial leads implanted through an open incision may have greater risk for infection than the straight percutaneous method.

A careful trial period of 5–7 days is advocated to decrease the risk of a failed implant. Patients are encouraged to pursue normal activities, with the exception of aggressive bending or twisting to prevent lead migration. Despite careful patient selection and introduction of improved and redundant multilead systems, which gives a host of varied stimulation options, clinical failures of SCS trials remain all too common. Prudent pain practitioners therefore must critically evaluate the trial outcomes and adhere to strict selection criteria. Even though most practitioners consider 50% or more of pain relief as indicative of a successful trial, other factors, such as functional improvement, increased activity level, and reduced analgesic intake should also be taken into account.

If the trial succeeds, the patient returns for permanent lead and generator placement. The technical challenges of permanent lead placement depend on (1) proper fixation and (2) lead redundancy. Consistent and reliable stimulation depends on applying an electric field over a small area of the spinal cord. SCS leads have a limited capacity for stretch, and certain body movements can stretch leads significantly and prompt lead migration. Although sclerotic changes in the epidural tissue surrounding the implanted leads stabilize them in the long run, during the acute phase, proper anchoring is a major factor in successful lead placement (Fig. 73.5).

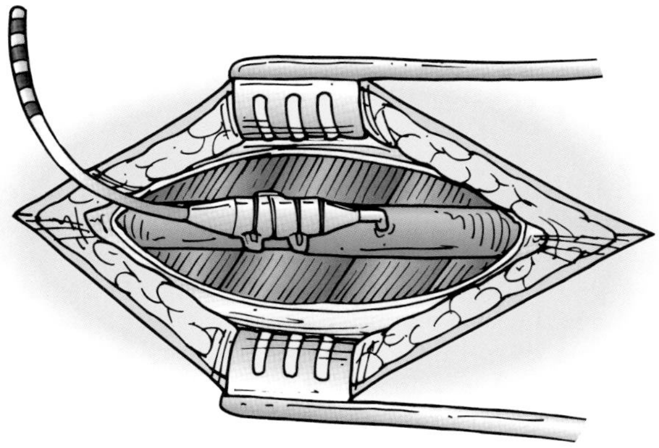

FIG. 73.5 Anchoring the lead. *(Courtesy Medtronic Inc.)*

In the event of minor lead migration, electrode redundancy is used to accommodate for minor shifts by using alternative electrodes to accommodate the desired electric field.

The generator unit is generally implanted in the lower abdominal area or in the posterior superior gluteal area (Fig. 73.6). For cervical or occipital leads, generators are often placed in between the scapula. In general, generators should be in a location the patient can access with his or her dominant hand for adjustment of settings or charging.

Placement of leads in the cervical spine should account for the fact that the spinal cord in the mid-to-lower cervical spine has high mobility, making it difficult to maintain constant paresthesias with tonic stimulation as the neck changes position.[11] This increased mobility also increases lead migration risk in the cervical region. In general, cervical lead placement involves entry into the epidural space between T1 and T4,[11] with percutaneous leads advanced to the appropriate level in the cervical spine.

In the thoracic region the spine is more fixed and immobile. This allows less vulnerability to lead migration. At the T5 level the CSF diameter is largest dorsally, and the spinal cord is smallest.[14,15] Thus stimulation thresholds are higher and postural changes are problematic when leads are placed at this level.[11]

Leads may be placed in the lumbar spine, and electrical currents directed to conus medullaris or cauda equina, when attempting to provide relief for pelvic, sacral, or foot pains.[16] With spinal nerves free-floating at these vertebral levels, stimulation is vulnerable to patient movement and can be suboptimal.[11,13]

COMPLICATIONS

Complications with SCS range from minor problems, such as lack of appropriate paresthesia coverage, to devastating complications, such as paralysis, nerve injury, and death. Overall complication rates from SCS range from 28% to 42%.[17] In a systemic review by Cameron the most common complication was found to be lead migration or breakage, which occurred in 22% of implanted cases.[17] Studies by Barolat and May reported lead revision rates due to lead migration of 4.5% and 13.6% and breakage of 0% and 13.6%, respectively.[18,19] The generator can also be a source of revision if changes in body habitus affect the source position.

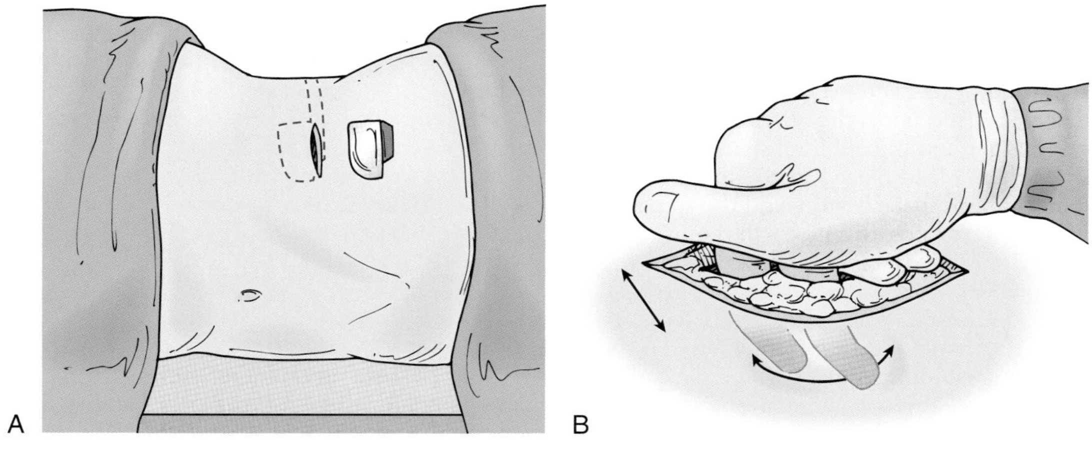

FIG. 73.6 (A and B) Permanent implant: pulse generator internalization. *(Courtesy Medtronic Inc.)*

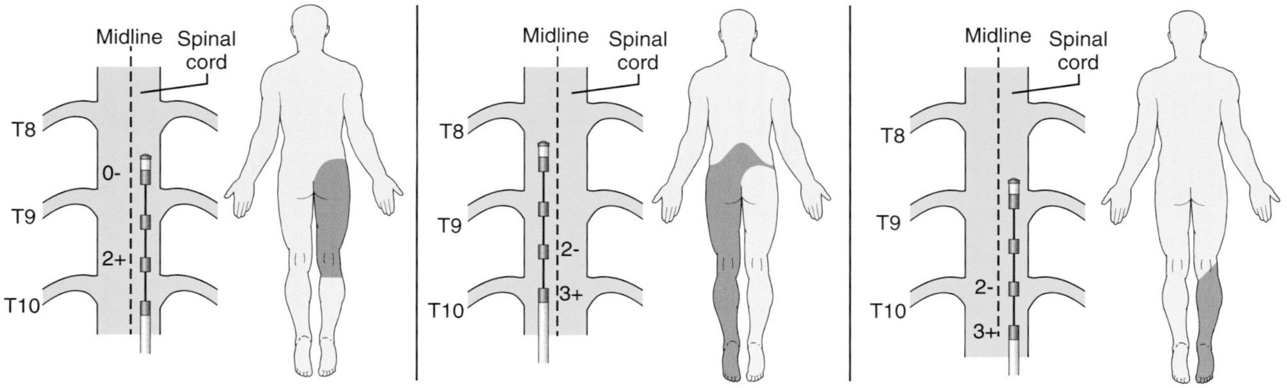

FIG. 73.7 Typical patterns of coverage using different anodal and cathode combinations. *(Courtesy Medtronic Inc.)*

Studies have demonstrated superficial infectious rates ranging from 2.5% to 7.5%, but fortunately only rarely these progressed to more serious infections (<0.1%).[7,18,20,21] To avoid infectious complications, proper sterility should be observed in the operating environment. In addition, the patient should be instructed on wound care and on recognition of signs and symptoms of infection. Many superficial infections can be treated with oral antibiotics, but more serious infection may require surgical exploration and removal of the device. Although less common, abscess of the epidural space can lead to paralysis and death if not identified quickly, so a high index of suspicion is warranted. *Staphylococcus aureus* is the predominant pathogen for percutaneous epidural catheter–related infections.[21]

PROGRAMMING AND TECHNICAL OVERVIEW

A full understanding of SCS requires appreciation of Ohm's law: $I = V/R$, current *(I)* equals voltage *(V)* divided by resistance *(R)*. In SCS circuit, voltage is supplied by the IPG and resistance is the impedance between the lead electrodes (determined by the tissues surrounding the electrodes including the dorsal columns), with these two variables determining the flow of current between the SCS electrodes.[4] Factors such as epidural fibrosis, a large epidural space or small spinal cord diameter at any particular level, and a thick CSF layer may increase resistance or impedance to current flow between the electrodes, requiring higher voltages by the IPG to maintain adequate stimulation.[4] An understanding of the anatomy of the spinal cord and particularly of the size/shape of the epidural space at varying levels is therefore important. Studies confirm that a lead placed in the cervical spine, where the spinal cord is larger and the epidural space narrow, has lower impedance than a lead placed in the lower thoracic spine, where the epidural space is large and the spinal cord diameter is small.[22] Increased resistance will require higher voltage to maintain optimal current flow. As power is directly proportional to voltage and current, appropriately manipulating these variables may allow for better power performance.[4] To date, the following factors have not been correlated with changes in impedance: age, spine surgery, number of leads, or model. However, males were found to have 21% higher impedance than women in the thoracic spine, without clear physiologic explanation.[4]

There are four basic parameters in traditional tonic neurostimulation, which may be adjusted to create stimulation paresthesia in the painful areas, thereby mitigating the patient's pain (Fig. 73.7). They are amplitude, pulse width, rate, and electrode selection.[23]

Amplitude is the intensity or strength of each individual pulse and can be controlled by voltage or current. There is no evidence of superiority for voltage or current control. However, current-control systems are theoretically more immune to changes in electrical resistance in the tissue due to sclerosis and patient positional changes. As such, mathematical modeling predicts more even paresthesia.[24] Amplitudes are variably optimized for each individual patient, but typical initial settings are 60%–90% of motor threshold.[6] Pulse width is the duration of a pulse measured in microseconds (μs). It is usually set between 100 and 400 msec. Similar to increasing the amplitude, a larger pulse width delivers more energy per pulse and typically provides broader coverage. Common initial settings are 0.2 msec.[6] Rate is measured in hertz (Hz) or cycles per second, between 20 and 150 Hz. At lower rates, the patient may feel myoclonic vibrations, whereas at higher frequencies, the feeling is more of a buzzing sensation. Higher frequencies (>500 Hz) are suggested to increase blood flow and decrease vascular resistance.[25]

Targets for lead placement is a complex topic. Barolat and colleagues mapped data of sensory response and coverage patterns based on lead location in the epidural space in 106 patients.[26] Most patients' stimulators are programmed with electrode selection such that the patient obtains anatomic coverage, and then the pulse width and rate are adjusted for maximal comfort.

Placement of the electrodes for a few important and frequently used targets includes the following:

- C2: lower half of face[13]
- C2-C4: neck, shoulder, hand[13]
- T5-T6: abdomen[13]
- T7-T9: back[13]
- T10-T10: leg[13]
- T12-L1: foot[13]
- L1: pelvis[13]

The lowest acceptable settings on all parameters are generally used to conserve battery life. Other programming modes that save battery life include a cycling mode during which the stimulator cycles full on/off at patient-determined intervals (minutes, seconds, or hours). The patients' programming may change over time and reprogramming needs are common.

SCS TYPES: TRADITIONAL, HIGH-FREQUENCY, AND BURST SCS

TRADITIONAL SCS

Thus far we have primarily addressed traditional SCS. Conventional SCS, in line with the gate theory, allows agreeable, therapeutic paresthesia to overlap the distribution of the patient's pain and thereby overwhelms the painful sensation. The IPG delivers stimuli by activating a constant voltage or constant current system and generally uses frequencies between 50 and 150 Hz.[4] The effective amplitude, which impacts the intensity of the paresthesia, is adjusted for the individual patient. This method mimics tonic firing patterns in the brain and is referred to as tonic stimulation.[27] Source-localized electroencephalogram (EEG) data indicate that tonic SCS stimulation mainly activates the lateral pain pathway, which accounts for the sensory-discriminatory components of pain.[27]

BURST SCS

Burst SCS uses unique waveform characteristics and offers minimal paresthesia to the patient. Burst stimulation delivers a train of five spikes at 500 Hz per spike, 40 times per second, with a pulse width of 1 millisecond and constant current.[28] This form of SCS mimics burst firing in the thalamic cells of the nervous system, and based on functional magnetic resonance imaging (fMRI) and source-localized EEG data, it is hypothesized to stimulate both the medial and lateral pain pathways.[27] The lateral pain pathway (affected in tonic and burst modes) is thought to be responsible for the discriminative component of pain, whereas the medial pathway (affected in burst mode) is thought to be responsible for the affective-motivational component of pain.[13] Despite the lack of paresthesia, burst SCS still necessitates the placement of the SCS leads in the appropriate location in the epidural space based on Borolat's mapping of sensory responses to electrical stimulation at varying spinal cord levels. Burst SCS has been claimed to provide superior pain control, as well as relief of axial back pain, which is traditionally hard to cover. It has been proposed to offer a rescue option to patients who fail tonic stimulation.

HIGH-FREQUENCY SCS

High-frequency SCS (HF-10) is a paresthesia-free SCS modality used for the relief of axial and radicular pain. HF-10 uses high-frequency (10 kHz), low-amplitude pulses (1–5 mA) of short duration (30 msec) in a charged balanced, biphasic waveform.[11] These pulses are applied via lead contacts positioned in the T8-T11 epidural space, most commonly with two stacked leads. The exact mechanism of pain relief with HF-10 is not entirely clear; however, based on rat and goat models, it is hypothesized that HF-10 reduces WDR dorsal horn neuron activity, attenuates nociceptive pain signal transmission, and mitigates overall excitability.[13] A study by Shechter and colleagues in a rat model supported frequency- and intensity-dependent analgesia and showed that high-frequency SCS allowed for greater inhibition of neuropathic mechanical hypersensitivity than traditional SCS.[29] HF-10 does not require the overlapping of paresthesia with painful areas; thus it eliminates the need for intraoperative paresthesia mapping and allows for deep sedation or even general anesthesia for the procedure.[13] It is hypothesized that HF-10 is more forgiving to lead migration when compared with tonic stimulation because precision lead placement in the epidural space is not necessary. The change in the intensity of paresthesia with change in body position and the subsequent need for adjustment of stimulation parameters by the patient, characteristic of tonic stimulation, is also eliminated with HF-10. This may prove key to patient satisfaction and adequate sleep.[13] High-frequency SCS has been claimed to provide superior relief of axial pain, and it provides an alternative for patients who experience painful or uncomfortable stimulation with conventional SCS.

DORSAL ROOT GANGLION STIMULATION

Dorsal root ganglion stimulation is a new avenue for more selective stimulation. Because another chapter is dedicated to this topic (Chapter 75), this will not be discussed further here.

OUTCOMES: CLINICAL STUDIES OF TRADITIONAL SCS

Outcomes research for SCS is evolving. Greater research is needed to refine the technology, pursue increased efficacy, and limit complications. Much of the initial evidence is observational in nature or are comparative effectiveness studies. This is due to the invasive nature of the modality and due to the fact that blinded or placebo treatment, especially in the case of traditional tonic stimulation with the necessity for paresthesia, is difficult. Important studies on outcomes of traditional SCS are detailed later and in Table 73.1.

FAILED BACK SURGERY SYNDROME

There are two notable randomized controlled trials (RCTs) on SCS for FBSS. North and colleagues selected 50 FBSS patients who were randomized to either repeat laminectomy or SCS, and crossover between the groups was permitted after 6 months.[31] Of the 26 patients who had undergone reoperation, 54% (14 patients) crossed over to SCS, and the 24 patients who had undergone SCS, 21% (5 patients) opted for crossover to reoperation. At average of 3 years, 90% of the patients were available for long-term follow-up and showed that, using standard measures, SCS was significantly more effective than reoperation.[31]

The second RCT was a multicenter international study that randomized 100 FBSS patients with neuropathic radicular pain to SCS plus conventional medical management (CMM) (SCS group) or CMM only for 6 months.[34] Primary outcome was 50% or greater reduction in pain,

TABLE 73.1 Clinical Outcomes Studies on Tonic Spinal Cord Stimulation

Study	Design Details	Significant Results	Analysis
Kemler and colleagues (2004)[30]	• $n = 54$ • Cohort: CRPS • Randomized 2:1 to SCS + PT or PT only • RCT • Prospective • 2-year follow-up	In SCS + PT group: • VAS ↓ by 2.1 (vs. no ↓ in PT only) • Patient satisfaction higher	• SCS for CRPS may allow for better pain reduction when combined with PT • 38% complications May reflect older equipment. Limitations: • Not blinded
North and colleagues (2005)[31]	• $n = 50$ • Cohort: FBSS • Radicular pain • $n = 45$ follow-up • SCS vs. reoperation • RCT, optional crossover • Prospective • 3-year mean follow-up	• Pain relief > 50%: • 9/19 in SCS group • 3/26 in reoperation group • SCS better than reoperation ($P < .01$) • More opioid use in reoperation group vs. SCS group ($P < .025$) • Patients less likely to crossover from SCS group ($P < .02$)	• SCS had better outcomes than reoperation for FBSS Limitations: • not ITT analysis (crossovers counted as outcome measures).[32] • some reoperation patients switched to SCS despite meeting success criteria • not blinded
Kumar and colleagues (2008)[33]	• $n = 100$ • Cohort: FBSS • Neuropathic pain • SCS + CMM vs. CMM only • RCT • Multicenter • Prospective • 2-year follow-up • 1-year results published separately (detailed in text)	• At 2 years ≥50% pain: • Modified ITT: 37% SCS group vs. 2% CMM ($P = .003$) • As treated analysis: 47% SCS group vs. 7% CMM ($P = .02$) • SCS group: Better secondary outcomes based on ODI, QOL, patient satisfaction • No difference in analgesic intake	• SCS + CMM was more effective than CMM alone for FBSS Limitations: • Not blinded • Comparison group not truly placebo controlled

CMM, *Conventional medical management;* CRPS, *complex regional pain syndrome;* FBSS, *failed back surgery syndrome;* ITT, *intention to treat;* ODI, *Oswestry Disability Index;* PT, *physical therapy;* QOL, *quality of life;* RCT, *randomized controlled trial;* SCS, *spinal cord stimulation;* VAS, *visual analog scale.*

and secondary outcomes included quality of life indicators, functional capacity, pain medication use, satisfaction, and complications. Crossover was permitted at the 6-month interval, with an intention-to-treat model, and patients were followed for an entire year. The results showed a statistically significant advantage of SCS and CMM over CMM only for the primary ($P < .001$) and secondary ($P \leq .05\%$) outcomes, except for decrease in pain medication use, which trended downward but was not statistically significant. After the study midpoint, 5 of 50 SCS patients crossed over to CMM versus 32 of 50 CMM to SCS. However, at the study conclusion, 32% of SCS patients experienced device-related complications.[34] The 2-year follow-up study results were published separately in 2008 and provided similar results. Forty-six patients randomized to SCS and 41 patients randomized to CMM were available for follow-up.[33]

There are three valuable systematic reviews on neurostimulation for chronic pain of spinal origin. Turner and colleagues completed a meta-analysis of articles on treatment of FBSS by SCS published from 1966 to 1994. Even though pain relief exceeding 50% was experienced by 59% of the patients, the authors concluded that there was insufficient evidence of effectiveness of SCS relative to no treatment or other treatments.[35] The review by North and Wetzel consisted of case-control studies and two prospective control studies. It concluded that patients reporting a reduction in pain of at least 50% during a trial and demonstrating improved or stable analgesic requirements and activity levels had significant benefit from permanent SCS.[36]

COMPLEX REGIONAL PAIN SYNDROME

High-quality research regarding SCS and complex regional pain syndrome (CRPS) is limited, but existing data are overwhelmingly positive in terms of pain reduction, quality of life, analgesic use, and function.

The International Association for the Study of Pain (IASP) has recommended that SCS be implemented within 12–16 weeks when conservative therapy does not provide successful outcomes.[11] The CRPS-I Task Force of the Dutch Society of Rehabilitation Specialists and the Dutch Society of Anesthesiologists was established in 2010 to provide evidence-based guidelines on CRPS-I treatment. After examining the available literature, the group concluded that SCS for CRPS-I led to long-term pain relief and improved quality of life but no improvement in function. They indicated that SCS was a reasonable treatment option for carefully selected CRPS-I patients who were refractory to other treatment modalities.[37]

Kemler and colleagues published a randomized comparative trial of SCS versus conservative therapy for CRPS. Patients with a 6-month history of CRPS of the upper extremities were randomized to either SCS plus physiotherapy versus physiotherapy alone.[38] At a 2-year follow-up, the patients in the SCS group had a significantly greater reduction in pain and had higher satisfaction.[30] The authors concluded that in the short term, SCS reduces pain and improves the quality of life for patients with CRPS involving the upper extremities. However, the 5-year follow-up data showed that the effect of SCS diminished over time.[39]

Several case series have been published on the use of neurostimulation in the treatment of CRPS. Calvillo reported on a series of patients with advanced CRPS treated with either SCS, peripheral nerve stimulator (PNS), or both. After a 3-year follow-up, patients with SCS had a statistically significant reduction in pain scores and improvement in return to work.[40] The authors concluded that in late stages of CRPS, neurostimulation (with SCS or PNS) is a reasonable option when alternative therapies have failed.[40]

Another case series reported by Oakley evaluated treatment response to SCS in CRPS patients.[41] The study followed 19 patients and analyzed the results using a sophisticated battery of outcomes tools (McGill Pain Rating Index, the Sickness Impact Profile, Oswestry Disability Profile, Beck Depression Inventory, and visual analog scale [VAS]). After an average follow-up of 8 months, all scales showed statistical benefits of SCS and all patients received at least partial pain relief, with 30% receiving significant pain relief.[41] A prospective, observational case series by Geurts and colleagues published in 2013 followed 79 CRPS-I patients who had SCS placed during the 11-year time period from 1997 to 2008. The authors found that 41% of patients experienced 30% or greater pain relief.[42]

Two long-term follow-up studies are available. In 2011 Kumar and colleagues published results (mean follow-up of 7 years) for 25 CRPS-I patients treated with cervical SCS.[43] They noted decreased need for analgesics and significant improvements in pain score, functional status, and quality of life. They found the highest success with patients under 40 years of age and when implant was within the first year of onset of disease.[43] Also in 2011 Sears and colleagues published results of 18 patients with CRPS who had SCS using implanted paddle electrodes. They reported significant pain reduction and high patient satisfaction at 5-year follow-up. However, the efficacy of the SCS did slightly decrease over time.[44]

A literature review by Stanton-Hicks of SCS for CRPS consisted of seven case series. These studies ranged in size from 6 to 24 patients. Results were noted as "good to excellent" in greater than 72% of patients over a time period of 8–40 months. The review concluded that SCS was a powerful tool in the management of patients with CRPS.[45]

PERIPHERAL ISCHEMIA AND ANGINA

Cook reported in 1976 that SCS successfully relieved pain associated with peripheral ischemia.[46] The results have been confirmed and noted to have particular efficacy in conditions associated with vasospasm, such as Raynaud disease. Studies have also shown efficacy of SCS in treating intractable angina with success rates greater than 80% in some of the studies.[47] The use of SCS for these indications is widespread outside of the United States. This active area of research has an expanding body of literature, and interested readers are encouraged to evaluate the literature themselves because it is beyond the scope of this chapter.

CLINICAL STUDIES OF BURST SCS

The literature for burst SCS is evolving because the burst mode of SCS allows for placebo-controlled, double-blinded trials more readily than traditional SCS due to the lack of paresthesia. Important studies are detailed next and in Table 73.2.

In 2010 De Ridder and colleagues published prospective data on 12 patients with neuropathic pain, the majority having FBSS.[51] The patients were trialed in random order with two, 1-hour sessions in tonic mode and an equal number/length of sessions in burst mode on a separate day. All patients preferred the burst mode. The patients reported significantly better suppression of axial and limb pain with burst mode than tonic mode based on VAS. Additionally, only 17% of the patients experienced paresthesia with burst mode of SCS compared to 91% of the patients with tonic SCS. At 1-year follow-up, the patients still experienced significant axial and limb pain reduction with the burst mode.[51] While this study had a small sample size and was not a placebo controlled, double-blinded trial, it highlighted the potential for paresthesia-free stimulation with burst SCS as well as the potential for axial pain relief.

In 2013, De Ridder and colleagues performed a prospective, randomized, double-blinded, placebo controlled study in 15 patients with mixed limb and axial back pain.[28] Burst SCS was studied against tonic SCS and placebo. Patients received each mode for 1 week, in a randomized sequence and VAS scores were measured. The authors showed that burst SCS was superior to placebo in decreasing VAS scores for axial, limb, and general pain. It was also superior to tonic SCS in suppressing axial and general pain, but there was no significant difference in limb pain.[28] Given that each mode was evaluated for only 1 week, the conclusions are restricted to short-term evaluation. The study was also limited by the small sample size and a skewed gender demographic because the sample consisted of 4 men and 11 women.[28]

In 2014 de Vos and colleagues prospectively studied 48 patients with neuropathic pain secondary to FBSS or painful diabetic neuropathy (PDN).[50] All had used tonic SCS for at least 6 months before the study. Three groups were created: (1) FBSS with good response to tonic SCS, 24 patients, (2) FBSS with poor response to tonic SCS, 12 patients, and (3) PDN, 12 patients. All groups were switched to burst mode for 2 weeks. Overall, 60% of the patients experienced better pain relief with burst SCS as compared with tonic SCS. Subgroup analysis showed that burst SCS allowed 44% more pain relief in PDN patients and 28% better relief in FBSS.[50] The study was not a randomized, placebo-controlled, double-blind study. In addition, it was limited by only 2 weeks of follow-up, failure of the cohort to isolate to one neuropathic pain state, and questionable washout interval between modes, potentially allowing for carry-over effects.

Also in 2014 Schu and colleagues performed a study that was similar in design to De Ridder's 2013 study but looked at FBSS patients who already had received tonic SCS stimulation for 3 months.[49] This was a prospective, randomized, double-blind, placebo-controlled study and tested burst SCS against tonic SCS and placebo. The patients received each mode for 1 week, in a randomized sequence. Numeric Rating Scale (NRS) pain intensity scores were measured, as were short-form McGill pain questionnaire (SF-MPQ) pain quality scores. Burst SCS significantly improved NRS and SF-MPQ scores compared with tonic SCS and placebo in FBSS patients who were already using tonic SCS.[49] However, it should be noted that each mode was only evaluated for 1 week, possible carry-over effects existed from the baseline tonic stimulation mode, and the study was small in scale.

TABLE 73.2 Clinical Outcome Studies on Burst Spinal Cord Stimulation

Study	Design Details	Findings	Analysis

De Ridder and colleagues (2014)[48]	• n = 102.
	  • Cohort: FBSS/PDN
	  • tSCS × 6 months before study
	  • 2 groups: responders vs. nonresponders to tSCS
	  • All switched to burst
	• Retrospective
	• Multicenter
	• tSCS vs. burst tested
		• 94.8% responders to tSCS had improved pain relief with burst
		  • Axial: burst 29% better than tSCS
		  • Limb: burst 31% better than tSCS
		• 62% nonresponders to tSCS "rescued" with burst
			• Burst may salvage nonresponders to tSCS
			• Burst provided greater relief than tSCS in both tSCS responders and nonresponders
			Limitations:
			• No control group
			• Follow-up only 2 weeks

Schu and colleagues (2014)[49]	• n = 20
	  • Cohort: FBSS
	  • All used tSCS × 3 m
	• Burst vs. tonic vs. placebo
	• Patients received each mode × 1 week each
	• Prospective, randomized, double-blind, placebo-controlled
		• 80% preferred burst
		• Burst ↓ NRS pain intensity score ($P < .05$) compared to other modes
		NRS:
		  • Burst: 4.7 ± 2.5
		  • Tonic: 5.6 ± 1.7
		  • Placebo: 8.3 ± 1.1
		• Burst pain ↓ SFMPQ scores ($P < .05$) indicating improved pain quality
		  • Burst: 19.5 ± 10.5
		  • Tonic: 25.0 ± 7.1
		  • Placebo: 33.5 ± 11.8
			Conclusions:
			• Burst improved pain intensity and pain quality scores compared to tonic and placebo in FBSS
			• Limitations:
			• Each mode only evaluated for 1 week
			• Possible carry-over effects
			• Small scale study

de Vos and colleagues (2014)[50]	• n = 48
	  • Cohort: Neuropathic pain (FBSS, PDN)
	  • All used tSCS for ≥6 months
	  • 3 groups: FBSS with good response to tSCS = 24, FBSS poor response to tSCS (PR) = 12, PDN = 12
	• Burst for 2 weeks
	• Prospective
		• Burst VAS ↓ from baseline:
		  • 77% in PDN, 57% in FBSS, 23% in PR (all p values < 0.05)
		• Burst vs. tSCS:
		  • Burst: 44% more relief in PDN patients ($P < .001$) and 28% more in FBSS ($P < .01$)
		  • No significant difference in poor responders
			60% of tSCS patients experienced better pain relief with burst SCS
			Limitations:
			• Only 2 weeks follow-up
			• Possible carry-over effects
			• Not randomized, placebo-controlled, double-blind study

De Ridder and colleagues (2013)[28]	• n = 15
	  • Cohort: Limb and axial back pain
	• Burst vs. tSCS vs. placebo
	• Patients had each mode × 1 week each
	• VAS score measurement
	• Prospective, randomized, double-blind, placebo controlled
		• All patients preferred burst
		• Pain relief:
		• Burst vs. placebo, VAS ↓ by
		  • Axial: 51.3% vs. 18.9%
		  • Limb: 52.7% vs. 11.7%
		  • General: 55.0% vs. 10.9%
		  • All $P < .05$
		• Burst vs. tSCS, VAS ↓ by
		  • Axial: 51.3% vs. 30.3%
		  • General: 55.0% vs. 30.9%
		  • Both $P < .01$
		• Paresthesia:
		  • tSCS—more paresthesia than burst and placebo ($P < .05$).
		  • No difference in paresthesia between placebo and burst
			• Burst SCS provided better pain relief for back and general pain than placebo and tonic, with reduced paresthesia
			Limitations:
			• Each mode only evaluated for 1 week
			• Possible carry-over effect
			• Small sample size
			• Sample with skewed gender demographic

De Ridder and colleagues (2010)[51]	• n = 12.
	  • Cohort: Neuropathic pain (11/12 FBSS, 1/12 PDN).
	• Prospective.
	• Paddle leads.
	• tSCS vs. burst tested with VAS during trial
	• Implanted with mode of choice and followed 1 year
		• All patients preferred burst
		• Pain relief at trial sessions
		  • Axial pain: VAS ↓ by
		    • tSCS: 1.83 pts ($P = .05$)
		    • Burst: 5.25 pts ($P < .001$)
		  • Limb pain: VAS ↓ by
		    • tSCS: 4.41 pts ($P < .001$)
		    • Burst: 7.29 pts ($P < .001$)
		• At 1 year with burst: significant pain relief (axial 58.7%, limb 70.2%)
		• Paresthesia: 17% burst, 91% tonic
			• Burst had better pain suppression and less paresthesia than tonic
			Limitations:
			• Not a placebo controlled, double-blind study
			• Small sample size

FBSS, *Failed back surgery syndrome;* NRS, *numeric rating scale;* PDN, *painful diabetic neuropathy;* PR, *poor responders;* SFMPQ, *short form McGill pain questionnaire;* tSCS, *tonic spinal cord stimulation;* VAS, *visual analog scale.*

TABLE 73.3 Clinical Outcome Studies on High-Frequency Stimulation

Study	Design Details	Findings	Analysis

Kapural and colleagues (2016)[52]	• n = 198
	  • Cohort: back ± leg pain
	  • n = 171 successful trial and implant
	  • Naive to SCS
	• Multicenter, prospective, randomized, controlled trial
	• Follow-up: 24 months
		• Responders—HF vs. tSCS:
		  • leg pain: 76.5% vs. 49.3%
		  • back pain: 72.9% vs. 49.3%
		  • $P < .001$
		• Degree of response—HF vs. tSCS:
		  • back pain: 66.9% ± 31.8% vs. 41.1% ± 36.8%
		  • leg pain: 65.1% ± 36% vs. 46% ± 40.4%
		  • $P < .001$
			• HF at 10 kHz better suppressed back and leg pain for more subjects than tonic SCS over long term.
			Limitations:
			• Not blinded
			• No placebo group

Tiede and colleagues (2013)[53]	• n = 24 • Cohort: back pain > leg pain • Multicenter case series • Prospective, open-label • Trialed with tSCS (4 days) and then with HF (4 days)	• 88% preferred HF to tSCS • 77% reduction of VAS for back pain and overall pain from baseline with HF ($P < .001$)	• HF at 10 kHz may be preferred by patients and effective for axial pain Limitations: • Not randomized or controlled • No placebo arm • Short duration • Small sample

Van Buyten and colleagues (2013)[54]	• n = 83
	  • Cohort: low back pain (81% FBSS)
	  • n = 72 for implant
	• Prospective, multicenter, open-label, observational
	• Follow-up: 6 months
		• VAS ↓ from baseline at 6 months:
		  • Back pain: 8.4–2.7
		  • Limb pain: 5.4–1.4
		  • $P < .001$ (both)
		• ODI ↓ by 17 points from baseline at 6 months ($P < .001$)
		• At 6 months, 75% with >50% pain relief
		• 11/14 who failed tSCS were rescued with HF
		• Similar safety to conventional SCS
			• HF at 10 kHz improved pain control for back/limb pain from baseline, and improved disability scored. May also salvage tSCS nonresponders.
			Limitations:
			• Not randomized or controlled
			• No placebo arm

Perruchoud and colleagues (2013)[55]	• n = 40
	  • Cohort: stable relief with tSCS
	  • Results for n = 33
	• Randomized, controlled, double blind
	• HF at 5 kHz (instead of 10 kHz) vs. placebo
	• 2-week duration
		• Mean benefit of HF at 5 kHz not statistically significant over placebo
		• Strong "period effect" ($P < .006$)
			Possible that HF at 10 kHz is efficacious, but HF at 5 kHz is not[11]
			Limitations:
			• Therapy applied subthreshold kHz
			• Short duration
			• Does not address patients naïve to SCS

HF, *High-frequency stimulation;* ODI, *Oswestry Disability Index;* SCS, *spinal cord stimulation;* tSCS, *tonic spinal cord stimulation;* VAS, *visual analog scale.*

Finally, De Ridder and colleagues published a retrospective, multicenter study on 102 patients with FBSS or PDN who had all used tonic SCS for at least 6 months prior to the study.[48] The patients were categorized into responders to tonic SCS group and nonresponders to tonic SCS group. Both groups were switched to burst mode SCS. Interestingly, 94.8% of responders to tonic SCS had improved pain suppression with burst stimulation. In addition, 62% of the nonresponders to tonic SCS were "rescued" with burst mode SCS. Thus it was concluded that (1) burst SCS may salvage nonresponders to tonic SCS and that (2) burst SCS may provide greater relief than tonic SCS in both tonic responders and nonresponders.[48] This study was limited due to its retrospective nature, the lack of control group, and short-term 2-week follow-up.

CLINICAL STUDIES OF HIGH-FREQUENCY SCS

Notable studies for high-frequency SCS are discussed next and summarized in Table 73.3. Most recently, in 2016, Kapural and colleagues published a multicenter, prospective, randomized, controlled trial of 198 patients with back and leg pain who were naïve to SCS.[56] The patients were randomly assigned to receive either tonic SCS or HF-10 in a 1:1 ratio, and success was defined as ≥50% axial pain reduction.[56] At 2 years, the HF-10 SCS suppressed back and leg pain in more subjects than tonic SCS did.[52] Limitations of the study included the lack of a placebo group and its nonblinded nature. This would have been difficult to accomplish with only one mode of SCS generating paresthesia.

Van Buyten and colleagues in 2013 published a prospective, multicenter, open-label, observational study of 83 patients with low back pain (81% FBSS), 14 of whom had failed traditional tonic SCS.[54] The HF-10 systems were implanted in 72 patients after a successful trial, and these patients were followed for 6 months, when 75% of the patients reported greater than 50% pain relief. The VAS score showed significant improvement from baseline for both back and limb pain, along with significant improvements in function (Oswestry Disability Index [ODI]) and sleep. Notably, of the 14 patients who had failed tonic SCS, 11 responded to the HF-10 SCS, and the authors suggested that nonresponders to tonic stimulation may be salvaged.[54] This study was not randomized or controlled, and it lacked a placebo group.

The efficacy of high-frequency SCS was challenged in a randomized, controlled, double-blind trial performed by Perruchoud.[55] This trial enlisted 40 patients with stable pain relief from tonic SCS who underwent high-frequency SCS at 5 kHz (instead of 10 kHz) with a 60 msec pulse width and low-intensity monophasic pulses as against placebo of 2-week duration. Data were available for 33 patients, and the mean benefit of SCS at these modified settings was not statistically significant over placebo. The results suggested that although high-frequency SCS at 10 kHz may be effective, at 5 kHz it was ineffective and its efficacy was similar to placebo.[55] As the patients all had a positive response to tonic SCS prior to the high-frequency SCS, it is possible that they associated paresthesia with the device working and that this preexisting notion could have confounded the results.[11] The limitations of this trial included the short duration and the failure to address patients who were naïve to SCS.

COST EFFECTIVENESS

The cost effectiveness of SCS for the treatment of chronic back pain was evaluated by Kumar and colleagues in 2002 and by Bala and colleagues in 2008. Kumar prospectively followed 104 patients with FBSS, of whom 60 were implanted with an SCS and the rest were treated conservatively.[57] Both groups were monitored over a 5-year period. The stimulation group's annual cost was $29,000 versus $38,000 in the control group. The higher costs in the nonstimulator group were associated with medications, emergency center visits, radiographs, and ongoing physician visits.[57] Bala and colleagues reviewed one RCT, one retrospective cohort study, and 13 case series and concluded that SCS was effective for treatment of FBSS and was less costly over the long term.[58] The findings of these studies consistently showed higher initial cost of the SCS, but the overall long-term cost effectiveness was greater than CMM.

Bell performed an analysis of the medical costs of SCS in patients with FBSS and compared it with an alternative regimen of surgeries and other interventions.[59] Even though no value was placed on pain relief or improvements in the quality of life that successful SCS therapy can generate, the authors concluded that SCS therapy can lower medical costs and on average it paid for itself within 5.5 years. In patients for whom SCS therapy was efficacious, the therapy paid for itself within 2.1 years.[59]

Kemler and colleagues showed that SCS was less costly than standard treatment protocols.[60] Even though in the first year, the treatment per patient was $4000 more in patients treated with SCS, over the lifetime the cost of SCS per patient was $60,000 cheaper than control therapy.[60]

PERIPHERAL, CORTICAL, AND DEEP BRAIN STIMULATION

Besides stimulation of the spinal cord, neurostimulation can successfully be used at other locations in the peripheral and central nervous systems to provide analgesia. Peripheral nerve stimulation was the first neuromodulation technique, introduced by Wall, Sweet, and others in the mid-1960s. This technique has shown efficacy for peripheral nerve injury pain syndromes, as well as CRPS, with the use of a carefully implanted paddle lead using a fascial graft to help anchor the lead without traumatizing the nerve.[61] Motor cortex and deep brain stimulation are techniques that have been explored to treat highly refractory neuropathic pain syndromes, including central pain, trigeminal neuralgia, and others. Deep brain stimulation has become a widely used technique for movement disorders and much less so for painful indications, even though there have been many case reports of its utility in treating highly refractory central pain syndromes.[62] Further discussion of these modes of neurostimulation are beyond the scope of this chapter.

RECOMMENDATIONS

The following (Table 73.4) are recommendations that the authors propose based on the available literature, clinical experience, and recommendations from the Neuromodulation Appropriateness Consensus Committee (NACC).[11]

KEY POINTS

- The relief of pain from SCS may be due to several mechanisms. In neuropathic pain the suppression of central excitability is the likely mechanism.[6] For ischemic pain, vasodilation and inhibition of sympathetic outflow are the more likely factors.[6]
- Appropriate patients for neurostimulation need to have the following criteria: (1) a diagnosis amenable to this therapy, (2) failed conservative therapy for at least 6 months, (3) significant psychological issues have been ruled out, (4) history of illicit drug abuse is not present, and (5) a trial has demonstrated pain relief.[7]
- It is hard to maintain constant paresthesia with leads placed in the cervical region because the spinal cord in the mid-to-lower cervical spine has high mobility.[11]
- In the thoracic region the spine is more fixed and immobile, allowing for less lead migration. At the T5 level the CSF diameter is largest dorsally and the spinal cord is smallest.[14,15] Stimulation thresholds are therefore higher and postural changes are problematic with leads placed at this level.[11]
- Conventional SCS allows therapeutic paresthesias to overlap the distribution of the patient's pain and thereby overwhelm the painful sensation.
- Burst SCS uses unique waveform characteristics and offers minimal paresthesia to the patient.
- Burst SCS has been claimed to provide superior pain control, as well as relief of axial back pain, which is traditionally hard to cover.
- High-frequency SCS (HF-10) is a paresthesia-free SCS modality, it uses high-frequency (10 kHz), low-amplitude pulses (1–5 mA) of short duration (30 msec) in a charged balanced, biphasic waveform.[11] Based on animal models, it is hypothesized that HF-10 reduces

TABLE 73.4 Spinal Cord Stimulation Trial and Implant Recommendations

Widely accepted indications	• Ongoing axial/radicular pain in FBSS (if no evidence of neurologic damage or progression that requires further surgery)[11] • Chronic radicular pain • Extremity neuropathic pain • CRPS I and II • Axial pain preferably by using burst or HF SCS • Ischemic pain, Raynaud syndrome
Contraindications	• Uncontrolled psychiatric conditions • Patients who cannot come off anticoagulants safely • Systemic infection • Unclear pain generator[11] • Unable to participate in own care • Unable to cognitively comprehend device
Hematology	• Platelets < 100 k • SCS trial and implant: "high bleeding risk" per ASRA 2015 interventional spine guidelines[63]

Preoperative care	• Preoperative antibiotics:
	  • cephalosporin (such as cefazolin)[4]
	  • clindamycin if β-lactam allergic[4]
	  • vancomycin if the patient is MRSA[4] positive
	• Obtain/review preoperative MRI to assess for anatomical changes
	• Optimize glucose control in diabetics
	• Pregnancy test when appropriate
	• Screening for MRSA/MSSA
	• Rule out active infection and treat as necessary
	• Urinalysis[11]
	• Collaborate with prescribing physician to discontinue antiplatelets/anticoagulants appropriately
	• Cardiac clearance in high-risk patients[11]
	• Determine where battery will be implanted
	• Patient/caregiver education

Implanter credentials	• Interventional pain management fellowship–trained physician or spine surgeon[11] • Has an implanter in mind before performing trials (self or other)[11] • Physicians with high rate of complications should obtain remedial training[11]
Caution encouraged	• Multiple pain generators (e.g., back and neck pain)[11] • Pacemakers/AICD: Proper intraoperative monitoring and cardiology evaluation necessary[11] • Patients requiring frequent MRIs for comorbid conditions: choose an MRI compatible system • Dominant axial back pain: consider paddle leads, burst, high-frequency systems • HIV neuropathy: look at medications and disease status[11] • Postamputation pain: unpredictable results[11] • Spinal cord injury • Pregnancy • Patients who wish to drive with SCS active[11]

AICD, *Automated implantable cardioverter-defibrillator;* ASRA, *American Society of Regional Anesthesia and Pain Medicine;* CRPS, *complex regional pain syndrome;* FBSS, *failed back surgery syndrome;* HF, *high frequency;* HIV, *human immunodeficiency virus;* MRI, *magnetic resonance imaging;* MRSA, *methicillin-resistant* Staphylococcus aureus; MSSA, *methicillin-sensitive* Staphylococcus aureus; SCS, *spinal cord stimulator.*

WDR dorsal horn neuron activity, attenuates nociceptive pain signal transmission, and mitigates overall excitability.[13]

- Controlled studies on traditional SCS showed its efficacy in FBSS, CRPS, and peripheral ischemia and angina.
- The results of studies on burst SCS in FBSS and PDN are promising.
- The initial studies on high-frequency SCS have not been uniform.

REFERENCES

Access the reference list online at ExpertConsult.com.

CHAPTER

74 PERIPHERAL NERVE STIMULATION

Moustafa Ahmed, MD ✪ Marc Alan Huntoon, MD

Chronic intractable neuropathic pain is increasingly common and results in impaired quality of life.[1] Standard neuropathic pain treatments may not be effective and have been thoroughly studied only for common syndromes, such as painful diabetic polyneuropathy.[2] For patients who fail conservative therapy, neuromodulation techniques may be considered and may improve quality of life.[3] Peripheral nerve stimulation (PNS) and spinal cord stimulation (SCS) have evolved at different rates, largely driven by available technologies with the latter predominating. However, technical advances have led to growth in PNS use for a wide variety of chronic pain disorders, such as limb mononeuropathies or entrapments, phantom limb and stump pains, complex regional pain syndrome, and regional pain not amenable to SCS.[4–8] PNS has been also tried in functional conditions such as, but not limited to, vagus nerve stimulation for obesity treatment; carotid sinus stimulation for resistant hypertension and heart failure; hypoglossal nerve stimulation for obstructive sleep apnea (OSA); sphenopalatine ganglion stimulation in neurovascular headaches/cluster headaches; peroneal nerve stimulation for foot drop; tibial nerve stimulation for overactive bladder and pelvic pain; and occipital nerve stimulation (ONS) for migraine.

This chapter will focus on PNS for neuropathic pain in the trunk, head, and limbs through stimulation of named peripheral nerves.

HISTORY AND PATHOPHYSIOLOGY

Electricity has been used to modulate pain since before the era of modern medicine, through various basic means.[3] The Egyptians were already using eels, catfish, or torpedo fish, which generated electrical discharges for the treatment of various medical conditions. Romans were prescribed contact with a living torpedo fish for analgesia, with one species capable of voltages as high as 220 volts.[9] With the publication of this book, the field of PNS in the modern era is officially 50 years old, following the original work of Wall and Sweet in 1967. They tested a small group of patients after first testing infraorbital nerve stimulation on themselves.[10] This first use of PNS was based on suppositions from the gate control theory, wherein large myelinated fiber stimulation might block transmission of smaller unmyelinated pain fiber transmission to the central nervous system.[11] Despite advances in the understanding of pain pathophysiology since that time, there is no current unifying theory of how neuromodulation affects chronic pain. In addition to gate control, suppressed firing of neuromas, selective modulation of pain-neurotransmitters, and spinal/supraspinal descending modulation are all possible.[12–15] Prolonged analgesia (minutes to hours) may occur after 30-minute applications of balanced-charge kilohertz frequency alternating current (KHFAC) that may lead to a true nerve conduction block wherein action potentials under the blocking electrode are desensitized (action potential progression is arrested).[4,16] More research is required to better understand the mechanisms of "standard frequency PNS" as compared with KHFAC.

EVIDENCE

In a prospective multicenter, randomized, double-blinded, partial crossover study performed by Deer and colleagues[8] a new technology that uses a flexible percutaneously inserted electrode using ultrasound (US) guidance was examined. The efficacy and safety of this new PNS device (StimRouter, Bioness) was demonstrated and is now US Food and Drug Administration (FDA) approved to treat patients with intractable neuropathic chronic pain of peripheral origin. One exciting use of this technology is for axillary nerve stimulation in chronic poststroke shoulder pain (see Fig. 74.1, Bioness StimRouter). In another trial of PNS, an experimental feasibility study for a novel KHFAC device was tested on lower extremity postamputation pain.[4] The trial tested various domains of pain, function, medication use, and patient satisfaction and suggested evidence of both safety and efficacy for both residual limb pain and phantom limb pain. This trial demonstrated the exciting finding of

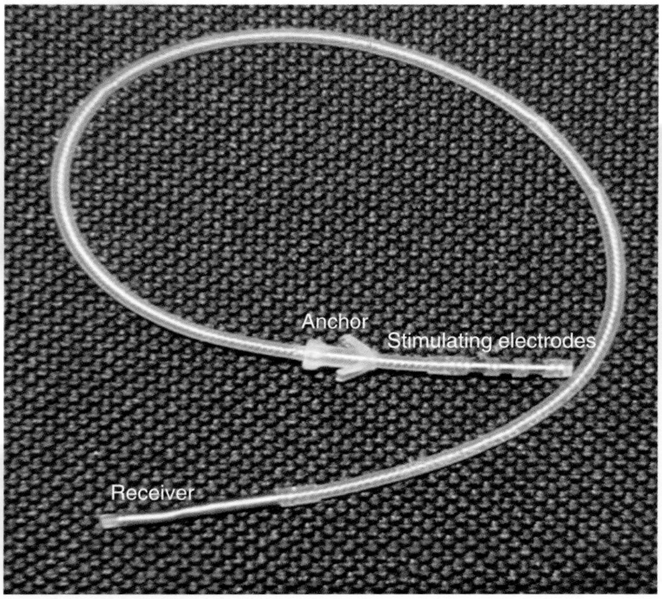

FIG. 74.1 The Bioness StimRouter peripheral neurotranstimulator Electrical Pulse Transmitter (EPT) showing Anchor, stimulating electrodes and receiver.

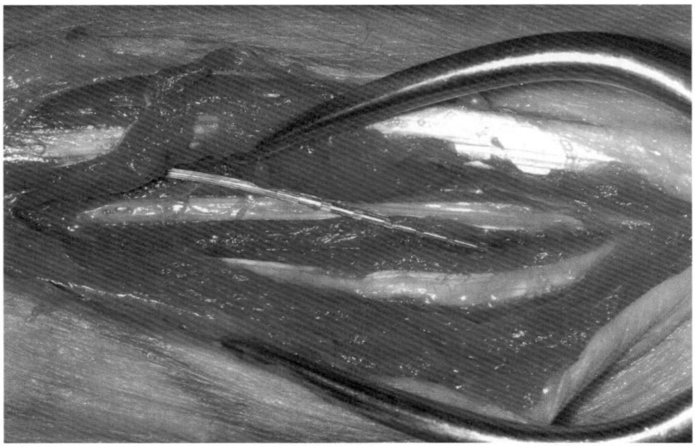

FIG. 74.2 Dissection of final placement of percutaneous electrode at median nerve in a fresh cadaver model.

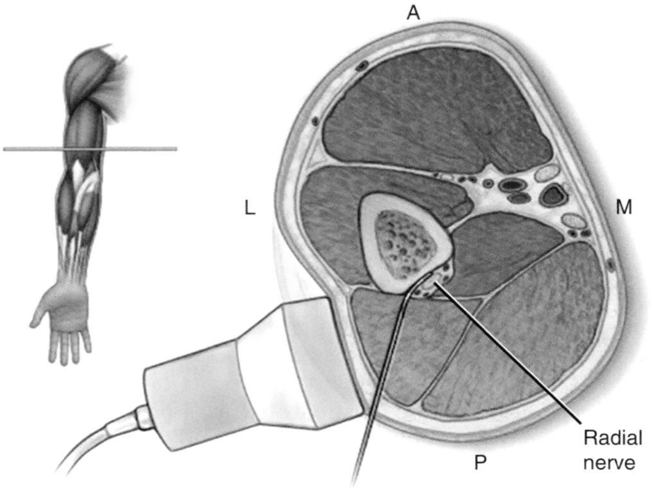

FIG. 74.3 A cartoon showing placement of a peripheral nerve stimulation electrode and needle with percutaneous ultrasound-guided technique. *A*, Anterior; *L*, lateral; *M*, medial; *P*, posterior. *(From Huntoon MA, Huntoon EA, Obray JB, et al: Feasibility of ultrasound-guided percutaneous placement of peripheral nerve stimulation electrodes in a cadaver model. Part I, lower extremity,* Reg Anesth Pain Med. *33:551-557, 2008.)*

an enduring analgesic effect, persisting despite cessation of the stimulation, for minutes to hours, suggesting that noncontinual use may be possible in selected pain syndromes.

TECHNICAL CONSIDERATIONS

For each of the limb nerves described in the anatomy sections later, there are universal considerations. Sunderland noted significant variability in fascicle number, location, and size within a given nerve trunk.[17] The complex fascicular arrangement of upper extremity nerves is an important consideration when attempting to stimulate a sensory fascicle. Briefly, a peripheral nerve will have one to several internal fascicles that routinely change locations within the nerve topography. Thus, if the desired fascicle is on the medial peripheral aspect of the nerve, it would be ideal to locate the target electrodes as close to that area as is feasible. Often, the location of these fascicles is an advantage of the percutaneous approach. An open neurosurgical approach allows only intraoperative motor testing with a nerve stimulator, unless the operator performs a wake-up test. In the upper extremity, peripheral nerves were mapped as to the variability in the internal structure of the nerves.[17,18] The key nerves of interest are usually superficial enough to be seen well under US. US also allows visualization of surrounding key soft tissue structures, and in each case, care should be taken to not pierce muscle compartments or vascular structures along the needle/lead path to the nerve.[19–21] For implantation cases the lead can be anchored to the superficial muscle fascia with a strain relief loop. As nerves will normally move within the neurovascular compartment as much as several millimeters, redundancy of available contacts or advanced programming capabilities are important (Fig. 74.2). Note that these technical considerations are merely examples and not intended to be all inclusive.

RADIAL NERVE

Anatomy: The radial nerve in the midhumeral area is very close to the lateral surface of the humerus, in a shallow groove called the radial groove (at a point 10–14 cm proximal to the lateral epicondyle). The deep branch of brachial artery runs lateral to the radial nerve.

Sonoanatomy: With the probe placed in the posterolateral midhumeral area, one will be able to identify the triceps muscle and immediately deep to the triceps muscle the hypoechoic shadow of the humerus. The radial nerve has a honeycomb appearance sandwiched between the triceps and humerus. Color power Doppler can be used to identify the deep brachial artery lateral to the radial nerve.

Scanning technique: Using linear 38-mm, high-frequency 10- to 12-MHz probe, optimize machine image by selecting the appropriate depth, gain, and focus range. Usually beginning at the lateral aspect of the elbow and, with the probe in short axis view (a transverse orientation to the arm), continue cephalic alignment (move the probe in the longitudinal axis to the scanned structure) moving the probe proximally until the desired view is identified (Fig. 74.3).

Needle insertion/electrode placement: The needle can be advanced in plane from posterolateral to anteromedial to lie between nerve and humerus. Piercing the lateral head of the triceps muscle may be unavoidable.

Potential patients could include those with posterior interosseous neuropathies or resistant lateral epicondylitis (tennis elbow) patients.

ULNAR NERVE

Anatomy: The ulnar nerve is superficial to the medial head of the triceps muscle. In anatomic feasibility studies, the nerve was easily identified at a point 9–13 cm proximal to the medial epicondyle in the medial/posterior arm.[20,21]

Sonoanatomy: With the probe placed in posteromedial midhumeral area you will be able to identify the medial head of triceps muscle immediately under the skin; the ulnar nerve is located, using color power Doppler to identify the vascular structures accompanying the ulnar nerve.

Scanning technique: Using linear 38-mm, high-frequency 10- to 12-MHz probe, optimize machine image by selecting the appropriate depth, gain, and focus range.

US scanning can commence at the elbow and, with the probe in a short axis view (transverse orientation to the arm), continues alignment (move the probe in the longitudinal axis to the scanned structure) of the probe proximally until the nerve fascicular arrangements can be well identified (honeycomb appearance).

Needle insertion/electrode placement: The needle may be advanced from posterior to anterior on the medial aspect of the arm to lie between nerve and humerus, staying superficial to the medial head of the triceps. Electrode orientation can be transverse or longitudinal depending on device specifics.

Ulnar nerve placements are perhaps the most facile of all the upper extremity nerves because the nerve lies superficial to the medial head of the triceps muscle. Caution is important to avoid injury to the medial cutaneous nerve of the arm, as well as the recurrent ulnar collateral artery.

MEDIAN NERVE

Anatomy: The median nerve enters the antecubital fossa medial to the biceps muscle and its tendon, medial to the brachial artery. The nerve passes between the two heads of the pronator teres muscle and then passes under the sublimis bridge of the two heads of the flexor digitorum superficialis. The common neural fascicular communications between the median and ulnar nerves in the forearm are an important consideration in terms of expected stimulation patterns.

Scanning technique: Using a linear 38-mm, high-frequency 10- to 12-MHz probe, optimize machine image by selecting the appropriate depth, gain, and focus range. US scanning can commence at the antecubital crease with the probe in a short axis view (transverse orientation to the arm); the brachial artery serves as a good landmark. Medial to the artery there is a hyperechoic honeycomb appearance (median nerve); continue to scan either distally[11] or proximally until the desired location is identified.

Needle insertion/electrode placement: Median nerve stimulation may be accomplished either superior to the elbow or inferior. In some cases, during anatomic testing, the US probe was placed in the longitudinal plane with the nerve to allow more electrode contact (see Fig. 74.1).

POPLITEAL AREA

COMMON PERONEAL NERVE AND POSTERIOR TIBIAL NERVE

Anatomy: The common peroneal nerve and posterior tibial nerve are branches of the sciatic nerve. Its branch point from the sciatic nerve is approximately 6–12 cm proximal to popliteal crease. From the point of branching, the common peroneal nerve follows the medial border of the biceps femoris running in a lateral and inferior direction and wraps around the neck of fibula when entering the lateral compartment of the leg. The tibial nerve is always associated superficially to the popliteal artery.

Sonoanatomy: With the probe placed approximately 5 cm proximal to the popliteal crease, there are two muscles in the medial aspect (semimembranosus and semitendinosus) and the biceps femoris is lateral. The popliteal artery and vein superficial can be identified using color power Doppler, and superior to the popliteal artery is the tibial nerve and lateral to it is the common peroneal nerve.

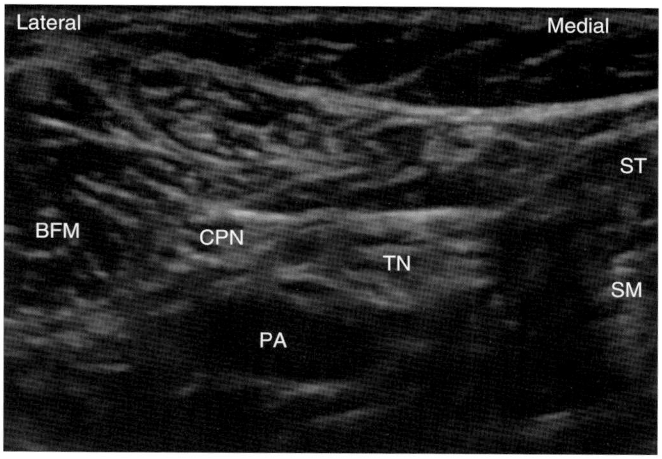

FIG. 74.4 Ultrasound image of the sciatic nerve at popliteal region with tibial nerve (TN) and common peroneal nerve (CPN) in one sheath posterior-superficial to popliteal artery (PA), medial to biceps femoris muscle (BFM), and lateral to semitendinosus muscle (ST) and semimembranosus muscle (SM).

Scanning technique: Using a linear 38-mm, high-frequency 10- to 12-MHz probe, optimize machine image by selecting the appropriate depth, gain, and focus range. US scanning usually commences at the popliteal crease and, with the probe in a short axis view (transverse orientation to the limb), identify the popliteal artery and vein; superficial to the artery a hyperechoic structure, which is the tibial nerve, is found. Then continue alignment proximally until the common peroneal nerve comes from the lateral aspect to join the tibial nerve to form the sciatic nerve (see Fig. 74.4). Ultrasound view of popliteal fossa near bifurcation of sciatic nerve into tibial and common peroneal components.

Needle insertion/electrode placement: Either transverse or longitudinal placement can be used, with transverse placement being more forgiving of movement, but a greater number of possible electrodes contacting the nerves with longitudinal placement. The needle may be advanced from posterolateral to anteromedial in a slightly oblique plane, attempting to avoid passing through the biceps femoris. In some cases, both the tibial and common peroneal nerves may be approached simultaneously, within the common subepineural sheath at the sciatic bifurcation. One must also scan thoroughly to see the sural branches to avoid injury. The popliteal area is highly rich in surrounding adipose tissue. The adipose provides a nice acoustic contrast when performing US.

SELECTED PERIPHERAL NERVE STIMULATION

OCCIPITAL NERVE STIMULATION FOR MIGRAINE

ONS for cervicogenic headache is explored in Chapter 22. In Chapter 19 the pharmacologic management of migraine is discussed. ONS has also been used for chronic migraine and was shown in a systematic review and meta-analysis to be more effective than placebo.[22] The randomized controlled trials (RCTs) that were included were either double blinded or single blinded[23–26] and open label.[27] The average effect size was noted to be modest and may have been exaggerated by bias secondary to blinding problems. The patients in three studies reviewed by Chen and colleagues were followed during the blinded portion of their study for 12 weeks then followed on an open label for 1–3 years.[23–25] One specific follow-up still showed improvement in terms of headache days, 30% and 50% reduction of pain intensity, disability assessments, and patient satisfaction.[28]

HYPOGLOSSAL NERVE STIMULATION FOR SLEEP APNEA

The relationship between OSA and loss of genioglossus muscle activation during sleep and upper airway closure led investigators to alleviate the condition with hypoglossal nerve stimulation. Published studies at this time are mostly case series. A systematic review and meta-analysis included six prospective studies with 200 patients.[29–34] At 12 months the pooled fixed effects analysis showed statistically significant reductions in apnea-hypopnea index, oxygen desaturation index, and Epworth Sleepiness Scale (Certal).[35] The authors concluded that hypoglossal nerve stimulation may be considered in patients with OSA who fail medical treatment; they also called for randomized controlled studies.[35]

ADVERSE EVENTS

Analysis of the device- and procedure-related adverse events in ONS for migraine showed that implantable pulse generator device pocket location closer to the lead (e.g., in the infraclavicular region) was associated with fewer side effects.[36] Stimulation- and hardware-related events such as lead migration, infection, and pain were less with greater implanter experience.

Abrecht and colleagues extracted the data on perioperative complications from the National Anesthesia Clinical Outcomes Registry (NACOR).[37] The registry contained 15,184 cases of PNS. The most common complication was urinary dysfunction, implant complication, defecation dysfunction, and painful bladder syndrome.

FUTURE APPLICATIONS OF PERIPHERAL NERVE STIMULATION

PERONEAL NERVE STIMULATION FOR FOOT DROP

Foot drop is common after stroke. The usual treatment is the use of an ankle foot orthosis. Functional electrical stimulation via foot drop stimulation, wherein branches of the common peroneal nerve are electrically stimulated to dorsiflex the foot during the swing phase of gait, has been tried as an alternative. A systematic review of the published studies showed efficacy of both the ankle orthosis and peroneal stimulation in increasing gait speed.[38] In the studies on electrical stimulation, the electrodes were applied subcutaneously. Foot drop after stroke is a possible application of PNS; future RCTs can examine the efficacy of direct stimulation of the peroneal nerve.

TIBIAL NERVE STIMULATION FOR FECAL INCONTINENCE, OVERACTIVE BLADDER, AND PELVIC PAIN

The effects of transcutaneous tibial nerve stimulation for fecal incontinence have been contradictory.[39,40] For overactive bladder, there have been reports of efficacy of posterior tibial nerve stimulation in controlling this bothersome condition.[41,42] The transcutaneous electrodes are placed cephalad to the medial malleolus. The rationale is that stimulation of the tibial nerve modifies the efferent responses in the lumbosacral spinal cord or it may have a direct effect on the bladder or a central effect on the micturition center. Stimulation of the tibial nerve delivers modulation to the pelvic floor through the sacral plexus.[41] Inhibition of detrusor activity may be the reason for reported efficacy of posterior tibial nerve stimulation in pelvic pain.[43] Pain medicine practitioners should keep abreast of these developments because directly stimulating the tibial nerve may provide better efficacy.

CONCLUSION

PNS is a promising "new" frontier in chronic and acute pain medicine. Studies undertaken for a variety of applications have been generally positive, although further trials are warranted as techniques and clinical applications evolve. Key questions that need to be addressed as the field moves forward follow:

- What is the long-term safety and durability of the percutaneous leads relative to flat surgical plate or cuff electrodes?
- Do percutaneous leads cause more fibrosis and epineurial scarring due to increased friction/movement?
- What are the optimal programming considerations for the percutaneous leads?
- How close to the nerve do the leads need to be to provide optimal stimulation characteristics?
- Do cross-sectional fascicle maps matter anymore with newer-generation stimulation algorithms and devices; that is, is unwanted motor stimulation still an issue?
- Where do PNS systems fit in comparison to dorsal root ganglion stimulation systems when a single nerve or territory is involved?

Pain physicians, with the assistance of US guidance, have the ability to identify important anatomy and accurately place leads. Future comparative studies and development of new electrodes may be helpful in furthering this minimally invasive technology. Some applications of PNS (lumbar field stimulation) may not require US, and other references provide appropriate technique descriptions.

KEY POINTS

- PNS systems can be trialed prior to permanent implantation with an US-guided placement. However, the simplicity of some new minimally invasive systems warrants initial permanent placement.
- The long-term safety of permanent implants of percutaneous electrodes is not yet known with certainty, but newer lead designs appear very promising.

- Although percutaneous US-guided PNS is similar to peripheral nerve catheter placement for perioperative nerve blockade, the use of larger needles, sheaths, guidewires, lead configurations, and anchoring principles are quite different. These differences mandate a very strict and disciplined approach to implementing these novel techniques into practice.
- Programming for peripheral nerve stimulator systems is changing as the techniques and available systems have evolved, such that both motor and sensory stimulation may be indicated (e.g., postcerebrovascular accident shoulder pain) and the potential use of conduction blockade with higher frequencies looms on the horizon.[4]
- A thorough knowledge of cross-sectional anatomy is desirable to avoid injury to surrounding structures when minimally invasive techniques are used.
- Adaptation of existing percutaneous SCS electrodes to PNS is less desirable as a long-term strategy unless key modifications occur with the advent of well-designed devices.

REFERENCES

Access the reference list online at ExpertConsult.com.

CHAPTER 75

Dorsal Root Ganglion Stimulation

Jean Pierre Van Buyten, MD, PhD

INTRODUCTION

Electricity has been used for the management of pain since ancient times. Perhaps most notably, the Greeks used the electric ray to numb the pain of childbirth and operations. In the Roman literature, we find referral to the use of torpedo fish for the treatment of headache and gout. Over the past 100 years, electricity has been used in different forms and applications for the management of pain.

The publication of the gate control theory by Melzack and Wall,[1] which postulates that activity in large diameter Aβ afferent fibers attenuates spinal ascending pain transmission by activating inhibitory interneurons in the dorsal horn of the spinal cord, is believed to be the starting point for the development of spinal cord stimulation (SCS). In 1967 Shealy reported the first cases of refractory cancer pain treated with dorsal column stimulation.[2] In 1989 SCS was approved by the US Food and Drug Administration (FDA). Since then, SCS has been used for the management of different chronic pain syndromes.

In a search for improving clinical outcomes and reducing complications, electrodes and pulse generators have progressively improved. The electrodes, initially applied directly to the dorsal column in a subdural location, were later inserted epidurally and even ventrally. The shape, size, and number of contacts were adapted to allow percutaneous lead placement and programmable stimulation.[3] The available data suggest benefit for the use of SCS for failed back surgery syndrome (FBSS),[4] complex regional pain syndrome (CRPS),[5] angina pectoris,[6] and nonsurgically correctable chronic critical leg ischemia.[7]

Clinically, tonic SCS targets specific segmental levels to produce paresthesias overlapping the painful area. However, the anatomic specificity is not exact, which makes the localization of the lead in the spinal canal difficult. Finding the exact balance between paresthesia coverage of the painful area and the acceptable level of tingling sensation may prove to be difficult. For example, this is the case when paresthesia is required in the foot, hand, or groin. Inadequate coverage is one of the major reasons for SCS treatment failure. Even when coverage is initially optimal, movement of the lead over time has been reported with consequent loss of effect.

Patients treated with tonic SCS may experience position-related changes in the perception of neurostimulation. Changes in position from upright to supine or prone may provoke an uncomfortable increase in stimulation or a loss of paresthesia. These changes in stimulation are mainly due to changes in the thickness of the cerebrospinal fluid (CSF) layer interposing the spinal cord and the epidurally placed electrodes.[8,9] Adapting stimulation parameters according to position can mitigate this problem. New stimulation paradigms, including the high-frequency SCS (10 KHz) and burst stimulation allow SCS without the need for paresthesias. Some reports demonstrate good results with these devices for neuropathic pain in the limbs.[10–12] Although tonic SCS has been reported to be effective in the management of different chronic neuropathic pain syndromes, difficulty in finding the correct lead placement and stimulation parameters has prompted the search for other stimulation targets.

DORSAL ROOT GANGLION "GATEKEEPER" IN PAIN TRANSMISSION

The dorsal root ganglion (DRG) has been compared with a gatekeeper, a railway marshaling station, and a highway intersection, among others. All of these terms indicate the key role the DRG plays in relaying sensory information from the periphery to the central nervous system (CNS).

ANATOMY OF THE DORSAL ROOT GANGLION

The right and left paired "mixed" spinal nerves carry autonomic, motor, and sensory information between the periphery and the spinal cord. These spinal nerves are composed of afferent sensory dorsal axons (dorsal root) and motor ventral efferent axons (ventral root). They emerge from the intervertebral neural foramina between adjacent vertebral segments.[13,14] The dorsal sensory roots exit the neural foramina to form the DRG.

The DRG is located bilaterally on the distal end of the dorsal root in the anterolateral epidural space. In humans, there are 8 paired cervical, 12 paired thoracic, 5 paired lumbar, and 4 paired sacral DRGs. The morphology of the DRG is longer and wider in more caudal locations. It typically lies within the intervertebral foramen, behind the vertebral artery, and is protected by the vertebrae. In healthy individuals the DRGs from L1 to L4 are mostly foraminal, and L4 DRG lies foraminal. At L5 the DRG lies intraforaminally or in a minority of the cases intraspinally.[15] At S1, most DRGs are intraspinal.

The DRG consists of a collection of bipolar cell bodies of primary sensory neurons surrounded by glial cells and the axons of the DRG sensory cells that form the primary afferent sensory nerve. The DRG neurons are pseudounipolar neurons composed of two branches, a distal and a proximal process, connected by an outgrowth cell body. The DRG contains the largest proportion of peripheral sensory nerves in the body. These cells are responsible for transducing visceral and somatic sensory information from the periphery and transmitting this information to the CNS. The cell bodies actively participate in the signaling process by sensing certain molecules and manufacturing other molecules that modulate the sensory transduction process.[16] They are surrounded by layers of satellite glial cells (SGCs). The DRG is not protected by a blood nerve barrier, allowing small and large molecules and even macrophages to cross the SGC wrap of the DRG neuron.[17]

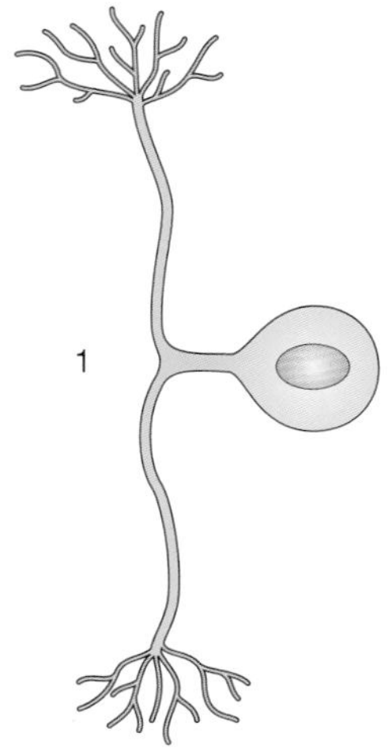

FIG. 75.1 Illustration of a pseudounipolar neuron, with one axon divided into two separate branches, one from the periphery to the body and one from the body to the spinal cord. *(From Krames ES. The role of the dorsal root ganglion in the development of neuropathic pain.* Pain Med. *2014;15:1669-1685, with permission.)*

SGCs form a functional unit of the sensory neuron within the DRG, and "instruct the nervous system what to do."[18] Stimulation of the DRG neuron triggers a delayed and long-lasting response via a pathway between glia, called the "sandwich synapse" (SS).[19] The receptors on the SGCs that bind such molecules as chemokines, cytokines, adenosine-5′-triphosphate (ATP) and bradykinins participate in the transmission process within the DRG. Glial cells change in morphology and biochemical function after a peripheral afferent fiber injury and participate actively in central and peripheral nervous system processes.

ROLE OF THE DORSAL ROOT GANGLION IN IMPULSE PROPAGATION

Primary sensory neurons start at the peripheral receptive field of the neuron, and their cell body resides in the DRG. A stimulus in the periphery alters the firing of the neuron and propagates into the CNS, beginning in the dorsal horn of the spinal cord and ending in the relevant portions of the thalamus and brain.[20] The pseudopolar neurons of the DRG lie within the DRG and have axons that split peripherally and centrally away from the soma (Fig. 75.1). At the branch point, the so-called T-junction of the DRG can act as an impediment to electrical impulse from the nociceptor to the dorsal root entry zone; specifically, it can alter the propagation of the electrical pulse by acting as a low-pass filter to electrical information from the periphery (Fig. 75.2).[21]

Thermomechanical reception occurs in small unmyelinated, nociceptive C-fiber cells in the DRG. These cells contain substance P or calcitonin gene-related peptide (CGRP), which function as neuromodulators and neurotransmitters. The terminals of the larger, myelinated A-fiber neurons are low-threshold mechanoreceptors.[21]

When primary sensory neurons are injured, Schwann cells and SGCs in the DRG release proinflammatory mediators, such as eicosanoids, bradykinins, serotonin, neurotrophins, cytokines (e.g., interleukins, tumor necrosis factor [TNF]-α), interferons, growth factors, chemokines, ATP, and reactive oxygen species.[21]

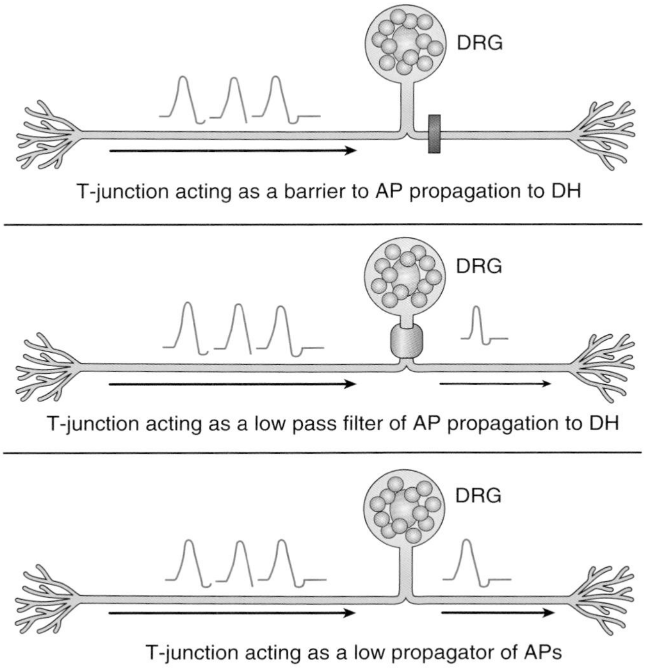

FIG. 75.2 Potential roles of the T-junction in the propagation of action potentials. *AP*, Action potential; *DH*, dorsal horn; *DRG*, dorsal root ganglion. *(From Krames ES. The role of the dorsal root ganglion in the development of neuropathic pain.* Pain Med. *2014;15:1669-1685, with permission.)*

Ion channels and receptors that are located in the primary sensory neurons have three functions: transduction, transmission, and modulation of sensory information. Transduction of noxious information to electrical signals at the peripheral terminals of the DRG include transient receptor potential channels, Na^+ channels, acid-sensing ion channels, and ATP-sensitive receptors.[22] Propagation of action potentials involves Na^+ and K^+ channels, whereas the modulation of synaptic transmission is performed by voltage-gated Ca^{++} channels and glutamate receptors. The latter are expressed on presynaptic membranes at the terminal of the primary afferents of the dorsal horn.

SOMATOTOPY OF THE DORSAL ROOT GANGLION

The cell bodies within the DRG are somatotopically organized. The topographic distribution of sciatic and femoral nerve sensory neuronal somata in the L4 DRG of the adult rat was mapped after retrograde tracing.[23] The tracers were applied to the proximal transected end of either nerve alone, or from both nerves in the same animal using separate tracers. Three-dimensional reconstructions of the distribution of labeled neurons were made from serial sections of the L4 DRG, which is the only ganglion that these two nerves share. The results showed that with little overlap, femoral nerve neurons distribute dorsally and rostrally, whereas sciatic nerve neurons distribute medially and ventrally (Fig. 75.3). This finding indicates the existence of a somatotopical organization for the representation of different peripheral nerves in dorsal root ganglia of adult animals.[23] Theoretically, this makes it possible for precision targeting.

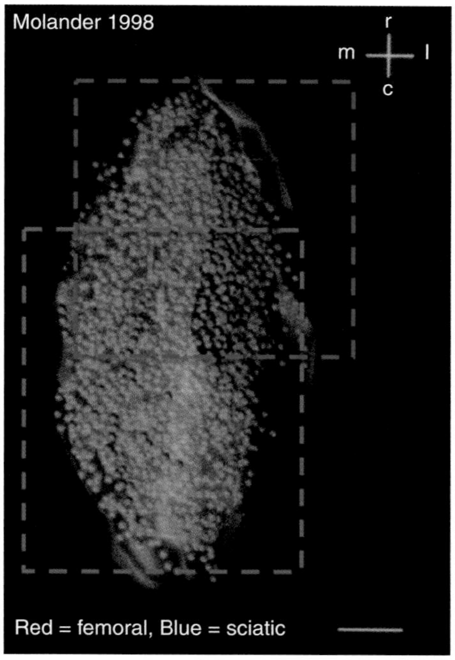

FIG. 75.3 Somatotopic organization of the rat sciatic nerve neurons. *(From Puigdellívol-Sanchez A, Prats-Galino A, Ruano-Gil D, Molander C. Sciatic and femoral nerve sensory neurones occupy different regions of the L4 dorsal root ganglion in the adult rat.* Neurosci Lett. *1998;251:169-172.)*

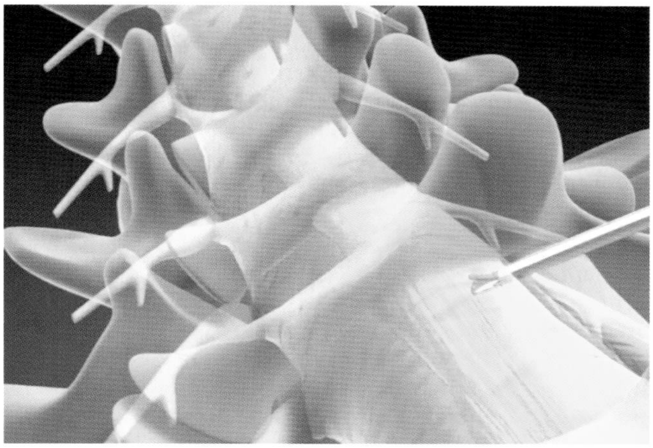

FIG. 75.4 Schematic representation of the epidural space giving access to the dorsal root ganglion.

DORSAL ROOT GANGLION AS TARGET FOR THE TREATMENT OF CHRONIC PAIN

The accessibility of the DRG and its critical role in the transmission and transduction of pain make it a preferred target for the treatment of chronic pain (Fig. 75.4).

DORSAL ROOT GANGLIONECTOMY

Dorsal root ganglionectomy was popular during the 1960s and 1970s. However, this technique has some limitations, which has curtailed its use. It requires open surgery and far lateral laminectomy and foraminotomy to expose the DRG. Even in settings of one level radicular pain, a single-level ganglionectomy is seldom efficacious because of the fact that peripheral pain afferents send fibers to multiple adjacent DRGs.[24] It has therefore been suggested that to improve outcomes, the DRG that somatotopically matches the pain distribution as well as ganglia rostal and caudal should be resected. This makes the procedure a large, multilevel, and potentially morbid operation. The outcomes for ganglionectomy have mainly been reported in case series and retrospective studies for the management of neuropathic pain conditions such as CRPS, chest wall pain, monoradicular sciatica, occipital neuralgia, and cervicogenic headache with a neuropathic component.[24] The quality of these studies does not allow one to formulate firm conclusions regarding the effectiveness of this intervention for the treatment of intractable pain. As alluded to earlier, a single-level ganglionectomy is not sufficient to control the pain because of convergence of sensory inputs. The complications of ganglionectomy include the occurrence of deafferentation pain, dysthesias, allodynia, and even CRPS.[25–27]

RADIOFREQUENCY TECHNIQUES ADJACENT TO THE DORSAL ROOT GANGLION

Radiofrequency (RF) treatment consists of the application of a high-frequency electrical current close to a nerve(s) or ganglion. The high-frequency current generates heat, which in turn results in destruction of the nerve tissue. RF treatment was initially thought to be selective for the small Aδ fibers. Several studies have evaluated conventional RF for the treatment of radicular pain. A well-designed randomized controlled trial failed to demonstrate the superiority of RF treatment compared with placebo for the management of lumbosacral radicular pain.[28] However, a smaller, earlier randomized controlled trial evaluating RF treatment adjacent to the cervical DRG showed a positive effect compared with placebo.[29] Another trial compared RF treatment at 67°C with RF treatment at 40°C and found clinical improvement in both groups.[30]

The possibility of heat-induced large nerve lesions resulting in deafferentation pain led to the development of pulsed radiofrequency (PRF), whereby the high-frequency current is applied in short bursts followed by a longer silent period. This allows for dissipation of the heat, thereby maintaining the electrode tip below the neuroablative temperature of 42°C. In a small, double-blind study performed in patients with chronic cervical radicular pain, PRF treatment adjacent to the cervical DRG was found to be superior to sham RF.[31] An uncontrolled, prospective study evaluating the treatment of lumbosacral radicular pain with PRF treatment adjacent to the lumbar DRG demonstrated a good clinical outcome in more than 50% of patients, lasting until 6 months after treatment.[32]

NEUROSTIMULATION OF THE DORSAL ROOT GANGLION

Neurostimulation is a minimally invasive, reversible treatment for chronic pain. Over the years the value of SCS for the treatment of chronic neuropathic pain syndromes has been documented in randomized controlled trials[33–35] and prospective and retrospective studies.

The drawbacks to this treatment option include the following:

- Some patients experience only partly or even no reduction in their pain.
- Achieving satisfactory paresthesia coverage of the painful area may be difficult.
- Even when paresthesia coverage is initially achieved, the lead may be displaced over time.
- Patients may experience position-related changes in stimulation that is bothersome and requires the stimulation program to be adjusted.

Stimulation of the DRG is an appealing alternative to SCS because stimulation at this site involves spinal and supraspinal mechanisms dependent on Aβ fibers. The DRG contains sensory neuron somata for all sensory modalities and fiber types, and stimulation of the sensory afferent units allows direct modulation of Aδ- and C-fibers. Sensory neuron stimulation diminishes neuronal excitability, thus interfering with pain pathogenesis.

IN VITRO STUDIES

In vitro studies have shown that ganglion field stimulation at 30 V or more generates an immediate response and elevated Ca^{++} levels throughout the treatment period, which returns to baseline, occurred within 60 seconds of terminating stimulation.[36]

Ganglion field stimulation suppresses action potential firing, which is maintained throughout the stimulation period.[36] The conduction velocity of slow-conducting fibers is significantly reduced after ganglion field stimulation. It has been speculated that clinical electrical stimulation of the DRG activates sensory neurons, causing Ca^{++} influx that triggers Ca^{++}-dependent processes, which in turn leads to decreased somatic excitability and increased filtration of high-frequency afferent action potential trains. This, combined with dorsal horn modulation of nociceptor input from activation of low-threshold units, may produce beneficial effects in humans with chronic pain.

DORSAL ROOT GANGLION STIMULATION IN HUMANS

TECHNICAL ASPECTS

The characteristics of the DRG and findings from in vitro pain models make it a logical target for neurostimulation. Case reports on cervicogenic headache, postherpetic neuralgia and discogenic pain describe significant pain reduction.[37,38] However, the conventional equipment used for midline dorsal column stimulation is not readily adaptable to placement at the DRG. The leads must be manually curved, and the dimensions, rigidity, and spaces between contacts may compress the DRG, thereby recruiting unwanted targets, including the dorsal root entry zone (DREZ) and motor fibers. Moreover, traditional epidural equipment often results in motor stimulation.[39] Therefore specialized and modified equipment are required.

The lead should be flexible and its form adapted to the curve of the DRG. The space between the contacts should allow adapted somatotopic stimulation and the system must enable the practitioner to make incremental changes in stimulation output so as to allow fine adjustments in current delivered to neural tissues. Considering the dermatomal and segmented anatomic distribution of sensory afferents, the pulse generator should allow multiple leads to be connected.

The St. Jude Medical Axium neurostimulator system consists of a stimulator device (an external trial neurostimulator [TNS] that is used for the trial period, followed by an implanted neurostimulator [INS] if successful), and up to four quadripolar percutaneous leads and wireless patient- and clinician-programmer devices. Both TNS and INS are constant voltage devices.

Under monitored sedation, leads are placed via an epidural approach, with access gained using the loss-of-resistance technique standard for this type of intervention. Leads are advanced in an anterograde or retrograde fashion and then steered under fluoroscopic guidance into the intervertebral foramen near the DRG. Appropriate lead position is determined through intraoperative device programming after the patient is awakened to confirm paresthesia overlap with the painful regions. If pain-paresthesia overlap is not achieved through programming, the leads are repositioned under fluoroscopy and programmed again. The DRG is in a consistent location anatomically; thus lead position should accurately reflect the ability to stimulate the ganglion. Due to the fact that cell bodies are present in the ganglion and not in the nerve root, and because many membrane alterations occur in the cell bodies of primary sensory neurons and not nerve roots, there are electrophysiologic differences between these structures. In part, generating an electrical field around a ganglion provides an enhanced ability to provide acute and specific subdermatomal coverage compared with a nerve root. Although prior investigators had tried DRG stimulation, there were limitations in both the logistics of lead placement, as well as the ability to provide tailored stimulation therapy.

There is a steep learning curve involved with the placement of DRG leads. Entry into the neuroforamen can be difficult, depending on the level at which one is implanting the lead. For example, entering the L4-5 or L5-S1 neuroforamen can be challenging in patients with foraminal stenosis or degenerative disc disease. Therefore many investigators perform the trial using an extension lead that can be converted to a permanent lead. Based on patient feedback on paresthesia coverage of the painful area during the procedure, the external nerve stimulator is programmed. The second phase consists of connecting the lead to the battery with or without an extension lead, depending on where the pocket site is (i.e., gluteal or abdominal). When strain relief loops are used, there is no need to anchor the lead (Figs. 75.5–75.9).

CLINICAL RESULTS

A pilot study in 10 patients with chronic back and extremity pain showed that DRG stimulation reduced pain by at least 30% in almost 90% of patients (Table 75.1).[40] More than 70% of patients reduced their consumption of analgesic medications. The authors observed pain relief in specific anatomic regions such as the leg, back, and foot that are typically difficult to cover with SCS.[40]

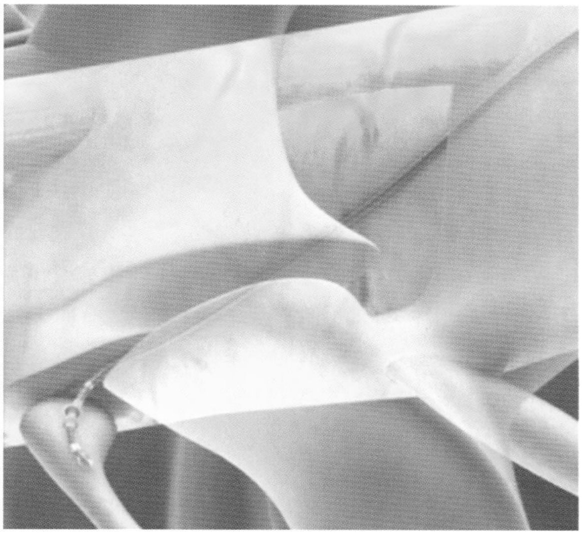

FIG. 75.5 Schematic representation of the lead position on the DRG. *DRG*, Dorsal root ganglion.

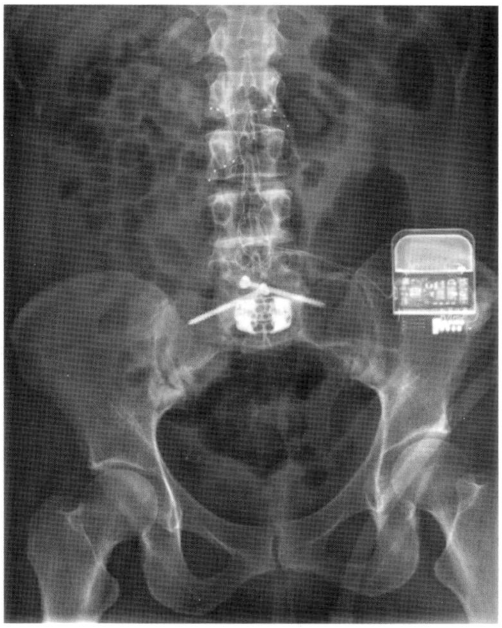

FIG. 75.6 DRG stimulation (three leads) for the management of failed back surgery syndrome. *DRG*, Dorsal root ganglion.

In a multicenter prospective study, 51 patients with chronic intractable pain underwent trial implantation.[41] At the end of the trial period, 39 reported more than 50% pain relief. Seven patients did not proceed to implanted stimulation. Two did not provide a reason for refusal, in one patient the pain did not recur after the trial, another patient had 100% pain relief in one foot but none in the other, and three patients were withdrawn for unrelated medical reasons. Therefore 32 patients received an implanted stimulator. All had chronic neuropathic pain of varying etiology, with the most frequent diagnoses being FBSS and CRPS involving anatomic regions. One week after permanent implantation, the patients' average pain was reduced from 77.6 mm (baseline) to 34.9 mm on a

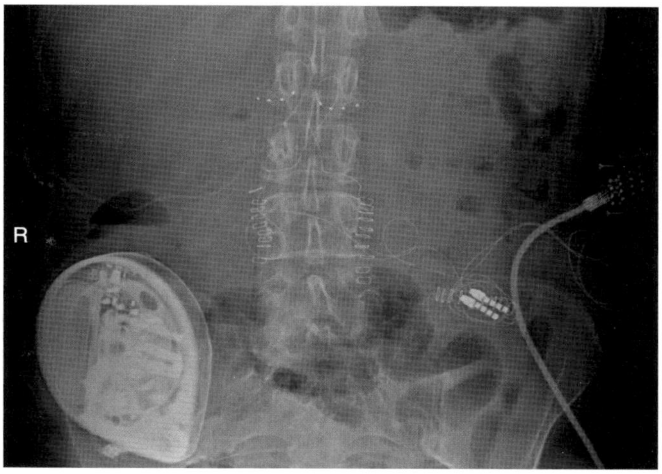

FIG. 75.7 Bilateral DRG stimulation for a patient who failed intrathecal therapy. *DRG*, Dorsal root ganglion.

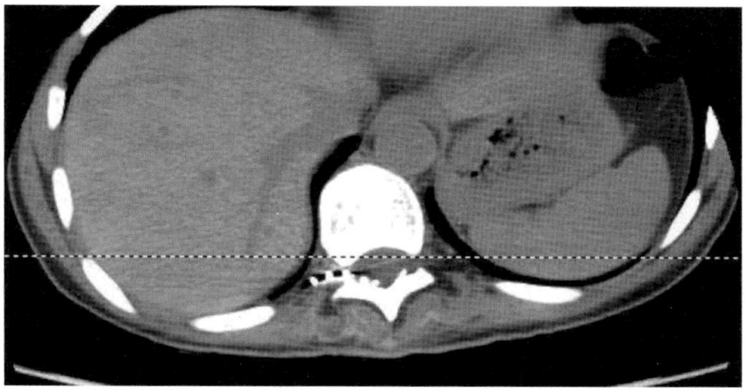

FIG. 75.8 Computed tomography scan of the lead for DRG stimulation. *DRG*, Dorsal root ganglion.

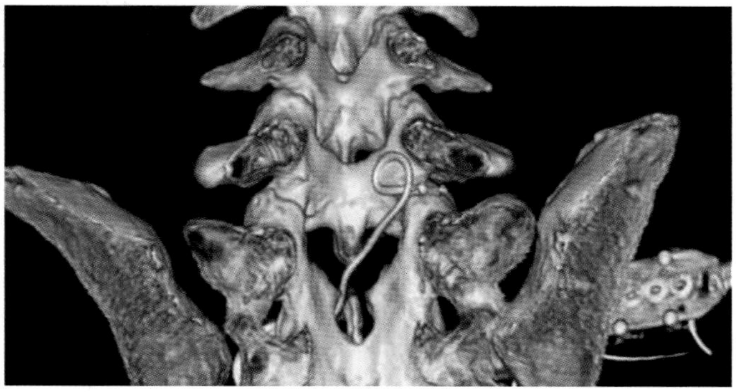

FIG. 75.9 Three-dimensional reconstruction of the spine with the lead for DRG stimulation in place based on the computed tomography scan (note the strain relief loop). *DRG*, Dorsal root ganglion.

100-mm VAS pain scale, with the average pain at 4 weeks being 36.6 mm. At the 4-week assessment, stimulation was suspended to verify intrasubject effectiveness. After 1 week without stimulation the patients reported that the overall pain returned to near-baseline levels. Stimulation was then restored and at 3 months post implant the average pain score was 38.4. At 6 months, pain relief continued to be maintained, with the mean pain score declining slightly to 33.5.[41]

TABLE 75.1 Selected Studies on Dorsal Root Ganglion Stimulation for Pain Control

Study	Intervention	Results	Comments
Deer et al.,[40] P, M; 10 patients, chronic intractable pain (DPN, LBP, PHN, peripheral neuropathy)	Study of a trial period of stimulation. Two to four leads inserted towards the lateral epidural space, near the DRG.	One patient dropped out due to illness. An average of 70% reduction in pain; 8 of 9 patients had >30% reduction of pain; 7 of 9 patients reduced their pain medication.	Adverse events included increased pain, device inactivation, lead migration, reaction to antibiotic.
Liem et al.,[41] P, M, 32 patients with chronic intractable pain (CRPS, FBSS, LBP, postsurgery pain)	Patients followed up for 6 months.	More than half of patients had 50% or better pain relief. At 6 months, overall pain ratings were 58% lower than baseline.	Pain returned to baseline when device was turned off. Paresthesia intensity not affected by body posture or position.
Liem et al.,[41] P, M, 32 patients (same patients as above but follow-up at 12 months)	Follow-up at 12 months	Overall pain reduction of 56%, 60% reported greater than 50% relief. QoL and mood improved.	DRG-SCS appears to be comparable to traditional SCS.
Van Buyten et al.,[42] P, CS, 11 patients with CRPS	8 of 11 patients had successful permanent implantation	All 8 patients experienced relief. At 1 month, average reduction in pain to 62% of baseline values; relief lasted 12 months.	Edema, trophic changes, and function improved in some patients.
Schu et al.,[43] R; 29 patients with groin pain herniorraphy, FBSS, femoral vascular access, other surgery	Leads implanted at DRGs between T12 and L4. Patients with >50% relief had permanent implantation.	25 patients had permanent implantation; average follow-up of 27.8 ± 4.3 weeks; average pain reduction of 71.4 ± 5.6%; 86% experienced >50% reduction of pain	Subanalysis of postherniorraphy cohort showed significant improvement.
Eldabe et al.,[44] R; 8 patients with phantom limb pain	After satisfactory response to a trial, implantation was performed.	At follow-up (average: 14.4 months), pain rating decreased from 85.5 to 43.5 mm. QoL and functional capacity improved.	Some patients reduced/eliminated their pain medication. Three patients had diminution of their pain relief.

CRPS, *Complex regional pain syndrome;* CS, *case series;* DPN, *diabetic painful neuropathy;* DRG, *dorsal root ganglion;* FBSS, *failed back surgery syndrome;* LBP, *low back pain;* M, *multicenter;* P, *prospective;* PHN, *postherpetic neuralgia;* QoL, *quality of life;* R, *retrospective;* SCS, *spinal cord stimulation.*

The 12-month follow-up of these patients was published in 2015.[45] Pain was reduced by 56%, with 60% of patients reporting greater than 50% improvement. Quality of life and mood were also improved, and patients reported a high degree of satisfaction. The good pain-paresthesia overlap at the time of implantation remained stable throughout the 12-month follow-up period.

CRPS is challenging. There is evidence showing the efficacy of SCS, but obtaining an adequate pain-paresthesia overlap may be difficult. A case report on DRG stimulation for the management of CRPS type I of the knee illustrates the possibility of obtaining complete coverage.[46] Implantation of a DRG stimulation lead at L3 did not result in entire coverage of the painful area. Implantation of an additional lead at L4 improved coverage, and following the implantation of a third lead at L2, coverage was almost complete. After 8 days of stimulation the patient reported substantial pain relief, although a spot on the lateral knee was not covered. The patient was satisfied with the degree of pain reduction during the trial from NRS 6 to 9 at baseline to 1; therefore a permanent pulse generator was implanted. At 1-month post implant the patient reported complete coverage of the painful area and an NRS pain score of 1–2. Switching off the stimulator resulted in the pain returning within minutes, but switching it back on produced recurring relief in less than 1 minute.

In a multicenter prospective trial, 11 patients with CRPS refractory to conservative treatment received a quadripolar percutaneous lead implantation near the DRG relevant to their pain distribution.[42] After the trial stimulation, the INS was switched off for 1 week. Patients who experienced a minimum of 50% pain relief during trial stimulation received a permanent implant. Stimulation was restarted at 4 weeks, at which point the stimulator was switched off for 1 week. The patients were followed for 12 months. The evolution of the pain intensity is illustrated in Fig. 75.10. In addition to pain reduction, patients reported a decrease in mood disturbances such as tension, depression, and anger. Fig. 75.11 provides an example of a sample patient's pain and paresthesia distributions before and post implant. Neurovascular changes and improvement in mobility were also reported.

Chronic groin pain may seriously impact the patient's quality of life and often proves to be refractory to pharmacotherapy and injections. Peripheral nerve stimulation and SCS have previously been used with varying success. Treatment failure is mainly due to difficulty in covering the painful area. In a case series on the management of neuropathic with DRG stimulation,[45] some patients with neuropathic groin pain were included. Finding the exact target level can be challenging because the sensory input to the groin is covered by nerve fibers derived from L3 up to T11.

In a case study a practical work-up using retrograde transforaminal paresthesia mapping was performed prior to DRG lead placement.[47] Under fluoroscopic control, a 22-gauge Sluijter-Mehta kit (SMK) needle was placed via

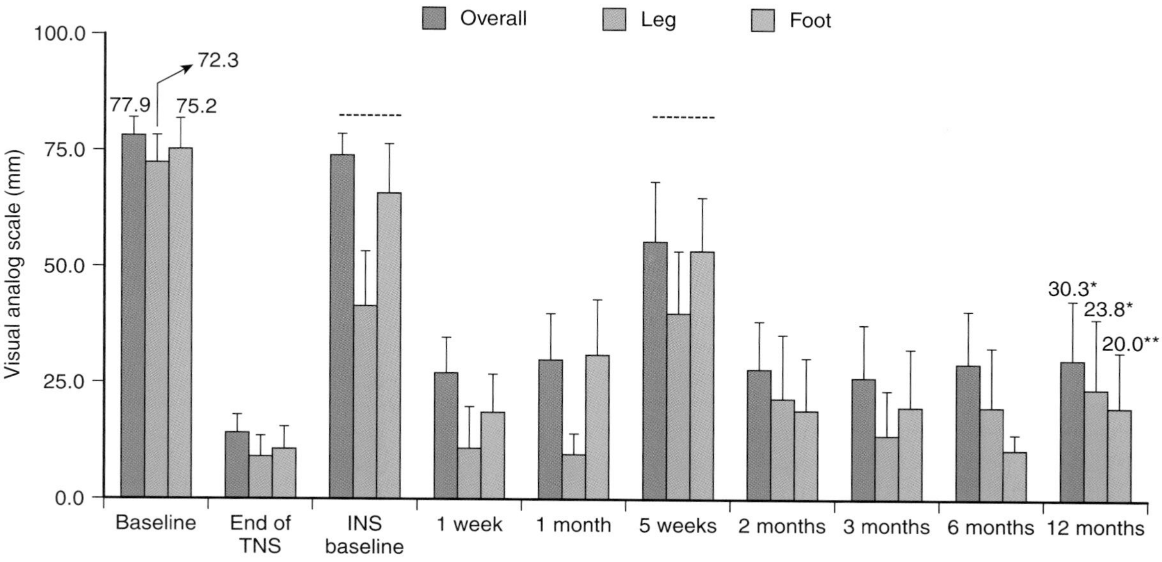

FIG. 75.10 Average overall, leg, and foot pain rating during the trial and implantation phases of treatment with dorsal root ganglia stimulation. Error bars indicate standard error of the mean. The dotted bars represent time points when stimulation was turned off. *$P < .05$ and **$P < .005$. INS, *Implanted neurostimulator*; TNS, *trial neurostimulator*. *(From Van Buyten JP, Smet I, Liem L, Russo M, Huygen F. Stimulation of dorsal root ganglia for the management of complex regional pain syndrome: a prospective case series.* Pain Pract. *2015;15:208-216, with permission.)*

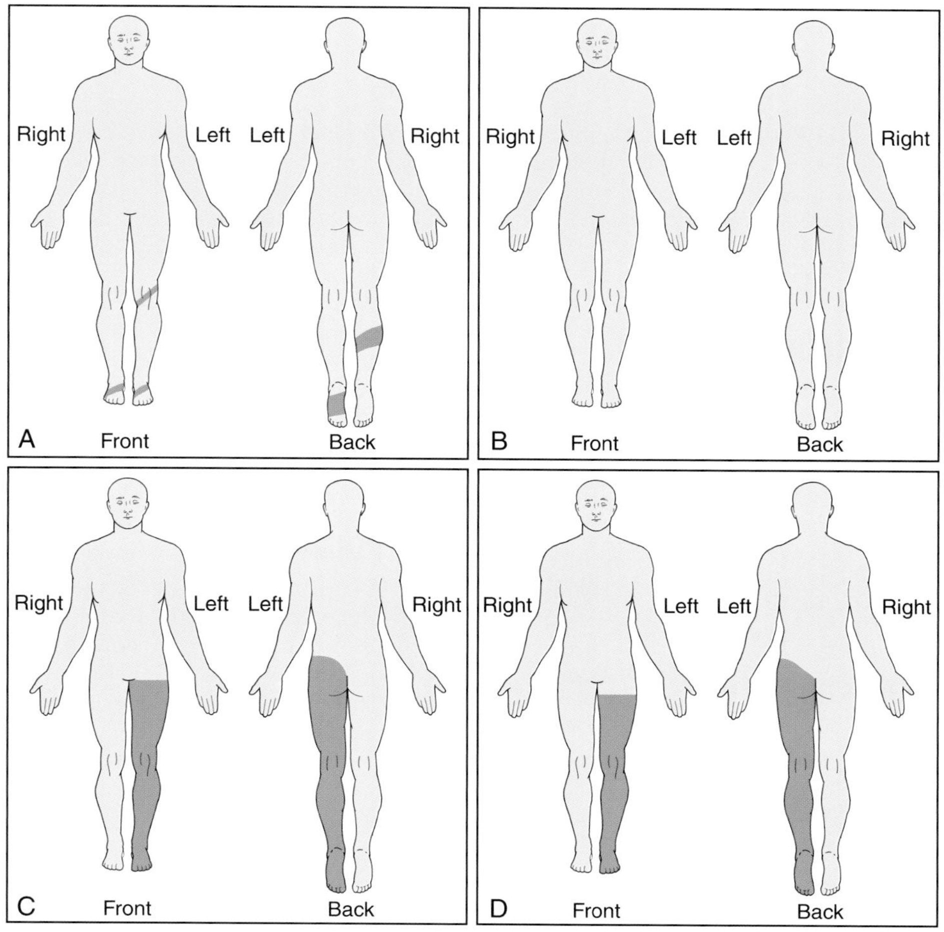

FIG. 75.11 Pain distribution at (A) baseline and (B) week 1 in a representative subject with a good treatment response. At 12 months, self-reported paresthesia distributions were identical whether the subject was (C) upright or (D) supine. *(From Van Buyten JP, Smet I, Liem L, Russo M, Huygen F. Stimulation of dorsal root ganglia for the management of complex regional pain syndrome: a prospective case series.* Pain Pract. *2015;15:208-216, with permission.)*

the retrograde transforaminal approach close to the DRG. After insertion of a thermocouple, paresthesias were elicited by electrostimulation at 50 Hz with 1 ms pulse width. Patients were asked to describe the location and percentage of the painful area covered. In the operating room the DRG lead was placed at the levels determined by preoperative paresthesia mapping. DRG stimulation of the preoperative paresthesia mapping was performed in three patients, all of whom reported >90% pain relief.

A retrospective chart review at 11 sites in Europe was performed in 29 patients with chronic neuropathic groin pain (12 had postherniorrhaphy pain) who were treated with DRG stimulation.[43] The patients received up to three leads to cover the painful area; 25 patients had a positive trial and received a permanent implant. The mean follow-up period was 27.8 weeks (range, 0–68 weeks). At follow-up, 80% of the patients experienced >50% pain reduction and 50% more than 80% improvement. The paresthesia coverage in this difficult patient group was precise, and extraneous stimulation was mostly avoided. Minimal changes in paresthesia coverage were noted over time.[43]

There are numerous treatment possibilities described for phantom limb pain, which is indicative of the refractory nature of the condition. Poor somatotopic specificity is suggested to be one important reason for the variable success rates obtained with SCS.

In a case series, DRG stimulation leads were implanted in eight patients with phantom limb pain after a positive trial period.[44] The mean baseline VAS pain score was 85.5 mm. At a mean follow-up period of 14.4 months, the average pain decreased to 43.5 mm. Patients perception of quality of life and functional capacity improved, and some patients were able to discontinue pain medications. Most patients reported precise concordance of paresthesias with the painful regions, including their phantom limb.[44]

SIDE EFFECTS AND COMPLICATIONS

Side effects and complications reported in the available trials are comparable to those known from tonic SCS. Infection is a serious complication associated with all interventional techniques. Lead migration has been reported, and although the available numbers do not allow for the calculation of incidence, it appears that this complication occurs less frequently than with dorsal column stimulation. The side effects and complication of neurostimulation of the DRG are listed in Box 75.1.

BOX 75.1 Complications and Side Effects of Dorsal Root Ganglion Neurostimulation

Infection
Bleeding, hematoma
Lead migration
Intermittent cramping
Discomfort from stimulation
Temporary cessation of stimulation
Ataxia
Formation of CSF hygroma
Temporary motor stimulation

CSF, Cerebrospinal fluid.

DORSAL ROOT GANGLION STIMULATION IN PERSPECTIVE

Tonic SCS has been documented to be effective in FBSS, CRPS, and other types of neuropathic pain. The major drawbacks are inadequate paresthesia coverage and positional changes in paresthesia requiring reprogramming of the stimulator.

Clinical experience suggests that DRG stimulation enables precise coverage of painful areas, even for individual toes. This is particularly appreciated in the management of CRPS and groin pain. The best indications for DRG stimulation seem to be dermatome-specific pain syndromes such as postherniorrhaphy pain, postthoracotomy pain, postradiation neuropathy, postmastectomy and breast surgery pain, posttraumatic foot pain, CRPS, and postherpetic neuralgia.

Placing leads in nonadjacent spinal levels results in broader coverage, as illustrated in Figs. 75.12 and 75.13.

With tonic SCS, patients often feel an uncomfortable increase in stimulation or a loss of paresthesias when they change from an upright to a supine or prone position and vice versa. These changes are primarily due to changes in the thickness of the CSF layer interposing the spinal cord and the epidurally placed leads. CSF layer thickness changes because the spinal cord moves inside the spinal canal.[48] In a substudy of a larger clinical trial, patients' paresthesia perception remained stable across all subjects and time points in the upright and recumbent positions.

Lead migration and problems with lead breakage are two of the major technical problems associated with tonic SCS. As noted earlier, the incidence of lead migration or other technical problems appears to be lower with the Axium SJM stimulation system. In summary, DRG stimulation represents an important tool in the armentarium of neurostimulation techniques for chronic refractory neuropathic pain and in the future may be considered as complementary to dorsal column stimulation. Further research should focus on refining patient selection criteria to optimize the use of DRG stimulation.

KEY POINTS

- Classic tonic SCS targets specific segmental levels to produce paresthesias overlapping painful areas. Because anatomic specificity is not exact, localization of the lead(s) in the spinal canal can be difficult.
- Patients treated with classic SCS may experience position-related changes in their perception of stimulation. Changes in their position from upright to supine or prone may provoke an uncomfortable increase in stimulation or a loss of paresthesias.
- The DRG are located bilaterally on the distal end of the dorsal root in the anterolateral epidural space. They consist of a collection of bipolar cell bodies of primary sensory neurons surrounded by glial cells and the axons of the DRG sensory cells that coalesce to form the primary afferent sensory nerve. The DRG contains the largest proportion of sensory nerves in the body.

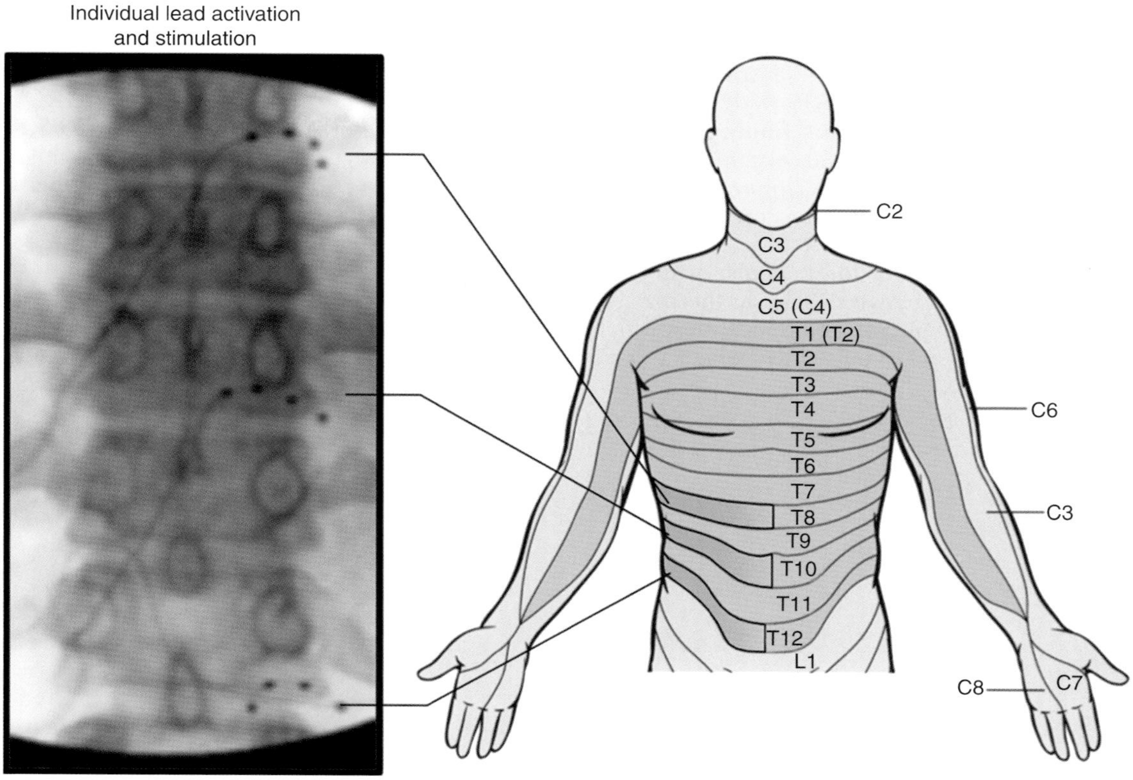

FIG. 75.12 Multisegmental stimulation of nonadjacent levels is often used to obtain coverage over a wide range of dermatomes, as illustrated in this patient with symptoms extending from T8 to T12.

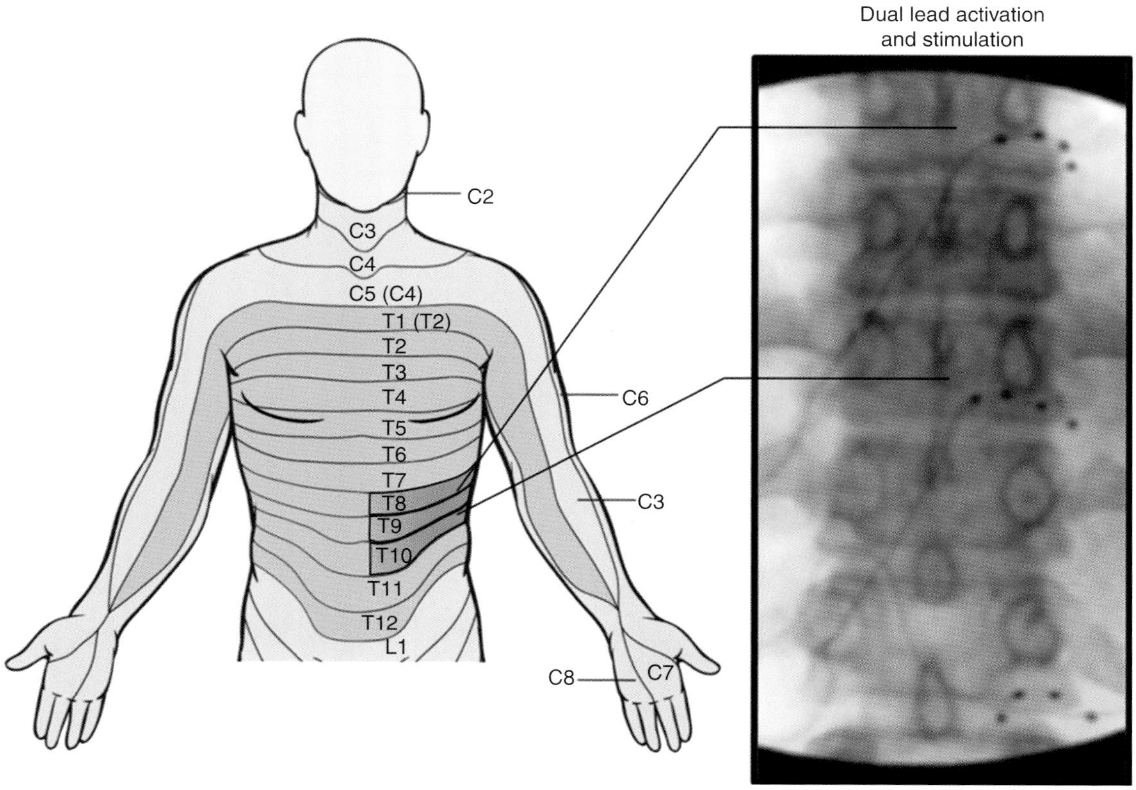

FIG. 75.13 Nonadjacent level stimulation at T8 and T10 can provide broader coverage.

- The cell bodies within the DRG are somatotopically organized. Mapping of the topographical distribution of sciatic and femoral nerve sensory neuronal somata in the L4 DRG in rats showed little overlap between the two nerves. This finding indicates the existence of a somatotopical organization for the representation of different peripheral nerves in DRG, raising the possibility of precision targeting in humans.
- RF applications to the DRG for radicular pain have shown beneficial results. However, classic thermal RF may be associated with neurolytic complications, which has led to a surge in the use of pulsed RF, which acts via a variety of mechanisms.
- Neurostimulation of the DRG requires specialized and modified equipment and is associated with a steep learning curve.
- Studies on neurostimulation of the DRG in patients with peripheral neuropathic pain, CRPS, groin pain, and phantom pain have reported varying degrees of efficacy. The published studies have either been retrospective or prospective case series.
- Randomized controlled studies are needed to establish the efficacy of DRG neurostimulation.

REFERENCES

Access the reference list online at ExpertConsult.com.

CHAPTER 76

Implanted Drug Delivery Systems for Control of Chronic Pain

David E. Jamison, MD ◦ Steven P. Cohen, MD ◦ Joshua Rosenow, MD, FAANS, FACS

INTRODUCTION

The delivery of medication into the cerebrospinal fluid (CSF) has a long history and can be traced to the spinal anesthetic works of Corning and Bier in the late 1800s.[1,2] With the discovery of opioid receptors in the central nervous system (CNS) in the 1970s, it was postulated that the CSF could provide a route not only for anesthesia but also for providing analgesia.[3,4] The use of intrathecal (IT) medications has expanded over the ensuing decades to involve several classes of medications, indications beyond chronic pain, and has benefited from advancements in implantable pump technology.

The primary rationale for instituting intrathecal drug delivery (IDD) is to achieve similar or superior therapeutic effect when compared with oral medications, while avoiding typical dose-dependent side effects. Some medications can safely be delivered long term via implantable pumps, whereas others are primarily indicated for single-shot applications in discrete pain conditions. The decision to proceed with IT therapy is based on several factors, and potential risks and benefits must be weighed carefully, as with any invasive treatment.

Selection criteria, as detailed next, should be used to identify patients that may benefit from IDD:

- Chronic pain or spasticity refractory to prior treatments
- Presence of prohibitive side effects with other medication delivery routes
- Lack of confounding psychological comorbidities
- Absence of systemic or surgical site infection
- Absence of coagulopathy
- Lack of CSF flow obstruction
- Life expectancy greater than 3 months
- Demonstrated efficacy with trial implantation

Patients meeting these criteria for therapy with an implantable pump should receive a trial to determine if the selected IT therapy will provide adequate clinical effect, although there are some experts who advocate for proceeding straight to implantation in well-selected patients with cancer pain.[5] Although epidural and IT single-shot trials are described, the preferred method involves placement of an IT catheter to best mirror potential implant conditions. Hospital admission is generally recommended to allow for dose titration while monitoring for adverse effects, mainly because of the possibility of delayed respiratory depression with rostral spread of opioids.

COMPLICATIONS

Potential complications of IDD may be procedurally or medication related. Procedural complications can occur after single-shot injection or pump implantation and include superficial and neuraxial infection, peripheral and neuraxial bleeding, postdural puncture headache, and catheter-tip granuloma formation. Infections or bleeding within the neuraxis are rare but carry the potential for catastrophic permanent sequelae. Suspected neuraxial hematoma or infection necessitates prompt imaging and neurosurgical evaluation. Anesthesia risks must also be considered prior to surgical pump implantation, particularly in patients with multiple comorbidities or advanced malignancy.

Patients with implantable pumps are also at risk of complications during required pump refills. Risks involve administration of incorrect medication, pump reprogramming error, and improper refill technique. Misidentification of the pump refill port can result in delivery of medication into the subcutaneous pocket rather than the pump itself, which can lead to catastrophic consequences. An inadvertent "pocket fill" creates a large depot of medication that can be absorbed into the body at a much greater than intended rate. A 2011 report from Medtronic cited 351 cases of pocket fills between 1996 and 2010, eight of which resulted in patient death.[6] Needle placement must be confirmed by adhering to recommended refill procedures, imaging via ultrasound or fluoroscopy should be used when the refill port cannot be palpated, and patients with suspected pocket fill should be closely monitored.

Withdrawal syndromes can also occur with pump malfunction or programming error, and the severity of symptoms varies with the class and dose of medication being delivered. Opioid withdrawal symptoms include increased pain, anxiety, sweating, diarrhea, and vomiting. Withdrawal from opioids, although unpleasant, is generally not life threatening and can be treated with supportive care and delivery of opioids via oral or parenteral routes.[7] A more serious clinical entity is represented by abrupt withdrawal from gamma-aminobutyric acid (GABA) agonists (benzodiazepines or baclofen). Sudden cessation of IT baclofen can result in a constellation of symptoms that includes increased spasticity, hyperthermia, seizures, coma, rhabdomyolysis, multisystem organ failure, and death.[8] Treatment of suspected cases of baclofen withdrawal involves initiation of oral baclofen, which is not always sufficient to prevent withdrawal, and investigation into the cause of interrupted IT delivery. A similar range of symptoms is seen in cases of benzodiazepine withdrawal,[9] but this syndrome is seldom encountered given the relatively infrequent use of benzodiazepines in long-term infusions.

Table 76.1 summarizes the common and serious adverse effects for classes of IT medications.

MEDICATION CLASSES

Although only morphine, baclofen, clonidine, and ziconotide are currently approved by the US Food and Drug Administration for use in implantable IDD systems,

TABLE 76.1 Class-Specific Adverse Effects

Class of Medication	Common Adverse Effects	Serious Adverse Effects
Opioids	Constipation, sweating, nausea, urinary retention, pruritis	Respiratory depression, granuloma with morphine or hydromorphone
Calcium channel blockers	Dizziness, nystagmus, confusion, fever	Psychosis, seizure, suicidal ideation
Local anesthetics	Weakness, edema	Paresis, bowel or bladder dysfunction
Gamma-aminobutyric acid agonists	Sedation, hypotonia, headache	Life-threatening withdrawal syndrome, respiratory depression with overdose
Alpha-2 adrenergic agonists	Hypotension, nausea, sedation, bradycardia	Hallucination, respiratory depression
Corticosteroids	Adrenal suppression with overuse	Adhesive arachnoiditis

TABLE 76.2 Conversion Guidelines Between Routes of Administration for Intrathecal Medications

Agent	Oral (mg)	Parenteral (mg)	Epidural (mg)	Intrathecal (mg)
Morphine	300	100	10	1
Hydromorphone	40–60	10	2	0.2
Fentanyl	—	1	0.1	0.01
Sufentanil	—	0.1	0.01	0.001
Baclofen	1	—	—	0.005
Midazolam	—	5	—	1–2

Note: Doses represent relative conversion factors for each agent, not equianalgesic conversion between agents.

a variety of other medications continue to see use as off-label adjuncts or sole agents delivered by subarachnoid injection. Combinations of several classes of medications are also used when monotherapy fails to provide adequate analgesia, most commonly in the form of mixed opioid and local anesthetic solutions.

OPIOIDS

Research regarding the analgesic properties of IT opioids began in the 1970s, and they remain the prototypical and most widely used IT analgesic. Originally reserved for treatment of cancer-related pain, IT opioids have increasingly been used for nonmalignant pain in correlation with rising rates of oral opioid use and spine surgery.

Compared with oral opioids, IT opioids can achieve a similar clinical effect at approximately 1/300th of the dose. This dramatic increase in effect is due to the high concentration of opioid receptors in the substantia gelatinosa of the spinal cord, where they synapse with ascending pain tracts. Binding of opioids to the Mu receptor results in presynaptic and postsynaptic effects that inhibit transmission of pain signals from the periphery to the brain.[10] Presynaptic binding leads to decreased release of pronociceptive neurotransmitters, whereas postsynaptic binding leads to decreased neuronal action potential.[11]

IT opioids must remain in the CSF to exert their effect on spinal Mu receptors, and their duration within the spinal fluid is primarily dependent on their degree of hydrophilicity. More hydrophilic medications, such as morphine and dilaudid, remain solubilized in the CSF for extended periods of time, resulting in an extended duration of action as well as spread within the CSF beyond the immediate location of the catheter tip. Conversely, lipophilic opioids, such as fentanyl or sufentanil, are poorly solubilized in the CSF and rapidly diffuse away from the spinal column. Consequently, lipophilic opioids have a shorter duration of spinal action and tend not to distribute within the CSF beyond the point of entry.[12] Table 76.2 summarizes the conversion ratios for commonly used opioids, baclofen, and midazolam.

The evidence supporting the use of IT opioids in the management of chronic pain is generally positive but is based mostly on uncontrolled prospective and retrospective studies. The lone randomized trial, published by Smith et al. in 2002, compared the effects of IDD plus conventional therapy with conventional therapy alone.[13] A total of 202 patients with refractory cancer pain were randomized to receive either IDD with opioid or conventional medical management, which consisted of all typical medical and interventional therapies excluding IDD and cordotomy. Primary outcome was at least a 20% decrease in pain as measured on a visual analog scale (VAS) coupled with at least a 20% decrease in drug toxicity at 4-week follow-up. Secondary outcomes included several measures, such as differences in individual drug toxicities, quality of life, and health care resource use. The results showed that a higher proportion of the IDD group achieved the primary outcome at 4 weeks (57.7% vs. 37.5%) and a lower percentage of patients achieved neither the threshold 20% reduction in VAS score nor the toxicity end point (11.3% vs. 23.6%). Interestingly, the IDD group also displayed a trend towards increased survival at 6-month follow-up (54% vs. 37%).

Nonrandomized studies have incorporated several types of trial designs but have generally shown good benefit with IT opioids for both malignant and nonmalignant pain. A large retrospective study by Paice et al. ($n = 429$) was conducted via surveys completed by patients undergoing IDD and their physicians.[14] Overall results showed a mean pain reduction of 61% with IDD, and 66.7% of patients reported that they were very satisfied with IDD. A high device malfunction rate was also noted (20.1%), which consisted mainly of catheter-related issues such as kinking and withdrawal. A similar study by Winkemüller and Winkemüller ($n = 120$) showed mean pain reductions of 67% at 6 months and 58% at 48-month follow-up.[15]

An advent in opioid IDD is the practice of "microdosing," wherein patients are weaned from all opioids prior to initiation of IT opioid therapy at much lower than typical doses. A 2011 case series reported experience in 20 patients with nonmalignant pain who were weaned from oral opioids and then maintained opioid free for 6 weeks prior to a trial of IT morphine.[16] The dose of morphine was initiated at 25 μg/day on day 1 of the trial and was increased sequentially until satisfactory analgesia was obtained. The average efficacious dose was 140 μg/day. Similar results were shown in the 2016 prospective study by the same researchers that also followed their preimplantation protocol.[17] Seventy-three patients with nonmalignant pain underwent weaning and a trial with microdose opioids, with 60 continuing to pump implantation. Patients were followed for 36 months, and over that time period the opioid dose increased from 221 μg/day of morphine equivalents to 325.4 μg/day, which still represented a substantial dose reduction from a typical IT regimen. The 2012 study by Hamza et al. also used microdosing of opioids in patients with nonmalignant pain, but patients were required to wean from only 50% of their opioids prior to the IT trial.[18] Those patients who had a positive response to trial infusion were then weaned completely from opioids over 3 to 5 weeks and remained opioid-free for 7 to 10 days prior to pump implantation. Significant pain relief was observed at 6-month follow-up, with average pain decreased from a baseline of 7.47 to 2.97. Mean morphine equivalent dose was approximately 1.4 mg/day at 6-month follow-up and had increased to approximately 1.58 mg/day at 36-month follow-up.

Despite these promising results, microdosing remains an area of controversy. It is unclear whether the requirement for pretrial and preimplant weaning leads to selection of patients who inherently require less opioids, or what the magnitude or duration of the wean should be. For example, the 1-week opioid-free period used in the Hamza et al. study is probably not sufficient for any opioid-induced hyperalgesic effect to wear off. The weaning requirement also likely precludes using microdosing in patients with malignant pain. Randomized trials comparing standard trialing methods and regular opioid dosing to microdosing are required.

Adverse effects with IT opioids include those effects also associated with other routes of opioid administration, including constipation, sweating, nausea, urinary retention, hypothalamic-pituitary axis suppression, and sedation.[19] These effects are generally dose dependent, and most are therefore less prevalent with IT versus other routes of delivery. Side effects that may be more frequent with IT opioids can include urinary retention, pruritis, and lower extremity edema. Respiratory depression may be dose dependent but can also occur at lower doses due to rostral spread of opioid to the respiratory centers in the brainstem. Delayed respiratory depression may occur within 24 hours even after a single bolus dose, but the risk appears to be elevated with doses greater than 0.2 mg or with catheter placement higher in the spinal column.[20]

IT morphine and dilaudid are also associated with the formation of inflammatory masses at their site of delivery into the IT space. These catheter-tip granulomas can result in catastrophic neurologic sequelae due to a mass effect on the spinal cord, and treatment can require surgical removal via laminectomy.[21,22] Granulomas appear to form due to an inflammatory process at the catheter tip and are composed of multiple types of immune cells to include eosinophils, macrophages, lymphocytes, and fibroblasts. Typical symptoms include those of cord compression, such as new or worsening neuropathic pain, neurologic deficits, and bowel or bladder dysfunction. Mild cases may improve with rotation to another opioid, replacement of the medication with saline, or caudad revision of the IT catheter, but more severe cases typically require neurosurgical consultation for consideration of granuloma resection. Given the time required for granuloma formation, they are more frequently observed in patients with nonmalignant pain, but the primary risk factors for formation are increasing dose and/or concentration of morphine or dilaudid. Lower daily doses and concentration appear to be protective, and the risk has been shown to be highest in patients receiving high daily doses of more concentrated solutions.[21] Table 76.3 summarizes recommended dose ranges for medications delivered via both infusion and single shot.

CALCIUM CHANNEL BLOCKERS

The calcium ion has several pronociceptive effects to include increased excitatory neurotransmitter release and activation of second messenger systems within the spinal cord and brain. Studies have identified the N- and T-type voltage-gated calcium channels as having the predominant influence over these excitatory effects, which has resulted in their targeting as a site for inhibition.[23,24]

Currently, the only calcium channel blocker approved for IT use is ziconotide, which is marketed under the trade name Prialt. Ziconotide is derived from the venom of a predatory marine snail and acts by blocking the N-type calcium channel in the dorsal horn of the spinal cord.[25] Given its ability to decrease pronociceptive excitation, ziconotide is indicated for use in a range of neuropathic pain and mixed somatic-neuropathic pain conditions.[26] Considering that ziconotide is synthesized from a highly potent neurotoxin, it is not surprising that adverse reactions include many CNS effects. Common reactions include confusion and dizziness, and more serious reactions include hallucinations, new or worsened depression, and suicidal ideation.[26] Ziconotide is contraindicated in patients with a history of psychosis.

Randomized trials have shown favorable results in treating neuropathic pain states. The 2004 trial by Staats et al. randomized 111 patients with chronic pain due to malignancy or acquired immunodeficiency syndrome (AIDS) to

TABLE 76.3 Dose Ranges for Intrathecal Infusion and Single-Shot Injection

Agent	Typical Infusion Dose	Typical Starting Dose	Typical Bolus Dose
Morphine	1–20 mg/day	0.1–1 mg/day	0.2–1.0 mg
Hydromorphone	0.5–10 mg/day	20–200 μg/day	40–200 μg
Fentanyl	20–300 μg/day	20–75 μg/day	25–75 μg
Sufentanil	2–100 μg/day	1–20 μg/day	5–20 μg
Bupivacaine	4–30 mg/day	1–4 mg/day	0.5–2.5 mg
Baclofen	50–1000 μg/day	50–200 μg/day	50–75 μg
Ziconotide	5–19 μg/day	0.5–2.4 μg/day	1–5 μg
Clonidine	30–1000 μg/day	30–100 μg/day	25–100 μg
Midazolam	n/a	n/a	1–2 mg
Dexmedetomidine	n/a	n/a	5–10 μg
Methylprednisolone	n/a	n/a	60 mg

n/a, *Not applicable.*

receive either IT ziconotide or placebo.[27] Results showed significantly better pain relief in the ziconotide group (52.9% vs. 17.5%) at 2 weeks. However, adverse effects were also significantly higher in the ziconotide group, with a higher percentage reporting any adverse effect (97.2% vs. 72.5%), and more than 3 times the number of control patients experiencing serious adverse effects (30.6% vs. 10.0%), approximately half of which involved the CNS. It should also be noted that the rate of ziconotide initiation was decreased from 0.4 μg/h to 0.1 μg/h or less after the first 48 patients due to an unacceptable rate of adverse effects.

The 2006 trial by Rauck et al. was performed not only to further detail the analgesic efficacy of ziconotide, but also to determine whether a slower titration schedule would decrease the incidence of adverse effects.[28] The study randomized 220 patients with poorly controlled pain despite medical management or nonziconotide IDD to receive either ziconotide or placebo for 3 weeks. Titration was started at 0.1 μg/h, and the target dose was reached slowly over a 3-week period to a mean dose of 0.29 μg/h. Analgesic efficacy was again superior in the ziconotide group, which demonstrated a greater decrease in VAS pain score (14.7% vs. 7.2%), and a higher percentage of patients reporting complete or "a lot" of satisfaction (28.4% vs. 12.1%). Although total reported adverse effects were higher with administration of ziconotide (92.9% vs. 82.4%), serious adverse effects occurred less frequently than in the previous study (11.6%) and were similar to those reported with placebo (9.3%). This study suggests that a lower starting dose and slower upwards titration may ameliorate some serious adverse effects. A retrospective report in 15 patients who received ziconotide therapy initiated at 0.05 μg/h yielded no serious adverse effects, which provides further evidence that slow initiation and titration are key in providing tolerable analgesia with this medication.[29]

The long-term effects of ziconotide are unclear given that it is a recent addition to the field of IT analgesia. The longest-term retrospective study followed 104 patients with malignant and benign pain enrolled in the Italian Registry of Ziconotide for up to 12 months.[30] The study's data revealed that only 43% of patients continued therapy with ziconotide for 12 months, but this subset of patients reported an average 36.9% decrease in pain scores and a stability of dose that suggests tolerance is not as prominent a factor as it is with opioids.

LOCAL ANESTHETICS

Local anesthetics have the longest history of IT use but were not used for treatment of chronic pain until the 1990s.[31] The analgesic effect of local anesthetics is accomplished through blockade of sodium channels, which inhibit nerve transmission by preventing development of an action potential. Local anesthetics are generally used as adjuncts in mixed IT infusions and require administration close to the desired spinal level(s). Potential side effects include dose-dependent local anesthetic effects, such as weakness, numbness, and bowel or bladder dysfunction.

Studies supporting the use of IT local anesthetics have generally focused on combination infusions that included bupivacaine and have shown particular benefit in neuropathic pain conditions.[32] Several prospective studies have also demonstrated an opioid-sparing effect when combination infusions were compared with monotherapy with opioids.[33–35]

The 1999 Van Dongen et al. study in 20 patients with chronic pain due to terminal cancer compared IT morphine with IT morphine plus bupivacaine.[34] The results showed a similar degree of pain relief in both groups, but those in the combination group required a significantly lower morphine dose. In addition, five patients in the morphine group switched to the combination group due to inadequate analgesia with morphine alone, and the only patient who required oral morphine supplementation was also allocated to morphine monotherapy. Similar results were demonstrated in the 2002 Deer et al. retrospective study that compared analgesia in 109 patients who were transitioned from morphine infusions to morphine-bupivacaine infusions.[35] Pain relief in these patients was significantly improved with the addition of bupivacaine, and secondary measures were also improved to include dose of oral opioids, number of pain clinic visits, and overall patient satisfaction.

GAMMA-AMINOBUTYRIC ACID AGONISTS

GABA is the primary inhibitory neurotransmitter in the CNS and exerts its actions at two receptor subtypes, $GABA_A$ and $GABA_B$. The $GABA_A$ receptor is a ligand-gated chloride channel, whereas the $GABA_B$ receptor is a G-protein–linked complex, but activation of either results in neuronal hyperpolarization and decreased excitability.[36]

$GABA_A$ agonists include substances from multiple classes to include ethanol, barbiturates, benzodiazepines, zolpidem, and esczopiclone. Among these disparate agonists, only midazolam has been advocated as an effective IT medication for treatment of pain.[37]

Literature supporting the use of IT midazolam is sparse and conflicting. Animal models have shown both benefit[38–40] and possible neurotoxicity,[41,42] whereas human data are gleaned mainly from studies using single-shot techniques in the perioperative period. A 1992 trial randomized 28 patients with axial low back pain to receive either epidural steroid or IT midazolam but did not include a placebo group.[43] There was improvement in both the steroid and midazolam groups, but the data are difficult to interpret given that steroid was suspended in 10 mL of normal saline and was also accompanied by IT injection of dextrose, whereas the IT midazolam injection was diluted in dextrose but was accompanied by epidural injection of 10 mL of normal saline. The 2010 Dureja et al. trial randomized 150 patients with chronic pain due to postherpetic neuralgia (PHN) to receive either (1) epidural methylprednisolone, (2) IT midazolam, or (3) both epidural methylprednisolone and IT midazolam.[44] Their results showed that pain relief was improved in both groups that received IT midazolam, but the effects were more pronounced when combined with steroid. Multiple trials have shown favorable results with the addition of midazolam to spinal anesthetics,[45–47] but its role in sustained infusions via implantable pump remains unclear.

$GABA_B$ receptor agonists are less common and include several experimental compounds, the rare amino acid isovaline, and baclofen. Of these, only baclofen is used clinically, and is FDA approved for IT treatment of spasticity. Activation of the $GABA_B$ receptor at the spinal level results in decreased release of excitatory neurotransmitters, which in turn yields muscular relaxation.[48] Although its precise mechanism for providing analgesia is unclear, several studies have shown an analgesic effect for baclofen in treatment of complex regional pain syndrome and central pain syndromes.

The 2000 van Hilten et al. trial was designed primarily to assess the effects of IT baclofen on dystonia in patients with CRPS.[49] All seven patients had IT catheters placed and received randomized daily injections of varying doses of baclofen or saline, after which they graded both their dystonia and level of pain. Higher doses of baclofen (50 or 75 μg) were associated with reductions in both dystonia and pain, and this effect persisted at 6-month follow-up. This result is supported by the 2002 Zuniga et al. case series, which showed significant improvement in two patients with pain related to CRPS who did not have features of spasticity or dystonia.[50] The results from a small randomized study that compared the effects of IT baclofen versus saline in nine patients with central pain showed significant improvement in dysesthetic pain with baclofen, but the improvement seemed to coincide with improvements in muscle spasm and dystonia.[51] Similar results were reported in the 1995 case series by Taira et al., who found significant decreases in allodynia and hyperalgesia in 9 of 14 patients with central pain with central pain due to stroke or spinal cord injury.[52]

Baclofen use is well supported for conditions that include an element of spasticity or dystonia, but its use in other pain conditions is less well established. A 2000 case series by Zuniga et al. describes the use of IT baclofen in five patients with chronic pain due to causes that included residual limb pain, postlaminectomy syndrome, and cerebral palsy.[53] Three patients had persistent pain despite receiving IT morphine via an implantable pump, one had pain despite implantation of a spinal cord stimulator, and one had previously undergone both spinal cord stimulation and IDD with morphine. All patients experienced significant improvement with transition to IT baclofen. Four of the patients were maintained on baclofen monotherapy, whereas one required a combination morphine-baclofen infusion. The 2010 randomized trial by Schechtmann et al. compared IT baclofen, clonidine, and saline infusions in patients with neuropathic pain and inadequate analgesia despite use of spinal cord stimulation.[54] Ten patients received daily injections of clonidine (25, 50, or 75 μg), baclofen (25, 50, or 75 μg), or saline, and pain was measured via VAS every 30 minutes until it returned to baseline. Results showed significant improvement with either baclofen or clonidine versus placebo, but the improvement with baclofen increased linearly with increasing dose, whereas relief with clonidine was best at 50 μg. Parameters further improved with the combination of IDD and the patient's existing spinal cord stimulator.

The risk of granuloma formulation with baclofen is unclear but likely low. Two cases of apparent granuloma formation in patients receiving baclofen monotherapy were reported in 2007, both of whom improved with catheter revisions.[55] Subsequent reevaluation of these cases suggested that precipitation of baclofen was the more likely cause of these catheter-tip masses given the reported precipitation of baclofen noted in in vitro studies.[56,57]

Table 76.4 summarizes the outcomes of randomized studies regarding the use of IT medications for chronic pain.

ALPHA-2 ADRENERGIC AGONISTS

Adrenergic receptors mediate many essential physiologic functions of the sympathetic nervous system and are found in locations throughout the central and peripheral nervous system. The alpha-2 receptor type is best known for its sympatholytic properties in the vasculature, but it also produces analgesia and sedation via its alpha-2A and alpha-2B receptor subtypes.[63] Alpha-2 receptor agonists produce their inhibitory effects by decreasing presynaptic neurotransmitter release and by increasing potassium conductance postsynaptically to cause hyperpolarization.

TABLE 76.4 Randomized Studies Evaluating Intrathecal Pain Medications

Study	Study Design	Technique	*(n)*, Pain Type	Efficacy	Comments
Smith et al. (2002)[13]	Morphine vs. medical management	Infusion	143; CA	84.5% with IDD achieved ≥20% reduction in either VAS or side effects compared with 70.8% with CMM at 4 weeks	Less side effects in IDD group.
Staats et al. (2004)[27]	Ziconotide vs. placebo	Infusion	111; CA or AIDS	Mean VAS improved 53.1% with ziconotide vs. 18.1% with placebo at 2 weeks	Short follow-up, more serious adverse effects in treatment group (30.6% vs. 10%).
Rauck et al. (2006)[28]	Ziconotide vs. placebo	Infusion	220; LBP	Mean VAS improved 14.7% with ziconotide vs. 7.2% with placebo at 3 weeks	Slower titration yielded less serious adverse effects (11.6%).
Van Dongen et al. (1999)[34]	Bupivacaine vs. morphine plus bupivacaine	Single shot	15, CA	Slightly superior pain relief with combination	Combination infusion resulted in lower morphine dose, slower dose increase.
Serrao et al. (1992)[43]	Midazolam vs. ESI	Single shot	28; LBP	Similar and significant pain relief in both groups at 2 months	Numeric data not detailed and no placebo group was used.
Dureja et al. (2010)[44]	Midazolam vs. ESI vs. midazolam plus ESI	Single shot	150; PHN	Best relief with combined injection at 12 weeks (19% with excellent relief compared to 5% with midazolam, 3% with ESI)	No placebo group.
van Hilten et al. (2000)[49]	Baclofen vs. placebo	Single shot	7; RSD	Mean VAS improved 54% points with baclofen 50 and 75 μg, 18% with baclofen 25 μg, 4%–8% with saline	5 daily injections (2 normal saline; baclofen 25, 50, and 75 μg).
Herman et al. (1992)[51]	Baclofen vs. placebo	Single shot	9; neuropathic pain	Mean VAS significantly lower with baclofen (approximately 1 vs. 9 with saline)	Baseline VAS not reported, individual VAS not detailed.
Schechtmann et al. (2010)[54]	Baclofen vs. clonidine vs. placebo	Single shot	10; neuropathic pain despite SCS	Improvement in all groups compared to placebo. baclofen best relief at 75 μg (40% VAS reduction), clonidine best at 50 μg (50% VAS reduction)	8 injections over 2 weeks (2 normal saline; clonidine 25, 50, and 75 μg; baclofen 25, 50, 75 μg).
Siddall et al. (2000)[58]	Clonidine vs. morphine vs. clonidine plus morphine vs. placebo	Single shot	15; SCI with neuropathic pain	Mean VAS reduction 37% with combined morphine-clonidine, 20% with morphine, 17% with clonidine, approximately 0% with saline	Patients initially randomized to saline, clonidine, or morphine daily injections for 3 days. All then received combined clonidine and morphine for 3 days.
Kikuchi et al. (1999)[59]	IT steroid vs. ESI	Single shot	25; PHN	92% of IT group reported good or excellent pain relief at 24 weeks compared with 16% patients with ESI	Weekly injections for 4 weeks. No placebo group.
Kotani et al. (2000)[60]	IT steroid plus LA vs. IT LA vs. no intervention	Single shot	277; PHN	91% of IT steroid/LA group with good or excellent relief at 24 weeks compared with 15% with LA, 4.4% in control group	Weekly injections for 4 weeks.
Rijsdijk et al. (2013)[61]	IT steroid plus LA vs. IT LA	Single shot	10; PHN	100% of IT steroid/LA group with increased pain at 8 weeks compared with 25% of LA group	Weekly injections for 4 weeks. Trial stopped early due to lack of effect.
Munts et al. (2010)[62]	IT steroid vs. placebo	Single shot	21; CRPS	No significant difference in any outcome measure at 6 weeks.	One injection, 1st follow-up at 6 weeks. Trial stopped early due to lack of effect.

AIDS, *Acquired immunodeficiency syndrome;* CA, *cancer;* CMM, *comprehensive medical management;* CRPS, *complex regional pain syndrome;* ESI, *epidural steroid injection;* IDD, *intrathecal drug delivery;* IT, *intrathecal;* LA, *local anesthetic;* LBP, *low back pain;* PHN, *postherpetic neuralgia;* RSD, *reflex sympathetic dystrophy;* SCI, *spinal cord injury;* SCS, *spinal cord stimulation;* VAS, *visual analog pain scale.*

Endogenous agonists include the catecholamines epinephrine, and norepineprhine, whereas exogenous IT medications include clonidine and dexmedetomidine.

Clonidine is one of the four medicines approved for IT use by the FDA, but it is most commonly used as an adjunct in combined IT infusions.[64] The potential adverse effects of IT clonidine are those associated with systemic sympatholysis, namely hypotension, bradycardia, and sedation. As with oral clonidine, abrupt discontinuation of IT clonidine can result in rebound hypertension.

The use of clonidine for neuropathic pain conditions is generally supported by animal and human studies, but some trials have yielded mixed results. The 2000 Siddall et al. trial compared the effects of IT clonidine, IT clonidine in combination with morphine, or IT saline in 15 patients with neuropathic pain following spinal cord injury.[58] Although the initial infusions were assigned randomly, all were switched to a combined infusion of clonidine and morphine on day 4 of the 6-day trial. Subgroup analysis was performed to compare analgesia attained with each type of infusion and revealed more significant reduction in VAS pain scores with the combination infusion (37%) than with morphine (20%) or clonidine (17%) monotherapy, or with IT saline (0%). Another short-term study compared pain response with intradermal capsaicin in 16 volunteers after receiving intravenous clonidine, 50 μg IT clonidine or 150 μg IT clonidine.[65] Results showed a significant decrease in pain magnitude only in the 150 μg IT clonidine group. Several randomized trials regarding use of clonidine in combination spinal anesthetics have also shown good effect and a lack of significant adverse effects.[66–68]

The risk of granuloma formation with IT clonidine is accepted to be less than with opioids but remains somewhat unclear. Animal models have shown a protective effect against granuloma formation when clonidine was added to opioid infusions,[69] but this effect has not been universally observed in human use. A 2005 case report described development of a granuloma in a patient treated with a morphine-clonidine infusion that improved with replacement of IT medications with saline.[70] A 2015 review of all patients who initiated IDD at two Swiss centers over an approximately 10-year time span identified granuloma formation in 13 of 204 total patients. Of these 13 patients, clonidine was used in 8, but always in combination with morphine at concentrations that ranged from 10 to 45 mg/mL.[71]

Dexmedetomidine is an alpha-2 adrenergic agonist that was approved for clinical use in 1999. Dexmedetomidine has a higher affinity for the alpha-2 receptor than clonidine and is used primarily as a sedative in the intensive care and ambulatory surgery settings.[72] This medication produces sedation via decreasing excitation in the brainstem, but it does not cause respiratory depression. The analgesic properties of dexmedetomidine have been illustrated in animal models,[73,74] but its long-term use in humans undergoing IDD has not been studied.

Numerous studies regarding the use of dexmedetomidine as an adjunct to bupivacaine for spinal anesthesia have been performed and generally show superior block characteristics to either monotherapy with bupivacaine or combinations with fentanyl or clonidine.[75–77] A 2016 meta-analysis reviewed the use of dexmedetomidine as an adjuvant for spinal anesthesia and found that it was well tolerated and was associated with faster onset and longer duration of sensory blockade.[78]

CORTICOSTEROIDS

A staple of pain medicine due to their potent antiinflammatory properties, corticosteroids have a limited IT role. Corticosteroids are produced by the adrenal cortex and include both glucocorticoids and mineralocorticoids. Glucocorticoids inhibit multiple proinflammatory mediators to include prostaglandins, leukotrienes, cytokines, and tumor necrosis factor alpha and may upregulate genes involved in the resolution of inflammation.[79] IT glucocorticoids were once used routinely for treatment of low back pain and radiculopathy, but this approach was abandoned in the 1980s, given an association with adhesive arachnoiditis.[80–82] The preservative polyethylene glycol is now thought to be the more likely cause of the reported cases of arachnoiditis,[83] but epidural administration remains the preferred method for steroid treatment of back pain and radiculopathy. IT glucocorticoids via single-shot injection have been advocated for treating the neuropathic pain associated with PHN and to a lesser extent complex regional pain syndrome, although the results of clinical trials are contradictory.

PHN is a painful sequela of herpes zoster, better known as "shingles," which is itself a potential sequela of prior infection with the varicella zoster virus.[84] After initial infection the varicella virus can lie dormant in the dorsal root ganglia for years before reactivating to cause an outbreak of shingles. Approximately 10% of patients with shingles will develop PHN, and the incidence is significantly higher in the geriatric population and in individuals with suppressed immune systems.[85] Treatment of PHN is challenging and typically relies on medical management with membrane stabilizers, antidepressants, topical agents, and opioids. Refractory cases may benefit from IT steroids, although careful consideration of the risks must be undertaken.

Randomized studies have shown mixed effect for IT steroids when treating refractory PHN. The 1999 trial by Kikuchi et al. randomized 25 patients with PHN to receive steroids either epidurally or intrathecally but was not placebo controlled.[59] All patients received weekly injections for 4 weeks and then were followed for up to 24 weeks. Results showed superior pain relief at all time periods in the IT group, with 12 of 13 patients reporting good or excellent pain relief at study completion, compared with only 2 of 12 patients in the epidural group. A subsequent study by Kotani et al. included a placebo-control group, randomizing 277 patients with refractory PHN to receive IT methylprednisolone with lidocaine, IT lidocaine, or no intervention.[60] Injections were received once per week for 4 weeks, and follow-up ranged up to 24 months. Results strongly favored the steroid group, with 91% reporting excellent or good pain relief at end of treatment, compared with approximately 15% in the lidocaine group and 4.4% in the control group. No serious adverse effects were reported, and serial CSF examination did not reveal potential markers of developing arachnoiditis. A similar 2013 trial by Rijsdijk et al. randomized patients with PHN to

TABLE 76.5 Recommendations Per Class of Medication

Class of Medication	Recommendation
Opioids	Strong for malignant pain, weak evidence for nonmalignant pain in patients on high-dose oral opioids
Calcium channel blockers	Strong for malignant or neuropathic pain, moderate for nonneuropathic pain
Local anesthetic	Moderate for use as adjunct in malignant or neuropathic pain
Gamma-aminobutryic acid agonist	Strong for use of baclofen in treating spasticity Moderate for baclofen in other pain states Weak for use of midazolam in neuropathic pain
Alpha-2 adrenergic agonist	Moderate for use of clonidine as an adjunct in neuropathic pain Weak for use of dexmedetomidine
Corticosteroid	Weak for use in postherpetic neuralgia

receive either IT methylprednisolone plus lidocaine or IT lidocaine.[61] Unlike the prior studies, not only was there no benefit in the six patients randomized to receive steroid, but their pain level was actually increased at 6-week follow-up. The study was stopped early due to an observed lack of efficacy. Poor results were also reported in a 2010 trial that randomized patients with CRPS to receive either IT methylprednisolone or placebo.[62] Patients received a single injection and were evaluated 6 weeks post injection. Results showed no significant improvement in pain with use of steroid, and the study was again halted early due an unacceptable risk-benefit ratio. Table 76.5 summarizes the strength of recommendation by class of medication.

CONCLUSION

When compared with other routes of administration, the delivery of medications into the CSF offers the potential for greater analgesia with fewer medication-related adverse effects. The field has benefited from advances in implantable pump technology and a steady expansion beyond the opioid and local anesthetic medication classes, but the potential benefits of this invasive therapy must be balanced by an awareness of the potential medication and procedural risks.

The body of literature supporting the use of IT pain medications as a whole is sparse, and contains few high-quality randomized trials. The use of opioids for cancer-related pain is strongly supported, but only weak evidence supports their use in nonmalignant pain states. There is strong evidence to support the use of baclofen in pain conditions that include a component of spasticity, and moderate evidence supporting its use in other neuropathic pain conditions. Ziconotide is associated with CNS side effects and has a narrow therapeutic window, but there is good evidence for its use in neuropathic pain conditions. There is good evidence that both clonidine and bupivacaine are effective adjuncts, and each has been shown to have opioid-sparing effects when used in long-term combination infusions. The evidence supporting the use of corticosteroids for PHN is weak and conflicting.

There are multiple areas for future research given the overall paucity of available literature, but efforts should focus on minimizing adverse effects and complications, maximizing cost effectiveness, and improving methods of patient selection.

KEY POINTS

- The primary rationale for instituting IDD is to achieve similar or superior therapeutic effect when compared with oral medications, while avoiding typical dose-dependent side effects.
- Potential complications of IDD may be procedurally or medication related. Procedural complications can occur after single-shot injection or pump implantation and include infection, bleeding, postdural puncture headache, and catheter-tip granuloma formation.
- Complications during pump refills include administration of incorrect medication, pump reprogramming errors, and improper refill technique. Misidentification of the pump refill port can result in delivery of medication into the subcutaneous pocket, which can lead to catastrophic consequences.
- Opioid withdrawal symptoms include increased pain, anxiety, sweating, diarrhea, and vomiting. A serious clinical entity is abrupt withdrawal from GABA agonists. Sudden cessation of IT baclofen can result in increased spasticity, hyperthermia, seizures, coma, rhabdomyolysis, multisystem organ failure, and death.
- The evidence supporting the use of IT opioids in the management of chronic pain is generally positive but is based mostly on uncontrolled prospective and retrospective studies.
- An advent in opioid IDD is the practice of "microdosing," wherein patients are weaned from all opioids prior to initiation of IT opioid therapy at much lower than typical doses. Another microdosing technique involves weaning the patient to 50% of their opioids prior to IT trial. Despite these promising results, microdosing remains an area of controversy.
- IT morphine and dilaudid are associated with the formation of inflammatory masses. Given the time required for granuloma formation, they are more frequently observed in patients with nonmalignant pain. The risk factors for formation are increasing dose and/or concentration of morphine or dilaudid.
- Ziconotide, a calcium channel blocker, is indicated for use in a range of neuropathic pain and mixed somatic-neuropathic pain conditions. Because ziconotide is synthesized from a highly potent neurotoxin, adverse reactions include many CNS effects.
- The addition of bupivacaine to IT morphine may yield better pain relief in some patients with lower body pain and result in a lower dose of IT opioids.
- Literature supporting the use of IT midazolam is sparse and conflicting. Animal models have shown both benefit and possible neurotoxicity, whereas human data are gleaned mainly from single-shot studies in the perioperative period.

- Baclofen use is well supported for conditions that include an element of spasticity or dystonia; its use in other pain conditions is less well established.
- Clonidine is most commonly used as an adjunct in combined IT infusions.
- An initial study on the use of IT steroid for PHN showed promising results. However, subsequent studies failed to replicate these findings.

REFERENCES

Access the reference list online at ExpertConsult.com.

CHAPTER 77

FLUOROSCOPY AND RADIATION SAFETY

Andrea L. Nicol, MD, MSc ◎ Brian A. Chung, MD ◎ Honorio T. Benzon, MD

The use of fluoroscopy has revolutionized interventional pain management. Fluoroscopy is required in advanced procedures where precise needle placement is required. These procedures include interventions for back and neck pain, such as epidural steroid injections, facet joint injections, facet joint nerve (medial branch) blocks and rhizotomy, sacroiliac joint injections, discography, placement of spinal cord stimulators, and the newer interventional procedures, such as biaculoplasty, nucleoplasty, and vertebral augmentation. Fluoroscopy is also used in lumbar paravertebral sympathetic blocks as well as visceral sympathetic blocks, such as celiac plexus blocks, superior hypogastric plexus blocks, and ganglion impar blocks. Blocks outside the vicinity of the spine also benefit from fluoroscopic guidance and include trigeminal nerve blocks.

Several studies on epidural steroid injections have shown the usefulness of fluoroscopy. Anatomic landmarks can be difficult to recognize especially in obese, elderly, or arthritic patients.[1] Access to the epidural space is not always straightforward, especially in the sacral region where surface landmarks are not clearly delineated in the adult patient. In addition, fluoroscopy can inform the physician of important details not clearly known to the patient. For example, a patient who was treated by one of the authors had a history of a laminectomy and fusion, and presented with a right L1 radiculopathy (Fig. 77.1). She did not realize that she had a bone stimulator in situ that was placed at the time of surgery. As the device was clearly evident on x-ray imaging, a right paramedian epidural steroid injection was safely performed with the needle insertion performed a safe distance from the bone stimulator (Fig. 77.2).

In a nationwide survey done in the United States in 2002, investigators found that there was wide variability in the use of fluoroscopy. At that time, private practitioners used fluoroscopy more than those in academic centers. In the cervical region 73% of private practitioners used fluoroscopy compared to only 39% in academic institutions.[2] The transforaminal approach to epidural injections was used in patients who had previous laminectomy by 61% of private practitioners compared to 15% of those in academic institutions.[2] Although these numbers may not be applicable at the present time, it shows that a fair number of pain practitioners do not use fluoroscopy for their spine interventions. For transforaminal epidural steroid injections, confirmation of correct needle placement and spread of the dye in the anterior epidural space can only be demonstrated by fluoroscopy or more advanced radiological imaging.

One of the earlier studies on epidural steroid injections showed that blind placements were accurate in 83 of 100 patients.[1] In this study, in which 85% of the injections were performed in the lumbar area, the anesthesiologists who performed the interlaminar epidural placements were well experienced, and yet the incidence of inaccurate placement was 17%. Another study in which the epidurals were again placed by experienced anesthesiologists and an orthopedic surgeon showed a 75% success rate with blind epidural placements.[3]

In cervical epidural placements a study noted that there was a 47% success rate on the first attempt of needle placement.[4] In 63% of the placements (24 of 38 epidurals), a second attempt was required. The lack of reliability of the loss-of-resistance technique may be partially due to the lack of continuity of the ligamentum flavum in the cervical area.[5] Another finding in the study[4] was a 51% incidence (19 of 38) of unilateral spread of contrast, although the authors inserted their needle slightly lateral to the midline. In addition to the slightly lateral insertion of the needle, the unilateral spread may also be caused by the plica mediana dorsalis, a thin septum dividing the posterior epidural space. The presence of the plica mediana dorsalis has not been demonstrated in the cervical region, but in the lumbar and thoracic levels the plica mediana dorsalis has been shown to divide the posterior epidural space into compartments hindering the free flow of the injected solution.[6–8] Knowledge that the contrast spread is unilateral can allow for readjustment of the needle tip. One of the more interesting findings in the study by Stojanovic et al.[4] is that the spread of the contrast in the ventral epidural space occurred in only 28% of the patients (11 out of 38 epidurograms). The spread of the injectate in the anterior epidural space is important since this is the location of herniated intervertebral disc(s) and the interface between the herniated disc and the nerve root. The placement of the drug in the anterior epidural space is the rationale for transforaminal epidural steroid injections (see Chapter 63).

Caudal epidural steroid injections are ideally performed under fluoroscopic guidance. Without image guidance, experienced radiologists incorrectly place the caudal needle 38% of the time.[9] Renfrew et al.[9] showed that the experience of the physician improved the success rate of blind caudal epidural placements. Physicians who performed less than 10 epidurals had a success rate of 48% compared to 62% by experienced physicians.[9] Another study showed that senior physiatrists successfully placed the caudal needle in 74% of their initial attempts.[10] Their success rate improved to 88% when landmarks were identified easily. It appears that the most common site of incorrect needle placement is in the subfascial plane posterior to the sacrum.[10] Correct placement of the caudal needle is intuitively improved when fluoroscopy is utilized. In a study of 116 caudal steroid injections done under fluoroscopy, radiologists found that the success rate was 97%.[11] In this study,[11] it was found that the injection of 9- to 15-mL volume reached the mid to upper lumbar spine except in those patients with a severely stenotic spinal canal.

In patients who have had a previous laminectomy, it was noted that the mean number of attempts to place the needle in the epidural space successfully is 2 ± 1.[12] The difficulties

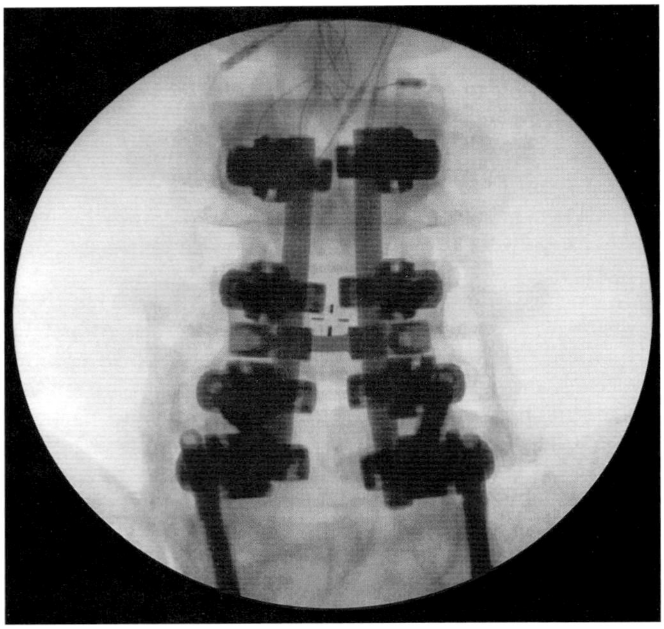

FIG. 77.1 Fluoroscopic image of a patient who had a lumbar laminectomy and fusion. In addition, a bone stimulator was placed.

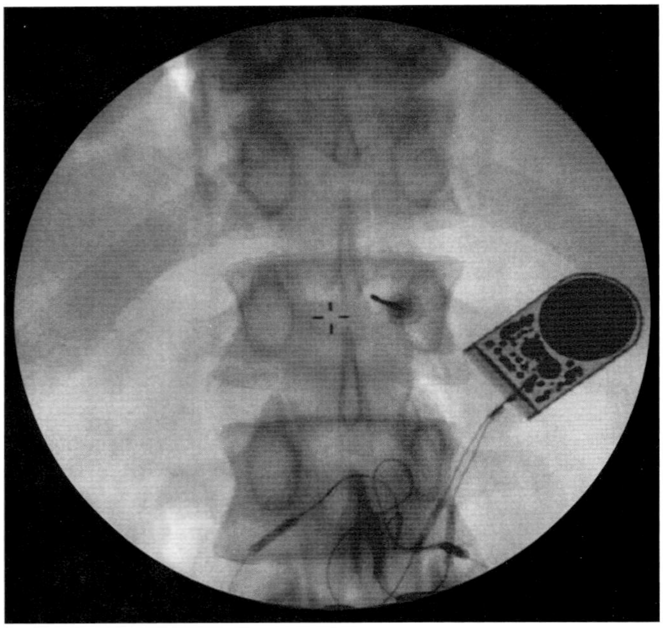

FIG. 77.2 Fluoroscopic image of the patient wherein a right T12–L1 paramedian epidural steroid injection was performed; the needle was inserted close to the bone stimulator. A lead wire is seen obscuring the L1–L2 interspace.

in placing the epidural needle may be due to the resection of the ligamentum flavum, as well as fibrosis and adhesions within the epidural space, rendering the loss-of-resistance technique equivocal. In a study by Fredman et al.[12] in 25 of 48 patients, the Touhy needle and epidural catheter were placed one or two intervertebral spaces above or below the desired level. The lack of reliability of surface landmarks may be due to the surgical removal of the posterior spinous process making the count of the vertebral levels difficult. When 5 mL of contrast medium was injected, the contrast reached the level of pathology in only 26% (12 of 47) of the patients. It has been postulated that this is due to postoperative adhesions that hindered the spread of the dye.[12] The success rates of needle placements in the studies[1,3,4,9–12] are shown in Table 77.1.

Manchikanti et al.[13] emphasized the necessity of using fluoroscopy in epidural steroid injections. The low incidence of contrast reaching the level of pathology during "blind" injections requires the use of fluoroscopy to eliminate the question of incorrect needle placement. Documentation of the spread of contrast can be correlated with the response of the patient. However, it should be noted that there are differences in the flow characteristics between the contrast media and the steroid solution, and that the flow of dye may not completely predict the flow of the steroid injectate. The steroid solution may be more limited in its distribution because it tends to precipitate in its diluent, which is typically either a local anesthetic or saline.

In addition to confirmation of the correct needle placement, the other main advantage of using fluoroscopy is the determination of the needle tip in an inadvertent location prior to injection. Unintentional intravascular or intrathecal injection may occur in spite of negative aspiration of blood or cerebrospinal fluid, respectively, through the needle. The vascular uptake of contrast can be detected when live fluoroscopy is used during injection, or can be suspected when there is immediate contrast disappearance after injection. Intravascular injections are especially hazardous via the transforaminal route as the radicular arteries accompanying the nerve root feed the spinal cord, depending on the level involved. Smuck et al.[14] performed a prospective observational study on the incidence of simultaneous epidural and vascular injection during cervical transforaminal epidural injections. They found that vascular-only injection had a 13.9% incidence where as a vascular and epidural injection occurred in 18.9% of their study patients. They recommended real-time use of fluoroscopy for contrast injection. A similar study was performed by the same group of authors at lumbosacral levels.[15] Although the incidence of vascular and vascular plus epidural injection was much lower than at cervical levels, they made the same recommendation for using live fluoroscopy during these procedures. Digital subtraction angiography (DSA) can further increase the sensitivity of real-time fluoroscopy for intravascular detection. McLean et al.[16] found that with live fluoroscopy alone, intravascular injection was detected in 17.9% of their study population. When DSA was employed, the rate rose to 32.8% (see Chapter 63).

Although not typically as catastrophic as injection into an artery, intrathecal injection of injectate needs to be detected as well. For example, the unintentional injection of 3 mL of lidocaine 1% into the intrathecal space is enough to cause a significant motor and sensory block with accompanying hemodynamic alterations. In addition, as the injectate is not placed in the epidural space, the intended therapeutic effect may be lacking. Recognizing the characteristic spread of contrast intrathecally can help to avoid this complication. One may look for a distinctive

TABLE 77.1 Success Rates in Epidural Placements

Route	Blind/Fluoroscopy	Physician	Experience/Faculty	Success Rate (%)	Reference
Cervical	Fluoroscopy	Anesthesiologists	Faculty/house staff	100[a]	4
Lumbar[b]	Blind	Anesthesiologists	Experienced	83	1
Lumbar	Blind	Anesthesiologists and orthopedic surgeons	Experienced	75	3
Lumbar, s/p surgery	Blind	Anesthesiologists	Attending	92	12
Caudal	Blind	Radiologists	Attending	48–62[c]	9
Caudal	Blind/fluoroscopy	Radiologists	Attending	74–88	10
Caudal	Fluoroscopy	Radiologists	Attending	97	11

[a] *Up to four attempts were made in successfully placing the needle in the epidural space.*
[b] *Eight-five percent of the injections were in the lumbar area.*
[c] *Experienced radiologists had a success rate of 62% compared to 48% for inexperienced anesthesiologists (see text).*

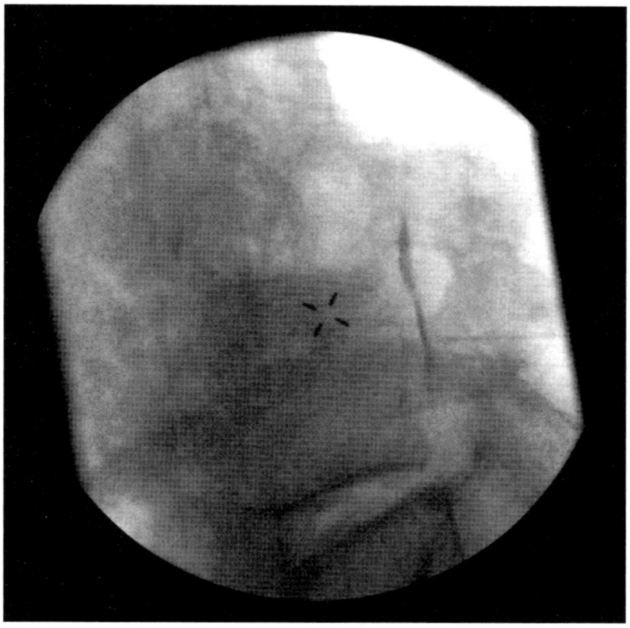

FIG. 77.3 Lateral fluoroscopic view showing placement of 25-gauge spinal needle intrathecally in a patient in the prone position. The contrast has a characteristic appearance in which the contrast border is uneven dependently (i.e., anteriorly) and essentially straight posteriorly at the contrast–cerebrospinal fluid interface.

contrast-fluid level seen on lateral imaging with the patient in the prone position (Fig. 77.3).

There are reasons for not utilizing fluoroscopy in epidural steroid injections. These include the avoidance of radiation; costs associated with the fluoroscopic equipment, its maintenance and technicians; inconvenient scheduling; location of the x-ray facility; and allergy to iodinated contrast agents (though this does not preclude fluoroscopy use, and there are other contrast alternatives that can be substituted). However, the substantial potential for incorrect needle location makes fluoroscopy desirable for epidural steroid injections, and necessary or strongly recommended for other procedures. The added benefits of fluoroscopy include the documentation of whether the spread of contrast is unilateral, located in the ventral epidural space, or whether it reached the desired level of pathology. The documentation of correct needle placement and ideal spread of the injectate eliminates technical factors as a cause of lack of response of the procedure in the patient. For these reasons, the use of fluoroscopy and contrast epiduroscopy is becoming the standard of care for epidural steroid injections as well as for other spinal procedures. The *Practice Guidelines for Spinal Diagnostic and Treatment Procedures* published by the International Spine Intervention Society (ISIS) mandates the use of fluoroscopy for the performance of transforaminal epidural steroid injections as well as medial branch blocks.[17,18] One final factor to consider when deciding whether to make the use of fluoroscopy standard during spine procedures is reimbursement. For example, in January 1, 2010, the established Current Procedural Terminology (CPT) codes for medial branch blocks were removed and replaced with codes that bundle together the medial branch block(s) and use of fluoroscopy for needle guidance. There is no longer a separate billable code for a medial branch block that has been performed without x-ray guidance.

The above discussions focused on the importance of fluoroscopy in epidural steroid injections. While one can do interlaminar epidural steroid injections (ESIs) without fluoroscopy, fluoroscopy is an integral part of facet and sacroiliac joint injections, and the other interventional pain procedures.

FLUOROSCOPY MACHINE

For medical imaging purposes, x-radiation can be produced with the aid of electricity. A current, which is measured in milliamperes (mA), passes from an electrically heated negatively charged filament (the cathode) to an anode under high voltage (kilovolt peak, kVp) within an x-ray tube.[19] The anode is typically tungsten, which has a high melting point.[20] As the electrons interact with the anode, energy is released as both heat and photons called x-rays. These x-rays will then exit the tube and either become absorbed by or pass through the patient. The energy that passes through the patient will enter an image intensifier where it is converted to a visible image that is displayed on a monitor screen and can be saved as part of the permanent medical record.

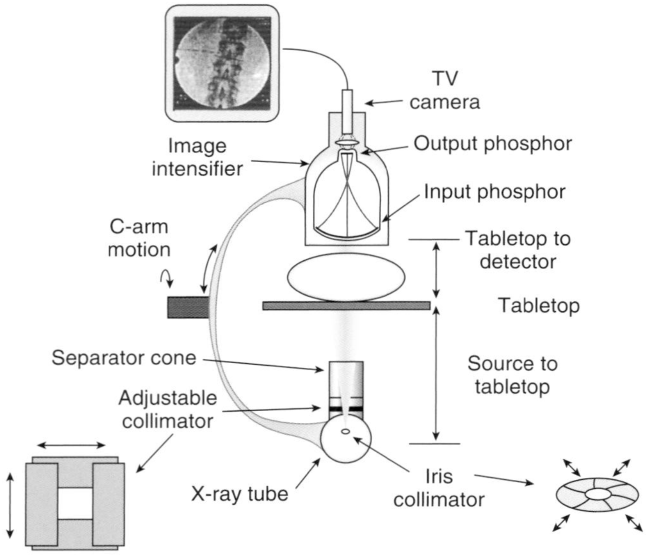

FIG. 77.4 General components of the C-arm fluoroscope. (Fishman SM, Smith H, Meleger A, et al: Radiation safety in pain medicine. *Reg Anesth Pain Med.* 27:296-305, 2002, with permission from the American Society of Regional Anesthesia and Pain Medicine.)

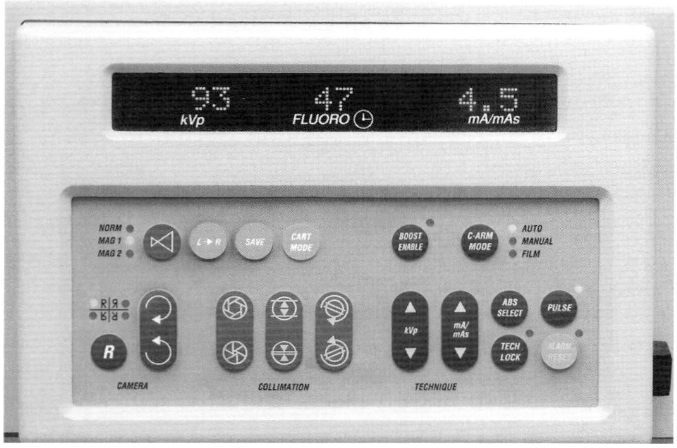

FIG. 77.5 Control panel of the fluoroscopy machine.

The important parts of the fluoroscopy machine include the x-ray tube, the image intensifier, the C-arm, and the control panel (Fig. 77.4).[21] The x-ray tube fires the beam of electrons through a high-voltage vacuum tube, forming x-rays that are emitted through a small opening. The image intensifier collects the electromagnetic particles and translates them into a usable image that can be viewed on a television monitor. The C-arm allows for the x-ray source and recording source (i.e., the image intensifier) to be on opposite sides of the patient. By its design, it will also facilitate the positioning of the fluoroscope for the physician to easily obtain anteroposterior, oblique, and lateral views of the patient. The control panel (Fig. 77.5) contains the controls for the technician to make adjustments either to the image itself or the settings used to create the x-ray image. For the latter, typically the "automatic brightness control," or ABC, system is employed (see below). Also located in the control panel are the controls for magnification and collimation of the image. Many machines also have the software required for DSA, which is useful to detect inadvertent vascular placement. The quality of image contrast depends on the balance between the tube voltage (or kVp) and the tube current.[21] The kVp is the voltage through which the electron beam passes in the x-ray vacuum tube. Increasing the kVp increases the penetrability of the x-ray beam through the patient and thereby decreases its absorption. This will act to produce brighter, more exposed images, but will decrease the contrast. The fluoroscopic examination of the spine of a normal-sized adult starts with the kVp set at ~75; larger patients require a higher kVp. The typical settings are 80–100 kVp for the back, 50 kVp for the hands, and 70 kVp for the abdomen. Broadman[19] recommends the highest kVp setting that produces the adequate contrast or grayscale ordering to minimize x-ray exposure for the patient and personnel. The x-ray (tube) current reflects the number of electrons fired through the high-voltage vacuum tube. Higher tube currents mean more x-rays are produced and emitted. The tube current is set between 1 and 5 mA; lower settings are adequate for most interventional fluoroscopy procedures.

The image contrast is obtained by balancing the tube voltage or kVp against the tube current.[19] Higher kVp settings reduce the number of x-rays absorbed and decrease exposure time. However, if the kVp settings are too high, the image will lack the necessary contrast to provide useful visualization. In terms of the resulting image, it can be likened to a photograph taken with an inappropriately bright flash in which all objects appear overexposed and the ability to distinguish features falters. A nice component of fluoroscopy machines is the ABC system in which the computer automatically analyzes the image contrast and makes the appropriate tube current adjustments, balancing image contrast and patient safety. It is recommended that the interventional pain physician leave the machine on the ABC system during the performance of most interventional procedures.

RADIATION SAFETY

The increasing use of fluoroscopy necessitates that the pain physician be aware of radiation safety to limit the radiation exposure to the patient and personnel.[22] Editorials, review articles, book chapters, monographs, and government publications are available to help the interventional pain physician better understand the concept of radiation safety.[19,21,23–28]

Radiation is the process by which energy, in the forms of waves or particles, is emitted from a source.[21] Radiation includes x-rays, gamma rays, ultraviolet, infrared, radar, microwaves, and radio waves. Radiation absorbed dose (rad) is the unit of measure that expresses the amount of energy deposited in tissue from an ionizing radiation source. Units of gray (Gy) are preferred, instead of rad, in the International System of Units (SI). A gray is defined as the quantity of radiation that results in an energy deposition of 1 joule per kilogram (1 J/kg) within the irradiated material; 1 Gy is equivalent to 100 rad and to 1000 mGy.

Different types of radiation may have similar absorbed doses but produce different biologic effects.[21] To predict occupational exposure from x-radiation, the rad is converted to radiation equivalent man (rem) in a 1:1 ratio. The unit of dose equivalent to rem in the SI system is the sievert (Sv); 1 rem is equivalent to 1 rad and 100 rem is equivalent to 1 Sv.

There remains a paucity of literature on ionizing radiation exposure and dose among interventional pain physicians. The majority of published reports use fluoroscopic or screening times as a proxy for radiation dose (Table 77.2). In general, published data have shown that fluoroscopic times were shorter in private practice[29–33] compared to university settings where supervision of trainees occurs.[34,35] Nevertheless, there is wide variation in fluoroscopy times and radiation dose in attending physicians in both private practice[30] and university settings.[34] Fluoroscopic times may further vary by mode used (continuous vs. pulsed), the experience of the radiographer, technician, or interventionalist, and difficulties in obtaining a satisfactory image given the severity of degenerative disease or patient body habitus. Overweight patients also appear to require significantly longer fluoroscopy times and have higher radiation exposure compared to normal-weight patients.[36,37]

Some studies have reported radiation exposure through dosimetry measurements for a variety of interventional pain management procedures. These studies, which were performed in both private practice and university settings, have shown that radiation dose levels in interventional pain physicians are within regulated acceptable dose limits, provided the appropriate radiation protection measures have been utilized (Table 77.3).[29–38] Interpretation of these results has its limitations, as each study utilized different modes of fluoroscopy, varying types of shielding, and measured effective dose over differing lengths of time and at variable locations. Ultimately, even though these studies provide some security that the overall exposure for these procedures is within safe limits, it may provide a false sense of security as the risks due to chronic and cumulative low-dose exposure have yet to be studied.[39]

There remains a significant dearth of published data on interventions to minimize cumulative radiation exposure in interventional pain physicians. In the small number of available studies, it does appear that procedural and equipment changes,[39] peer-based education,[40] coaching,[41] and shielding improvements[31] effectively reduce radiation dose in this population.

RADIOBIOLOGY

The biologic effects of radiation are caused either by the direct disruption of macromolecules such as DNA or by the ionization of water molecules within cells, producing highly reactive free radicals that then damage the macromolecules. Acute effects (nonstochastic or deterministic) occur at relatively high dose levels, such as those given during radiotherapy treatments or in accidents. The term *acute* refers not only to the short time course, but also to the high dosage involved. Chronic effects are the results of long-term, low-dose effects. The severity of these effects is unrelated to the dose as there is a threshold effect. Hence chronic effects are termed stochastic or nondeterministic. Doses lower than 1 Gy generally do not cause noticeable acute effects other than slight cellular changes. However, there is an increased probability of induced cancer or leukemia in the exposed individual. A radiation dose equivalent of 25 rem (0.25 Sv) may lead to measurable hematologic depression.[21,25] A whole body total radiation dose exceeding 100 rem (1 Sv) may lead to nausea, fatigue, radiation dermatitis, alopecia, intestinal disturbances, and hematologic disorders. The average annual radiation dose from medical x-rays is only approximately 40 mrem (0.4 mSv).[21,25]

MAXIMUM PERMISSIBLE DOSE

The maximum permissible dose (MPD) is the upper limit of allowed radiation dose that one may receive without the risk of significant side effects. The annual whole-body dose limit for physicians is 50 mSv. Table 77.4 shows the annual maximum permissible dose per target area.[21] For the fetus, the annual maximum permissible dose is 0.5 rem or 5 mSv. Assuming proper techniques and well-functioning equipment, the scattered radiation dose to the patient and the medical personnel should be less than the above radiation doses. Reduction of the amount of radiation implies proper selection of the type of examination and imaging modality in order to minimize the exposure to the patient and personnel. These include knowledge of the value of the radiologic examinations and the views that are necessary, selection of the equipment to be as dose-efficient as possible, and proper installation and regular maintenance of the equipment. The principle involved in reducing the amount of radiation dose is as low as reasonably achievable (ALARA) or as low as reasonably practicable (ALARP). This implies that in the process of obtaining good, usable images for the procedure, all steps are taken to minimize extraneous radiation exposure.

RADIATION PROTECTION OF THE PATIENT

Several precautions should be employed to minimize the exposure of the patient to radiation. The beam-on time should be reduced since radiation exposure increases linearly with time, and total exposure is equal to the exposure rate multiplied by the time. It is recommended that the fluoroscopy machine be equipped with a laser pointer, which is attached to the image intensifier (Fig. 77.6). The laser pointer allows the technician to "mark" the area of interest externally before an image is taken. This will reduce the number of scout fluoroscopy views required before the actual area of interest is encountered. The x-ray tube should be kept as far away from the patient as possible. Increasing the distance between the x-ray tube and the patient reduces radiation to the patient. It will also necessarily move the patient closer to the image intensifier leading to a sharper and higher quality image. It has been recommended that the x-ray tube be at least 30 cm away from the patient. The image intensifier should be positioned as close to the patient as possible while still maintaining the necessary space required to perform the procedure. Collimation should be used to reduce the area being irradiated, thereby reducing the amount of x-rays received by the patient. Collimation may also increase the quality of the image by a reduction in radiation scatter.

TABLE 77.2 Average Fluoroscopy Time Per Interventional Pain Procedure

	Fluoroscopy Time Per Procedure (Seconds)											
	Facet Joint Nerve Block		Lumbar Facet Joint Injection	Facet Denervation	Caudal Epidural	Translaminar Epidural	Transforaminal Epidural		Sympathetic Block		Sacroiliac Joint Injection	SCS Trial
	Cervical	Lumbar					Cervical	Lumbar	SGB	LSB		
Manchikanti et al.[29]	5.9 ± 0.07	5.7 ± 0.09	—	12.7 ± 1.49	3.75 ± 0.13		8.8 ± 0.78	10.9 ± 0.72	6.5 ± 0.68	12.0 ± 1.49	—	—
Manchikanti et al.[30]	5.8 ± 0.11		—	—	3.7 ± 0.29		10.6 ± 0.60		7.4 ± 1.09		—	—
Manchikanti et al.[31]	4.5 ± 0.07		—	—	2.7 ± 0.27		8.4 ± 0.5		4.0 ± 0.35		—	—
Botwin et al.[32]	—	—	—	—	12.55	—	—	—	—	—		—
Botwin et al.[33]	—	—	—	—	—	—	—	15.16	—	—	—	—
Zhou et al.[34]	81.5 ± 12.8				—	46.6 ± 4.2			—	—	50.6 ± 41.9	—
Wininger et al.[38]	—	—	—	—	—	—	—	—	—	—	—	133.4 ± 84
Hanu-Cernat et al.[36]	—	28.41 ± 18.5	29.50 ± 17.39	38.23 ± 13.33	16 ± 6.98		—	—	—	—	43 ± 20.73	—

LSB, *Lumbar sympathetic block;* SCS, *spinal cord stimulator;* SGB, *stellate ganglion block.*

Reprinted, with permission, from: Nicol AL, Benzon HT, Liu BP. Radiation exposure in interventional pain management: we still have much to learn. Pain Pract. *15(5):389-392, 2015.*

TABLE 77.3 Radiation Exposure During Interventional Pain Procedures

Study	Procedure	Ring Badge	Glasses Badge	Outside Apron Badge	Inside Apron Badge	Average Fluoroscopy Time (seconds)
Botwin et al.[32]	Caudal ESI	4.10 mrem	2.47 mrem	3.98 mrem	0.15 mrem	12.55
Botwin et al.[33]	Lumbar TF ESI	0.7 mrem	0.4 mrem	0.3 mrem	ND	15.16
Manchikanti et al.[29]	Caudal & IL & TF ESIs, facet injections, intercostal blocks, sympathetic blocks, percutaneous adhesiolysis	—	—	0.748 mrem	0 mrem	7.7 ± 0.21
Manchikanti et al.[30]	Same as above	—	—	0.834 mrem	NA	7.5 ± 0.27
Manchikanti et al.[31]	Same as above	—	—	0.362 mrem	0 mrem	4.9 ± 0.11

Readings are average exposure per procedure in mrem.
Manchikanti et al.[29]: No protective measures in the lower part of the body.
Manchikanti et al.[31]: Protective measures including lead shielding from table to floor.
ESI, *Epidural steroid injection;* IL, *interlaminar;* ND, *none detectable;* TF, *transforaminal.*
Reprinted, with permission, from: Nicol AL, Benzon HT, Liu BP: Radiation exposure in interventional pain management: we still have much to learn. Pain Pract. *15(5):389-392, 2015.*

TABLE 77.4 Annual Maximum Permissible Radiation Dose by Target Organ

Organ/Area	rem	mSv
Whole body	5	50
Lens of eye	15	150
Thyroid	50	500
Gonads	50	500
Extremities	50	500

Source: Fishman SM, Smith H, Meleger A, et al: Radiation safety in pain medicine. Reg Anesth Pain Med. *27:296-305, 2002, with permission.*

The use of live fluoroscopy should be minimized, and freeze frames should be relied on as frequently as possible. Many machines have the capacity to use pulsed, live fluoroscopy. This will create a choppier moving image as opposed to a smooth image from continuous fluoroscopy, but significantly reduces exposure. Some machines also have a low-dose mode, which provides grainier images that lack the fine detail that would be provided if a higher dose of radiation were used (Fig. 77.7). These settings may be used in those circumstances in which a high-quality or smooth moving image is not required. Finally, magnification should be limited, since magnifying the image by a factor of 1 increases the amount of radiation 2.25 times, while magnifying the image by a factor of 2 increases the amount of radiation 4 times.[21]

As stated earlier, the MPD to the fetus is 5 mSv per year. An old theory is the "10-day rule," wherein it was thought that x-ray examination of the abdomen in a woman of childbearing age should be carried out within 10 days of the onset of menstruation, since this time represents the least likelihood window of conception taking place. However, if conception did take place during this period, it was thought that the embryo would be most sensitive to the effects of radiation. The "10-day rule" is probably erroneous. The period when the fetus is most sensitive to radiation is between 8 and 15 weeks' gestation, when the rate of proliferation of DNA within the brain is at a maximum.[23] Any significant deleterious effect of radiation during the first few weeks of conception will likely lead to spontaneous abortion.

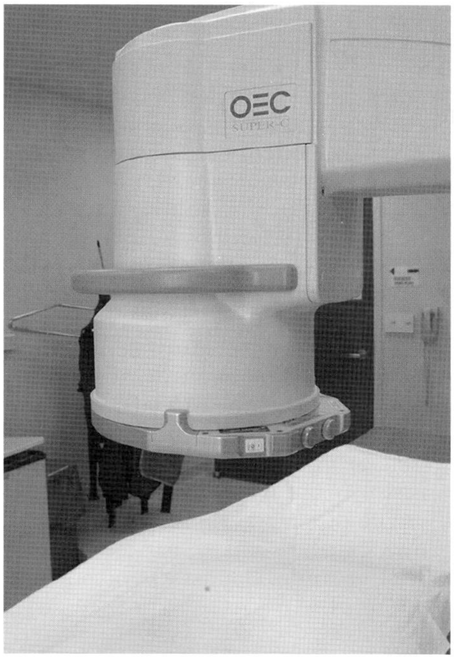

FIG. 77.6 A laser pointer is attached to the image intensifier. The *red dot* corresponds with a target (such as an "X") on the fluoroscopic image.

RADIATION PROTECTION OF PERSONNEL

The factors affecting radiation exposure to personnel include the time or duration of x-ray exposure, the distance from the source of the x-rays, and protection from

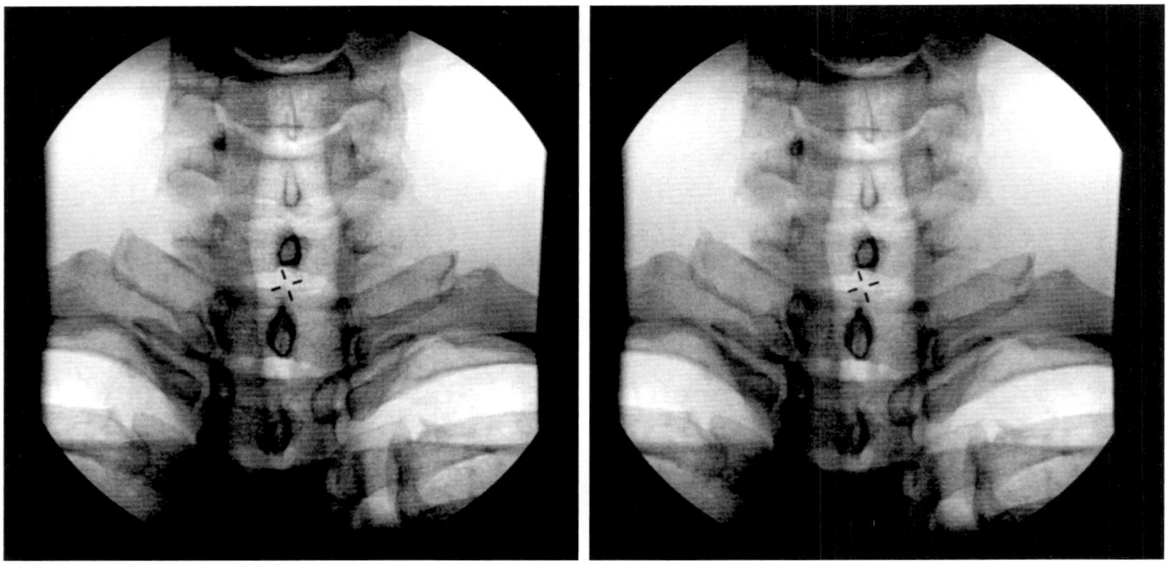

FIG. 77.7 On the *left* is an image using the standard automatic brightness control setting (kVp 71, 2.2 mA); on the *right* is an image using the low-dose setting (kVp 75, 0.84 mA). The differences in this image are subtle with the low-dose image differing notably by a blurring of the edge margins.

the radiation. It should be noted that the major source of radiation to personnel is the patient or fluoroscopy table, which serves as a conduit for scattered radiation. The radiation dose to the patient and subsequent scatter can be reduced by using the lowest tube current (mA) compatible with a good x-ray image. The beam-on time should be kept to a minimum; there is a 5-minute alarm on most fluoroscopy machines. Only essential personnel should be present in the fluoroscopy room. Personnel should be notified each time before fluoroscopy is used. The personnel should step back from the field whenever possible when the fluoroscopy machine is used. The intensity of ionizing radiation decreases exponentially as the distance from the source is increased. The inverse square law shows that the radiation is inversely proportional to the square of the distance (the space between the individual and the x-ray source). Therefore, as the distance is doubled, the exposure rate is reduced by one-fourth.[21] Finally, barriers or screens can be employed; these are utilized mostly in orthopedic, urology, and radiology suites.

UNDERCOUCH AND OVERCOUCH FLUOROSCOPY

The conventional undercouch fluoroscopy arrangement occurs when the x-ray tube is located beneath the fluoroscopy table and the image intensifier is above the table (Fig. 77.8). In this arrangement, and with the table horizontal, most of the scattered radiation is in the downward direction and absorbed in the floor or the side panels of the table. In the overcouch fluoroscopy arrangement, the positions of the x-ray tube and image intensifier are reversed, or the oblique and lateral views are employed. In this arrangement, it is more difficult to adequately shield medical personnel. The maximum amount of scattered radiation is normally backwards from the entrance surface of radiation on the patient receiving most of the primary beam (i.e., the side of the x-ray tube). Scattered radiation is 2–3 times higher on the side of the x-ray tube compared to the image intensifier. The physician should preferably stand on the side of the image intensifier when lateral views are taken; care must be taken to ensure that the x-ray tube and image intensifier are at the same (not

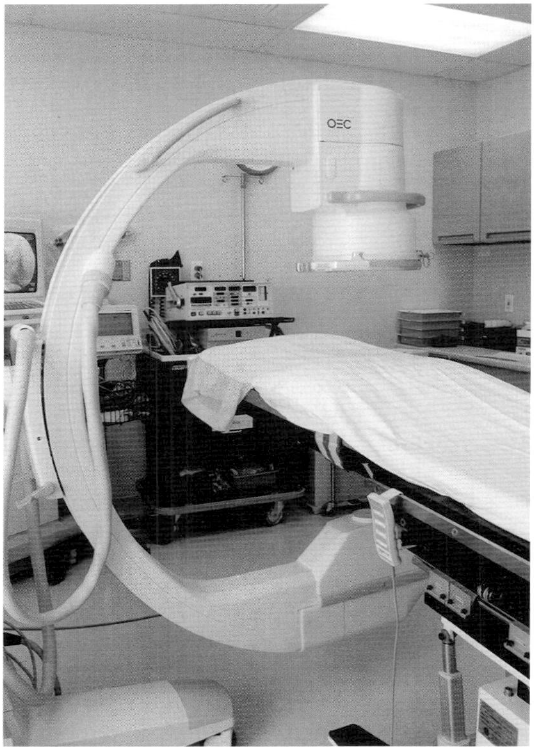

FIG. 77.8 A conventional undercouch fluoroscopy arrangement wherein the x-ray tube is located beneath the fluoroscopy table and the image intensifier is above the table.

TABLE 77.5 Percentage Primary X-Ray Beam Transmission for Kilovoltages and Lead Aprons, Single-Phase Generator (1 or 2 Pulse)

Lead Thickness (mm)	75 kVp	100 kVp	125 kVp
0.22	4.5	12.1	12.8
0.44	0.7	3.7	5.1
0.5	<0.1	3.1	4.4
0.72	<0.1	1.4	2
1	<0.1	0.3	0.6

Source: Robinson A: Diagnostic protection and patient doses in diagnostic radiology. In Grainger RG, Allison D, editors: Grainger & Allison's Diagnostic Radiology: A Textbook of Medical Imaging, *New York: Churchill-Livingstone, 1997, pp 169-189.*

above) level of the patient. The image intensifier also has a lead-plastic apron attached to its edge, which serves to absorb much of the scattered radiation that emerges from the patient and shield the physician from some of the scattered radiation.

TABLE 77.6 Ten Measures for Minimizing Risks From Fluoroscopic X-Rays

1. Dose rates are greater and dose accumulates faster in larger patients, so extra precautions may be warranted.
2. Keep the tube current as low as possible.
3. Keep the kVp as high as possible (and mA as low as possible) to achieve the appropriate compromise between image quality and low patient dose.
4. Keep the patient at maximum distance from the x-ray tube.
5. Keep the image intensifier as close to the patient as possible.
6. Do not overuse geometric or electronic magnification.
7. If the image quality is not compromised, remove the grid during procedures on small patients or when the image intensifier cannot be placed close to the patients.
8. Always collimate down to the area of interest.
9. Personnel must wear protective aprons, use shielding, monitor their doses, and know how to position themselves and the machines for minimum exposure.
10. Keep beam-on time to an absolute minimum.

Source: Wagner LK, Archer BR: Minimizing Risks from Fluoroscopic X-Rays, *ed 3, Woodlands, TX, RM Partnership, 2000.*

BARRIERS AND SHIELDING

Shielding refers to radiation protection afforded by equipment that absorbs x-rays. The categories of shielding include fixed, mobile, and personal shielding.[23] Fixed shielding includes the thickness of walls, which should have a lead equivalence of 1–3 mm, the doors, and protective cubicles. Mobile shielding is appropriate during fluoroscopy procedures whereby a member of staff needs to remain near the patient. Personal shielding includes lead aprons, gloves, thyroid shields, and glass spectacles.

Lead Aprons

For reasons of weight, lead aprons generally have shielding equivalence equal to a 0.25–0.5-mm lead barrier, and will only attenuate the radiation. Lead aprons absorb 90%–95% of scattered radiation that reaches them (Table 77.5). "Wrap-around" lead aprons are useful when medical personnel spend a lot of time with their backs turned away from the patient. When wrap-around aprons are not used, the personnel wearing them should not turn their unshielded backs toward the x-ray beam. Lead aprons should be worn and stored properly. They should not be folded or thrown on the floor since it may produce creases that develop into breaks in the protective barrier. The integrity of lead aprons should be assessed annually.

Lead Rubber Gloves and Leaded Glasses

Lead rubber gloves usually have a minimum lead equivalence of 0.25 mm since thicker leaded gloves make manipulations that require dexterity difficult. The protection offered by "radiation-resistant" gloves may not be significant, providing a false sense of security. The use of leaded gloves may actually increase the x-ray exposure when the fluoroscopy machine is in the ABC mode. In this scenario, the machine senses the poor contrast between the bones of the gloved hand and the surrounding soft tissue, and the ABC system automatically adjusts the tube current setting to produce better contrast at the expense of a higher radiation dose.

The use of leaded glasses with side shields may reduce the risk of cataract formation. However, the effectiveness of glass spectacles may be overrated, and ordinary eyeglasses may provide adequate reduction in the radiation dose that reaches the eye. A single dose of 200 rem (2 Sv) or a total exposure of 800 rem (8 Sv) has been related to cataract formation, with the latent period between the radiation exposure and the appearance of cataracts being approximately 8 years.[21,25]

MINIMIZING AND MONITORING RADIATION

Wagner and Archer recommended 10 measures to reduce risks from fluoroscopic x-rays (Table 77.6).[27] Federal and state regulations in the United States require that anyone who works in a station where he or she may receive over 25% of the allowable quarterly limit (1.25 rem or 1250 mrem) must be supplied with monitoring equipment or a radiation or film badge. A radiation badge is a pack of photographic film that measures radiation exposure for personnel monitoring. It measures the quantity and the quality of radiation (beta or gamma radiation). It is read with a densitometer and the amount of darkening of the film is proportional to the amount of radiation absorbed by the film. The film inside the badge is easily damaged by pen or moisture, and the badge cannot be used for periods exceeding 8 weeks because the image fades.

There are usually two badges worn by the physician during the fluoroscopy procedure. The "collar badge" is worn outside the apron on the upper portion of body, usually on the upper edge of the thyroid shield. This badge approximates radiation exposure to the lens of eye. The "behind

NORTHWESTERN MEM HOSP
251 E HURON
RADIATION SAFETY OFC
GALTER RM 8-138
CHICAGO IL 60611

LANDAUER®
Landauer, Inc. 2 Science Road Glenwood, Illinois 60425 - 1586
Telephone: (708)755-7000 Facsimile: (708)755-7016
www.landauerinc.com
RADIATION DOSIMETRY REPORT

luxel®

ACCOUNT NO.	SERIES CODE	ANALYTICAL WORK ORDER	REPORT DATE	DOSIMETER RECEIVED	REPORT TIME IN WORK DAYS	PAGE NO.
79397	ATH	0126800010	10/04/01	09/25/01	7	1

** DUPLICATE **

PARTICIPANT NUMBER	NAME: ID NUMBER	BIRTH DATE	SEX	DOSIMETER	USE	RADIATION QUALITY	DOSE EQUIVALENT (MREM) FOR PERIODS SHOWN BELOW: DEEP DDE	EYE LDE	SHALLOW SDE	QUARTERLY ACCUMULATED DOSE EQUIVALENT (MREM): DEEP DDE	EYE LDE	SHALLOW SDE	YEAR TO DATE DOSE EQUIVALENT (MREM): DEEP DDE	EYE LDE	SHALLOW SDE	LIFETIME DOSE EQUIVALENT (MREM): DEEP DDE	EYE LDE	SHALLOW SDE	RECORDS FOR YEAR	INCEPTION DATE (MM/YY)
FOR MONITORING PERIOD:							08/10/01 – 09/09/01			QTR 3			2001							
07377				P	COLLAR		M	M	M										8	07/99
			M	P	WAIST		M	M	M											07/99
					ASSIGN		M	M	M	M	M	M	18	11	13	18	14	18		
					NOTE		ASSIGNED DOSE BASED ON EDE 1 CALCULATION													
07379				P	COLLAR		M	M	M										8	07/99
			M		NOTE		ESTIMATED													
				P	WAIST		M	M	M											07/99
					NOTE		ESTIMATED													
					ASSIGN		M	M	M	M	M	M	13	10	11	13	10	13		
					NOTE		ESTIMATED													
					NOTE		ASSIGNED DOSE BASED ON EDE 1 CALCULATION													
07380				P	COLLAR		M	M	M										9	07/99
			M		NOTE		ESTIMATED													
				P	WAIST		M	M	M											07/99
					NOTE		ESTIMATED													
					ASSIGN		M	M	M	M	M	M	14	34	34	14	198	208		
					NOTE		ESTIMATED													
					NOTE		ASSIGNED DOSE BASED ON EDE 1 CALCULATION													
07507				P	COLLAR		M	M	M										8	02/00
			M	P	WAIST		M	M	M											02/00
					ASSIGN		M	M	M	M	M	M	15	9	10	16	10	11		
					NOTE		ASSIGNED DOSE BASED ON EDE 1 CALCULATION													

M: MINIMAL REPORTING SERVICE OF 1 MREM   QUALITY CONTROL RELEASE: **VG**   2S - PR 7326 - RPT130 - N1 C   - 09552

Accredited by the National Institute of Standards and Technology through NVLAP *

FIG. 77.9 Printout sample of radiation exposure of medical personnel.

the apron" badge is worn behind the apron, usually on the waist of the physician. The x-ray reading in this badge represents the actual dose to the gonads and the major blood-forming organs. The film badges should be placed correctly and worn consistently. It is not uncommon for the physician to interchange the placement of the badges, resulting in a gross error in the interpretation of the x-ray risk to the physician.

The badges should be returned on time: Old badges give inaccurate results. It should be realized that all the radiation badges from all departments in the hospital (e.g., radiology, cardiology, operating rooms, etc.) are sent for readings at the same time and that a delay in returning the badges from one department unnecessarily delays the reading of all badges. The reports are usually issued in the form of monthly computer printouts (Fig. 77.9).

ORGANIZATION OF RADIATION PROTECTION

Each hospital has a radiation safety office. The office usually has a clinical director, a radiation adviser, and a radiation protection supervisor.[23] The clinical director is usually a radiologist or clinician responsible for establishing protocols and procedures for the examination of patients, who is involved in the selection of equipment as well as day-to-day decisions. The radiation protection adviser (RPA) is usually an experienced physicist who gives advice on the design of x-ray rooms, monitoring of doses to patients and staff, and who performs calibration and safety checks on radiology equipment. The radiation protection supervisor (RPS) is usually an experienced full-time member of the radiology staff who will, in collaboration with the RPA, write local rules and ensure their compliance by the staff, ensure that the staff wear radiation monitoring devices, and report to the department chair, administration, or RPA any incident in the hospital that is related to radiation safety.

RADIOLOGICAL CONTRAST MEDIA

Iodine is the only element that has proved satisfactory for general use as an intravascular radiological contrast medium. Its radio-opacity is conferred by its high molecular weight. The maximum recommended concentration of iodine is 300 mg iodine per mL and the maximum recommended dose is 3 g of iodine. The absorption of iodine is variable. Its mean half-life is 12 hours and 80%–90% is excreted via the kidneys within 24 hours. There are two kinds of contrast media with respect to their osmolality: the high-osmolality contrast

TABLE 77.7 Contrast Media, Iodine Concentrations, and Osmolalities

Contrast Medium	Iodine (mg/mL)	Osmolality
HOCM		
Diatriazoate Na (Hypaque)	300	1522–1550 (Delete: Hypaque)
Diatriazoate Na	292	1422–1539
(8%)-meglumine	—	—
(52%) (Renografin)	—	—
Iothalamate meglumine	282	1400
(60%) (Conray)	—	—
LOCM		
Iohexol (Omnipaque)	300	709
Iopamidol (Isovue)	300	616
Ioversol (Optiray)	320	702
Ioxaglate sodium	320	600
(19.6%)-meglumine	—	—
(39.3%) (Hetabrix)	—	—

Source: Drug reviews from the formulary. Intravascular contrast media. Hosp Pharm. *26:275-278, 1991.*

media (HOCM) and the low-osmolality contrast media (LOCM) (Table 77.7).[42,43] The HOCM are ionic monomers and include various concentrations of sodium, meglumine, or sodium-meglumine salts of diatrizoic and iothalamic salts. They are also called first-generation agents. These media provide three iodine atoms for two ions, giving an iodine:particle ratio of 3:2; their osmolalities range between 433 mOsm/kg and 2400 mOsm/kg.[42] The LOCM are nonionic monomers, that is, molecules that do not dissociate in solution. They are also called second-generation agents, and are by far the most common type of contrast agent used today. The LOCM provide an iodine:particle ratio of 3:1 and their osmolalities range between 411 mOsm/kg and 796 mOsm/kg.[42] The LOCM cause less nausea and vomiting, produce less pain on peripheral arterial injection, and are associated with a lower incidence of mild, moderate, and severe adverse reactions compared to the HOCM (the incidence of adverse reaction rate with LOCM is 0.03% compared to 0.36% with HOCM). There are formulations of LOCM that are Food and Drug Administration-approved for intrathecal use (e.g., Isovue-M 200 and 300, Omnipaque 180 and 210). Only these agents should be used for spine procedures, as any planned injection may be inadvertently deposited in the intrathecal space.

ADVERSE REACTIONS TO CONTRAST MEDIA

The concerns regarding the use of contrast media include adverse reactions. Patients considered at greater risk of an adverse reaction to the contrast media are listed in Table 77.8.[42] Patients who have a history of allergic reaction to the radiologic contrast media should be premedicated. Greenberger and Patterson[44] have recommended that the patient be given three doses of oral prednisone 50 mg at 13, 7, and 1 hours before the procedure. It has also been recommended that oral diphenhydramine (Benadryl) 50 mg be given 1 hour before injection of the contrast.[27] Lasser et al.[45] have recommended two oral doses of methylprednisolone 32 mg given at 12 and 2 hours before the procedure.

TABLE 77.8 Patients at Greater Risk of a Severe Adverse Reaction to Radiologic Contrast Media

Patients with history of a previous adverse reaction to radiologic contrast media (excluding mild flushing, nausea)
Asthmatic patients
Allergic and atopic patients
Cardiac patients with decompensation, unstable arrhythmia, recent myocardial infarction
Renal failure, diabetic nephropathy
Feeble infants and the elderly
Patients with severe general debility or dehydration
Patients with metabolic hematologic disorders

Source: Grainger RG: Intravenous contrast media. In Grainger RG, Allison D, editors: Grainger & Allison's Diagnostic Radiology: A Textbook of Medical Imaging, *New York, Churchill-Livingstone, 1997, pp 35-45.*

GADOLINIUM AS AN ALTERNATIVE TO IODINATED RADIOGRAPHIC CONTRAST MEDIA

Gadolinium chelates (e.g., gadopentate dimeglumine (Magnevist)), are intravenous contrast agents used to enhance vascular structures during diagnostic magnetic resonance imaging. Gadolinium chelates have been used successfully in place of iodinated contrast media for image-guided spine interventions and have become an alternative to iodinated contrast agents in patients with known contrast allergy. The radio-opacity of gadolinium is less than that of iodinated contrast agents, which results in a less distinct appearance on fluoroscopic images. Regardless, the injection of 1–3 mL of undiluted gadopentate dimeglumine (Magnevist) has been used to successfully identify the placement of the needle in the epidural space and at other target sites. Gadolinium chelates also appear to be safe when administered directly into the cerebrospinal fluid (CSF) (i.e., a "wet tap" during epidural steroid injection).[46] A rare but catastrophic risk associated with gadolinium-based contrast agents is the possible development of nephrogenic systemic fibrosis in patients with renal disease.[47] The risk depends on the degree of renal dysfunction, the dose of contrast agent, and the severity of concomitant illness; it varies from negligible in healthy patients up to 2%–5% in high-risk patients. The use of gadolinium-based contrast is contraindicated in patients with a glomerular filtration rate (GFR) < 30 mL/min per 1.72 m^2, and caution is recommended in patients with moderately reduced kidney function (30–60 mL/min).[48] Given the small amount of gadolinium used in most fluoroscopically-assisted pain interventions, the risk of renal toxicity is negligible.

KEY POINTS

- Studies have shown the usefulness of fluoroscopy in pain interventional procedures as landmarks can be difficult to recognize in the obese, the elderly, and those with spinal stenosis.
- ABC is the system wherein the computer automatically analyzes the image contrast and makes appropriate tube current adjustments, balancing image contrast and patient safety. It is advisable that the physician leaves the ABC system on during procedures. However, the system can increase radiation when the physician wears lead gloves. Sensing a poorly imaged interventionalist's hand, the system will automatically increase the voltage to improve the image.
- Other than lead aprons, measures to improve radiation safety include increased distance between the patients and the x-ray tube, the use of pulse mode, intermittent fluoroscopy, collimation, limited use of magnification, and greater distance between the physician and the x-ray tube.
- LOCM are the most commonly used as they cause fewer side effects compared to the high-osmolality contrast media.
- Patients with a history of allergic reaction to contrast media should be prepped with a steroid, with or without diphenhydramine.
- Gadolinium-based contrast agents can be used in patients with a history of contrast allergy as allergic reactions to these agents are extremely rare. It may cause nephrogenic systemic fibrosis and should not be used in patients with renal insufficiency.

REFERENCES

Access the reference list online at ExpertConsult.com.

CHAPTER 78

Efficacy of Interventional Procedures for Neuropathic Pain

Jiang Wu, MD · Brett Stacey, MD · Srinivasa N. Raja, MD

INTRODUCTION

Neuropathic pain (NP) has recently been defined as "pain caused by a lesion or disease of the somatosensory system."[1] It has an estimated prevalence of 7% to 9.8% of the adult population, and up to 20% of patients with chronic pain may have neuropathic characteristics.[2,3] Moreover, NP is reported to be severely debilitating, and is associated with negative impacts on health-related quality of life, including significant anxiety, depression, and high economic burden.[4–6] Unfortunately, NP is often refractory to pharmacologic and noninterventional treatment as only a minority of people who receive these treatments experience meaningful analgesic benefit,[7] leaving many patients with high levels of pain and distress, and in need of alternative treatment approaches.

Interventional treatments, defined as "invasive procedures involving delivery of drugs into targeted areas, or ablation/modulation of targeted structures for the treatment of persistent pain,"[8] provide an alternative treatment strategy for patients with refractory NP. With increasing knowledge of pain mechanisms, technical advances, and technique refinement, interventional pain approaches remain attractive treatment options for people living with refractory NP.

Unfortunately, the literature supporting interventional procedures for chronic pain treatment is limited due to the numerous barriers to placebo-controlled or comparative clinical trials in general, and for neuropathic pain in particular.[9,10] Additionally, the currently available evidence is difficult to analyze due to variations in study methodology, varied patient populations, inconsistent outcome measures, lack of consensus regarding what constitutes a successful treatment response,[11] and limited attention to demonstrating the impact of these interventions on health-related quality of life, including physical and emotional functioning.[12,13] Therefore, the literature interpreting the available clinical evidence and describing the roles of these interventions is controversial and inconsistent.[14–18] Given this lack of quality data and consensus, there are no strong recommendations that can be made on interventional management of neuropathic pain. However, there is sufficient evidence to support consideration of specific interventional options for selected neuropathic pain states, particularly for patients with pain that has not responded adequately to other treatment efforts.

Examples of peripheral NP states include herpes zoster, postherpetic neuralgia (PHN), traumatic or postsurgical neuropathy, peripheral painful diabetic neuropathy (PPDN), and other peripheral neuropathies including compression neuropathy. The prime examples of central NP are central poststroke pain and spinal cord injury pain. We also included two diagnoses that may not be considered to be purely neuropathic: complex regional pain syndrome (CRPS) and persistent pain following spine surgery, commonly known as "failed back surgery syndrome" (FBSS).

In this chapter, we present an up-to-date summary of the scientific evidence on the efficacy of neural blockade and neurolytic procedures for managing NP. The evidence for efficacy is, at best, moderate, and is often limited or conflicting. A detailed discussion of the risk-benefit analysis and cost effectiveness of the interventional techniques is beyond the scope of this chapter. Due to an emerging body of evidence for spinal cord stimulation (SCS) and intrathecal drug delivery therapies for neuropathic pain, these will be discussed in detail in separate chapters (see Chapters 73 and 76).

NEURAL BLOCKADE TECHNIQUES

THE DIAGNOSTIC VALUE OF NEURAL BLOCKADE

In patients with focal peripheral neuropathic pain, diagnostic nerve blocks may be used to determine if a particular nerve is involved in the patient's symptoms by either signaling the pain from innervated tissues, or being the source of ectopic activity that leads to neuropathic pain. Although technical advances, such as direct visualization with advanced image guidance, allow the accurate delivery of small volumes of local anesthetics (typically without steroids when injected for diagnostic purposes) to the targeted nerve, interpretation of even properly performed diagnostic blocks is not always straightforward. Information obtained from blocks may be helpful in confirming a clinical impression, for selecting among different treatment options (the choice of medicines, therapeutic blocks, or surgical therapy), or predicting the response to neuroablative therapies. Examples include blocks of the median, ulnar, or radial nerve for pain in the hand, intercostal nerves for pain after thoracotomy/mastectomy, and ilioinguinal and iliohypogastric nerve blocks for pain after hernia repairs. The value of diagnostic blocks in confirming a diagnosis, formulating a treatment plan, or predicting the response of a subsequent treatment have not been carefully examined for most procedures.

The utility of diagnostic nerve blocks is best established in nonneuropathic axial spine pain, specifically with medial branch blocks for cervical and lumbar zygapophysial (facet) joint pain. Studies to support diagnostic blocks for neuropathic pain are growing for peripheral nerve blocks in mononeuropathies, including median nerve compression (carpal tunnel syndrome), occipital neuralgia, or selective nerve root blocks for radiculopathy. Nevertheless, there are no clear standards for many details of diagnostic procedures specifically for neuropathic pain, including guidance technique, needle placement, injectate (medication and volume), the need for controlled or repeated procedures, or comparison with other diagnostic techniques. These deficiencies need to be recalled as we review these techniques.

Radiculopathy

The selective nerve root block was developed as a technique to identify the source of intractable radicular symptoms, particularly when the clinical symptoms are not well localized, and imaging studies indicate multilevel degenerative changes with possible compression of several roots. While these techniques may be used for surgical decision making, there are only limited data (primarily retrospective) to support their use for prediction.[19] Therefore, the use of diagnostic or prognostic selective nerve root blocks needs to be put in a careful individualized context.

Retrospective studies have investigated the ability of selective spinal nerve blocks to diagnose disease and to predict surgical outcome. The positive predictive value (fraction of patients with injection indicating radiculopathy, in whom surgery confirmed radicular pathology at the level indicated by the test) ranged from 87% to 100%.[20–23] The negative predictive values (percentage of patients with a negative injection test and confirmed at the surgery to have normal nerve roots) were reported as 20% and 38% of the small number of patients operated upon, despite negative tests.[20,21] Bear in mind that such "diagnostic" injections are typically only considered when the information will be acted upon, meaning surgical intervention is viewed as a viable treatment option.

The role of injected steroids in addition to local anesthetic in a diagnostic block is a controversial topic. However, a retrospective report of the ability of a steroid-containing injection of the spinal nerve to predict surgical outcome showed that the false positive rate (percentage of patients with failed surgery who had a favorable response to injection) was 5%, and the false negative rate (percentage of surgical successes who had no response to steroids) was 35%. These observations suggest that patients with radicular pain who are unlikely to benefit from surgery can be reliably identified by a lack of response to epidural steroid injections (ESIs), but some patients who may benefit from surgery could be missed by this diagnostic test.[24]

Peripheral Neuropathic Pain

The main diagnostic tools in peripheral neuropathies are electromyography, ultrasonography, computed tomography, and/or magnetic resonance imaging, which are interpreted in the context of clinical findings. At times, an injection might provide valuable information if more standard testing has led to ambiguity. A case report on the role of diagnostic ultrasound-guided selective common peroneal nerve block in a patient with classic neuropathic pain after below-knee amputation suggested that successful diagnostic, ultrasound-guided, selective peripheral nerve block may be performed to help in the diagnosis and subsequent surgical resection of a painful neuroma to relieve severe neuropathic pain.[25] A multicenter retrospective study examined the role of diagnostic nerve blocks in evaluating pulsed radiofrequency (PRF) for occipital neuralgia. It reported that about half of the subjects experienced a positive outcome (≥50% pain relief coupled with procedure satisfaction lasting at least 3 months), and variables associated with a positive outcome included a traumatic inciting event and lower diagnostic block volumes.[26]

BOX 78.1 Comments on Diagnostic Nerve Blocks in Neuropathic Pain

Neuropathic Pain	Comments
Radiculopathy	The 35% false negative rate response to steroid injections suggests that patients who do not experience relief will not respond to surgery
Peripheral neuropathic pain	There is paucity of data on the efficacy of diagnostic blocks
Complex regional pain syndrome (CRPS)	Data on the efficacy of sympathetic blocks in CRPS is weak

Complex Regional Pain Syndrome

Given the possible involvement of the sympathetic nervous system in the initiation or maintenance of pain in CRPS, sympathetic blocks have a unique and long tradition in the dual roles of both diagnostic and therapeutic tools in the management of CRPS. Despite this history, the data supporting them is limited with weak evidence to support the diagnostic role of the classic stellate ganglion block (SGB) and lumbar sympathetic block (LSB) to differentiate sympathetically independent pain from sympathetically maintained pain (SMP).[27]

Specific comments on the value of diagnostic nerve blocks are in Box 78.1.

Summary: Diagnostic Value of Neural Blockade

- Diagnostic nerve blocks have a potential role in the management of chronic neuropathic pain, as they can help determine the anatomical source of pain, and a target for treatments.
- Specificity of the diagnostic nerve blocks may be enhanced by advanced imaging guidance using the lowest volume of injectate, preferably with local anesthetic alone rather than steroids.
- The classic SGB and LSB that remain in most CRPS treatment algorithms in order to differentiate sympathetically independent pain from sympathetically maintained pain need to be interpreted with caution.

THE THERAPEUTIC VALUE OF NEURAL BLOCKADE

NP has multiple etiologies, but nerve entrapment/compression in tissue planes and trauma to nerves are important causes.[28] Nerve injury has been shown to activate the secretion of inflammatory mediators and to increase ectopic discharge from injured primary afferents,[29,30] thereby contributing to the development of NP.[31,32] Peripheral damage may lead to changes in central pain processing and central sensitization.[33] Many physicians have observed improved pain in response to a series of local anesthetic injections with steroids in patients with chronic neuropathic nonmalignant pain. The exact mechanism of this seeming reversal of adverse neuroplastic changes is unknown. Corticosteroids have anti-inflammatory effects and immunosuppressant actions. Application of steroids to injured nerve fibers is presumed to suppress both of these mechanisms, alleviating edema, and resulting in a reduction of both spontaneous and evoked pain.[34] Although botulinum toxin (BTX) is only FDA-approved for chronic migraine in pain medicine, the literature strongly suggests its efficacy for several NP conditions.

Peripheral Compression or Trauma-Related Neuropathic Pain

Perineural steroids are often used to treat chronic peripheral NP that is secondary to trauma or compression,[35,36] and Morton's neuroma.[37] Some randomized controlled trials (RCTs) showed that combining steroids with local anesthetic (LA) may increase efficacy,[38] and LA injections without steroids may confer long-term analgesic benefits.[39] A recent systemic review concluded that the change in mean pain scores following the injection of steroids represented a modest, but significant, reduction from baseline (25%).[18] The analgesia resulting from steroid injection is possibly dose-dependent. A double-blind, placebo-controlled study in patients with peripheral nerve compression or trauma-related NP showed that 40–80 mg of methylprednisolone or triamcinolone (these steroids are equipotent)[40] had a beneficial effect in reducing pain at 1–3 months after injection when compared with LA injection or Conventional Medical Management (i.e., no injections). A larger reduction in pain scores was observed in RCTs that used higher doses of steroids (methylprednisolone 80 mg) and recorded pain scores at 3 months,[41,42] when compared with trials that used lower doses of steroids (methylprednisolone or triamcinolone 40 mg) and recorded pain scores earlier (at 1–2 months).[38,43,44] Studies with a high risk of bias[38,42,44] were associated with a significant analgesic effect in favor of perineural steroids. Other studies indicate that the placebo analgesic effect is strong and that some of the analgesic benefits from perineurally injected steroids may be due to systemic uptake of the drug.[45] Multiple subsequent injections are probably justified if substantial clinical benefit is obtained from the first injection; however, there is no evidence to support the contention that multiple injections will generate long-term relief.

Carpal tunnel syndrome is a common focal peripheral mononeuropathy caused by compression of the median nerve in the carpal tunnel at the wrist. Local anesthetic and steroid injections are commonly used to provide short-term symptomatic relief and to improve functional status as a step before more definite surgical decompression. This approach is supported by three high-quality RCTs: Clinical improvement for carpal tunnel syndrome at 1 month or less following local corticosteroids was demonstrated in a total of 141 participants compared with placebo injection,[46,47] and significantly more improvement was observed in the corticosteroid injection group compared with the oral corticosteroid group within 8 weeks.[48] Although more than one (two injections vs. one) injection of local corticosteroid did not provide further clinical improvement,[49] prior local steroid injection does not prejudice the outcome of subsequent surgery.[50]

Technically, more accurate localization of the median nerve with ultrasound guidance might lead to better outcomes. A Bayesian network meta-analysis of 10 studies with 633 patients compared the clinical effectiveness of local corticosteroid injections using the distal to flexor crease approach, the proximal to flexor crease approach, an ultrasound-guided in-plane injection, and an ultrasound-guided out-of-plane injection. Based on the clinical response, the change in symptom severity scale, and the change in the functional status scale before or near 8 weeks, the study concluded that the ultrasound-guided in-plane approach was the most effective among the above four injection techniques for carpal tunnel syndrome.[51]

The prognostic value of local corticosteroid injections in predicting surgical outcomes in carpal tunnel syndrome was evaluated in a prospective study, which concluded that longer relief of symptoms after steroid injection correlated with better results of surgical treatment.[52]

The effectiveness of intradermal injection of botulinum neurotoxin-A (BTX-A) for either surgical trauma-related or nonsurgical trauma-related nerve injuries was also studied. A randomized, prospective, double-blind, parallel group study in 25 patients assessed the effectiveness of intradermal injection of BTX A and reported significant improvement in average pain scores, brush allodynia, and cold pain threshold despite transiently aggravating immediate postprocedural pain.[53]

Herpes Zoster

Studies of neural blockade in herpes zoster vary in the method, number, frequency, and duration of the blocks, and hence, are difficult to interpret. An RCT suggested that epidural blocks with local anesthetics combined with steroids soon after the onset of herpes zoster can result in decreased pain and allodynia.[54] Another RCT reported that a single epidural injection of methylprednisolone and bupivacaine within 7 days of the onset of herpes zoster resulted in a modest benefit at 1 month (48% with pain in epidural steroid group vs. 58% with standard therapy). However, the prevalence of chronic pain over a 6-month follow-up period was not significantly reduced.[55]

An RCT found that repetitive paravertebral injections (the paravertebral block with local anesthetics and steroids every 48 hours for 1 week plus acyclovir and analgesics) for acute herpes zoster resulted in only 13% of patients reporting zoster-related pain versus 45% in participants allocated to standard therapy (acyclovir and analgesics) at 1 month posttherapy. At 3, 6, and 12 months posttherapy, the incidence of PHN continued to be significantly lower in the paravertebral group than in the standard therapy group.[56]

The results of RCTs suggest that repetitive epidural injections of local anesthetics and steroids early in herpes zoster may prevent PHN.[54,56] These results are consistent with the results of several previous observational and cohort studies evaluating epidural local anesthetics alone or combined with steroids in herpes zoster.[57]

Postherpetic Neuralgia

The literature on the efficacy of intrathecal methylprednisolone acetate (IT MPA) in NP patients is contradictory in three published RCTs. In the first small study in which 25 patients were divided into two arms, IT administration of MPA was more effective than epidural administration.[58] Later, the same researchers reported the efficacy of four IT injections of MPA and lidocaine (89 subjects) performed over a 1-month period was superior compared with lidocaine alone (91 subjects) and a no-treatment control group (90 subjects) on 1–2 years follow-up.[59] In order to confirm the results obtained from this trial, an independent research group attempted to replicate the findings. This trial was terminated early because an increase in pain was experienced at 8 weeks in all six patients randomized to IT MPA compared to one of four people in the control group.[60] The lack of reproducibility of the results of this single RCT, along with lack of biological plausibility[61–65] and the potential risks of adhesive arachnoiditis[66–68] and fungal meningitis, have raised concerns over the use of IT MPA.

Several nonrandomized trials assessing sympathetic blockade in PHN have failed to demonstrate any benefit, and since there are very few data available to suggest a beneficial effect, it is difficult to recommend this as a viable treatment option.[57,69,70]

In contrast, two double-blind, randomized studies support the efficacy of BTX-A in the treatment of PHN. The first study compared subcutaneous, gridlike, 1-cm interval injections of BTX-A, lidocaine, and saline (20 people in each of the three groups) into the region of tactile allodynia, and reported better pain relief, improved sleep hours, and reduced opioid consumptions in the BTX-A group over a 3-month follow-up.[71] The favorable outcomes—improvement in visual analogue scale (VAS) pain score and quality of sleep—were reproduced in a subsequent study comparing the effect of subcutaneous, "chessboard manner" injection of BTX-A with placebo in 30 adult subjects with PHN.[72] The efficacy of BTX-A treatment for PHN from blinded observations are further supported by two retrospective observational studies in small numbers of patients.[73,74]

Lumbosacral and Cervical Radiculopathy

An epidural injection of steroids to treat radicular pain can be accomplished by many techniques with varied success and risks. The most commonly studied approaches are the interlaminar (IL), transforaminal (TF), and caudal routes. A comparative study among IL, TF, and caudal steroid administration concluded that the TF route is more effective than the caudal or IL routes.[19] Using a TF approach, the injectate spreads to the ventral epidural space in almost all cases (close to the intervertebral disk),[75] while the injectate using the IL approach can miss the targeted ventral epidural space in up to 40% of cases.[76] Three systematic reviews and meta-analysis of RCTs concluded that a TF ESI offered short-term positive pain-reducing benefits (>2 weeks but <12 months) for patients with acute or subacute radicular pain.[15,77,78] A comprehensive evidence-based review of RCTs on ESIs concluded that a modest benefit lasting up to 3 months was more likely when the TF technique was used (>70%) compared to the caudal (60%) and interlaminar (50%) techniques. In addition, the specialty of the author heavily influenced the results of both RCTs and review articles, with greater than 75% of RCTs and reviews authored by pain physicians being positive, compared to only 30% of RCTs and review articles conducted by nonpain physicians.[19] In light of the potential catastrophic complications associated with the TF approach, the parasagittal interlaminar route was investigated in a double-blind RCT and found to result in comparable ventral epidural spread, pain relief, and functional improvement, while being associated with a lower risk of complications.[79] Factors other than route may be associated with a less robust response to ESI. In a prospective cohort study, pain duration greater than 12 months, prior surgery, and heightened anxiety all decreased the odds of achieving a minimum clinically important difference in the Oswestry Disability Index 3 months after lumbar epidural steroids injection (LESI).[80]

Interestingly, ESIs might represent a relatively safe and inexpensive option to facilitate functional recovery or avoid surgery. A double-blind RCT, authored by an orthopedic spine group, evaluated the operative rate in surgically amenable patients with herniated disk or spinal stenosis. It found that 29% of patients in the ESI group underwent surgery, which favorably compared with a 67% operative rate in the control group without ESI at follow-up periods ranging between 13 and 28 months; the avoidance of surgery persisted in most patients available at a subsequent 5-year follow-up.[81] A recent meta-analysis and systematic review of randomized trials evaluating the efficacy of ESI found that epidural steroids have a small preventive effect on the need for surgery in the short term (<1 year), but not the long term.[82] Another orthopedic RCT performed in 200 patients who were followed for 2 years after lumbar discectomy reported a 2-day reduction in hospital stay (from 8 to 6 days, $P = .0001$) and a reduction in the number of patients with neurological signs (70% vs. 44%, $P = .0004$) in the group who received ESI following discectomy, although no difference in reoperation rates was noted.[83]

Failed Back Surgery Syndrome With Prominent Radicular Symptoms

Persistent pain after spinal surgery, often referred to as FBSS, represents an important and heterogeneous group of chronic pain patients, many of whom have an NP component with a variety of potential pathophysiologic mechanisms.[16] Patients with prominent radicular symptoms associated with FBSS represent one group who are frequently referred for ESIs. Unfortunately, there are no high-quality studies of ESIs specifically in this patient population, but a prospective web-based registry study suggests decreased efficacy in these patients. This study of 239 consecutive patients undergoing LESI for back-related disability, back pain, and leg pain associated with degenerative spine pathology concluded that prior surgery decreased the odds of achieving a minimum clinically important difference in the Oswestry Disability Index after LESI.[80]

Complex Regional Pain Syndrome

Based on the evidence for possible involvement of the sympathetic nervous system in the initiation or maintenance of pain in CRPS, a sympathetic nerve block (SNB) is commonly used for pain relief, and to provide a "window of opportunity" for more aggressive rehabilitation therapy.[84] The potential benefits of sympathetic blockade with local anesthetics in patients with CRPS have been systematically reviewed.[85,86] In patients who respond favorably to an SNB, the pain relief generally outlasts the effects of the local anesthetic and may be long lasting in some cases.[87,88] A randomized crossover study of seven subjects showed modest benefits 3 days after a local anesthetic SNB.[87] An RCT of SGB versus "active control" (in the form of guanethidine IV regional block) reported improvement in both groups, but without significant differences between groups.[89] A long-term, randomized, double-blinded, active-control study evaluated the efficacy of a thoracic sympathetic block (TSB) for upper limb type I CRPS at the 12-month follow-up in 36 patients. Scores from average pain items, pain dimensions (McGill Pain Questionnaire), evoked-pain symptom subscores, and depression scores were significantly lower in the TSB group compared to the control group.[90] Furthermore, a case series of 25 subjects who underwent three SGBs at weekly intervals for upper-extremity CRPS reported that 40% of patients had complete pain relief, 36% had partial pain relief, and 24% had no pain relief over a 6-month observation period.[91]

Given the role of the proliferation of adrenergic receptors and depolarization of nociceptors by increasing catecholamine release at the cholinergic nerve terminals as a possible molecular basis underlying SMP, BTX was introduced to prolong the duration of SNB. A double blind, cross-over RCT evaluated the duration of analgesia by LSB with BTX in nine patients with SMP of the lower extremity caused by CRPS. The study reported the median time to analgesia failure was 71 days after LSB with BTA, compared with less than 10 days after standard LSB. They concluded that BTA profoundly prolonged the analgesia from SNB in this pilot study.[92] An effective and durable sympathetic blockade with the mixture of local anesthetics and BTX was reported again in a small case report of LSB on two patients with CRPS in the lower extremity. Pain intensity and the neuropathic symptoms and signs score were significantly reduced, allodynia and coldness disappeared, and skin color returned to normal.[93] In agreement with these observations, another single case report described similar favorable outcomes after a subcutaneous injection of BTX-A in a patient with CRPS in the upper extremity.[94]

Due to the ease of application, the relative safety, and the limitations of alternative treatment options for CRPS, SNB—particularly when used in the context of a comprehensive treatment strategy—is a reasonable treatment option to consider for patients with CRPS refractory to pharmacologic and nonpharmacologic noninterventional treatments, especially when conducted early in the disease course, and when the patient favors such treatment before consideration of more invasive options, such as SCS.[84]

Trigeminal Neuralgia and Trigeminal Neuropathy

Most of the evidence for the efficacy of BTX-A in treating NP comes from trigeminal neuralgia (TN). There are 20 reports (including three double-blind[95–97] and one single-blind studies[98]) describing favorable effects and no serious side effects. A 13-week, randomized, parallel design, double-blind, placebo-controlled study assessed the subcutaneous injection of BTX-A in dosages up to 75 U in the trigeminal area affected, and demonstrated significant reduction in pain frequency and intensity. There were a higher number of pain responders in the interventional group (21 subjects) compared to the saline group (19 subjects), with some side effects, such as mild facial asymmetry and local facial swelling.[95] Two years later, the same group of authors compared the effects of low-dose (25 U) and high-dose (75 U) BTX-A to saline in a similar patient population. The study again reported the efficacy of BTX-A, with comparable efficacy between the groups, but fewer side effects in the low-dose group.[96] A third study evaluated 50 U of BTX-A and found marginal improvement at 2 months, but significant improvement in VAS pain scores at 3 months after injection in the interventional group (20 patients) compared to the placebo group (16 patients).[97] The reduction in pain intensity is clinically significant, as highlighted in a single-blind, randomized control study of 20 subjects, which compared subcutaneous injection of 40–60 U of BTX-A with placebo. This study demonstrated a reduction of 6.5 points on the VAS, compared with three points in the placebo group.[98]

Due to the lack of RCTs or prospective cohort studies, there are few systematic reviews based on uncontrolled case series of interventional treatments with local anesthetics in patients with medically refractory TN.[65,99–103] Although the evidence is not robust, evidence-based reviews conclude that percutaneous procedures delivering a local anesthetic at the trigeminal ganglion can play a role in the management of selected patients.

Painful Diabetic and Other Peripheral Neuropathies

Recently, three placebo-controlled, blinded studies and a meta-analysis have appeared in the literature supporting the efficacy of BTX-A for metabolic-induced painful peripheral neuropathies like PDN, although there are still no controlled studies assessing its efficacy in drug-induced and chemotherapy-related painful neuropathies. One double-blind, crossover study of 18 patients in which 4 U per site of Botox were injected intradermally into the hyperesthetic and allodynic foot regions reported improvement in pain reduction and sleep quality at 12 weeks.[104] Another study with a similar size and design reported a marked decrease in both tactile perception and mechanical pain

BOX 78.2 Results of Published Studies on the Effects of Therapeutic Nerve Blocks in Neuropathic Pain

Neuropathic Pain	Comments
Peripheral compression (NP)	Studies showed the efficacy of perineural local anesthetic and steroid injections in peripheral compression syndrome
Herpes zoster	Two RCTs on the efficacy of epidural steroids in preventing postherpetic pain, given within 1 week of the onset of rash, showed different results
Postherpetic neuralgia	The benefit derived from intrathecal steroid injections was not confirmed in a subsequent study
Lumbosacral and cervical radiculopathy	Transforaminal ESIs appear to be more effective than interlaminar ESI in unilateral one-level radiculitis
FBSS	There are no high-quality studies on ESIs in FBSS
Trigeminal neuralgia	Studies showed that the subcutaneous BTX-A reduces the frequency and intensity of pain in trigeminal neuralgia
PDN	The intradermal injection of BTX-A appears to reduce the hyperesthesia and allodynia in PDN

BTX-A, Botulinum toxin A; *ESI,* epidural steroid injections; *FBSS,* failed back surgery syndrome; *NP,* neuropathic pain; *PDN,* painful diabetic neuropathy; *RCTs,* randomized controlled trials.

in the interventional group at weeks 1, 4, 8, and 12 after treatment compared with baseline.[105] A third controlled trial assessing the safety and efficacy of repeated subcutaneous administration of BTX-A up to 300 U in 66 patients with NP showed a sustained analgesic effect over 24 weeks from the first administration in the interventional group (34 subjects) compared to the placebo group (32 subjects), with pain on injection being the only adverse effect reported.[106] A meta-analysis that included two studies on PDN showed improvement of 1.96 VAS points following treatment with BTX-A, suggesting a correlation between BTX-A and the improvement in pain scores.[107] General comments on the value of therapeutic nerve blocks are shown in Box 78.2. The results of BTX injections in TN are shown in Table 78.1. The results of BTX injections in PDN are shown in Table 78.2.

Summary: Therapeutic Value of Neural Blockade

- Perineural steroids can provide symptomatic relief of chronic peripheral NP from traumatic or compressive etiologies;
- Epidural or paravertebral local anesthetic and steroid nerve blocks provide symptomatic relief of acute pain associated with herpes zoster;
- Epidural steroids are a viable treatment option for acute radiculopathy for short-term benefit, and ESI might facilitate recovery and reduce the need for surgical intervention;
- Percutaneous procedures directed at the trigeminal ganglion are a treatment option for refractory TN;
- Local corticosteroid injection for carpal tunnel syndrome provides short-term clinical improvement in symptoms;
- The use of intrathecal methylprednisolone or sympathetic nerve blocks in PHN should generally be avoided[108];
- A short series of sympathetic blocks is a reasonable treatment option for patients with CRPS refractory to pharmacologic and nonpharmacologic noninterventional treatments, especially when conducted early in the disease course and combined with rehabilitation efforts. A BTX-A injection may prolong the analgesia of a local anesthetic from a sympathetic ganglion block;
- A BTX-A injection could provide prolonged symptomatic pain relief for refractory TN, PHN, posttraumatic neuralgia, and PDN; a repetitive injection at monthly intervals could provide long-term pain relief with mild and transient side effects.

NEURAL DESTRUCTIVE TECHNIQUES, PULSE RADIOFREQUENCY

Once the nociceptive pathways have been identified, and in certain rare instances (e.g., if pain is experienced within the sensory territory of a single nerve and that nerve is both distal and purely sensory in function, or if a neuroma has formed as a result of nerve injury), ablative procedures, including chemical denervation (phenol or alcohol), cryoneurolysis or cryoablation, and radiofrequency ablation of a peripheral nerve, may be of long-term benefit for chronic NP.[109,110]

Recently, a new mode of radiofrequency, PRF, has been appearing in the literature. PRF was conceived as a novel, potentially safer mode of administration of radiofrequency (RF) energy, as the PRF technique is considered to be nondestructive, exposing the neural tissue to a high-frequency electric field without raising the temperature of the electrode tip beyond 42°C, thereby avoiding nerve injury.[111,112] For this reason, PRF is often used to treat refractory NP conditions.

Neural ablative modalities should be cautiously considered for severe nonmalignant NP only after other treatment modalities have been attempted without success. For example, with the possible exception of cryoablation,[113] neuroablative therapies are rarely used to treat NP because an additional insult/injury to the nervous system carries a risk of increasing the pain from a preexisting nervous system injury.[114] An exception to this rule is in the treatment of terminal cancer pain, given that the pain relief of the neurolytic procedure will generally outlast the life of the patient. In other words, the time it takes for the additional injury from the neurolytic procedure to cause pain is longer than the life of the patient.

Postherpetic Neuralgia

A double-blind RCT compared PRF versus sham therapy in 96 patients with PHN affecting thoracic dermatomes (T2–T11).[115] The intercostal nerve at the level of the zoster lesion, and the segments above and below received PRF treatment once a week for 3 weeks. Postprocedure pain scores and tramadol use in the PRF group were significantly lower, and several health-related quality-of-life measurements were significantly improved through 6 months after treatment, compared to the sham group. An open-label, prospective study assessed the efficacy of PRF treatment of the affected cervical, thoracic, or lumbar dorsal root ganglion (DRG) for 49 patients with refractory PHN, and demonstrated

TABLE 78.1 Results of Randomized Controlled Trials on Botulinum Toxin Injection for the Treatment of Trigeminal Neuralgia

Author, Year	Study Design	Number of Patients	Results	Comments
Wu et al. (2012)[95]	Randomized, parallel design, double-blinded, placebo-controlled	Intradermal and/or submucosal injection of BTX-A 75 U (*n* = 21) vs. saline injection (*n* = 19)	Significant reduction in pain frequency and intensity, and a higher number of pain responders in the interventional group	Reports safety and efficacy of BTX-A
Zhang et al. (2014)[96]	Randomized, double-blinded, placebo-controlled	Subcutaneous injection of saline (*n* = 28) vs. BTX-A 25 U (*n* = 27) vs. BTX-A 75 U (*n* = 29)	Reports safety and comparable efficacy between low-dose (25 U) and high-dose (75 U) groups in 8 weeks	Reports safety and efficacy of BTX-A
Zuniga et al. (2013)[97]	Randomized, double-blinded, placebo-controlled	Subcutaneous injection of BTX-A 50 U + saline (*n* = 20) vs. saline injection (*n* = 16)	Marginal improvement at 2 months, but significant improvement in VAS pain scores at 3 months	Reports safety and efficacy of BTX-A
Shehata et al. (2013)[98]	Randomized, single blinded	Subcutaneous injection of 40–60 U of BTX-A (*n* = 10) vs. saline (*n* = 10)	A reduction of 6.5 points on the VAS, compared with 3 points in the placebo group	Reports clinically significant pain reduction with BTX-A

BTX-A, *Botulinum neurotoxin-A;* VAS, *visual analogue scale.*

TABLE 78.2 Results of Randomized Controlled Trials on Botulinum Toxin Injection for the Treatment of Diabetic Painful Neuropathy

Author, Year	Study Design	Number of Patients	Results	Comments
Yuan et al. (2009)[104]	Double-blind crossover	Intradermal injection of BTX-A (4 U/site) (*n* = 18)	Improvement in pain reduction and sleep quality at 12 weeks	Reports safety and efficacy of BTX-A
Chen et al. (2013)[105]	Double-blind crossover	Subcutaneous injection of BTX-A (*n* = 18)	A marked decrease in both tactile perception and mechanical pain in the interventional group at weeks 1, 4, 8, and 12 treatment compared with baseline	Reports safety and efficacy of BTX-A
Attal et al. (2016)[106]	Randomized, double-blinded, placebo-controlled	Subcutaneous injection of BTX-A (up to 300 U) (*n* = 34) vs. saline injection (*n* = 32)	A sustained analgesic effect over 24 weeks from the first administration	Reports safety and efficacy of BTX-A
Lakhan et al. (2015)[107]	Systemic review and meta-analysis	—	Improvement of 1.96 VAS points following treatment with BTX-A	Suggest a correlation between BTX-A and improvement of pain scores

BTX-A, *Botulinum neurotoxin-A;* VAS, *visual analogue scale.*

a 55% reduction in pain score (from baseline mean pain score 7.2 ± 1.7 to postprocedure pain score 3.4 ± 1.5) at 4 weeks after PRF, which was maintained at the subsequent 12-week follow-up.[116] Although these preliminary studies are promising, the results need to be confirmed by controlled trials.

Cervical and Lumbosacral Radiculopathy

Percutaneous conventional RF techniques are applied for the palliation of lumbosacral and cervical radiculopathy, and the efficacy of DRG rhizotomy in radicular pain has been examined.[117–119] The results of the RCTs did not support the role of RF lesioning of the DRG for lumbosacral radiculopathy. A double-blind RCT compared RF lesioning of the DRG to sham therapy in 83 patients with lumbosacral radicular pain and failed to demonstrate any significant benefit.[120] In contrast, the favorable safety profile and beneficial effect of PRF therapy has been described in the treatment of lumbosacral radiculopathy in a clinical audit, as well as a systemic review.[121,122]

PRF treatment of DRG in cervical radicular pain was examined in two RCTs. One reported a significant reduction in the VAS pain score and improvement in other multidimensional outcome parameters in the PRF group 2 months after treatment compared to sham therapy in 20 patients.[123] Another study observed a significant and identical reduction in VAS scores (3 or more points out of 10) in two groups with electrode tip temperatures of 40°C and 67°C 3 months after therapy in 61 patients.[124] The short-term efficacy of PRF treatment of the cervical DRG and segmental nerve roots was reproduced in two clinical trials. A pilot case series[125] and subsequent small RCT[126] by the same group of investigators suggested 3 months of beneficial effect in 23 patients with cervical brachialgia. Furthermore, an RCT performed in 27 patients with lumbosacral radicular pain reported long-term pain reduction (up to 12 months after treatment) compared to a control group that received nerve root blocks with local anesthetics.[127]

Sympathetically Maintained Pain

Sympathetic ablation techniques have been advocated for many years, mainly by surgeons, in an effort to produce a permanent interruption in the transmission of sympathetically maintained pain. Multiple nonsurgical techniques have also been employed to accomplish this, including chemical neurolysis (usually performed with phenol or alcohol), and percutaneous radiofrequency ablation.

RF ablative techniques are much more controllable than neurolytic solution injections and are less invasive than surgical ablation. Percutaneous RF techniques have been described in a large case series that included 148 procedures performed on 110 patients to ablate the upper thoracic sympathetic supply. A series of three lesions created with 18-gauge RF electrodes oriented rostrocaudally was employed to destroy the entire fusiform ganglion. Lesion effectiveness was observed, such that the sympathetic activity in 91% of operated limbs at 3-year follow-up continued to be completely or largely interrupted, though there was no reported assessment of clinical analgesic or functional outcomes.[128]

The available literature describing these sympathetic ablation techniques consists of either uncontrolled case series or poorly controlled comparison studies.[86] Preliminary reports in the form of case series are promising with regard to short-term outcomes, but neurodestructive techniques have fallen out of favor due to significant problems, such as deafferentation syndromes, recurrence of former symptoms or postsympathectomy neuralgia 6 months to 2 years postsympathectomy. The reported incidence of postsympathectomy neuralgia was 44% in one series evaluating open sympathectomy for causalgia.[129] These postablation pain conditions are often worse than the original pain.[114] The same holds true for neurolytic blocks utilizing alcohol or phenol, which have largely been relegated to the terminally ill. To date, there are no published data on pulsed RF sympathetic ganglion techniques.

Summary

- There is accumulating evidence for the efficacy of PRF of the intercostal nerve(s) and DRG in the treatment of PHN.
- There is limited evidence for the beneficial effects of PRF of DRG, and no evidence of benefit for RF lesioning in the treatment of lumbar radiculopathy.[130]
- There is limited evidence of a potential short-term benefit for PRF therapy of the DRG and segmental nerve roots in the treatment of chronic cervical radicular pain.
- Ablative sympathectomy techniques have been available for many years, but to date, no high-level evidence exists to support their widespread use, while postablation pain remains a real concern.
- It might be prudent that these ablative techniques generally be avoided given the weak evidence of their success, and the potential for serious associated sequelae.

REFERENCES

Access the reference list online at ExpertConsult.com.

SECTION IX

OTHER NERVE BLOCKS IN PAIN MEDICINE

SECTION OUTLINE HEAD

CHAPTER 79

Ultrasound-Guided Procedures for Pain Management: Spine Injections and Relevant Peripheral Nerve Blocks

Anuj Bhatia, MBBS, MD, FRCA, FFPMRCA, FIPP, FRCPC, EDRA, CIPS
Philip Peng, MBBS, FRCPC, Founder (Pain Med)

INTRODUCTION

Ultrasound (US) is a relatively new modality for guiding interventional procedures to provide pain relief. Traditionally, anatomic landmarks, fluoroscopy, computed tomography (CT), and nerve stimulation have been used for procedural guidance in pain management, but these modalities are associated with several limitations that can be overcome with US. US can enhance the accuracy and safety of procedures while eliminating exposure to ionizing radiation associated with fluoroscopy and CT and painful muscle contractions elicited by nerve stimulators. Imaging in real time, portability, and ability to see anatomic structures (e.g., nerves, muscles, blood vessels) are distinct advantages of US over other procedural guidance modalities.[1]

There are also some limitations with US guidance. Image quality is compromised with increase in depth of scanning and bony structures, and there are no validated surrogates for contrast-enhanced visualization of injectate available with fluoroscopy-guided techniques. A limited field of view and dependence of image quality on skill of the operator, who has to focus simultaneously on both image acquisition and procedural performance, are some of the other challenges with US.

US-guided procedures for relieving pain can be anatomically classified broadly into two categories, axial (spine-related)[2] and peripheral structures (nerves and muscles).[3] We present information on procedures in each of these two categories under the following headings: Anatomy, Sonoanatomy, Indications, Technique, and Pearls. This is preceded by discussion of US physics and knobology. Knowledge of these is a necessary prerequisite for performing procedures accurately, safely, and with minimal discomfort to the patient.[4]

BASICS OF ULTRASOUND

Medical US refers to use of sound waves at frequencies higher than the upper audible limit of human hearing. The usual range of medical US for procedural guidance is 1–18 MHz. US waves are generated by a transducer (also called a probe), a device that uses the piezoelectric effect to convert electrical energy to acoustic energy. The waves are propagated through the tissue and reflected back to the transducer from tissue interfaces that differ in density. A reverse piezoelectric effect is used to generate images from the reflected waves. The speed of sound waves through the tissues is a function of wavelength and frequency. Higher frequency is associated with shorter wavelengths and vice versa. Shorter wavelengths (i.e., higher frequencies) result in higher resolution (the ability to discriminate between two adjacent structures). Therefore high-frequency linear transducers (range 6–18 MHz) produce images with a better resolution of structures located in a relatively narrow area, which corresponds to footprint of the probe at a maximum depth of 6–7 cm, while low-frequency curved/curvilinear transducers (range 2–5 MHz) are used to visualize deeper structures with a wider field of view but with poorer resolution. Depth and focus of the ultrasonic waves can be adjusted by the operator using controls on the US machine panel as can be Gain, a feature that allows adjustment of intensity of the image. Time gain compensation (TGC) is an additional feature that reduces impact of wave attenuation by tissues through increased intensity of the received signal in proportion to the depth. This reduces artifacts in the image. US can also be used to assess tissue movement by using the color Doppler function (change in frequency of sound waves as an object moves toward or away from the receiver). This is a useful feature for US-guided pain procedures because it helps to detect the presence of small blood vessels, thereby reducing the probability of vascular puncture and injection. A "color" function is available on most US machines that provides directional information with red color indicating movement towards and blue color indicating movement away from the transducer. The power Doppler function is more sensitive to movement but it does not provide directional information.

The operator should be aware of various artifacts that can affect the interpretation of images produced by US machines. These include anisotropy and reverberation. *Anisotropy* refers to the change in characteristics of the image as a result of the change of the US probe angle relative to the structure of interest. It is often seen with tendons and can result in an incorrect diagnosis of a tear in the tendon. *Reverberation* is a phenomenon when a smooth structure (e.g., pleura, metallic implant, or fluid trapped within gas) reflects the sound beams back and forth between itself and the probe, causing linear echoes deep to the structure. It is often referred to as "comet tail" artifacts. Reverberation artifacts can be reduced by changing the angle of insonation (i.e., the angle between the probe and the skin).

In summary, the anesthesiologist or pain interventionalist should at least consider the following prior to performing a US-guided procedure: transducer type, depth, gain, and Doppler function. Angle of insonation can be adjusted by heel-toe or toggling movements to reduce reverberation.

Finally, ergonomics in terms of positioning the patient, US machine, transducer grip, and injectate assembly (needle, extension tubing syringe, syringe) should be optimized.

AXIAL PROCEDURES

INJECTION OF THE CERVICAL FACET JOINT NERVE SUPPLY

Anatomy

Cervical medial branch nerves that innervate the facet joints arise from the cervical dorsal rami and innervate the cervical facet joints (CFJs). CFJs receive dual innervation from two medial branches, one above and one below the joint. As an example, the CFJ between the inferior articular process of the third cervical vertebra and the superior articular process (SAP) of the fourth cervical vertebra (C3–C4) is innervated by the third and the fourth cervical medial branches. After their origin, the cervical medial branches travel transversely along the "waist" of the facetal pillar (approximately halfway between the joints) with the exception of innervation of the C2–C3 FJ. The C3 dorsal ramus has two medial branches, a deep medial branch that passes around the waist of the C3 articular pillar and supplies the C3–C4 FJ and a superficial medial branch, the third occipital nerve (TON). The TON curves around the lateral and then the posterior aspect of the C2–C3 FJ and contributes articular branches to the joint.

Sonoanatomy

In the longitudinal plane on the lateral aspect of the neck, scanning is initiated behind the ear over the mastoid process. Sliding the probe caudally and posteriorly brings the lateral tip of the transverse processes (TPs) of C1 and, further caudad, C2 into view. The pulsation of the vertebral artery can also be visualized between these two levels. Caudad and posterior from the tip of the TP of C2, a wavy hyperechoic shadow with a series of "peaks and troughs" is identified (Fig. 79.1). This represents the surface of the cervical articular pillars, with the peaks representing the CFJ and the troughs representing the "waist" of the articular pillars, where the cervical medial branches transverse in an anterior-to-posterior direction. The first of these peaks is the C2–C3 FJ; a "drop-off" toward the cranial side represents the downslope of the inferior articular process, and the absent SAP of the C2 can be identified. The medial branches can be visualized in the trough as round or oval structures under the overlying semispinalis capitis muscle. An artery (usually a branch of ascending cervical artery) can often be visualized adjacent to the nerve.

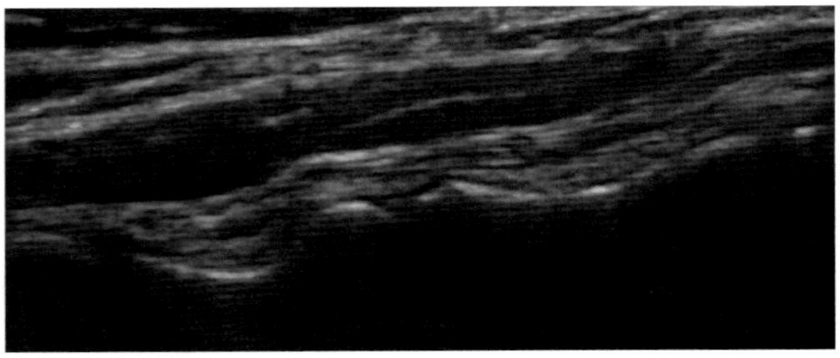

FIG. 79.1 Ultrasound image of the cervical facetal column in the longitudinal view. Hyperechoic cervical medial branch nerves can be seen at the deepest part of the troughs on both sides of the cervical facet joint (seen as a "break" in the wavy outline of the facetal column). (*Image courtesy of Dr. Anuj Bhatia.*)

Indications

Cervical medial branch injections are performed for the diagnosis and treatment of cervicogenic headaches and/or CFJ-related neck and shoulder pain not responsive to conservative therapy. Patients often present with a history of whiplash injury or clinical and/or radiologic evidence of CFJ arthritis.

Technique

The patient is positioned in the lateral decubitus position with the neck in a neutral position (a small pillow under the head helps to achieve this goal). The side of the procedure is kept nondependent and the interventionalist faces the patient. It is advisable to perform a color Doppler scan of the injection site prior to inserting the needle to avoid penetrating any blood vessels during injection. The targets for these injections are medial branch nerves at the "troughs" on either side of the CFJ. A high-frequency linear US probe with a small footprint is oriented longitudinally over the cervical facet column with the cephalad edge of the probe over the tip of the mastoid bone behind the ear. For injection a 25-gauge needle (4 or 8 cm long) is inserted out of plane from the anterior side of the probe. The needle is then advanced slowly until it penetrates the fascia of the semispinalis capitis; its tip is then placed adjacent to the nerve (or, if it is not visualized, the deepest part of the trough). Turning the US probe to a longitudinal orientation visualizes the needle in plane. The tip of the needle should be over the most prominent aspect of the facetal pillar and dorsal to the posterior tubercle of the TP. Note that the TON is located at the surface of the C2–C3 FJ, and it is usually hyperechoic. The volume of local anesthetic injected per level is 0.5 mL.

Pearls

- The exiting cervical nerve root can be visualized anterior to the posterior tubercle; care should be taken to ensure that the injectate does not flow toward it.
- This is an out-of-plane technique (at least during needle insertion), and the needle tip or shaft will be visualized only when it crosses the US beam. An extension tubing connected to a syringe of saline may be used for hydrodissection to locate the needle tip. Only small volumes (0.1 mL at a time) should be used for this purpose.
- US-guided cervical medial branch injection is an "advanced" technique because of the proximity of the medial branch nerves to vertebral and other arteries and neural foramina. It is recommended that interventionalists gain experience with other, more superficial nerve or musculoskeletal US-guided procedures before attempting this procedure.

INJECTION OF THE CERVICAL NERVE ROOT

Anatomy

The cervical nerve roots emerge between the anterior and posterior tubercles of the TPs at each cervical level (except the C7, since there is no anterior tubercle at this level). The nerve roots occupy the lower part of the cervical intervertebral foramen with the epiradicular veins in the upper part. Vertebral, ascending cervical, and deep cervical arteries are also in proximity to the cervical spinal nerve roots, and these arteries often give branches that contribute to radicular arteries perfusing the spinal cord. One third of these vessels enter the foramen posteriorly, potentially forming a radicular or segmental feeder vessel to the spinal cord, making it vulnerable to inadvertent injury or injection.

Sonoanatomy

It is vital to identify the appropriate level for injection. Two anatomic features of the cervical spine are useful in this regard. The transverse process of the C6 vertebra has a prominent anterior tubercle (usually larger than the posterior tubercle), and the C7 vertebra possesses only a posterior tubercle and no/rudimentary anterior tubercle. To locate the level of interest, one must slide the probe caudally until the TP of the C7 is identified (it appears as a gently sloping structure with the posterior tubercle at its peak) and then count up from there. At the C7 level, the emerging cervical nerve root can be identified immediately ventral to the posterior tubercle as a hypoechoic round structure, and the vertebral artery can be identified anterior to it by its pulsation. Moving the probe cephalad to the TP of the sixth cervical vertebra (C6) will bring the prominent anterior and smaller posterior hyperechoic tubercle into view. Similarly, the TPs of the fifth, fourth, and third cervical vertebrae can be identified by their tubercles, which are usually of equal size/prominence (unlike the C6) (Fig. 79.2). The US probe may have to be rotated slightly from the transverse position to visualize both tubercles because the anterior tubercle is often slightly cephalad to the posterior tubercle.

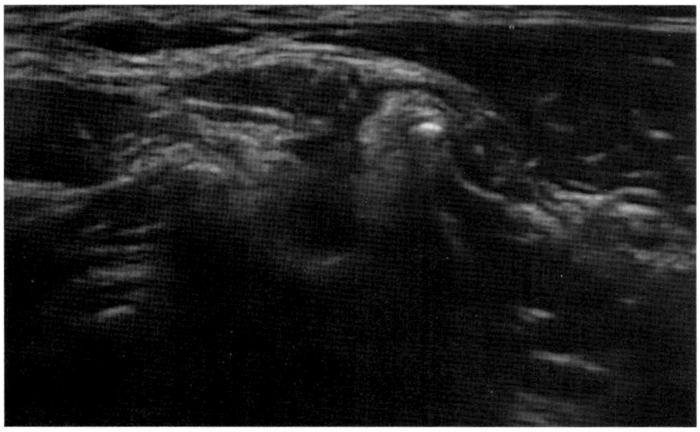

FIG. 79.2 Ultrasound appearance of the anterior (on the *right*) and posterior (on the *left*) tubercle of the sixth cervical transverse process and the emerging spinal nerve root between the two tubercles. (*Image courtesy of Dr. Anuj Bhatia.*)

Indications

Compression of an exiting cervical spinal nerve by a herniated intervertebral disc or foraminal stenosis can cause radicular pain. Injection of local anesthetics and/or steroids around compressed cervical nerve roots can provide analgesia; this intervention can also be used to prognosticate the analgesic outcome of cervical discectomy or decompression-fusion surgery.

Technique

The patient is placed in the lateral decubitus position with the neck in a neutral position with the procedure side nondependent. The operator should stand behind the patient. A high-frequency linear transducer is placed over the cricoid cartilage and then moved laterally to the side of interest. The lateral lobe of the thyroid gland is visualized wrapped around the lateral wall of the trachea, followed by the common carotid artery, internal jugular vein, and the muscles (superficial: sternocleidomastoid; deep: anterior and middle scalene, longus colli, and capitis). A more lateral and posterior position of the US probe will bring the prominent anterior and a smaller posterior tubercle of the cervical TP of the C6 and the emerging nerve roots between the two tubercles into view (see Fig. 79.2). The appropriate nerve root to be blocked is now identified. A color Doppler scan of the injection site is performed to avoid penetrating any blood vessels in proximity of the nerve root during the injection. A 22- or 25-gauge blunt needle (4–8 cm long) is introduced in plane from the dorsal side of the probe (i.e., the side closer to the operator) at an angle of 30 degrees to the skin. This approach is used because there is less probability of encountering blood vessels posterior to the nerve root as compared to the anterior aspect. The target for the tip position is immediately posterior to the emerging nerve root. Following a negative aspiration to rule out intravascular placement of the needle, up to 1 mL of the injectate is slowly injected around the nerve root.

Pearls

- The vertebral artery usually enters the foramen transversarium below the C6 in most patients, but it may be outside this foramen at the C6 level in up to 10% of patients. A thorough preprocedure scan to identify any aberrant blood vessels in proximity of the target nerve root is recommended.
- Failure to visualize spread of the injectate around the nerve root during the injection may be due to intravascular injection or incorrect orientation of the US probe.

INJECTION OF THE LUMBAR FACET JOINT NERVE SUPPLY

Anatomy

Lumbar medial branch nerves arise from the lumbar dorsal rami and innervate the lumbar facet joints (LFJs). Each LFJ receives dual innervation from two medial branches, one above and one at the level of the joint. As an example, the LFJ between the inferior articular process of the third lumbar vertebra and the SAP of the fourth lumbar vertebra (L3–L4) is innervated by the second and third lumbar medial branches that cross the grooves between the L3

SAP and TP and the L4 SAP and TP, respectively. The L5 dorsal ramus, located at the junction of the sacral SAP and the sacral ala, is targeted for blocking the nerve supply to L4–L5 or L5-sacral FJs. As opposed to the thoracic FJ, each LFJ is dorsal to the lumbar TPs.

Sonoanatomy

The patient is placed in prone position with pillows underneath the abdomen. Minimizing the lordosis is important to open up the interlaminar space and enable the US beam to strike the LFJ perpendicularly. A low-frequency curvilinear probe is used to scan the lumbosacral spine. The lumbar spinous processes are large and tend to reflect most of the US beam. The upper margin of the spinous process of a lumbar vertebra corresponds to the lower level of the TPs of the level above. A US scan at the midline in the sagittal plane reveals an undulating shadow that represents the tip of the lumbar spinous processes with minimal transmission of the US beam deeper to the spinous processes. The most caudal (also continuous) shadow in this view is the sacral median crest. A paramedian sagittal scan with the probe tilted medially reveals laminae and interlaminar spaces where the posterior and anterior dura can be identified (Fig. 79.3A). The spinal level should be counted and indicated on the skin with a marker using this view. Orienting the US probe perpendicularly at this spot (i.e., removing the medial tilt) reveals the "sawtooth" appearance of the articular processes and the LFJ (see Fig. 79.3B). Moving the probe further laterally while maintaining the perpendicular orientation allows the TPs to be visualized at a greater depth compared with the LFJ (see Fig. 79.3C), while moving it slightly medially from this point shows the junction of the articular process and the TP (see Fig. 79.3D). Rotating the probe transversely and scanning in the midline cranially from the level of the upper sacrum initially reveals the flat appearance of dorsal sacrum, with the prominent median sacral crest ("flying seagull" sign) followed by an interlaminar view between the sacrum and the fifth lumbar vertebra. Further cranial scanning helps confirm the counting of the intervertebral spaces, which was performed with the US probe in the sagittal orientation. The anterior and posterior dura can be visualized in the middle with the "two steps" of the inferior articular process (first step) and the TP (second step) (see Fig. 79.3E). The SAP is often difficult to visualize because it is oriented parallel to the US beam. The visualized medial edge of the TP (signifying the groove between it and the SAP) is the target for the medial branch nerve block.[5]

Indications

Diagnosis and treatment of axial back pain not responsive to conservative therapy in patients with historical, clinical, and/or radiologic evidence of LFJ arthritis.

Technique

The patient is positioned prone with a pillow under the abdomen to reduce lumbar lordosis. Intervertebral spaces are identified as described earlier (under Sonoanatomy), and the US probe is positioned at the level of interest. The "two-steps" scan is obtained and the probe is moved laterally toward the side of the intended target. A 22- or 25-gauge needle (8 or 11 cm long) is introduced lateral to the probe and advanced in an in-plane fashion and lateral-to-medial direction. The needle tip should contact bone at the perceived junction of the TP (or sacral ala) and the SAP. To further confirm the needle position, the probe is rotated to a longitudinal orientation (thereby causing the needle to assume an out-of-plane orientation) while jiggling the needle. The correct needle position should be in the cranial edge of the TPs. Adjust the needle if required and then inject 0.5 mL of the local anesthetic.

Pearls

- Anatomic variations of the lumbar spine that can make visualization of the targets difficult include scoliosis, spondylolisthesis, a sixth lumbar vertebra, or four lumbar vertebrae with a sacralized fifth vertebra. Reviewing imaging studies (x-rays, CT, or magnetic resonance imaging [MRI] scans) prior to performing the procedure can help to avoid some of these pitfalls.
- Do not advance the needle if bone is not contacted at the depth of the perceived TP. The intertransverse ligament is often echogenic and can be incorrectly identified as the TP. However, this ligament will not halt progress of the needle and further advancement may injure an exiting spinal nerve root.
- The L5 dorsal ramus block can be technically challenging due to a high iliac crest, especially in male patients. If the iliac crest is obscuring the view, the injection may be done using an out-of-plane approach or an in-plane approach with an oblique tilt to the transversely oriented probe, thereby causing the lateral edge of the probe to be cranial in relation to its medial edge.

INJECTION OF THE SACROILIAC JOINT

Anatomy

The sacroiliac joint (SIJ) is responsible for transmitting the weight of the upper segment of the body to the lower segment. It has the characteristics of a synovial joint in its inferior aspect. A fibrous capsule covers the joint posteriorly and the posterior sacroiliac, sacrotuberous, and sacrospinous ligaments stabilize the joint.

Sonoanatomy

The inferior part of the posterior SIJ is targeted for intraarticular injections. The posterior surface of the sacrum with the median and lateral crests is visualized as a "flying seagull"–shaped hyperechoic line, but the ilium is harder to visualize lateral to the joint because its inclined surface is a poor reflector of the US beam. The posterior sacral foramina are visualized as disruptions in the contour of the posterior surface of the sacrum immediately medial to the lateral sacral crest. The synovial part of the SIJ is located at and caudal to the second posterior sacral foramen and the posterior aspect of the SIJ is medial to the anterior aspect.

Indications

Diagnosis and treatment of SIJ dysfunction secondary to ankylosing spondylitis or arthritis causing low back pain, with referral to the buttock and posterior thigh.

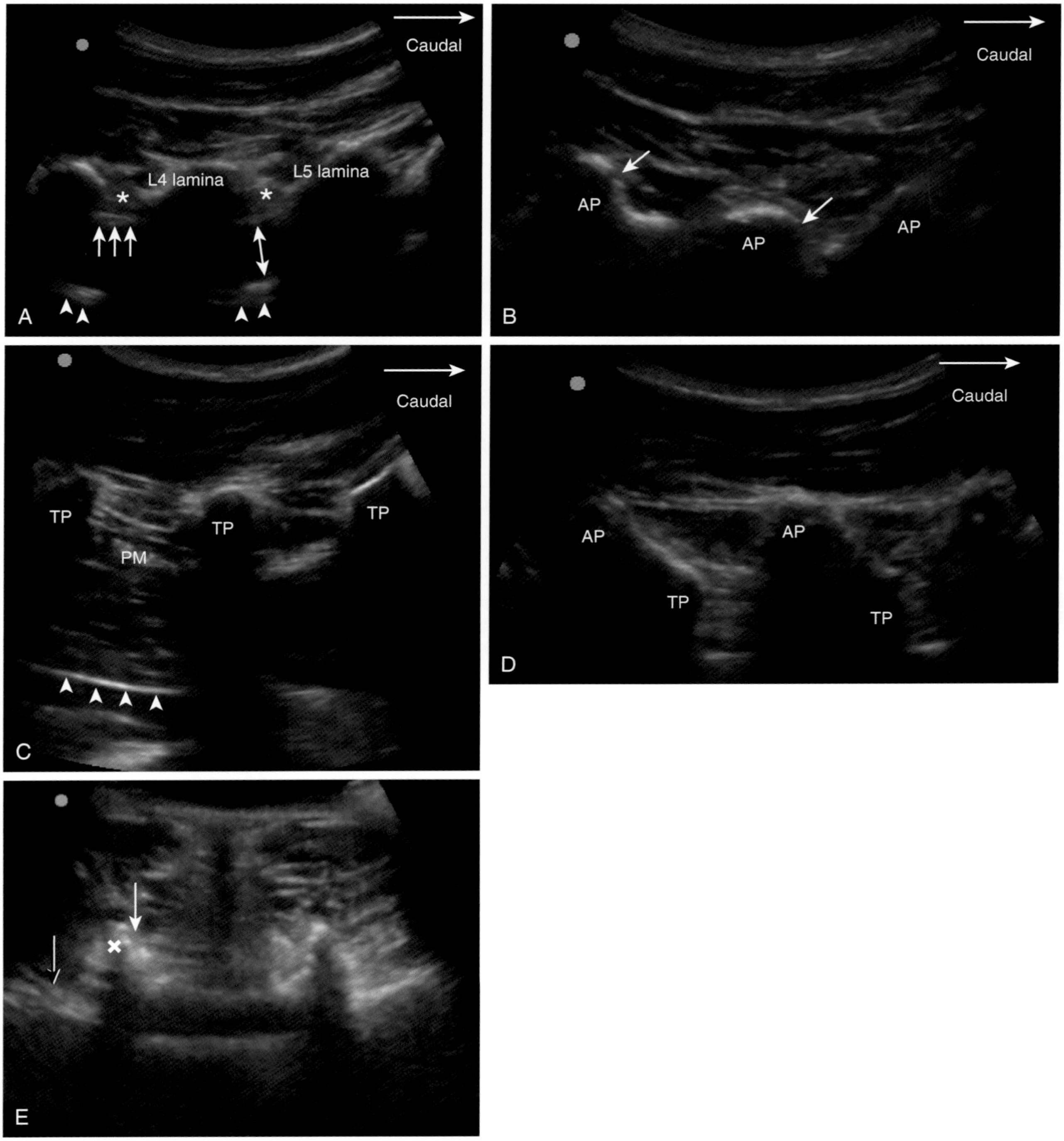

FIG. 79.3 Sonoanatomy of the lumbar spine. (A) Paramedian sagittal scan showing laminae and interlaminar spaces with dorsal dura (indicated by *arrows*) and anterior complex (anterior border of vertebra, posterior longitudinal ligament, and ventral dura; indicated by *arrowheads*); *, ligamentum flavum; the spinal canal is indicated by the *bidirectional arrow*. (B). "Sawtooth" appearance of the articular processes and the facet joints (*AP*, Articular process; *arrows* point to facet joints). (C) Lumbar vertebral transverse processes (*PM*, Psoas major muscle; *TP*, transverse process; *arrowheads* indicate peritoneum). (D) Paramedian view of articular and transverse process junction (E). Axial view of the "two steps": inferior articular process (first step, *white arrow*), transverse process (second step, *black arrow*), and facet joint *(white cross)*. (*Reproduced with permission from Philip Peng Educational Series.*)

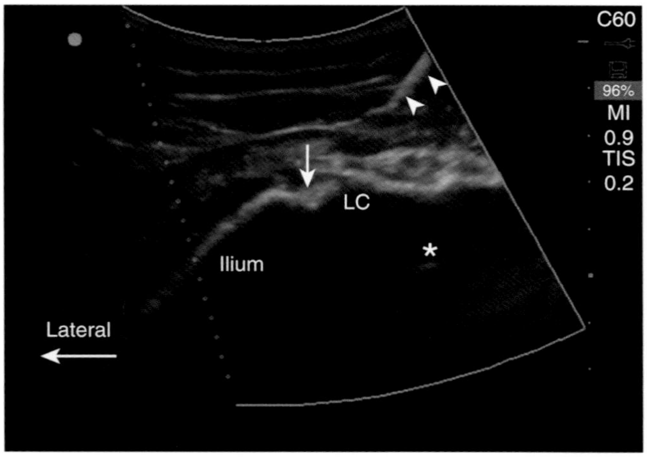

FIG. 79.4 Ultrasound image of injection into the lower part of sacroiliac joint. (*LC*, Lateral crest; *bold arrowheads*, needle; *, drop shadow of second sacral foramen; *line arrow*, sacrolilac joint). (*Reproduced with permission from Philip Peng Educational Series.*)

Technique

The patient is positioned prone with a pillow under the abdomen to reduce lumbar lordosis. A low-frequency curved probe is placed transversely at the level of the posterosuperior iliac spine and moved in a caudal direction. The first posterior sacral foramen can often be identified at this level. The ilium gradually becomes deeper and the joint cavity can be identified between the sacrum and the ilium. The probe is then moved caudally until just past the second posterior sacral foramen. The ilium disappears from view at the level of the greater sciatic notch. The probe is now moved cranially until the SIJ is visualized again. Finally the probe is positioned caudally to reveal the synovial part of the SIJ for injection. At this point an 8-cm needle can be introduced out of plane or in plane (from a medial-to-lateral direction; Fig. 79.4). The needle pierces the ligament complex on the posterior surface of the joint and a loss of resistance is often felt as the needle tip accesses the SIJ. The injectate (2 mL local anesthetic with or without steroid) can be injected, but "leakage" into the posterior periarticular tissues is often noticed toward the end of the injection.[6]

Pearls

- Avoid accessing the joint above the second posterior sacral foramen.
- There is a higher probability of periarticular (rather than intraarticular) injection with US-guided techniques compared to fluoroscopic or CT-guided SIJ injections, but the analgesic outcomes are similar with all image-guided techniques.

CAUDAL EPIDURAL INJECTION

Anatomy

The dural sac ends inferiorly at the level of the second (or occasionally third) sacral segment. The epidural space can be accessed through the sacral hiatus—a defect in the sacrum due to incomplete fusion of the fourth and fifth sacral segments. The sacral hiatus is bounded dorsally by the sacrococcygeal ligament, laterally by the two sacral cornua, and anteriorly by the posterior surface of the sacrum. The caudal epidural space contains sacral and coccygeal nerve roots, the filum terminale, and the epidural venous plexus.

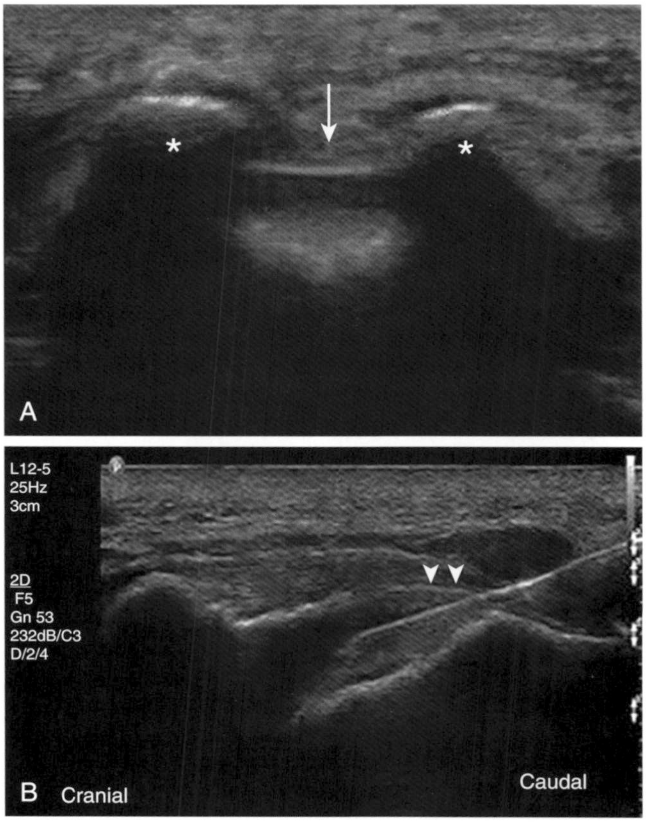

FIG. 79.5 Sonoanatomy of the caudal epidural space. (A) Transverse view; the *asterisk* (*) indicates the sacral cornu and the *arrow* indicates the sacrococcygeal ligament. (B). Long-axis view of the caudal canal showing the sacrococcygeal ligament *(arrowheads)*, anterior and posterior wall of sacral canal, and a needle in the caudal epidural space deep to the sacrococcygeal ligament. (*Reproduced with permission from Philip Peng Educational Series.*)

Sonoanatomy

Placement of the US probe over the two sacral cornua reveals these two hyperechoic structures, with the sacrococcygeal ligament in the intervening space (Fig. 79.5A). A long-axis view of the caudal canal shows the prominent sacrococcygeal ligament and the anterior and posterior walls of sacral canal (see Fig. 79.5B).

Indications

The caudal epidural space is accessed with US guidance for the diagnosis and treatment of lumbar and sacral spinal pain conditions when previous spine surgery (e.g., laminectomy) or spinal stenosis presents challenges for accessing the epidural space safely at the lower lumbar levels, especially in patients with a high body mass index in whom palpation of the cornua is difficult.

Technique

The patient is positioned prone and a high-frequency linear US probe is placed in the long axis of the caudal canal between the cornua. The epidural needle (18-, 20-, or 22-gauge; 8 cm long) is introduced in a caudal-to-cranial direction with an in-plane orientation (see Fig. 79.5B). A distinct loss of resistance is felt as the needle penetrates the sacrococcygeal ligament. The needle is then advanced gradually until its tip begins to disappear below the sacral bone. Injection should be made at this point or a catheter introduced and advanced.

Pearls

- Needles and catheters cannot be visualized with US inside the sacral epidural space. Precautions to detect inadvertent intravascular or subarachnoid placement of needles/catheters include checking by aspiration, injection of contrast under fluoroscopic guidance, and the use of test doses of injectate.
- The presence of turbulence during injection within the caudal space, as detected by color-flow Doppler mode on US, has been proposed as a reliable indicator of correct epidural injection, as the absence of turbulence suggests intravascular placement of the needle.

PERIPHERAL PROCEDURES

INJECTION OF THE CERVICOTHORACIC SYMPATHETIC CHAIN (STELLATE GANGLION) (DISCUSSED IN MORE DETAIL IN CHAPTER 84)

Anatomy

Cell bodies of preganglionic neurons located in the anterior lateral horn of the first and second thoracic spinal cord segment contribute to the peripheral sympathetic nerve supply of the head and neck regions. Axons arising from these cell bodies pass via the anterior roots of the spinal nerves at the same levels through the rami communicantes to join the three cervical sympathetic ganglia: superior, middle, and inferior. In 80% of the population, the inferior cervical and first thoracic ganglion are fused to form the stellate ganglion, which extends from the level of the head of the first rib to the inferior border of the TP of the seventh cervical vertebra. It lies immediately adjacent to the dome of the pleura and posterior to the subclavian artery. The postganglionic fibers from the stellate ganglion to the seventh and eighth cervical nerves and the first thoracic nerve provide sympathetic innervation to the upper limbs. The stellate ganglion (or the cervicothoracic sympathetic chain) is located on the anterolateral surface of the longus colli muscle and dorsal to the posterior fascia of the carotid sheath. It is embedded in the prevertebral fascia.

Sonoanatomy

Refer to the sonoanatomy section under Injection of the Cervical Nerve Root for information regarding identification of the TP and anterior tubercle of C6. The longus colli muscle is located anterior to the TP and medial to the anterior tubercle and is around 1 cm thick. The prevertebral fascia on the anterior surface of the muscle and the thickening representing the cervical sympathetic chain are then identified. Other important structures to recognize include the lateral lobe of the thyroid gland, blood vessels (common carotid artery, internal jugular vein, inferior thyroid artery, branches of the ascending cervical artery), esophagus, and exiting cervical nerve roots that may be in the planned path of the injecting needle.

Indications

Injection of the cervicothoracic sympathetic chain is performed for the management of a variety of pain conditions, including complex regional pain syndrome, refractory angina, and ischemic pain in the upper limb from peripheral vascular disease.

Technique

The patient is placed in the semilateral position with the procedure side nondependent and the neck in slight extension. A high-frequency linear US probe is placed transversely on the neck at the level of cricoid cartilage and the TP of C6 with the longus colli muscle identified. A preinjection Doppler scan is advised to check for any vessels in the intended path of the needle. A lateral-to-medial in-plane approach is used to advance the 22- or 25-gauge needle 4 or 8 cm long. The scan view is adjusted to remove C6 from the view; this reduces the probability of encountering the nerve root while the needle is advanced. The internal jugular vein can be avoided by "pushing" away with the needle, but it may have to be traversed. The needle tip is positioned deep to the prevertebral fascia (to avoid spread along the carotid sheath) but superficial to the fascia investing the anterolateral surface of the longus colli muscle (to avoid injecting into the muscle substance). Hydrodissection with 0.9% saline is recommended to ensure that the needle is in the correct plane (Fig. 79.6). This is followed by slow injection of a maximum of 5 mL of 0.5% bupivacaine in 1:200,000 epinephrine. This volume has been shown to be adequate for spread from the fourth cervical to the first thoracic vertebral level.

Pearls

- Visualization of the spread of injectate under real-time scanning is important, as its absence may suggest unsuspected intravascular injection. Continuous hemodynamic and respiratory monitoring (electrocardiography, blood pressure, pulse oximetry) is recommended during and for 5–10 minutes after the injection. A small volume (0.5 mL) should be injected initially. Correct placement of the needle will result in a significant spread of injectate across the fascia. The injection should be monitored in real time to make sure that there is no intravascular spread and the patient should be assessed for signs of local anesthetic toxicity.

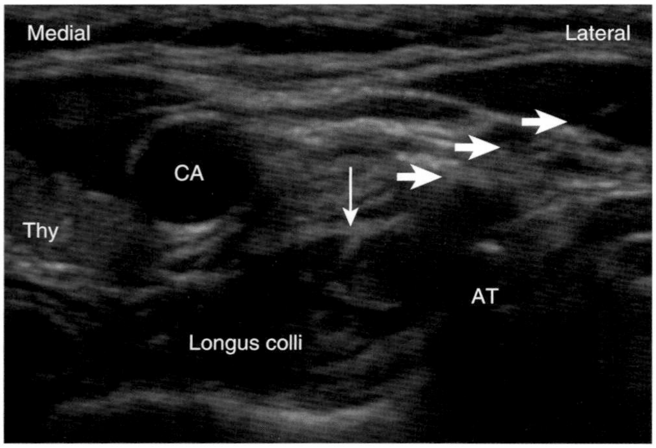

FIG. 79.6 Ultrasound-guided injection of the cervical sympathetic trunk at the level of the sixth cervical (C6) vertebra. The carotid artery (CA) is seen medially, the longus colli muscle deep to it, and the injection site *(arrow)* on surface of the muscle lateral to the artery and medial to the anterior tubercle (AT) of the C6 vertebra *(arrowheads* indicate needle shaft). *(Image courtesy of Dr. Anuj Bhatia.)*

- Skin temperature probes should be placed on both upper limbs prior to the procedure if the procedure is performed for relieving sympathetically mediated pain in the upper extremity, then. An increase of 1°C–3°C is usually accepted as a sign of adequate sympathetic blockade, although this has been contested in recent literature.

INJECTION OF THE GREATER OCCIPITAL NERVE (DISCUSSED IN MORE DETAIL IN CHAPTER 82)

Anatomy

The greater occipital nerve (GON) is the medial branch of the dorsal ramus of the second spinal nerve (C2); it provides cutaneous innervation to the major portion of the posterior scalp. It emerges below the posterior arch of the atlas, curls around the lower border of the obliquus capitis inferior muscle (OCIM), and passes cranially superficial to this muscle across the roof of the suboccipital triangle. It then turns dorsally to pierce the semispinalis capitis, after which it runs a short distance rostrally and laterally, lying deep to the trapezius muscle. The GON becomes subcutaneous slightly inferior to the superior nuchal line by passing above an aponeurotic sling. This sling is composed of insertions from the trapezius and sternocleidomastoid muscles. At this point, the GON is immediately medial to the occipital artery.

Sonoanatomy

A linear high-frequency US probe is moved in a caudal direction from the external occipital protuberance in the midline. The smooth posterior arch of the first cervical vertebra (C1) is identified, followed by the bifid spinous process of the second cervical vertebra (C2) (note that the spinous process of the third cervical vertebra can also be bifid). Moving the US probe laterally and tilting the lateral edge of the probe over the TP of the C1 allows visualization of the hyperechoic lamina of the C2 with the overlying OCIM. This muscle originates from the spinous process of the C2 and inserts onto the TP of the C1. The GON can be visualized as a hyperechoic oval structure in the fascial plane between the OCIM and the more superficial semispinalis capitis. Moving the probe superiorly from this point reveals the gradual medial course of the nerve as it proceeds cranially to pierce the trapezius.

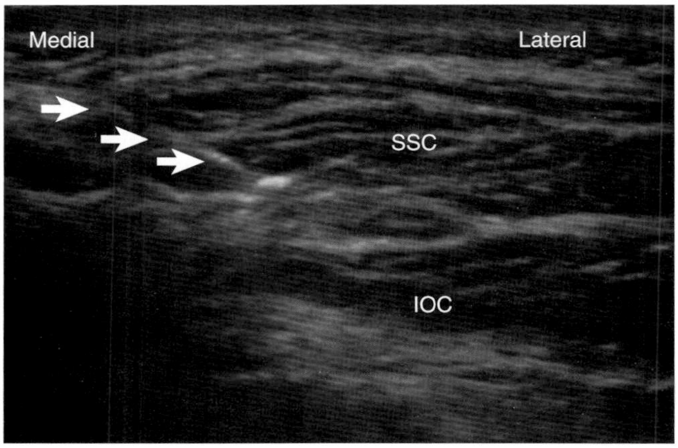

FIG. 79.7 Ultrasound-guided injection of the greater occipital nerve. The needle is seen in-plane (indicated by *arrows*) and the injectate is observed around the greater occipital nerve in the fascial plane between the inferior oblique capitis (IOC) and semispinalis capitis (SSC) muscles. *(Image courtesy of Dr. Anuj Bhatia.)*

Indications

GON block is performed to treat occipital neuralgia and cervicogenic headache. Occipital neuralgia is characterized by a paroxysmal jabbing pain in the distribution of the GON accompanied by diminished sensation or dysesthesia in the affected area. It is often associated with tenderness over the affected nerve. Occipital neuralgia may also present in the context of migraine or cluster headaches with associated signs and symptoms.

Technique

The patient is positioned prone and the medial edge of a linear US probe is placed over the bifid spinous process of the C2. The GON is identified in the fascial plane between the OCIM and the semispinalis capitis muscles. A 25-gauge needle 4 or 8 cm long is introduced in plane from a lateral-to-medial direction. The needle tip is placed adjacent to the nerve and 1–2 mL of local anesthetic (with or without steroid) is injected (Fig. 79.7).

Pearls

- The vertebral artery lies laterally and slightly cranial to the level of injection as it travels between the foramina transversaria of C2 and C1. A lateral-to-medial insertion of the needle reduces the probability of the needle tip penetrating this artery.

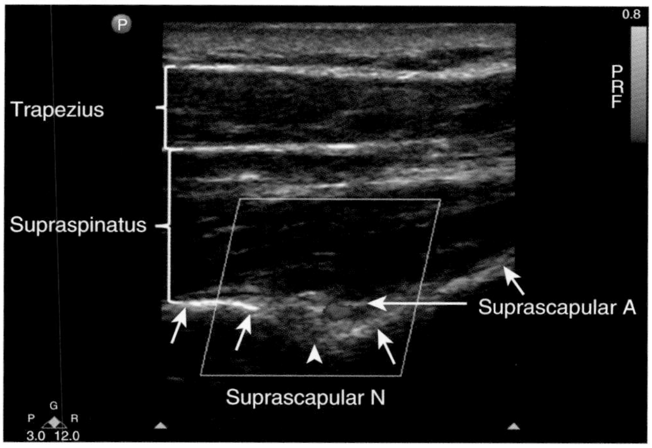

FIG. 79.8 Suprascapular nerve (indicated by *arrowhead*) on the floor of the supraspinous fossa (indicated by *arrows*) with the thick supraspinatus and thinner trapezius muscles overlying it. (*Reproduced with permission from Philip Peng Educational Series.*)

- The TON often lies in the same fascial plane but it is medial (i.e., closer to the spinous process of the C2) to the GON.

INJECTION OF THE SUPRASCAPULAR NERVE (ALSO DISCUSSED IN CHAPTER 83)

Anatomy

The suprascapular nerve arises from the ventral rami of fifth and sixth cervical nerves, which form the upper trunk of the brachial plexus. It lies under the inferior belly of the omohyoid muscle in the posterior triangle of the neck and then travels through the suprascapular notch under the superior transverse scapular ligament and enters the supraspinous fossa. It then takes a dorsolateral course toward the spinoglenoid notch to enter the infrascapular fossa. In the suprascapular fossa, the nerve is in direct contact with the floor in its course between the two notches and is accompanied by the suprascapular artery in this location. It innervates the supraspinatus and infraspinatus muscles; it also provides sensory innervation to the glenohumeral and acromioclavicular joints, coracohumeral ligament, subacromial bursa, and the scapula, but it does not innervate the skin overlying the shoulder joint.

Sonoanatomy

The optimal location at which to inject around the nerve using US guidance is the supraspinous fossa. The nerve lies on the floor of the fossa with the thick supraspinatus and the thinner trapezius muscles overlying it (Fig. 79.8). The suprascapular artery can be visualized in proximity to the nerve at this location. The US probe should be oriented to optimize the short-axis view of the nerve.

Indications

The suprascapular nerve is injected for both acute and chronic pain conditions. Acute pain indications include trauma or surgery to the shoulder joint. Chronic pain syndromes include degenerative conditions (arthritis), inflammatory pathologies (bursitis), and tears of the rotator cuff muscles.

Technique

The subject is placed in a sitting position. The US probe is positioned medial to the acromion. The suprascapular nerve is visualized on the floor of the supraspinous fossa with the suprascapular artery lateral to it. A 22- or 25-gauge needle (8 cm long) is inserted in an in-plane fashion from the medial edge of the probe. The needle tip is positioned adjacent to the nerve and 5 mL of injectate is delivered.

Pearls

- Injection around the suprascapular nerve should not be attempted at the suprascapular notch because it is technically challenging to inject the nerve in this location and the proximity of the pleura makes pneumothorax a possibility.

INJECTION OF THE INTERCOSTAL NERVE (ALSO DISCUSSED IN CHAPTER 83)

Anatomy

The intercostal nerves are ventral rami of the thoracic nerve roots. Each nerve gives off a lateral cutaneous branch before continuing as the anterior cutaneous branch. Injections performed medial to the angle of the rib (or the posterior axillary line) will allow coverage of innervation territory of the lateral branch because this branch takes off lateral to the angle of the rib. There are 11 intercostal nerves, with the ventral rami of the 12th thoracic nerve root, also known as the subcostal nerve. The intercostal nerves supply innervation to the skin and musculature of the chest and abdominal walls. Although the nerves are traditionally believed to travel in the groove at the inferior aspect of the rib along with the intercostal arteries and veins, the nerves can also lie in between the ribs. The intercostal nerves are located deep to the internal intercostal muscle layer and superficial to the pleura. Each intercostal space is innervated by the intercostal nerve running in the space and the nerves in the two adjacent spaces (above and below).

Sonoanatomy

A high-frequency linear US probe is used for procedural guidance. Important structures to be identified include ribs, external and internal intercostal muscles, and the pleura. The intercostal space can be identified in the short axis by placing the length of the probe perpendicular to the space or in the long axis when the probe is parallel to the space. In the short-axis view, ribs and intercostal spaces are counted from below upward and the levels of interest are identified. The pleura, internal intercostal muscles, and the plane for injection deep to this muscle layer are identified. The ribs appear as short linear hyperechoic segments, and the pleura has a shiny, shimmering appearance deeper to the ribs, and it appears to slide with respiration. Tilting the US probe cranially and using the color Doppler function

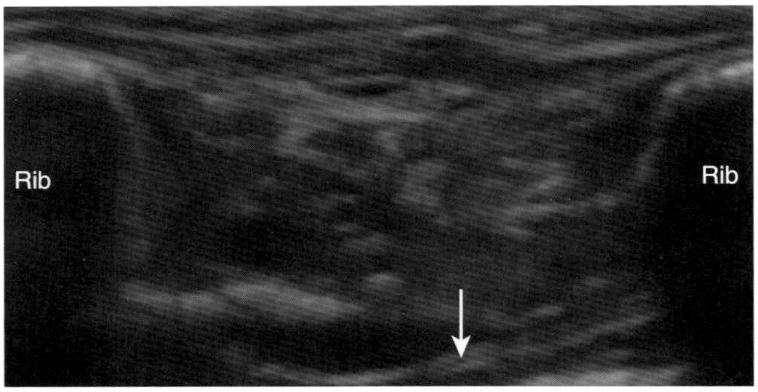

FIG. 79.9 Ultrasound image of an intercostal nerve block. Note that the pleura *(arrow)* is pushed down by the injectate and assumes a "scalloped" appearance. (*Image courtesy of Dr. Anuj Bhatia.*)

can reveal pulsation of the intercostal artery under the inferior aspect of the upper rib.

Indications

Intercostal nerve blocks are performed for both acute and chronic pain conditions. Acute pain conditions include pain from rib fractures and surgical procedures on the chest. Chronic pain indications include intercostal neuralgia as a sequela of herpes zoster infection, surgical procedures, or cancer involving the chest and/or abdominal wall.

Technique

The patient is positioned prone with a roll placed under the chest. The injection can be performed with a short- or long-axis view and the needle can be introduced in or out of plane. The short-axis view with the in-plane approach is often used because of its technical ease. After identifying the intercostal space of interest by counting the ribs, the two ribs and intervening pleura are placed in the center of the screen. The thicker external and thinner internal intercostal muscles are identified in the intercostal space. A 22- or 25-gauge needle (4 or 8 cm long) is introduced from the caudal edge of the probe in an in-plane fashion. Hydrodissection is recommended to identify the needle tip, which is placed immediately deep to the internal intercostal muscle. At this point 0.5–2 mL of injectate is delivered.[7] The pleura is often pushed down by the injection and takes on a "scalloped" appearance (Fig. 79.9).

Pearls

- To avoid pneumothorax, a serious complication of this procedure, an in-plane technique and hydrodissection should be used to ensure that the operator is aware of the position of the needle tip at all times. If out-of-plane technique is used, hydrolocation is essential.
- Narrow intercostal spaces make in-plane injection with short-axis visualization difficult. An alternative option in these situations is to obtain a long-axis view of the intercostal space and then perform the injection in or out of plane. The ribs and pleura have a similar appearance in the long-axis view. Preprocedural scanning helps differentiate the more superficial ribs from the relatively deeper pleura.

INJECTIONS OF THE ILIOINGUINAL AND ILIOHYPOGASTRIC NERVES (ALSO DISCUSSED IN CHAPTER 83)

Anatomy

The ilioinguinal (II) and iliohypogastric (IH) nerves arise from ventral rami of the 12th lumbar and the 1st lumbar spinal nerves and provide sensory innervation to the skin between the thigh and the abdomen. The nerves emerge at the lateral border of the psoas muscle before traveling inferolaterally onto the anterior surface of the quadratus lumborum muscle. Further laterally and superior to the anterior superior iliac spine, the nerves pierce the transversus abdominis (TA) muscle to lie in the fascial plane between this muscle and the more superficial internal oblique (IO) muscle, with the IH nerve superolateral to the II nerve. The deep circumflex iliac artery travels in the same plane in proximity to the two nerves. The IH nerve then pierces the IO muscle to lie in the plane between the internal and external oblique muscles and then pierces the external oblique aponeurosis above the superficial inguinal ring. It gives off lateral and anterior cutaneous branches that provide sensation to the skin of the gluteal region and over the hypogastric region, respectively. The II nerve pierces the IO at its lower border, passes between the crura of the superficial inguinal ring (anterior to the spermatic cord), and provides sensory fibers to the skin over the root of penis and scrotum (mons pubis and labium majus in females) and superomedial thigh region.

Sonoanatomy

With a high-frequency linear US probe placed cranial and dorsal to the anterosuperior iliac spine and the long axis of the probe pointing to the contralateral shoulder, both II and IH nerves are seen in the fascial plane between the TA and IO muscles (Fig. 79.10). The peritoneum is deeper to the TA; it is distinguished by peristalsis of the underlying bowel. The fascial plane of the II and IH nerves is easier to recognize by identifying muscles from the TA toward the skin. The two nerves can usually be identified individually, but they may travel as a single neural bundle.

Indications

II and IH nerves are injected for the treatment of acute and chronic pain. Acute pain indications include analgesia for open inguinal hernia surgery, whereas chronic pain indications include persistent postoperative pain following surgery on the abdominal or pelvic wall (open hernia repair, abdominal hysterectomy, cesarean section) and abdominal wall neuropathic pain associated with visceral inflammatory conditions (inflammatory bowel disease, endometriosis, interstitial cystitis).

Technique

The patient is placed in the supine position. The US probe is positioned at the midpoint between the 12th rib and the iliac crest with the long axis of the probe pointing toward the contralateral shoulder. The lateral edge of the probe is positioned on the iliac crest (note that the probe is cranial and dorsal to the anterosuperior iliac spine). The

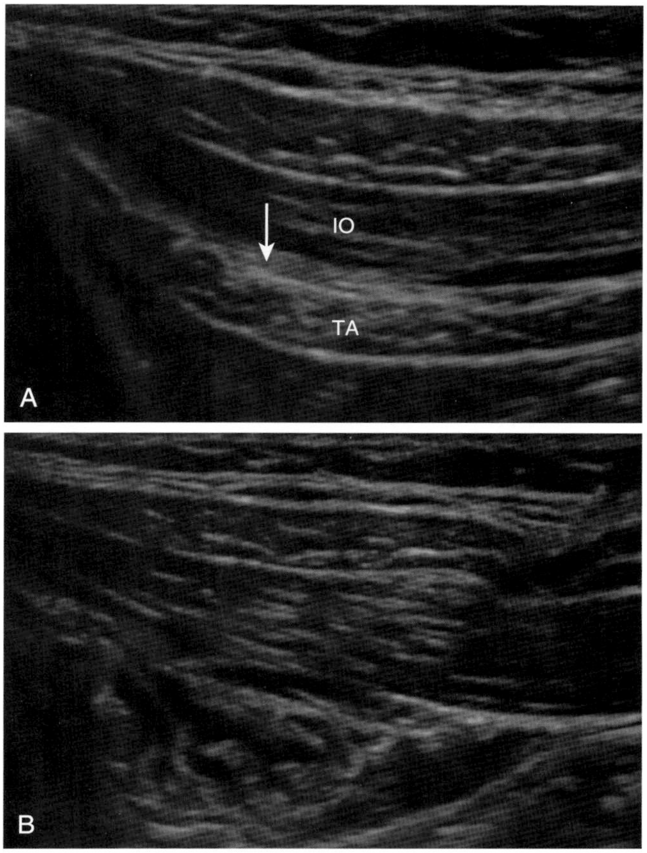

FIG. 79.10 Ultrasound image of ilioinguinal and iliohypogastric nerves before (A) and after (B) injection in the fascial plane *(arrow)* between the transversus abdominis (TA) and internal oblique (IO) muscles. *(Image courtesy of Dr. Anuj Bhatia.)*

peritoneum and underlying bowel are identified, followed by the fascial plane between the TA and IO muscles where the II and IH nerves are located. A color Doppler scan to identify the deep circumflex iliac artery in this fascial plane aids in identifying II and IH nerves adjacent to it and in avoiding vascular puncture. A 22-gauge needle (8 cm long) is used for the injection. An out-of-plane technique with hydrodissection to confirm that the needle tip is in the appropriate fascial plane is often used for this injection. Injection results in opening up of this fascial plane with an injectate volume of 5–8 mL (see Fig. 79.10).

Pearls

- Make sure that the needle tip is in the correct fascial plane and not in the IO or the TA muscles.
- Angling the US probe caudally (i.e., as if looking into the pelvis) often improves visualization of the nerves.

INJECTION OF THE LATERAL FEMORAL CUTANEOUS NERVE (ALSO DISCUSSED IN CHAPTER 83)

Anatomy

The lateral femoral cutaneous nerve (LFCN) is a sensory nerve that originates from dorsal divisions of the second and third lumbar nerves. It provides innervation to the anterolateral aspect of the thigh up to the knee and part of the skin over the gluteus through its anterior and posterior divisions. After emerging from the lateral border of the psoas muscle, it travels obliquely downward on the surface of the iliacus. It then makes an acute turn and travels on the anterior surface of the sartorius. At or below the level of the inguinal crease, it is found consistently in the groove between the sartorius and tensor fascia lata and is deep to the fascia lata.

Sonoanatomy

The LFCN can be located in the thigh as an oval hyperechoic structure in the subfascial plane between the sartorius and tensor fascia lata muscles. This is usually at a distance of 5–8 cm inferior to the anterosuperior iliac spine. The nerve can then be followed proximally as it nears the anterosuperior iliac spine.

Indications

Injections can be performed around the LFCN for acute and chronic pain management. LFCN block is performed for perioperative analgesia for skin graft or muscle biopsy procedures in the area of its innervation. Injections are also performed for the diagnosis and treatment of meralgia paresthetica, a chronic pain syndrome from entrapment, injury, or stretching of the LFCN.

Technique

The patient is positioned supine and a linear high-frequency probe is placed inferior to the inguinal crease with the center of the probe on the intermuscular groove between sartorius and tensor fascia lata. The nerve is located and an attempt is made to follow the nerve as far proximally as possible. A 25-gauge needle (4 or 8 cm long) is inserted in plane from lateral to medial at the most proximal location where the nerve is visualized. Hydrodissection is performed in the interfascial plane between the fascia lata and underlying muscle fascia if the nerve is not visualized prior to insertion of the needle. The needle tip is then placed in proximity to the nerve and 2–4 mL of injectate is delivered around the nerve (Fig. 79.11).

Pearls

- The LFCN can be difficult to identify because of its small size. Hydrodissection with saline in the intermuscular groove can aid identification.
- The sartorius muscle is easier to visualize in the proximal thigh than near the anterosuperior iliac spine, where the muscle is small in size because of its origin. The LFCN is also flatter and more hypoechoic at this level compared with its appearance in the proximal thigh.
- The LFCN can split into its divisions close to the anterosuperior iliac spine. It then takes on an appearance of multiple small bubbles.

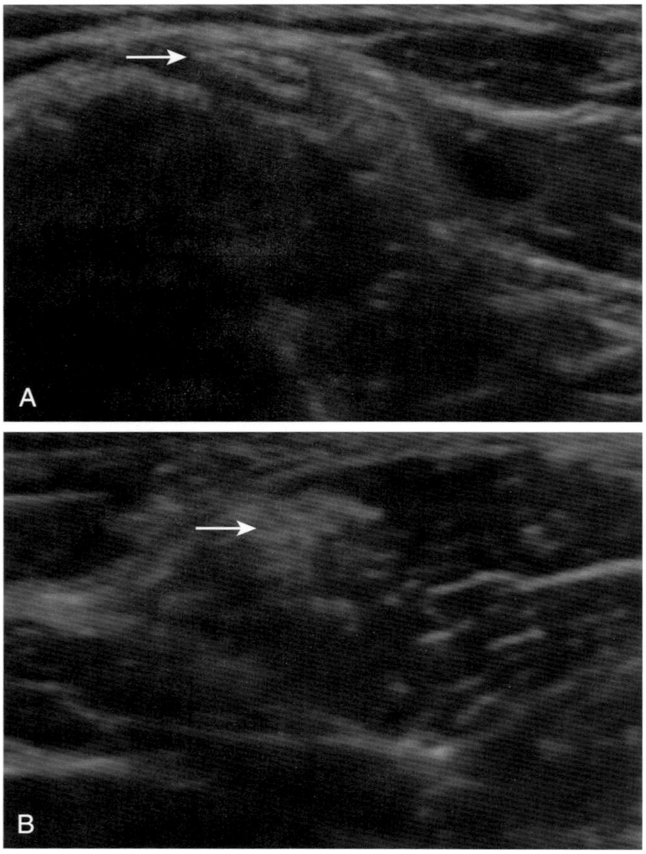

FIG. 79.11 Ultrasound image of lateral femoral cutaneous nerve (LFCN) in proximity to the anterior superior iliac spine (A, *arrow* indicates LFCN) and between the tensor fascia lata and sartorius (B, *arrow* indicates LFCN). The left side of both images is lateral. The LFCN is seen as an oval hyperechoic structure superficial to the sartorius muscle. (*Image courtesy of Dr. Anuj Bhatia.*)

KEY POINTS

- Image quality with US is compromised with increase in depth of scanning and bony structures, and there are no validated surrogates for contrast-enhanced visualization of injectate available with fluoroscopy-guided techniques.
- The usual range of medical US for procedural guidance is 1–21 MHz.
- Higher frequency is associated with shorter wavelengths and vice versa. Shorter wavelengths (i.e., higher frequencies) result in higher resolution (the ability to discriminate between two adjacent structures).
- High-frequency linear transducers (range 6–18 MHz) produce images with a better resolution of structures located in a relatively narrow area that corresponds to the footprint of the probe at a maximum depth of 6–7 cm, whereas low-frequency curved/curvilinear transducers (range 2–5 MHz) are used to visualize deeper structures with a wider field of view but with poorer resolution.
- Anisotropy is the change in characteristics of the image as a result of the change of the US probe angle relative to the structure of interest.
- Reverberation is a phenomenon when a smooth structure (e.g., pleura, metallic implant, or fluid trapped within gas) reflects the sound beams back and forth between itself and the probe, causing linear echoes deep to the structure. Reverberation artifacts can be reduced by changing the angle of insonation (i.e., angle between the probe and the skin).
- US-guided spine injections are "advanced" techniques. It is recommended that interventionalists gain experience with more superficial nerve or musculoskeletal US-guided procedures before attempting this procedure.

REFERENCES

Access the reference list online at ExpertConsult.com.

CHAPTER 80

Deep Muscle Injections: Piriformis, Scalene Muscle, Iliopsoas Injections

Ariana Nelson, MD ◌ Honorio T. Benzon, MD ◌ Juan Francisco Asenjo, MD, FRCPC

INTRODUCTION

Pain syndromes that can be attributed to deep muscles are often caused by mechanical impingement of the muscular tissue upon traversing neurovascular structures. The most common of these disorders include piriformis syndrome, in which the piriformis muscle may compress the sciatic nerve, and thoracic outlet syndrome (TOS), in which the scalene musculature compresses the brachial plexus. In contrast, iliopsoas-related pain is not related to compression or irritation of a nerve. However, all three of these pathophysiologic states can be managed through conservative measures, injection therapy, or surgical intervention.

PIRIFORMIS SYNDROME

Although piriformis syndrome is rare, occurring in only 5%–6% of patients that are referred for back or leg pain, the syndrome is often underrecognized and should therefore be considered in the differential diagnosis of patients that present with unilateral buttock and leg pain. A more detailed discussion of the syndrome may be referenced in Chapter 67.

DIAGNOSIS

There are no standardized diagnostic criteria for piriformis syndrome, and the pattern of pain produced is very similar to other more common pain generators such as lumbar facet arthropathy or herniated intervertebral disc. As such, piriformis syndrome is not only a clinical diagnosis but also a diagnosis of exclusion. It should be considered in the differential diagnosis of patients with unilateral buttock/leg pain, but clinical suspicion may be increased in the presence of several signs on physical exam. In contrast to other sources of lower extremity pain, typically patients with true piriformis syndrome do not exhibit low back pain. Common symptomatology includes an aching pain that localizes to the buttock, is unilateral, and radiates down to the posterior aspect of the leg, occasionally into the calf or foot. Piriformis syndrome may be more common in the setting of an aberrant relationship between the piriformis muscle and the sciatic nerve. Six different relationships exist; these are described in Chapter 67. Aberration from the typical anatomy is also thought to decrease the likelihood that piriformis injections will be effective.[1] Diagnosis of the syndrome is based on symptoms, physical examination findings, and a favorable response to a local anesthetic injection into the piriformis muscle.

CONSERVATIVE TREATMENT

As with all pain syndromes, conservative management is attempted first for piriformis syndrome. Antiinflammatory agents and muscle relaxants used in conjunction with physical therapy are the first line of treatment in piriformis syndrome.[2,3] Improved outcomes have been noted in patients that receive piriformis injection compared with those that receive only conservative management with physical therapy and medications.[4] Therefore if a patient's symptoms are not adequately treated with conservative measures, injection therapy is recommended as the next step in management.

INJECTION TREATMENT

Injection without the assistance of an imaging modality is technically challenging because the piriformis muscle is small in size and deep in anatomic location. Common methods of image guidance include ultrasound and fluoroscopy, which may be used alone or in tandem with electromyography (EMG).[5–7] Techniques for injection using computed tomography (CT) have also been described but are not as useful clinically, given increased radiation exposure to the patient and increased duration of procedure.[4] Regardless of choice of technique, the patient is placed in the prone position and vital signs are monitored throughout the procedure. A 20–22-gauge needle is used for the procedure, with an echogenic needle being preferable for ultrasound-guided technique and a stimulating needle if EMG is to be utilized. For all techniques, the area to be injected is cleansed with an alcohol-based cleaning solution and then the site of skin insertion and deeper tissues are anesthetized with 1% lidocaine.

FLUOROSCOPIC INJECTION TECHNIQUES

The piriformis muscle can be injected either in its belly or its tendon. When injecting into the tendon, fluoroscopy in the anterior-posterior (AP) orientation is used to identify the proximal end of the femur. After appropriate sterile preparation, draping, and administration of local anesthesia, a needle is advanced to the insertion edge of the piriformis muscle on the greater trochanter. Contrast agent is then injected and observed to spread into the tendon, and after negative aspiration, a 5-mL volume of local anesthetic and steroid is administered.

There are two methods of injection into the belly of the muscle: sacroiliac joint landmark and acetabular landmark.

Sacroiliac Joint Landmark

The fluoroscope is positioned to view the sacroiliac joint (SIJ) in AP orientation. An area 2–3 cm caudal and 2–3 cm lateral to the inferior margin of the SI joint is marked and anesthetized with lidocaine. A needle is placed at this mark and inserted 5–7 cm into the musculature in coaxial alignment with the fluoroscope (Fig. 80.1A). The needle is then advanced in lateral view to the anterior margin of the sacrum and contrast medium is injected (see Fig. 80.1B). An appropriate myogram outlining the piriformis is verified in AP view (see Fig. 80.1C), and after negative aspiration, the steroid and an additional volume of local anesthetic is injected.[8]

Acetabular Landmark

An alternative technique also targets the muscle belly but at a slightly more lateral location. The fluoroscope is initially positioned in AP view, with the center of the scope approximating the superomedial margin of the acetabulum. In coaxial orientation, the needle is advanced toward the anatomic "X" marking the junction of the line descending inferiorly from the greater sciatic notch and the curvature of the pelvic brim. The proceduralist must ensure that the needle tip remains lateral to the curvature of the pelvic inlet (Fig. 80.2). The procedure is then conducted as described previously. Using this method, the needle is advanced toward bone, which is an added level of safety compared to the SIJ method, in which the needle is advanced through the pelvic inlet and care must be taken to avoid injury to soft tissue structures.

COMBINATION FLUOROSCOPIC AND NERVE STIMULATION TECHNIQUE

The piriformis muscle can be approached using the landmarks described previously (i.e., 2–3 cm caudal and 2–3 cm lateral to the inferior margin of the SI joint) or at the "X" junction of the pelvic brim and the ridge descending inferiorly from the greater sciatic notch. When using EMG in addition to fluoroscopic guidance, the 6–10-cm stimulating needle is connected to a nerve stimulator with settings of 2 Hz and 1 mA. Contraction of the gluteal muscles indicates that the needle is close and superficial (posterior) to the sciatic nerve and piriformis muscle. Proximity of the tip of the needle to the sciatic nerve results in plantar flexion, dorsiflexion, eversion, or inversion. The presence of one of these evoked motor responses at 0.2–0.4 mA implies close proximity of the needle tip to the nerve. The needle is withdrawn 2 mm to ensure that the needle is not intraneural, and 5 mL of steroid and saline (to avoid leg numbness) is injected. The needle is then withdrawn 1 cm and 1–3 mL contrast is injected, which should ideally outline the belly of the piriformis. Another 5 mL of steroid and local anesthetic is then injected.

Another technique involves drawing a line from the greater trochanter to the middle of the sciatic notch, and a mark is made at the midpoint of this line. The needle is inserted in a slightly lateral to medial trajectory and advanced until the needle tip makes contact with the ilium. The needle is withdrawn 1 cm and attached to a nerve stimulator set at 1 mA, 2 Hz, 0.2 ms. The needle is then manipulated with very small movements until the appropriate motor response, dorsiflexion, plantar flexion, eversion, and inversion of the ipsilateral foot is noted. The subsequent steps are then similar to the previously described technique.[2] This technique is most often used when imaging methods are not accessible, but given the increasing availability of fluoroscopes

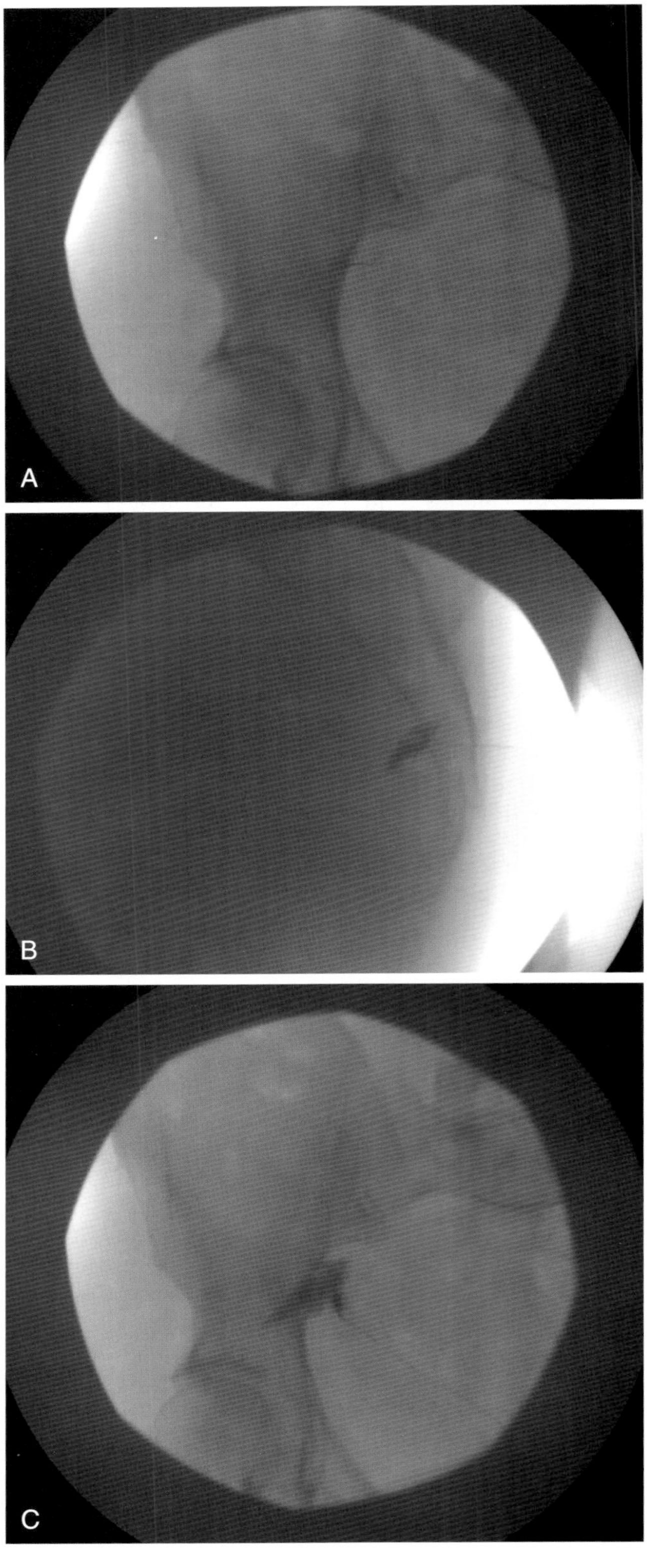

FIG. 80.1 Fluoroscopy-guided piriformis muscle injection—sacroiliac joint (SIJ) landmark technique. This may be performed with or without electromyographic guidance. (A) Needle is advanced in coaxial orientation to a site 2–3 cm lateral and 2–3 cm inferior to the inferior pole of the SIJ. (B) Contrast dye spread within the piriformis muscle in lateral view. (C) Myogram outlining the piriformis muscle in anterior-posterior view.

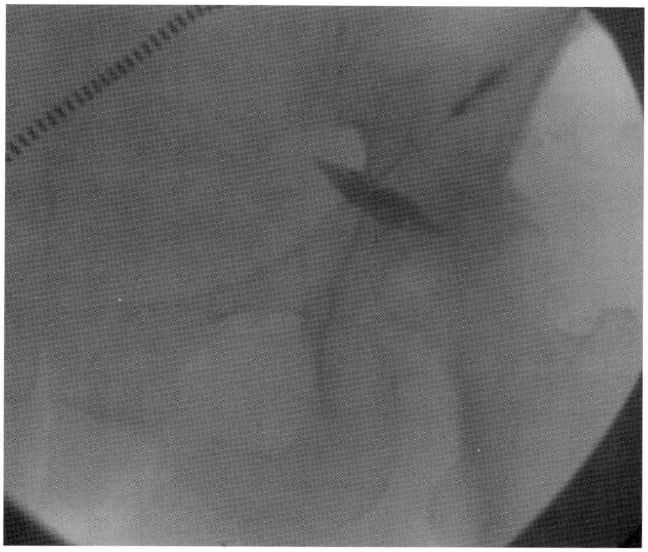

FIG. 80.2 Fluoroscopy-guided piriformis muscle injection—acetabular landmark technique This image demonstrates a myogram outlining the piriformis in AP view. Needle is advanced toward the intersection point of the ridge descending from the greater sciatic notch with the pelvic brim. Care should be taken to maintain the needle superior to the osseous surface, and thus slightly lateral to the pelvic brim.

and ultrasound machines, image guidance is now used in the majority of procedures.

ULTRASOUND-GUIDED TECHNIQUE

As previously stated, the ultrasound-guided technique allows visualization of soft tissue, such as vasculature, the piriformis muscle itself, and the muscle's relationship to the sciatic nerve.[9] The ultrasound machine should ideally be equipped with a Doppler and be positioned on the contralateral side to the patient's affected limb. Although the flat, high frequency transducer may be used in thin patients, a curved, low frequency (2–6 MHz) ultrasound probe is used more frequently to ensure adequate visualization of these deep structures.

Localizing the Piriformis Muscle

Method 1: To visualize the small, spindle-shaped piriformis muscle, the transducer is typically positioned in the short axis (transverse) view (Fig. 80.3A) over the sacroiliac joint, with the sacrum in view on the medial portion of the ultrasound screen and the ilium/gluteus maximus visible on the lateral view of the screen. Given that the muscle lies horizontally between the sacrum and greater trochanter of the femur, the transducer is then moved caudally such that the sacroiliac joint remains in the center of the screen but the lateral view of the ilium is out of view. This signifies that the transducer is positioned directly over the greater sciatic notch and the hyperechoic lateral aspect of the sacrum can be visualized medially. The operator should observe the large gluteus maximus muscle spanning the center of the image and, deep to this, the small, sardine-sized, piriformis muscle originating from the anterolateral sacral edge. If the transducer is manipulated inferiorly and rotated (clockwise if the injection is performed on the left and counterclockwise if the injection is performed on the right), then the sciatic nerve will become visible deep to the medial aspect of the piriformis (see Fig. 80.3B). The inferior gluteal artery, medial to the sciatic nerve and anterior to the piriformis, should be identified and avoided during needle insertion. The ischium appears initially as a curved hyperechoic line (posterior acetabulum) and will then appear as a flat line deep to the piriformis as the probe is moved caudally.

Method 2: An alternate method of locating the piriformis involves drawing a line connecting the greater trochanter and ischial tuberosity. The transducer is positioned over this line to identify the sciatic nerve. The nerve is followed cephalad until the gluteus maximus and piriformis are visualized superficial to the sciatic nerve.[2,9,10]

Confirmation of Visualization

With the piriformis muscle in the center of the ultrasound screen, flex the ipsilateral knee to 90 degrees and rotate the hip both internally and externally. This maneuver will cause the piriformis to glide over the ischium while the gluteus maximus remains motionless. Other muscles that are similar in size and may be confused with the piriformis should be identified to ensure that the appropriate muscle is targeted for injection. A relatively simple way to make this distinction is visualization of the ischial spine, as only the gemelli and obturator muscles insert onto this anatomic landmark.

Needle Insertion

An area 3–4 cm from the lateral aspect of the transducer should be anesthetized with lidocaine. The echogenic needle is advanced, in plane with the ultrasound probe, in a lateral to medial and posterior to anterior direction into the gluteus maximus and the medial half of the piriformis. If the needle tip is difficult to visualize due to loss of resolution with increasing depth, hydrodissection may assist in confirming depth. When the needle is positioned in the piriformis muscle (see Fig. 80.3C), then the injectate may be administered. If desired, the needle may then be advanced at a shallow angle and positioned in the fascial plane separating the piriformis from the sciatic nerve (see Fig. 80.3D), where additional injectate may be administered.[9,10]

ULTRASOUND AND ELECTROMYOGRAPHIC GUIDANCE

After identification of the presumptive piriformis muscle using the technique described previously, EMG may be used to verify placement in the piriformis rather than surrounding musculature. If EMG is to be used concomitantly with ultrasound guidance, hydrodissection must be conducted with a nonelectrolyte solution, such as 50% dextrose, whereas normal saline may be used in a strictly ultrasound-guided procedure.[11]

Postprocedure Monitoring

Patients may develop weakness/numbness in the distribution of the sciatic nerve following this injection. The patient should

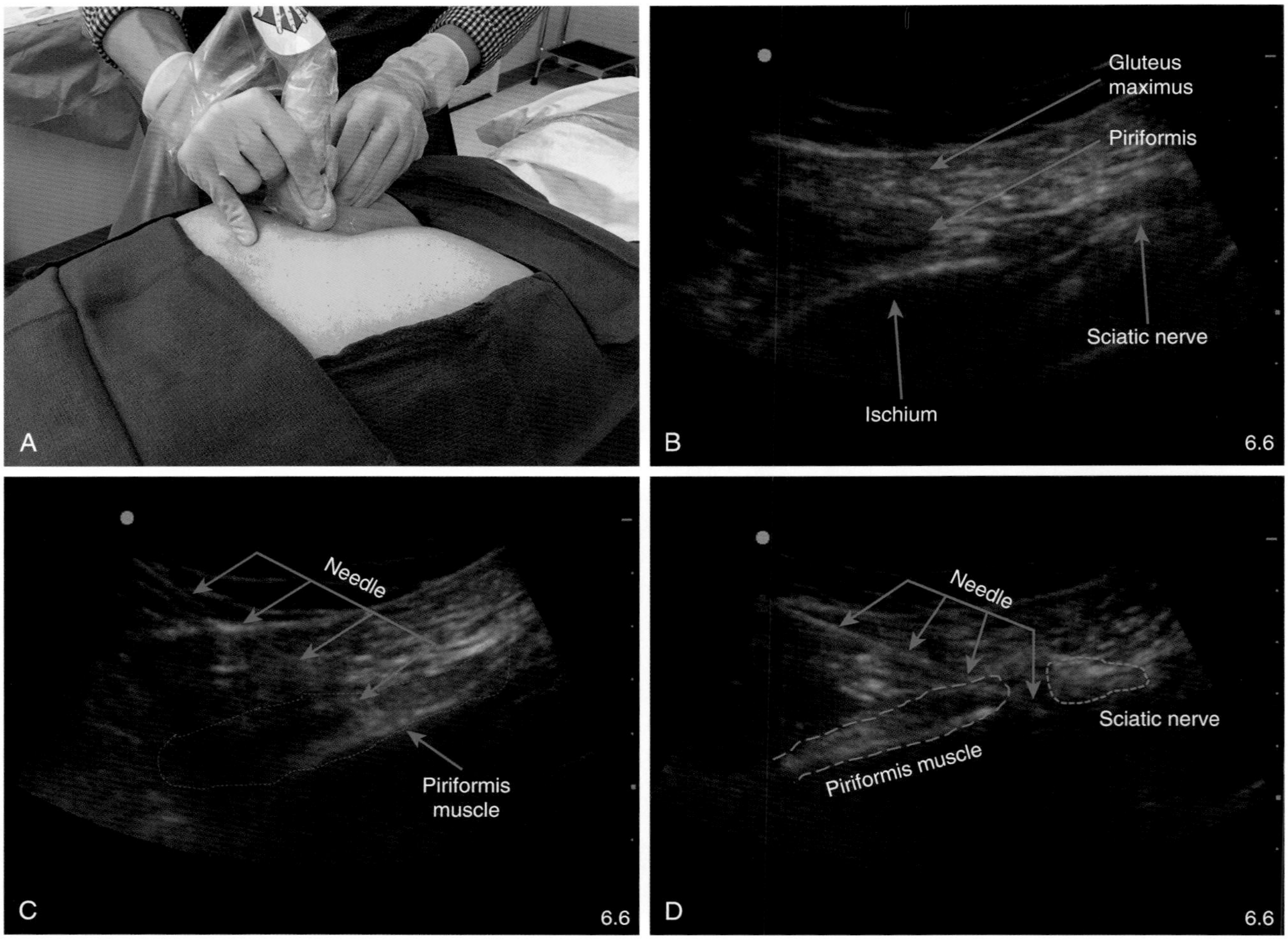

FIG. 80.3 Ultrasound-guided piriformis muscle injection. (A) External view of the position of the ultrasound probe prior to piriformis injection. (B) The relationship between the piriformis muscle, gluteus maximus muscle and sciatic nerve as visualized under ultrasonography. (C) Optimal needle position immediately prior to intramuscular piriformis injection. (D) Shallow needle entry and advancement medially to position the needle tip for perineural injection of the sciatic nerve.

be cautioned that they have an increased risk of fall for the expected duration of the local anesthetic used and that they should not operate motor vehicles. The patient should also be advised that bleeding/bruising at the injection site may be normal. Adverse outcomes include local infection, bleeding/bruising, and other neurologic symptoms such as bowel/bladder incontinence. Signs and symptoms of these should prompt medical staff to send the patient to the emergency room.

Comparison of Techniques

Ultrasound-guided and fluoroscopic techniques for piriformis injection have not been shown to differ in terms of patient outcome measures, complication rate, or duration of procedure.[12] However, this may be difficult to assess, given the already low rate of complications for these procedures. The advantage of ultrasound guidance includes visualization of soft tissue structures (e.g., vasculature), but resolution attenuates when attempting to visualize deeper structures such as the piriformis. This poor visualization is exacerbated by obesity or large body habitus, causing increased tissue depth between the ultrasound probe and the deep musculature.

INJECTATE

Injection of the piriformis muscle is deemed a trigger point injection when providers bill for the procedure, despite the more technically difficult nature of the injection. Often the injection is advertised as proffering analgesic efficacy for several months, but this duration will vary based on many patient factors, the number of injections in the series, and the injectate used. Common options include local anesthetic, steroid, and botulinum toxin. A common injection includes approximately 5 mL of 1% lidocaine with 40 mg of a particulate form of steroid, either methylprednisolone or triamcinolone. Water-soluble forms of steroid, such as dexamethasone or betamethasone, are another injectate option. Lastly, botulinum toxin may be administered, ordinarily as the sole agent, with a typical dose of 100 mouse units in 2 mL of normal saline.[7] See Table 80.1 for a summary of injection studies for deep musculature.

LOCAL ANESTHETIC AND STEROID

The most common injectate undoubtedly for piriformis syndrome includes local anesthetic, typically lidocaine, and

TABLE 80.1 Results of Injection Therapy—Summary of Studies

Muscle Injected	Author, Year of Publication	Number of Patients	Type of Study	Image Guidance	Injectate	Outcome
Piriformis	Porta, 2000[7]	23 7 10	RCT	CT	Methylprednisolone 80 mg or Btx-A 100 U piriformis 150 U iliopsoas 80 U ant. scalene	Improved pain in Btx-A group 60 days postinjection
	Fanucci et al., 2001[64]	30	Prospective	CT	(ona) Btx-A 100 U	Improved pain with either 1 or 2 injections
	Fishman et al., 2002[5]	21	RCT double blind parallel	EMG	(abo) Btx-A 200 U	Majority of patients had >50% pain reduction
	Childers et al., 2002[19]	9	RCT double blind crossover	EMG + FL	(ona) Btx-A 100 U	Improved pain, distress, spasm, and functional status with Btx-A
	Fishman et al., 2004[20]	27	Prospective	EMG	Btx-B	Most patients had >50% relief at 3 months
	Lang, 2004[21]	20	Prospective open-label	EMG	Btx-B 5000 U	Improved pain 16 weeks postinjection
	Yoon et al., 2006[22]	20	Prospective	CT	(abo) Btx-A 150 U	Improvement in pain and functional status at 12 weeks
	Naja et al., 2009[23]	19	RCT double blind parallel	EMG CT verified	Clonidine 150 mcg + bupivacaine vs. bupivacaine alone	Clonidine improves pain compared to bupivacaine alone at 6 months
	Masala et al., 2012[4]	23	Prospective	CT	Methylprednisolone 40 mg	Improvement in pain at 12 months compared with control
	Michel et al., 2013[65]	122	Prospective	EMG	(ona) Btx-A 50–100 U	Most patients had good or very good results from injection
	Al-Al-Shaikh et al., 2015[18]	12	Retrospective	Ultrasound/CT	(ona) Btx-A	Improvement in pain
	Albayrak et al., 2015[8]	28	Prospective	FL	Methylprednisolone, unknown dose	Improvement in pain and functional status
	Jeong et al., 2015[47]	63	Retrospective	Ultrasound	40 mg of triamcinolone	Improvement in pain in majority of patients
	Misirlioglu et al., 2015[67]	47	RCT double blind	Ultrasound	Lidocaine 2% vs. Lidocaine + betamethasone	Improvement in pain in both groups

Continued

TABLE 80.1 Results of Injection Therapy—Summary of Studies—cont'd

Muscle Injected	Author, Year of Publication	Number of Patients	Type of Study	Image Guidance	Injectate	Outcome
Iliopsoas	Porta, 2000[7]	7	RCT	CT	Methylprednisolone 80 mg or Btx-A 100 U piriformis 150 U iliopsoas 80 U ant. scalene	Improved pain in Btx-A group 60 days postinjection
	Nunley et al., 2009[24]	19	Retrospective	FL	Triamcinolone 40 mg + local anesthetic	Improvement of pain in the majority of patients
	DeAndres et al., 2013[49]	27	RCT	FL	Btx-A 50 U	Improvement in pain at 3 months
	Liu et al., 2014[40]	37	RCT	US	Btx-A, weight-based dosing (pediatric study)	Improvement in motor function and gait compared to PT alone
	Rosseaux et al., 2014[66]	11	Prospective open label	EMG	(ona) Btx-A 300 or 400 U	Improvement in comfort, hypertonia, and passive ROM
	Agten et al., 2015[26]	39	Prospective	FL	Triamcinolone 40 mg	Improvement in pain, functional status at 1 month

Muscle Injected	Scalene Targeted	Author Year of Publication	Number of Patients	Type of Study	Image Guidance	Injectate	Outcome
Scalene	Anterior	Porta et al., 2000[7]	10	RCT	CT	Methylprednisolone 80 mg or Btx-A 100 U piriformis 150 U iliopsoas 80 U ant. scalene	Improved pain in Btx-A group 60 days postinjection
	Anterior	Jordan et al., 2000[61]	22	Prospective open label	EMG + FL	Btx—unspecified	Majority of patients had pain relief > 1 month
	Anterior and middle	Jordan et al., 2007[62]	245	Retrospective	EMG + FL EMG + Ultrasound	Btx-A 12 U to ant scalene 12–15 to mid scalene	Improvement in pain, average duration 5 months. No difference in method of image guidance.
	Anterior	Torriani et al., 2009[55]	29	Prospective	Ultrasound	0.5% bupivacaine	Improvement in pain in majority of patients
	Anterior	Christo et al., 2010[60]	27	Prospective	CT	Btx 20 U	Improvement in pain at 3 months
	Anterior and middle	Benzon et al., 2012[54]	12	Retrospective	Ultrasound	0.25% bupivacaine	Pain relief is not related to blockade of brachial plexus
	Anterior	Lum et al., 2012[59]	159	Retrospective	Ultrasound	Lidocaine or Btx	Pain relief from diagnostic scalene injection correlates with good surgical outcome for TOS
	Anterior and middle	Kim et al., 2016[63]	20	RCT crossover	Ultrasound	20 mg triamcinolone into each muscle	Improvement of pain compared with physical therapy

Although there is considerable variety in quality, the listed studies universally demonstrate a benefit in patient pain or other outcome measure.
Btx, *Botulinum toxin;* CT, *computed tomography;* EMG, *electromyography;* FL, *fluoroscopy;* RCT, *randomized controlled trial.*

a steroid particulate formulation, most often methylprednisolone or triamcinolone. Bupivacaine is not the preferred local anesthetic because it is the most myotoxic of all the local anesthetics. Also, bupivacaine can result in prolonged numbness if it leaks out of the piriformis muscle into the area of the sciatic nerve. Although botulinum toxin may lead to longer term relief, local anesthetic and steroid carries a lower risk of side effects or adverse outcomes and has been shown to provide up to a 50% reduction in pain at 10 months.[13]

BOTULINUM TOXIN

Although largely known as a paralytic acting to block release of acetylcholine at the neuromuscular junction,[14] botulinum toxin has now been shown to have direct analgesic effects, even in neuropathic pain states.[15,16] This may be due to direct inhibition of inflammatory mediators and neurotransmitters known to participate in pain pathways. Botulinum injection has no benefit when injected to nonspecific trigger points,[17] but in piriformis syndrome an injection to the muscle significantly reduces pain and is likely superior to steroid and local anesthetic.[5,6] The mechanism for this is most likely due to atrophy and increased fatty infiltration that occurs after denervation of the muscle.[18] Botulinum toxin has been shown to have significantly greater pain relief than steroid injection for more than 2 months postinjection in small randomized controlled trials.[7,19] In other uncontrolled studies, botulinum toxin has also proffered months of pain relief to patients with piriformis syndrome.[20–22]

CLONIDINE

This antihypertensive is a direct alpha-2 agonist and has a long history of use as an adjuvant analgesic. A double-blinded RCT demonstrated at least 6 months of benefit in piriformis syndrome after injection.[23]

ILIOPSOAS PAIN

Iliopsoas pain is an uncommon cause of anterior hip pain, lower back, and groin or thigh pain. The symptoms can occur after total hip arthroplasty (THA) due to impingement of the iliopsoas tendon[24] or iliopsoas bursitis.[25] In the nonsurgical population, iliopsoas pain may be due to rheumatoid arthritis, osteophytic overgrowth of the anterior joint, or anterior labral tears, or may occur in the context of overuse injuries in athletes.[26] Pain due to iliopsoas dysfunction may be myofascial, originating in the muscle itself, or due to bursitis, especially after total joint replacement. An additional syndrome, "snapping hip," the descriptive name for coxa saltans, describes the audible or sensory perception of a snap over the hip with movement that may or may not be associated with pain. One subtype of snapping hip is termed "internal snapping hip" and is due to iliopsoas dysfunction. This is most often caused by snapping of the iliopsoas tendon over the iliopectineal eminence, which is an osseous ridge located where the iliac and pubic bones articulate. Also, after THA, snapping may occur over the acetabular prosthesis or in native hips, over the femoral head or a paralabral cyst. Snapping may also occur when a portion of the iliacus becomes intercalated within the iliopsoas tendon and pelvic bone during a return to neutral from a position of abduction and external rotation. Iliopsoas pain may be more likely after resurfacing surgeries or metal-on-metal THA, because the femoral heads are larger than conventional THA, theoretically leading to greater disruption of the iliopsoas musculotendinous unit.[27] Lastly, a bifid iliopsoas tendon may also cause a snapping hip due to the medial head flipping over the lateral head.[28] Most commonly, inflammation of either the tendon or the bursa will cause pain and inflammation in the unaffected portion of the anatomy. Therefore most often both the tendon and the bursa are pain generators in iliopsoas syndrome.[29]

DIAGNOSIS

Common symptoms include pain with ascending stairs, exiting or entering vehicles, or standing from seated position. The diagnosis can be made with dynamic sonographic imaging, which permits static and dynamic visualization of the psoas muscle and bursa during manipulations in instances of snapping hip,[30] or MRI in other instances of iliopsoas-related pain.[31] Sonographic evidence of bursitis or tendinitis is usually absent and is better imaged with MRI, although the snapping motion of the iliopsoas tendon is usually evident on ultrasound.[28,32]

RELEVANT ANATOMY

The iliopsoas musculotendinous unit is located in the retroperitoneal space and is composed of the psoas major and iliacus, which have a common tendon that inserts on the lesser trochanter of the femur.[31] The psoas major originates along the transverse processes and discs from the T12 to L5 vertebral levels, and the iliacus originates at the iliac fossa. The psoas is innervated by the lumbar plexus via the anterior rami of L1, L2, and L3, and the iliacus is innervated by the femoral nerve, specifically the anterior rami components of L2 and L3.[33] The iliopsoas courses anterolaterally below the inguinal ligament and anterior to the hip joint, a trajectory that makes it the major flexor of the hip joint. There is controversy regarding its function as a hip rotator or trunk stabilizer, but its function as the major hip flexor is irrefutable. In 60% of adults, a psoas minor muscle arises from T12 to L1 and courses along the medial aspect of the psoas major.[31] However, this muscle does not insert upon the lesser trochanter of the femur like the iliopsoas; instead, it attaches to the innominate bone and the iliac fascia at the pelvic brim and therefore is not responsible for hip flexion but rather weak spine flexion.[34] Lastly, the iliopsoas muscle does possess a bursa in order to reduce friction between the muscle and surrounding bone of the iliopubic eminence. It is located anterior to the hip joint, posterior to the iliopsoas tendon and femoral nerve, and lateral to the femoral vasculature.[25] This synovial bursa is relatively large but thin, which makes it difficult to detect on many imaging modalities other than magnetic resonance imaging (MRI). This bursa rarely communicates with the normal hip joint, but trauma, inflammation, or surgical exploration significantly increase the incidence of such a relationship.[29] Iliopsoas impingement may be a cause of anterior labral pathology of the hip, in which case endoscopic surgery is often required.[35] Because iliopsoas impingement, bursitis, and tendinopathy are difficult to discern on physical exam and often exist concomitantly, they are collectively known as iliopsoas syndrome.[36,37]

CONSERVATIVE MANAGEMENT

As with most pain conditions, conservative treatment with physical therapy and medications is appropriate in the acute phase immediately after onset of symptoms. A 3-month course of hip strengthening is often highly effective in treating iliopsoas syndrome.[38] Ultrasound as a modality of physical therapy has also been used, although limited evidence exists for its benefit.[28] Standard physical therapy measures are typically the only intervention required for iliopsoas dysfunction, but in recalcitrant cases, injection therapy can be instituted.[29,36,37]

ILIOPSOAS INJECTIONS

Image guidance for iliopsoas injections, much like piriformis injections, may be fluoroscopic, EMG, or ultrasound guided. Iliopsoas injections have been shown to provide pain relief in patients with native hip joints and in patients who are post-THA, although the injection is often more challenging due to the presence of hardware.[24]

FLUOROSCOPIC-GUIDED TECHNIQUE

The patient is placed supine and the fluoroscope is positioned in the anteroposterior view. The lateral femoral head is identified, and the area above this is cleansed and draped. The site of insertion and the projected tract is anesthetized with lidocaine. A 22-gauge 3–5-inch spinal needle is most often used for fluoroscopically guided techniques.

Medial Portion of Iliopsoas

The needle is advanced, coaxial to the fluoroscopic beam, until it makes contact with the osseous surface of the acetabulum over the center of the femoral head. The needle is then "walked" medially until it is approximately 0.5 cm from the medial edge of the acetabulum, as visualized on fluoroscopy. Contrast dye is injected to ensure that the needle tip is inside the bursa, and then the injectate is administered (Fig. 80.4A).[39]

Inferior Portion of Iliopsoas

In coaxial orientation, the needle is advanced until it comes in contact with the osseous surface of the lesser trochanter. Contrast dye is injected to ensure that the needle tip is inside the bursa and then the injectate is administered (see Fig. 80.4B).

Superior Portion of Iliopsoas

The needle is advanced toward the superomedial aspect of the acetabulum, which targets the course of the iliopsoas muscle closer to its origin. Contrast dye is injected to ensure appropriate spread outlining the muscle, and then the injectate is administered (see Fig. 80.4C).

ELECTROMYOGRAPHIC-GUIDED TECHNIQUE

In order to localize the iliopsoas muscle with EMG, the pulse frequency should be set at 3 Hz and a current intensity of 10–15 mA. This is used initially to scan the area of the inguinal crease for the point at which the lowest intensity of current triggers the most significant hip flexion. This area is marked at the skin and then prepped with sterile solution and draped in typical fashion. After this, the current is decreased to 3 mA with the same pulse frequency and the insulated needle is inserted in the musculature; the needle is then adjusted until the minimum current is required for maximal muscle contraction. At that point the medication can be injected.[40]

ULTRASOUND-GUIDED TECHNIQUE

Ultrasound guidance can be complex in the psoas compartment: Three methods have been described. Ultrasound affords the operator the added safety of visualizing soft tissue structures and vasculature, but it is much more technically challenging.

Axial Probe Position

With the patient in lateral decubitus position (Fig. 80.5A), place the curved ultrasound probe in cross-sectional view over the lateral part of the abdomen facing the spine (see Fig. 80.5B). The probe is moved superiorly and inferiorly to identify the lateral view of the vertebral bodies, the kidney, the psoas, the quadratus lumborum, and the posterior paravertebral muscles. At the L3–L4 area, the transducer is placed just above the iliac crest. The skin is anesthetized posterior to the probe and lateral to the spinous processes (see Fig. 80.5C). The needle is inserted using the in-plane technique 4 cm medial/posterior to the medial/posterior portion of the transducer (between the spinous processes and the transducer). The needle is advanced into the psoas muscle, while crossing from posterior to anterior, the skin, fat, posterior paravertebral muscles, intertransverse muscles, and enters the psoas in the posterolateral portion (see Fig. 80.5D), which is located lateral to the vertebral body and anterior to the transverse process. Care should be taken to avoid the segmental artery and the nerve root. The pulsation of saline may be administered to verify the location of the needle tip. In our experience this approach is only recommended in patients with a BMI less than 35. Larger patients with increased subcutaneous fat will obscure the visualization of the needle.[41]

Sagittal Probe Position

The patient lies prone with a pillow under the abdomen, and the ultrasound probe is positioned longitudinally over the spinous processes at the L3–L4 level. The probe is then moved laterally to show the laminae, facet column, and the transverse processes of L2–L3–L4, which will have the appearance of a trident on the monitor. At this point the patient presses the ipsilateral knee against the examination table, causing the psoas muscle fibers between the transverse processes to contract and move. After cleansing and anesthetizing the skin, the needle is inserted using in-plane technique, to cross between the transverse processes

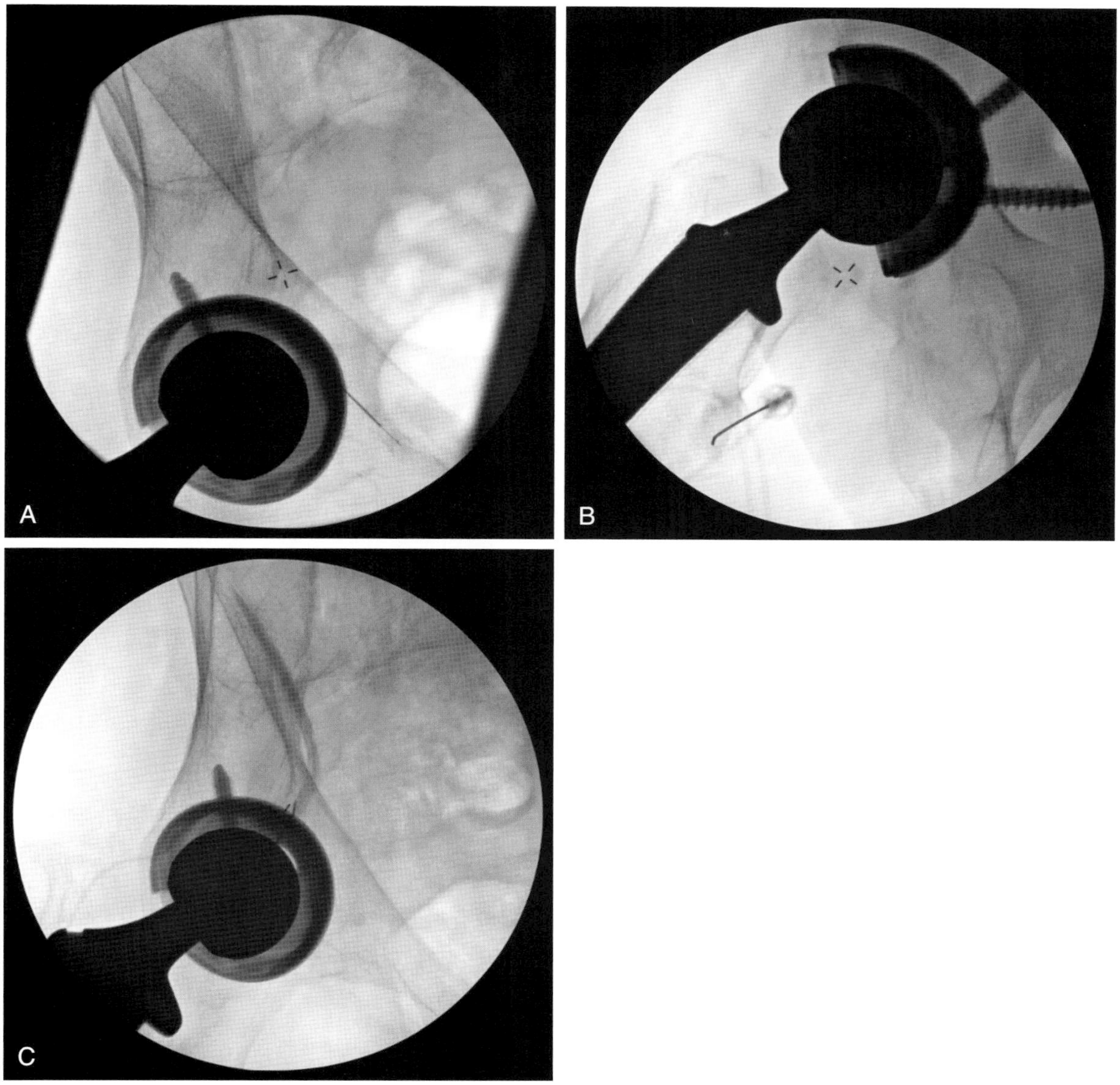

FIG. 80.4 Fluoroscopy-assisted iliopsoas muscle injection (A) Medial injection. The needle tip is positioned at the medial aspect of the acetabulum with contrast dye outlining the psoas muscle. (B) Inferior injection. The target is the lesser trochanteric bursa, insertion site of the iliopsoas, and contrast dye in the image is visualized outlining the inferior portion of iliopsoas. (C) Superior injection. Needle is positioned at the superomedial aspect of the acetabulum, with contrast dye outlining the superior portion of iliopsoas.

of L3 and L4. The needle is advanced 1.5 cm deeper to the posterior aspect of the transverse processes. While injecting, the provider should ensure that no liquid fills the area superficial to the transverse processes.[42]

Supine Patient

With the hip in neutral position, the transducer is placed parallel and just inferior to the inguinal ligament. The operator should maintain a clear ultrasonographic view of the femoral head to ensure that the injection does not enter the hip joint. The needle is inserted from lateral to medial using the in-plane technique relative to the transducer.[43]

Possible side effects are as follows: If the injection is too anterior with the first technique described, the injectate may enter the aorta or vena cava. This adverse event is, of course, less likely with ultrasound guidance. If the patient experiences unilateral lower extremity weakness, this indicates that a lumbar plexus block has occurred along with a true iliopsoas injection. If the bilateral lower extremities are weak, this indicates the injection was epidural or spinal due to either a medial location of the needle tip or an excessively large volume of injectate.

RESULTS OF TREATMENT OF PIRIFORMIS AND ILIOPSOAS INJECTIONS

Several studies have established the efficacy of interventional techniques, with a range of invasiveness from trigger point injections in conjunction with physical therapy to image-guided

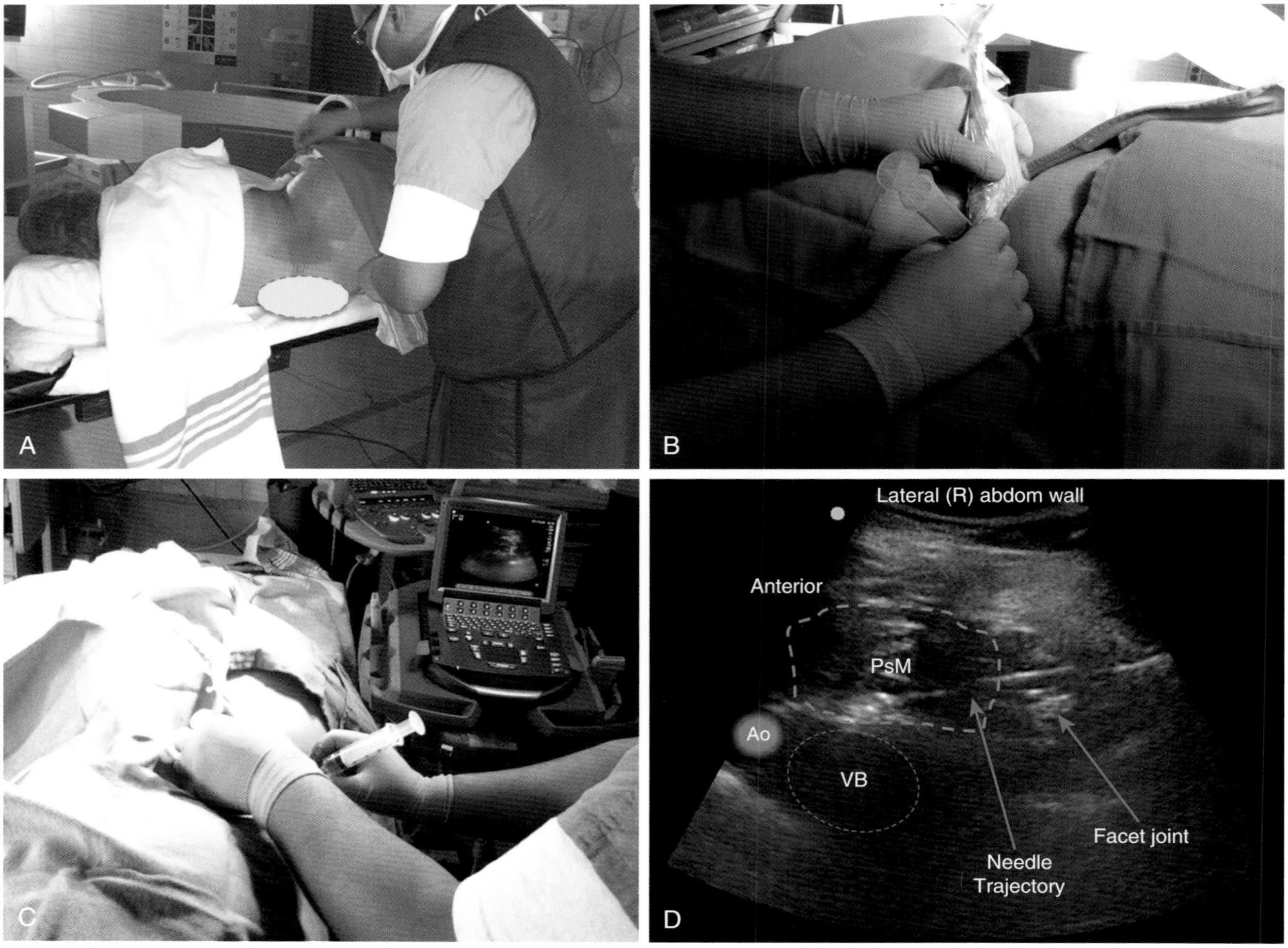

FIG. 80.5 Ultrasound-assisted iliopsoas muscle injection. (A) Patient in lateral position with affected side up, area of injection is cleansed and draped in sterile fashion. (B) Transducer positioned on the lateral part of the abdomen and scanning towards the center of the trunk. (C) Needle insertion 3–4 cm posterior to the posterior aspect of the transducer. (D) Visualization of sonoanatomy demonstrating the needle trajectory for axial probe technique to inject the psoas compartment. *Ao*, Aorta; *PsM*, psoas major muscle; *VB*, vertebral body.

piriformis injections. Although studies performed in this area vary greatly in quality, most reveal an improvement in piriformis syndrome pain with injection treatment.[2,4,6,8,9,11,13,21,44–48] However, there is conflicting evidence regarding the relative efficacy of different injectates, with some studies reporting the superiority of botulinum toxin over steroid/local anesthetic[6] and another showing no difference between botulinum and local anesthetic injection.[49] Another case series extols the virtues of dry needling performed in combination with stretching.[32] If the patient responds to neither conservative management nor injection therapy, then surgical lengthening or endoscopic release can be considered.[37] See Table 80.1 for a summary of evidence-based medicine regarding the efficacy of deep muscle injections.

THORACIC OUTLET SYNDROME

Scalene muscle injections are used to diagnose or treat TOS, which is an uncommon disease caused by compression of the brachial plexus, subclavian artery, and subclavian vein as they pass through the cervicoaxillary canal. TOS has three etiologies, with neurogenic TOS accounting for greater than 95% of cases and the remaining cases being attributed to venous (2%–3%) or arterial compression (>1%).[50] Neurogenic TOS is most amenable to injection treatment because it is due to the compression of the brachial plexus by the scalene muscles. Venous or arterial TOS is not amenable to injection treatment and often requires surgical first rib resection.[51] Trauma, such as whiplash injuries or repetitive motion stress, is implicated in up to two-thirds of neurogenic TOS cases, and the remaining cases are due to abnormalities in the scalene musculature, bone abnormalities, and rarely due to metastases or osteomyelitis.[50] Trauma to the scalene muscles, most often from a single incident but occasionally from small repetitive trauma, causes scarring and spasm, which then compress the brachial plexus, leading to pain and paresthesia in the unilateral upper extremity.[52]

DIAGNOSIS

Thoracic outlet syndrome can be difficult to distinguish from various other pathologies that create similar

TABLE 80.2 Special Tests for Diagnosis of Thoracic Outlet Syndrome

Special Test	Execution of Test
Roos test	(1) Abduct arm 90 degrees, (2) flex elbow 90 degrees and hold posterior to midline of the thorax, (3) open and close hand slowly. Positive test = reproduction of symptoms, heaviness, weakness.
Upper limb tension test	(1) Abduct arm 90 degrees, (2) flex elbow 90 degrees, (3) dorsiflex the wrist, (4) laterally flex neck to ipsilateral side. Positive test = ipsilateral pain with steps 1 and 2. Contralateral pain with step 3.
Adson's test	(1) Rotate head toward test shoulder, (2) extend neck while examiner laterally rotates and extends shoulder and elbow, (3) take a deep breath and hold. Positive test = loss of radial pulse and reproduction of symptoms.

Here we describe several specific maneuvers that assist in the diagnosis of TOS. The Roos test and Adson test should be used for diagnosis of vascular TOS, and the upper limb tension test is most useful for diagnosis of neurogenic TOS.[52]
TOS, *Thoracic outlet syndrome.*

symptoms of pain, muscle weakness, and sensory changes in a unilateral upper extremity. No specific diagnostic criteria exist, and imaging studies are either entirely or relatively insensitive for thoracic outlet syndrome.[51] Patients will most often report unilateral pain, paresthesia, or cold intolerance in the upper extremity, frequently in the ulnar distribution. There are a variety of special tests that can aid in the diagnosis (Table 80.2). Imaging rarely identifies the abnormalities in soft tissue structures that cause TOS but is often indicated to rule out other sources of the symptoms, such as rotator cuff tear, presence of a cervical rib, or ominous pathologic processes such as osseous fracture, tumor, or osteomyelitis. Due to the broad differential for patients with this constellation of symptoms, injections to the anterior and middle scalene muscles can be very useful in the diagnostic process as well. Although a decision to proceed with surgery is often definitively indicated in arterial or even venous etiologies of TOS, it is more challenging if the patient has neurogenic TOS. The variable recovery of patients after neurogenic TOS may be due to inappropriate diagnosis,[53] and injection of scalene muscle will have diagnostic value in distinguishing TOS from other causes of upper extremity symptoms. After injection, the scalene muscles relax, which causes the first rib to move inferiorly, and the relief is not simply due to brachial plexus blockade, because the relief can be sustained.[54] In fact, the relief can even be comparable to surgical treatment, and with considerably less risk to the patient.[55]

RELEVANT ANATOMY

Typically the scalene musculature consists of three paired muscles: the anterior, middle, and posterior scalene muscles. Occasionally a fourth muscle, the scalene minimus, is present or the muscle fascicles of the others may be fused, resulting in considerable variation in the origin and insertion site. The anterior scalene originates from the anterior tubercles of the C3–6 vertebral bodies and inserts on the scalene tubercle of the first rib. It is proximal and anterior to the subclavian artery. The middle scalene originates from the posterior tubercles of C2–7 and inserts on the first rib posterolaterally to the anterior scalene and posterior to the subclavian artery. Actions of the scalene muscles include forward and lateral flexion of the neck. In addition, they are accessory muscles of respiration, causing elevation of the first and second ribs during deep inspiration.[56,57] The anterior and middle scalene muscles form the interscalene triangle, in which the brachial plexus courses, which is the basis for the distribution of pain symptoms in TOS.[52] This anatomical relationship is both the reason for the anterior and middle scalene as injection targets and the cause of the common effect of brachial plexus anesthesia after injections that use local anesthetic.

SCALENE MUSCLE INJECTION

Given the neurovascular structures in close proximity to the injection site, a blind technique for injection is not recommended, and injections are most commonly guided by ultrasonography, fluoroscopy, or computed tomography (CT). As the ultrasound technique permits visualization of the carotid artery, jugular vein, brachial plexus, and thyroid gland, it is currently the preferred method for injection.

ULTRASOUND-GUIDED TECHNIQUE

The patient lies supine with the neck rotated 15°–20° contralateral to the painful site. A flat ultrasound probe is selected and the frequency is set to 12 MHz.

Medial to Lateral Approach

The probe is positioned over the cricoid cartilage and moved laterally from the trachea, identifying the carotid artery and jugular vein en route, until the scalene muscles come into view. The brachial plexus can be identified between them.

Inferior to Superior Approach

The probe is placed just superior to the clavicle and lateral to the sternocleidomastoid muscle. The brachial plexus is then identified and followed superiorly until the point at which it courses between the anterior and middle scalene muscles.

Injection

A 25-gauge, 1.5-cm length echogenic needle should be selected and advanced either in-plane or out-of-plane while the ultrasound probe is held in transverse orientation across the neck. The anterior and middle scalene muscles are injected separately, without penetrating the fascia which separates them, to ensure avoidance of brachial plexus blockade. Techniques have been described that inject only the anterior scalene muscle or both the anterior and middle scalene muscles.[54,55] Injection of both muscles is the most commonly performed procedure, as both muscles can compress the brachial plexus (Fig. 80.6).

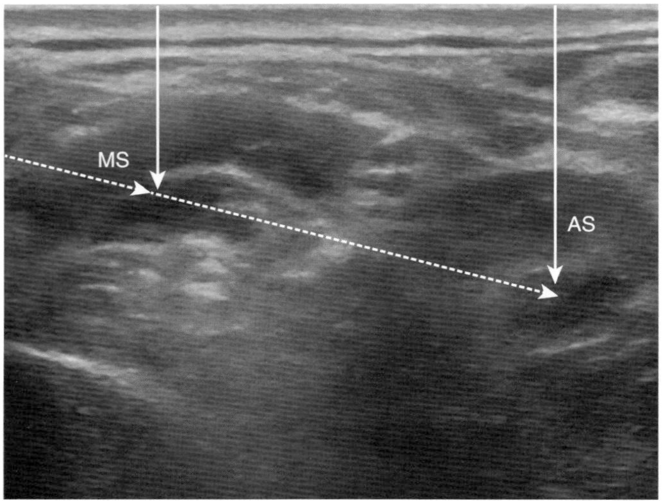

MS = Middle scalene muscle, AS = Anterior scalene muscle
Arrows display location of injection: Solid line = Out-of-plane technique
Dashed line = In-plane technique

FIG. 80.6 Ultrasound-assisted scalene muscle injection. Injection of the middle scalene muscle with the needles in-plane and out-of-plane. (*From Benzon HT, Rodes ME, Chekka K, Malik K, and Pearce W: Scalene muscle injections for neurogenic thoracic outlet syndrome: case series.* Pain Practice. *2012;12(1):66-70.*)

RESULTS OF INJECTION

As previously stated, scalene muscle injections are often performed for diagnostic and therapeutic purposes. Although a true "gold standard" for diagnosis of TOS does not exist, if the patient's symptoms of thoracic outlet syndrome are relieved, even transiently, by a scalene muscle injection, then this predicts a good outcome after surgical management of TOS such as scalenotomy or first rib resection.[58,59] When injections performed include steroid and local anesthetic, they are often performed as a series of three injections performed at 2–3-week intervals. This may extend the duration of relief from the common result of 1 week of relief to a full 4 weeks of relief after a series.[54] However, if this is insufficient and the patient requires escalating therapy, then botulinum toxin may be considered. A single injection of botulinum toxin has been shown to reduce pain scores for over 3 months.[60] The dose of botulinum toxin injection has been described as 15 units per scalene muscle,[60–62] which is a relatively low dose. For a more prolonged effect, one of the authors (Honorio T. Benzon) empirically injects 30–40 units for the anterior scalene and 40–50 units for the middle scalene muscles. If local anesthetic is included in the injection, the patient may have significant arm weakness, given that the brachial plexus courses directly between the anterior and middle scalene muscles. Therefore if the local anesthetic is injected outside or diffuses out of the fascia surrounding these muscles, the patient may lose motor function in the unilateral upper limb. If this occurs, the patient should be provided with a sling upon discharge for both safety and comfort. The common inclusion of local anesthetic when injecting the scalene musculature has resulted in some speculation that the relief resulting from these injections may be in part due to blockade of the brachial plexus. However, it was noted that the presence and duration of relief is not related to the occurrence of numbness. A recent study using steroid as monotherapy for injection did show greater improvement in patients with thoracic outlet syndrome compared with patients treated with medication and physical therapy.[63]

KEY POINTS

- Deep muscle injections are commonly performed on the piriformis muscle, iliopsoas muscle, and scalene muscles.
- Pain syndromes that result from deep muscles are often due to mechanical pressure from the muscle that is exerted upon neurovascular or articular structures.
- Because the injection targets are not superficial, these injections are typically not performed blind or with the use of landmarks alone.
- Deep muscle injections may be performed with image guidance from fluoroscopy, ultrasonography, or even CT. Occasionally an EMG has been used as well.
- These injections may be diagnostic or therapeutic, or have dual function.
- Typical initial injectate includes a combination of deposit form of steroid combined with local anesthetic.
- If the patient enjoys good but transient benefit from the steroid/local anesthetic injections, then botulinum toxin may be injected to provide more long lasting relief.
- Injections are often one component of a multimodal treatment plan, including medication administration, and a course of physical therapy.

REFERENCES

Access the reference list online at ExpertConsult.com.

CHAPTER 81 ULTRASOUND-GUIDED MUSCULOSKELETAL INJECTIONS—SHOULDER, HIP, AND KNEE

Sadiq Bhayani, MBBS, FRCA ◎ Philip Peng, MBBS, FRCPC, Founder (Pain Med)

Pain originating from the musculoskeletal (MSK) system is among the major global causes of disability and one of the most common reasons for patients to visit primary and tertiary care practitioners.[1,2] The application of ultrasound for MSK examination and injection is increasingly popular and well established. The anatomy and sonoanatomy relevant to the injection of shoulder, hip, and knee joints is described in this chapter.

SHOULDER

The shoulder is more prone to injuries or attrition and therefore it is the most common region where ultrasound-guided MSK injections are performed. Common sites of intervention in the shoulder include the acromioclavicular joint (ACJ), long head of the biceps (LHB), subacromial subdeltoid bursa (SASDB), and glenohumeral joint (GHJ).

The shoulder girdle is composed of the scapula, clavicle, and proximal humerus, all functioning as a single biomechanical unit. There are three joints (glenohumeral, acromioclavicular, and sternoclavicular) and two gliding planes (subacromial and scapulothoracic), providing the greatest range of movement of any joint in the body.[3]

ACROMIOCLAVICULAR JOINT

Osteoarthritis of the ACJ is a common source of shoulder pain; it is often ignored by clinicians due to the higher prevalence of rotator cuff pathology. The proper diagnosis of ACJ osteoarthritis requires a thorough physical examination, plain-film radiograph, and diagnostic local anaesthetic injection. The main indication for ACJ injection is osteoarthritis of this joint.[4]

The ACJ is a small synovial joint with the articular surfaces separated either partly or completely by a wedge-shaped fibrocartilaginous disk (Fig. 81.1). The capsule of the ACJ is reinforced by the acromioclavicular ligaments in its superior, inferior, anterior, and posterior aspects.[5] Caudally it is also reinforced by fibers from the coracoacromial ligament, which blends with the undersurface of the ACJ. The coracoclavicular ligament, composed of the conoid and trapezoid ligaments, anchors the lateral aspect of the clavicle to the coracoid process and plays a crucial role in maintaining the vertical stability of the ACJ (Fig. 81.2). The inferior surface of the joint is in direct contact with the subacromial bursa and rotator cuff and may play a role in the development of the impingement syndrome (see Fig. 81.1).

Sonoanatomy of the Acromioclavicular Joint

The joint can be simply reviewed with a high-frequency linear probe over the joint in the coronal plane (long-axis of joint) or sagittal plane (short-axis of joint). In a young healthy patient, a fibrocartilaginous disk is usually seen as a slightly hyperechoic wedge-shaped structure attached to the superior joint capsule (Fig. 81.3). The hyperechoic ends of the acromion and the distal clavicle may not appear at the same level in 16% of patients because of the variable obliquity of the joint.[6]

Injection Technique for the Acromioclavicular Joint

The main indication for ACJ injection is osteoarthritis of this joint.[7] The patient's position can be either sitting or supine. The arm should be in the neutral position, as the deep joint space is the widest in this position.[8] A linear probe with high frequency is used because the structures are superficial. The probe is placed over the medial side of the acromion in line with the clavicle. The ACJ can thus be visualized with the capsule covering the two hyperechoic structures, acromion and clavicle (Fig. 81.4). In young patients, the fibrocartilage can be seen interposing the ACJ.

Both out-of-plane and in-plane techniques have been described, but out-of-plane is preferred as the joint space is very superficial. The needle should be directed almost parallel to the probe. The depth of the joint is small and overzealous insertion of the needle can result in puncturing the

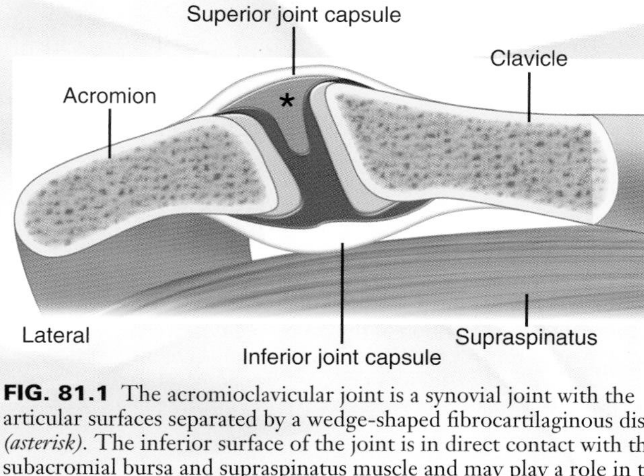

FIG. 81.1 The acromioclavicular joint is a synovial joint with the articular surfaces separated by a wedge-shaped fibrocartilaginous disc (*asterisk*). The inferior surface of the joint is in direct contact with the subacromial bursa and supraspinatus muscle and may play a role in the development of the impingement syndrome. (*Reprinted with permission from Philip Peng Educational Series.*)

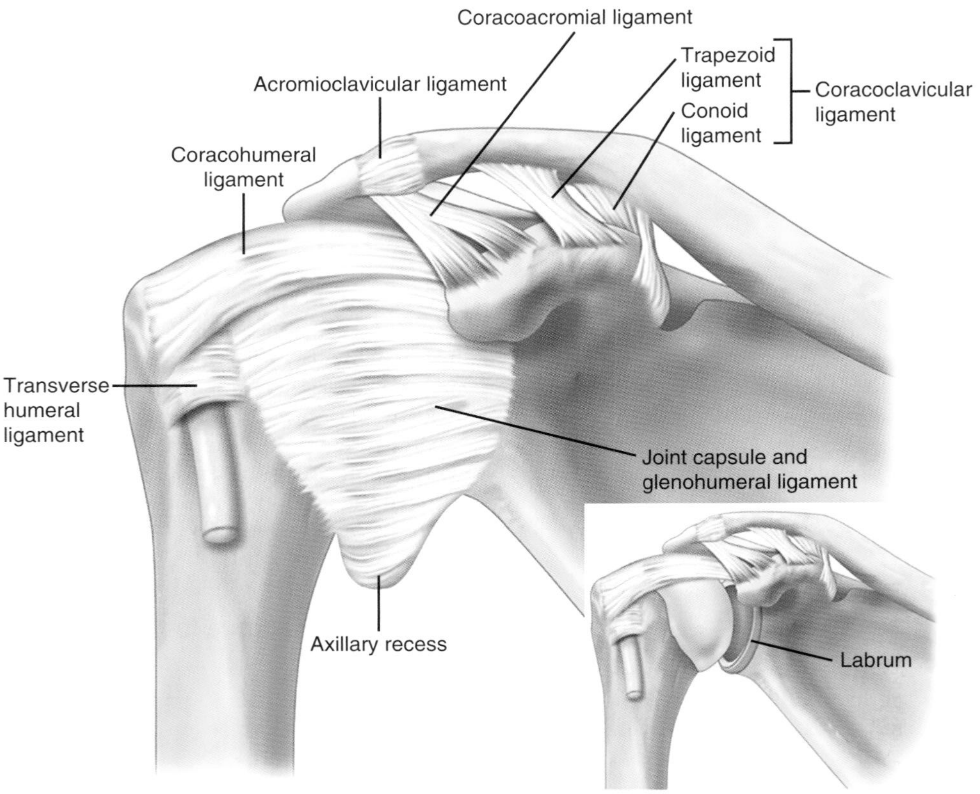

FIG. 81.2 The glenohumeral joint with various ligaments and the joint capsule. The anterior capsule is reinforced by the superior, middle, and inferior glenohumeral ligaments. The *insert* shows the articular surface, glenoid process, and labrum. (*Reprinted with permission from Philip Peng Educational Series.*)

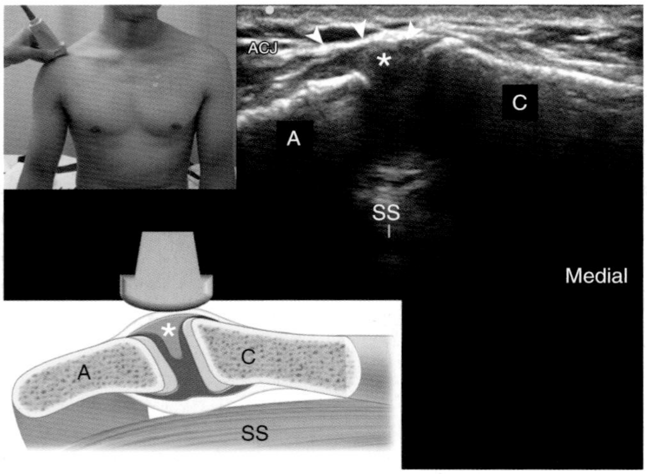

FIG. 81.3 Ultrasound image of the acromioclavicular joint (ACJ). The *upper insert* shows the position of the probe and the patient; the *lower insert* shows the position of the probe and the structures underneath. *A*, Acromion process; *C*, clavicle; *SS*, supraspinatus muscle; *, wedge-shaped fibrocartilaginous disc. *Arrowheads* point to the superior joint capsule. (*Reprinted with permission from Philip Peng Educational Series.*)

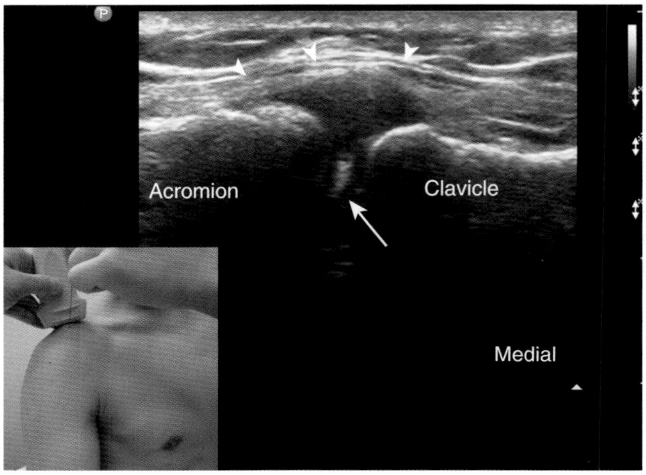

FIG. 81.4 The *insert* shows the position of the ultrasound probe and the needle with the out-of-plane technique. The corresponding ultrasound image shows the acromioclavicular joint with the image of the needle *(solid arrow)*. The *arrowheads* outline the superior joint capsule. (*Reprinted with permission from Philip Peng Educational Series.*)

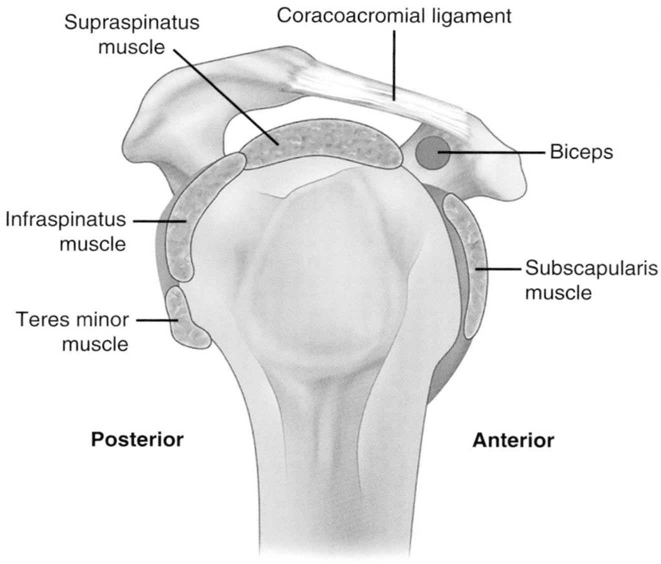

FIG. 81.5 A schematic diagram showing the arrangement of the four rotator cuff muscles: subscapularis, supraspinatus, infraspinatus, and teres minor. (*Reprinted with permission from Philip Peng Educational Series.*)

deep capsule and entering the subacromial space. The volume of injectate is usually 2 mL, and a successful injection is indicated by elevation of the capsule and widening of the joint space under real-time scanning. With the use of ultrasound, the accuracy was high (95%–100%) in cadaver studies.[9,10]

LONG HEAD OF THE BICEPS TENDON AND ROTATOR CUFF INTERVAL

The LHB tendon arises from the supraglenoid tubercle and the superior labrum. The proximal part of this tendon is intraarticular but extrasynovial.[11,12] The tendon travels obliquely over the anterosuperior aspect of the humeral head and exits the joint within the bicipital groove formed by the greater and lesser tuberosities on the lateral and medial sides, respectively (Figs. 81.5 and 81.6). In the bicipital groove, an extension of the synovial lining of the GHJ invests the LHB tendon down to approximately 3–4 cm beyond the distal end of the groove (Fig. 81.7). Thus fluid distension within the sheath usually reflects an underlying GHJ disease. In the bicipital groove, the LHB tendon is accompanied by the ascending branch of the anterior circumflex artery and is covered by the transverse humeral ligament, a weak ligament formed by the superficial fibers of the subscapularis (SSC) tendon.

The rotator cuff interval is a triangular space that occupies the area between the tendons of SSC and supraspinatus (SS) and the base of the coracoid process.[13,14] It is roofed by the rotator cuff interval capsule, which is principally made up of the CHL (Fig. 81.8) and contains the tendon of the LHB and the superior glenohumeral ligament (SGHL).[15] The combination of the CHL and SGHL has a complex relationship to the LHB tendon, which act together to prevent the tendon from subluxing in the anterior direction.[15] The rotator cuff interval is a space where the GHJ synovial lining extends around the biceps tendon and the arthroscope enters the GHJ to avoid damaging the cuff tendons.[16,17] Thus this is an entry site in which the interventionalist can access the GHJ.

Sonoanatomy of the Long Head of the Biceps Tendon and Rotator Cuff Interval

To examine the LHB tendon, the patient is placed in the sitting position with the arm placed in a neutral or slight internal rotation position, the elbow bent, and the palm facing up. A high-frequency linear probe is placed approximately at the level of coracoid process (Fig. 81.9A). A short-axis view of the humerus reveals the greater and lesser tuberosities and the bicipital groove, where the LHB tendon is found. The greater tuberosity has a rounder look, whereas the lesser tuberosity assumes a pointed shape (see Fig. 81.9B). Because of the anisotropic nature of the biceps tendon in this short-axis view, the tilting of the probe is important (see Fig. 81.9B). Doppler imaging of the area reveals the ascending branch of the anterior circumflex artery, which is usually on the lateral side of the tendon. In the bicipital groove, the tendon is invested by its synovial sheath and the effusion at this level should be noted.

Moving the ultrasound probe more proximally along the orientation of the LHB tendon reveals the rotator cuff interval (see Fig. 81.9C). The LHB tendon appears as a hyperechoic elliptical structure at this level and is sandwiched between the SS tendon laterally and SSC tendon medially. The coracohumeral ligament (CHL) forms the roof of the interval.

Injection Technique for the Long Head of the Bicep Tendon

The main indication for injection around the LHB tendon is biceps tendinopathy, which involves a spectrum of pathology ranging from inflammatory tendinitis to degenerative tendinosis.[4,18] Ultrasound is a useful tool that can reliably diagnose complete rupture, subluxation, or dislocation of the LHB tendon.[19] To perform the injection, the patient is placed in a sitting position. A high-frequency linear probe is placed over the bicipital groove (approximately midway between the clavicle and anterior axillary fold) to reveal the short-axis view of the LHB tendon. A color Doppler scan is used to locate the anterior circumflex artery. An out-of-plane approach is used with a 25-gauge needle inserted from the medial side through the transverse humeral ligament (Fig. 81.10). Methylprednisolone 10–20 mg diluted in local anesthetic with a total volume of 4 mL is used as an injectate. A well-directed injection will show the local anesthetic surrounding the LHB tendons at the bicipital groove (see Fig. 81.10).

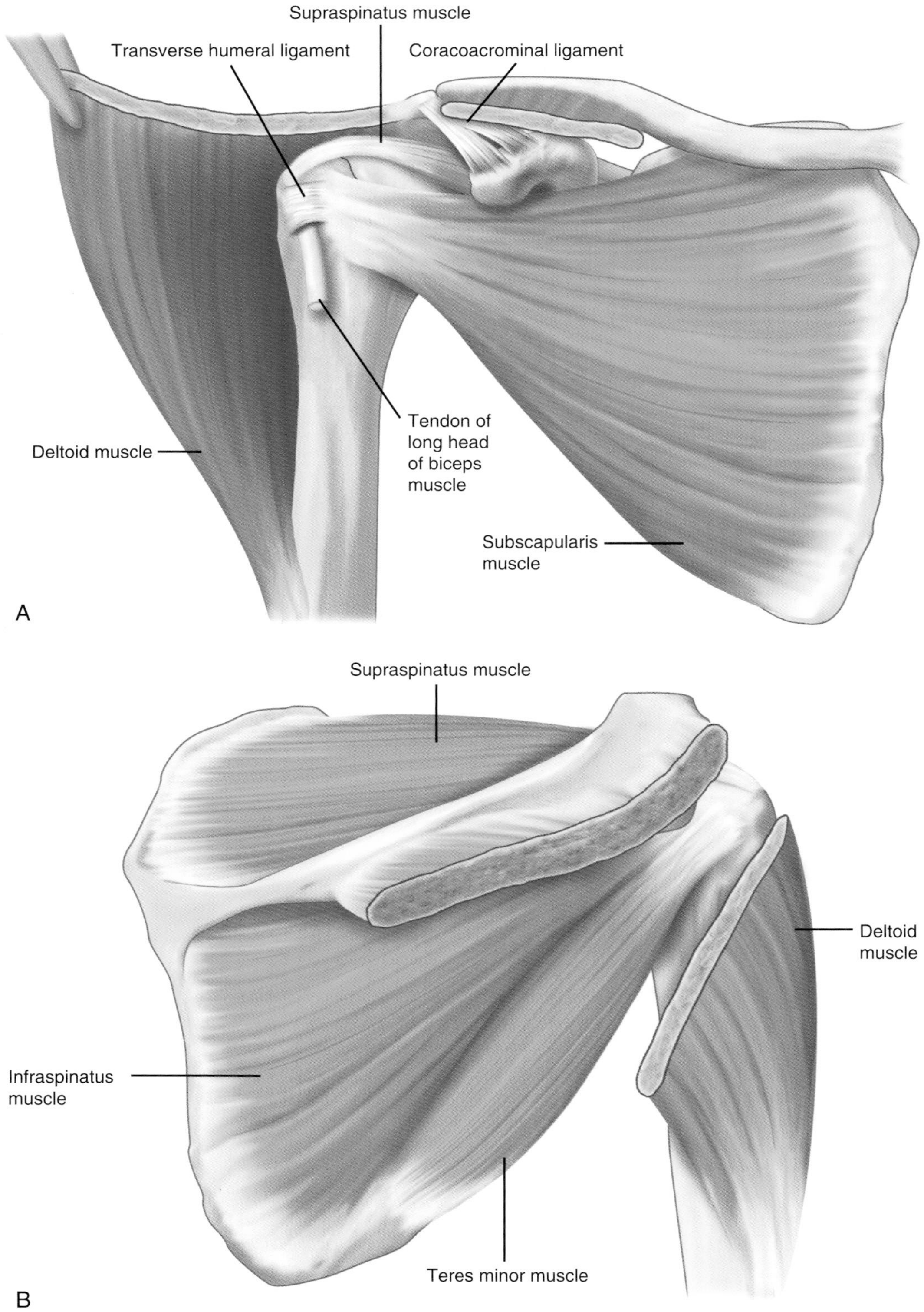

FIG. 81.6 (A) Anterior view of the shoulder showing the subscapularis and supraspinatus muscles. The anterior portion of the deltoid muscle was reflected to show the underlying rotator cuff muscle. (B) Posterior view of the shoulder showing the infraspinatus and teres minor muscles. The posterior portion of the deltoid muscle was partially removed to show the underlying muscle. (*Reprinted with permission from Philip Peng Educational Series.*)

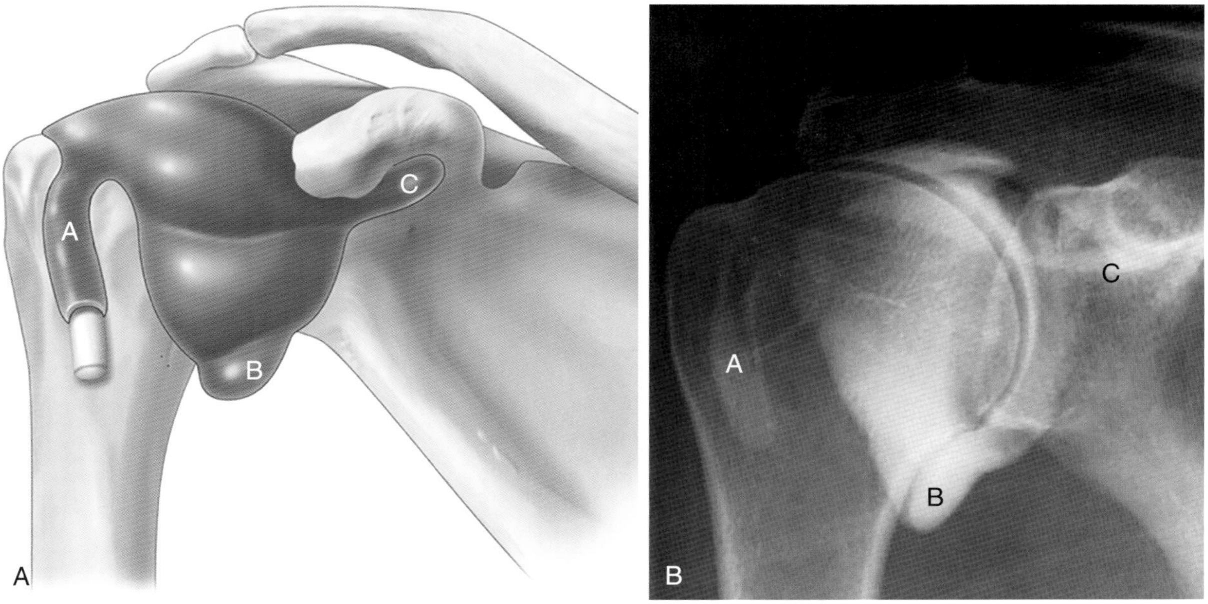

FIG. 81.7 Drawing of the three main recesses of the joint *(left)*: (A) the biceps tendon sheath, (B) the axillary pouch, (C) the subscapular recess, and the corresponding radiographic (arthrogram) appearance *(right)*. (*Reprinted with permission from Philip Peng Educational Series.*)

SUBACROMIAL SUBDELTOID BURSA

The SASDB, the largest bursa in the body, is located underneath the acromion, the coracoacromial ligament (CAL), and the deltoid muscle. The main role of the SASDB is to minimize attrition of the cuff against the coracoacromial arch (acromion and CAL) and the deltoid muscle during movement of the arm. It overlies the superior aspect of the SS tendon and also extends anteriorly to cover the bicipital groove and medially to the coracoid process (subcoracoid bursa). The lateral border may reach approximately 3 cm below the greater tuberosity.[20]

Sonoanatomy of the Supraspinatus Tendon and Subacromial Subdeltoid Bursa

A high-frequency linear probe is placed in the long axis of the SS tendon, which is parallel to the LHB tendon. The medial aspect of the probe is placed over the lateral part of the acromion to obtain the long-axis view of the SS tendon (Fig. 81.11A).[4] Only the distal portion of the SS tendon can be seen with the arm in neutral position. The SS tendon looks like a convex, beak-like structure attached to the greater tuberosity. Dynamic assessment of subacromial impingement is possible, with the patient abducting the arm while in internal rotation. With this maneuver, the SS tendon can be seen passing deep to the coracoacromial arch. A modified Crass position (patient's arm extended posteriorly with the palm on the superior aspect of the iliac wing) is recommended to provide more complete visualization of the tendon (see Fig. 81.11B).[21,22] Under normal circumstances, the synovial lining of the SASDB cannot be visualized but its presence can be estimated from the peribursal fat in between the deltoid muscle and the SS tendon and the use of dynamic scanning (see Fig. 81.11).

Injection Technique for the Subacromial Subdeltoid Bursa

The main indication for the SASDB injection is subacromial impingement syndrome,[4,23] which covers a constellation of conditions: partial- and full-thickness rotator cuff tear and rotator cuff tendinopathy.[24] The injection can be performed in either the supine or sitting position, with the ipsilateral arm in the modified Crass position. With this position, the SASDB is outlined by the peribursal fat between the deltoid muscle and the SS tendon (Fig. 81.12). An in-plane approach is preferred, with the needle inserted from a lateral-to-medial direction. In some slim individuals, the probe can be better stabilized by turning it 90 degrees. The needle can be inserted in plane from an anterior-to-posterior direction (see Fig. 81.12).

The total volume of 4–6 mL of local anesthetic with 40 mg of methylprednisolone or triamcinolone is used as the injectate.

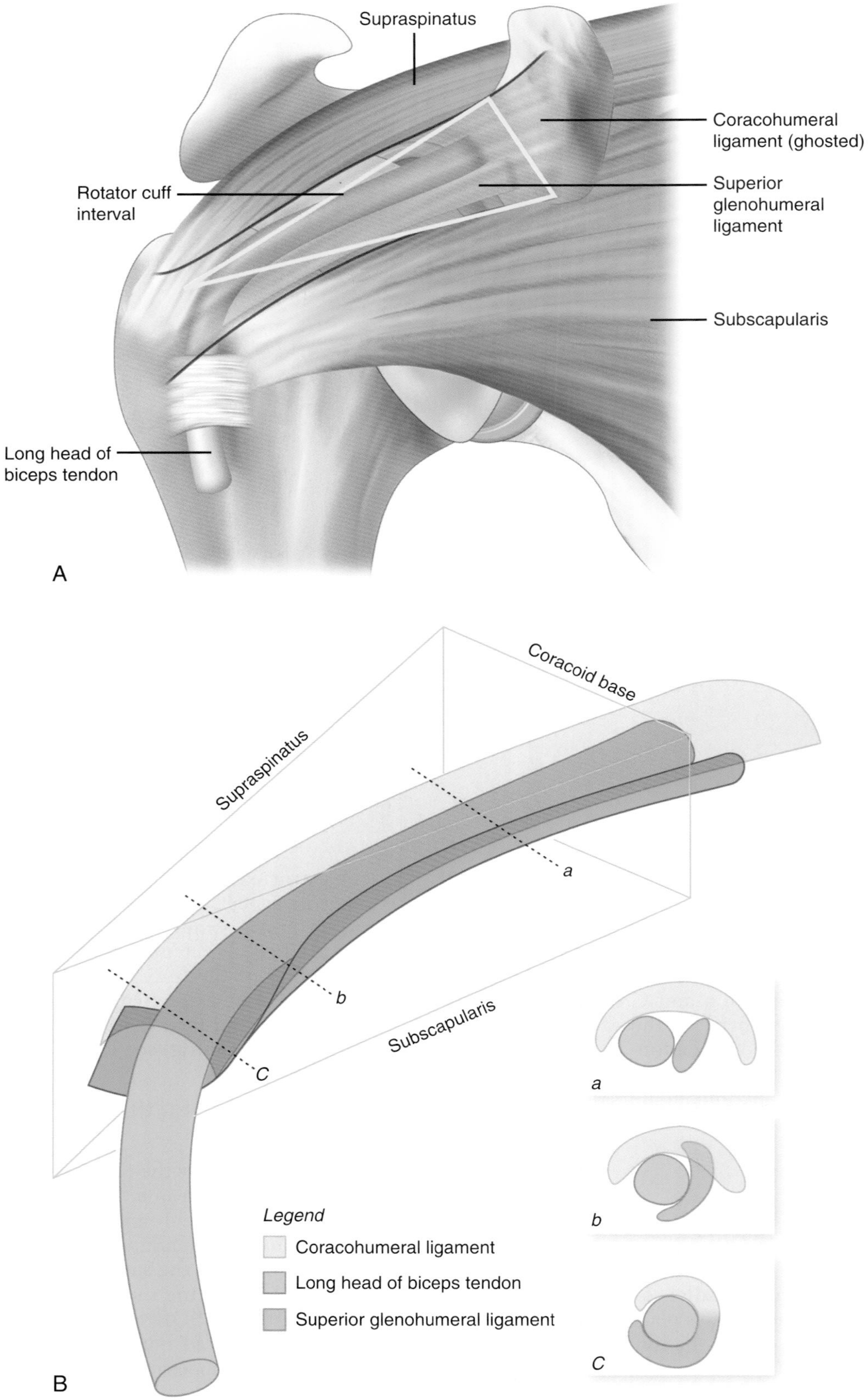

FIG. 81.8 (A) Anterosuperior view of the rotator cuff interval, which is a triangular space between the tendons of the subscapularis (anterior) and supraspinatus (posterior) muscles and the base of the coracoid process. The roof is the coracohumeral ligament *(ghosted)* and the contents are the long head of biceps tendon *(blue)* and superior glenohumeral ligament *(green)*. (B) The cutout of the rotator cuff interval shows the content. The superior glenohumeral ligament, a focal thickening of the glenohumeral joint capsule, runs anterior to the tendon of the long head of the biceps (LHB) tendon initially (position *A*). The superior glenohumeral ligament maintains a close relationship with the long head of biceps tendon and subsequently inserts into a small depression above the lesser tuberosity (position *B*), contributing to the biceps reflection pulley (position *C*) to prevent dislocation of the LHB tendon. (*Reprinted with permission from Philip Peng Educational Series.*)

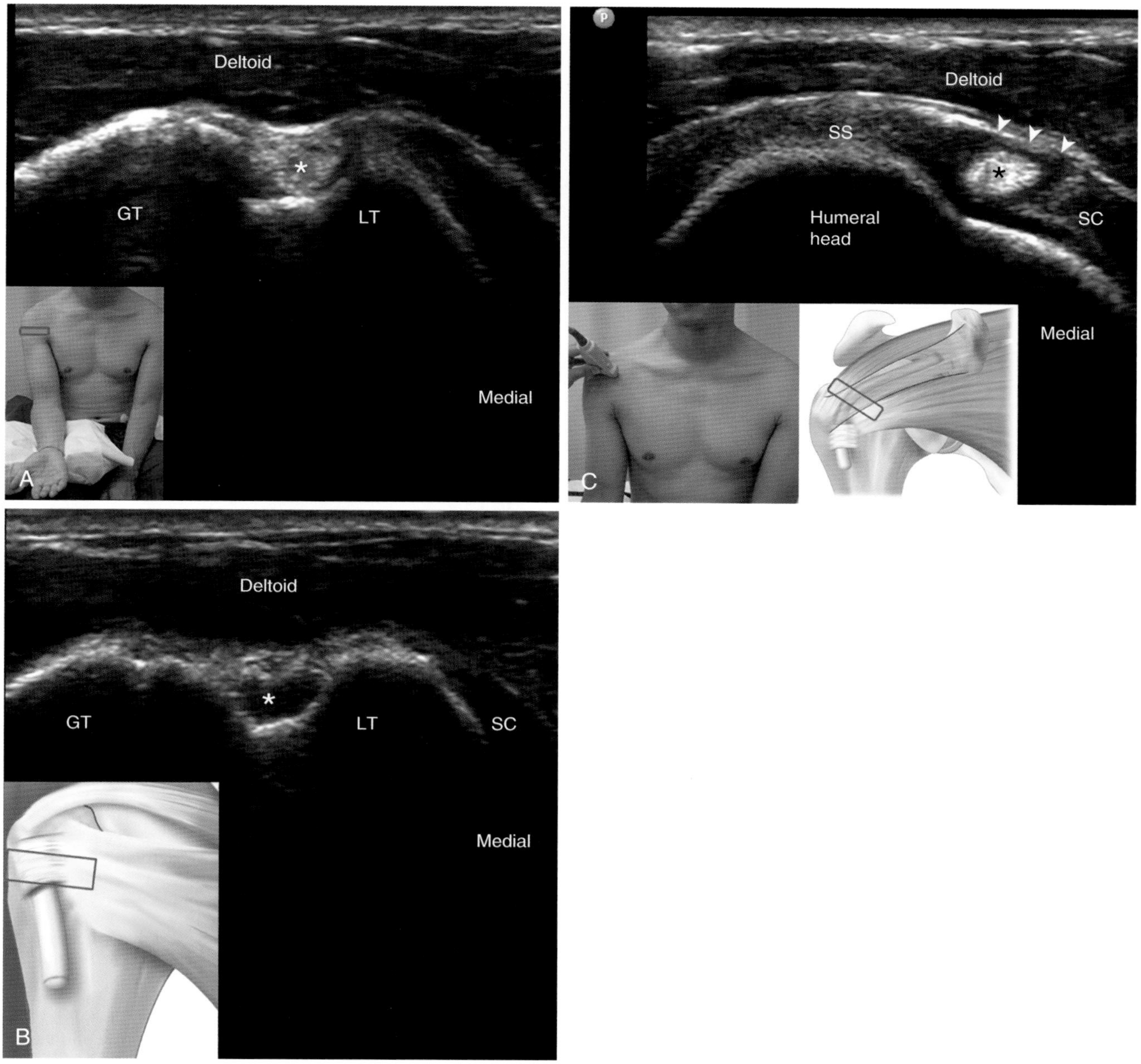

FIG. 81.9 (A) Ultrasound image showing the long head of the biceps (LHB) tendon *(asterisk)* within the bicipital groove. The *insert* shows the position of the patient and the linear ultrasound probe. Note that the LHB tendon appears hyperechoic. (B) Ultrasound image similar to *A* with a different tilt of the ultrasound probe. The image illustrates the anisotropy with the LHB tendon *(asterisk)* changed from a hyperechoic to a hypoechoic structure. The *insert* shows the position of the probe and the corresponding anatomic structures underneath. (C) By moving the ultrasound probe more proximally along the orientation of the LHB tendon, a view of rotator cuff interval is obtained. The LHB tendon *(asterisk)* is always hyperechoic at this level, and sandwiched between the supraspinatus (SS) tendon laterally and the subscapularis (SC) tendon medially. The coracohumeral *(arrowheads)* forms the roof of the interval. The *insert* on the left shows the orientation and position of the probe, and the *insert* on the right shows the probe position and the structures underneath it. *GT*, Greater tuberosity; *LT*, lesser tuberosity. (*Reprinted with permission from Philip Peng Educational Series.*)

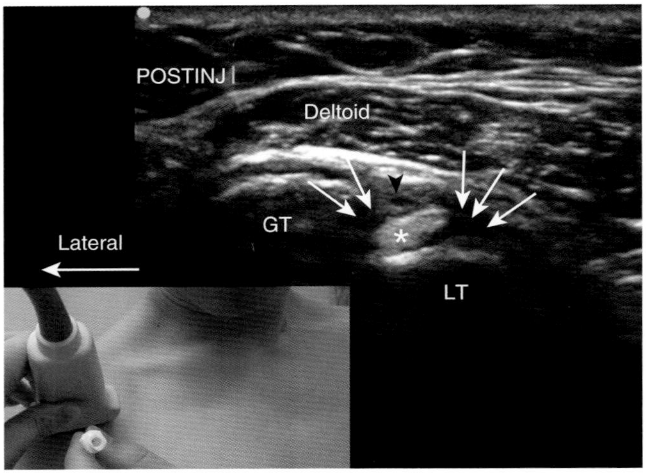

FIG. 81.10 The *insert* shows the position of the ultrasound probe and the needle with the out-of-plane technique. The local anesthetic is seen surrounding the bicep tendons (*) in the bicipital groove *(line arrows)*. The *black arrowhead* points to the anterior circumflex artery. *GT*, Greater tuberosity; *LT*, lesser tuberosity. (*Reprinted with permission from Philip Peng Educational Series.*)

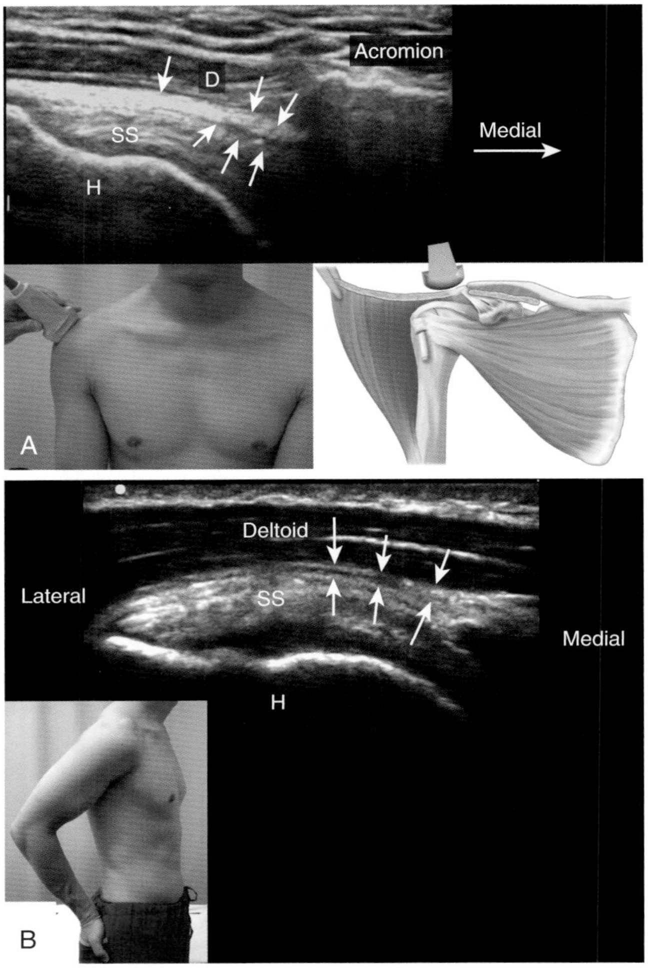

FIG. 81.11 (A) Ultrasound image of the subacromial subdeltoid bursa (SASDB). The supraspinatus (SS) tendon is seen attached laterally onto the greater tuberosity of the humeral head (H). The *insert* on the left shows the position of the patient and the ultrasound probe; the one on the right shows the probe and the structures underneath: deltoid muscle (D) and SS muscle. (B) Ultrasound image of the SS tendon when the arm is put in the modified Crass position. Note that the portion of the SS tendon lateral to the acromion process is significantly increased by this maneuver. The *insert* shows the position of the modified Crass position. *Line arrows* outline the peribursal fat of the SASDB. (*Reprinted with permission from Philip Peng Educational Series.*)

GLENOHUMERAL JOINT

This ball-and-socket synovial joint is composed of a round humeral head and a relatively small, flat, pear-shaped glenoid fossa. The fibrocartilaginous rim, the glenoid labrum, widens the glenoid cavity (see Fig. 81.12). Only one third of the humeral head is covered by the glenoid cavity. Although this allows the shoulder the widest range of movement, it also confers inherent instability to the shoulder, making it susceptible to subluxation and dislocation.[25–27] The joint capsule is attached medially to the margin of the glenoid cavity extending to the base of the coracoid process and laterally to the anatomic neck of the humerus (see Fig. 81.12). The synovial membrane lines the capsule on its deep surface and overlies the LHB tendon. From there, three recesses are formed: the biceps tendon sheath anteriorly, the SSC recess medially, and the axillary pouch inferiorly (see Fig. 81.6). The stability of the GHJ is maintained by the ligaments, the rotator cuff tendons, and the deltoid muscle. The glenohumeral ligaments (GHLs) are three weak bands of fibrous tissue (superior GHL [SGHL], middle GHL, and inferior GHL) that strengthen the front of the capsule. The CHL is a strong band of fibrous tissue arising from the coracoid process and inserting onto the greater and lesser tuberosities to reinforce the capsule (see Fig. 81.2).

Sonoanatomy of the Glenohumeral Joint

The GHJ can be examined with either the anterior or posterior approach. Only the posterior approach is discussed here because there are fewer stabilizers (such as GHL) and no important articular structures (such as capsulolabral complex); there is also less extravasation. The patient is placed in the sitting or lateral position, with the ipsilateral arm touching the contralateral shoulder. A high-frequency ultrasound probe is placed over the infraspinatus (IS) tendon caudal to the scapular spine (Fig. 81.13A). With this probe position, the posterior part of the humeral head, glenoid process, and labrum are visualized. Medial to the GHJ, the spinoglenoid notch is usually visualized (see Fig. 81.13B). The suprascapular nerve, accompanied by the suprascapular artery, curves around this notch to supply the IS muscle in the IS fossa.

Injection Technique for the Glenohumeral Joint

The indications for GHJ injection are mainly glenohumeral arthrosis and adhesive capsulitis. Glenohumeral arthrosis is characterized by progressive and irreversible articular destruction and frequent involvement of the surrounding soft tissues.[28] The exact prevalence is not well documented.[29]

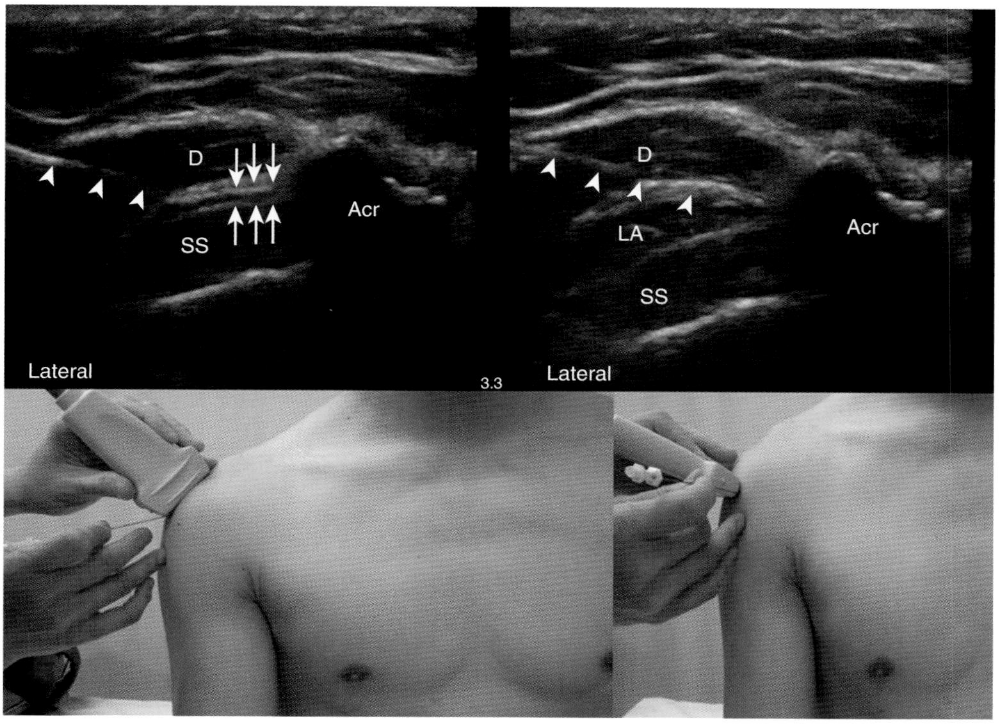

FIG. 81.12 The *insert* on the left shows the position of the ultrasound probe and the needle with the in-plane technique. Note that the medial end of the ultrasound probe is placed over the acromion (Acr). However, in a patient with a slim body build, the probe can be placed in another orientation as shown in the right *insert*. The ultrasound image on the left shows the needle *(arrowheads)* inserted with in-plane technique to the subacromial subdeltoid bursa, as highlighted by the peribursal fat *(line arrows)*. The image on the right shows the presence of local anesthetic following the injection, with the separation of the deltoid muscle (D) and supraspinatus (SS) tendon. (*Reprinted with permission from Philip Peng Educational Series.*)

The patient is positioned either in sitting or semiprone position with the ipsilateral hand crossing the chest. A 20- or 22-gauge needle is inserted in plane from the lateral aspect of the probe and directed between the free edge of the labrum and the hypoechoic articular cartilage of the humeral head (Fig. 81.14). With the injection of normal saline (hydrolocation), the posterior joint capsule is seen displaced. If there is a resistance on injection, either the bevel of the needle can be rotated or the needle can be withdrawn for a small distance. A volume of 5 mL of local anesthetic with 40 mg of methylprednisolone or triamcinolone is used as the injectate.

HIP

The hip is a ball-and-socket synovial joint formed by the articulation of the femoral head and the acetabulum. The acetabular labrum, a fibrocartilaginous ring attached directly to the rim of the acetabulum, increases the depth and surface of the acetabular cavity (Fig. 81.15). Approximately 40% of the articular surface of the femoral head is covered by the acetabulum in any position of hip.[30] The joint capsule surrounds the outer surface of the labrum and inserts distally to the intertrochanteric region and posterior aspect of the femoral neck. The anterior joint capsule is composed of two layers, anterior and posterior, separated by the anterior recess of the joint space (Fig. 81.16). Each layer is of considerable thickness (2–4 mm) and lined by only a minute synovial membrane.[31] The anterior layer runs caudally and inserts on the intertrochanteric line, where it blends with the periosteum. The trochanters (greater and lesser) and the lateral third of the posterior femoral neck are extraarticular.[30] The ligamentum teres femoris, an intracapsular ligament, is attached to the acetabular notch and a depression on the femoral head called the fovea capitis.[32] From medial to lateral the structures in the anterior aspect of hip are as follows: pectineus muscle, femoral neurovascular bundle, iliopsoas muscle and tendon, and sartorius and rectus femoris muscles (Fig. 81.17).

SONOANATOMY OF HIP JOINT

The patient is placed supine with the hip in neutral position and the groin exposed. A curvilinear probe is used and placed over the infrainguinal region. The femoral neurovascular bundle is visualized in the first scan (Fig. 81.18A).[33] The probe is then positioned along with the axis of the femoral neck to reveal the anterior recess (see Fig. 81.18B).[33,34] The scan is then optimized to visualize the femoral head, neck, and joint capsule.

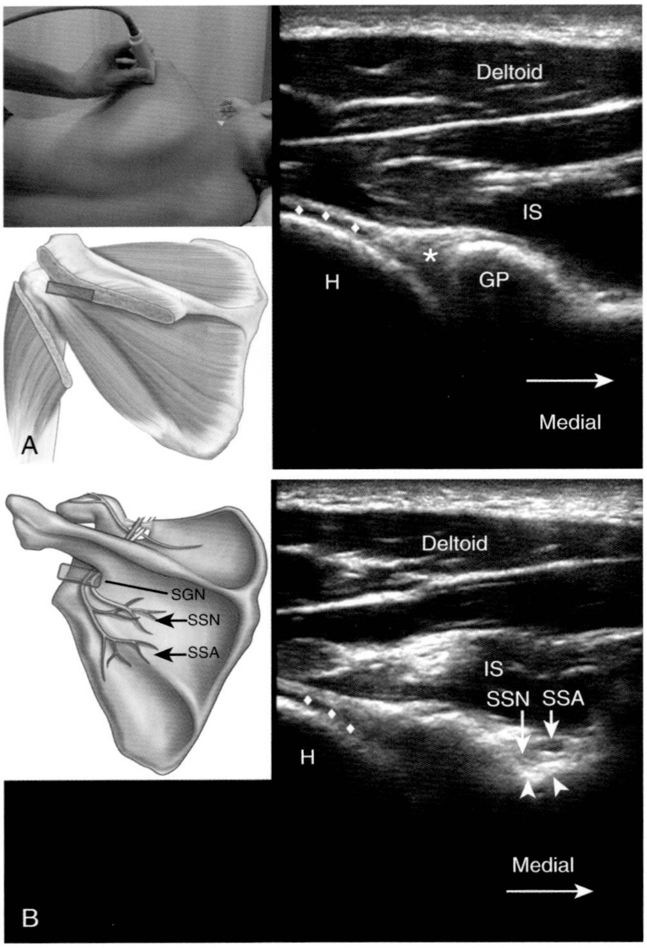

FIG. 81.13 (A) Ultrasound image of the posterior glenohumeral joint. The glenoid process (GP) and humeral head (H) both appear as hyperechoic structures with anechoic shadows. The *insert* at the top shows the position of the patient and the ultrasound probe, whereas the one below shows the probe position and the structures underneath. (B) Ultrasound image of the spinoglenoid notch obtained by moving the ultrasound probe slightly medially. The *insert* shows the position of the probe and the spinoglenoid notch as well as the suprascapular neurovascular bundle. *IS*, Infraspinatus; *SSN* and *SSA*, suprascapular nerve and artery *(line arrows in ultrasound image)*; *SGN*, spinoglenoid notch *(arrowheads)*. *, Glenoid labrum; ♦, articular cartilage of the humeral head. (*Reprinted with permission from Philip Peng Educational Series.*)

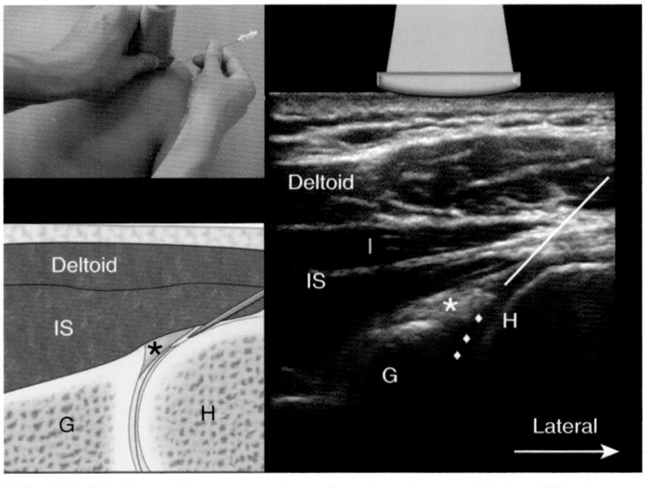

FIG. 81.14 Posterior approach to the glenohumeral joint. The *insert (upper left)* shows the position of the ultrasound probe and the needle with the in-plane technique. The corresponding ultrasound image *(right)* is shown with the line representing the needle path, which was directed between the free edge of the labrum (*) and the hypoechoic articular cartilage (♦) of the humeral head (H). *G*, Glenoid; *IS*, infraspinatus. *Insert* at the lower left shows an anatomic drawing of the ultrasound image. (*Reprinted with permission from Philip Peng Educational Series.*)

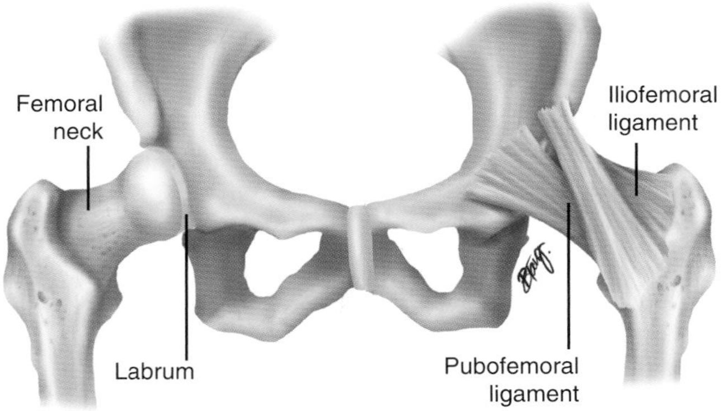

FIG. 81.15 Front view of hip joint, the labrum *(left)*, and the hip ligaments. Ischiofemoral ligament cannot be seen from this view because of the posterior location. (*Reproduced with permission from Philip Peng Educational Series.*)

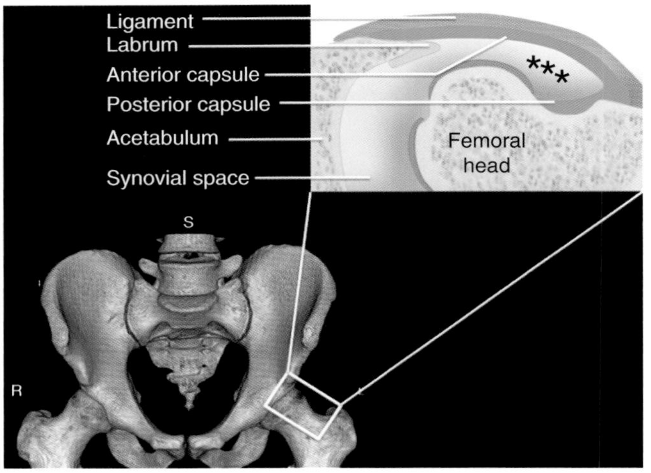

FIG. 81.16 The anterior synovial recess (***). Under normal circumstances the amount of synovial fluid in the recess is kept to a minimum. This figure shows a hip with effusion for demonstration. (*Reproduced with permission from Philip Peng Educational Series.*)

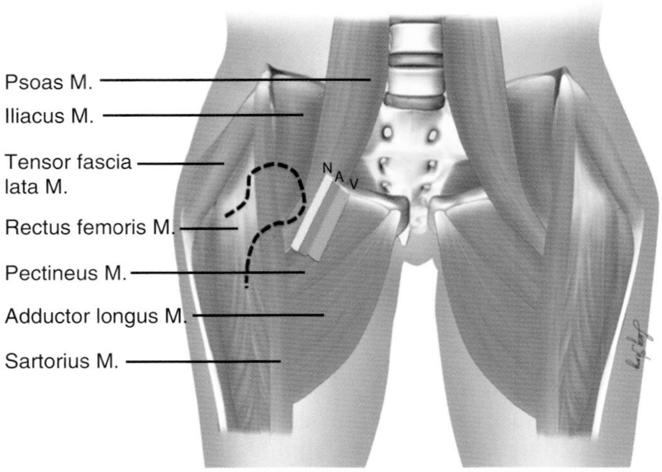

FIG. 81.17 Muscles (M) around hip joint. The femoral head and neck *(in dotted line)* and the schematic of femoral neurovascular bundle are shown here for reference. *A*, Femoral artery; *N*, femoral nerve; *V*, femoral vein. (*Reproduced with permission from Philip Peng Educational Series.*)

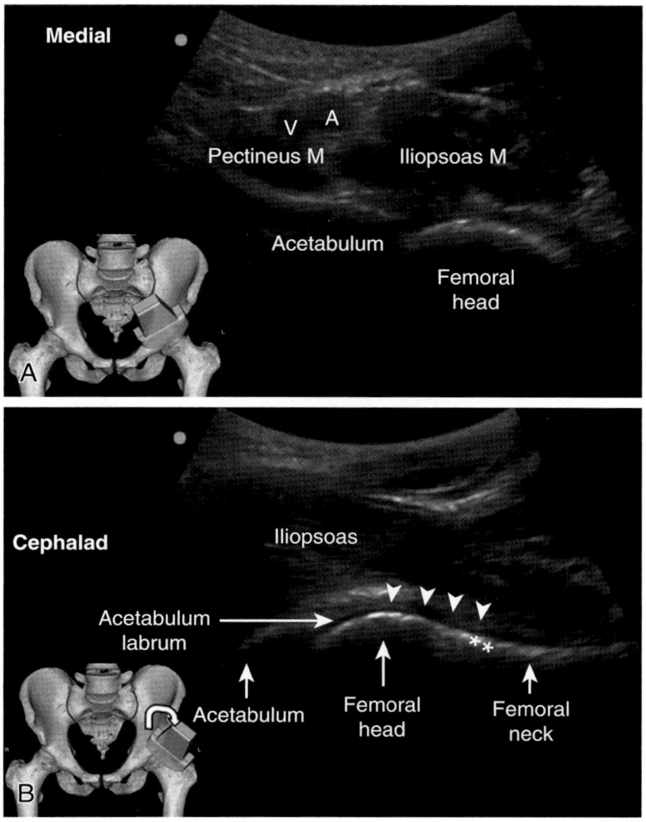

FIG. 81.18 (A) Sonoanatomy of the infrainguinal hip region. The position of the transducer is shown in the *insert*. **, The target of the needle placement; *A*, femoral artery; *V*, femoral vein. (B) Sonoanatomy of the anterior hip region when the transducer is placed in the long axis of the femoral neck. The *arrowheads* indicate the anterior recess. The position of the transducer is shown in the *insert*. (*Reproduced with permission from Philip Peng Educational Series.*)

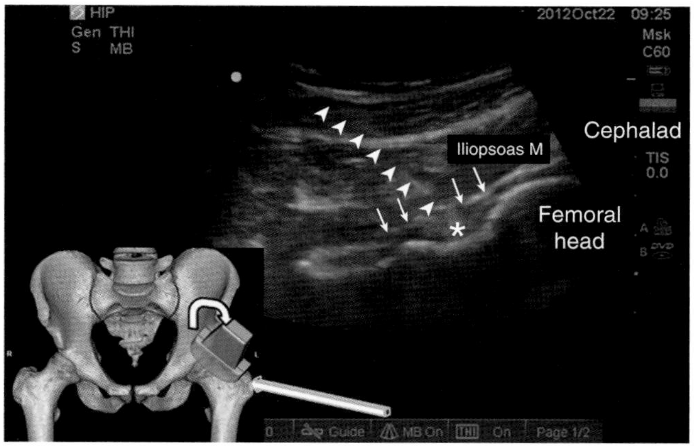

FIG. 81.19 Ultrasonography shows the anterior recess (*) as the target. *Small arrows* outline the joint capsule, and *arrowheads* indicate the needle. The *insert* shows the position of the transducer and the needle. (*Reproduced with permission from Philip Peng Educational Series.*)

INJECTION TECHNIQUE

Intraarticular hip joint injection has both diagnostic and therapeutic value. One of the main indications for hip injection is osteoarthritis. The target is the synovial recess underneath the joint capsule between the femoral head and neck (Fig. 81.19).[33,34] Before a needle is inserted, a Doppler scan for any unsuspected vessel in the needle path is performed. A 22-gauge, 3.5-inch spinal needle is inserted in plane from lateral to medial to the junction between the femoral head and neck. The needle is inserted until bone is contacted and is then withdrawn 1 mm to avoid engaging the needle tip in the posterior capsule. The spread of the injectate is monitored in real time throughout the procedure; this is important to make sure that the injectate is spread within the joint space. A total volume of 5 mL including local anaesthetic and steroid is used.

KNEE JOINT

The knee joint is a complex structure consisting of three components: the femorotibial, patellofemoral, and superior tibiofibular joints. The femorotibial joint is composed of two compartments: medial and lateral (Fig. 81.20).[35] The fibrocartilaginous medial and lateral menisci increase the surface area of contact between the convex femoral condyles and flat tibial plateau (see Fig. 81.20).[35] The various structures surrounding the joint reinforce the articular capsule. These structures include muscles and tendons, retinaculum, and ligaments. Anteriorly, they are the quadriceps and patella tendons, medial and lateral patellofemoral ligaments, and retinaculum from the vastus medialis and lateralis. Medially, this structure is reinforced by the medial collateral ligament. Laterally, it is strengthened by the iliotibial band, lateral collateral ligament, and bicep tendons and their fascial expansion. There are many recesses in the femorotibial joint, but the widest is the suprapatellar recess (SPR; see Fig. 81.20), which originates from the fusion of the subquadriceps bursa with the joint cavity and allows access for injection into the joint cavity. Isometric contraction of the quadriceps or the application of pressure in the parapatellar space to squeeze the synovial fluid will distend the SPR with the synovial fluid even if its scanty.[36]

SONOANATOMY OF THE KNEE JOINT

The knee joint can be examined with ultrasound using a high-frequency linear ultrasound probe. The knee is lightly flexed 20–30 degrees by placing a pillow or a bolster under it. The ultrasound probe is placed longitudinally above the patella to evaluate the quadriceps femoris tendon (Fig. 81.21A).[35] The prefemoral fat pad can be found over the femur and the suprapatellar fat pad underneath the quadriceps tendon. Just beneath the tendon of the quadriceps femoris is the suprapatellar bursa, appearing as a thin hypoechoic line between these two fat pads (see Fig. 81.21B and C). This is a commonly chosen site for knee joint injection.

INJECTION TECHNIQUE FOR KNEE JOINT

The main indication for intraarticular knee injection is osteoarthritis of the knee. A suprapatellar approach to the knee joint is the best-studied approach and has the greatest efficacy[35]; hence that approach is described here. With the knee slightly flexed and supported, a high-frequency linear

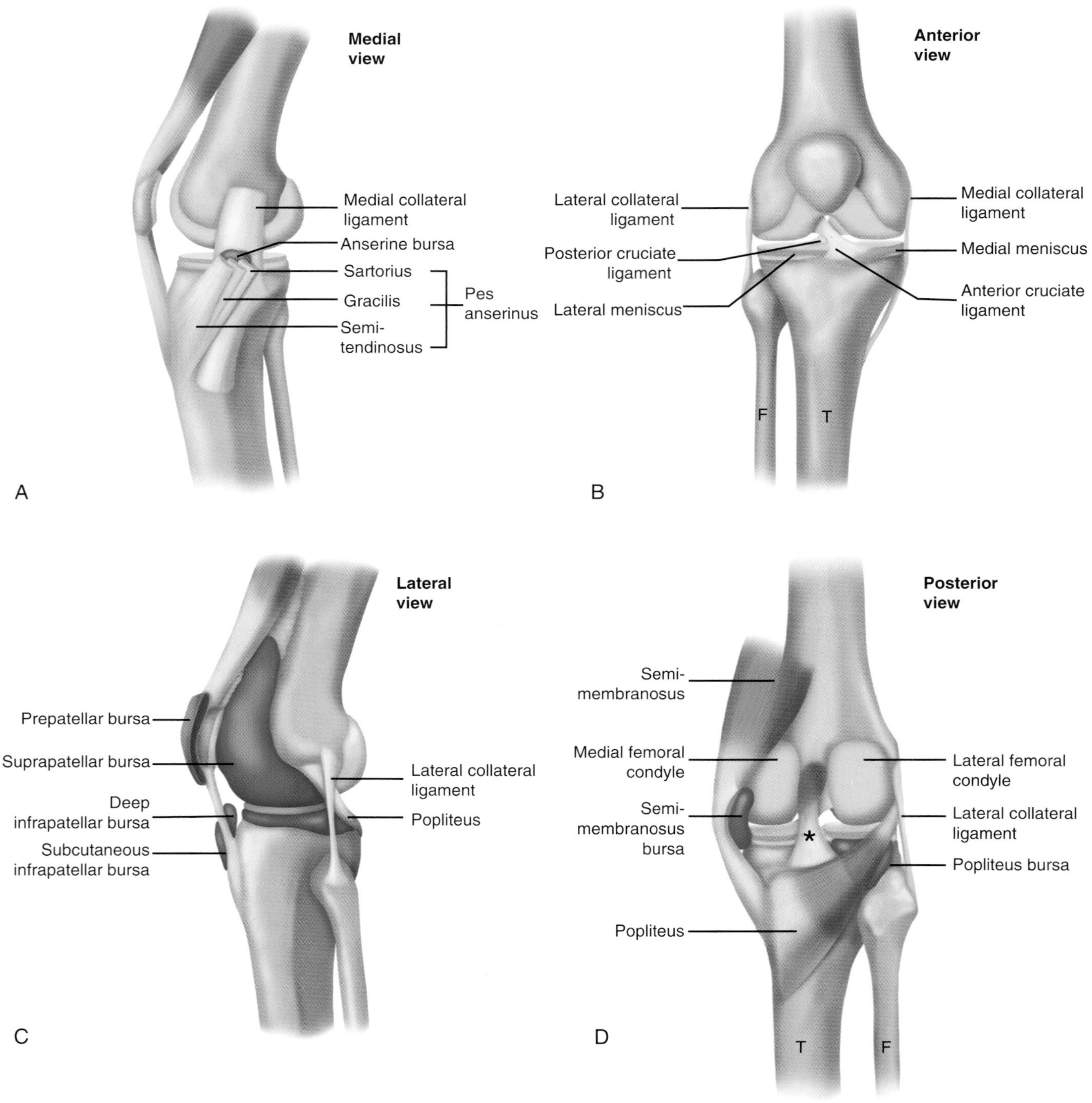

FIG. 81.20 Four views of the knee showed the ligaments and bursae. (A) Medial view. (B) Anterior view. (C) Lateral view. (D) Posterior view. In the posterior view, the medial head of gastrocnemius was removed to reveal the intraarticular structures. *F*, Fibula; *T*, tibia. (*Reproduced with permission from Philip Peng Educational Series.*)

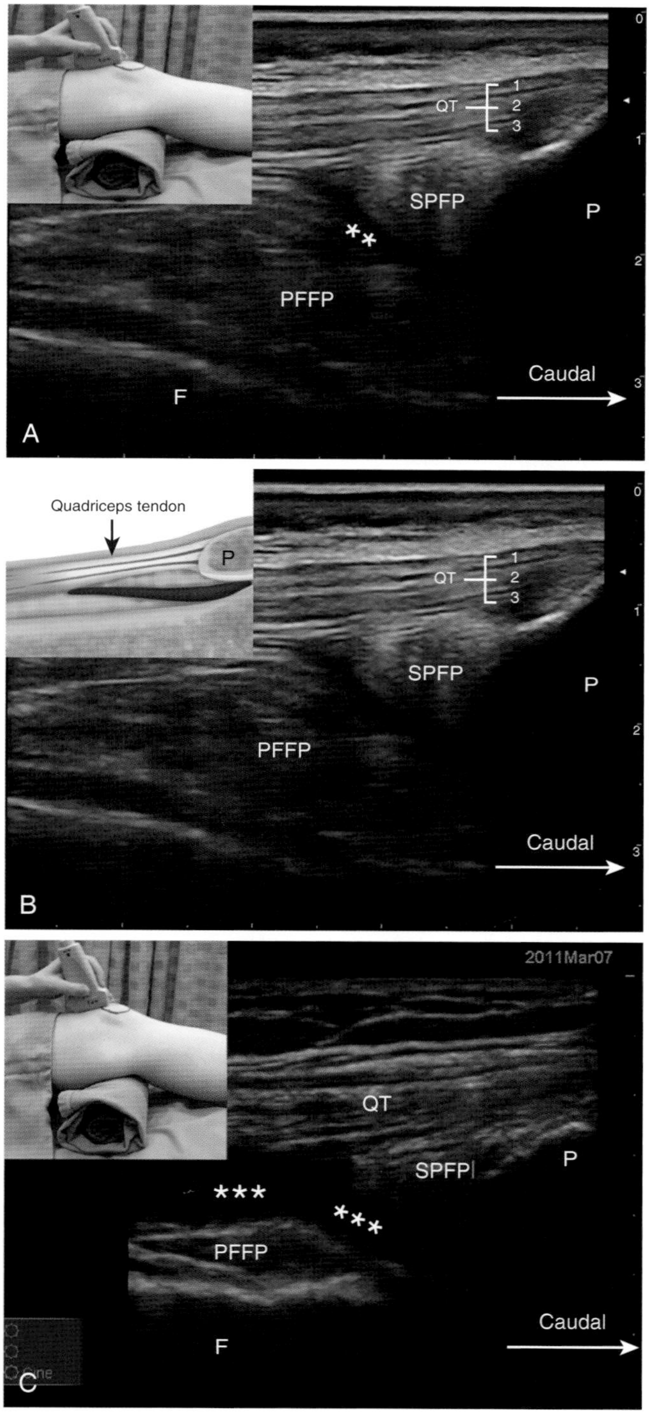

FIG. 81.21 (A) Sonographic suprapatellar view of a normal knee. The *insert* shows the position of the patient and the ultrasound probe. (B) Sonogram showing the details of the quadriceps tendon (QT). (C) Sonographic suprapatellar view of a knee with effusion. Note the presence of effusion fluid filling the space between prefemoral fat pad and quadriceps tendon. *F*, Femur; *P*, patella; *PFFP*, prefemoral fat pad; *SPFP*, suprapatellar fat pad; ** or ***, suprapatella recess. (*Reproduced with permission from Philip Peng Educational Series.*)

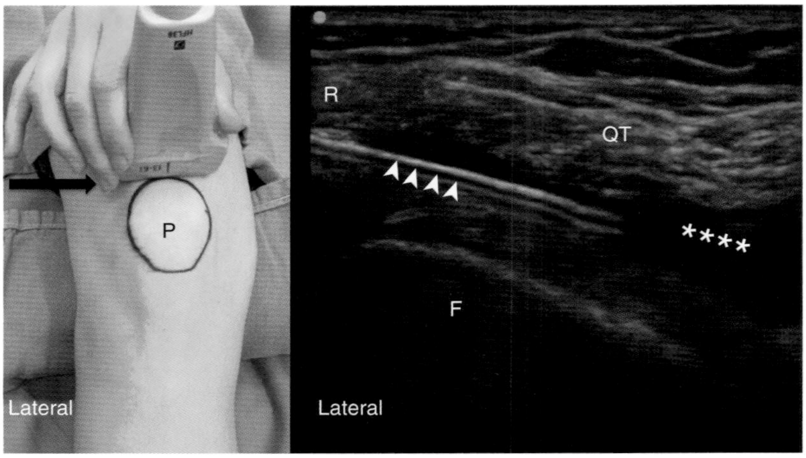

FIG. 81.22 Illustration of the injection technique. The ultrasound probe is placed between the patella and quadriceps tendon initially and then turned 90 degrees upon visualization of the suprapatella recess (SPR). The needle is then approached from lateral to medial to avoid puncturing the quadriceps tendon. The needle is indicated by the *arrowheads* and the SPR by asterisks (****). *F*, Femur; *QT*, quadriceps tendon; *R*, retinaculum. (*Reproduced with permission from Philip Peng Educational Series.*)

probe is placed over the patella and quadriceps tendon (Fig. 81.22). With proper positioning, the SPR between the suprapatellar and prefemoral fat pads can be visualized. Once the SPR is seen, the ultrasound probe is rotated 90 degrees above the patella. A 20- or 22-gauge needle is inserted from lateral to medial by the in-plane technique toward the SPR. Aspiration of synovial fluid should always be considered. A total volume of 5 mL, including local anesthetic and steroid, is used as the injectate.

KEY POINTS

- Use of ultrasound for MSK interventions offers many advantages over the traditional radiologic imaging modalities.
- Ultrasound not only avoids the radiation and risks associated with the use of contrast but also allows visualization of soft tissue and vascular structures, thus improving accuracy.
- Intraarticular major joint injections can be reliably performed using ultrasound. In contrast, the landmark-based technique is not as reliable and subjects the patient to the risk of soft tissue or nerve injury.

REFERENCES

Access the reference list online at ExpertConsult.com.

CHAPTER 82

Head and Neck Blocks

Miles Day, MD ◎ Rafael Justiz, MD ◎ Antoun Nader, MD

Nerve blocks of the head and neck can be rewarding procedures for any anesthesiologist or pain management practitioner. The blocks can be used for regional anesthesia and postoperative pain control as well as for diagnostic and therapeutic purposes for managing chronic pain. In the algorithm for treating chronic pain, the blocks are indicated when pharmacologic therapy is partially effective or ineffective in alleviating a patient's pain. Detailed knowledge of the relevant anatomy and the use of fluoroscopy and ultrasound will theoretically improve efficacy and minimize complications.

INDICATIONS AND CONTRAINDICATIONS

Specific indications are listed with the individual blocks. Informed consent prior to the block is a necessity. Absolute contraindications include patient refusal, local infection, sepsis, and increased intracranial pressure (trigeminal ganglion block). Relative contraindications are coagulopathy, anticoagulant therapy, history of facial and neck trauma (potential for altered anatomy), and preexisting neurologic deficits. Prior to stopping any anticoagulant therapy, consult the prescribing physician for guidance. Drug-eluting cardiac stents should also be considered. Allergy to medications used can be absolute or relative depending on the severity of the allergy. Pretreatment with H1 and H2 receptor blockers plus corticosteroids may be necessary.

TRIGEMINAL NERVE AND GANGLION

ANATOMY

The trigeminal ganglion resides in the middle cranial fossa.[1–3] It is situated in a fold of dura mater that forms an invagination around the posterior two-thirds of the ganglion. This region is referred to as Meckel's cavity and contains cerebrospinal fluid. The ganglion is bound medially by the cavernous sinus and optic and trochlear nerves, superiorly by the inferior surface of the temporal lobe of the brain, and posteriorly by the brain stem. The ganglion is formed by the fusion of a series of cell bodies that originate at the midpontine level of the brain stem. The ganglion has three major divisions: ophthalmic (V1), maxillary (V2), and mandibular (V3). The ophthalmic division is located dorsally, the maxillary branch intermediate, and the mandibular branch ventrally. The ophthalmic division leaves the ganglion and passes into the orbit through the superior orbital fissure. It further divides into the supraorbital, supratrochlear, and nasociliary nerves, which innervate the forehead and nose.[3] The maxillary division exits the middle cranial fossa via the foramen rotundum, crosses the pterygopalatine fossa, and enters the orbit through the inferior orbital fissure. Branches include the infraorbital, superior alveolar, palatine, and zygomatic nerves, which carry sensory information from the maxilla and overlying skin, the nasal cavity, palate, nasopharynx, and meninges of the anterior and middle cranial fossa.[3] The mandibular division exits through the foramen ovale and divides into the buccal, lingual, inferior alveolar, and auriculotemporal nerves. These nerves carry sensory input from the buccal region, the side of the head and scalp, and the lower jaw, including teeth, gums, anterior two-thirds of the tongue, chin, and lower lip. The motor component of V3 innervates the masseter, temporal, medial, and lateral pterygoid muscles. The ganglion interfaces with the autonomic nervous system via the ciliary, sphenopalatine, otic, and submaxillary ganglia. It also communicates with the oculomotor, facial, and glossopharyngeal nerves (GNs).[4]

PROCEDURES

OPHTHALMIC NERVE BLOCK

Two of the terminal branches of the ophthalmic division can be blocked as they exit their respective foramina for pain in the forehead. The supratrochlear nerve exits its foramen on the medial aspect of the superior orbital ridge, whereas the supraorbital nerve exits its foramen in the middle of the superior orbital ridge. After sterile prep, palpate the foramen and subcutaneously inject 1–2 mL of local anesthetic over the foramen. If the pain is alleviated, cryoneurolysis of the nerve or nerves can provide long-lasting relief.

MAXILLARY NERVE BLOCK

Diagnostic and therapeutic blocks of the maxillary nerve are performed similarly. Fluoroscopy is not always necessary, but it may be used when external landmarks are not easily palpated or when a neurolytic technique is planned. The most common indication for this block is regional anesthesia for surgery of the upper jaw, but it is also effective for acute postoperative pain control. In the pain management arena, it is indicated for the diagnosis and treatment of chronic pain in the distribution of the maxillary division of the trigeminal nerve.

For localized pain, the infraorbital nerve can be blocked as it exits its foramen below the inferior orbital ridge. After sterile prep, palpate the foramen subcutaneously and inject 1–2 mL of local anesthetic over the foramen.

To block the maxillary division, place the patient in the supine position. Palpate the mandibular notch located below the zygoma and anterior to the temporomandibular joint. Under sterile conditions, anesthetize the skin over the notch. Insert the block needle (usually a 22-gauge 8–10-cm short-bevel or a same-size curved blunt needle)

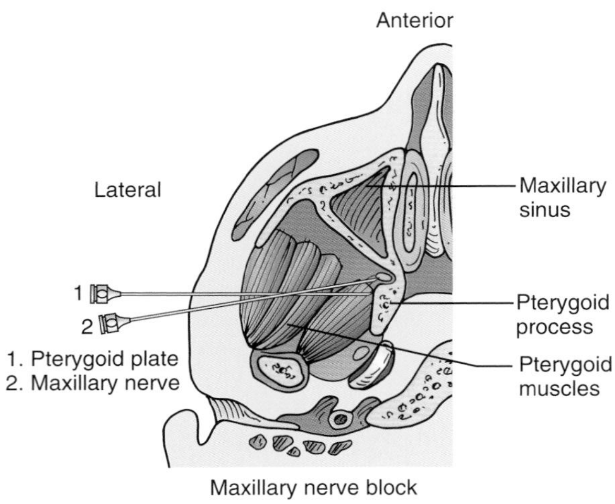

FIG. 82.1 Maxillary nerve block, transverse section.

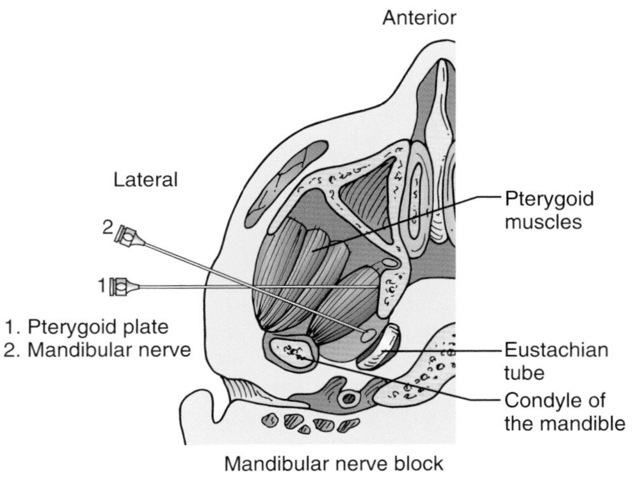

FIG. 82.2 Mandibular nerve block, transverse section.

in a horizontal plane through the mandibular notch until bone (lateral pterygoid plate) is touched (typically 4–5 cm) (Fig. 82.1). If a blunt needle is used, an 18-gauge 1.25-inch angiocatheter is inserted first. Withdraw the needle and redirect it anteriorly and superiorly through the pterygomaxillary fissure into the pterygopalatine fossa. Advance the needle approximately 0.25–0.5 cm, at which depth a paresthesia is usually perceived in the upper lip or teeth.[5] If this procedure is performed under fluoroscopy, the needle is angled toward the superior portion of the pterygopalatine fossa, which appears as a "V" on the lateral image. On an anteroposterior image, the needle tip should be above the level of the middle turbinate. At this point inject 3–5 mL of local anesthetic. If fluoroscopy is used, 0.5–1.0 mL of contrast can be injected first to rule out intravascular placement of the needle. Remove the needle and apply an ice pack to the cheek.

Neurolytic blocks can be done with 6% phenol or absolute alcohol. After appropriate placement of the needle, up to 1.0–1.5 mL of the neurolytic solution is injected in 0.1-mL aliquots. The needle should then be flushed with 0.5 mL of saline prior to removal. Pulsed radiofrequency lesioning can also be performed after a successful diagnostic block. Sensory stimulation is performed at 50 Hz, 1 V. Paresthesia in the upper teeth should be perceived at less than 0.3 V. Once confirmed, two or three 120-second pulsed radiofrequency cycles are administered at 45 V.

MANDIBULAR NERVE BLOCK

Diagnostic and therapeutic blocks of the mandibular nerve are both performed in the same manner. Fluoroscopic guidance is not a necessity but is encouraged when a therapeutic block is planned, as it can facilitate needle positioning. Indications are similar to those for the maxillary nerve block except that the area to be anesthetized or treat pain is the lower jaw and tongue.

The procedure is performed identically to the maxillary nerve block except for the following: once the lateral pterygoid plate has been touched with the block needle, withdraw it and redirect in a slightly caudal and posterior direction until a paresthesia is produced in the lower lip, lower jaw, or ipsilateral tongue or ear (Fig. 82.2).[6] The depth should not be more than 0.1–0.25 cm beyond the depth at which the lateral pterygoid plate was contacted.[7] The total distance should not exceed 5.5 cm. If a paresthesia is not elicited at a depth of 5.5 cm, the needle should be withdrawn and redirected.

After proper positioning, inject 2–3 mL of local anesthetic, remove the needle, and apply an ice pack to the side of the face. If using fluoroscopy, start with a lateral view and proceed using the same technique as already described. Since this technique involves blocking the nerve as it exits the foramen ovale, a submental oblique view can be obtained (described later in this chapter under Trigeminal Ganglion Block) in order to verify the position of the needle tip in relation to the foramen ovale. The needle tip should be adjacent to, or overlie, the shadow of the foramen ovale. To rule out intravascular or intrathecal injection, inject 0.5–1.0 mL of contrast. If negative, inject the aforementioned volume of local anesthetic.

Chemical neurolysis can be achieved using 6% phenol, 50% glycerol, or absolute alcohol. After a successful diagnostic block and after proper positioning of the needle, up to 1.0 mL of the neurolytic solution is injected in 0.1-mL increments. Flush the needle with 0.5 mL normal saline before removing it.

For pulse radiofrequency lesioning, perform sensory and motor stimulation at 50 Hz, 1 V, and 2 Hz, 2 V, respectively, to check needle position. Paresthesia should be obtained at less than 0.3 V and masseter contraction should be apparent at less than 0.6 V. There is no consensus on the number of pulse cycles that should be performed, but 2–4, 120-second cycles should be carried out at 45 V.

TRIGEMINAL GANGLION

Tic douloureux is the most common indication for trigeminal ganglion blockade.[8] The block is indicated for patients who have failed conventional pharmacologic therapy and are deemed noncandidates for surgical microvascular decompression. Secondary trigeminal neuralgias from injury to the major divisions or the distal branches of the ganglion are a frequent indication.[4] Palliation of cancer-related pain has been accomplished through blockade of the trigeminal ganglion or its divisions. This block has also found a niche in the treatment of chronic, intractable cluster headaches.[9–13] Persistent idiopathic facial pain (formerly called atypical facial pain) also responds to ganglion blockade and neurolysis.[14]

As with most current fluoroscopically guided block techniques, the original description of the trigeminal ganglion block utilized external landmarks and a blind approach. The pupil in the midline and the external auditory meatus helped guide the practitioner to the target. Since the use of fluoroscopy is stressed in this chapter to improve the accuracy and success of the block as well as to decrease the chance of complications, the blind approach is not discussed, but knowing the external landmarks can be helpful if the foramen ovale is hard to visualize. The description of this block focuses on the use of a 20- to 22-gauge curved blunt needle, but sharp spinal or block needles are also acceptable.

Obtain intravenous access. Place the patient on the table in the supine position with the head slightly extended. Light sedation with midazolam and fentanyl is usually required, but propofol may be necessary. Using sterile procedure, prepare and drape the appropriate side, leaving the eye exposed. Utilizing continuous or pulsed fluoroscopy, locate the foramen ovale by rotating the C-arm image intensifier obliquely away from the nose approximately 20–30 degrees and then angle the C-arm image intensifier approximately 30–35 degrees in the caudocephalad direction to bring the foramen ovale into view. Subtle adjustments of the C-arm angles may be necessary. Raise a skin wheal directly over the shadow of the foramen, which will be approximately 2–2.5 cm lateral to the corner of the mouth. Insert a short, 16- or 18-gauge angiocatheter through the skin wheal and advance to the hub. Insert a gloved finger into the oral cavity to confirm that the buccal mucosa has not been breached. Reglove before proceeding. Insert a 20- or 22-gauge, curved blunt block needle through the angiocatheter and advance a few centimeters. Obtain a fluoroscopic image to check the trajectory of the needle. The goal is to advance the needle in a coaxial fashion toward the foramen ovale (Fig. 82.3). Corrections in trajectory can be made by turning the needle tip in the appropriate direction. With respect to external landmarks, the trajectory of the needle will be in a plane slightly superior to the external auditory meatus and medially toward the pupil in the midline. Advance the needle in 1- to 2-cm increments until bone is touched. Obtain a lateral image to check the position of the needle. If the foramen has not been traversed, adjust the needle tip (usually posterior) and advance through the foramen a distance of 0.5–1.0 cm (Fig. 82.4). Do not advance the needle tip past the shadow of the clivus. The depth of the needle tip is not as important with a local anesthetic block as it is for a neurolytic procedure. After a negative aspiration for cerebrospinal fluid or blood, inject 0.5–1.0 mL of nonionic water-soluble contrast to confirm position and filling of Meckel's cavity. Any vascular runoff requires repositioning of the needle. If cerebrospinal fluid is obtained, the needle tip can be withdrawn until fluid is no longer appreciated. If an abundant cerebrospinal fluid leak is present, the remainder of the procedure should be halted. With a significant leak, a high spinal block can be caused with even low volumes of local anesthetic. A small leak of cerebrospinal fluid may or may not cause a high spinal block; if such is present, the pain practitioner should proceed with caution. Inject local anesthetic in volumes of 0.25–0.5 mL at a time, up to 1–2 mL, and observe for effect. Remove the needle and apply an ice pack to the cheek to decrease swelling.

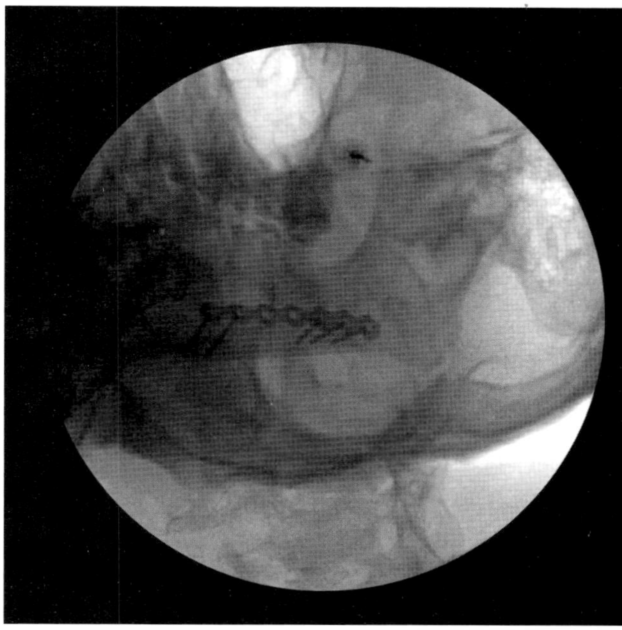

FIG. 82.3 Submental oblique coaxial fluoroscopic image of the block needle through foramen ovale.

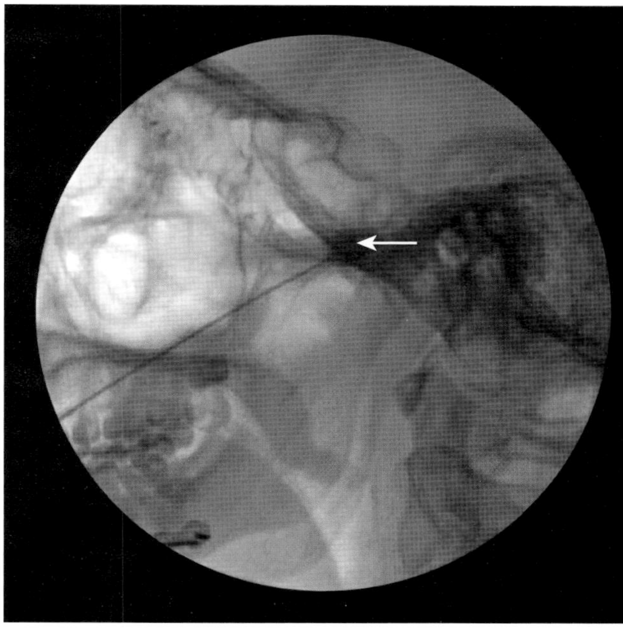

FIG. 82.4 Lateral fluoroscopic image of the block needle residing in the middle cranial fossa. The *arrow* indicates the tip of the needle.

NEUROLYTIC TECHNIQUES

After a successful diagnostic block, a neurolytic procedure can be planned. Needle placement for all neurolytic procedures except balloon microcompression is performed in the same manner as for the local anesthetic block. Heavier sedation may be required for radiofrequency techniques.

CONVENTIONAL RADIOFREQUENCY

For conventional radiofrequency lesioning, a 3- to 5-mm active-tip needle is placed. The target depth of the needle tip depends on the division of the trigeminal nerve that is to be lesioned. The mandibular division is rostral and lateral; the maxillary division is intermediate; and the ophthalmic division is mostly cephalad and medial. Location of the needle tip on the appropriate division or divisions is determined by the response to sensory and motor stimulation (50 Hz, 1 V, and 2 Hz, 2 V, respectively) of the ganglion. Paresthesia should be perceived at less than 0.3 V, with little to no muscle contraction of the masseter muscle at 0.6–1.0 V.[4] If no contraction is seen, then the tip of the needle is on the ophthalmic or maxillary divisions. Once the patient senses paresthesia in the painful area, inject 0.5 mL of 0.25% bupivacaine or 0.2% ropivacaine with steroid.[11] Wait 30–60 seconds and begin lesioning at 60°C for 90 seconds. If the patient cannot tolerate the lesioning, stop and wait an additional 30 seconds, then try again or add another 0.5 mL of local anesthetic prior to resuming lesioning. If more than one branch of the trigeminal nerve is affected, perform several lesions of the ganglion. Reposition the needle and repeat the stimulation test to get paresthesia in the desired site. For lesioning of the ophthalmic division, assess the corneal reflex during and after each lesion. Lesioning is typically started at temperatures of 55°C–65°C to preserve this reflex. One or two lesions are recommended. If the corneal reflex diminishes, lesioning should be stopped.

PULSED RADIOFREQUENCY

Pulsed radiofrequency is not a temperature-dependent technique. It is a nondestructive method of providing long-term pain relief.[15] After proper positioning of the needle tip, perform 2–4 pulsed radiofrequency cycles for 120 seconds each at 45 V. The temperature of the needle tip rarely exceeds 42°C; thus local anesthetic is not required. If significant masseter contraction is noted during pulsing, inject 1–2 mL of local anesthetic to diminish this, or hold the patient's mouth closed with your hand while the cycles are completed.

CHEMICAL NEUROLYSIS

Chemical neurolysis has been performed with phenol and alcohol in the past, but their use is not currently recommended if radiofrequency lesioning is available. Glycerol is the chemical neurolytic of choice. Once through the foramen ovale, advance a sharp needle until cerebrospinal fluid is observed returning through the needle. Place the patient in a semisitting position with the neck flexed. Inject water-soluble nonionic contrast solution in 0.1-mL aliquots (up to 0.5 mL) into the trigeminal cistern.[6] Failure of visualization or diffusion of the contrast requires repositioning the needle. Once the cistern is visualized, draw back the contrast material by free flow. The flow of contrast is slower than that of cerebrospinal fluid. Inject the same amount of glycerol into the cistern. Flush the needle with 0.5 mL of saline prior to removal. Keep the patient in a semisitting position for 2 hours. During the procedure, patients often report pain, burning, or paresthesia in the affected divisions.[16]

COMPLICATIONS

With the exclusion of sensory loss (an expected side effect), radiofrequency thermal lesioning had the highest number of complications (29.2%), followed by glycerol rhizotomy and balloon compression at 24.8% and 16.1%, respectively, for all neurolytic techniques.[17] Retrobulbar hematoma is possible if the needle is advanced into the retrobulbar space. Exophthalmos develops secondary to bleeding in the retrobulbar space. Cheek hematoma can occur if a blood vessel is punctured during placement of the needle. Masseter weakness can develop, especially with lesioning of the mandibular division. The incidence is highest with balloon microcompression (66%) and less for radiofrequency lesioning and glycerol rhizotomy (24% and 1.7%, respectively), but it usually resolves after 12 months.[6,18] Loss of the corneal reflex, keratitis, ulceration, and hypesthesia are observed in 3%–15% of patients after a neurolytic procedure.[8] Keratitis has been more likely to occur after radiofrequency lesioning and glycerol neurolysis.[17] Corneal anesthesia was highest for radiofrequency rhizotomy at 7% and was observed with glycerol rhizotomy and balloon compression at 3.7% and 1.5%, respectively.[6] Anesthesia dolorosa (deafferentation pain) occurs in up to 4% of patients who have undergone RFTC, followed by glycerol, where it occurs in 2% of cases.[6] Other complications include meningitis, dural arteriovenous fistulas, rhinorrhea, transient cranial nerve deficits, tissue sloughing, and even death.[17,19] Postprocedure trigeminal nerve sensory loss is an expected occurrence after a properly performed neurolytic procedure. The incidence of this with radiofrequency rhizotomy is as high as 98%, followed by balloon compression (72%) and glycerol neurolysis (60%).[20]

ULTRASOUND GUIDED TRIGEMINAL NERVE BLOCK

The branches of the trigeminal nerve, especially the second (maxillary, V2) and the third (mandibular, V3), can be blocked after they exit from the base of the skull through their respective foramina. The maxillary nerve (V2) exits the base of the skull through the foramen rotundum to travel laterally through the pterygopalatine fossa and enter the infraorbital fissure. Injecting a small amount of local anesthetic in the pterygopalatine fossa in close proximity to the foramen rotundum will result in a retrograde spread of the injectate to the gasserian ganglion, which results in blockade of the branches of the trigeminal nerve.[21–23] In addition, all the contents of the fossa will be blocked, including the sphenopalatine ganglion.

The pterygopalatine fossa is bounded anteriorly by the maxillary bone, superiorly by the sphenoid bone, and posteriorly by the lateral pterygoid plate; it is covered laterally by the lateral pterygoid muscle. The upper head of the lateral pterygoid muscle originates from the infratemporal portion of the sphenoid bone and inserts on the capsule of

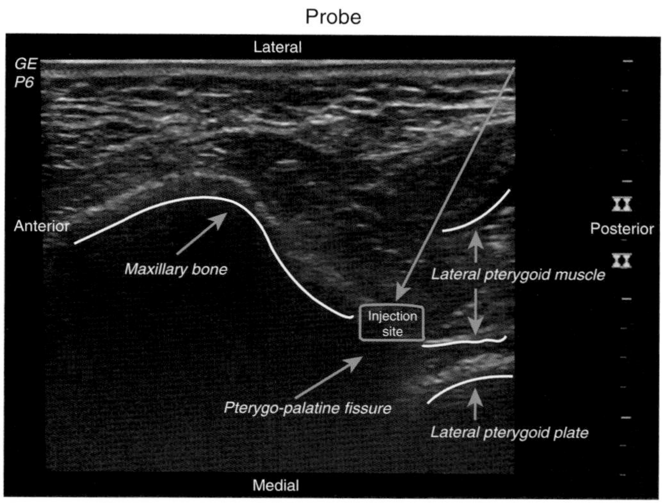

FIG. 82.5 Ultrasound view for trigeminal nerve block.

the temporomandibular joint. Injection of local anesthetic posterior to the maxilla, anterior to the lateral pterygoid plate, and deep to the lateral pterygoid muscle through the pterygopalatine fissure will result in blockade of the trigeminal nerve.

Ultrasound guidance provides excellent visualization of these bony and muscular structures. In addition, the tortuous maxillary artery and vein, which accompany the maxillary nerve, can easily be identified and spared.

TECHNIQUE

The patient is placed in the lateral decubitus position and standard American Society of Anaesthesiologists (ASA) monitoring is applied. The area below the zygomatic bone is cleaned and prepped. A high-frequency small-print linear probe is selected. If the patient exhibits any signs of facial allodynia, an intravenous access is secured and sedation administered. The infrazygomatic area is scanned anterior to the condylar process in the coronoid notch. The acoustic reflections of the maxillary bone and lateral pterygoid plate are identified (Fig. 82.5). The upper head of the lateral pterygoid muscle is identified. The maxillary artery is identified. The needle is directed from lateral to medial and from posterior to anterior toward the pterygopalatine fissure. The needle tip is placed at the fissure. At this point the entire needle trajectory can be visualized. A total of 5 mL of local anesthetic and steroid is injected through the pterygopalatine fissure below the lateral pterygoid muscle. The patient is monitored for 20 minutes for signs of local anesthetic toxicity or extensive local anesthetic spread. Pulsed radiofrequency ablation of the maxillary nerve has been described using this approach.[24]

COMPLICATIONS

Although no major complications have been reported from this technique, injection of local anesthetic near the pterygopalatine fossa can result in an intravascular injection, worsening of the symptoms due to an intramuscular injection (lateral pterygoid muscle), or extensive spread of the local anesthetic to basal structures of the brain. Damage to the maxillary artery can result in jaw atrophy. Repeated steroid injection can result in deleterious side effects including atrophy at the injection site.

SPHENOPALATINE GANGLION

ANATOMY

The ganglion resides in the pterygopalatine fossa. The fossa is bordered anteriorly by the maxillary sinus, posteriorly by the medial pterygoid plate, medially by the palatine bone, and superiorly by the sphenoid sinus. The pterygomaxillary fissure allows passage of a needle into the fossa, while the pterygopalatine foramen is located medial to the ganglion and is just posterior to the middle turbinate. The fossa is approximately 1 cm wide and 2 cm high and appears as a V-shaped structure on a lateral fluoroscopic image. A large venous plexus overlies the fossa. The foramen rotundum and pterygoid canal are located on the superolateral and inferomedial aspects of the fossa, respectively. The maxillary artery resides in the fossa. The ganglion is "suspended" from the maxillary nerve by the pterygopalatine nerves and is medial to the maxillary nerve. Posteriorly the ganglion is connected to the vidian nerve, which is formed by the deep petrosal (sympathetic from the upper thoracic spinal cord) and greater petrosal (parasympathetic from the superior salivatory nucleus) nerves. The ganglion has efferent branches and forms the superoposterior lateral nasal and pharyngeal nerves. Caudally, the greater and lesser palatine nerves exit the ganglion. Sensory fibers arise from the maxillary nerve, pass through the sphenopalatine ganglion (SPG), and innervate the upper teeth, nasal membranes, soft palate, and some parts of the pharynx. A small number of motor nerves are believed to travel with the sensory trunks.

PROCEDURE

Indications for sphenopalatine ganglion block and neurolysis include sphenopalatine neuralgia, trigeminal neuralgia, migraine headaches, cluster headaches, atypical facial pain, and cancer of the tongue and floor of the mouth. Other reported but not yet mainstream therapeutic uses include sinus arrest in postherpetic neuralgia, vasomotor rhinitis, complex regional pain syndrome of the lower extremity, low back pain, and posttraumatic headache.[25–29]

INTRANASAL APPROACH

The intranasal SPG block can be safely performed in an office setting. The location of the SPG in relation to the middle turbinate as well as the lateral nasal mucosa allows absorption of local anesthetic from a cotton-tipped applicator inserted into the nares. Four percent cocaine is the local anesthetic of choice secondary to its inherent vasoconstrictor property. If this is not available or contraindicated, 1% or 2% lidocaine or 0.25%–0.5% bupivacaine or ropivacaine can be used instead. If these are chosen, the practitioner can pretreat the nares with neosynephrine to produce vasoconstriction. Place the patient in the supine position. Estimate the depth of insertion by externally measuring the distance from the opening of the nares to the mandibular notch. Place a mark corresponding to this depth on the shaft of the cotton-tipped applicator. Soak the applicators in the local anesthetic for several minutes. Slowly insert the applicator into the nares and advance in a line parallel to the zygoma with the tip angled laterally. Do not advance the applicator in a cephalad direction. The endpoint should be the depth marked on the applicator. Place a second applicator into the nare using the same technique, except advance it approximately 0.5–1 cm deeper and superior to the first. If resistance is encountered at any time, slightly withdraw and redirect the applicator. The second applicator is not a necessity and the nares of some patients may not accommodate it. Leave the applicator or applicators in for 30–45 minutes. Signs of a successful block of the SPG include ipsilateral tearing, conjunctival injection, and nasal congestion. If the SPG is a pain generator or transmitter, analgesia should also be apparent. If after 20–30 minutes there are no signs of a block or the patient has not received any pain relief, additional local anesthetic may be needed and can be trickled down the shaft of the applicator. Remove the cotton-tipped applicators after 45 minutes even if there are no signs of block or analgesia, in which case the SPG may be too deep to be blocked by this technique or is not involved in the transmission of pain. Regardless, the infrazygomatic approach should be performed to rule out both of the aforementioned scenarios.

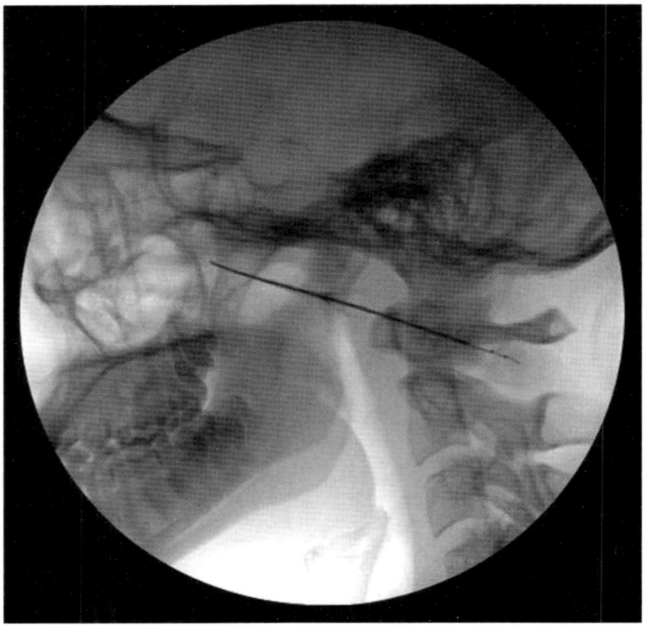

FIG. 82.6 Lateral fluoroscopic image of the block needle in the mid-portion of the pterygopalatine fossa.

INFRAZYGOMATIC APPROACH

The infrazygomatic approach to SPG blockade is technically challenging. Therefore fluoroscopic guidance is highly recommended, as this will improve the success of the block as well as the speed at which it is performed; it will also decrease potential complications. Noninvasive monitors should be used to record vital signs. Light sedation with midazolam and fentanyl can be used, but on occasion deeper sedation may be necessary for radiofrequency lesioning. For pulsed radiofrequency ablation, heavy sedation is not required.

Place the patient in the supine position. Using sterile procedure, prep and drape the appropriate side of the face. Obtain a lateral fluoroscopic image. Palpate the mandibular notch and anesthetize the skin. If the notch is not palpable, identify the notch on a lateral fluoroscopic view. Identify the pterygopalatine fossa (which appears as a "V") on the lateral image and superimpose the right and left fossae (see Fig. 82.5). This is accomplished by manipulating the C-arm or the head. The block can be performed with a 4.5-inch, 22-gauge short-bevel needle with the distal tip bent at a 30-degree angle or with a curved blunt 10-cm, 20- or 22-gauge needle. The description of the technique reflects the use of a blunt needle. Anesthetize the skin and insert a 1.25-inch 16-gauge angiocatheter through the skin; advance it until it is just medial to the ramus of the mandible. This can be checked on an anteroposterior (AP) image. Pass the block needle through the angiocatheter and advance it medially, anteriorly, and slightly cephalad. Obtain a lateral image to check the direction of the needle. Your target is the middle to upper portion of the pterygopalatine fossa (Fig. 82.6). Get an AP view and advance the needle toward the middle turbinate, stopping when the tip is adjacent to the palatine bone (Fig. 82.7). If resistance is encountered at any point, withdraw and redirect the needle. Given the small size of the fossa, frequent AP and lateral images may be required to redirect the needle. Once in the fossa, inject 0.5–1 mL of nonionic water-soluble contrast and observe for intravascular spread and/or intranasal placement of the needle. Once correct placement has been confirmed, inject 2 mL of local anesthetic with or without steroids.

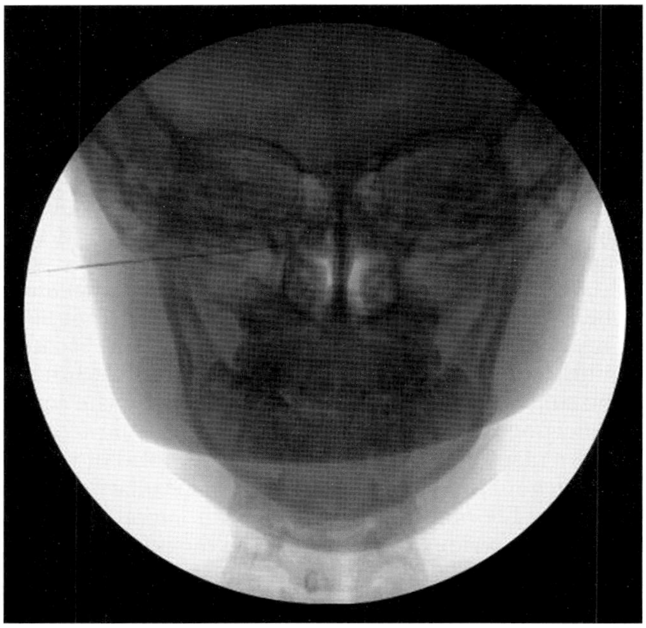

FIG. 82.7 Anteroposterior fluoroscopic image of the block needle adjacent to the palatine bone at the level of the middle turbinate.

RADIOFREQUENCY AND PULSED RADIOFREQUENCY THERMOCOAGULATION

After a successful diagnostic block, two therapeutic choices are available: conventional radiofrequency lesioning (radiofrequency thermocoagulation [RFTC]) and pulsed electromagnetic field radiofrequency (P-EMF) thermocoagulation. An insulated RF needle with a 3- or 5-mm active tip is placed using the infrazygomatic approach. Once in place, sensory stimulation is performed at 50 Hz up to 1 V. If the tip of the needle is adjacent to the SPG, the patient should perceive a paresthesia at the root of the nose at less than 0.3 V. If the paresthesia is felt in the hard palate, the needle should be redirected cephalad and medial. A paresthesia in the upper teeth indicates stimulation of the maxillary nerve, in which case the needle should be placed more caudally and medially. Motor stimulation is not necessary. After appropriate sensory stimulation, RFTC can be performed at 67°C–80°C for 90 seconds times 2 cycles. Before lesioning, 2–3 mL of local anesthetic should be injected. To avoid inadvertent lesioning of other nerves around the SPG, a 3-mm active tip is a better choice. For P-EMF, the size of the active tip is not important, as the electromagnetic field is projected from the tip of the needle and not from the shaft. With P-EMF lesioning, 2–4, 120-second lesions are performed at 45 V. Local anesthetic is not required for P-EMF. The choice of whether to do an RFTC or P-EMF lesioning after a successful block is up to the discretion of the pain practitioner.

COMPLICATIONS

Complications include bruising, bleeding, infection, damage to nerves, proptosis from retrobulbar hematoma, dysesthesias, paresthesias, and/or numbness from RFTC. Bradycardia (the Konen reflex) has been noted during RFTC and P-EMF and can be prevented with pretreatment with atropine or glycopyrrolate.[30]

OCCIPITAL NERVE BLOCK

Occipital headaches, known as occipital neuralgia, can present from multiple sources. The term *occipital neuralgia* was initially introduced in 1821 to describe a headache originating from the occipital and suboccipital region.[31,32] The term describes an irritation of the greater occipital nerve (GON) and/or the lesser occipital nerve (LON). The International Headache Society defines occipital neuralgia as a paroxysmal jabbing pain in the distribution of the greater or LONs or of the third occipital nerve (TON), sometimes accompanied by diminished sensation or dysesthesia in the affected area. It is commonly associated with tenderness over the nerve in question and the pain is often relieved with a local anesthetic block.[33]

Recognized causes of occipital neuralgia include trauma to the greater and LONs, compression of the greater and/or LONs or C2 and/or C3 nerve roots by degenerative cervical spine changes, cervical disc disease, myofascial pain, referred pain from an ipsilateral trigeminal distribution, and tumors involving the C2 and C3 nerve roots.[34]

Treatment options vary depending on the etiology of the pain. Management usually begins with conservative treatment such as physical therapy, massage, nonsteroidal antiinflammatory drugs (NSAIDs), muscle relaxants, tricyclic antidepressants, and anticonvulsants. When occipital neuralgia has a structural basis then treatment is aimed at the cause, and surgery may be warranted such as decompression or resection. Structural lesions are rare, and most patients who suffer from occipital neuralgia are usually treated with local anesthetic blocks, botulinum toxin injections, medications, and occipital nerve stimulators.

Several authors have reported improvement in pain associated with occipital neuralgia following occipital nerve blocks. Tobin and Flitman performed a literature review and concluded that occipital nerve block is an effective treatment for cervicogenic headache, cluster headache, and occipital neuralgia.[35] Anthony evaluated 796 patients with idiopathic headache, of which 128 were found to be suffering from cervicogenic headache. Injections of depot methylprednisolone into the region of the GON and LON produced complete relief of headache in 169 out of 180 patients with cervicogenic headaches for a period ranging from 10 to 77 days.[36]

ANATOMY

The cutaneous innervation of the posterior head and neck is from the cervical spine nerves. In the treatment of occipital neuralgia, it is essential to understand the course of these cervical nerves, as their muscular investment may be a source of entrapment, leading to compression and irritation. The GON arises from the dorsal ramus of the second cervical nerve and to a lesser extent the dorsal ramus of third cervical nerve. This nerve passes between the inferior capitis oblique and semispinalis capitis muscles and ascends to pierce the semispinalis capitis and the trapezius superiorly. At this point it travels with the occipital artery to provide cutaneous innervation to the posterior scalp as far anterior as the vertex of the skull. Medially and over the occiput, this nerve communicates with the TON and laterally with the LON. The LON is composed of branches from the ventral ramus of the second and third cervical nerves and ascends toward the occiput by running parallel to the posterior border of the sternocleidomastoid muscle. Near the scalp it perforates the deep fascia and is continued superiorly over the occiput, where it supplies the skin over the posterolateral portion of the scalp and above the ear. The TON arises deep to the trapezius from the medial branch of the dorsal ramus of the third cervical nerve. This nerve ascends medial to the GON and is connected to it both over the occiput and as the GON rounds the inferior edge of the inferior capitis oblique. The medial terminal branch of the TON supplies the skin over the rostral end of the neck and the occiput near the external occipital protuberance (Fig. 82.8).[37]

TECHNIQUE

The patient is placed in a sitting or prone position with the head slightly flexed downward. The following landmarks are then identified: occipital protuberance, superior nuchal ridge, occipital artery, and mastoid process. The location of the GON is typically medial to the occipital artery one third the distance between the occipital protuberance and the mastoid process on the nuchal ridge. The LON is often found two thirds the distance from the occipital protuberance and the mastoid process on the nuchal ridge. When the occipital artery is palpated, the GON should be located just medial to the artery. However, anatomy may vary and the GON may be located just lateral to the occipital

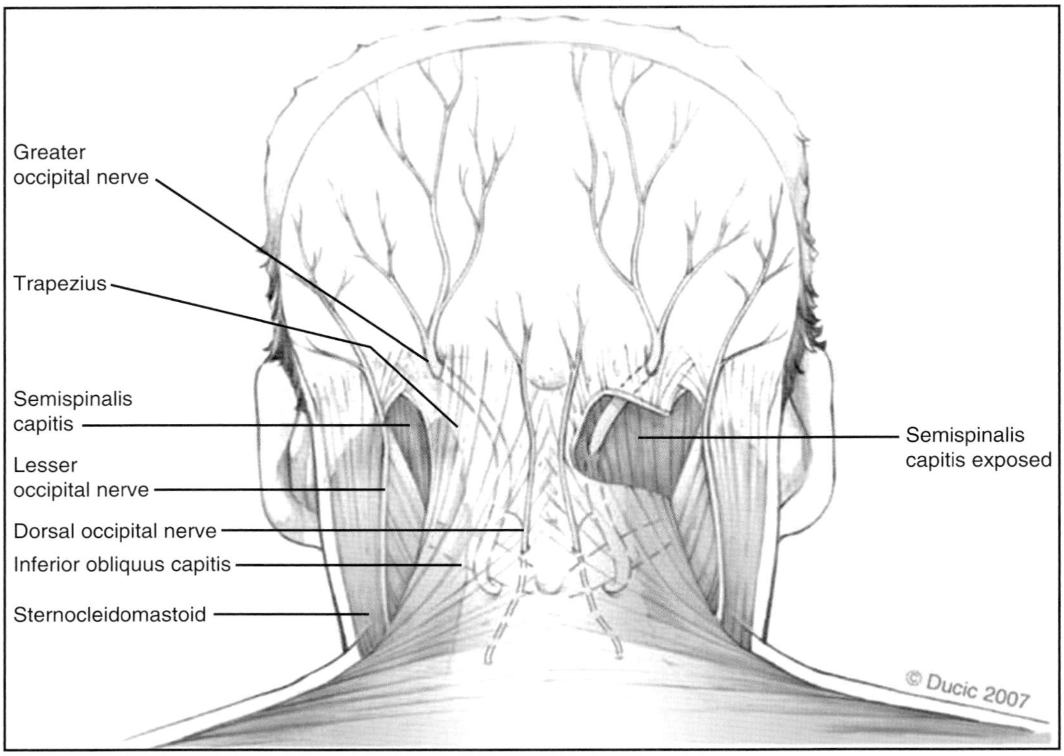

FIG. 82.8 Occipital triangle cartoon showing the innervation of the occiput by the occipital nerves.

artery. At the nuchal ridge a 1½-inch 22- or 25-gauge B-bevel needle is inserted in the skin at the nuchal ridge and advanced until bony contact is made. The needle is then slightly withdrawn just short of the bone and, after negative aspiration, a total of 3–5 mL of local anesthetic is injected. Many authors advocate a fanlike approach when injecting local anesthetics. We recommend avoiding the fanlike approach, as this can puncture the occipital artery. Instead, withdraw the needle slightly and after negative aspiration, inject the local anesthetic. If a diagnostic block is planned, a small volume (1–1.5 mL) should be used, to avoid any confusion in distinguishing greater occipital neuralgia from myofascial pain. The LON block is performed in a similar fashion at its location. The most serious complication is piercing the occipital artery and causing bleeding. Compression of the occipital artery is usually effective in avoiding significant problems.

INJECTION OF THE SUBOCCIPITAL COMPARTMENT

Numerous causes have been attributed with multiple interventions aimed for the treatment of occipital headaches. However, there is no clear consensus on the best approach to diagnosis and treatment. Treatment of occipital neuralgia is theorized on the basis of neural entrapment within the muscle and fascia of the suboccipital compartment and the posterior occiput. The traditional approach to blocking the GON has been to infiltrate local anesthetic with or without steroid into the subcutaneous tissue around the course of the nerve after it has penetrated the trapezius muscle. The goal of infiltration at this point along the course of the nerve is the pharmacologic blockade of nociceptive transmission. This treatment is effective when the entrapment is superficial, but it fails when the entrapment occurs deeper within the suboccipital triangle. Currently other treatment options include conservative medical management, physical therapy, nerve stimulators, C2 gangliectomy, C2–C3 rhizotomy/root decompression, radiofrequency lesioning, and sectioning of the inferior oblique muscle. Although many of the aforementioned treatments have shown good results, the benefits are usually short-lived, lasting for only weeks to months. In contrast, procedures such as surgical decompression of the nerves in the suboccipital compartment have proven effective for longer periods of time.[38,39] Although surgery has shown better outcomes compared with nonsurgical treatment, there are increased risks, with higher rates of morbidity and mortality. Currently there is an alternative approach to treating occipital neuralgia caused by neural entrapment within the suboccipital triangle. The suboccipital compartment injection, introduced in 1980 by Racz, has become popular over the last 5 years. Recently Justiz et al. performed a retrospective study of 29 patients with confirmed occipital neuralgia using the suboccipital compartment injection. This study showed (by numerical rating scale) that the procedure was effective in reducing headaches more than 50% at 6-month follow-up in 58% of patients. At 1-year follow-up, 34.5% of patients still showed significant pain relief.[40] Lauretti et al. compared the classical versus subcompartmental GON block techniques for cervicogenic headaches.[41] The classical GON technique resulted in 2 weeks of analgesia and less rescue analgesic consumption compared with 24 weeks after the subcompartmental technique ($P < .01$). Quality of life improved at 2 and 24 weeks after the classical and suboccipital techniques, respectively

($P < .05$). The data revealed that the groups were similar regarding analgesia when compared with volume of injection ($P > .05$). Given that this is one of the most common sites of entrapment within the suboccipital triangle, this less invasive approach for treatment has been implemented without the complications associated with surgery.

ANATOMY

The suboccipital triangle is a region of the posterior cervical neck that has the potential for neural structures to become entrapped at multiple locations. The triangle is composed of bony articulations, ligaments, and fibrofatty tissue; it is bounded by three muscles: the rectus capitis posterior major, the obliquus capitis inferioris (inferior oblique), and the obliquus capitis superioris. The triangle comprises the suboccipital nerve as well as the GON, TON, and vertebral artery. As these nerves enter and exit the triangle, their courses can be tortuous, with anatomic variation among individuals.[42] As they travel past the muscles that enclose the triangle, there is a potential for impingement, especially of the GON. The most common site of entrapment within the triangle is the inferior oblique muscle and, outside the triangle, the trapezius.

Initially the GON begins within the suboccipital triangle and courses downward and lateral in a posterior direction at the lower edge of the inferior oblique muscle, where it bends around the muscle and ascends in a superior and medial direction above the rectus capitis toward the head of the semispinalis muscle. Here the nerve forms another bend from its upward orientation in a deep to a superficial direction as it begins to move laterally. As the nerve courses upward and laterally, it moves between the dorsal aspect of the semispinalis muscle and deep to the trapezius muscle. Here the nerve may pierce the semispinalis muscle or just continue upward until it pierces the trapezius muscle and travels subcutaneously upward toward the base of the occiput.

TECHNIQUE

The patient is placed in a prone position with the neck slightly flexed. The superior nuchal ridge is palpated and the occipital protuberance identified. Two to three centimeters lateral to the occipital protuberance, at the nuchal ridge, the skin is anesthetized with 1% lidocaine. Thereafter a 22-gauge, 1.5- to 3.5-inch sharp or blunt Stealth (Epimed International, New York) needle is advanced in a posteroanterior direction perpendicular to the skin toward the arch of C1 (Fig. 82.9). Once the needle has been advanced 2–3 cm into the tissue, a lateral view is obtained. While in the lateral view, the needle is further advanced under live fluoroscopy toward the arch of C1. As the needle is advanced, you should note two to three distinct pops as each muscle fascial layer is penetrated (Fig. 82.10). Once the needle tip is positioned at posterior arch of C1, contrast material is injected in the lateral radiographic view. The contrast spread should be limited around the muscle layers that enclose the suboccipital compartment with no vascular uptake (Fig. 82.11). After successful needle position is confirmed, a total of 5–10 mL of local anesthetic (0.2% ropivacaine or 0.25% bupivacaine) and steroid (20 mg methylprednisolone or 4 mg dexamethasone) is injected. Complications are rare; patients may complain of slight dizziness immediately after the procedure.

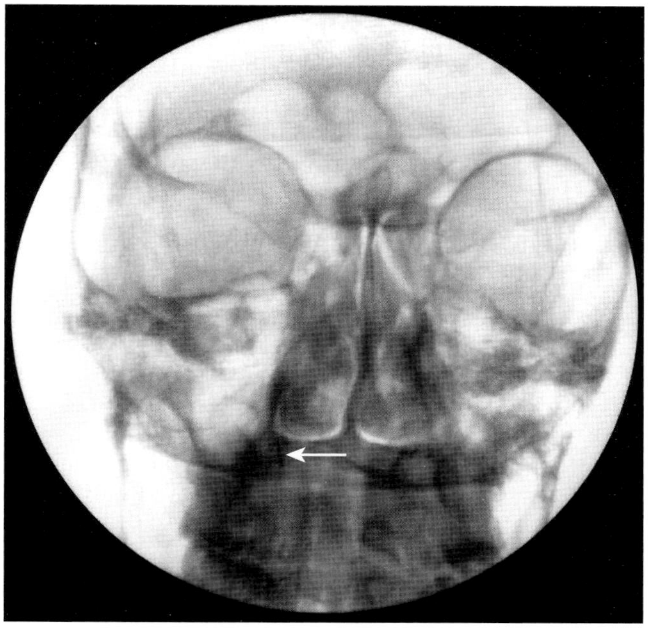

FIG. 82.9 Anteroposterior fluoroscopic image of the block needle. The *arrow* indicates the needle.

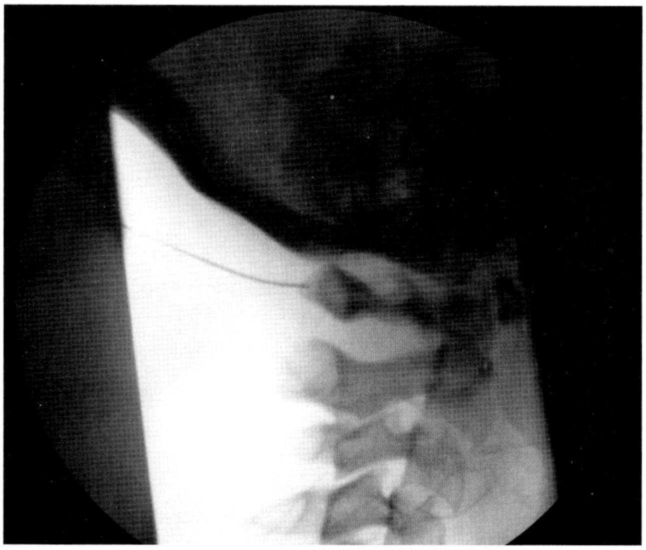

FIG. 82.10 Lateral fluoroscopic image of the block needle with the tip at the level of the posterior arch of C1.

ULTRASOUND-GUIDED OCCIPITAL NERVE BLOCK

ANATOMY

The posterior division of second cervical nerve and its main branch, the GON, can be blocked between the obliquus capitis inferior and the semispinalis muscle in the suboccipital triangle. After emerging from the spinal cord between the arch of the first cervical vertebra and the lamina of the second vertebra, the posterior division of C2

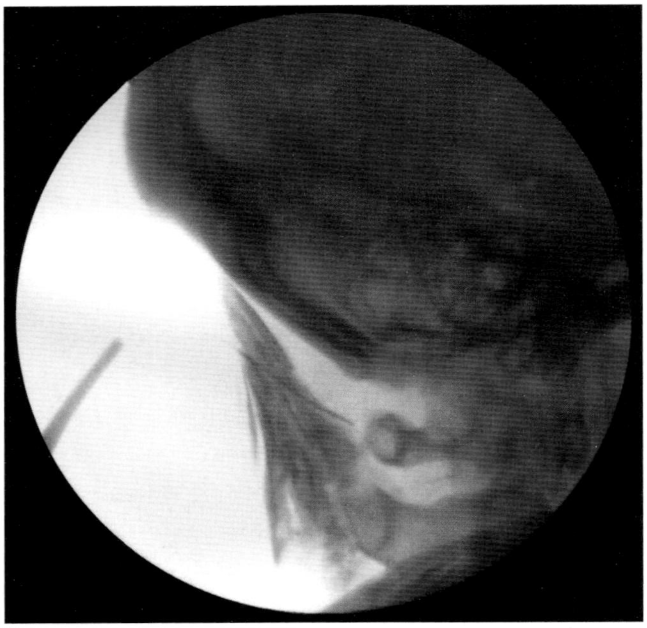

FIG. 82.11 Lateral fluoroscopic image after injection of nonionic water-soluble contrast.

travels in a cephalad direction between the obliquus capitis inferior and the semispinalis capitis, where it can blocked. The belly of the obliquus capitis inferior can easily be identified at this level as it originates from the spinous process of C2 and inserts on the lateral mass of the atlas.[43] The vertebral artery should be identified as it lies deep to the lateral border of this muscle. The TON (posterior branch of C3), which solely innervates the C2–C3 joint, travels from lateral to medial in the same fascial plane[44]; a communicating branch from the first cervical nerve and the lateral third cervical nerve can be found in the same plane laterally.

TECHNIQUE

The patient is placed in the sitting position. Standard ASA monitoring is applied. The area below the nuchal line is cleaned and prepped. A high-frequency small-print linear probe is selected. If the patient is anxious or bradycardic, an intravenous access is secured and light sedation is administered. The obliquus capitis inferior muscle is identified between the spinous process of C2 and transverse process of C1. The semispinalis muscle is identified just superficial to the obliquus capitis inferior muscle. The vertebral artery is identified deep to the lateral part of the muscle. The GON is identified in the plane separating both muscles. The needle is inserted from medial to lateral toward the nerve. A total of 1–3 mL of local anesthetic and steroid is injected. Injection of local anesthetic in this fascial plane results in analgesia in the distribution of the greater and lesser occipital nerves and TON (C2–C3 joint).

COMPLICATIONS

Although the most common complication of this injection is a vasovagal syndrome, injection in this fascial plane can results in an intravascular injection, worsening of the symptoms owing to an intramuscular injection or extensive spread of the local anesthetic to the brain stem.

GLOSSOPHARYNGEAL NERVE BLOCK

ANATOMY

The GN originates from the cranial part of the medulla oblongata. Its rootlets form one root that courses forward laterally until it reaches the jugular foramen. As it exits the jugular foramen, it joins with the vagus and spinal accessory nerve and passes between the internal jugular vein (IJV) and the internal carotid artery (ICA). It continues to descend anterior to the ICA and dips medially behind the styloid process in close proximity to the vagus nerve, accessory nerve, and IJV, emerging beneath the tip of the styloid and continuing to its terminal branches. The GN is a mixed nerve containing sensory, motor, and autonomic fibers. It provides sensation to the posterior one third of the tongue, middle ear, palatine tonsils, and mucous membranes of the mouth and pharynx above the vocal cords. Additionally it innervates the carotid sinus and the carotid bodies. The motor fibers innervate the stylopharyngeous muscle, and its autonomic functions are related to the parotid gland via the otic ganglion.

The GN lies in close relation to the vagus and spinal accessory nerves. Specifically they are in close approximation until they diverge at the midpoint of the styloid process. There have been reported cases of GN paroxysms with associated bradycardia and asystole. This phenomenon is due to the close connection between the vagus and the GN.[45] Lesions arising from the GN can send afferent impulses via the tractus solitarius to the dorsal motor nucleus of the vagal nerves, resulting in reflex bradycardia or asystole.[46] Although there are no reported adverse events associated with the spinal accessory or hypoglossal nerve, there can be complications following blockade of the GP nerve. There is a potential of pharyngeal and trapezius weakness due to unwanted blockade of the closely situated nerves.

INDICATIONS

Blockade of the GN is used for the treatment of glossopharyngeal neuralgia (GPN). GPN is a rare facial pain syndrome characterized by paroxysms of excruciating pain in the sensory distribution of the auricular and pharyngeal branches of glossopharyngeal (IX) and vagus (X) cranial nerves. The block can be done with local anesthetics as a diagnostic tool to determine if the patient truly has GPN, or it can be performed with the addition of steroids for therapeutic treatment. The procedure can also be used for surgical anesthesia or as an adjunct to depress the gag reflex in an awake endotracheal intubation or endodontic procedure. If a neurolytic procedure is considered, the block can be used prior to neurolysis as a prognostic indicator.

TECHNIQUE

Extraoral Approach

Ensure appropriate monitoring and intravenous access prior to proceeding. Two major landmarks must first be identified: the angle of the mandible anteriorly and the mastoid process posteriorly. The patient is placed supine and the head is turned slightly opposite the direction of the affected side. Once in correct position, a lateral fluoroscopic view is obtained to visualize the angle of the mandible and the mastoid process. Once identified and marked, a line is drawn between those two points inferior to the ear and the styloid process should lie midway between both points. When the target is identified, a small skin wheal with 1% lidocaine is applied to the skin and a 22-gauge 1.5-inch needle is advanced perpendicular toward the styloid process. Bony contact is typically obtained at 3 cm. After contact, the needle is slightly withdrawn and walked approximately 0.5 cm off the styloid process in an anterior direction. Inject 1 mL of contrast agent under continuous fluoroscopy. This permits real-time imaging of the contrast medium to look for any irregular patterns indicating that a vascular structure has been punctured. After injecting the contrast, 2–3 mL of local anesthetic (0.2% naropin [Ropivacaine]) and steroid (4 mg dexamethasone) is injected.

Intraoral Approach

This approach is popular when there is an anatomic distortion externally by previous surgery or tumor. The patient is placed in a supine position with the mouth wide open and the tongue is retracted downward and medially using a tongue depressor or a laryngoscope blade. The nerve will be located at the inferior portion of the tonsillar pillar and is accessed via the palatoglossal fold. Once the fold has been identified, a topical local anesthetic spray or pledget with 1 mL of saline with epinephrine is applied for hemostasis. A 22- or 25-gauge needle with a slight distal bend (25 degrees) is advanced to a depth of no more than 0.5 cm into the mucosa. After negative aspiration 2–3 mL of local anesthetic (0.2% ropivacaine) and steroid (4 mg of dexamethasone) is injected (Figs. 82.12 and 82.13).[47]

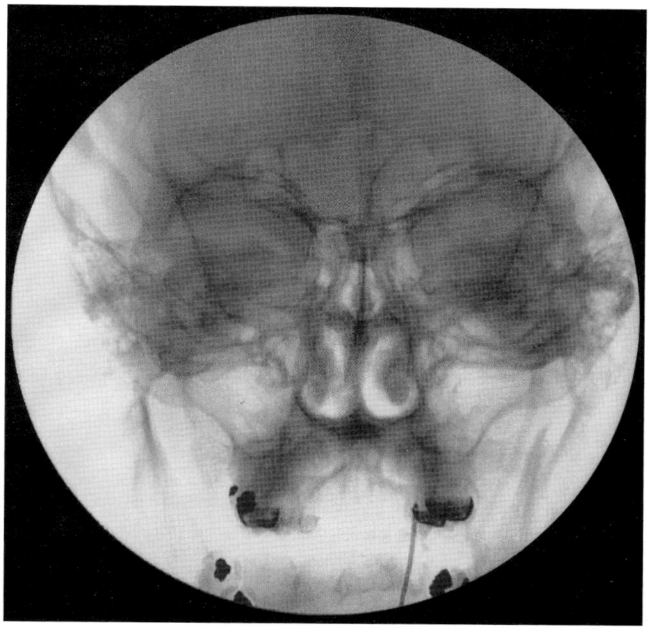

FIG. 82.12 Anteroposterior fluoroscopic image of the block needle in position for a glossopharyngeal nerve block.

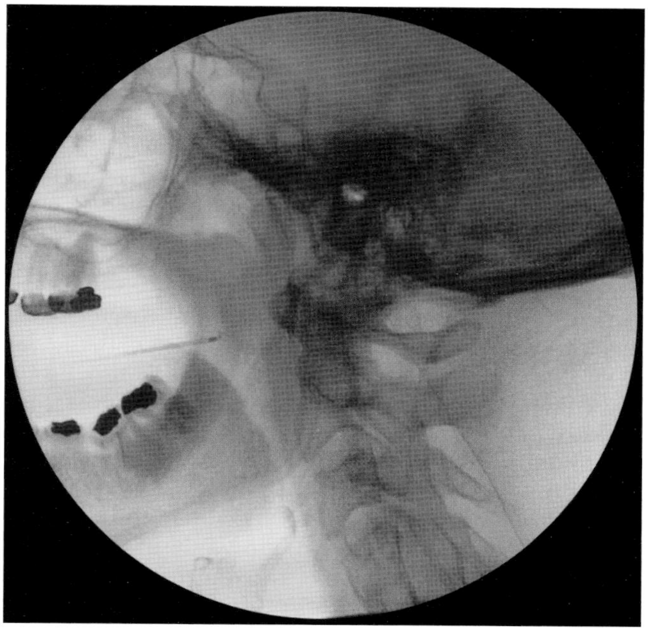

FIG. 82.13 Lateral fluoroscopic image of the block needle in position for a glossopharyngeal nerve block.

COMPLICATIONS

Multiple complications can occur with this procedure and care must be taken in performing it. Such complications will vary depending on the approach used for the blockade. The extraoral approach can be inherently more difficult and may lead to complications secondary to the close proximity of cranial nerves IX, X, XI, and XII to the styloid process.

There can be an accidental puncture of the vessels, leading to vessel trauma and hematoma formation. Also inadvertent intravascular injection of the ICA or IJV may lead to seizures or even cardiovascular collapse. With the intraoral approach, there is a potential for vessel trauma and neurotoxicity, but much less than with the extraoral approach.

Other complications can occur with unwanted blockade of cranial nerves X, XI, and XII. As mentioned earlier, these complications will vary by approach. With the extraoral approach, there is the potential for unwanted blockade of the aforementioned nerves. Blockade of the vagus can lead to bradycardia, asystole, reflex tachycardia, and syncope as well as dysphonia secondary to ipsilateral vocal cord paralysis. Blockade of cranial nerves XI and II can result in temporary weakness of the trapezius muscle and the tongue. These complications can be minimized with small amounts of local anesthetic but not necessarily avoided. Most complications of the affected nerves will gradually resolve as the local anesthetic wears off.

CERVICAL PLEXUS BLOCK

The cervical plexus block is performed for anesthesia and analgesia involving the head and neck region. The cervical plexus is formed by the anterior divisions of the first four upper cervical nerves (C1–C4) and the lower four nerves (C5–C8) together with the first thoracic ventral ramus

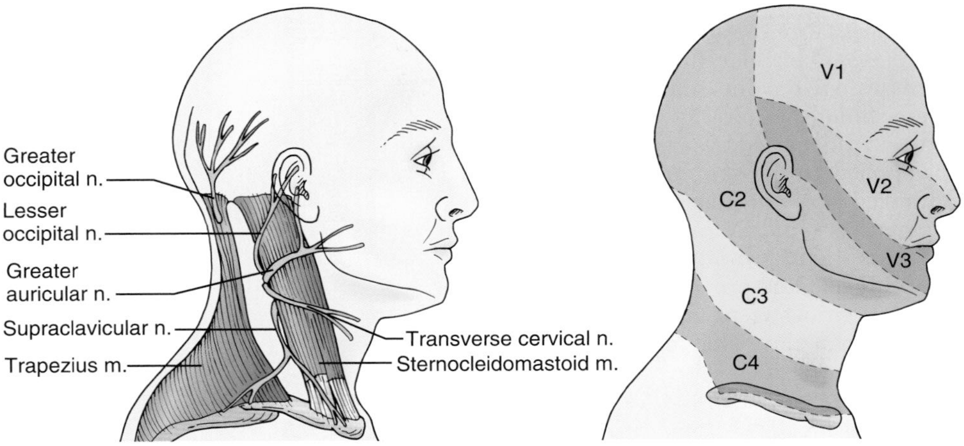

FIG. 82.14 Peripheral cutaneous *(left)* and dermatomal *(right)* innervation of the head and neck, including the branches of the superficial cervical plexus and the greater occipital nerve.

(T1), forming the brachial plexus. The cervical plexus lies deep to the IJV upon the levator scapulae and scalene muscles and underneath the sternocleidomastoid muscle. The plexus is divided into two separate rami, each dividing into an ascending (superficial cervical plexus) and descending (deep cervical plexus) branch; except for the first ramus, these form loops at each level with the corresponding nerves.

The first cervical ramus (suboccipital nerve) is thought to be primarily a motor nerve. Even though it lacks cutaneous innervation, it does have some sensory function and communicates sensory information to deeper muscles in the suboccipital region as the suboccipital nerve. C1 is often not affected by a cervical plexus block owing to its posterior and deeper location.

The second, third, and fourth cervical nerves leave their respective transverse processes anteriorly and surface lateral to the vertebral artery. C2 and C3 continue on and emerge at the midpoint of the posterior border of the sternocleidomastoid muscle and travel toward to their destination. C2 moves upward along the sternocleidomastoid toward the posterior and lateral part of the scalp. It provides cutaneous innervation to the posterior scalp behind the ear and the upper and posterior auricle as well as the mastoid and angle of the mandible as the lesser occipital and great auricular nerve. C3 bifurcates into anterior and descending portions. The anterior branch runs in an anterior oblique direction, where it gives cutaneous innervation to the lateral neck from the chin to the sternum as the transverse cervical nerve. The descending branch continues along the sternocleidomastoid muscle into the posterior triangle of the neck beneath the platysma and deep cervical fascia and joins the fourth cervical nerve. Here these nerves provide cutaneous innervation to the upper trapezius, shoulder, and pectoral region as the supraclavicular nerves (Fig. 82.14).[48]

The deep branches of the cervical plexus divide into medial and lateral branches. The medial branches supply the anterior and lateral neck muscles and gives rise to the phrenic nerve via the fourth cervical nerve as the main contributor. The lateral deep branch forms communicating branches between the C1 and C2 rami to the vagus and hypoglossal nerves. Additionally, the deep cervical plexus gives rise to several muscular branches. These branches supply the rectus capitis lateralis (C1), rectus capitis anterior (C1, C2), longus capitis (C1–C3), and longus colli (C2–C4). The lateral branches communicate with the spinal accessory nerve and supply the deep surface of the trapezius via the communicating branches. The muscular branches are distributed to the sternocleidomastoid (C2–C4), trapezius (C2, C3), levator scapulae (C3, C4), and scalene medius (C3, C4).[48]

INDICATIONS

The cervical plexus block is a regional technique that is a safe alternative to general anesthesia for procedures involving the anterior-lateral portion of the neck, upper shoulder, and posterior scalp. Its potential indications are many and include superficial neck procedures, neck dissection, thyroglossal and brachial cyst surgery, thyroidectomy, lymph node dissection, cervical node biopsy, carotid endarterectomy, and other head and neck neuralgias. The sensory and motor components of the cervical plexus can each be blocked separately or together. A deep cervical plexus block provides motor and sensory blockade while a superficial plexus block blocks only the sensory component of the plexus.[49]

Blockade of the superficial cervical plexus provides anesthesia and analgesia for the posterior and anterior auricular scalp region, lateral and anterior neck, and upper shoulder region. The superficial cervical plexus block is useful for postoperative pain relief, reducing nausea and vomiting with surgeries involving the tympanic-mastoid region, and for simple superficial procedures such as those involved with plastic surgeries or superficial biopsies involving the neck. Additionally, this block is sometimes performed for carotid endarterectomy and thyroid surgery. The branches blocked by the superficial cervical plexus block include the lesser occipital, great auricular, transverse cervical, and supraclavicular nerves. For blockade of the deeper structures and the motor components, a deep cervical plexus block is warranted.

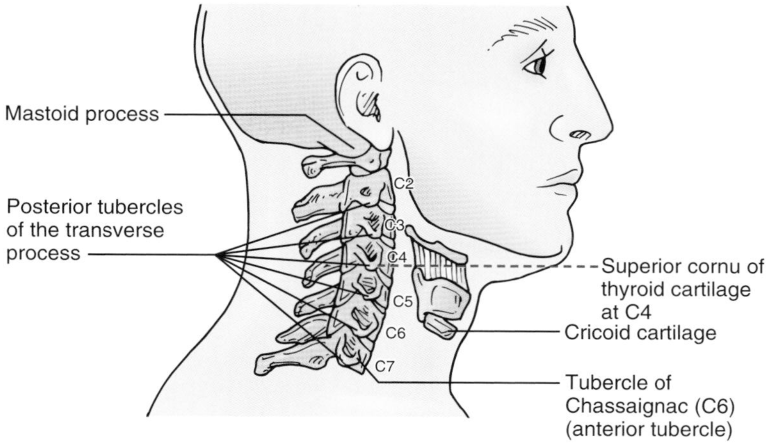

FIG. 82.15 Bony landmarks for deep cervical plexus block. (*From Raj PP, Pai D, Rawal N: Techniques of regional anesthesia in adults. In: Raj PP, editor:* Clinical Practice of Regional Anesthesia, *New York: Churchill Livingstone, 1991, p 271.*)

Blockade of the deep cervical plexus provides anesthesia and analgesia of the superficial and the deeper muscles within the anterior and lateral neck up to the upper shoulder region. Both the motor and sensory components of the aforementioned regions are interrupted as the nerve roots are anesthetized prior to the branching of the motor and sensory components. This technique can be used for surgical anesthesia, postoperative pain relief, and the diagnosis and treatment of painful conditions involving the neck, posterior scalp, and upper shoulder region. This block is performed for procedures such as thyroidectomy, tracheostomy, and laceration repairs under local anesthesia or any procedure that requires relaxation of the neck muscles. One of the most common indications is for awake carotid endarterectomy. This helps with instant feedback to the surgeon and anesthesiologist in the event of any neurologic compromise so that they can act appropriately without delay.[50] One of the more uncommon indications is for the treatment of intractable hiccups, as the deep branches innervate the muscle of the diaphragm.

TECHNIQUE

SUPERFICIAL CERVICAL PLEXUS BLOCK

The essential component of this procedure is identification of the sternocleidomastoid muscle. The patient is placed in a supine position with the head turned away from the side that is going to be blocked. Once this has been done, it is important to identify the posterior border of the sternocleidomastoid muscle. This can be done one of two ways. Two landmarks must be identified: the mastoid process and Chassaignac's tubercle at C6. A line is drawn from the mastoid process to Chassaignac's tubercle over the sternocleidomastoid muscle. Alternatively, the patient can lift the head and the sternocleidomastoid muscle will be identified. The drawn line should overlie the path of the superficial cervical plexus over the posterior border of the sternocleidomastoid muscle. The point of needle entry will be in the middle of a line drawn from the mastoid process to Chassaignac's tubercle. This is where the branches of the superficial plexus appear behind the posterior boundary of the sternocleidomastoid muscle. A 22- or 25-gauge 4- to 5-cm needle is inserted subcutaneously 2–3 cm deep at the midpoint of the posterior border of the sternocleidomastoid muscle and 3–5 mL of local anesthetic is injected. The needle is then withdrawn and redirected subcutaneously in a superior direction toward the mastoid process while injecting 3–5 mL of local anesthetic in a fanlike fashion. The needle is then redirected in an inferior direction subcutaneously toward Chassaignac's tubercle, injecting 3–5 mL of local anesthetic in a fanlike fashion. This technique should provide adequate blockade of all four major branches of the superficial plexus.

DEEP CERVICAL PLEXUS BLOCK

The deep cervical plexus block is performed in much the same manner as the superficial plexus block with some distinct differences, as the transverse processes of C2–C4 will be targeted. The patient is placed in a supine position with the head turned away from the side that is going to be blocked. Once this has been done, two landmarks are identified: the mastoid process and Chassaignac's tubercle at C6 (see Fig. 82.14). A line is drawn from the mastoid process to Chassaignac's tubercle overlying the sternocleidomastoid muscle. Once the sternocleidomastoid has been identified, the transverse processes of C2, C3, C4, and C6 must be identified. This is achieved by first identifying the cricoid cartilage. Once identified a line is drawn from the inferior aspect of the cricoid to the sternocleidomastoid. The point where these two lines intersect at a right angle is the C6 transverse process. Next the thyroid notch and superior cornu is palpated. Once these have been located, a line is drawn to the sternocleidomastoid and the transverse process of C4 is identified at the point where the two lines intersect. Once the C4 transverse process has been located, the transverse processes of C2 and C3 can easily be identified. This is done by taking half the distance between C4 and C6. This measurement will be the distance between the transverse processes at each level. Once the intertransverse process distance has been determined, it is plotted along the original line drawn from the mastoid to Chassaignac's tubercle. Beginning at the C4 transverse process, the distance is plotted upward toward the mastoid process; it should identify the C3 transverse process. When the same distance is plotted from C3 to the mastoid, the C2 transverse process will be identified (Fig. 82.15). The intertransverse process distances will typically measure some 2 cm from each other. Some authors advocate drawing a second line 1 cm posterior to the original line from the mastoid to Chassaignac's tubercle, as the transverse processes may vary in location. After drawing out the points of interest, the neck is prepped, cleaned, and draped in sterile fashion.

The block is performed by using a 22-gauge 1.5-inch needle. The transverse processes are located by entering the skin in a perpendicular fashion. The needle is always directed in a medial caudal direction to avoid any unintentional vertebral artery, epidural, subdural, or spinal injection. The needle is advanced slowly until the transverse process is contacted, which is typically 1.5–2.5 cm. The depth of the transverse process will vary with the body habitus of the patient. In general, as you proceed inferiorly, the other transverse processes will appear more superficial. If a paresthesia is obtained, the needle should be redirected slightly posteriorly, as the spinal nerves are located just in front of the transverse process. When bony contact is made, withdraw the needle 1 cm and, after negative aspiration, 3–5 mL of local anesthetic is injected slowly. The needle is then removed and the entire procedure is repeated at the other two transverse processes. Failure to contact the transverse process can be a problem with this procedure. When insertion of the needle does not result in bony contact, the needle should be withdrawn and redirected in a caudal inferior manner approximately 15 degrees until the transverse process is contacted. If this does not work, the needle should be withdrawn and the landmarks reassessed. Never attempt to redirect the needle in a cephalad direction or to go deeper than 3 cm, as you may risk inadvertently injuring the cervical spinal cord.

CHOICE OF LOCAL ANESTHETICS

There are several choices of local anesthetic, depending on the length of surgery and the duration of the blockade desired. For shorter procedures 2% lidocaine and mepivacaine may be preferred, as this can achieve blockade up to 4 hours. For longer procedures, ropivacaine or bupivacaine can be used; this may prolong the block up to 8 hours. Higher concentrations of local anesthetic will also prevent required supplemental infiltrations from the surgeon. Umbrain and colleagues have shown that a 0.75% concentration of ropivacaine was more effective in duration compared with 0.5% or 0.375%.[51] Onset times will vary with the local anesthetic used. Lidocaine will have faster onset times than mepivacaine, ropivacaine, or bupivacaine.[52] Additionally, the neck is a highly vascular area and there is a potential for toxicity that must be considered in performing this block. The total local anesthetic given in superficial plexus block and a deep cervical block will vary depending on each individual block or if combined. A total amount of 0.4 or 0.5 mL/kg (30 mL) is usually considered sufficient to perform either the superficial or deep block or a combination of both.[53] Furthermore, toxicity and systemic absorption can be decreased with the addition of epinephrine to the local anesthetics. Epinephrine will decrease the systemic absorption of bupivacaine and lidocaine by 20% or more.[54] Another adjunct used with local anesthetics is clonidine. Clonidine used with lidocaine has not been as successful as epinephrine. Adding clonidine 5 mg/mL does not change onset time or block duration and may lead to potential toxicity with lidocaine.[55] However, clonidine used with ropivacaine has been shown to decrease onset time of block and improve surgical anesthesia in patients undergoing elective carotid endarterectomy.[56]

COMPLICATIONS

Several complications can occur when a cervical plexus block is being performed. With careful attention and a good knowledge of the cervical anatomy, this procedure can be done with minimal complications. If complications do arise, they can be minimized with appropriate care and knowledge of the possible reactions that may occur.

As with many interventional procedures, there is always a risk of infection when a needle punctures the skin. The risk of infection, albeit low, is present and can be avoided with strict aseptic technique. There is always the risk of hematoma when a cervical plexus block is being performed. To reduce the risk of arterial puncture, you should minimize multiple needle insertions or passes if the initial attempt is unsuccessful. If a hematoma does develop, you should hold constant pressure over the site for 5 minutes and evaluate the airway for possible compromise by an expanding hematoma. If airway compromise does occur, an emergent airway and surgical consultation may be indicated.

Temporary diaphragmatic paresis will invariably occur with the deep cervical plexus block. Blockade of the phrenic nerve cannot be avoided with this block. For that reason this procedure should never be performed in a bilateral fashion. Patient selection in performing this procedure is essential and should be carefully considered in patients who suffer from chronic respiratory disease. These patients may not be suitable candidates, as they will experience diaphragmatic hemiparesis and possibly compromised breathing. The superficial plexus block will not cause blockade of the phrenic nerve.

Local anesthetic toxicity is something always to be considered with any type of regional technique but especially in relation to a cervical plexus block, due to the high vascularity of the neck region. Intravascular injection may occur into either a vein or an artery. Puncture of the vertebral or carotid artery is possible due to their close proximity to the block site. The vertebral artery is typically located 0.5 cm below the tip of the transverse process. Intravascular injection of local anesthetics can lead to central nervous system (CNS) or cardiac side effects. The CNS effects can vary and will most likely consist of perioral numbness, sedation, tinnitus, or even seizures. Cardiac effects can occur but are usually seen with higher blood levels of local anesthetic. These complications can be minimized with careful and frequent aspiration prior to injecting the local anesthetic and constant communication with the patient during the procedure to look for signs of CNS toxicity.

Nerve injury is another complication that can occur and can be avoided with careful attention while performing the procedure. Try to avoid multiple passes of the needle. After two unsuccessful attempts, reassess the anatomic landmarks prior to proceeding. Also never inject the local anesthetic if the patient complains of severe pain with injection or if you experience high resistance with injection. This may indicate that the needle has been placed into the nerve

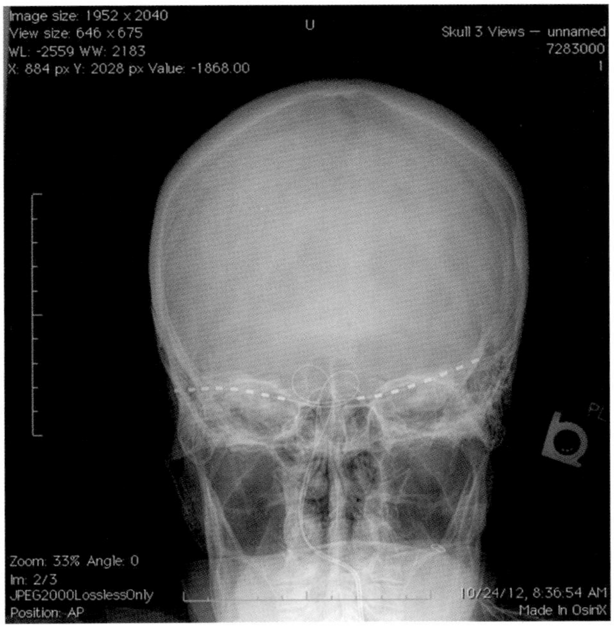

FIG. 82.16 Anteroposterior view of two percutaneous eight-contact occipital nerve stimulator leads.

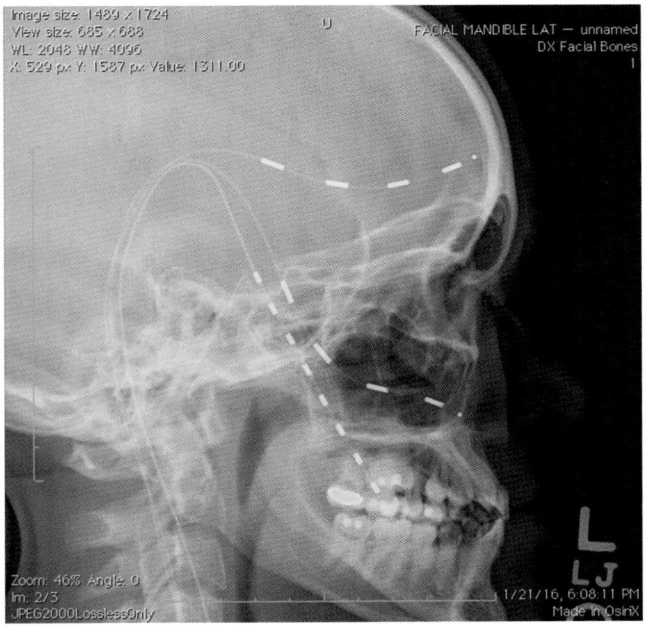

FIG. 82.17 Lateral view of percutaneous, peripheral nerve stimulator leads for pain in the three branches of the trigeminal nerve.

or nerve sheath, in which case injection of local anesthetic may lead to nerve ischemia and permanent damage.

Lastly, a high spinal block is a potential complication of this procedure. Avoid inserting the needle too deep, as there is a possibility of injecting a cervical nerve or the spinal canal. As mentioned earlier, avoid injecting with high resistance. The injection of local anesthetics within the dural sleeves around the nerves can cause some of the volume to backtrack into the epidural space and even the subarachnoid space, leading to a high spinal block. This will present as hypotension and loss of consciousness. Treatment will involve airway control and cardiovascular support until the local anesthetic is metabolized from the CNS.

NEUROMODULATION

Infrequently, pain management practitioners will encounter patients who have pain that is not adequately treated with medical management and advanced nerve block procedures. Fortunately, over the last several years, occipital nerve stimulation and peripheral field stimulation have been utilized with some success. A trial is performed with percutaneous or paddle leads, which are placed in the location of the peripheral nerve (Fig. 82.16). These provide paresthesias in the area of pain and hopefully analgesia. A 2015 systematic review by Sweet et al. classified occipital nerve stimulation as a level III (recommended) procedure for medically refractory occipital neuralgia.[57] This strength of recommendation was based on evidence from case series, comparative studies with historical controls, case reports, and expert opinion as well as significantly flawed randomized controlled trials. Occipital nerve stimulation has also been used successfully for medically refractory migraine and cluster headaches and for refractory headache in those with the Chiari malformation.[58–60] Stimulation of the peripheral branches of the trigeminal nerve has been used for the treatment of postherpetic neuralgia, posttraumatic trigeminal neuropathic pain, and idiopathic facial pain (Fig. 82.17).[61] Lead migration is the most common complication with these devices. Chapter 74 provides a more detailed discussion of peripheral nerve stimulation.

CONCLUSION

When noninvasive treatment is no longer effective, minimally invasive blocks can be incorporated into the treatment of head and neck pain. Knowledge of the relevant anatomy is key and will increase the success of the block as well as decrease potential complications. Neuromodulation should be considered for the most refractory cases.

KEY POINTS

- Branches of the trigeminal nerve can be blocked blindly or with fluoroscopic guidance. The trigeminal nerve can be blocked with ultrasound.
- The sphenopalatine ganglion can be blocked intranasally or through a fluoroscopy-guided infrazygomatic approach.
- The occipital nerve can be blocked blindly lateral to the greater occipital protuberance. With ultrasound, it can be blocked at the nape at the region of the oblique capitis muscle.
- The GN lies in close proximity to the vagus and spinal accessory nerve. As such, the extraoral approach to blocking this nerve is associated with more complications.
- A deep cervical plexus block results in both motor and sensory blockade, whereas a sensory block is associated with blockage of the superficial cervical plexus only.

REFERENCES

Access the reference list online at ExpertConsult.com.

CHAPTER 83

Truncal Blocks: Paravertebral, Intercostal, Pectoral Nerve, Suprascapular, Ilioinguinal, Iliohypogastric Nerve, and Transversus Abdominis Plane Blocks

Rohit Rahangdale, MD ◎ Luminita Tureanu, MD ◎ Honorio T. Benzon, MD

Truncal blocks are commonly employed for perioperative and chronic pain management. In this chapter, we will describe paravertebral (PV), intercostal, and transversus abdominis plane (TAP) blocks. The interpleural block will not be reviewed since this block is rarely used today. Pectoral nerve blocks appear to be promising for perioperative and chronic pain control, and will be analyzed. Suprascapular, ilioinguinal, and iliohypogastric nerve blocks will also be discussed since they are used to relieve pain in the trunk. In our discussions, comments on efficacy of the blocks, especially in the perioperative setting, will be minimal, and focus will be placed on the performance of the block.

PARAVERTEBRAL BLOCK

Regional anesthetic techniques involving truncal neural blockade have enjoyed a resurgence in recent years, particularly with the introduction of ultrasound guidance techniques. PV blocks, when compared to epidural analgesia for patients undergoing thoracotomy, demonstrated no difference in opioid consumption or pain scores at 4–8, 24, and 48 hours, with fewer side effects including pulmonary complications, hypotension, urinary retention, and nausea and vomiting. Rates of failed blocks and complication rates were lower as well.[1]

ANATOMY

The PV space is a wedge-shaped area adjacent to the vertebral column that contains the sympathetic chain, the dorsal and ventral (intercostal) roots of the spinal nerve, the white rami communicantes, as well as fatty tissue and intercostal vessels (Fig. 83.1). The base of the wedge constitutes the medial border of the PV space and is formed by the vertebral body and the intervertebral disc where there is communication with the epidural space via the intervertebral foramen. The posterior border of the PV space is the superior costotransverse ligament, which extends laterally to become continuous with the aponeurosis of the internal intercostal muscle. This internal intercostal membrane runs between the ribs, whereas the superior costotransverse ligament runs from the inferior border of the transverse process (TP) above to the superior border of the rib tubercle below. As the wedge tapers off laterally, it is continuous with the intercostal space. Anterior and lateral to the PV space is the parietal pleura. Within the PV space, the spinal nerves themselves do not have a fascial sheath and are easily susceptible to local anesthetic blockade. However, there is the endothoracic fascia, which is the deep investing fascia of the thoracic cavity, within the PV space, which can affect the spread of injected solutions.[2]

TECHNIQUES

Conventional Technique

Conventional techniques have described a loss-of-resistance approach to reach the PV space. A small-gauge Tuohy needle is inserted 2.5 cm lateral to the superior edge of the spinous process perpendicular to all planes, and is advanced until contact is made with the TP. The needle is then withdrawn to the skin, redirected caudad or cephalad by 15 degrees and advanced deep to the superior costotransverse ligament at which point a loss of resistance is achieved. To avoid pleural puncture, the needle is advanced 1 cm (and no further than 1.5 cm) past the point at which the TP was contacted. It is best to avoid medial angulation of the needle to minimize the risk of local anesthetic injection into a dural sleeve. It is also prudent to avoid lateral angulation given that the PV space is narrower laterally, increasing the risk of pleural puncture.

Ultrasound Guidance Technique

The addition of ultrasound guidance has been used to facilitate the thoracic PV in determining needle insertion sites, depth to TP and pleura, and needle tip location. A linear,

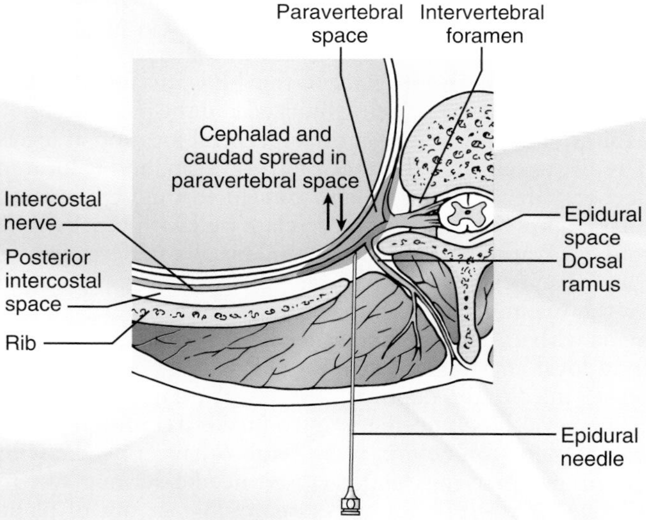

FIG. 83.1 The paravertebral space is contiguous with surrounding spaces. *Arrows* depict the spread of local anesthetic to the intercostal, epidural, and inferior and superior paravertebral spaces. (*From Chan VW, Ferrante FM: Continuous thoracic paravertebral block. In: Ferrante FM, Vade Boncoeur TR, editors:* Postoperative Pain Management, *New York: Churchill-Livingstone, 1993, p 408.*)

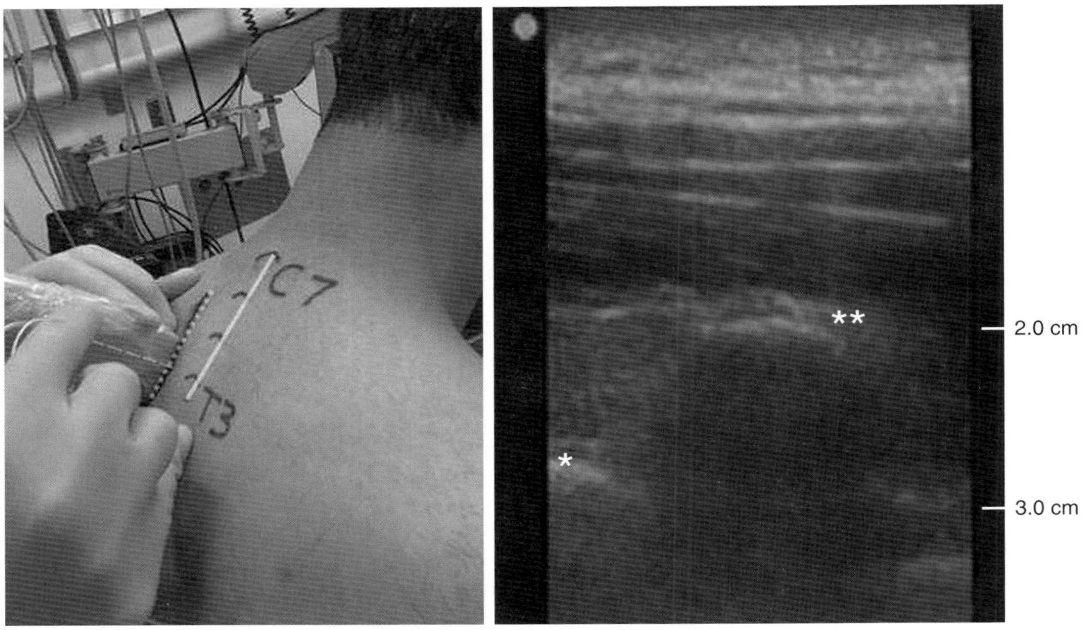

FIG. 83.2 Paravertebral block. Solid line, Midline of spinous process; dashed line represents 2.5 cm lateral of midline; *, parietal pleura; **, transverse process.

high-frequency probe can be used, and in some instances, a curvilinear probe may offer a better approach to the PV space. Several major ultrasound-guided approaches have been described.

One approach utilizes ultrasound primarily to identify the TP. Once the TP is contacted under ultrasound guidance, the conventional loss-of-resistance technique is utilized. To visualize the TP, the ultrasound probe is placed in a longitudinal parasagittal plane 2.5 cm from the midline. Generally, a 5- to 10-degree tilt laterally is needed to best visualize the TP, which appears as a concave hyperechoic structure approximately 1 cm wide with anechoic space deep to it. This is commonly referred to as a "thumbprint sign." The parietal pleura can be visualized approximately 1 cm deep to the TP on either side as a sharp hyperechoic line (Fig. 83.2). The distance to the TP is variable depending on the level that is being blocked and the patient's body habitus. The TP is at its most superficial location at levels T3–T5, usually at a distance of 1.5–2.5 cm, and is located deeper at levels cephalad and caudad to this. Ultrasound imaging has been shown to correlate well with the distance to the TP and the PV space,[3,4] and usually underestimates these distances by 0.3–0.7 mm due to skin compression by the scanning head. Initial contact with the TP can be made with a 22-gauge finder needle that can serve to infiltrate local anesthetic. Once the TP is contacted with the seeker needle, the depth is noted, and a Tuohy needle or blunt-bevel block needle is introduced. To minimize the risk of pleural puncture, it is useful to have a needle with centimeter markings and a closed needle-syringe system relative to atmospheric pressure. Using an out-of-plane needle approach and similar to the conventional technique, the TP process is contacted and then redirected caudad 1 cm (and no more than 1.5 cm) past the TP. Loss of resistance to saline is confirmed and local anesthetic injection is performed by an assistant with intermittent aspiration while maintaining ultrasound visualization. It is important to note that loss of resistance can be very subtle and does not invariably occur. With ultrasound, downward movement of the parietal pleura is visualized as confirmation of correct local anesthetic placement. If a Tuohy needle was used, a catheter may be placed while maintaining lateral or cephalad needle tip orientation. One should expect slight resistance while passing the catheter. If no resistance is encountered, it is possible that the needle tip is in the intrapleural space.

Another approach is a slight variation of the first and utilizes an in-plane or out-of-plane approach to the PV space.[5] The probe is in the identical longitudinal parasagittal plane as described above and the PV space is approached directly without first contacting the TP process. In utilizing this approach, precise needle tip visualization is important. If the needle tip is difficult to visualize, local anesthetic or saline can be injected incrementally to track needle tip advancement by hydrodissection. Again, a "pop" may be felt when the posterior costotransverse ligament is traversed with a corresponding loss of resistance.

Still another approach, the TP is initially imaged with a similar longitudinal parasagittal view, and the probe is then rotated obliquely to allow for the best view of the posterior costotransverse ligament and the PV wedge. The needle is advanced carefully utilizing an in-plane needle approach (Fig. 83.3).[6,7]

In an excellent review with elegant illustrations, Krediet et al. discussed the different approaches to PV block.[8] The ultrasound is either placed in transverse or parasagittal direction with the needle either in-plane or out-of-plane. The "lateral approach" is aimed close to the tip of the TP or inbetween the ribs while the "medial approach" is performed medial to the costotransverse joint. The anatomical landmarks of all the approaches are the same: TP, rib, and pleura. For the novice, the authors recommended a parasagittal position of the

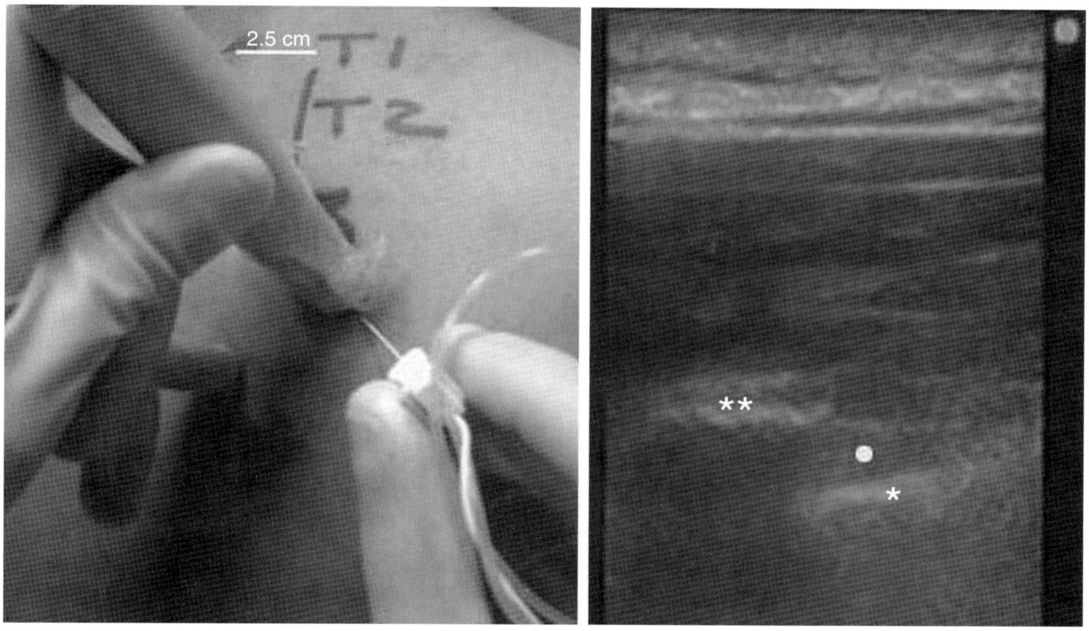

FIG. 83.3 Paravertebral block. *, parietal pleura; **, transverse process; *dot*, paravertebral space.

transducer 2 cm lateral to the midline. An in-plane approach may require a steep angle of needle insertion due to the small distance between the adjacent TPs. Therefore, sometimes an out-of-plane approach may be necessary. For skilled practitioners, an in-plane transverse technique is an option. The needle is passed using an in-plane lateral to medial approach with the needle tip passing through the internal intercostal membrane. The final injection point is typically at the junction of the intercostal and PV spaces immediately ventrolateral to the tip of the corresponding TP. This approach allows for excellent needle visualization because it is typically more lateral than the parasagittal approach, and thus more superficial. However, if this technique is performed using a more medial injection site, where the PV space is larger, there are the associated increased risks of epidural or intrathecal spread, which the practitioner must consider.

The presence of the endothoracic fascia within the PV space can affect spread of injected solutions, and therefore some authors have suggested nerve stimulation in addition to the loss of resistance technique. Nerve stimulation can allow for more accurate placement of local anesthetic within the PV space; that is, anterior to the endothoracic fascia.[9,10] Additionally, by injecting in this anterior location within the PV space, better craniocaudal spread in the PV "gutter" may be achieved and the need for multiple level injections obviated. This technique has not been studied in conjunction with ultrasound use. Conversely, other experts have argued that needle readjustment within the PV space may lead to a higher incidence of intravascular injections and pneumothorax,[11] and that multiple-level PV injections allow for true graduated dosing of local anesthetic, and result in a more reliable spread of injectate within the PV space.[12]

DOSING

A single injection of 15 mL can be expected to provide analgesia over 3–4.6 dermatomes in the thoracic region.[12] Spread is initially at the level of injection and along the intercostal nerve, and progresses in the PV "gutter" to cover one dermatome above and two dermatomes below. Most studies have shown a preferential caudad spread of injectate.[12] Analgesia typically ranges from 6 to 12 hours for a single injection. If a catheter is placed, infusion of ropivacaine 0.2%–0.5% at rates of 4–8 mL/h may be used. Blood levels are similar to those seen with an epidural catheter.

COMPLICATIONS

Pneumothorax is estimated to occur in up to 0.5% of patients, yet most are not clinically significant and can be managed conservatively. Contrary to popular belief, violation of the parietal pleura does not result in aspiration of air unless the visceral pleura is also punctured or atmospheric air has entered the thoracic cavity. Instead, most patients will present with a sudden irritating cough or sharp pain in the chest. If the parietal pleura is violated, the block can be converted to an intrapleural block. It is important to remember that loss of resistance is not a consistent sign of entry into the PV space, and it is in these patients that ultrasound guidance should be of particular value. Also of note, patients with previous thoracotomy may have adhesions in the PV space, making PV catheter placement difficult.[9]

Life-threatening complications from PV blocks have occurred as a result of bolus dosing. A bolus dose can accidentally be injected into the intrathecal or epidural space, or into a blood vessel. Many authors have argued that it is bolus dosing with subsequent intrathecal or intravascular spread—and not pneumothorax—that is the greatest risk associated with this procedure.[13] Unilateral epidural spread is known to occur in 70% of patients; however, the majority of injectate remains confined to the PV and intercostal spaces.[14,15] Bilateral epidural spread can occur through the ipsilateral epidural space or the prevertebral space and is usually associated with bolus dosing or medial angulation of the needle. Vascular puncture has been reported to occur in up to 3.8% of patients.[14] Thus, graduated dosing either through a catheter or multiple injection points is recommended. Placement of PV blocks in the anticoagulated patient remains controversial and should probably be avoided, given that the space is in direct communication with the epidural space and not compressible.

INTERCOSTAL NERVE BLOCK

In patients with spinal anomalies, trauma, or previous spine surgery that have altered epidural or PV anatomy, intercostal blocks can be used to provide chest wall analgesia.

ANATOMY

As nerves leave the PV space, they enter the intercostal space and lie between the innermost intercostal muscle and the pleura. Lateral to the PV muscles, the prominent angles of the ribs are palpable as the primary landmark for intercostal nerve block. At the angle of the rib, the nerve lies between the innermost intercostal muscle and the inner intercostal muscle. Also, at this location, the thickness of the rib is approximately 8 mm and the costal groove is known to be the widest.[15] Classically, the intercostal nerves have been thought to lie caudad to the intercostal vein and artery, on the inferior portion of the rib. However, a cadaver study found that the intercostal nerve remained in a classic subcostal position only 17% of the time.[16] It was shown to be in a midcostal location most frequently (73%), and it was supracostal in some cadavers (10%). The intercostal nerves are the primary rami of thoracic nerves T1–T11. Most of the T1 nerve fibers combine with C8 to form the lower trunk of the brachial plexus. Fibers from T2 and T3 form the intercostobrachial nerve that supplies the upper chest wall along with cervical fibers from the brachial plexus. Intercostal nerves T4–T11 supply the thoracoabdominal wall from the nipple line to below the umbilicus. The T12 nerve is actually a subcostal nerve that contributes branches to the iliohypogastric and ilioinguinal nerves.[17]

TECHNIQUE

The ideal patient position is prone, with a pillow under the abdomen and both upper extremities hanging over the sides of the table, which maximizes retraction of the scapulae away from the upper ribs. This allows for bilateral blockade and posterior access to the angles of the ribs to enhance safety and success of the procedure. The lateral decubitus position is also quite satisfactory for unilateral blockade after rib fractures and lateral thoracotomy, as well as for chest tube placement. The supine position may also be utilized for bilateral block at the level of the midaxillary line; however, the rib and intercostal space are narrower here.

Classic techniques have described locating the angle of the rib (~8 cm lateral to the midline) and using a 22-gauge, short-bevel needle to walk off 3-mm deep to the lower costal margin, and repeating this at the desired levels. More recently, ultrasound-guided approaches have been proposed.[18,19] Ultrasound imaging is used to identify the space between the internal and innermost intercostal muscles 8 cm lateral to the spinous process, and D5W or saline can be injected to confirm needle tip position in the fascial plane and anterior pleural displacement. In a case report by Ben-Ari et al. the intercostal space was identified as described above, followed by placement of 19-gauge, wire-bound catheters.[18] The catheters were then advanced 7 cm to the PV space, achieving a spread of five dermatomes.

DOSING AND COMPLICATIONS

A single-shot intercostal block can be expected to provide analgesia for only 6–8 hours. Perineural catheter placement can provide for longer-lasting analgesia, and as described above the catheter can be advanced into the PV space. Total spinal anesthesia by injection into a dural sleeve is a rare but dangerous complication.[20] Local anesthesia toxicity as a result of bolus dosing may occur due to rapid uptake from the well-vascularized intercostal space. Also, pneumothorax and liver subcapsular hematoma formation are potential complications. Ultrasound guidance may aid in maintaining better needle tip control and minimizing the occurrence of these complications.

PECTORAL NERVE BLOCKS

Pectoral nerve blocks, also known as Pecs blocks, are suited for perioperative pain control and management of chronic pain after breast surgery. The blocks were initially described by Blanco et al. It consists of the Pecs block type I and type II blocks.[21,22] The type I block appears to be suited for breast expander surgery and prosthesis insertion, when the pectoralis minor muscle is mainly affected. The type II block is employed for mastectomy and axillary dissection since the long thoracic and thoracodorsal nerves are involved.[23] Another block, the serratus fascial plane block, was described to block the thoracic intercostal nerves primarily and provide analgesia to the lateral part of the thorax.[24]

ANATOMY

The pectoralis major muscle inserts superiorly into the inferior clavicle, supero-laterally into the proximal humerus, and medially into the sternum. It extends down to the seventh rib. The pectoralis minor muscle inserts supero-laterally into the coracoid process of the scapula and infero-medially into the third, fourth, and fifth ribs. The innervation for the pectoralis major comes from C5 to T1. The lateral and medial pectoral nerves, which branch off the brachial plexus, innervate the pectoralis major. They course between the pectoralis major and minor muscles after branching from the brachial plexus.[25]

TECHNIQUE

The original technique of the Pecs type I block involves insertion of the needle into the fascial plane between the pectoralis major and minor muscles (Fig. 83.4). The ultrasound probe is placed below the clavicle, similar to an infraclavicular nerve block. The pectoral branch of the thoraco-acromial artery is identified. As the lateral pectoral nerve is consistently located adjacent to the artery, 10 mL of local anesthetic (e.g., 0.25% bupivacaine) is injected in the area.[21] A variation of the original approach involves placement of the ultrasound probe below the outer third of the clavicle, transverse to the axis of the body (Fig. 83.5A).[26] As in the original approach, the pectoralis major and minor muscles, and the thoracic-acromial artery and cephalic vein are identified. The needle is inserted in-plane, from medial to lateral direction, until the tip is in the interpectoral plane. Advantages of this approach include decreased incidence of vascular and pleural puncture and easier identification of the lateral border of the pectoralis minor muscle.

The Pecs type II block was designed to block the intercostobrachial; third, fourth, and fifth intercostal nerves, and the long thoracic nerves. In this approach, the ultrasound probe placement is placed similar to the Pecs I block. The probe is moved towards the axilla until the serratus anterior muscle is identified above the second, third, and fourth ribs. The needle is inserted into the fascial plane between the pectoralis minor muscle and serratus anterior muscle; 20 mL of local anesthetic is injected (see Fig. 83.5B). In the serratus facial plane block, the ultrasound probe is placed over the midclavicular region in a sagittal plane. At the level of the fifth rib in the midaxillary line, a 22-G 50-mm needle is inserted in-plane and the tip placed into the plane between the more superficial latissimus dorsi and the serratus anterior muscle. A total of 20–25 mL of local anesthetic is injected between the two muscles and deep to the serratus anterior muscle, before the external intercostal muscle.[24]

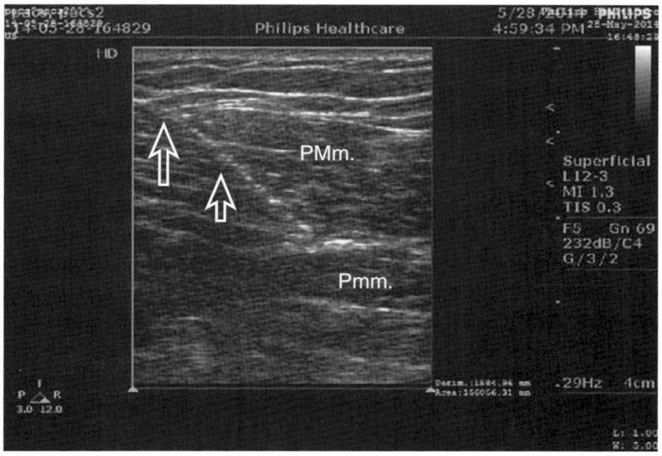

FIG. 83.4 Pectoralis (Pecs) type I block showing the needle tip in the fascial plane between the pectoralis major and minor muscles. *PMm,* Pectoralis major muscles; *Pmm,* pectoralis minor muscles. (*Reprinted with permission from Bashandy GM, Abbas DN: Pectoral nerves I and II blocks in multimodal analgesia for breast cancer surgery. A randomized clinical trial.* Reg Anesth Pain Med. *40:68-74, 2015.*)

CLINICAL APPLICATIONS

The Pecs I block has been employed effectively to manage pain after submuscular insertion of breast tissue expanders or after breast augmentation.[25] The Pecs I and II blocks were found to be better than PV blocks, in terms of pain scores and postoperative morphine consumption, after modified radical mastectomy.[23] The Pecs I and II blocks were also noted to be beneficial after unilateral modified radical mastectomy. Compared to a control group, the blocks resulted in diminished intraoperative fentanyl requirements, lower pain scores, less postoperative morphine consumption, decreased incidence of postoperative nausea and vomiting, and shorter postanesthesia care unit

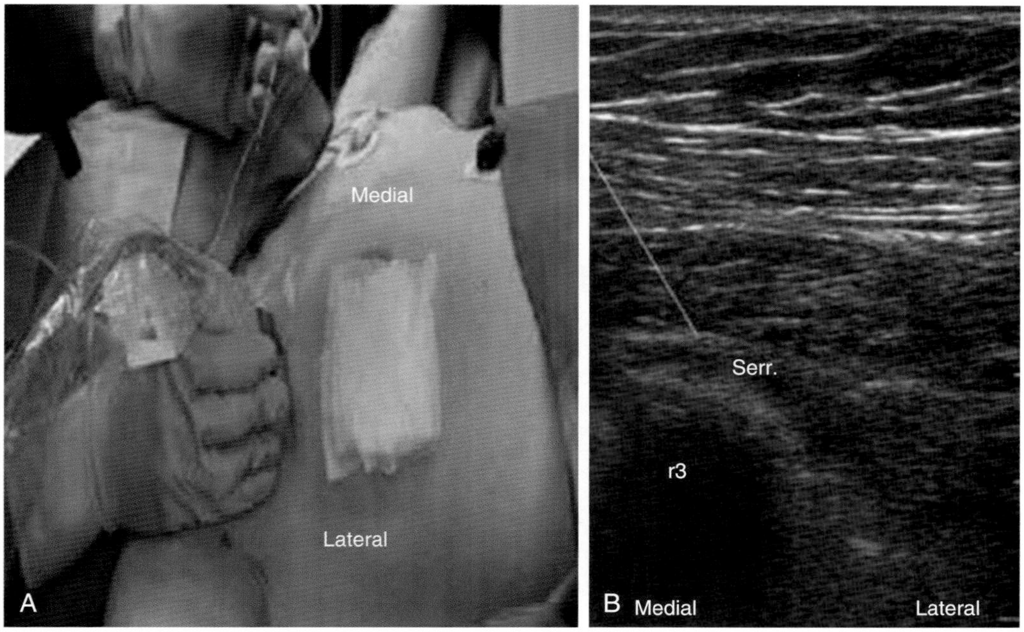

FIG. 83.5 Pectoralis (Pecs) type I block. (A) Image showing the ultrasound probe position. (B) Image showing needle placement with the tip below the pectoralis minor and above the serratus anterior. *r3,* Third rib; *Serr,* serratus anterior muscle. (*Reprinted with permission from Bashandy GM, Abbas DN: Pectoral nerves I and II blocks in multimodal analgesia for breast cancer surgery. A randomized clinical trial.* Reg Anesth Pain Med. *40:68-74, 2015.*)

and hospital stays.[27] At the present time, more definitive studies on the Pecs I and II and serratus plane blocks for breast surgery are ongoing. Although definitive evidence is lacking, the blocks offer a new modality in the perioperative care of patients who undergo breast surgery.

SUPRASCAPULAR NERVE BLOCKS

Suprascapular nerve block (SSNB) is indicated for relief of acute and chronic pain in the shoulder, which may be due to bursitis, capsular tear, periarthritis, or arthritis. Its use in recalcitrant shoulder pain secondary to malignancy has been recently reported as well.[28] In a study of 34 patients with frozen shoulder, the patients received a series of three weekly SSNBs using 10 mL 0.5% bupivacaine or saline. A 64% reduction in the McGill Pain Questionnaire multidimensional pain descriptors score was observed in the treatment group, versus 13% in the placebo group, after 1 month.[28] In another randomized controlled trial, 83 patients with chronic shoulder pain due to arthritis received a single SSNB, for a total of 108 affected shoulders, using either 10 mL of 0.5% bupivacaine with 40 mg of methylprednisolone acetate or saline. Clinically significant improvements in all VAS pain scores, the shoulder pain disability index, the Short Form-36, and in some range of movement scores were seen at weeks 1, 4, and 12 in the treatment group compared to placebo.[29] In conjunction with physical therapy, the SSNB increases the range of motion of the involved shoulder. In a prospective, randomized controlled trial where ultrasound-guided pulse radiofrequency ablation of SSN was performed in patients with adhesive capsulitis, the intervention group had significantly greater improvement in pain and disability scores, and range of motion.[30]

When SSNB was compared with interscalene nerve block for shoulder arthroscopy in a prospective, randomized, blind study, the SSNB was found to be an appropriate alternative.[31] SSNB was used as a method of preemptive analgesia in patients who had various arthroscopic surgeries, and provided significant benefits on days 1–3 after surgery.[32] More recently, the SSNB has been used in conjunction with axillary nerve block to provide shoulder anesthesia and analgesia for shoulder surgery, including total shoulder arthroplasty.[33,34]

ANATOMY

The suprascapular nerve originates from the superior trunk of the brachial plexus (C4–C6), crosses the posterior triangle of the neck, and passes deep to the trapezius muscle. The nerve traverses the suprascapular notch and descends deep to the supraspinatus and the infraspinatus muscles, supplying the two muscles and about 70% of the shoulder joint. Sensory innervation includes the posterior and posterosuperior regions of the shoulder joint and capsule, and the acromioclavicular joint.

TECHNIQUE

The patient is positioned sitting, preferably with the arms folded across the abdomen. A line is drawn along the spine of the scapula from the tip of the acromion to the scapular border. The midpoint of this line is noted, and a vertical line, parallel to the vertebral spine, is drawn through it. The angle of the upper outer quadrant is bisected with a line; the site of insertion of the needle is 2.5 cm from the apex of the angle. A 3-inch (7.5-cm), 22-gauge needle is inserted perpendicular to the skin in all planes. After contacting bone (i.e., the area surrounding the suprascapular notch) at approximately 5–6.5 cm, the needle is slightly withdrawn and redirected as needed until it slides into the notch. Up to 10 mL of local anesthetic is injected. No skin analgesia results from the block. Weakness of external shoulder rotation also confirms a successful block.[35] Pneumothorax may occur in less than 1% of cases.

A modified lateral approach has been described as well.[36] In this technique, the point of insertion was determined in the angle of the lateral end of the clavicle, acromion, and the spine of the scapula. The needle is directed towards the medial, dorsal, and caudad direction. The entire supraspinous fossa is filled with 5–10 mL of local anesthetic.[36] Various guidance modalities, including fluoroscopy, fluoroscopy with nerve stimulation, computed tomography guidance, and real-time ultrasound guidance have all been used. The ultrasound technique is less expensive, is readily available, and is devoid of radiation exposure for both personnel and patient.

ULTRASOUND GUIDANCE

The patient is positioned sitting. A high-frequency ultrasound probe is placed over the scapular spine in transverse orientation, and the suprascapular fossa with the supraspinatus muscle above it are scanned. Slight lateral movement will bring into view the suprascapular notch. The SSN is visualized as a hyperechoic structure beneath the transverse scapular ligament in the suprascapular notch (Fig. 83.6).[37] High-frequency ultrasound has also been used to evaluate the suprascapular notch. The superior scapular ligament and the artery-vein complex, using color Doppler, were also visualized, in 96% and 86% of volunteers, respectively.[38]

A new ultrasound-guided approach has been described by Siegenthaler et al. where the SSN is visualized in the supraclavicular region, under the omohyoid muscle. Of note in this location, the SSN is in close proximity to the brachial plexus and the pleura.[39]

ILIOINGUINAL AND ILIOHYPOGASTRIC NERVE BLOCKS

Ilioinguinal and iliohypogastric nerve blocks may be used in the diagnosis and treatment of chronic suprapubic and inguinal pain after lower abdominal surgery or hernia repair. They may be combined with genitofemoral nerve block. These blocks may be applied in the management of patients with neuralgias and nerve entrapment syndromes. Iliohypogastric and ilioinguinal nerve blocks are also important components of regional anesthesia of the inguinal region, typically performed for inguinal herniorrhaphy. In a recent randomized, controlled, double blind study of 60 male patients, Baerentzen et al. showed that when ultrasound-guided nerve blocks were performed for postoperative analgesia, they resulted in a statistically

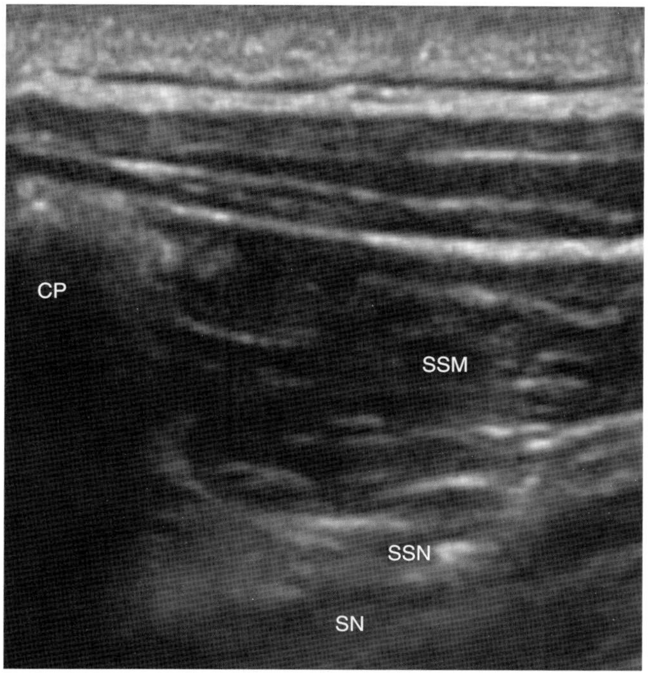

FIG. 83.6 Ultrasonography of the suprascapular nerve. *CP*, Coracoid process; *SN*, suprascapular notch; *SSM*, supraspinatus muscle; *SSN*, suprascapular nerve.

significant decrease in pain scores in the postanesthesia care unit (PACU), both at rest and with movement.[40] Bilateral ilioinguinal nerve block with 0.5% bupivacaine also decreased analgesic requirements and pain scores for 24 hours after cesarean sections performed under general anesthesia.[41] A recent randomized, double-blind, placebo-controlled trial also showed that in patients postcesarean section, bilateral ilioinguinal iliohypogastric blocks using a multilevel technique were able to decrease their morphine consumption; however, there was no reduction in the opioid-related side effects.[42] These blocks do not provide visceral analgesia.

ANATOMY

The iliohypogastric (T12–L1) and ilioinguinal (L1) nerves emerge from the lateral border of the psoas major muscle, travel around the abdominal wall, and penetrate the transverse abdominal and the internal oblique muscles to innervate the hypogastric and inguinal areas. The anterior cutaneous branch of the iliohypogastric nerve passes through the internal oblique muscle just medial to the anterior superior iliac spine (ASIS) to lie next to the external oblique muscle. It then passes through the external oblique above the superficial inguinal ring, and supplies the suprapubic area. The ilioinguinal nerve remains between the deeper two muscle layers; it travels through the inguinal canal and supplies the upper medial thigh and superior inguinal region. An effective block of both nerves performed medial to the ASIS must be made at multiple depths, in various fascial planes. The genitofemoral (L1–L2) nerve passes through and along the anterior surface of the psoas major muscle, and it divides into genital and femoral branches above the inguinal ligament. Its genital branch travels with the spermatic cord and innervates the genitalia inferior to the area supplied by the ilioinguinal nerve.

TECHNIQUE

The patient is positioned supine, with a pillow under knees. The primary anatomic landmark is the ASIS, identified by palpation. The injection site is about 2 inches medial and 2 inches cephalad to the ASIS. A 25-gauge, 1.5-inch needle is inserted perpendicular to the skin, noting the double pop feeling when each layer of fascia is penetrated. Infiltration with about 10 mL of local anesthetic is performed at each depth and, subsequently, fanned in the area. Supplemental infiltration of the incision and/or field block may be needed for surgery of the inguinal region. The genital branch of the genitofemoral nerve block can be blocked by the infiltration of 5–10 mL of local anesthetic, using a 25-gauge, 1.5-inch needle inserted just lateral to the pubic tubercle and below the inguinal ligament. Infiltration around the spermatic cord at its exit from the inguinal canal is also an effective technique.[43]

Using anatomic landmarks in the setting of what is rather a field block can lead to variable results, not to mention the risk of visceral perforation in thin patients, especially in children.[44]

Ultrasound guidance allows a precise localization of nerves and surrounding sonoanatomy, the visualization of injectate spread and increased safety with visualization of the peritoneum, bowels, and vascular structures. Schmutz et al. showed that these nerves cannot be blocked selectively under ultrasound guidance, even when small volumes are used.[45] Ultrasound-guided approaches have been described both in children[46] and adults.[47] In a cadaver study, Eichenberger et al. had a simulated block success rate of 95%, when the nerves were targeted at 5 cm cranial and posterior to the ASIS.[48] Ultrasound guidance also allowed for finding the optimal local anesthetic volume needed for this block, of only 0.075 mL/kg.[49] The use of ultrasound-guided serial ilioinguinal nerve blocks has been recently reported for the treatment of chronic inguinal neuralgia in adolescents.[50] However, in a 2012 randomized, double bind, placebo-controlled study, Bichoff et al. found that blocking these nerves under ultrasound guidance did not make a difference in either the diagnosis or treatment of chronic inguinal postherniorrhaphy pain.[51]

ULTRASOUND GUIDANCE

The patient is positioned supine, and a high-frequency ultrasound probe is placed superior and medial to the ASIS, on an imaginary line uniting the ASIS and the umbilicus. The nerves are usually visualized between the internal oblique and transversus muscles. An in-plane technique provides optimal access to the ilioinguinal and iliohypogastric nerves; hydrodissection may be useful to better delineate the narrow fascial plane. Small vessels, including the deep circumflex iliac artery, identified with color Doppler, may be present in the fascial plane. Deep to the transversus muscle the parietal peritoneum and bowel can be identified (Fig. 83.7).

COMPLICATIONS

A few complications can occur with these blocks, including ecchymosis, hematoma, visceral perforation, local anesthetic toxicity, and infection. Accidental block of the lateral femoral cutaneous nerve and partial block of the femoral nerve may also occur.

TRANSVERSUS ABDOMINIS PLANE BLOCK

ANATOMY

The TAP block, first described by McDonnell in 2007, uses anatomic landmarks to approach the plane through the triangle of Petit.[52] The triangle of Petit is bordered by latissimus dorsi posteriorly, the external oblique muscle anteriorly, and the ASIS as the base of the triangle. The innervation of the anterior abdominal wall is provided by the anterior rami of the T7–T12 and L1 nerves, whose terminal branches are coursing in the fascial plane between the internal oblique and the transversus abdominis muscle, the TAP.

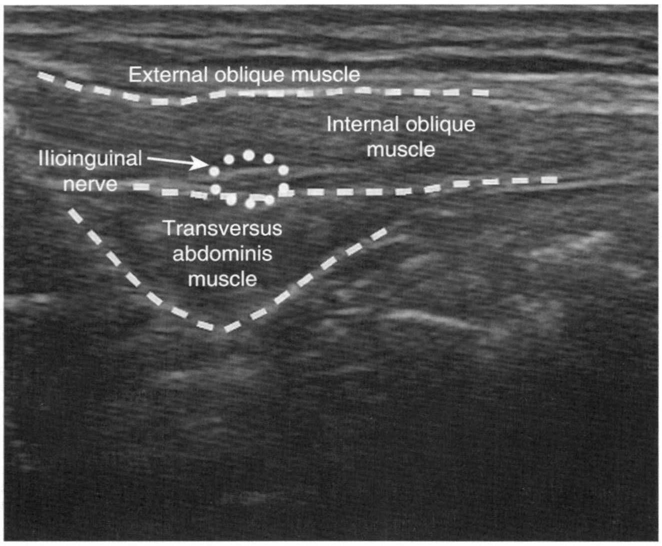

FIG. 83.7 Ultrasonography of the ilioinguinal nerve.

TECHNIQUE

Using anatomic landmarks, the TAP is accessed through the triangle of Petit. A "double-pop" technique is used to confirm the needle passage through the external oblique fascia, followed by the passage through the fascial plane between the internal oblique and the transversus abdominis muscles.

ULTRASOUND GUIDANCE

The three muscle layers, the external oblique, internal oblique, and transversus abdominis, and the needle insertion plane, between the internal oblique and transversus abdominis muscles, can be easily visualized when the probe is placed above the ASIS.[53]

An in-plane or out-of-plane technique can be used. Hydrodissection of the plane may facilitate accurate placement of the needle. Typically, 15–20 mL of local anesthetic are used on each side (Fig. 83.8).

Ultrasound-guided TAP blocks have been used to provide postoperative analgesia for lower abdominal surgeries, including inguinal hernia repair, open total abdominal hysterectomy,[54] cesarean section,[55] and retropubic prostatectomy.[56] A subcostal approach has been described for laparoscopic cholecystectomy.[57] It has also been used to provide postoperative analgesia for other upper abdominal surgeries, including laparoscopic surgeries, such as appendectomy and incisional hernia repair.[58]

Cadaver studies have confirmed T9–L1 spread,[59] and T9–T11 with the subcostal approach.[60] Radiologic studies have confirmed spread beyond the TAP into the PV and intercostal space. The TAP block is devoid of any hemodynamic effects, and provides no visceral analgesia.

Interestingly, Stoving et al. in a randomized, placebo-controlled trial in volunteers found that the cutaneous sensory block area was nondermatomal.[61] Instead, they noted

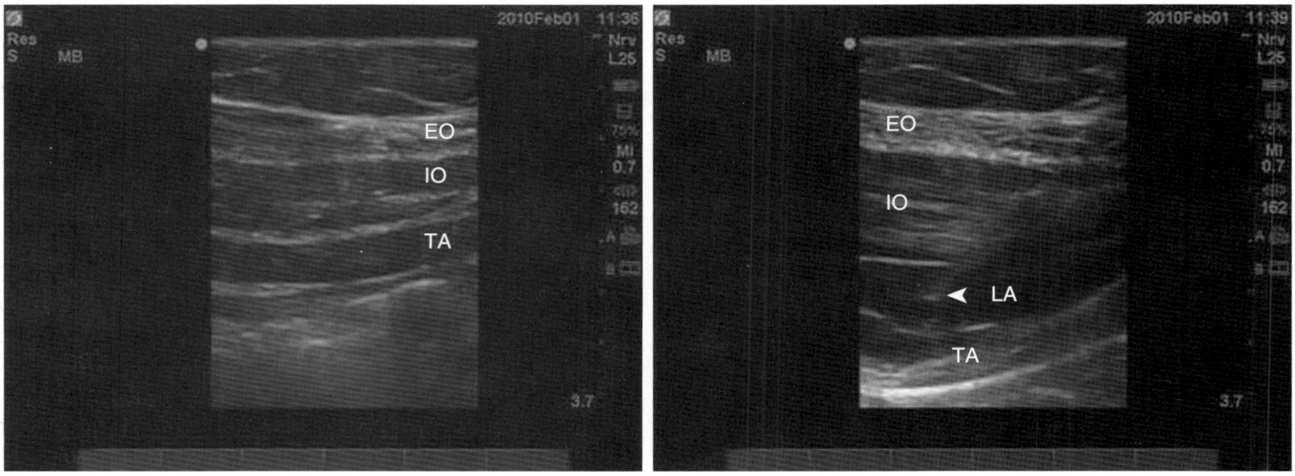

FIG. 83.8 Ultrasonography of the transversus abdominis plane. *EO*, External oblique muscle; *IO*, internal oblique muscle; *LA*, local anesthetic in transversus abdominis plane; *TA*, transversus abdominis muscle; *arrow*, needle tip in transversus abdominis plane.

a large caudal and lateral involvement, associated with significant muscle relaxation of the lateral abdominal wall, and with an average duration of 10 hours.

Continuous TAP block catheters have been used as part of multimodal analgesia for a variety of abdominal surgeries, with the sparing of opioids consumption and increased patient satisfaction.

A new application of TAP block has been described in chronic pancreatitis patients presenting with an acute flare, raising the question of possible coverage of visceral pain as well.[62]

Neurolytic TAP block with alcohol has been reported as being effective in three patients with chronic abdominal pain secondary to metastatic disease of the abdominal wall.[63] The volumes and concentrations of alcohol injected were 12 mL of 67% alcohol and 13 mL of 75% alcohol (the alcohol was diluted with local anesthetic) in patient 1; 25 mL of 60% alcohol in patient 2; and 15 mL of 33% in patient 3. Satisfactory pain control was attained for 50 days, 6 months, and 17 days, respectively, until the patients died.

KEY POINTS

- When compared to epidural analgesia for thoracotomy, PV blocks with catheters provide equipotent analgesia with a lower incidence of pulmonary complications, hypotension, urinary retention, nausea and vomiting, and failure rate.
- A single injection of 15 mL in the thoracic PV space can be expected to provide analgesia over 3–4.6 dermatomes, with a preferential caudad spread of the injectate.
- Ultrasound imaging usually underestimates the distance to the TP and PV space by 0.3–0.7 mm because of skin compression by the scanning head.
- Total spinal anesthesia by injection into a dural sleeve is a rare but dangerous complication of both PV and intercostal nerve blocks.
- Pecs nerve blocks type I and II appear to be effective in the management of pain after breast augmentation and in the perioperative management of unilateral radical mastectomy.
- SSNB has proven efficacy for significant pain relief and functional improvement in patients with shoulder arthritis or frozen shoulder.
- Ultrasound guided ilioinguinal nerve block does not seem to be effective in the diagnosis or treatment of chronic inguinal pain after hernia repair.
- The ultrasound-guided TAP block is an attractive component of multimodal analgesia for various abdominal and pelvic surgeries.
- Neurolytic TAP block may be effective in helping attain satisfactory pain control in patients with abdominal wall pain secondary to metastasis in the abdominal wall.

REFERENCES

Access the reference list online at ExpertConsult.com.

CHAPTER 84

Fluoroscopy and Ultrasound-Guided Sympathetic Blocks: Stellate Ganglion, Lumbar Sympathetic Blocks, and Visceral Sympathetic Blocks

Michael Gofeld, MD ◎ Hariharan Shankar, MD ◎ Honorio T. Benzon, MD

INTRODUCTION

Analgesic and neurolytic blockade of the autonomic (sympathetic) nervous system was introduced in the beginning of the previous century. The frequently observed autonomic phenomena in different acute and chronic painful conditions prompted physicians to investigate and invent methods of interruption of the sympathetic pathways with the purpose of alleviating chronic pain. Though the use of the paravertebral analgesic blockade was primarily developed for surgical anesthesia, the method was introduced for the diagnosis and treatment of visceral pain. Eventually, the definition of "paravertebral blockade" evolved. The interventions targeting sympathetic ganglia and nerves were christened as "the sympathetic nerve blocks."

The sympathetic blocks are anatomically subdivided according to the corresponding spinal segments, vis à vis cervical, thoracic, lumbar, and sacral. The abdominal autonomic ganglia (e.g., celiac, mesenteric) are surrounded by visceral and vascular structures and situated ventrally from the vertebral column; special analgesics and neurolytic techniques have been developed.

There has been confusion regarding the type and structure of nerve cells and fibers—the blockade of which produces an analgesic effect. While the efferents have strict dichotomy to preganglionic and postganglionic fibers, the afferents, bearing pain signals may or may not make ganglionic connections. Aside from the purely autonomic pathways, sensory sympathetic unmyelinated fibers accompany somatic nerves making connections with the prevertebral or cranial ganglia. Therefore, blockade of a large mixed somatic nerve would inevitably result in certain autonomic phenomena. The detailed discussion of the autonomic nervous system anatomy and taxonomy is beyond the scope of this chapter. It is sufficient to mention that either autonomic ganglia or traversing fibers are blocked; the end result is abolition of the sympathetic tone (e.g., vasodilation, dry skin or mucosa, increased temperature) and alleviation of the sympathetically maintained pain that is typically described in terms of burning, diffuse, and annoying.

STELLATE GANGLION AND CERVICAL SYMPATHETIC CHAIN BLOCKADE

Cervical sympathetic analgesic and neurolytic blockade are commonly used in the diagnosis and management of sympathetically mediated pain and vascular insufficiency of the upper extremities. In addition, the stellate ganglion block has been advocated for the treatment of a variety of medical conditions, such as phantom pain, postherpetic neuralgia, cancer pain, cardiac arrhythmias, orofacial pain, and vascular headache. Recently, cervical sympathetic blockade has been suggested as an effective method for the prevention and treatment of the cerebral vasospasm, as well as the posttraumatic stress disorder.[1]

The stellate ganglion, also known as the cervicothoracic ganglion, represents a fusion of the inferior cervical and first thoracic ganglions of the sympathetic trunk. It can be found in about 80% of the population. Anatomy and position of the stellate ganglion have been investigated by dissection, magnetic resonance imaging (MRI), and computed tomography (CT).[2–6] It is usually situated at the lateral border of the longus colli muscle anterior to the neck of the first rib. It lies posteriorly to the vertebral vessels and is separated from the cervical pleura by the suprapleural membrane inferiorly. It measures 1–2.5 cm long, about 1 cm wide, and 0.5 cm thick, and may be fusiform, triangular, or globular.

Although a C7 approach to stellate ganglion has been described, the blockade is routinely performed at the C6 level according to the following anatomic landmarks: prominent anterior tubercle of the transverse process (the Chassaignac's tubercle), cricoid cartilage, and carotid artery. Given that only traversing sympathetic fibers or middle cervical ganglia can be found at the C6 level, the procedure should more accurately be named the *cervical sympathetic block*. The middle cervical ganglion or traversing sympathetic fibers are located anterolateral to the belly of the longus colli muscle. Conceivably, such a "convenient" position makes it easily accessible for either the diagnostic or the therapeutic blockade.

Cervical sympathetic block has been traditionally performed as a surface anatomy-based (also known as a "blind") injection, even though fluoroscopic verification has been strongly recommended. Practitioners are typically taught to palpate Chassaignac's tubercle, gently retract the carotid artery, and then insert the needle paratracheally until it contacts bone surface. The needle is then withdrawn 1–5 mm, and a solution injected. This maneuver was assumed to be sufficient to position the needle outside the longus colli muscle, where the stellate ganglion was thought to be situated. However, this "blind" paratracheal injection technique has been associated with unreliable results and multiple side effects and complications, including intravascular injection, bleeding, temporary paralysis of the recurrent laryngeal nerve, discitis, and esophageal injury.

A "blind" injection at the C6 level on the left side may cause inadvertent esophageal puncture. Hematoma formation is likely related to penetration of the vascular thyroid gland or damage of the inferior thyroid artery.[7] Postprocedural hoarseness is attributable to an injury, although fortunately transient, of the recurrent laryngeal nerve.

Fluoroscopic guidance reduces overall risk associated with the "blind" technique. It has the advantage of identifying bony anatomy, although the anatomic position of the cervical sympathetic trunk (CST) may be only approximately correlated with the X-ray image. CST is completely surrounded by soft prevertebral tissues (e.g., longus colli muscle, fascia, carotid artery). Preliminary injection of a contrast agent should produce a "honey-comb" longitudinal spread along the longus colli muscle. Nevertheless, often the spread is rather intramuscular and inconsistent. Ostensibly, neither "blind" nor fluoroscopy-guided injection can guarantee a desirable result and prevent adverse outcomes.

Injection of local anesthetics at the C6 level has a long history and evolution, but the reliability of achieving blockade of the stellate ganglion has only recently been tested. The success or failure of the cervical sympathetic block is contingent on precise needle placement, and is therefore entirely dependent on the anatomic location of the CST and the thickness of the longus colli muscle. Several clinical and cadaver trials have been performed in an attempt to elucidate the pattern of spread when solutions are injected at the C6 level. These studies reported conflicting results. The discrepancies were probably related to differences in research design: cadavers versus live subjects, low volume versus high volume of injectate, and CT versus fluoroscopy control. One cadaver experiment was suggestive that only deposition of a solution into the prevertebral "interlaminar space" provides reliable spread to the stellate ganglion.[8] The cervical prevertebral fascia is attached to the base of the skull and extends over the prevertebral muscles (longus capitis, rectus capitis, and longus colli muscles) to the T4 vertebra, just beyond the longus colli muscle. This positioning of the fascia forms a plane along which the injected fluid can flow.

Although some anatomic and imaging studies indicate a subfascial position of the sympathetic chain, other sources relate the path of the CST to the suprafascial plane. Two published studies unequivocally demonstrated the true anatomical pathway of CST.[9,10] One utilized cadaver dissections and showed *subfascial* position of the stellate ganglion. This study described a highly variable thickness of the longus colli muscle, which may lead to failed "blind" injection.[9] The second study was designed as a step-by-step methodology validating of a new ultrasound-guided approach (described below); a *subfascial* position of the sympathetic trunk was discovered by three-dimensional (3D) ultrasonography and confirmed by cadaver dissections. In addition, this study measured the thickness of the longus colli muscle at the C6 level, and proved that the muscle is 2–10 times thicker than was previously suggested in the regional anesthesia literature.[10] As such, routine injection by the traditional method most certainly ends up as an intramuscular injection, although CST will be eventually blocked by an overflow or diffusion of the injectate. Even the CT guidance may not assure the precise needle position between fascial layers (Fig. 84.1).

Ultrasound guidance is a logical solution to ensure accurate injection when soft tissues are involved. Conspicuous muscles, fasciae, blood vessels, viscera, and bone surface make ultrasonography superior to fluoroscopy for image-guided CST block. In 1995, Kapral and colleagues described an ultrasound-guided technique in a case series.[11] Compared with "blind" injection, the authors found that the ultrasound-guided stellate ganglion block required a smaller quantity of local anesthetic (5 mL vs. 8 mL), was not associated with the formation of a hematoma (whereas three patients in the blind injection group had a hematoma), and produced a more rapid onset of Horner's syndrome. However, because tissue visualization was probably not feasible below the C7, the authors concluded that a local anesthetic depot was limited to the C4–C7 levels and speculated that the abolished sympathetic response in the upper extremity was not related to the blockade of the stellate ganglion *per se.* Their findings agreed with those published by Hogan and Erickson,[5] but these observations and conclusions have been refuted by Gofeld and colleagues, who observed the contrast agent spread between the C4 and T1 levels in all patients, occasionally reaching the T2 level.[10]

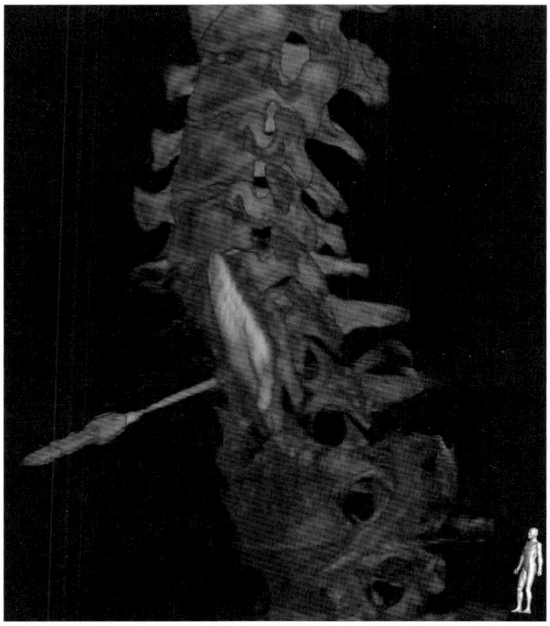

FIG. 84.1 Three-dimensional reconstruction of the stellate ganglion block. The contrast agent spread is intramuscular.

Shibata and colleagues were the first to suggest that subfascial injection would result in a better spread of the injectate and more reliable sympathetic blockade[12]; however, the published image in that study was more consistent with an intramuscular injection. Such an injection may be a limiting factor in the onset and spread of the blockade. In a study by Gofeld and colleagues, 5 mL of local anesthetic injected beneath the fascia, but superficial to the longus colli muscle, ensured consistent spread of the solution to the stellate ganglion.[10] More recently, experimental clinical studies endorsed the ultrasound-guided technique and found it superior to the fluoroscopy-controlled technique.

TECHNIQUE

There are two ultrasound-guided approaches to the CST: the modified "anterior" paratracheal out-of-plane

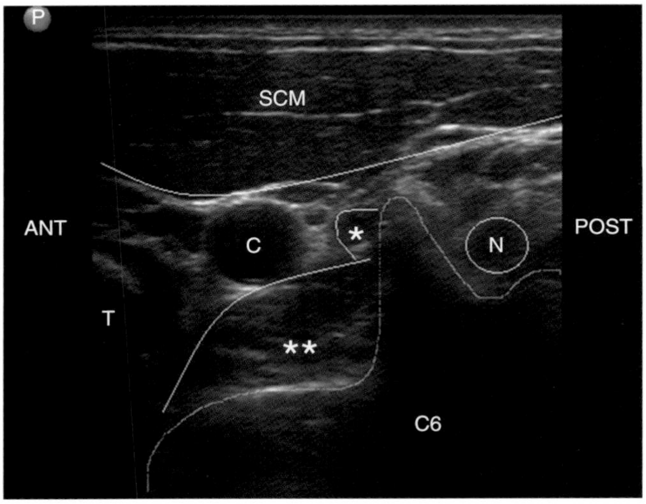

FIG. 84.2 Linear transducer positioned at the cricoid cartilage level *(right);* sonogram. *Asterisk*, longus capitis muscle; *C*, carotid artery; *C6*, C6 vertebra; *double asterisk*, longus colli muscle; *N*, exiting C6 nerve root; *SCM*, sternocleidomastoid muscle; *T*, trachea.

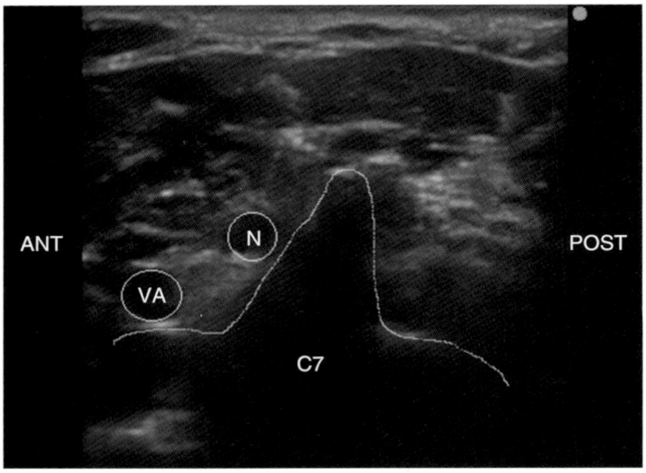

FIG. 84.3 Sonogram at C7 vertebral level. *C7*, C7 vertebral body; *N*, exiting C7 nerve root; *VA*, vertebral artery.

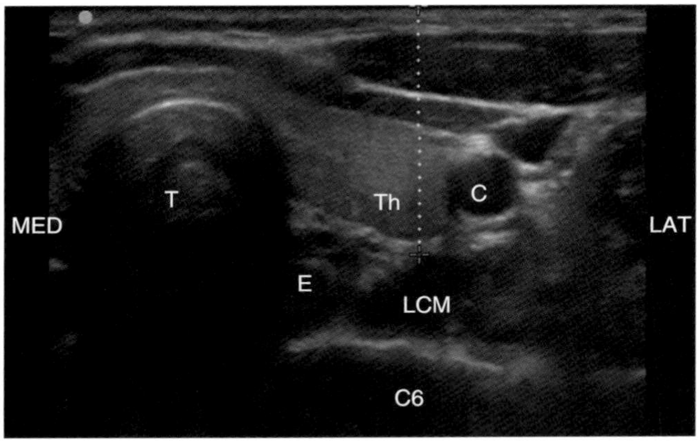

FIG. 84.4 Sonogram of anterior neck obtained with gentle transducer pressure. *C*, Carotid artery; *C6*, C6 vertebral body; *E*, esophagus; *LCM*, longus colli muscle; *Th*, thyroid gland; *T*, trachea; *white dotted line*, skin to target distance (2.2 cm).

approach, and the newer "lateral" in-plane method. Both techniques can be performed using either low-frequency curvilinear or high-frequency linear ultrasound transducers. Low-frequency sonography provides a wide-angle field of view and facilitates needle entry planning, while a high-frequency transducer allows better resolution of the pertinent anatomy and fascial planes.

Anterior Approach

The patient is positioned supine. A pillow can be placed under the lower neck to achieve an extension. The head may be slightly rotated contralaterally to the injection side, thereby increasing the distance between the carotid artery and trachea and improving the sonographic view. After skin preparation and dressing, sterile ultrasonic gel is applied. The transducer is covered by a sterile adhesive transparent dressing or sleeve. Ultrasonography of the anterior neck is performed with initial transducer placement at the level of the cricoid cartilage, anterior to the sternocleidomastoid muscle. Short-axis ultrasonography reveals the typical appearance of the C6 transverse process—the prominent anterior tubercle, the short posterior tubercle, and the exiting C6 nerve root (Fig. 84.2). Scanning caudally and dorsally brings the C7 transverse process into the view. The C7 transverse process has no anterior tubercle. The C7 nerve root is situated just anterior to the posterior tubercle (Fig. 84.3). At the C6 level, the longus colli muscle is seen as an oval structure adjacent to the base of the transverse process and vertebral body (see Fig. 84.2). Sometimes the caudal portion of the longus capitis muscle can be seen as well. The CST is visualized as a spindle-shaped structure (the mid-cervical ganglion), which is typically situated at posterolateral surface of the longus colli muscle; if the CST cannot be identified, some widening of the tissue plane underneath the prevertebral fascia is typically seen. Once the desired target is localized, the surrounding anatomical structures are identified and the feasibility of the "anterior" approach should be determined. Often the distance flanked by the carotid artery, and the trachea is wide enough and, therefore, only thyroid tissue and superficial neck muscles are seen between the needle entry and the surface of the longus colli muscle. Gentle pressure may effectively decrease the skin-to-target distance and visually further separate the carotid artery from the trachea. Additional scanning should be performed to confirm that the inferior thyroid artery is not traversing the planned needle trajectory. The injection is performed as a short-axis out-of-plane approach (Fig. 84.4). The skin is anesthetized immediately caudad to the transducer. The injection is performed using a spinal needle (22–25 gauge and 2–3.5 inches long) with a three-way stopcock and extension tubing connecting two syringes, one with NaCl 0.9% and another with a local anesthetic. The needle is inserted under continuous ultrasound guidance, directed to the anterior surface of the longus colli muscle using a short-axis out-of-plane approach. When the needle tip is visualized, either directly or indirectly (tissue movement), approaching the target, 1–2 mL of saline is injected to confirm placement of the needle under the prevertebral fascia, which is appreciated as a separation of the tissue planes by the anechoic fluid (Fig. 84.5). If the injectate is observed

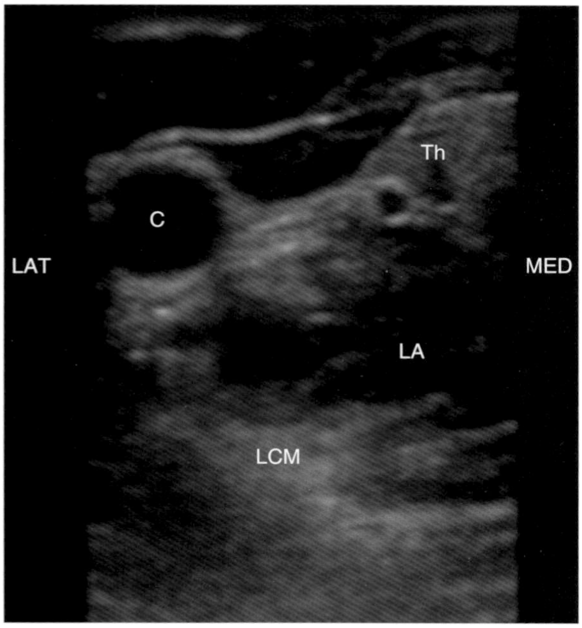

FIG. 84.5 The local anesthetic *(LA)* injected superficially to the longus colli muscle *(LCM)* and underneath of the prevertebral fascia. The longus colli muscle is compressed by the injectate and appears "hyperechoic." *C*, Carotid artery; *Th*, thyroid gland.

above the fascia or within the muscle, the needle must be carefully repositioned. If the spread is appropriate, 5 mL of local anesthetic is injected, and the needle is withdrawn.

The "anterior" approach must be abandoned and an alternative "lateral" approach may be attempted if any of the following conditions are present: (1) the anterior sonogram shows narrow distance between the carotid artery and the thyroid; (2) the inferior thyroid artery cannot be eliminated from the view; (3) the esophagus is seen above the longus colli muscle (left side); or (4) thyroid cysts are evident.

Lateral Approach

The patient is placed in the semilateral decubitus position, with the side to be treated uppermost. Preparation and ultrasonography is performed as previously described. However, the transducer is centered at the C6 transverse process and not at the anterior neck. It is of utmost importance to localize the C6 nerve root and the anterior process. With the transducer properly placed, only the anterior tubercle of the C6 transverse process is visible adjacent to the projected entry point of the needle without visceral or neural elements between the entry site and the anterolateral surface of the longus colli muscle. The needle tract should be entirely intramuscular, passing through the sternocleidomastoid muscle or the anterior scalene muscle, or both. Occasionally the internal jugular vein is seen within the projected needle tract, but it can be readily collapsed by light pressure on the transducer. Skin anesthesia is performed immediately posterior to the ultrasound transducer. Under continuous ultrasound guidance, the needle is inserted using the short-axis in-plane approach (Fig. 84.6). The advantage of the lateral approach, in addition to avoiding the trespass through the thyroid, is in the in-plane control of the needle insertion from the skin entry point to the target. Verification of the needle position and the rest of the procedure are the same as that for the anterior approach. An injection of 5 mL of a local anesthetic typically results in C3–T1 prevertebral spread and the complete blockade of the CST and the stellate ganglion (Fig. 84.7). If anesthetic blockade of the upper cervical ganglion is not desirable, it will be prudent to limit volume of the injectate to 3 mL.

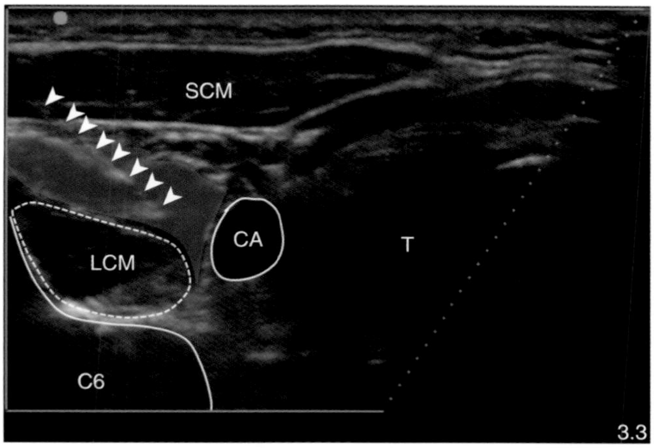

FIG. 84.6 In-plane insertion of the block needle *(arrowheads)* superficially to the longus colli muscle *(LCM)*. Injectate *(blue)* is wrapping LCM. *C6*, C6 vertebra (note: only the anterior tubercle is seen); *CA*, carotid artery; *SCM*, sternocleidomastoid muscle; *T*, thyroid gland.

Fluoroscopy-Guided Approach

The patient is positioned supine. A pillow can be placed under the lower neck to achieve some extension. The head may be slightly rotated contralaterally to the injection side increasing the distance between the carotid artery and the trachea. The image intensifier is positioned in such way that the cervical spine anteroposterior view is obtained. Additional adjustments are made to eliminate misalignment of the lower cervical intervertebral discs and to correct orientation of the spinous processes. After skin preparation and dressing, the target—junction between C6 transverse process and the vertebral body—is localized. Skin anesthesia is performed and the block needle inserted utilizing "tunnel view" until the bone surface is contacted. Prior to the needle placement, the anterior neck is palpated to verify absence of the carotid pulse at the entry point. If the carotid pulse is appreciated, the image intensifier may be slightly axially rotated or "tunnel view" may be abandoned. Once the bone surface is contacted, the needle is gently retracted for 3–5 mm and injection of a contrast agent is performed. Although, a "honey-combed" longitudinal spread has been reported as a confirmation of interfascial flow along the CST, most commonly the spread is intramuscular (Fig. 84.8). Although the needle tip is not directly located at the CST, injection of 10 mL of bupivacaine 0.25% or another local anesthetic will typically result in the facial and upper extremity sympathetic blockade in 10–15 minutes. This characteristic delay is attributable to a secondary spread onto the CST.

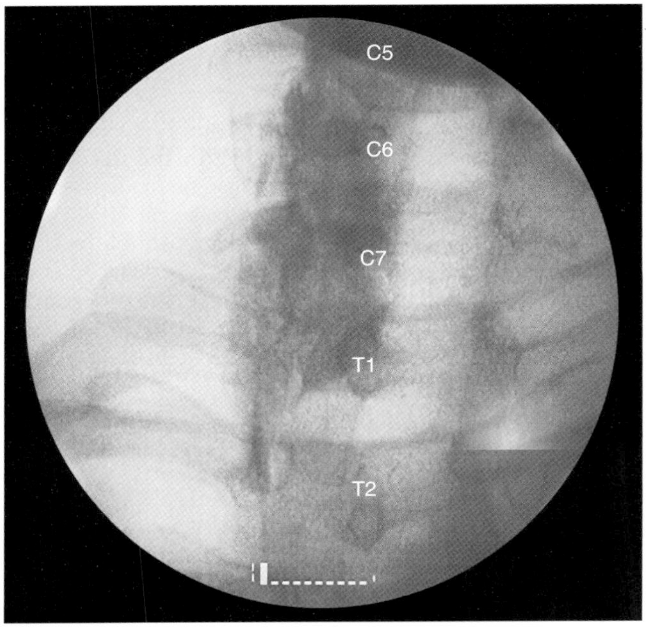

FIG. 84.7 Anteroposterior X-ray of the cervical spine. The contrast dye is clearly seen between C5 and T2 spinal levels as an interfascial (nonmuscular) pattern.

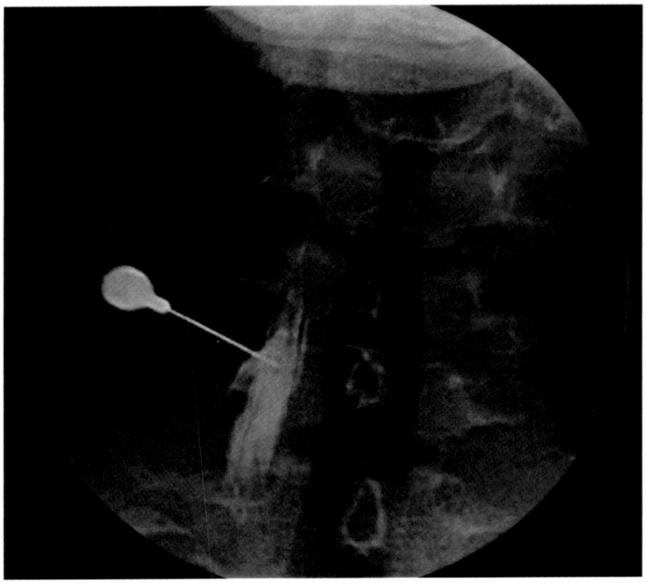

FIG. 84.8 Anteroposterior fluoroscopy demonstrates correct needle placement, and an intramuscular spread of injected contrast agent.

COMPLICATIONS

The blind paratracheal technique produces unreliable results, and is associated with a variety of side effects and complications, such as intravascular injection, formation of hematomas, temporary paralysis of the recurrent laryngeal nerve, discitis, and esophageal injury.[7,13,14] Fluoroscopy guidance may prevent adverse outcomes related to intravascular, nerve root or neuroaxial injections. However, soft tissue, parenchymal, and vascular injury may occur.[15]

CONCLUSIONS

Current literature and trends in clinical practice have made ultrasonography the preferred imaging guidance for CST block. A 5-mL injection into the correct fascial plane may reliably produce the sympathetic blockade. Ultrasound guidance may prevent complications and adverse outcomes associated with either blind or fluoroscopy-guided techniques.

KEY POINTS

- The stellate ganglion is usually situated at the lateral border of the longus colli muscle anterior to the neck of the first rib.
- Given that only traversing sympathetic fibers or middle cervical ganglia can be found at the C6 level, the *stellate ganglion block* should more accurately be named the *cervical sympathetic block*.
- At the lower neck, the sympathetic trunk is typically situated underneath the prevertebral fascia at posterolateral surface of the longus colli muscle.
- Ultrasound-guided block is a standard approach as it allows real-time visualization of pertinent anatomy, needle insertion, and spread of local anesthetic.

LUMBAR SYMPATHETIC BLOCK

Historically the first reported lumbar sympathetic block (LSB) was done by Brunn and Mandl,[16] who, in 1924, described a technique of injecting the lumbar sympathetic nerves as a component of their paravertebral approach blocking the mixed spinal outflow in the lumbar region. Kappis also described a technique of the LSB and surgical resection of the lumbar sympathetic nerves around that time.[17] During the 1950s, Bonica described in detail the importance of the lumbar sympathetic blockade, particularly in the treatment of the causalgia and posttraumatic reflex dystrophies in servicemen after World War II.[18]

There are two paravertebral sympathetic trunks located symmetrically at each side of the vertebral column. The thoracolumbar sympathetic fibers originate in the dorsolateral region of the anterior column and extend within the ventral roots of all the thoracic and the upper two or three lumbar spinal nerves. These preganglionic fibers form the rami communicantes that connect to the sympathetic chain. Some rami communicantes bypass the prevertebral plexuses and connect to the collateral ganglia (e.g., the celiac plexus). The cell bodies responsible for vasoconstriction in the lower limbs are in the lower three thoracic and first three lumbar segments. Each lumbar sympathetic chain enters the retroperitoneal space under the right and left crus of the diaphragm, continuing inferiorly in the interval between the anterolateral aspect of the vertebral bodies and the origin of the psoas muscle to enter the pelvis and the L5–S1 disc. Posteriorly, the periosteum overlies the vertebral bodies and the fibro-aponeurotic origin of the psoas muscles and their fascial coverings. The parietal reflection of the peritoneum is anterior, the aorta lying anteromedial to the left trunk, and the vena cava anterior to the right trunk. It should be noted that the white and gray rami communicantes pass to their respective ganglia beneath the fibrous arcades of the psoas attachments alongside the middle of the vertebral bodies.

The sympathetic ganglia of the lumbar sympathetic chain are variable in both numbers and position. Rarely, all five ganglia are found on each side in the same individual. In most cases, only four are found. The L1 and L2 ganglia are usually fused in most patients, and ganglia are aggregated at the L2–L3 and L4–L5 discs.[19] Also, there is considerable variability in the size of the ganglia, some being fusiform and as long as 10–15 mm, and others being round and approximately 5 mm long.

The indications for LSB may be divided into three broad categories:

1. Circulatory insufficiency in the leg, including arteriosclerotic vascular disease, diabetic gangrene, Buerger disease, Raynaud's phenomenon and disease, and reconstructive vascular surgery after arterial embolic occlusion
2. Pain from renal colic, complex regional pain syndrome types I and II, intractable urogenital pain, postamputation stump pain, phantom pain, and frostbite
3. Other conditions, such as hyperhidrosis, erythromelalgia, and acrocyanosis.

Although the mechanism contributing to pain relief remains unclear, blocks of the sympathetic nervous system may have two actions: (1) interruption of preganglionic and postganglionic sympathetic efferents may influence the function of the primary afferent neuron; or (2) the afferents from deep structures in the leg that travel with the sympathetic nerves may be blocked.

FLUOROSCOPY-GUIDED APPROACH

With the patient in a prone position, the C-arm is placed first in the anteroposterior and then ipsilateral to the injection side oblique view. The injection is typically performed at L3 level. The degree of the obliquity is judged based on appearance of the L3 spinous process. It has to overlay the contralateral facet joint. When the L3 transverse process is aligned with the center of lateral L3 vertebral body, the C-arm is tilted to eliminate the transverse process from the view and assure an unobstructed needle path. Skin and subcutaneous tissues are anesthetized. A 22-gauge 5- to 7-inch needle is then introduced in a tunnel view and advanced until it contacts the vertebral body (Fig. 84.9). Fluoroscopy in two planes should confirm its position and the angle to guide redirection of the needle to its final position at the anterolateral aspect of the vertebral body. With the fluoroscopy positioned laterally, final adjustments can be made to ensure the needle tip lies exactly at the anterolateral edge of the vertebral body. A contrast dye of 3–5 mL should confirm the location of the correct tissue plane (Fig. 84.10). If the contrast spread was limited to one segment, the procedure is then repeated with the second needle at the L2 or L4 vertebral body. The dye should spread to form a line conforming to the anterolateral margin of the vertebral bodies.

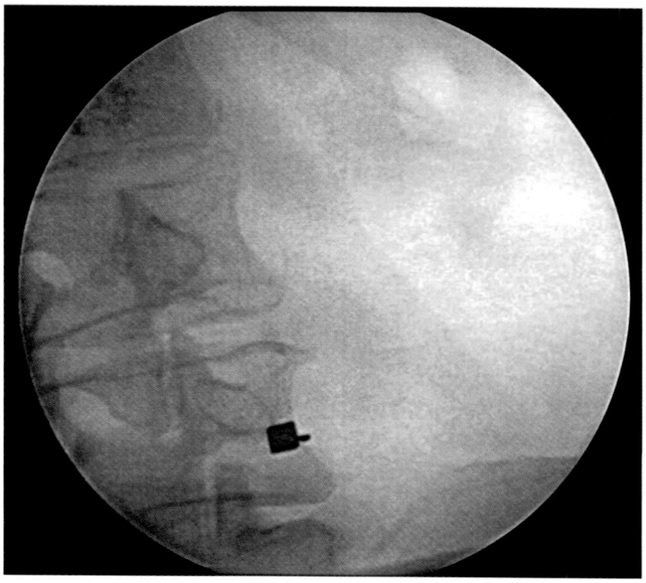

FIG. 84.9 Utilizing a steep oblique view, the block needle is inserted in tunnel view aiming for the anterolateral L3 vertebral body.

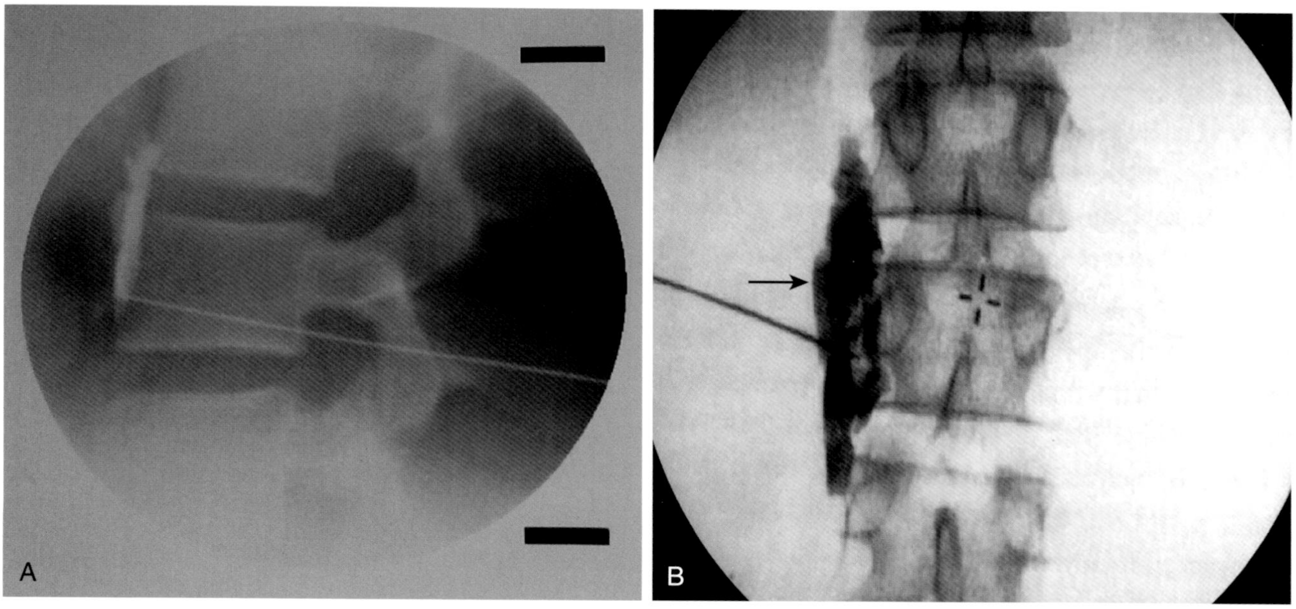

FIG. 84.10 Fluoroscopy performed in lateral (A) and anteroposterior (B) views confirmed prevertebral spread of the contrast dye *(black arrow)*.

A short-acting local anesthetic is commonly used for diagnostic sympathetic blocks. A long-acting agent, such as bupivacaine or ropivacaine, is advantageous for both therapy and prognosis, because it gives the patient a longer time to evaluate the effects of sympatholysis and any effect this might have on the pain. A concentration of 0.375% bupivacaine or 0.5% ropivacaine gives optimal duration without the need for an added vasoconstrictor.

ULTRASOUND-GUIDED APPROACH

Fluoroscopic guidance remains the standard approach to LSB with the sympathetic chain lying in an anterolateral location to the lumbar vertebra. While ultrasound-guided interventional procedures are in their infancy, they have benefits over the established fluoroscopically and CT-guided procedures in the reduction of radiation exposure and the ability to visualize soft tissue structures. Ultrasound-guided LSB was described by Kirvelä and colleagues in 1992.[20] Unfortunately, the description of the technique was unclear and the image quality was poor.

TECHNIQUE

The patient is positioned prone and spinal sonography, with a curved array transducer, is performed for identification of spinal level and target. The injection target is the most ventral and medial part of the L3 vertebral body. After sterile preparation and administration of local anesthesia, a 20-g or 18-g Touhy needle is inserted utilizing an in-plane approach contacting the lateral L3 vertebral body (Fig. 84.11). A loss of resistance technique is used to advance the needle deeper. Prevertebral space is reached usually after 1–2 cm, and an injection of 5–10 mL of 1% lidocaine is performed. Due to the limited visualization, ultrasound guidance for the neurolytic LSB cannot be currently recommended.

COMPLICATIONS

Because the LSB is a procedure that involves a deep paravertebral placement of the block needle, complications related to the injury of exiting nerve roots, kidney, and viscera have been reported. Other complications, such as total spinal block and priapism, are probably related to an inadvertent spread of the injected local anesthetic. Neurolytic agents may cause damage of the genitofemoral and lateral femoral cutaneous nerves.

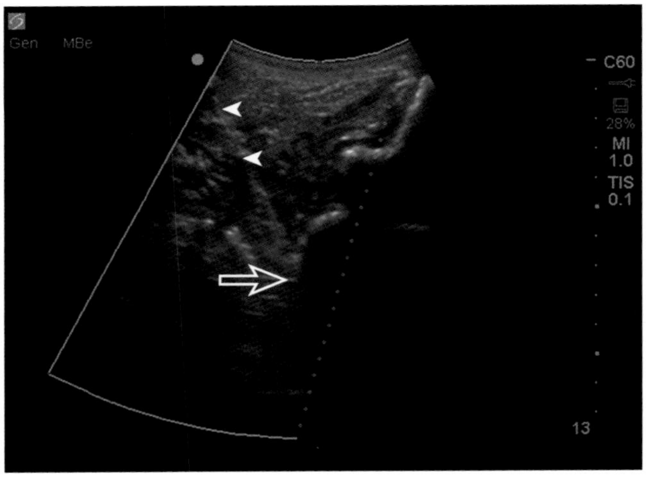

FIG. 84.11 Short-axis ultrasonography of the L3 vertebra and paraspinal anatomy. The needle *(arrowheads)* is inserted until it contacted the anterolateral surface of the vertebral body *(arrow)*.

CONCLUSIONS

LSB is indicated for variety of painful and painless conditions that are deemed to be alleviated by a decrease of sympathetic tone.

Currently fluoroscopy guidance is recommended as the standard of care.

KEY POINTS

- The cell bodies responsible for vasoconstriction in the lower limbs are in the lower three thoracic and the first three lumbar segments.
- A fluoroscopy-guided injection is performed at L3 level.
- The injected contrast agent should be observed at least two vertebral levels to achieve a reliable sympathetic blockade.

ABDOMINAL SYMPATHETIC BLOCKADE

CELIAC PLEXUS BLOCK

Chronic visceral pain is a common ailment in the general population. Main etiologies include functional gastrointestinal disorders, visceral malignancies, and chronic pancreatitis. Management options available for these painful conditions are both pharmacologic and interventional. Chronic visceral pain secondary to cancer of the pancreas, stomach, duodenum, and proximal small bowel may be alleviated by neurolytic celiac plexus block (NCPB).[21] There are also reports of NCPB benefits in the management of abdominal pain due to the chronic pancreatitis.[22] The most extensively studied painful condition ameliorated with NCPB is pancreatic cancer.[23–25] Approximately 75% of pancreatic cancer patients complain of moderate to severe pain that has a significant negative effect on physical functioning and quality of life. NCPB complements medical management and is considered the standard component of palliative care.

Clinically Relevant Anatomy

Located approximately at the level of the 12th thoracic and/or 1st lumbar vertebra, the celiac plexus is composed of two to five celiac ganglia with its network of nerve fibers. The plexus surrounds the celiac trunk and the superior mesenteric artery at its root. It is located in front of the aorta and the crura of the diaphragm, and posterior to the stomach and omental bursa. The presynaptic sympathetic fibers to the plexus are provided by the greater, lesser, and least splanchnic nerves, which originate from the paravertebral sympathetic ganglia T5–T12. The plexus, in turn, supplies the various abdominal viscera through multiple smaller plexi and nerve fibers accompanying the arteries. In addition, the plexus also receives parasympathetic supply from the vagus. The various structures that are supplied include the diaphragm, liver, stomach, spleen, suprarenal glands, kidneys, ovaries, testis, small intestine, and colon up to the splenic flexure. The celiac plexus also sends branches to the superior and inferior mesenteric plexuses.

Indications

NCPB may provide relief of pain originating from tumors of the stomach, liver, pancreas, spleen, and proximal small bowel besides adrenals.[26] Neurolytic or local anesthetic CPB has also been attempted for relief of chronic pancreatitis pain and during biliary interventions.

Available Techniques and Approaches

Landmark-based percutaneous CPB was introduced by Kappis in 1919.[17] With the introduction of fluoroscopy, CT, sonography, and MRI, the need for imaging for the safe conduct of CPB became obvious, although there is no study comparing the different imaging modalities. The various techniques include endoscopic transduodenal ultrasonography-guided CPB, intraoperative CPB, and percutaneous CPB.[27–29] Anterior and posterior approaches to the plexus have been described. The anterior approach is used during percutaneous and endoscopic ultrasound-guided CPB and with intraoperative CPB.[30] Fluoroscopic, MRI, and landmark-based injections approach the CPB posteriorly. CT-guided CPB may be performed through an anterior or posterior approach, although the posterior approach is commonly preferred. Fluoroscopy and CT carry the risk of increased radiation exposure. CT may provide finer details about the plexus, the celiac artery, and the neighboring structures for improved safety and better targeting.[31] By using surrogate bone landmarks, fluoroscopy guidance has a risk for soft tissue damage. CT and MRI require equipment that is costly and not readily available, limiting their utility in the routine clinical setting. MRI has been used with approximately 57% success for CPB, which is evidently unsatisfactory.[32] Endoscopic ultrasound-guided CPB has been safely performed with clear visualization of the ganglia, but requires deep sedation and a gastroenterology interventional setting. Nevertheless, endoscopic CPB may be more cost effective when compared to CT-guided CPB. Percutaneous sonographic guidance has been used successfully for CPB for many years. Ultrasound-guided percutaneous CPB has several advantages. It is cost effective, portable, may be performed at the bedside, and spares radiation exposure. In addition, the supine position is more comfortable for the patient. The abdominal aorta, celiac trunk, and mesenteric vessels are clearly visualized. It permits real-time visualization of the injectate spread. The disadvantages include poor visualization of deeper structures, including the pancreas and the acoustic interference produced by stomach or intestinal air. Similarly to CT guidance, it may cause injury to the visceral hollow organs, the pancreas, or the liver.

A variety of techniques and approaches have been described in the literature, including retrocrural, antecrural, transcrural, transdiscal, transaortic, and splanchnic nerves.[27,28,33,34] It can be done as a single- or two-needle technique. Each technique has its proponents and opponents claiming advantages and disadvantages. The cancer spread as seen on CT may dictate the approach. NCPB is usually performed with either phenol 6%–10% or alcohol 50%–100% following a diagnostic local anesthetic injection despite the low, negative, predictive value of the diagnostic block.[35]

Evidence for the Use of Neurolytic Celiac Plexus Block

NCPB has been shown to be effective in improving pancreatic cancer pain and, combined with other modalities, it is effective in about 80% of patients. The pain relief provided by NCPB seems to be better when performed at an earlier stage of the disease. A reduction in opioid consumption following NCPB has also been demonstrated.[36,37] Improving survival following NCPB has been suggested, but was found statistically insignificant. It is possible that statistical strict criteria may have prevented detection of small differences. The effect of NCPB on the quality of life is still unresolved, as some randomized controlled trials reported benefit while others did not.[38–40] A positive outcome following NCPB correlates with preexisting opioid use; patients with lower opioid consumption benefit more. For a more detailed discussion of this subject, please refer to Chapter 71.

Posterior Transcrural Fluoroscopy-Guided Approach

The patient is positioned prone on the fluoroscopic table. Usually, bolsters have to be placed under the chest and pelvis to alleviate abdominal discomfort, which may not be tolerated by patients. To prevent a sudden decrease in the blood pressure related to visceral vasodilation, 500 mL of an isotonic intravenous fluid is administered. After the usual sterile preparation, throracolumbar spine fluoroscopy is performed and the L1 vertebra is placed at the center of the scout image. Next, the image intensifier is rotated to an oblique position. The degree of obliquity is usually judged by observing the contralateral move of the spinous process. It has to be aligned with the contralateral facet joint. In addition, cephalad or caudad tilt is performed to “eliminate” the L1 transverse process from the view. The radiological target is the middle of the L1 vertebral body. Local anesthesia is performed and a 20- or 21-gauge Chiba-type needle is inserted and advanced in a coaxial view (Fig. 84.12). It has to contact the L1 vertebral body just 1–2 mm medially to the lateral edge of L1, in case further advancement will be difficult. Some practitioners manually bend the needle tip to obtain a 10- to 15-degree angle to improve steering. After bone is contacted, the image intensifier is rotated into the lateral position and further needle progress is performed under this view. It is also advisable to remove the stylet and use a loss-of-resistance device filled with either NaCl 0.9% or air. Typically, once the needle is advanced about 1 cm past the anterior L1 vertebra, the resistance drastically decreases and prevertebral/preaortic longitudinal contrast spread is observed (see Fig. 84.12). On the anteroposterior view a “honey comb” contrast shadow is seen (see Fig. 84.12).

In a similar fashion, the procedure is performed on the contralateral side. If the arterial blood is obtained or injected contrast produces an aortogram, the procedure may be converted into a transaortic single-needle technique. In such a case, the needle is advanced through the anterior aortic wall, and additional contrast dye is injected. Its spread should be confined to the retroperitoneal compartment. Once the needle’s position was verified, 5–10 mL of a local anesthetic mixed with contrast is injected and the patient is closely

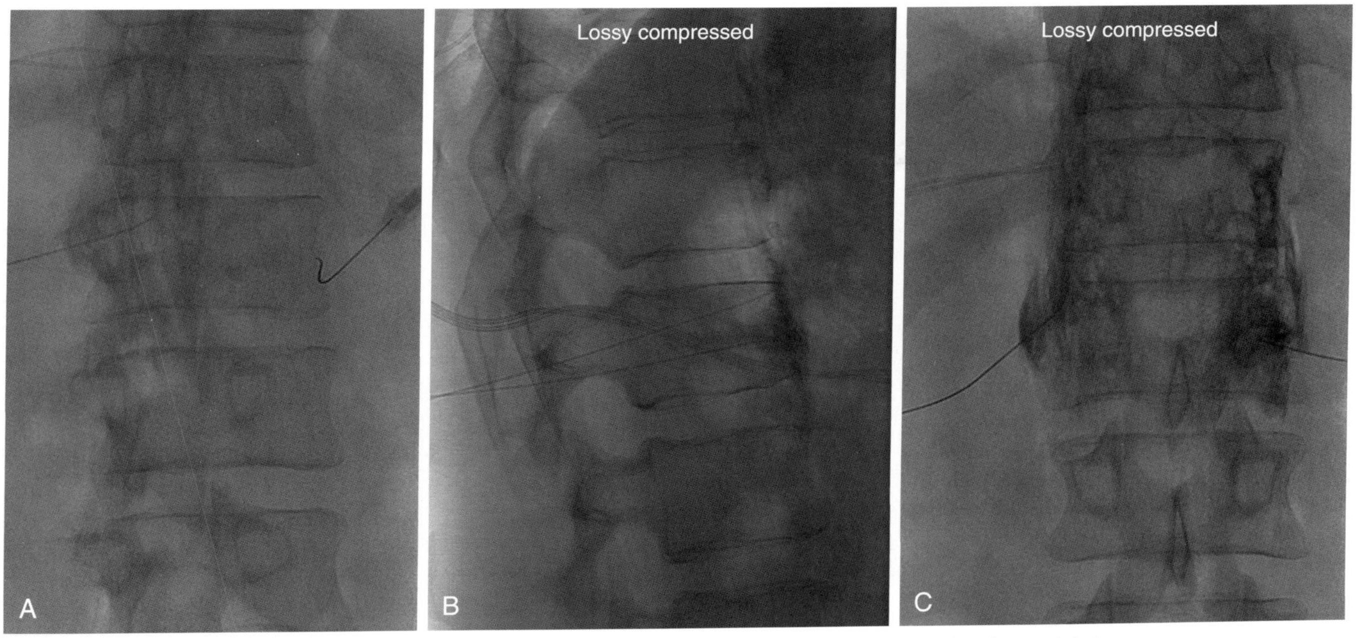

FIG. 84.12 Fluoroscopy-guided celiac plexus block. (A) The Chiba needle inserted in the coaxial view on the right. Radiopaque contrast was injected on the left. (B) The lateral view shows longitudinal prevertebral contrast spread. (C) "Honeycomb" appearance of the contrast on the anteroposterior view.

monitored for the signs of intravascular injection or neuroaxial blockade. After 3–5 minutes, 20–40 mL of 50%–80% alcohol is slowly injected. Alcohol can be mixed with the contrast to further assure an accurate injection.

Posterior Transcrural (Classic) Computed-Tomography-Guided Approach

The patient position and preparation is similar to the fluoroscopy-guided approach.

CT guidance can be performed by utilizing a standard planning grid or by using 3D reconstruction and cone-beam guidance. In the former, CT planning is completed, paying attention to the direction and depth. The patient is removed from the scanner, a needle is placed, and a second CT is erformed to confirm the final needle position. If the placeent is satisfactory, the contrast is injected and further conmed with CT, or an ancillary fluoroscopy is performed, neurolytic solution is slowly injected (Fig. 84.13). If the lle placement is inaccurate, the process is repeated. This od is definitely time consuming and is associated with icant radiation exposure.

vel cone-beam CT utilizes 50%–70% less radiation nventional CT scanners and combines the capabili- CT-scanner and a fluoroscopy. The procedure is sing specialized software showing the needle entry ction, and depth (Fig. 84.14). Next, the proceformed under live fluoroscopy guidance overlaid ging. This radiological method may effectively tion exposure and minimize procedure time icing technical accuracy (Fig. 84.15).

Percutaneous Ultrasound-Guided Block

itioned supine. A routine procedural mon- peripheral intravenous line is established.

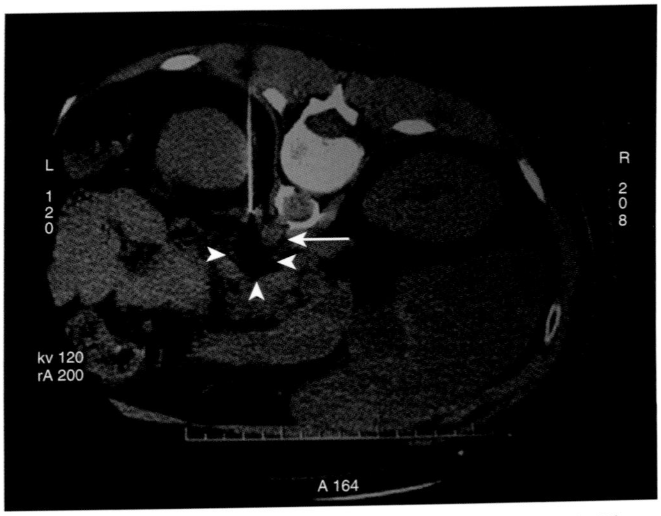

FIG. 84.13 Computed-tomography-guided celiac plexus block. The needle is positioned adjacent to the aorta, and alcohol is injected (*white arrowheads* are pointing to the *black shadow*); *white arrow*, celiac trunk.

The patient may be instructed to control his/her respiration at certain times during the procedure. Typically, a low-frequency, curved-array, 3- to 5-MHz transducer is used. A short-axis scan is performed starting from the epigastrium and moving caudad to visualize the aorta, the vertebral body, and the liver (Fig. 84.16). Once the celiac trunk is visualized, color flow Doppler is turned on to verify the location of the vessels (Fig. 84.17). Following this, the transducer is turned longitudinally, and the celiac trunk and the superior mesenteric artery are visualized (Fig. 84.18). Color flow Doppler is again used to verify the vessels. The target is a typically appearing hyperechoic (gray) zone surrounding the celiac trunk cephalad and/or laterally to the celiac trunk. The neurolytic agent spread may be determined more by the regional anatomy affected by cancer and previous surgeries

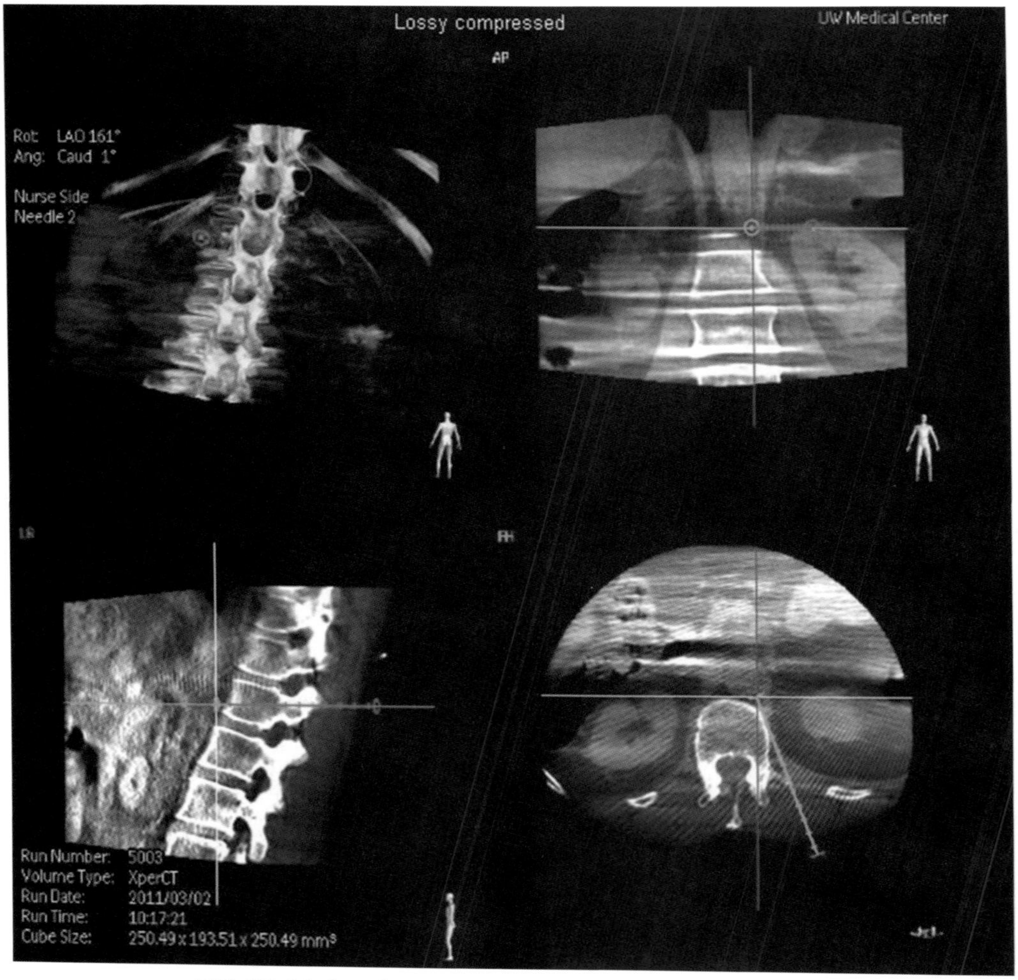

FIG. 84.14 Cone-beam computed tomography procedural planning.

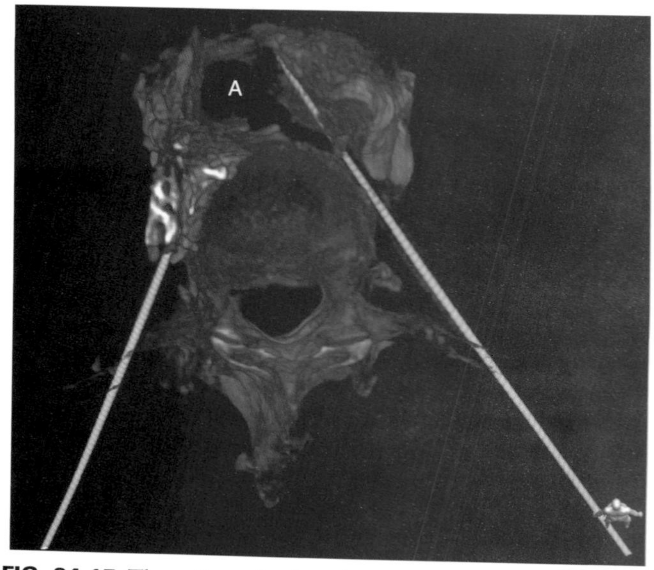

FIG. 84.15 Three-dimensional axial reconstruction. The contrast dye encircles the aorta *(A)*.

than the needle position. The scout scan also helps i ning the approach, based on the structures in the pa needle.

Following the scout scan, the area is p draped. With the transducer in a sterile slee is once again identified. A 22-gauge, 15- needle is advanced just cephalad to the longitudinal view. The needle may al short-axis to the aorta in-plane vie through the liver (Fig. 84.19) Th the safest path to the target area ence of the physician. An exte the needle. After negative asp of lidocaine with epinephri intravascular uptake. Subs the neurolytic agent in The typical volume of mL. The concentrat to 100%. With ph 6% to 10%. The anesthetic at the track of the re

An alternat duction of the nee ducer, and the celiac

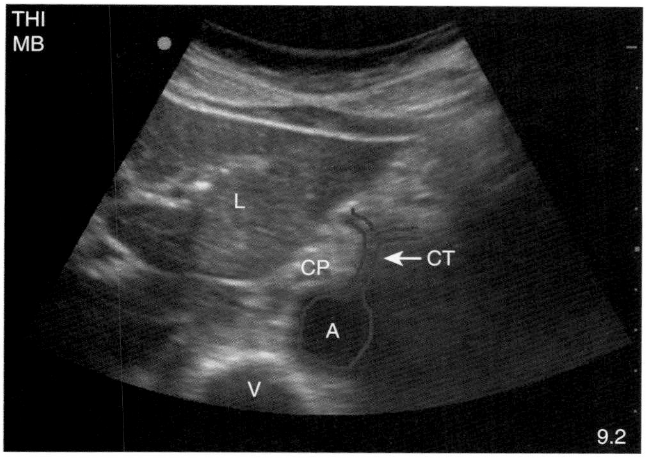

FIG. 84.16 Transverse ultrasound picture over the hypogastrium showing the various structures in relation to the celiac trunk. *A*, Abdominal aorta, *CP*, right celiac plexus; *CT*, celiac trunk; *V*, vertebral body.

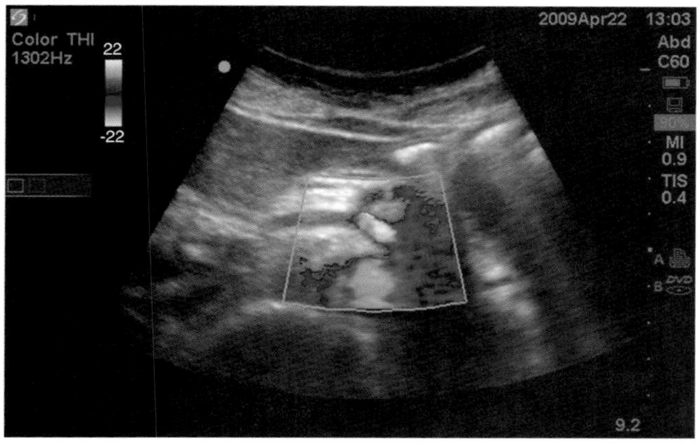

FIG. 84.17 Transverse ultrasound view of the celiac trunk and abdominal aorta with color Doppler.

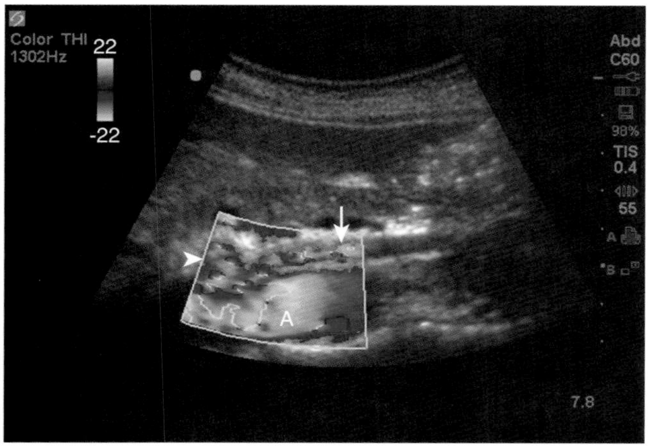

FIG. 84.18 Longitudinal ultrasound view of the celiac trunk and superior mesenteric artery. *Arrow*, Superior mesenteric artery; *arrowhead*, celiac trunk.

view. The injectate appears to be better visualized with this approach. Percutaneous neurolysis of the celiac plexus under sonographic guidance is noted to be effective in relieving the pain from abdominal tumors or pancreatitis.[41]

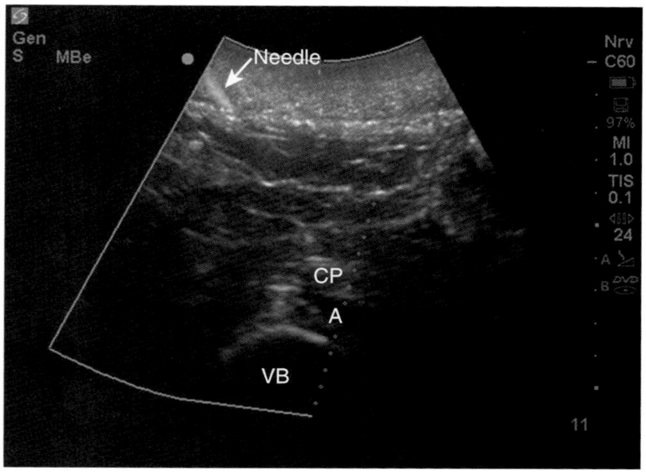

FIG. 84.19 The block needle is advanced through the liver aiming for the abdominal aorta *(A)* and the hyperechoic celiac plexus *(CP)*. *VB*, Vertebral body.

COMPLICATIONS

Side effects, such as orthostatic hypotension and transient diarrhea, are known to occur after CPB in approximately 38% and 44% of patients, respectively. One of the frequently reported complications is pain at the injection site, occurring in about 90% of cases. Other rare complications are retroperitoneal hematoma, penetration of the pleura and lung leading to pneumothorax, injury to kidneys and intestines, and paraplegia secondary to neurolytic solution injection into the epidural or spinal canal, or due to accidental injection into the artery of Adamkiewicz—all of which have been reported in less than 1% of cases. Superior mesenteric vein thrombosis has been reported after the injection of alcohol.[42] An intravascular injection of a neurolytic agent or a local anesthetic may result in cardiovascular collapse and seizures.[43]

CONCLUSIONS

Fluoroscopy or CT-guided CPB is a standard recommended technique. Ultrasound-guided CPB is a safe, real-time procedure, and may be performed at the bedside using an anterior approach. It may be especially useful in patients who have difficulty lying prone or immobile. The main difficulties include planning a safe trajectory, adjusting the breathing and aortic pulsation, and the steep needle angle. Supplementary technical aids, such as needle navigation software or brackets, may improve accuracy and increase confidence.

KEY POINTS

- Celiac plexus is supplied by the greater, lesser, and least splanchnic nerves originating from the T5 to the T12.
- Celiac plexus is made up five ganglia and interconnecting nerves, and is located adjacent to the junction of the celiac artery and the aorta.
- Ultrasound guidance for the performance of NCPB permits an anterior approach with relative safety and without radiation.
- The anterior approach eliminates the risk of an accidental neurolytic injection into the posterior structures including neuraxis.

- The target is the hyperechoic tissue surrounding the celiac trunk.
- Neurolytic celiac plexus block provides substantial pain relief in chronic visceral pain, specifically the pain in pancreatic cancer.

SUPERIOR HYPOGASTRIC PLEXUS BLOCK

The superior hypogastric plexus (SHGP) is retroperitoneal and lies anterior to the caudal third of the L5 and the cephalad third of the S1 vertebral bodies. The SHGP is a continuation of the bilateral paravertebral sympathetic chain. It belongs to "visceral sympathetic blocks" because the procedure is indicated primarily for the alleviation of lower abdominal pain related to pelvic malignancies.

SHGP is located anteromedially to the psoas muscle and caudally to the bifurcation of the iliac vessels. It is formed by multiple unmyelinated branches from the aortic plexus and the lumbar splanchnic nerves.[44] It continues on as the hypogastric nerves that form the inferior hypogastric plexus. The SGHP branches into multiple extensions to various smaller plexi supplying sympathetic efferent innervation to the pelvic viscera except the ovaries. In addition, SHGP includes the parasympathetic branches from the sacral outflow tracts. Sensory afferents pass to the dorsal spinal column visceral pathway along the sympathetic fibers without synapsing in the ganglia.

Blockade of the SHGP to manage pelvic pain was first described by Plancarte and colleagues in 1990 as a fluoroscopy-guided, posterior, two-needle technique, targeting the anterior portion of the L5 vertebral body.[45] Subsequently, other methods, including a single-needle technique, posterior transdiscal and anterior approaches utilizing fluoroscopy, and ultrasound guidance, have been described.[46–49] CT-guided techniques have been reported, but two publications only involved either one or two patients.[50,51] The one study that had 30 patients showed the CT-guided technique to take a shorter length of time and to result in better patient satisfaction.[52]

Mishra and colleagues described an ultrasound-guided SHGP block in 2008, using a transabdominal approach targeting the anterior-most portion of the L5 vertebral body.[53] They clinically validated the ultrasound-guided technique in a prospective, randomized, controlled study testing the method on 54 patients with advanced gynecological malignancy, and compared it against oral morphine analgesia. Recently, an imaging cadaver study confirmed the accuracy of the ultrasound-guided transabdominal technique and suggested technical pearls assuring procedural success.[54]

FLUOROSCOPY-GUIDED TRANSDISCAL APPROACH

Posterior fluoroscopic-guided transdiscal approaches were described by Erdine and colleagues in 2003 and Turker and colleagues in 2005.[55,56] Both techniques used the anterior border of the L5/S1 disc as the preferred target. The transdiscal technique has been validated against the originally described technique, highlighting the ease and speed of technique and safety, with similar reductions in the visual analogue pain scores and morphine consumption. The transdiscal approach has also been used as a rescue for those who failed to obtain pain relief when the original two-needle technique was used. However, the transdiscal method carries the risk of discitis, disc rupture, or disc herniation, although no cases have yet been reported in the literature.

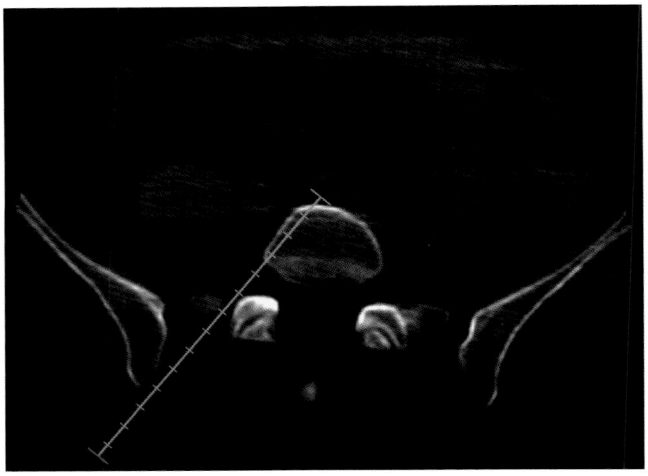

FIG. 84.20 Computed tomography axial image correlative to the oblique fluoroscopy view. A block needle inserted at 30 degrees oblique C-arm position is expected to exit anteriorly at the middle of the L5/S1 disc.

FLUOROSCOPY-GUIDED TECHNIQUE

The patient is positioned prone on the fluoroscopy table. If possible, a pillow or bolster is placed under the abdomen to alleviate lumbar lordosis. Antibiotic prophylaxis is provided by intravenous antibiotics (clindamycin 600 mg or vancomycin 1 g) administered 30 minutes prior to the procedure. Meticulous field and C-arm sterility as well as full surgical attire are mandatory. Conscious sedation is desirable because the procedure may be quite painful.

In order to facilitate C-arm oblique rotation and better procedural conditions, the right-sided entry point is usually selected by right-handed interventionists. After the elimination of double contours of the L5/S1 disc, the C-arm is rotated away from the operator to assume an oblique view. The degree of this rotation is dictated by the distance between S1 superior articular process (SAP) and the iliac bone. Often the "window" between these structures will be eliminated with only moderate rotation. The goal is to observe 1–1.5 cm of the L5/S1 disc laterally to S1 SAP (Fig. 84.20). After skin and deep tissue anesthesia is completed, a needle (e.g., Chiba needle 22-gauge 5–7 inches) is inserted and advanced through the disc. We do not recommend using intradiscal antibiotics and/or contrast, although others suggest such options. Optionally, a coaxial system can be used to add more protection from infection and to facilitate accuracy. A larger needle (introducer) is inserted first and advanced to the posteriolateral annulus fibrosis, then a smaller needle is placed through the introducer and steered through the disc. Regardless of the method, once the block needle has pierced the disc, the C-arm is rotated to the lateral view. The needle is advanced until it exits the anterior edge of the disc. Anteroposterior X-ray is obtained. Ideally the needle tip should be at the middle of the disc.

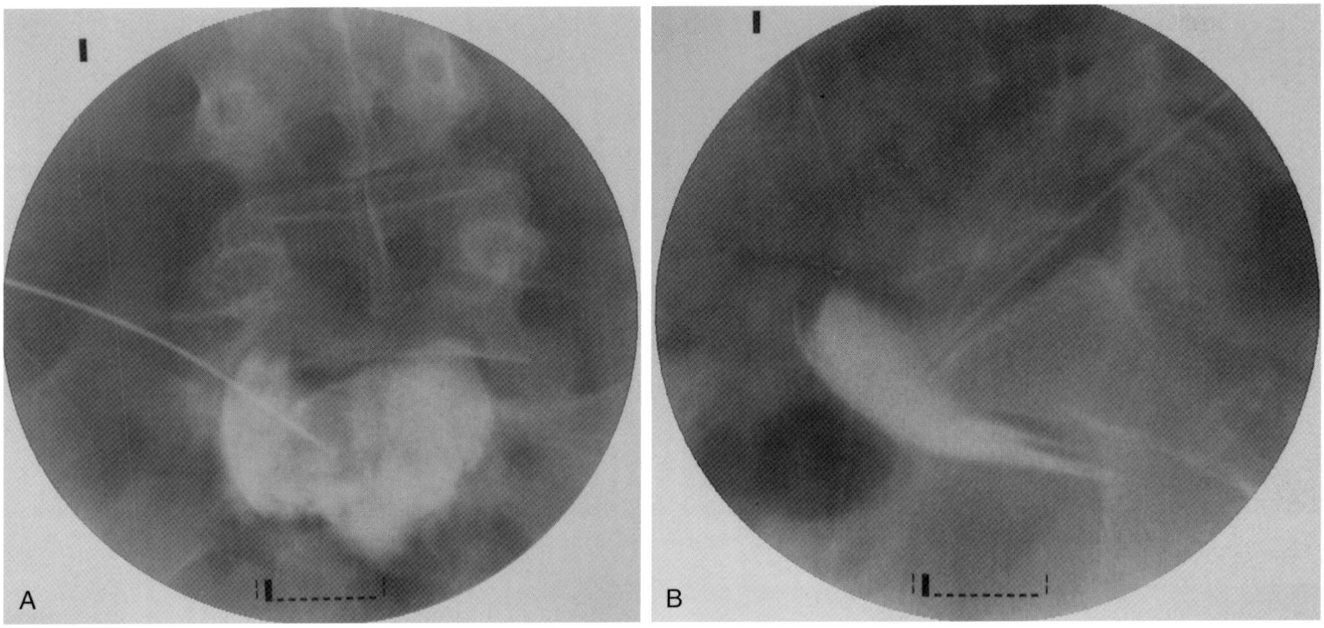

FIG. 84.21 Anteroposterior (A) and lateral (B) views of the L5/S1 spinal segment with injected contrast dye.

After verification of the needle tip position 1–3 mL of a contrast agent (e.g., iohexol 240 mgI/mL) is injected. The spread should be seen as a loose deposit covering the lower third of the L5 vertebral body and extending to the sacrum. On the lateral view, it should be confined to the prevertebral tissue plane (Fig. 84.21). After that, 10–20 mL of a local anesthetic or neurolytic solution is slowly injected (Fig. 84.22).

ULTRASOUND-GUIDED APPROACH

Based on the published experimental and clinical studies, the suggested technique is as follows.[54,57]

The patient must urinate prior to the procedure. Administer prophylactic antibiotics (e.g., cephazolin). The patient is positioned supine with a slight Trendelenburg tilt to displace bowels cephalad. A curvilinear low-frequency ultrasound transducer is used. The sagittal long-axis scanning to map out the L5/S1 disc is performed (Fig. 84.23). Once the L5/S1 disc is identified, the transducer is rotated 90 degrees. The disc appears as a hypoechoic convex structure. The anterior longitudinal ligament may sometimes be visible as a hyperechoic layer. Color Doppler must be used to identify prevertebral vessels to prevent an inadvertent damage or intravascular injection. With proper patient preparation and positioning, only abdominal wall structures are sandwiched between the transducer and the target: the center of the L5/S1 disc. The needle is introduced in-plane targeting the anterior surface of the L5/S1 disc. Once the needle tip is seen at the middle of the disc surface, 10 mL of analgesic or neurolytic solution is injected (Fig. 84.24). Real-time observation of the injectate to ensure bilateral spread is recommended. If a unilateral spread is identified, then the needle tip should be manipulated to ensure the bilateral spread. Alternatively, half of the solution can be delivered unilaterally, and then, the needle tip manipulated to deliver the remaining solution contralaterally. Upon completion, the needle is withdrawn and an adhesive dressing to cover the injection site is applied.

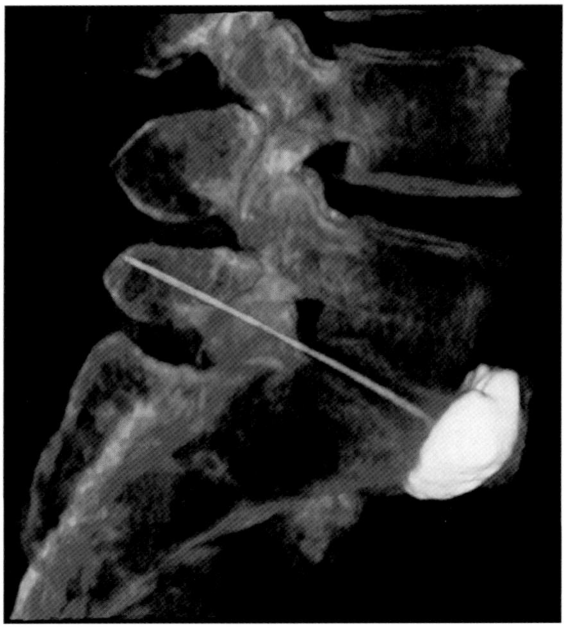

FIG. 84.22 Three-dimensional reconstruction after injection of the contrast dye.

COMPLICATIONS

Intravascular injection, inadequate spread, incomplete pain relief, and prolonged sensory and motor deficits have all been reported. Other potential complications include discitis with the transdiscal approach, dislodgment of atheromatous plaques from the major vessels, retroperitoneal hematoma, and bowel or urinary bladder perforation with the anterior approach.

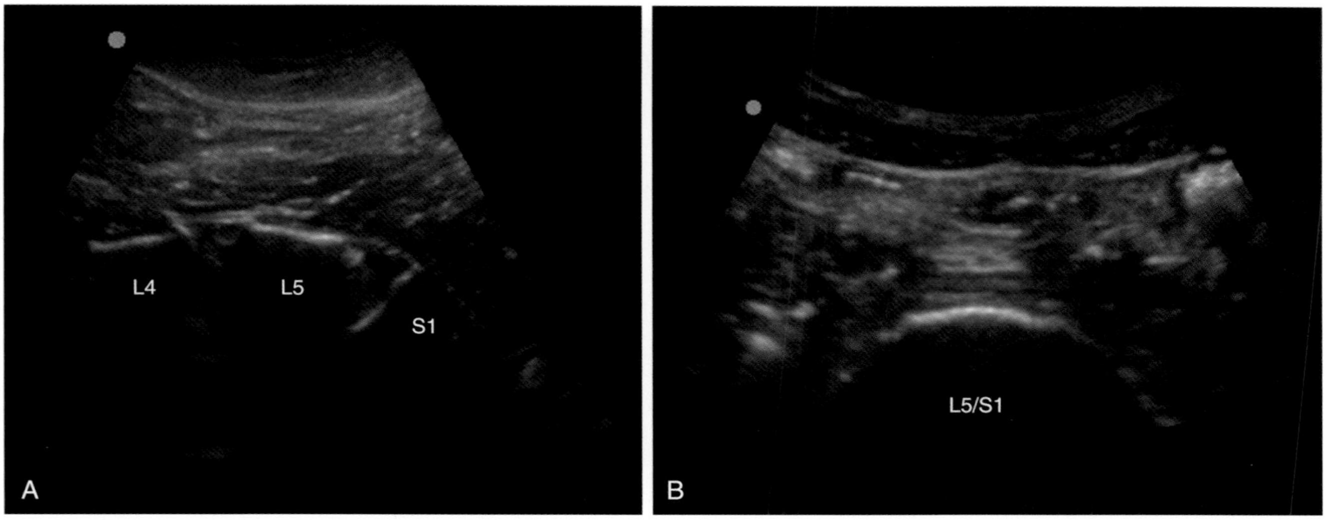

FIG. 84.23 Ultrasonography of the lumbosacral spine in the midline sagittal (A) and axial (B) planes.

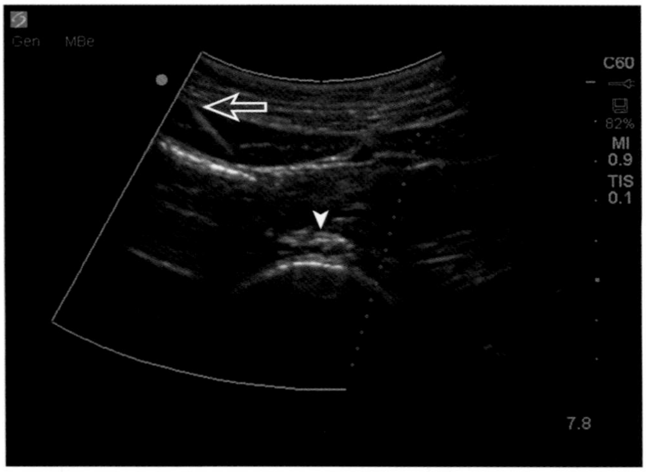

FIG. 84.24 The block needle *(arrow)* is inserted in-plane aiming for the center of the L5/S1 disc anterior surface. The injectate *(arrowhead)* is deposited at the center of the disc surface. Phenol typically produces a hyperechoic appearance. Local anesthetic would be seen as an anechoic signal.

CONCLUSIONS

SHGB is a useful intervention for managing intractable low abdominal visceral pain of pelvic malignancies. Both fluoroscopy- and ultrasound-guided approaches facilitate accurate and safe delivery of injected anesthetic or neurolytic solutions.

KEY POINTS

- The SHGP is retroperitoneal and lies anterior to the caudal third of the L5 and the cephalad third of the S1 vertebral bodies.
- The fluoroscopy-guided transdiscal approach is faster and easier than the traditional two-needle technique.
- The ultrasound-guided anterior approach is a reliable and readily available alternative.

GANGLION IMPAR BLOCK

The bilateral paravertebral sympathetic chain terminates anteriorly as the midline single-fused ganglion impar (the ganglion of Walther), which supplies sympathetic innervation to the perineum. Relief of perineal pain by ganglion impar block was originally described by Plancarte in 1990.[58] His original description of the landmark-based injection fell into disfavor because of the potential for rectal perforation and the high failure rate. Interest in this block has since regained with the increasing use of image guidance.

CLINICALLY RELEVANT ANATOMY

The ganglion impar is an irregularly shaped terminal ganglion of the sympathetic chain, which is usually located close to the midline. The varied shape ganglion is approximately 4 mm long. It may be located anywhere from the anterior surface of the sacrococcygeal junction to the lower coccygeal vertebral bodies. The exact location follows the Gaussian distribution centering on the first to second coccygeal vertebra. The rectum is located anterior to the ganglion. Fibers from the ganglion travel to the sacral spinal nerves along the gray rami communicantes.

INDICATIONS

The ganglion impar block is indicated for sympathetically mediated pain in the region of the anus, and distal parts of rectum, urethra, and vagina.[59–61] Coccygodynia following trauma, infection, degenerative changes, and subluxation has also been reported to respond to this block.[62]

EVIDENCE FOR THE USE OF GANGLION IMPAR BLOCK

Much anecdotal evidence exists for the usefulness of this block as demonstrated in the various techniques used for the performance of this block. Greater than 50% pain relief was obtained following a ganglion impar block with fluoroscopic guidance using a transsacrococcygeal approach in a variety of perineal pain disorders. Retrospective reviews of CT-guided ganglion impar blocks showed a greater than 75% decrease

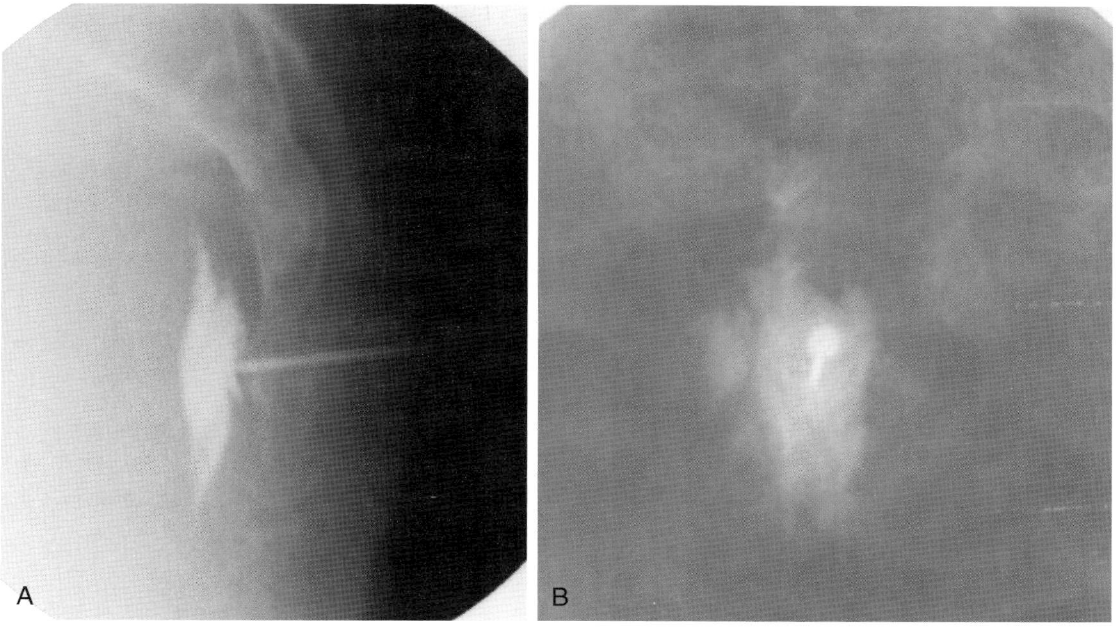

FIG. 84.25 Fluoroscopic image of the sacrum and coccyx (A, lateral and B, anteroposterior) with needle in a transcoccygeal approach showing contrast dye spread along the anterior surface of the coccyx.

in pain scores for up to 6 months. No adverse events have been reported. More recently, ultrasound guided and fluoroscopy have confirmed that ganglion impar blocks have also been found to be successful.[63,64]

AVAILABLE TECHNIQUES AND APPROACHES

The initial description of the ganglion impar block was a blind technique using a bent needle through the anococcygeal ligament with a finger in the rectum to detect perforation. Image guidance provides markedly increased technical success. Fluoroscopy facilitated further developments including the transcoccygeal, transarticular, transdiscal, intracoccygeal, and paracoccygeal approaches.[65–71] Combined with the use of contrast agents to visualize the spread of injectate, these techniques provided a modicum of safety. But, rectal gas shadow sometimes hinders proper visualization. Other limitations include the inability to visualize adjacent soft tissues, including tumor infiltrates and radiation exposure. CT-guided techniques using a lateral approach provide visualization of the ganglion and soft tissues. Ultrasound-guided techniques provide the advantage of real-time visualization and avoidance of radiation. To enhance safety, most practitioners using ultrasound guidance recommend fluoroscopic confirmation of contrast spread, as the needle tip cannot be visualized with ultrasound alone due to the bony coccyx, prior to injecting neurolytic agents. Several modifications in the design of the needle, including arc and double-bent needles, followed the initial bent needle design with their proponents claiming safety. The disadvantages of bent needles include the inability to perform cryoablation or radiofrequency ablation, and difficulty in extracting the stylet after proper needle positioning. A needle-in-needle technique may avoid trauma to the disc and coccyx, as well as decrease needle breakages during the transcoccygeal approach.[72] It may also decrease introducing perineal flora into osseous structures. Following diagnostic local anesthetic injections, neurolytic injection, cryoablation, or radiofrequency ablation of the ganglion may be performed.[73,74]

COMPLICATIONS

Potential for the perforation of the rectum, anus, and vascular structures in the neighborhood exist, which may lead to infection in the needle tract, including discitis. In addition, because of its location in the perineum, contamination from perineal flora always exists.

TECHNIQUE OF FLUOROSCOPY-GUIDED GANGLION IMPAR BLOCK

The patient is comfortably positioned prone with a pillow underneath the pelvis, and the hips externally rotated to provide exposure of the perineum. Fluoroscopy image intensifier is placed in the lateral view and the sacrococcygeal segment is identified. Subsequently, the area is prepped with a suitable antiseptic solution and draped in a sterile manner. Skin, subcutaneous tissues and periosteum are anesthetized with 1% Lidocaine at the point of needle entry. A short large-bore hypodermic needle is inserted through the first intercoccygeal joint. Once the tip is advanced anteriorly to the ventral bone surface, the anteroposterior fluoroscopy is performed to assure its midline position. Some practitioners prefer to place a second coaxial needle, for example, 2-in 22G Quincke, through the first needle. Further confirmation is provided by the lateral fluoroscopic view, where the needle tip should be seen just anteriorly to the coccyx bone. Using fluoroscopy, 0.5–1 mL of contrast agent is injected to confirm proper spread of the dye (comma sign) prior to injecting a local anesthetic, a steroid, or a neurolytic (Fig. 84.25). It is the authors' practice to inject local anesthetic first to confirm pain reduction with this procedure prior to steroid injection or neurolytic intervention. The total volume required is usually about 2–4 mL.

CONCLUSIONS

The ganglion impar block is now regaining its popularity among pain practitioners for the management of perineal visceral pain. Ultrasound guidance during the performance of this block provides real-time visualization and markedly decreases the radiation dose.

KEY POINTS

- Ganglion impar is the terminal midline sympathetic ganglion.
- The location of the ganglion impar is commonly over the first coccygeal vertebral body and the sacrococcygeal junction.
- The ganglion impar block provides relief in coccygodynia and pain of the lower part of the rectum, anus, urethra, and vagina.
- Image guidance for the performance of this block is provided by fluoroscopy, CT, and ultrasound—each with its own inherent advantages and disadvantages.

REFERENCES

Access the reference list online at ExpertConsult.com.

CHAPTER

85

INTERVENTIONAL PAIN PROCEDURES IN PATIENTS ON ANTICOAGULANTS

Honorio T. Benzon, MD

INTRODUCTION

The American Society of Regional Anesthesia and Pain Medicine (ASRA) has published guidelines on regional anesthesia in patients on anticoagulants. These guidelines have been used by clinicians in the United States and as a template for guidelines of regional anesthesia organizations in other countries.[1] The latest edition (the third edition) of the regional anesthesia guidelines was published in 2010 and is presently being updated. In the absence of guidelines on interventional procedures to guide them, pain physicians have used the ASRA regional guidelines in their practice. Unfortunately, there have been case reports of spinal anesthesia after epidural steroid injections (ESIs) or spinal cord stimulator placements not only when the regional anesthesia guidelines were followed but also when coagulation studies were normal (Table 85.1).[2–14]

The occurrence of spinal hematoma even when the coagulation studies were normal or when the ASRA guidelines were adhered to is due to several reasons. Pain patients are elderly, a known risk factor in exaggerated response to anticoagulants. Older patients have spinal stenosis wherein the epidural space is decreased.[15–17] Smaller amounts of hematoma can result in compression of the spinal cord, and progression of symptoms can be more rapid because of the diminished epidural space. The presence of numbness and/or weakness in patients with radiculitis, before the injection, confuses the clinical picture of spinal hematoma. Low back pain patients who had laminectomy can have scarring, further limiting the space where the hematoma can spread. With regard to the placement of spinal cord stimulators, large-bore needles are placed and several advancements and retractions are required to optimally place the electrodes. These result in a higher risk of trauma to the vascular structures. Finally, pain clinic patients may be on medications usually considered as not altering the clotting of blood. These drugs include the anticonvulsants carbamazepine, oxcarbazepine, valproate, and levetiracetam, and the selective serotonin reuptake inhibitors (SSRIs).[18–23] In addition to these medications, elderly pain patients may be on antiplatelets for cardiovascular or central nervous system (CNS) thrombotic/embolic prophylaxis. The intake of several antiplatelet drugs is a known risk of spinal hematoma after a neuraxial injection.[24]

Aware of the case reports of spinal hematoma when their guidelines on regional anesthesia were adhered to, the Board of Directors of the ASRA commissioned a Writing Committee to promulgate guidelines that are applicable to interventional pain procedures. These guidelines were endorsed by the European Society of Regional Anesthesia and Pain Therapy, American Academy of Pain Medicine, International Neuromodulation Society, North American Neuromodulation Society, and the World Institute of Pain.[25]

In this chapter, the following topics will be discussed: stratification of the risks of bleeding according to the type of procedure, antiplatelet medications, older anticoagulants, novel oral anticoagulants (NOACs), antidepressants, and herbal medications. Differences between the ASRA regional and interventional pain procedures will be pointed out. The GPIIb/IIIa inhibitors will not be discussed, as at present the use of these drugs is rare and, if used, the patients are usually placed on P2Y12 inhibitors for maintenance therapy.

STRATIFICATION OF RISKS

One distinguishing feature that the pain guidelines offer, in contrast to the regional guidelines, is stratification of the risks of bleeding according to the type of pain procedure (Table 85.2). This is because the risks of bleeding, progression, and consequence of the hematoma from lack of compressibility vary with the different procedures. On one hand, the abdominal and pelvic sympathetic blocks are close to large vascular structures, cannot be easily compressed, and symptoms associated with hematoma from these injections are vague. Intravertebral and perivertebral procedures are associated with compression of the spinal cord with devastating consequences. On the other hand, trigger point injections, joint injections, and superficial nerve blocks (e.g., occipital nerve blocks in the scalp) are avascular, superficial, and associated with minor bleeding complications. Mild anticoagulation is probably acceptable when the risk and consequences are small. This is to prevent the patient from having a stroke, myocardial infarction, or venous thromboembolism (VTE).

ASPIRIN PHOSPHODIESTERASE INHIBITORS AND NONSTEROIDAL ANTIINFLAMMATORY DRUGS

There are several mechanisms of aspirin's antiplatelet effect. Aspirin preferentially blocks COX-1 over COX-2. It irreversibly inactivates COX-1 through the acetylation of the amino acid serine.[26,27] By inactivating COX-1 and blocking thromboxane production, aspirin inhibits platelet activation, platelet aggregation, and thrombosis. Aspirin inactivates the COX-1 in the megakaryocytes in the bone marrow, and megakaryocytes are responsible for platelet production. The drug also influences coagulation through non-TXA2-mediated effects. These include impairment of secondary hemostasis and stability of the thrombus by acetylating fibrinogen and enhancing fibrinolysis.[28] Unlike nonsteroidal antiinflammatory drugs (NSAIDs), aspirin decreases thrombin formation.[29] At higher doses, aspirin prevents endothelial cell prostacyclin production by

TABLE 85.1 Reports of Spinal Hematoma After Epidural Steroid Injections or Spinal Cord Stimulator Placements

Report	Patient Profile	Outcome	Other Drugs; Comment
Williams et al.[9]	63, male, CESI	Full recovery	Indomethacin and allopurinol
Ghaly[10]	57, male, CESI	Full recovery	Diclofenac, amitriptyline
Reitman and Watters[11]	62, female, CESI	Partial recovery	Normal coagulation studies
Ain and Vance[12]	85, female, LESI	Motor recovery, residual numbness of left toes	Warfarin resumed the night after ESI, enoxaparin restarted 24 h later, INR 1.2 the next day
Xu et al.[13]	78, female, LESI	Full recovery	Warfarin restarted 8 h after ESI, enoxaparin resumed 30 h later
Giberson et al.[2]	2 cases: 53, male; 70, male	Patient 1: Residual left leg weakness Patient 2: Complete recovery	Patient 1 took aspirin the day the leads were pulled; patient 2 had not taken aspirin for 7 days before the trial
Buvanendran and Young[3]	73, female	Complete recovery	Took low-dose aspirin daily
Takawira et al.[4]	52, male	Spontaneous recovery	Patient not on anticoagulant. Symptoms on third day of trial; hematoma possibly from lead migration.
Smith et al.[5]	2 cases: 44, male; 66, female	Patient 1: No recovery Patient 2: Residual numbness below T8	Coagulation studies normal
Kloss et al.[6]	50, male	Partial recovery	No mention of medications or recovery

CESI, *Cervical epidural steroid injection;* LESI, *lumbar epidural steroid injection.*

TABLE 85.2 Pain Procedures According to the Potential Risks for Serious Bleeding[a]

High-Risk Procedures	Intermediate-Risk Procedures	Low-Risk Procedures
SCS trial and implant	Interlaminar ESIs	Peripheral nerve blocks
IT catheter and pump implant	Facet MBB and RFA	Peripheral joints and musculoskeletal injections
Vertebroplasty, kyphoplasty	Paravertebral blocks	Trigger point and piriformis injections
Epiduroscopy and epidural decompression	Intradiscal procedures	Sacroiliac joint injections
	Sympathetic blocks	Sacral LBBs
	Pocket revision and IPG/ITP replacement	

ESIs, *Epidural steroid injections;* IPG, *intrathecal pump generator;* LBB, *lateral branch block;* MBB, *medial branch block;* RFA, *radiofrequency ablation.*
[a]*Patients who are at high risk for bleeding undergoing low- or intermediate-risk procedures should be treated as intermediate or high risk, respectively. Patients with high risk for bleeding include the elderly, concurrent use of anticoagulants, low body weight, or advanced liver and renal disease.*

inhibiting COX-2.[28] Prostacyclin not only inhibits platelet coagulation but also stimulates vasodilation.

Aspirin (ASA) is rapidly absorbed from the gastrointestinal tract, peak levels occur 30 minutes after ingestion, and significant platelet inhibition is present at 1 hour.[30,31] For enteric-coated aspirin, peak plasma levels may be delayed until 3–4 hours after ingestion.[28,32] COX activity does not return for 48 hours after aspirin intake, and this has been interpreted as the duration of effect of aspirin on megakaryocytes.[33,34] The average lifespan of a platelet is 7–10 days.[35,36] Approximately 10% of the circulating platelet pool is replaced every day.[37] This means that at 5 days, approximately 50% of the circulating platelets are not affected by the aspirin.

Similar to the ASRA guidelines on regional anesthesia, the patient can continue to take the aspirin when low-risk pain procedures are performed. However, the two guidelines have different recommendations with regard to neuraxial injections. Whereas the regional guidelines allow neuraxial injections, the pain guidelines do not. This is in view of the case reports of spinal hematoma after ESI in patients on aspirin (see Table 85.1). The length of discontinuation depends on the reason for the patient's taking the aspirin: 6 days for primary prevention (aspirin in patients with no overt cardiovascular disease) and 4 days for secondary prophylaxis.[25,38] The drug can be resumed 24 hours later.

The commonly used phosphodiesterase (PDE) inhibitors are dipyridamole and cilostazol. These drugs impede PDE isoenzymes expressed by platelets.[39] PDE inhibitors thwart cyclic adenosine monophosphate (cAMP) and cyclic guanosine monophosphate (cGMP) levels. PDE-3 inhibitors increase cAMP levels, whereas PDE-5 inhibitors increase cGMP levels. Cilostazol inhibits PDE-3, while dipyridamole inhibits PDE-3 and PDE-5; dipyridamole has been combined with aspirin for a more pronounced effect. By blocking the secondary messengers cAMP, cGMP, and PDEs, these drugs reduce platelet aggregation and increase vasodilatation. These drugs decrease platelet aggregation by approximately 40%.[40] Dipyridamole has a half-life of 10 hours. The extended-release dipyridamole, used in combination with aspirin, has a half-life of 13.6 hours.[41] Cilostazol reaches peak plasma concentrations at 2 hours, and maximum platelet aggregation occurs at 6 hours.[39,42] Similar to dipyridamole, cilostazol has an elimination half-life of 10 hours. Five half-lives, where 97% of the drug is eliminated,[43] is equivalent to 50 hours. A discontinuation of 2 days should thus be adequate, and the drugs can be resumed 24 hours later.

NSAIDs, like aspirin, inhibit the COX enzyme. Such a blockade is reversible, compared with the irreversible effect of aspirin. The Writing Committee used the drug's half-life to guide the duration of discontinuation of the NSAID before a pain procedure.[44–47] As noted

TABLE 85.3 Duration of Discontinuation of Aspirin, Phosphodiesterase Inhibitors, and Nonsteroidal Antiinflammatory Drugs

Drug	Half-Life (Hours)	Discontinuation, in Days, Based on Five Half-Lives
Aspirin	20–30 min[a]	4 for secondary prophylaxis, 6 for primary prophylaxis
Cilostazol	10 h	2
Dipyridamole	10 h	2
Diclofenac	1–2	1
Ibuprofen	2–4	1
Ketorolac	5–6	1
Etodolac	6–8	2
Indomethacin	5–10	2
Naproxen	12–17	4
Meloxicam	15–20	4
Namebutone	22–30	6
Oxaprozin	40–60	10
Piroxicam	45–50	10

[a]*Aspirin has an irreversible effect on platelets; stoppage of drug is based on platelet recovery.*
From Patrick J, Dillaha L, Armas D, Sessa WC: A randomized trial to assess the pharmacodynamics and pharmacokinetics of a single dose of an extended-release aspirin. Postgrad Med. *127:573–580, 2015.*

previously, an interval of five half-lives is adequate, as this represents 97% elimination of the drug.[43] This results in a discontinuation of 1–2 days for ibuprofen, diclofenac, ketorolac, and indomethacin; 4 days for naproxen and meloxicam; 6 days for namebutone; and 10 days for oxaprozin and piroxicam. The drug can be resumed a day after the procedure (Table 85.3).

P2Y12 INHIBITORS CLOPIDOGREL, PRASUGREL, AND TICAGRELOR

The P2Y12 receptors are mostly found on the surface of platelets. ADP released from platelet-dense granules binds to two platelet G-protein-coupled receptors, the $P2Y_1$ and $P2Y_{12}$ receptors. $P2Y_1$ is a Gq-coupled receptor that initiates ADP-induced platelet aggregation via the stimulation of phospholipase C and phosphatidylinositol-signaling pathway. $P2Y_{12}$ is a Gi-coupled seven-transmembrane domain receptor, which mediates platelet activation by inhibiting the adenylate cyclase-mediated signaling pathway and decreasing intracellular cAMP levels. The decrease in intracellular cAMP levels and activation of the GPIIB/IIIa receptor results in reduced platelet aggregation and increased vasodilation.[48] $P2Y_{12}$ is also involved in platelet secretion induced by strong agonists. The significant role of the $P2Y_{12}$ receptor in platelet activation and formation of a stable thrombus has made it an important target in the management and prevention of arterial thrombosis. The P2Y12 inhibitors include clopidogrel, prasugrel, ticagrelor, and cangrelor. Patients who have cardiovascular problems are usually prescribed combined P2Y12 inhibitor and aspirin, the so-called "dual antiplatelet therapy," complicating the stoppage of these drugs before a pain procedure.

Clopidogrel and prasugrel are irreversible P2Y12 inhibitors. Both are prodrugs, requiring a two-step metabolism to be converted to their active metabolite. Clopidogrel is susceptible to genetic polymorphisms, and 9% of patients do not respond to the drug. Clopidogrel causes a 60% inhibition of platelets, while prasugrel results in 90% inhibition.[49] For this reason, a 7-day stoppage is recommended for medium and high-risk procedures (Table 85.4).[50] For clopidogrel specifically, the European and Scandinavian guidelines respectively recommended a 7- and 5-day stoppage of clopidogrel before regional anesthesia.[51,52] A 5-day duration may be reasonable, as a study showed that most patients have no platelet inhibition after 5 days, and the rest had minimal inhibition.[53] Since a trial of spinal cord stimulator entails several days, most pain clinicians stop the clopidogrel for 5 days. A test of platelet activity should be performed if only a 5-day stoppage is observed to document that platelet recovery is significant. The commonly used tests of antiplatelet activity of the P2Y12 receptors include either the VerifyNow P2Y12 assay or the platelet mapping portion of the thromboelastography.

TABLE 85.4 Recommended Intervals Between Stoppage and Resumption of the P2Y12 Inhibitors and Medium- and High-Risk Pain Procedures

Drug	Interval Between Discontinuation and Pain Procedure	Resumption of the Drug
Clopidogrel	7 days, 5 days if platelet function studies show adequate recovery	12 h when loading dose is given, 24 h for the usual maintenance daily dose
Prasugrel	7 days	24 h
Ticagrelor	5 days	24 h
Cangrelor	1–2 h	[a]

[a]*Patients who are given cangrelor are usually maintained on oral P2Y12 inhibitors.*

Ticagrelor, in contrast to clopidogrel and prasugrel, is a direct-acting P2Y12 inhibitor. It inhibits the aggregation of platelets by 90%; platelet function recovery is adequate 5 days after stopping the drug.[54] Cangrelor, another direct P2Y12 inhibitor, is given intravenously. The drug is approved for clinical use in patients undergoing percutaneous coronary intervention.[55] It has a fast onset of a few minutes, and its half-life is 3–7 minutes. Platelet function has been shown to normalize 1 hour after it is stopped. If a pain procedure has to be done, at least a 1-hour interval should be observed. This situation is rarely encountered, as patients are usually maintained on oral P2Y12 inhibitors.

Prasugrel and ticagrelor should be resumed 24 hours after the procedure, as these drugs take effect within 2–4 hours. Clopidogrel, if given in its usual 75-mg dose, can be started 12 hours after the pain procedure, since it takes 1 or 2 days to take full effect. However, a 300–600-mg loading dose of clopidogrel takes effect after a few hours and should be started 24 hours later.

OLDER ANTICOAGULANTS: WARFARIN, HEPARIN, LOW-MOLECULAR-WEIGHT HEPARIN, FIBRINOLYTIC AGENTS

Warfarin inhibits the γ-carboxylation of the vitamin K–dependent coagulation factors. These factors have different half-lives: 6–8 hours for factor VII, 20–24 hours for factor IX, 20–42 hours for factor X, and 48–120 hours for factor II.[56,57] The inhibition of clotting factor VII causes the initial anticoagulation from warfarin. This effect, however, is antagonized by a decrease in anticoagulant protein C,[57] making the International Normalized Ratio (INR) unreliable during the early phase of warfarin therapy.[57,58] The full anticoagulant effect of warfarin does not occur until 4 days later, when the levels of factor II are significantly decreased. Concentrations of clotting factors of 40% or more are considered adequate for hemostasis[59]; levels below 20% are associated with bleeding.[60] While warfarin is used in the United States, acenocoumarol is prescribed in Europe. The difference is the normalization of the INR between the two drugs: 5 days for warfarin and 3 days for acenocoumarol.

The ability of warfarin to affect the extrinsic pathway of the coagulation cascade (by inhibiting the activity of factor VII), the intrinsic pathway (factor IX), factor X (junction of the two pathways), and the end product of coagulation (factor II) makes it a powerful anticoagulant. However, warfarin is difficult to dose, as it has a narrow therapeutic index, there is wide interpatient dosing variability, and genetic factors account for a large proportion of the variations in dose requirements.[61] Although patients with variations in their CYP2C9 and/or VKORC1 require lower doses of warfarin, studies on genetic-based dosing were not uniform in their findings.[62–64] The American College of Cardiology recommended against pharmacokinetic-based dosing, pending clinical studies.[58]

In patients who have not taken warfarin, an INR of 1.4 is acceptable for neuraxial injections. However, in patients who took warfarin, the ASRA guidelines recommend normalization of the INR (1.2 or less) after stoppage of warfarin for 5 days before medium- and high-risk procedures are performed.[25] This is in contrast to the European and Scandinavian guidelines that accept an INR of 1.4 or less as long as the warfarin was stopped for 5 days.[51,52] A slightly prolonged INR of 1.3–1.4 may not be safe, as a study showed the levels of clotting factor X and II to be below 40% in two patients.[65]

A low-molecular-weight heparin (LMWH) "bridge" therapy may be considered in patients who are at high risk for VTE. A study in patients who had atrial fibrillation, however, showed that the discontinuation of warfarin without bridge therapy was noninferior to bridge therapy with dalteparin.[66] The incidence of arterial thromboembolism was not different between the two groups, while the incidence of major bleeding was significantly higher in the bridging group. This study may only be applicable to patients who have atrial fibrillation, the subject of the study, and not to patients with prosthetic cardiac valves. Another study showed patients who were bridged before their total hip arthroplasty had a slower healing time (in terms of their wounds) and also had a longer hospital stay.[67]

Heparin inactivates thrombin (factor IIa), factor IXa, and Xa.[1] The anticoagulant effect of intravenous heparin is immediate, whereas subcutaneous heparin takes 1 hour.[68] Its therapeutic effect ceases 4–6 hours after its administration. The half-life of heparin increases with increased dose: 30 minutes for the 25 U/kg dose, 60-minute half-life of 100 U/kg, and 150 minutes for the 400 U/kg dose.[69,70] Monitoring is via the activated partial thromboplastin time (aPTT), and therapeutic anticoagulation is achieved when the aPTT is 1.5–2.5 times the initial value.[71] Reversal is achieved with protamine, with the dose being 1 mg of protamine per 100 U of heparin.

The performance of pain procedures in patients on *intravenous* heparin should be avoided, since interventional pain procedures are usually elective procedures. Noninterventional procedures such as medications (opioids, anticonvulsants, antidepressants) and adjunctive therapy can be performed to alleviate the patient's pain. If an interventional procedure has to be done, it can be done at least 5 hours after the IV heparin is stopped. The 5-hour interval is based on the five half-lives (60-minutes) of the usual 100 U/kg clinical dose of *intravenous* heparin. As the half-lives of intravenous heparin varies with the dose, the interval between the last *intravenous* heparin dose and the interventional pain procedure should be adjusted accordingly.

The ASRA guidelines on regional anesthesia allow the continued use of *BID subcutaneous* heparin, while the pain guidelines recommended that interventional procedures not be performed until at least 8 hours after the subcutaneous heparin was given. This 8 hours is longer than the five-half-life (5–6 hours) of the drug. This was to accommodate patients with exaggerated response to heparin and the slightly more prolonged absorption of subcutaneous administration.[72] The drug can be restarted a minimum of 2 hours after the procedure. Interventional pain procedures are not recommended in patients on *TID subcutaneous* heparin. Two studies showed the probable safety of doing neuraxial interventions with patients on subcutaneous TID heparin. No epidural hematomas occurred after removal of epidural catheters in 714 patients on TID heparin, and 20 patients had PTTs greater than 35 seconds when their epidurals were removed.[73] Another study showed no spinal hematoma after thoracic epidurals in 928 patients; activated thromboplastin time was greater than 40 seconds in 115 patients.[74] The small number of patients in these two studies is not adequate to change the recommendations.

For LMWH, the ASRA pain (and regional) guidelines recommend a 12-hour interval between stoppage of prophylactic dose of enoxaparin and interventional pain procedures. For therapeutic doses of enoxaparin (i.e., 1 mg/kg) and for dalteparin, a 24-hour interval is recommended. The drug can be resumed 4 hours after a low-risk pain procedure, an interval similar recommended by a recent FDA Drug Safety Communication.[75]

In cases where the moderate- or high-risk procedures are bloody, the resumption of warfarin, heparin, and LMWH should be delayed for 24 hours after the procedure (see Table 85.5). As in the regional anesthesia guidelines, drugs that affect hemostasis (antiplatelet, NSAIDs, SSRIs, and other anticoagulants) should preferably not be concomitantly used in patients on these anticoagulants.

Fibrinolytic agents dissolve fibrin clots. Intravascular fibrin clots are dissolved by plasmin, which is derived from its inactive precursor plasminogen. These drugs include streptokinase and urokinase that dissolve thrombus band activate plasminogen, and alteplase and tenecteplase that are more fibrin-selective and have minimal effect on plasminogen. The half-life of fibrinolytic agents is only a few hours, but fibrinogen and plasminogen are decreased up to 27 hours. Therefore surgery or other interventions that may involve the puncture of noncompressible vessels

TABLE 85.5 Recommended Intervals Between Stoppage and Resumption of the Old Anticoagulants Interventional Pain Procedures

Drugs	Drug Discontinuation and Pain Procedure	Resumption of Drug
Warfarin	5 days, INR back to normal	24 h
IV heparin	4 h	2–24 h
BID subcutaneous heparin	8–24 h	2–4 h
TID subcutaneous heparin[a]	—	
LMWH, prophylactic dose	12 h	4–24 h
LMWH, therapeutic dose	24 h	4–24 h
LMWH, dalteparin	24 h	4–24 h
Fibrinolytic agents[a]	—	

[a]*Interventional pain procedures not recommended.*

have been advised against for up to 10 days.[1] The ASRA guidelines on regional anesthesia are vague because there is very little data on regional anesthesia in patients who had fibrinolytic agents. On the other hand, the ASRA pain guidelines recommended that interventional pain procedures be avoided in these patients. If a pain procedure has to be done, then a minimum of 48 hours should elapse from the time the drug was given to the time the procedure is performed. The 48-hour-interval is a little longer than the Scandinavian guidelines that recommended a 24-hour interval between the stoppage of the drug and a neuraxial block.[52] Longer intervals are preferable in view of the absence of data on these patients.

CLOTTING FACTOR INHIBITORS: FONDAPARINUX AND THE NOVEL ORAL ANTICOAGULANTS

Clotting Factor X sits at the junction of the intrinsic and extrinsic pathways of the coagulation cascade. Fondaparinux is a synthetic Factor Xa inhibitor. The NOACs, also called direct oral anticoagulants (DOACs), that are Factor X inhibitors include ribaroxaban, apixaban, and edoxaban (Fig. 85.1). The other NOAC is dabigatran, a direct thrombin inhibitor. Thrombin is the end product of coagulation. Factor X inhibitors and direct thrombin inhibitors have become the focus of development by the pharmaceutical companies. Several review articles on the pharmacology, indications, pharmacokinetics, and reversal of the drugs have been published over the last few years.[76–85] There are no published studies on the safety of NOACs in regional anesthesia and pain interventional procedures. To ensure that the plasma levels of the anticoagulant are low, the ASRA pain guidelines recommended a five half-life interval. The next edition of the ASRA regional anesthesia guidelines will base their recommendations on five half-lives of the drugs.

Fondaparinux is a synthetic anticoagulant that specifically blocks clotting factor Xa. Maximum concentration is attained within 2 hours of administration, its half-life of 17–21 hours.[86] In one study, no complications were noted in

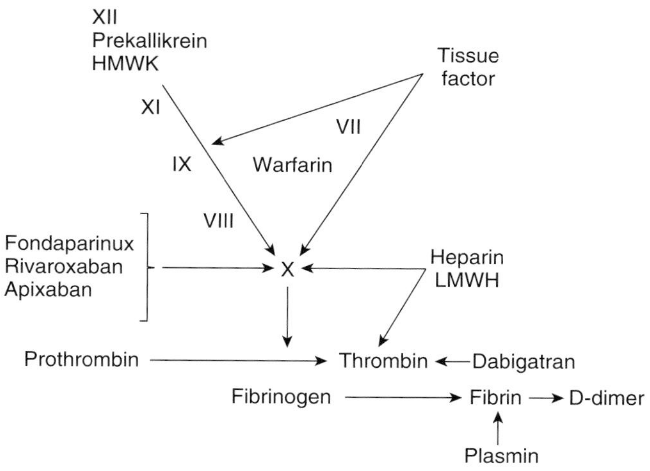

FIG. 85.1 Sites of inhibition by the anticoagulants in the coagulation cascade.

1603 patients who had neuraxial catheters or deep peripheral nerve catheters.[87] In that study, the protocol was quite strict and does not replicate actual clinical conditions. No more than three neuraxial attempts were allowed; patients were excluded if they were taking an antiplatelet medication, if there was bleeding with the neuraxial procedure, or if the plan was to remove the epidural catheter the day after the surgery. At any rate, 2.5 mg fondaparinux was given 6–12 hours after surgery, the catheters were removed 36 hours after the last dose of fondaparinux, and redosing was 12 hours after catheter removal.[87] The 36-hour interval corresponds to two half-lives of the drug. This can be risky in patients with spinal stenosis and those who had postlaminectomy scarring. The ASRA guidelines recommended a five-half-life interval or 3–4 day discontinuation before a medium- or high-risk interventional pain procedure is performed. The drug can be resumed 24 hours later.

Dabigatran is approved for the prevention of stroke in patients with nonvalvular atrial fibrillation in the United States, Canada, and Europe. It is also indicated for the prevention of VTE after knee or hip arthroplasty in Europe and Canada but not in the United States. This discrepancy is because studies in Europe showed it to be effective,[88] but studies in the US showed it to be inferior to twice-daily enoxaparin[89] in preventing VTE after total joint surgery. Dabigatran is a prodrug with an onset of 1.5–3 hours and a half-life of 14–17 hours.[90] It is 80% eliminated by the kidneys; the presence of renal insufficiency results in the doubling of its half-life, from 14 to 28 hours.[91] Five half-lives, corresponding to 4 days, is the recommended interval between stoppage of the drug and performing a pain procedure (Table 85.6). A longer interval, 6 days, should be observed in patients with renal problems. The drug can be resumed 24 hours after the procedure.

Rivaroxaban is approved for the prevention of stroke in nonvalvular atrial fibrillation, prophylaxis and treatment of VTE, and prevention of VTE after orthopedic surgery in the United States, Europe, and Canada.[78] A Factor Xa inhibitor, peak concentrations of rivaroxaban are reached 2.5–4 hours after intake, and its half-life is 6–9 hours.[92,93] One-third of the drug is eliminated by the kidneys, one-third by the fecal/biliary route, and the final third is

TABLE 85.6 Recommended Intervals Between Stoppage and Resumption of the New Anticoagulants and Interventional Pain Procedures, Laboratory Tests, and Reversal

Drug	Drug Discontinuation and Pain Procedure	Resumption of Drug	Laboratory Test	Reversal
Fondaparinux	4 days	24 h		
Dabigatran	4 days (6 days in renal patients)	24 h	Dilute TT ECT	Dialysis Activated charcoal within 2 h
Rivaroxaban	3–5 days	24 h	PT Anti-Xa assay	Activated charcoal within 8 h Four-factor PCC
Apixaban	3 days	24 h	Anti-Xa assay	Activated charcoal within 3 h
Edoxaban[a]	3 days (6 days in renal patients)	24 h	Anti-Xa assay	

ECT, *Ecarin clotting time (not readily available)*; PCC, *prothrombin complex concentrate*; PT, *prothrombin time*; TT, *thrombin time*.
[a]*Basis for resumption of the anticoagulants.*

changed to inactive metabolites. A five half-life interval, or 3 days, is recommended between discontinuation of the drug and medium- and high-risk procedures. The drug may be resumed 24 hours later.

Apixaban is a Factor Xa inhibitor drug and is indicated for the prevention of stroke in patients with nonvalvular atrial fibrillation and for VTE prophylaxis after hip and knee arthroplasty (Europe and Canada). Peak plasma concentrations are attained within 2 hours; it has a half-life of 13 ± 9 hours.[94,95] There have been few pharmacokinetic studies on the drug, resulting in a wide variation in its half-life (13 ± 9 hours). In patients who are not at high risk for bleeding, 3 days is recommended between stoppage of the drug and medium- and high-risk interventional pain procedures. For patients who are more susceptible to the effect of anticoagulants (elderly, low body weight, liver, and renal problems), a longer interval of 4–5 days should be considered. The drug can be resumed 24 hours later.

Edoxaban is a Factor Xa inhibitor that is approved for the prevention of stroke in patients with atrial fibrillation and for the treatment of deep venous thrombosis and pulmonary embolism. Maximum concentration is attained 2 hours after intake, the drug is 60% bioavailable, and 50% is excreted by kidneys. Its half-life is 8.75–10.4 hours.[96] Five half-lives (55 hours or 2.5 days) means a 3-day discontinuation before interventional procedures in patients without a renal problem. As it is significantly eliminated by the kidneys, a longer interval (e.g., 5–6 days) should be considered in patients with renal disease. The drug can be resumed 24 hours later (see Table 85.6).

The ASRA pain guidelines recommended that the anticoagulant can be resumed 24 hours after an interventional procedure. This is in contrast to the European regional guidelines that suggest 6–8 hours is adequate.[51] The 6–8-hour interval was based on the assumption that a clot is stable after 8 hours.[78] Studies support this interval. Clot resolution has been demonstrated to be complete after 7 hours.[97] The efficacy of thrombolytics to lyse a cerebral embolic clot was largely driven by patients who were treated within 3 hours of stroke onset, implying that anticoagulants do not contribute to clot lysis after 8 hours.[98,99] Enoxaparin given within 24–48 hours after intracerebral hemorrhage does not lead to enlargement of the hematoma.[100] Other experts, however, recommended a more conservative approach on the timing of resumption of anticoagulants, because the reinstitution of antithrombotic therapy within 24 hours after a major procedure might increase the risk of periprocedural bleeding.[77] Liew and Douketis[80] recommend a minimum of 24 hours in patients with low bleeding risk, and 48 hours in those with a high bleeding risk. Overall, a 24-hour interval is probably adequate.

LABORATORY TESTS AND REVERSAL OF THE NOVEL ORAL ANTICOAGULANTS

The more widespread use of the NOACs has been hampered by the lack of laboratory tests to monitor their effect. Even now, appropriate monitoring is not available, except in more advanced academic medical centers. For the novel anticoagulants, coagulation tests should be interpreted relative to the last administered dose, drug pharmacokinetics, and renal function. Each NOAC requires an analyte-specific test—that is, the test for apixaban will not give correctly calibrated results for rivaroxaban and vice versa. The anti-FXa chromogenic assay for monitoring the direct Xa inhibitors includes testing analyte-specific calibration and quality controls, assessing patient correlations with known samples, establishing standard operating procedures, training and development of test ordering in the laboratory information system, and notification of other departments, including medical services and pharmacy.[101]

The aPTT is prolonged after dabigatran, but the relationship between the test and the drug is not linear: there is a greater than linear increase at lower concentrations (at or below 200 ng/mL) and a linear relationship at higher concentrations (>200 ng/mL; see Table 85.6).[81,82] The thrombin time (TT), also known as thrombin clotting time (TCT), is highly sensitive to the effects of dabigatran.[82,83,102] A dilute TT (hemoclot thrombin inhibitory assay) has become available in some centers and has linearity across pharmacologically relevant plasma dabigatran concentrations.[81,83] The ecarin clotting time (ECT) directly measures thrombin generation. (Ecarin is a commercially available snake venom that converts prothrombin to meizothrombin, is prolonged by dabigatran, and is linearly and dose-dependently related to dabigatran concentrations.[81,90,102,103]) In summary, the prothrombin time

(PT) is the least sensitive test while the dilute TT and the ECT are the tests of choice for dabigatran.[81]

A linear correlation was observed between the effects of rivaroxaban and the PT, especially when neoplastin was used as the test reagent (see Table 85.6).[82,102] There is marked variability in the sensitivity of PT reagents to rivaroxaban, so every laboratory should calibrate the PT specifically for rivaroxaban to determine the effect of the drug on the test.[104] The INR is not recommended to monitor rivaroxaban, because the INR is dependent on the thromboplastin reagent, and thromboplastins vary greatly in their sensitivity to rivaroxaban. The aPTT lacks adequate sensitivity to determine the anticoagulant effect of rivaroxaban; the drug does not prolong the ECT.[82,102] The inhibition of Factor Xa may also be a surrogate for the plasma concentrations of rivaroxaban.[105] Overall, the PT and the anti-Xa are the tests best suited to monitor the effects of rivaroxaban.[81]

Compared to rivaroxaban, apixaban has little effect on the PT when given in the usual clinical doses.[82] Similar to rivaroxaban, each laboratory should specifically calibrate the sensitivity of their PT assay to apixaban. The dilute PT assay, wherein the thromboplastin reagent is diluted 16 times, has much better sensitivity compared with the conventional PT.[82] There is a linear correlation between anti-Xa activity and low, intermediate, or high plasma concentrations of apixaban; hence, the drug can be evaluated by the anti-Xa assay (see Table 85.6).[106] The anti-Xa assay is more sensitive than the PT and as sensitive as the dilute PT assay, and is the best choice for monitoring of the anticoagulant effect of apixaban.[81]

Edoxaban prolongs the PT in a dose-dependent linear fashion, but the assay is not adequately sensitive.[107] The drug also prolongs the aPTT in a dose-dependent manner. The PT is more sensitive than the aPTT, but there is interreagent variability, and some PT assays are not sensitive at troughlike concentrations. A prolonged PT in the absence of other explanation in a patient who is being treated with edoxaban indicates the presence of the drug; however, a normal PT does not exclude the possibility of edoxaban's effect. The thrombin generation assay (TGA) is more sensitive than the PT or aPTT but is not widely available. Anti-Xa activity increases in a dose-dependent linear fashion with edoxaban; the test provides the best correlation with plasma concentration of edoxaban.[107]

REVERSAL OF THE NOVEL ORAL ANTICOAGULANTS

Activated charcoal prevents absorption of the drug within the intestine, but it needs to be given within 2 hours of dabigatran ingestion (see Table 85.6). Dialysis speeds elimination of the drug but may not be clinically appropriate. Recombinant Factor VIIa (NovoSeven, Princeton, New Jersey) has been recommended to control hemorrhage,[80] but there is little clinical experience with this agent. Prothrombin complex concentrates (PCCs) are concentrated pooled plasma products that contain either three (Factors II, IX, and X) or four (Factors II, VII, IX, and X) clotting factors. While the use of four-factor PCCs has been suggested,[83,102] a trial of this concentrate did not reverse the in vitro anticoagulant effect of dabigatran in healthy volunteers.[108] There is a risk of thrombosis with the use of recombinant Factor VII and PCCs.

Idarucizumab is a monoclonal antibody fragment that that binds with free and thrombin-bound dabigatran.[109] Initial studies showed efficacy of the drug in reversing dabigatran in healthy and elderly volunteers.[110,111] A prospective cohort study of 90 patients showed idarucizumab to normalize the elevated ECT in 88%–98% of patients within minutes.[112] In that study, hemostasis was restored at a median of 11.4 hours in the group who had serious bleeding. In the other group that required an urgent procedure, normal intraoperative hemostasis was noted in 33 of 36 patients, and mildly or moderately abnormal hemostasis was noted in one and two patients, respectively. The dose of idarucizumab was 5 g intravenously, administered as two 50-mL bolus infusions, 2.5 mg each dose, given no more than 15 minutes apart.[112] Idarucizumab has recently been approved by the FDA.

Activated charcoal to decrease the absorption of rivaroxaban has been recommended, but it must be given within 8 hours of rivaroxaban ingestion.[102] Activated charcoal, given within 3 hours of apixaban ingestion, may be effective. The use of recombinant Factor VIIa has been shown to be effective in reversing the effect of fondaparinux[102] but has no demonstrated efficacy for reversing bleeding from the new oral anticoagulants. Because of the risk of thrombogenicity, the FDA issued a black box warning on the use of rFVIIa outside its approved indications. A four-factor PCC, although not effective in dabigatran overdose, has been shown to reverse the in vitro anticoagulant activity of rivaroxaban in healthy volunteers.[102] Whether PCCs would be effective in controlling clinical bleeding due to apixaban has not been adequately assessed.

Andexanet is a recombinant modified human Factor Xa decoy protein that binds and sequesters Factor Xa inhibitors within the vascular space, restoring the activity of the endogenous Factor Xa. The activity of the anticoagulant is decreased, as evidenced by measurement of thrombin generation and Factor Xa activity.[113] A two-part randomized placebo controlled study was recently conducted in older healthy volunteers.[114] In the apixaban-treated patients, antifactor Xa activity was reduced by 94% after andexanet, compared with 21% in the placebo group. Among the rivaroxaban-treated patients, antifactor Xa activity was reduced by 92% after andexanet, compared with 18% in the patients who received placebo.[114] In the study, andexanet was administered as a 400-mg intravenous bolus (30 mg per minute) or as a 400-mg intravenous bolus followed by a continuous infusion of 4 mg per minute for 120 minutes (total of 480 mg). In a multicenter, prospective, open-label, single-group study, patients who had major bleeding within 18 hours after administration of a Factor Xa inhibitor were given andexanet.[115] After andexanet, the median antifactor Xa activity decreased by 89% from baseline in the patients who had rivaroxaban and by 93% in the patients who received apixaban. Twelve hours after andexanet infusion, clinical hemostasis was judged as good or excellent in 37 of 47 patients (79%). Andexanet is presently undergoing additional phase 4 clinical trials in the United States.

ANTIDEPRESSANTS

The tricyclic antidepressants and nonserotonergic antidepressants appear not to be associated with increased bleeding.[25] In contrast, the serotonin reuptake inhibitors (SRIs) have antiplatelet effects. These SRIs decrease platelet serotonin reuptake in the blood, deplete the serotonin content of the platelet, and inhibit the serotonin-mediated platelet aggregation.[21,22,116,117] Increased bleeding has been noted in patients on SRIs.[116–119] Although the antiplatelet effect of SRIs is minimal—that is, equivalent to a low-dose ibuprofen—a lot of pain patients take other antiplatelet medications, and the potentiating interaction when antiplatelet drugs are combined should be considered.

HERBAL MEDICATIONS

Herbal medications can affect clotting. Garlic affects platelet aggregation, and doses as small as 25 mg/day can inhibit the aggregation of platelets.[120] A case report noted spontaneous spinal hematoma in an elderly man who was taking 2000 mg/day of garlic.[121] Garlic, when taken in large amounts, should be stopped for 7 days before a pain procedure. Dong quai potentiates the effect of warfarin, while danshen decreases the elimination of warfarin, so the INR should be checked in patients taking these drugs before an interventional procedure. Gingko biloba inhibits platelet activation factor, and a 36-hour discontinuation has been recommended.[25]

SUMMARY AND CONCLUDING STATEMENTS

The ASRA guidelines on interventional pain procedures in patients on anticoagulants were prompted by occurrences of spinal hematoma when the ASRA guidelines on regional anesthesia were followed. In some cases, spinal hematoma occurred in the presence of normal coagulation studies. An important feature of the pain anticoagulation guidelines is that they stratified the procedures according to the degree of risk of bleeding, allowing the continued use of some anticoagulants when the risk is minimal. In contrast to the regional anesthesia guidelines, aspirin and NSAIDs were recommended to be stopped before medium- and high-risk procedures. The two guidelines are mostly similar in their recommendations with respect to the older anticoagulants warfarin, LMWH, fibrinolytic agents, and fondaparinux. For the NOACs, a five half-life interval between discontinuation of the drug and performance of the interventional pain procedure is recommended. Tremendous advances on the monitoring and reversal of the NOACs have been made recently resulting in better patient care. Observance of the recommendations by ASRA and the other organizations should balance the avoidance of spinal hematoma and prevention of VTE.

REFERENCES

Access the reference list online at ExpertConsult.com.

CHAPTER 86

Interventional Pain Procedures and the Risk of Infection

David A. Provenzano, MD ◎ Michael C. Hanes, MD ◎ Timothy R. Deer, MD

INTRODUCTION

Infections related to interventional pain procedures and implantable devices vary considerably based on the target location, responsible pathogens, anatomical structures involved, collateral damage, and severity. Surgical site infections (SSIs) have been shown to significantly increase mortality, prolong hospital length of stay, and reduce health-related quality of life.[1,2] In addition, SSIs cost the US health care system an estimated $3.5–$10 billion annually.[3] The total cost of a single spinal cord stimulator (SCS) infection has been estimated to range from $28,500 to $54,500 in the United States.[4]

Recently there has been a global emphasis by national and international agencies and societies to create and promote recommended best practices to reduce SSI rates.[5–10] Despite these efforts, SSI rates have not significantly declined.[11] SCS infection rates are higher than those of other implantable devices, including cardiac pacemakers and total joint replacements.[12] A recent international survey of 506 physicians who perform SCS implants was conducted to examine compliance rates for the Centers for Disease Control and Prevention (CDC), National Institute for Health and Care Excellence (NICE), and Surgical Care Improvement Project (SCIP) infection control practice recommendations.[5,7,10] Only four of the 15 questions had compliance rates ≥80%, thus further highlighting the need for physician education in the field. Both current infection rates for implantable pain devices and survey responses suggest a need for improved education for interventional pain physicians on infection control practices.

This chapter will summarize the current literature and recommendations for commonly performed interventional pain procedures, with a distinction made between implantable device surgery including SCS and intrathecal drug delivery systems (IDDS) and nonimplantable device procedures including epidural steroid injections, facet blocks, neuraxial and peripheral nerve blocks, joint injections, sympathetic blocks, radiofrequency, discography, and vertebral augmentation (Tables 86.1 and 86.2). For implantable pain therapies, more detailed recommendations for the entire perioperative process (preoperative, intraoperative, and postoperative) will be provided.

DEFINITION OF SURGICAL SITE INFECTION

SSI has been defined by the CDC.[5] Identification of an SSI is based on physical exam findings of localized pain/tenderness, swelling, erythema, heat, or purulent drainage, as well as cultures and radiologic findings (Fig. 86.1). Superficial SSIs involve the skin and subcutaneous tissues, while deep SSIs involve the fascia and muscle layers. Superficial and deep SSIs occurring in the absence of an implantable device are defined as occurring within 30 days after the operation. When a device is implanted, a deep SSI is defined as occurring within 1 year post implant.

PATHOGENS ASSOCIATED WITH SURGICAL SITE INFECTIONS

Organisms causing SSIs can be categorized as coming from an endogenous or exogenous source. The most common

TABLE 86.1 Pain Procedure Classifications to Guide Infection Control Measures

A	B	C	Implantable Therapies
Trigger point injections	Interlaminar epidural steroid injections (C, T, L, S)	Intradiscal procedures (C, T, L)	Intrathecal catheter and pump implants/revisions
Peripheral nerve blocks	Transforaminal epidural steroid injections (C, T, L, S)	Peripheral nerve stimulation trials	Peripheral nerve stimulation trials/implants
	Facet joint and medial branch nerve block injections and radiofrequency ablation	Spinal cord stimulation trials	Spinal cord stimulation implants/revisions
	Musculoskeletal and joint injections	Indwelling catheters (epidural, intrathecal)	
	Sacroiliac joint injections and sacral lateral branch blocks	Vertebral augmentation (vertebroplasty and kyphoplasty)	
	Paravertebral blocks (C, T, L) Sympathetic blocks (stellate, thoracic, splanchnic, celiac, lumbar, hypogastric)		
	Single-shot intrathecal drug trials		
	Intrathecal pump refills		

C, *Cervical;* L, *lumbar;* S, *sacral;* T, *thoracic.*

TABLE 86.2 Surgical Site Infection Risk Reduction Technique Summary of Recommendations Based on Procedure Type

Risk Reduction Techniques #	A	B	C	Implantable Therapies
Identification and optimization of patient risk factors	X	X	X	X
Staphylococcus aureus screening and decolonization for carriers			Implantable trials[a]	X
Preprocedural intravenous antibiotics			X	X
Hand-washing with soap and water or an alcohol-based hand rub	X	X	X	X
2–5-minute surgical hand scrub			X	X
Do not wear hand or arm jewelry		X	X	X
Sterile gloves	X	X	X	X
Double gloving				X
Sterile surgical gown			X	X
Surgical cap and mask		X	X	X
Patient skin antisepsis with chlorhexidine	X	X	X	X
Full-length body drape			X	X
Use of styletted needle		X	X	X
Sterile C-arm cover			X	X
Sterile ultrasound probe cover and gel	X	X	X	X
Wound irrigation with sterile saline				X

[a]*Only recommended for consideration for implantable pain therapy trials.*
Refer to Table 86.1 for procedure classification.

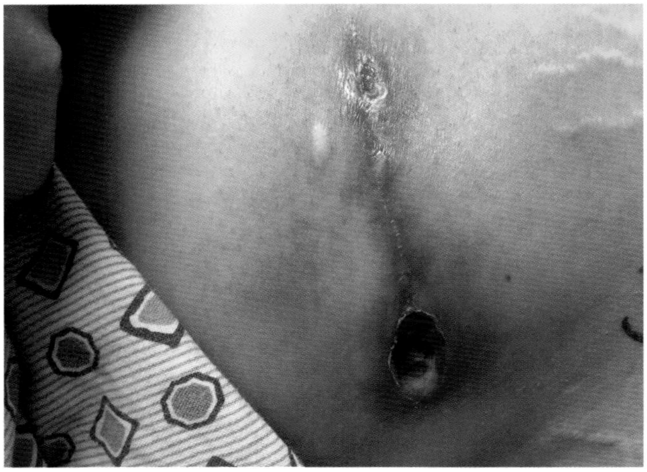

FIG. 86.1 A surgical site infection of an intrathecal pump abdominal incision.

pathogens in descending order are *Staphylococcus aureus*, *Staphylococcus epidermidis*, *Streptococcus*, *Escherichia coli*, and *Pseudomonas aeruginosa*. The most common source of infection is from the patient's own flora.[8,13,14] It has been shown that pathogenic *S. aureus* isolated from an infected wound matches cultures from the patient's nares 80%–85% of the time.[15]

SCOPE OF INTERVENTIONAL PAIN PROCEDURES AND RISK OF INFECTION

Interventional pain procedures and surgeries vary considerably based on the pain syndrome being treated, practitioner technique, and surgical theater environment. The invasiveness of procedures varies, and thus different infection control practices must be considered. Recommendations for the prevention of SSIs have been published by the CDC, NICE, and SCIP (Table 86.3).[5,8,10,16]

INFECTION RATES

Despite an emphasis to reduce SSIs, the rate of infections has remained relatively stable over the past two decades. In the United States, approximately 500,000 SSIs occur annually, accounting for 17% of all nosocomial infections. The relative risk of central nervous system infection following paraspinal injections has been estimated to be about 1/1000 (0.1%).[17] The risk of developing an epidural abscess from an indwelling catheter for postoperative analgesia has been reported to be 1 in 1930 catheters (0.05%).[18] Infection rates associated with single-shot peripheral nerve blocks are also low. A retrospective study examining 7476 patients who received an ultrasound-guided single injection peripheral nerve blockade using a low level disinfection technique in combination with a sterile transparent film transducer barrier reported no indications of block-related infections.[19] Although the overall rate of bacterial colonization with peripheral nerve block catheters is high, the risk of reported infection is low.[20] There have only been a few reports of infectious complications related to facet injections; thus the true incidence is unknown.[21–26] Incidence of disc infection with discography has been estimated to be 0.15% per patient and 0.08% per disc injected.[27] Published systematic reviews on SCS and IDDS report infection rates ranging from 3.4% to 10% and 2.4% to 4.6%, respectively.[28–32]

TABLE 86.3 Preoperative, Intraoperative, and Postoperative Centers for Disease Control and Prevention, National Institute for Health and Care Excellence, Surgical Care Improvement Project, and Author Recommendations

86.3.1 Preoperative Recommendations

Recommendations	CDC Evidence Rankings	SCIP Process of Care Performance Measures	NICE Guidelines	Authors' Additional Recommendations
Identify and treat all remote infections	IA			
Identify patient risk factors				✓[13,33,36]
Optimize glucose control	IB			
Discontinue tobacco use	IB			
Require patients to shower or bathe with an antiseptic agent prior to surgery	IB			
Preoperative screening and decolonization for SA carriers				✓[44,45,52,54,55]
Do not routinely use nasal decontamination for SA			✓	
Appropriate selection of intravenous antibiotic prophylaxis based on hospital pathogens and type of surgery/procedure	IA	✓	✓	
Weight-based antibiotic dosing				✓[62,63]
Appropriate prophylactic antibiotic received within one hour prior to surgical incision (two hours for vancomycin)	IA	✓	✓	
Appropriate agent selection for skin antisepsis (povidone-iodine or chlorhexidine)	IB		✓	
Vancomycin should not routinely be used	IB			
Preoperative surgical scrub for at least 2–5 min using an appropriate antiseptic. Scrub the hands and forearms up to the elbows	IB		✓	
Keep nails short and do not wear artificial nails	IB		✓	
Sterile gown and gloves	IB			
Do not wear hand or arm jewelry	II		✓	
Do not use hair removal routinely	IA		✓	
If hair is removed, use electric clippers immediately before surgery	IA	✓	✓	
Evaluate for skin lesions or areas of local infection				✓
Apply preoperative antiseptic skin preparation in concentric circles moving toward the periphery	II			
Wide prep and drape				✓

86.3.2 Intraoperative Recommendations

Recommendations	CDC Evidence Ranking	SCIP Process Care Performance Measures	NICE Guidelines	Authors' Additional Recommendations
Wear a surgical mask in the OR if sterile instruments are exposed	IB			
Wear a cap or hood to fully cover hair in the OR	IB			
Wear two pairs of sterile gloves when there is a high risk of glove perforation and the consequences of contamination are high			✓	✓[88]
Use sterile surgical gowns that are effective barriers when wet	IB		✓	

TABLE 86.3 Preoperative, Intraoperative, and Postoperative Centers for Disease Control and Prevention, National Institute for Health and Care Excellence, Surgical Care Improvement Project, and Author Recommendations—cont'd

86.3.2 Intraoperative Recommendations

Recommendations	CDC Evidence Ranking	SCIP Process Care Performance Measures	NICE Guidelines	Authors' Additional Recommendations
If an incise drape is used, use an iodophor-impregnated drape			✓	
Laminar flow and HEPA filters in OR	IB			
Limit OR traffic	II		✓	
Keep OR doors closed during procedure	IB			
Adhere to principles of asepsis when placing spinal or epidural catheters	IA			
Limit tissue trauma, maintain hemostasis, eradicate dead space, and avoid the electrocautery at tissue surface	IB		✓	
Vigorous wound irrigation with bulb syringe				✓[100,102]
Limit surgical time				✓[38,93]

86.3.3 Postoperative Recommendations

Recommendations	CDC Evidence Ranking	SCIP Process of Care Performance Measures	NICE Guidelines	Authors' Additional Recommendations
Prophylactic antimicrobial discontinued within 24 h of surgery		✓		
Occlusive dressing for a minimum of 24–48 h	IB		✓	
Do not routinely use topical antimicrobial agents for surgical wounds that are healing by primary intention			✓	
Continued comorbidity optimization				✓
Close postoperative wound surveillance				✓[28]
When SSI is suspected, prescribe an antibiotic that covers the likely causative organisms. Consider local resistance patterns and the results of microbiological tests in choosing an antibiotic.			✓	
Consult an infectious disease specialist if any sign or warning signals of infection are present				✓[163,164]
Wash hands before and after dressing changes	IB			
Use sterile technique for dressing changes	II		✓	
Educate patient and family on proper incision care, symptoms of SSI, and importance of reporting symptoms	II		✓	

CDC, *Centers for Disease Control and Prevention;* HEPA, *high-efficiency particulate air;* NICE, *National Institute for Health and Clinical Excellence;* OR, *operating room;* SCIP, *surgical care improvement projects;* SSI, *surgical site infection.*
CDC Recommendation Ranking Categories:
IA: Strongly recommended for implementation and supported by well-designed experimental clinical or epidemiological studies.
IB: Strongly recommended for implementation and supported by some experimental, clinical, or epidemiological studies and strong theoretical rationale.
II: Suggested for implementation and supported by suggestive clinical or epidemiological studies or theoretical rationale.

PREOPERATIVE RISK REDUCTION

PATIENT RISK FACTORS

Physicians should identify patient-related risk factors prior to performing a procedure, and efforts should be made to correct any modifiable risk factors (Table 86.4).[33–36] Postmarket surveillance data on SCS and IDDS implants revealed 38% and 70% of patients with SCS and IDDS infections, respectively, had a medical comorbidity that increased their risk of infections.[13] Smoking has been associated with an increased risk of SCS infections, likely secondary to the development of microvascular disease, leading to tissue ischemia and poor wound healing.[29,37] Although the biological effects of cancer and chemotherapeutic

TABLE 86.4 Patient-Related Risk Factors for Surgical Site Infection

Older age
Poor nutritional status
Diabetes mellitus
Smoking
Obesity
Coexisting infections at a remote body site
Colonization with *Staphylococcus aureus*
Altered immune status

Modified from Mangram AJ, Horan TC, Pearson ML, Silver LC, Jarvis WR: Guideline for prevention of surgical site infection, 1999. Hospital Infection Control Practices Advisory Committee. Infect Control Hosp Epidemiol. *20:250–278, 1999; quiz 279-280.*

drugs can weaken host immunity, a retrospective study demonstrated that implantable pain therapies can still be utilized in cancer patients without significantly increasing the risk of SSI when appropriate infection control measures are taken.[38]

Preoperatively, a thorough history and physical exam should be performed to identify patient risk factors. Many measures can be taken to reduce the risk of SSIs, such as glucose optimization, tobacco cessation (for at least 4 weeks), optimization of viral load in HIV patients, minimizing/avoiding perioperative steroids, and treatment of remote infections (e.g., urinary tract). Nonmodifiable risk factors need to be documented, and a discussion with the patient regarding the associated increased risk of infection should occur prior to the pain intervention.

STAPHYLOCOCCUS AUREUS CARRIERS

Staphylococcus aureus is the leading cause of SSIs, accounting for approximately 20% of all SSIs, 30% of implantable cardioverter-defibrillator (ICD) implants, and 60% of all prosthetic joint infections.[33,39–42] Greater than 80% of nosocomial *S. aureus* infections are endogenous, and the number of cases of methicillin-resistant *S. aureus* (MRSA) SSIs is increasing.[5,43] *S. aureus* nasal colonization rates have been reported from 20% to 80%, depending on the population studied.[44–48]

Methicillin-sensitive *S. aureus* (MSSA) and MRSA carriers have been shown to have a significantly higher risk for developing an SSI (two to nine times higher).[48–50] Therefore identification of carriers followed by decolonization protocols is critical in reducing SSI rates and has been recommended as an infection control measure.[28,44,45,51–53] Decolonization of *S. aureus* carriers has also been shown to be a cost-effective treatment.[45]

Decolonization protocols have described the application of mupirocin 2% nasal ointment applied twice daily, combined with chlorhexidine gluconate soap total-body washes daily for a duration of 5 days immediately preceding surgery.[44,54] Utilization of decolonization protocols in individuals that are colonized reduces the rate of postoperative infections by greater than 50%.[44,55,56] No data exist to support the use of routine decolonization protocols in patients who do not test positive for *S. aureus* colonization.[49]

ANTIBIOTIC PROPHYLAXIS

Preoperative antibiotic prophylaxis has been shown to significantly reduce the risk of SSIs, and the incidence of wound infection by approximately 50%, regardless of the type of surgery.[57] Antibiotic prophylaxis (Table 86.5) is recommended for implantable pain therapies (i.e., trials and implant stages). Proper antibiotic selection, route of administration, dosing, and timing are critical, as suboptimal implementation has been found to increase the risk of infection twofold to sixfold.[58,59] Cephalosporins are recommended as first-line agents. If a patient has a β-lactam allergy, clindamycin or vancomycin are alternative antibiotics. In individuals colonized with MRSA or at high risk for MRSA (e.g., institutions that have a high rate of MRSA infections), vancomycin is recommended.[7,60]

In order for antibiotic prophylaxis to be effective, minimum inhibitory concentrations (MIC) must be reached prior to surgical incision and maintained throughout the duration of the surgery. Preoperative antibiotics should be administered intravenously (IV) prior to incision time (30–60 minutes prior to incision or 120 minutes of incision for vancomycin). Cefmetazole 2 g IV administered immediately prior, 15 minutes prior, and 60 minutes prior to incision all showed MIC90 in blood and tissue samples throughout surgical procedures, lasting on average 2.1–2.4 hours.[61] In order to reach MIC, weight-based dosing is needed.[62,63] Weight-based dosing (2 g of cefazolin in morbidly obese patients) prior to gastroplasty was shown to decrease SSI rates to 5.6%, compared with 16.5% when 1 g of cefazolin was administered.[63]

The kidneys excrete the majority of antibiotics used for surgical prophylaxis. The exception is clindamycin, which is primarily excreted via the biliary system. Therefore creatinine clearance must be taken into account prior to antibiotic dosing. Redosing is needed when the duration of surgery is longer than two half-lives of the administered antibiotic (see Table 86.5).

The continuation of antibiotics in the postoperative period is not recommended beyond 24 hours for clean surgical wounds. Prolonged antibiotic use in the postoperative period does not improve outcomes and may result in poorer outcomes.[64,65] Specifically, the continuation of antibiotics in the postoperative period has been associated with delayed normalization of body temperature and elevation of the C-reactive protein (CRP) level.[64] The SCIP guidelines recommend the discontinuation of antibiotics within 24 hours of surgery.[7]

There are no recommendations or evidence for the use of antibiotic prophylaxis in the majority of routine interventional pain procedures (i.e., epidural steroid injections, facet blocks); however, for those that are considered higher risk for infection (i.e., indwelling catheters, and device trials/implants), antibiotic prophylaxis is recommended.[5,8] For discography and other intradiscal procedures, controversy exists on the need for IV and/or intradiscal antibiotic administration.[8,66] Intravenous antibiotics do not reliably achieve adequate intradiscal concentrations. Therefore intradiscal antibiotics have been recommended. However, ex vivo studies examining the effects of high antibiotic concentrations on cultured human intervertebral disc annular cells demonstrated

TABLE 86.5 Prophylactic Antibiotic Recommendations

Antibiotic	Standard Intravenous Dosing	Timing Prior to Incision	Redosing Interval	Indications
Cefazolin	1 g ≤ 80 kg 2 g > 80 kg 3 g > 160 kg	Within 30–60 min	3–4 h (CrCl > 50 mL/min) 8 h (CrCl 20–50 mL/min) 16 h (CrCl < 20 mL/min)	(1) First-line
Clindamycin	600 mg ≤ 80 kg 900 mg > 80 kg 1200 mg > 160 kg	Within 30–60 min	6 h (CrCl > 50 mL/min) 6 h (CrCl 20–50 mL/min) 6 h (CrCl < 20 mL/min)	(1) β-lactam allergy
Vancomycin	1 g ≤ 80 kg 2 g > 80 kg 3 g > 160 kg	**Within 120 min**	8 h (CrCl > 50 mL/min) 16 h (CrCl 20–50 mL/min) None (CrCl < 20 mL/min)	(1) β-lactam allergy (2) Known MRSA colonization

Modified from Bratzler DW, Houck PM, Surgical Infection Prevention Guidelines Writers W, et al: Antimicrobial prophylaxis for surgery: an advisory statement from the National Surgical Infection Prevention Project. Clin Infect Dis. *38:1706–1715, 2004; and Alexander JW, Solomkin JS, Edwards MJ: Updated recommendations for control of surgical site infections.* Ann Surg. *253:1082–1093, 2011.*

deleterious effects on cell survival, cell proliferation, and metabolic rates.[67] Bogduk et al. demonstrated with pooled data that the prevalence of discitis when antibiotic medications are not used is 0.24% (95% confidence intervals: 0.11%–0.37%), which is higher than the reported overall incidence of 0.15% per patient.[27,68]

SURGICAL HAND-WASHING

Appropriate surgical scrubbing of the hands and forearms is a CDC Category IB and NICE recommendation.[5,10] Commercially available antiseptic solutions in the United States contain alcohol, chlorhexidine, and/or povidone-iodine. There is evidence that chlorhexidine-based scrubs reduce the number of colony-forming units compared with povidone-iodine scrubs; however, the data supporting its clinical relevance are lacking. The duration of the surgical scrub appears to be the most important factor to ensure adequate hand hygiene and limit bacterial counts. Surgical hand-washing lasting between 2 and 5 minutes results in statistically fewer CFUs when compared with hand-washing techniques of lesser duration.[70]

The removal of hand and wrist jewelry prior to surgical scrub is a CDC Category II and NICE recommendation, as well as an American Society of Regional Anesthesia and Pain Medicine (ASRA) recommendation when performing regional anesthesia. The presence of hand jewelry increases bacterial counts on the hands of health care workers, even after hand-washing.[5,10,16,71]

The method of hand hygiene required to minimize the risk of infections associated with interventional pain procedures has not been clearly established. Hebl recommended thorough hand-washing with an alcohol-based antiseptic prior to performing regional anesthetic techniques, but did not recommend a specific method or duration.[16] For implantable devices and indwelling catheters, a full surgical scrub is recommended.

APPROPRIATE HAIR REMOVAL

The CDC Category IA and NICE do not recommend routine removal of hair to reduce the risk of SSI, and if hair is removed clippers are the method of choice.[5,10] Timing and method of hair removal appear to be the most important factors to consider. A meta-analysis looking at hair removal techniques concluded that there is no difference in SSI rates when comparing no hair removal to hair removal with chemical or clipper methods; however, shaving methods do increase the risk of SSIs.[72] Both clipping and shaving hair 24 hours or more before an operation significantly increases the risk of SSI.[5,73,74] There are no data to evaluate the efficacy of hair removal strategies prior to interventional pain procedures.

INTRAPROCEDURAL RISK REDUCTION

PATIENT SKIN PREPARATION IN THE OPERATING ROOM

Antiseptic solutions containing isopropyl alcohol, povidone-iodine, and/or chlorhexidine gluconate are most commonly used for patient skin preparation. Prior to application of a skin antiseptic, gross contamination around the incision site should be removed (CDC Category IB).[5] A randomized controlled trial and meta-analyses have shown that the use of chlorhexidine significantly reduces the rate of SSIs and results in cost savings compared with povidone-iodine.[75–77]

For interventional pain procedures, the US Food and Drug Administration has not approved the use of chlorhexidine for neuraxial procedures due to a lack of clinical safety trials. However, the use of chlorhexidine for spinal anesthesia has not been shown to increase neurologic complications.[78] The use of chlorhexidine prior to epidural catheterization has been shown to be superior to povidone-iodine in reducing catheter colonization rates.[79] Although there are no studies directly comparing infection rates with the use of chlorhexidine gluconate versus povidone-iodine for interventional pain procedures, based on extrapolation of data from other surgical subspecialties, chlorhexidine-based products may offer improvement in infection control rates.

DRAPING

The role of plastic surgical adhesive drapes and impermeable paper drapes in reducing SSI rates is unclear.[80] However, traditional cloth drapes are not recommended for implantable device surgery and have been shown to allow for increased bacterial penetration when wet.[5,81]

Iodophor-impregnated drapes may reduce the number of positive postprocedural skin cultures.[82–84] However, there are no data to support their routine use for the reduction of SSIs.[85,86] While the use of iodophor-impregnated drapes may be considered for high-risk patients, universal usage is not supported by the literature.

SURGICAL ATTIRE

Maximal sterile barrier precautions (surgical cap, mask, and sterile gloves and gowns) for surgical procedures are recommended by the CDC Category IB, NICE, and SCIP. In 2004, the CDC and Healthcare Infection Control Practices Advisory Committee (HICPAC) released a statement recommending the use of facemasks for neuraxial procedures after eight cases of bacterial meningitis following neuraxial procedures were linked to practitioners who were not wearing masks.[87]

The use of sterile gloves is recommended for interventional pain procedures and implantable therapies. While there are no studies directly comparing the risk of SSIs with single versus double gloving techniques, double gloving has clearly been shown in multiple studies to reduce the number of inner glove perforations.[88] Therefore double gloving should be considered for implantable device surgeries to both reduce the risk of SSI as well as to protect the practitioner.

SURGICAL TECHNIQUE AND PROCEDURAL EFFICIENCY

Electrocautery has not been directly found to affect SSI rates, and NICE guidelines specifically state not to use electrocautery as a means to reduce the risk of SSI.[10] However, studies have shown that it is associated with decreased intraoperative blood loss, incision time, and postoperative pain.[89,90] While electrocautery should be avoided at the tissue surface, it may be beneficial to maximize hemostasis and reduce surgery time, which have both been shown to be associated with increased SSI rates.[91]

Careful tissue handling is important not only to optimize healing, but it also may reduce SSI rates. Gentle tissue handling and minimization of devitalized tissue is a CDC Category IB recommendation.[5]

Appropriate surgical training and efficiency have also been shown to assist in the reduction of SSIs. Inadequate physician experience, low procedural volumes, and extended operative times have been suggested as possible risk factors for SSIs.[92–94] Specifically for implantable pain therapies, a retrospective review on IDDS and SCS implants for cancer patients suggested that extended operative times may be a risk factor SSIs.[38] Thus an attempt should be made to limit surgical time.[28] In addition, recent survey data for SCS demonstrated a significant inverse relationship between procedural volume and operative times.[95] The Neuromodulation Appropriateness Consensus Committee (NACC) has signaled for improvements in neuromodulation implantation training. The NACC recommends that during formal training, future implanters should ideally perform 10 supervised cases at a minimum during training as the primary implanter.[96]

WOUND IRRIGATION

Prior to closure, wound irrigation can be utilized to clean the surgical bed. The efficacy of wound irrigation depends on several factors, including delivery method, volume, and type of solution and additives delivered. Controversy exists regarding the use of high-pressure and low-pressure pulsatile lavage, as they may result in deep seeding of bacteria into exposed tissues and impair wound healing.[97] There is no consensus on the optimum volume of irrigation to use; however, animal studies suggest that larger volumes are superior.[98]

Irrigation solutions typically consist of normal saline, detergents, or antibiotics. Animal studies suggest that castile soap is more effective in preventing *P. aeruginosa* infections, while benzalkonium chloride is most effective in preventing *S. aureus* infections.[99] However, both benzalkonium chloride and bacitracin have been associated with impaired wound healing.[100,101] Bacitracin solution has not been shown to be superior to normal saline for reducing the presence of wound bacteria.[100,102] If wound irrigation is performed for implantable therapies, it is recommended to use normal saline through a bulb syringe.

TOPICAL ANTIMICROBIALS

Topical antimicrobials for SSI prophylaxis have been studied in the form of impregnated dressings, topical powders, and device envelopes. Randomized controlled trials using chlorhexidine-impregnated dressings for epidural catheters have shown a greater than sevenfold reduction in catheter-site bacterial colonization, with a mean catheter duration of 3.6 days.[103–105] The use of chlorhexidine-impregnated dressings should be strongly considered in any procedure where a catheter/lead is left exposed for an extended period of time in a patient at high risk for SSI (i.e., SCS trials, IDDS catheter trials, indwelling epidural catheters).

Intrasite vancomycin powder has gained popularity, specifically in spine surgery.[106] However, the FDA does not currently approve its use. The reported efficacy of vancomycin powder for SSI reduction is conflicting.[107–113] Meta-analyses and systematic reviews suggest that intrasite application of vancomycin powder is effective in preventing SSIs, specifically when hardware is implanted.[114–117] Amrani reported a significant decrease in SSIs with its use for paddle SCS implants, while Ghobrial et al. reported higher infection rates with its use in baclofen pump implants.[118,119] Currently, further studies are warranted prior to supporting the routine use of vancomycin powder for implantable pain therapies.

In 2008, the FDA approved the antimicrobial envelope (TYRX, Medtronic, Dublin, Ireland) for use in ICD implants, and in 2013 it gained approval for its use in neuromodulation implants. The antimicrobial envelope is a bioabsorbable, polypropylene mesh that releases minocycline and rifampin. It has been shown to reduce ICD infection rates by 60% when used empirically, and by more than 87% when used selectively in patients considered at high risk for SSI.[120–122] There is currently no specific data to support its use in SCS and IDDS implants; however, its use could be considered for patients considered at high risk for SSI.

OPERATING ROOM ENVIRONMENT

Ventilation and OR traffic likely affect SSI rates. Laminar-flow ORs and high-efficiency particulate air (HEPA) filters have been shown to reduce SSIs and wound contamination when compared with conventional airflow systems.[123–125]

Personnel are the major source of contamination in the OR.[126] The number of personnel as well as traffic flow rates in the OR positively correlate with the degree of airborne contamination.[127] Education, preoperative planning, communication, and limiting surgical time are the most effective measures to decrease traffic flow.

There are many potential sources of contamination from equipment within the OR (i.e., light handles, fluoroscopic C-arm, ultrasound probe; Fig. 86.2). The contamination of sterile light handles has been reported to be as high as 14.5%; therefore, the handling of OR lights should be minimized.[126,128] Biswas et al. evaluated the sterility of 25 C-arm drapes placed with aseptic technique after their use during spine surgery.[129] All locations were contaminated at the end of the surgical case. The front, top half and the superior end of the image intensifier were associated with higher contamination rates. All OR personnel should avoid contact with the C-arm.

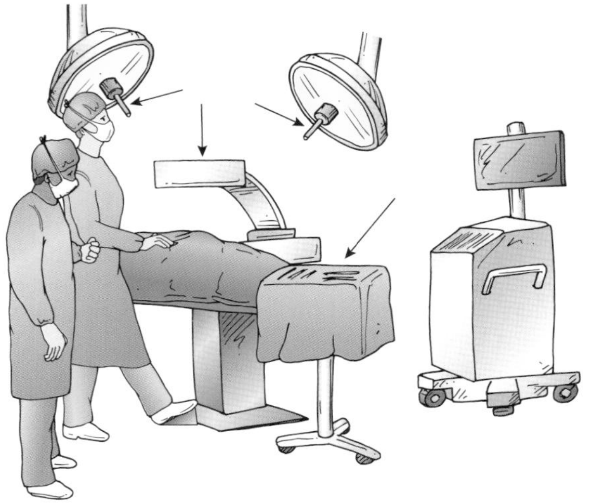

FIG. 86.2 Schematic of operating room demonstrating potential sources of contamination, including personnel, C-arm, light handles, and instrument stand.

WOUND CLOSURE

It is important to minimize dead space during wound closure. Dead space allows for the accumulation of serous fluid and blood, which can serve as mediums for bacterial growth. Layered closure techniques also help minimize dead space and tissue tension, which also promotes wound healing.[130] Certain suture types and materials are thought to promote bacteria colonization. For example, multifilament sutures (i.e., silk, vicryl) may promote bacterial colonization in between filaments. However, there is a lack of evidence to support the use of one type of suture over another for reducing SSIs.[131,132]

There is conflicting evidence on the benefit of closure method (suture vs. staples), whether staples increase the risk of SSI compared with sutures.[133] A meta-analysis of randomized controlled trials in obstetric/gynecology, general, head/neck, and vascular operations suggested that staples were associated with significantly fewer SSIs.[134] A Cochrane review concluded that there was insufficient evidence to suggest a difference in SSI rates when comparing suture versus staple closures for leg wounds after vein graft harvesting during cardiopulmonary bypass surgery.[135]

NEEDLE CONTAMINATION

Contamination of needles occurs despite adequate skin preparation. Epidural needle contamination rates have been reported as high as 35%, despite adequate skin preparation with 10% povidone-iodine.[136] Higher rates of discitis following discography using a nonstyletted, single-needle technique compared with a styletted, double-needle technique (1.4% vs. 0.4% per disc) have been reported.[14] Styletted needles should be used for all neuraxial procedures to reduce the risk of needle coring that can introduce skin bacteria into the injection site, and a double-needle technique should be considered in procedures that are considered to place patients at higher morbidity following infectious complications (i.e., intradiscal procedures). For discography, minimizing intradiscal needle time has been suggested to reduce the incidence of discitis.[137]

ULTRASOUND GUIDED REGIONAL ANESTHESIA AND PAIN PROCEDURES

Both the US gel and the probe can serve as vectors for infection. Individuals performing US-guided regional anesthesia and pain procedures should take steps to minimize infection and cross-contamination through US gel and probe.

Contaminated US gel has been implicated in a number of nosocomial infections, which led to a FDA safety communication calling for the use of sterile US gel for transthoracic echocardiography (Table 86.6).[138–145] Guidelines by Health Canada were published in 2004 recommending the use of sterile gel in all procedures that pass a device through tissue.[146] Recently in the United States, recommendations based on expert opinion have been proposed to minimize clinical risk (Table 86.7).[142] These recommendations build on the Health Canada recommendations recommending the use of single-use sterile gels for invasive procedures involving neonates, for all procedures involving sterile equipment or nonintact skin, and for procedures surrounding mucous membranes. In addition, several expert opinion publications have recommended the use of sterile gel for all interventional pain procedures.[142,147–150] Nonsterile packaged US gel typically contains parabens; however, antimicrobial resistance to parabens has been described, and bacterial and fungal contamination of US gel packaged in bottles has been shown to be present prior

TABLE 86.6 Case Reports of Contaminated Ultrasonography Coupling Gel Causing Nosocomial Infection

Author	Gel Used	Antimicrobial Agent	Identified Microorganism	Source of Contamination	Associated Procedure	Type of Noscomial Infection
Chittick et al.[149]	Other-Sonic; Pharmaceutical Innovations, Inc., Newark, NJ	Not indicated	Pseudomonas aeruginosa	In-use and unopened gel bottles	Transesophageal echocardiography	Respiratory tract infection
Olshtain-Pops et al.[141]	250-mL unidentified gel bottle	Not indicated	Achromobacter xylosoxidans	250-mL in-use gel bottles	Transrectal prostate biopsy	Bacteriuria and septicemia
Marigliano et al.[145]	Not indicated	Methylchloroisothiazolinone and methylisothiazolinone	Burkholderia cepacia	Not indicated	Echocardiographic procedures	Not indicated
Jacobson et al.[138]	250-mL gel bottles from 4 unidentified manufacturers	Propyl and methyl parabens	Burkholderia cepacia, Klebsiella oxytoca, Stenotrophomonas maltophilia, Ralstonia pickettii, Pantoea agglomerans, Enterobacter ictaluri, Burkholderia stabilis	250-mL in-use gel bottles	Diagnostic ultrasonography	Respiratory tract infection, bacteriuria, skin wound
Hutchinson et al.[140]	250-mL unidentified gel bottles, 5-L opened stock bottles	Methyl paraben	Burkholderia cepacia, Enterobacter cloacae	Intrinsically contaminated gel during the manufacturing process	Transrectal prostate biopsy	Urinary tract infection and septicemia
Weist et al.[143]	500-mL unidentified gel bottle	Not indicated	Methicillin-susceptible *Staphylococcus aureus*	Dispensing spatula and 500-mL in-use gel bottle	Neonate hip-joint sonography	Pyoderma
Gaillot et al.[139]	250-mL Sonecho gel bottles; Echos Contacts, Eragny, France	Not indicated	Klebsiella pneumoniae producing extended spectrum β-lactamase	Wide-mouthed bulk container	Emergency room ultrasound scan	Urinary tract infection and skin lesion
Keizur et al.[150]	Not indicated	Not indicated	Pseudomonas cepacia	Portable dispensing bottles and opened bulk dispensers	Transrectal prostate biopsy	Urinary tract infection

Used with permission from Provenzano DA, Liebert MA, Steen B, et al: Investigation of current infection-control practices for ultrasound coupling gel: a survey, microbiological analysis, and examination of practice patterns. Reg Anesth Pain Med. *38:415–424, 2013.*

to patient use.[148] Single-use, sterile US gel packets are recommended for use in interventional pain and regional anesthesia procedures.[147]

Ultrasound equipment can also serve as a potential vector for nosocomial infection.[151–153] While there are no data evaluating the efficacy of sterile probe covers or adhesive transparent dressings for reducing procedure infection rates, their use is recommended for interventional pain and regional anesthesia procedures.[147]

MEDICATION VIALS

The misuse of single-use vials (SUVs) for multiple patients has resulted in outbreaks of *S. aureus* infections. In 2012, the CDC issued a statement emphasizing the importance of proper usage of SUVs due to an outbreak of *S. aureus* infections in 10 patients treated with interventional pain procedures.[154] The final recommendations were (1) contents of an SUV should be withdrawn using a sterile syringe in an aseptic manner, (2) contents should be used promptly, (3) the vial and any remaining contents should be disposed of, (4) SUVs should not be used on multiple patients, and (5) if SUVs are used on multiple patients, the medication should only be separated from an unused SUV into SUVs or syringes by qualified health care personnel under a laminar-flow hood using strict adherence to *US Pharmacopeia* 797 standards.[155]

POSTOPERATIVE RISK REDUCTION

WOUND DRESSINGS

The CDC and NICE recommend the use of sterile occlusive dressings for 24–48 hours for incisions closed by primary intention (Category IB).[5] Early studies suggested occlusive dressings augment wound healing and decrease the rate of SSI.[156,157] However, more recent meta-analyses claim insufficient evidence for the use of occlusive dressings, advanced wound dressings (i.e., hydrocolloid, soft polymer), antimicrobial dressings, or leaving wounds uncovered to reduce SSI rates.[158,159] The efficacy of occlusive dressings beyond 48 hours is undetermined.

TABLE 86.7 Guidelines for Infection Control Practice for Ultrasound-Guided Procedures

- Follow the Centers for Disease Control and Prevention's guidelines for disinfection and sterilization in health care facilities for reprocessing ultrasound transducers.
- Prior to performing ultrasound scanning, confirm that the equipment was cleaned and disinfected appropriately.
- Use a sterile ultrasound sheath or sterile adhesive transparent dressing.
- Single-dose sterile ultrasound transmission gel should be used for the following procedures:
  1. Performing a biopsy or puncture
  2. Procedures involving mucous membranes
  3. Scanning nonintact skin
  4. Scanning near a surgical wound
  5. Scanning neonates and critically ill pediatric patients
- Nonsterile ultrasound gel may be used for low-risk, noninvasive procedures on intact skin and for low-risk patients.
- Seal multidose, nonsterile gel containers and replace when empty.
- Do not reuse ultrasound gel containers and replace when empty.
- When warming ultrasound gel, dry heat is the preferred method.

Modified from Oleszkowicz SC, Chittick P, Russo V, Keller P, Sims M, Band J: Infections associated with use of ultrasound transmission gel: proposed guidelines to minimize risk. Infect Control Hosp Epidemiol. *33:1235–1237, 2012; and Narouze SN, Provenzano D, Peng P, et al: The American Society of Regional Anesthesia and Pain Medicine, the European Society of Regional Anaesthesia and Pain Therapy, and the Asian Australasian Federation of Pain Societies Joint Committee recommendations for education and training in ultrasound-guided interventional pain procedures.* Reg Anesth Pain Med. *37:657–664, 2012.*

PATIENT EDUCATION AND POSTOPERATIVE WOUND SURVEILLANCE

During the postoperative period, optimization of medical comorbidities should continue, including tobacco cessation and glucose control. Patients and family members should be educated on signs and symptoms of an emerging SSI, incision care, and the importance of reporting any signs of infection. Patients should be seen within 10–14 days of surgery to evaluate for appropriate wound healing and signs of SSI.[28] Any evidence of a developing SSI requires closer follow-up.

INFECTION MANAGEMENT

Prompt recognition of an infection is the most important step in appropriate management of an SSI. Laboratory tests such as white blood cell (WBC) count, C-reactive protein (CRP), and erythrocyte sedimentation rate (ESR) can aid in the identification process. Following implantable surgeries, WBC counts, ESR, and CRP all rise transiently in the postoperative period due to the body's stress response to surgery. Systemic diseases such as malignancy and rheumatologic disorders can affect baseline ESR and CRP levels. CRP levels rise four to six hours after acute tissue injury, peaking around the second or third postoperative day following total joint arthroplasty and spine surgery.[160,161] ESR levels rise more slowly, peaking around the fourth or fifth postoperative day. CRP also returns to normal more rapidly (14–21 days) and predictably compared with ESR.[161,162] Postoperative CRP kinetics are more responsive to and predictive of infection.[161] Therefore failure for CRP levels to normalize or an unexpected rise in CRP is a highly sensitive predictor of an SSI. Likewise, a normal CRP is highly sensitive for lack of an SSI.

If any purulent drainage is identified, samples should be sent for culture and sensitivities. For neuraxial procedures and implantable pain therapies, imaging is often recommended to determine if an infection exists in the epidural space. If the implantable device still exists in the body, then MRI compatibility of the implantable system should be determined prior to initiating an MRI. Magnetic resonance imaging with and without gadolinium is the imaging modality of choice.

Except for superficial infections that in some cases should be managed with appropriate wound care and antibiotics, infections often require the removal of the implantable devices. When the device is removed, the leads/catheter should be sent for cultures and sensitivity. The formation of biofilm makes the eradication of an infection involving any hardware very difficult. Relapse of infection has been reported to occur in more than half of patients with ICDs left in place when generator pocket infections were identified.[163] Similarly, conservative management of deep brain stimulator infections is successful in less than 40% of cases.[164] Therefore consultation with an infectious disease physician is recommended. Empiric antibiotic therapy is initiated and then further refined once the pathogen is identified. In addition, reimplantation should only be considered when complete resolution of the infection is established.

CONCLUSION

Surgical site and procedural infections are associated with significant patient morbidity, clinical consequences, and economic costs. It is imperative that physicians performing interventional procedures understand and implement appropriate infection control guidelines. When infections occur, prompt recognition and appropriate treatment is required. In addition, further research is warranted specifically for interventional pain procedures to further define guidelines and recommendations.

KEY POINTS

- SCS infection rates are higher than those of other implantable devices, including cardiac pacemakers and total joint replacements.
- Identification of an SSI is based on physical exam findings of localized pain/tenderness, swelling, erythema, heat, or purulent drainage, as well as cultures and radiologic findings.
- The most common pathogens in descending order are *S. aureus*, *S. epidermidis*, *Streptococcus*, *E. coli*, and *P. aeruginosa*. The most common source of infection is from the patient's own flora.
- Postmarketing surveillance revealed 38% and 70% of patients with SCS and IDDS infections, respectively, had a medical comorbidity that increased their risk of infection. Smoking has been associated with an increased risk of SCS infections; the biological effects of cancer and chemotherapeutic drugs can weaken host immunity.

- Preoperative antibiotics should be administered IV prior to incision time (30–60 minutes prior to incision or 120 minutes of incision for vancomycin). The continuation of antibiotics in the postoperative period is not recommended beyond 24 hours for clean surgical wounds.
- Appropriate surgical scrubbing of the hands and forearms is a CDC Category IB and NICE recommendation.
- The CDC Category IA and NICE do not recommend routine removal of hair to reduce the risk of SSI, and if hair is removed, clippers are the method of choice.
- The use of chlorhexidine significantly reduces the rate of SSIs and results in cost savings compared with povidone-iodine.
- Maximal sterile barrier precautions (surgical cap, mask, and sterile gloves and gowns) for surgical procedures are recommended by the CDC Category IB, NICE, and SCIP.
- Personnel are the major source of contamination in the OR. There are many potential sources of contamination from equipment within the OR (i.e., light handles, fluoroscopic C-arm, ultrasound probe).
- Laboratory tests such as WBC count, CRP, and ESR can aid in identifying SSIs.

REFERENCES

Access the reference list online at ExpertConsult.com.

INDEX

Page numbers followed by *f* indicate figures; *t*, tables; *b*, boxes.

B

C

D

E

H

L

M

O

Q

R